THE EAR

COMPREHENSIVE OTOLOGY

THE EAR
COMPREHENSIVE OTOLOGY

Edited by

Rinaldo F. Canalis, M.D., F.A.C.S.

Professor
Division of Head and Neck Surgery (Otolaryngology)
and The Victor Goodhill Ear Institute
University of California, Los Angeles, School of Medicine
Los Angeles, California
Chief
Division of Head and Neck Surgery (Otolaryngology)
Harbor-UCLA Medical Center
Torrance, California

Paul R. Lambert, M.D., F.A.C.S.

Professor and Chair
Department of Otolaryngology-Head and Neck Surgery
and Communication Sciences
Medical University of South Carolina
Charleston, South Carolina

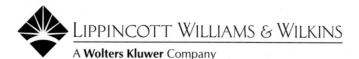

LIPPINCOTT WILLIAMS & WILKINS
A **Wolters Kluwer** Company
Philadelphia · Baltimore · New York · London
Buenos Aires · Hong Kong · Sydney · Tokyo

Acquisitions Editor: Danette Knopp
Developmental Editor: Stephanie Harris
Production Editor: Elaine Verriest
Manufacturing Manager: Tim Reynolds
Cover Designer: Mark Lerner
Compositor: Lippincott Williams & Wilkins Desktop Division
Printer: Maple Press

© 2000 by Lippincott Williams & Wilkins
227 East Washington Square
Philadelphia, PA 19106-3780 USA
LWW.com

Printed in the USA

Library of Congress Cataloging-in-Publication Data

The Ear : comprehensive otology / edited by Rinaldo F. Canalis, Paul R. Lambert.
   p.   cm.
   Includes bibliographical references and index.
   ISBN 0-7817-1558-X
   1. Otology. 2. Ear—Diseases.   I. Canalis, Rinaldo F.   II. Lambert, Paul R.
   [DNLM: 1. Ear Diseases—diagnosis.   2. Ear—physiology.   3. Hearing Disorders—diagnosis.
   4. Otolaryngology—history.   WV 210 E12 2000]
   RF121.E367   2000
   617.8—dc21
   DNLM/DLC   99-16731
   for Library of Congress   CIP

---

10 9 8 7 6 5 4 3 2 1

To my family and most especially to my wife Sandra,
whose love and support have been essential for the completion
of this and so many other large and small projects in my life.
                                                    —Rinaldo F. Canalis

To my family: my parents Paul Sr. and Helen; Marie;
my wife Debbie; and my children Lara, Paul, and Leslie.
Their encouragement and love are a constant source of inspiration
and happiness. I am also eternally grateful to the Lord,
for His blessings of grace, wisdom, and health.
                                                    —Paul R. Lambert

Then they brought to Him one who was deaf and had an impediment in his speech, and they begged Him to put His hand on him. And He took him aside from the multitude, and put His fingers in his ears, and He spat and touched his tongue. Then, looking up to heaven, He sighed, and said to him **"EPHPHATHA,"** that is, be opened. Immediately his ears were open, and the impediment of his tongue was loosed, and he spoke plainly.

Mark 7:32–35 *NKJ*

Contents

VI. The Cochlea

VII. Rehabilitation of the Hearing Impaired

VIII. The Vestibular System

IX. The Facial Nerve

X. Trauma

XI. Temporal Bone Neoplasias and Dystrophies

XII. Looking Ahead

Contributing Authors

Elliot Abemayor, M.D., Ph.D.   *Professor and Vice Chief, Division of Head and Neck Surgery, University of California, Los Angeles, School of Medicine, Center for the Health Sciences, 10833 Le Conte Avenue, Los Angeles, California 90095-1624*

Kedar K. Adour, M.D.   *Director of Research, Cranial Nerve Research Clinic, Department of Head and Neck Surgery, Kaiser Permanente Medical Center, 280 W. MacArthur Boulevard, Oakland, California 94611-5693*

Jayne B. Ahlstrom, M.S.   *Instructor, Department of Otolaryngology and Communicative Sciences, Medical University of South Carolina, 171 Ashley Avenue, Charleston, South Carolina 29425*

James C. Andrews, M.D., F.A.C.S.   *Professor, Division of Head and Neck Surgery, UCLA Medical Center, 10833 Le Conte Avenue, Los Angeles, California 90095*

Gregory A. Ator, M.D.   *Otologic Center, Inc., Otology/Neurotology, 3100 Broadway, Kansas City, Missouri 64111*

Robert W. Baloh, M.D.   *Professor, Departments of Neurology and Surgery (Head and Neck), University of California, Los Angeles, School of Medicine, 710 Westwood Plaza, Los Angeles, California 90095-1769; Director, Department of Neurology, UCLA Medical Center, Los Angeles, California 90095*

Kamran Barin, Ph.D.   *Assistant Professor, Department of Otolaryngology, The Ohio State University, 456 W. 10th Avenue, Columbus, Ohio 43210*

Donald P. Becker, M.D.   *Professor and Chief, Division of Neurosurgery, University of California, Los Angeles, School of Medicine, Los Angeles, California 90095*

Sanjay A. Bhansali, M.D.   *Atlanta Ear, Nose, and Throat Associates, 5555 Peachtree Dunwoody Road N.E., Atlanta, Georgia 30342-1703*

Dennis I. Bojrab, M.D.   *Associate Professor, Department of Otolaryngology, Wayne State University, Michigan Ear Institute, 27555 Middlebelt Road, Farmington Hills, Michigan 48334; Chief, Department of Otolaryngology-Head and Neck Surgery, Beaumont Hospital, 3601 W. 13 Mile Road, Royal Oak, Michigan 48075*

Alexandra R. Borges, M.D.   *VTG Assistant Professor, Department of Neuroradiology, UCLA Medical Center, 10833 Le Conte Avenue, Los Angeles, California 90095; Assistente Hospitalar, Department of Radiology, Instituto Portugues de Ongologia, R. Prof. Lima Basto, Lisboa 1070, Portugal*

Patrick E. Brookhouser, M.D.   *Director, Boys Town National Research Hospital; Father Flanagan Professor and Chairman, Department of Otolaryngology and Human Communication, Creighton University School of Medicine, 555 N. 30th Street, Omaha, Nebraska 68131-2136*

Stacy L. Butts, M.A., C.C.C.-A.   *Instructor/Clinical Audiologist, Department of Otolaryngology, University of Miami Ear Institute, 1666 N.W. 10th Avenue, Miami, Florida 33136*

Rinaldo F. Canalis, M.D., F.A.C.S. *Professor, Division of Head and Neck Surgery (Otolaryngology) and The Victor Goodhill Ear Institute, University of California, Los Angeles, School of Medicine, Los Angeles, California 90095-1624; Chief, Division of Head and Neck Surgery (Otolaryngology), Harbor-UCLA Medical Center, 1000 W. Carson Street, Torrance, California 90509; Co-director, Benign Brain Tumor and Skull Base Surgery Program (Neurosurgery), UCLA Medical Center, Los Angeles, California 90095*

Mack L. Cheney, M.D., F.A.C.S. *Associate Professor, Department of Otolaryngology, Harvard Medical School; Director, Division of Facial Plastic and Reconstructive Surgery, Massachusetts Eye and Ear Infirmary, 243 Charles Street, Boston, Massachusetts 02114*

Jeffrey T. Corwin, Ph.D. *Professor, Departments of Otolaryngology-Head and Neck Surgery and Neuroscience, University of Virginia School of Medicine, Charlottesville, Virginia 22908*

Donald D. Dirks, Ph.D. *Professor Emeritus, Division of Head and Neck Surgery, University of California, Los Angeles, School of Medicine, Hilgard and LeConte, Los Angeles, California 90095; Research Audiologist, Department of Veterans Affairs, Veterans Affairs Medical Center-Los Angeles, Wilshire and Sawtelle, Los Angeles, California 90025*

Shelly Dolan-Ash, M.S. *Department of Otolaryngology, University of Miami, 1666 N.W. 10th Avenue, Miami, Florida 33129*

Judy R. Dubno, Ph.D. *Professor, Department of Otolaryngology and Communicative Sciences, Medical University of South Carolina, 171 Ashley Avenue, Charleston, South Carolina 29425*

John D. Durrant, Ph.D. *Professor, Departments of Communication Science and Disorders and Otolaryngology, University of Pittsburgh, Forbes Tower 4033, Pittsburgh, Pennsylvania 15260; Professeur Associé en Physiologie, Otorhinolaryngology, Université Claude Bernard (Lyon 1), Hôpital Edouard Herriot, Place d'Arsonval, 69003 Lyon, France*

Bruce M. Edwards, M.A. *Audiologist, Department of Otolaryngology-Head and Neck Surgery, University of Michigan Health System, 1500 E. Medical Center Drive, TC 1904, Ann Arbor, Michigan 48109-0312*

Laurie S. Eisenberg, Ph.D. *Associate Scientist, Children's Auditory Research and Evaluation Center, House Ear Institute, 2100 W. Third Street, Los Angeles, California 90057*

John A. Ferraro, Ph.D. *Professor and Chairman, Department of Hearing and Speech, University of Kansas Medical Center, 3901 Rainbow Boulevard, Kansas City, Kansas 66160-7605*

Bruce L. Fetterman, M.D. *Clinical Assistant Professor, Department of Otolaryngology-Head and Neck Surgery, University of Tennessee, Memphis, Tennessee; Shea Ear Clinic, 6133 Poplar Pike, Memphis, Tennessee 38119*

Bruce J. Gantz, M.D. *Professor, Department of Otolaryngology-Head and Neck Surgery, University of Iowa; Head, Department of Otolaryngology-Head and Neck Surgery, The University of Iowa Hospitals and Clinics, 200 Hawkins Drive, Iowa City, Iowa 52242-1078*

George A. Gates, M.D., F.A.C.S. *Professor, Department of Otolaryngology-Head and Neck Surgery, University of Washington; Director, Virginia Merrill Bloedel Hearing Research Center, 1959 N.E. Pacific Street, Seattle, Washington 98195-7923*

Kenneth M. Grundfast, M.D., F.A.A.P., F.A.C.S. *Professor of Otolaryngology and Pediatrics and Interim Chairman, Department of Otolaryngology-Head and Neck Surgery, Georgetown University School of Medicine, 3800 Reservoir Road, N.W., Washington, D.C. 20007*

A. Julianna Gulya, M.D., F.A.C.S. *Clinical Professor, Department of Surgery (Otolaryngology-Head and Neck Surgery), The George Washington University, Washington, D.C. 20037*

Steven D. Handler, M.D. *Professor, Department of Otolaryngology-Head and Neck Surgery, University of Pennsylvania School of Medicine, 3400 Spruce Street; Associate Director, Department of Pediatric Otolaryngology, The Children's Hospital of Philadelphia, 34th Street and Civic Center Boulevard, Philadelphia, Pennsylvania 19104*

Irwin Harris, M.D., F.A.C.S. *Clinical Professor, Department of Surgery, Division of Head and Neck Surgery, University of California, Los Angeles, School of Medicine, 200 UCLA Medical Plaza, Los Angeles, California 90095-6959; Attending, Department of Surgery, Division of Head and Neck, UCLA Medical Center, 10833 Le Conte Avenue, Los Angeles, California 90024-2771*

George T. Hashisaki, M.D. *Assistant Professor, Department of Otolaryngology-Head and Neck Surgery, University of Virginia Medical Center, Charlottesville, Virginia 22908*

David S. Haynes, M.D. *Director of Otology and Neurotology, Department of Otolaryngology, Vanderbilt University Medical Center, 1301 22nd Avenue, Nashville, Tennessee 37232-5555; St. Thomas Hospital, Medical Plaza E., Nashville, Tennessee 37205*

Annelle V. Hodges, M.D. *Associate Professor, Department of Otolaryngology-Head & Neck Surgery, University of Miami Medical Center, 1666 N.W. 10th Avenue, Miami, Florida 33129*

Akira Ishiyama, M.D. *CHS, Division of Head and Neck Surgery, University of California, Los Angeles, School of Medicine, 10833 Le Conte Avenue, Los Angeles, California 90095*

C. Gary Jackson, M.D., F.A.C.S. *Clinical Professor, Department of Otolaryngology-Head and Neck Surgery, Otology and Neurotology, Vanderbilt University School of Medicine, 1211 22nd Avenue South, Nashville, Tennessee 37203; Department of Otolaryngology Head and Neck Surgery, Georgetown University Medical Center, 3800 Reservoir Road N.W., Washington, D.C. 20007-2197; Department of Surgery, Division of Otolaryngology Head and Neck Surgery, Otology and Neurotology, University of North Carolina School of Medicine, Chapel Hill, North Carolina 27599; Otologist/Neurotologist, Department of Surgery, Baptist Hospital, 2000 Church Street, Nashville, Tennessee 37203*

Herman A. Jenkins, M.D. *Professor, The Bobby R. Alford Department of Otolaryngology and Communicative Sciences, Baylor College of Medicine, One Baylor Plaza; Attending Physician, Active Staff, Otolaryngology-Head and Neck Surgery Service, The Methodist Hospital, 6565 Fannin, Houston, Texas 77030*

Gary D. Josephson, M.D., F.A.A.P. *Assistant Professor, Department of Otolaryngology and Pediatrics, University of Miami; Chief, Division of Pediatric Otolaryngology-Head and Neck Surgery, University of Miami, Jacksonville Hospital, 1666 N.W. 10th Avenue, Miami, Florida 33136*

Jack M. Kartush, M.D. *Academic Professor, Department of Otology/Neurotology, Wayne State University; Director, Department of Otology/Neurotology, Providence Hospital, 16001 W. Nine Mile Road, Southfield, Michigan 48075*

Paul R. Kileny, Ph.D., F.A.S.H.A. *Professor, Otolaryngology-Head and Neck Surgery, University of Michigan; Director, Audiology/Electrophysiology, Department of Otolaryngology-Head and Neck Surgery, University of Michigan Health System, 1500 E. Medical Center Drive, Ann Arbor, Michigan 48109-0312*

Mark Kriskovich, M.D. *Department of Otolaryngology-Head and Neck Surgery, University of Utah School of Medicine, 50 N. Medical Center Drive, Salt Lake City, Utah 84132*

Thomas C. Kryzer, M.D. *Clinical Assistant Professor, Department of Surgery, University of Kansas School of Medicine—Wichita, 1010 N. Kansas; Wichita Ear Clinic, 427 N. Hillside Street, Wichita, Kansas 67214-4917*

Paul R. Lambert, M.D., F.A.C.S. *Professor and Chair, Department of Otolaryngology-Head and Neck Surgery and Communication Sciences, Medical University of South Carolina, Charleston, South Carolina 29425*

Robert B. Lufkin, M.D. *Professor, Department of Radiology, University of California, Los Angeles, School of Medicine, 10833 Le Conte Avenue, Los Angeles, California 90095-1721*

Dennis R. Maceri, M.D. *Associate Professor, Department of Otolaryngology-Head and Neck Surgery, University of Southern California School of Medicine, 9621 Jellico Avenue, Northridge, California 91325*

Thomas M. Magardino, M.D. *Chief Resident, Department of Otolaryngology, University of Pennsylvania Medical Center, 3400 Spruce Street; Chief Resident, Department of Pediatric Otolaryngology, The Children's Hospital of Philadelphia, 34th Street and Civic Center Boulevard, Philadelphia, Pennsylvania 19104*

Charles D. Martinez, M.A.   *Department of Audiology, West Los Angeles VA Healthcare Center, 11301 Wilshire Boulevard, Los Angeles, California 90073*

Samuel Marzo, M.D.   *Associate Professor, Department of Otolaryngology, Loyola University Medical Center, 2160 South First Avenue, Maywood, Illinois 60153*

Jennifer L. Maw, M.D.   *Michigan Ear Institue, 27555 Middlebelt Road, Farmington Hills, Michigan 43334*

Amy McConkey Robbins, M.S., C.C.C.-Sp.   *Speech-Language Pathologist, Communication Consulting Services-Indianapolis, 8512 Spring Mill Road, Indianapolis, Indiana 46260*

Cliff A. Megerian, M.D., F.A.C.S.   *Associate Professor, Department of Otolaryngology, University of Massachusetts Medical School; Director of Otology and Neurotology, Department of Otolaryngology, University of Massachusetts Memorial Medical Center, 55 Lake Avenue North, Worcester, Massachusetts 01655*

Richard T. Miyamoto, M.D.   *Arilla Spence DiVault Professor and Chairman, Department of Otolaryngology-Head and Neck Surgery, Indiana University School of Medicine, Riley Hospital, 702 Barnhill Drive, Indianapolis, Indiana 46202*

Edwin M. Monsell, M.D., Ph.D.   *Head, Division of Otology and Neurotological Skull Base Surgery, Department of Otolaryngology-Head and Neck Surgery, Henry Ford Health System and Henry Ford Health Sciences Center, 2799 W. Grand Boulevard, Detroit, Michigan 48202*

Donald E. Morgan, Ph.D.   *Vice President of Clinical Research and Medical Affairs, Decibel Instruments, Inc., 3857 Breakwater Avenue, Fremont, California 94555*

Anita N. Newman, M.D.   *Faculty, Department of Head and Neck Surgery, University of Southern California School of Medicine; University Hospital, School of Medicine, 1510 San Pablo Street, Los Angeles, California 90020*

Douglas Noffsinger, Ph.D.   *Clinical Associate Professor, Department of Surgery (Head and Neck), University of California, Los Angeles, School of Medicine, 10833 Le Conte Boulevard, Los Angeles, California 90095; Professional Department Chair, Department of Audiology and Speech Pathology, West Los Angeles VA Healthcare Center, 11301 Wilshire Boulevard, Los Angeles, California 90073*

Michael M. Paparella, M.D.   *Otopathology Laboratory, Department of Otolaryngology, University of Minnesota, Minneapolis, Minnesota; Minnesota Ear, Head, and Neck Clinic, 701 25th Avenue South, Minneapolis, Minnesota 55454*

Dennis G. Pappas, Sr., M.D.   *Pappas Ear Clinic, P.C., 2937 Seventh Avenue South, Birmingham, Alabama 35233*

Brian P. Perry, M.D.   *Fellow Associate, Department of Otolaryngology, The University of Iowa, 200 Hawkins Drive, Iowa City, Iowa 52242*

Eduardo H. Rubinstein, M.D., Ph.D.   *Professor, Department of Anesthesiology, University of California, Los Angeles, School of Medicine, Center for the Health Sciences, Los Angeles, California 90095*

Jay T. Rubinstein, M.D., Ph.D.   *Assistant Professor, Department of Otolaryngology, The University of Iowa Hospitals and Clinics, 200 Hawkins Drive, Iowa City, Iowa 52242*

Robert O. Ruder, M.D.   *Department of Head and Neck Surgery, UCLA Medical Center, Beverly Hills, California 90024; Head and Neck Surgery, Cedars Sinai Medical Center, Los Angeles, California 90211-1715*

Roger A. Ruth, Ph.D.   *Professor, Department of Otolaryngology-Head and Neck Surgery, University of Virginia School of Medicine; Director, Department of Communication and Balance Disorders, University of Virginia Health System, Primary Care Center, Charlottesville, Virginia 22906-0008*

Hamed Sajjadi, M.D., F.A.C.S.   *Clinical Faculty, Neurotology Fellowship Program, Minnesota Ear, Head, and Neck Clinic, 701 25th Avenue South, Minneapolis, Minnesota 55454*

Joel A. Sercarz, M.D.   *Associate Professor, Department of Surgery-Head and Neck, University of California, Los Angeles; Attending Surgeon, Department of Surgery, UCLA Medical Center, 10833 Le Conte Avenue, Los Angeles, California 90095*

Clough Shelton, M.D., F.A.C.S.   *Division of Otolaryngology-Head and Neck Surgery, University of Utah Medical Center, 50 N. Medical Drive, Salt Lake City, Utah 84132-0001*

Neil T. Shepard, Ph.D.   *Professor, Department of Otorhinolaryngology, University of Pennsylvania; Director of Audiology, Speech Pathology and Balance Center, Department of Otorhinolaryngology, Hospital of the University of Pennsylvania, 3400 Spruce Street, Philadelphia, Pennsylvania 19104*

Lucy Shih, M.D.   *Assistant Clinical Professor of Otolaryngology, University of Southern California School of Medicine, Los Angeles, California 90033*

Joel B. Shulman, M.D.   *Otosurgical Group, 2080 Century Park East, Los Angeles, California 90067*

Marshall E. Smith, M.D.   *Assistant Professor, Division of Otolaryngology-Head and Neck Surgery, University of Utah School of Medicine, 50 N. Medical Drive, Salt Lake City, Utah 84132; Attending Physician-Active Staff, Division of Otolaryngology-Head and Neck Surgery, Primary Children's Medical Center, 100 N. Medical Drive, Salt Lake City, Utah 84113*

Ian S. Storper, M.D.   *Assistant Professor, Department of Otolaryngology-Head and Neck Surgery, College of Physicians and Surgeons, Columbia University, New York, New York; Department of Otolaryngology/Head and Neck Surgery, Columbia University, 630 W. 168th Street, New York, New York 10032*

Barry Strasnick, M.D., F.A.C.S.   *Associate Professor, Department of Otolaryngology, Eastern Virginia Medical School, 825 Fairfax Avenue, Norfolk, Virginia 23507; Chief, Department of Otolaryngology, DePaul Medical Center, 110 Kingsley Lane, Norfolk, Virginia 23505*

Steven A. Telian, M.D.   *John L. Kemink Professor, Department of Otolaryngology-Head and Neck Surgery, University of Michigan Medical Center; Director, Division of Otology/Neurotology, Department of Otolaryngology-Head and Neck Surgery, University of Michigan Health System, 1500 E. Medical Center Drive, Ann Arbor, Michigan 48109-0312*

J. Pablo Villablanca, M.D.   *Assistant Professor, Department of Radiological Sciences/Neuroradiology, UCLA Medical Center, 10833 Le Conte Avenue, Los Angeles, California 90095-1721*

Phillip A. Wackym, M.D., F.A.C.S.   *Professor and Chairman, Department of Otolaryngology and Communication Sciences, Medical College of Wisconsin; Chief, Department of Otolaryngology-Head and Neck Surgery, Froedtert Memorial Lutheran Hospital, 9200 W. Wisconsin Avenue, Milwaukee, Wisconsin 53226*

Mark D. Wilson, M.D.   *Department of Otolaryngology-Head and Neck Surgery, Henry Ford Health System and Henry Ford Health Sciences Center, 2799 W. Grand Boulevard, Detroit, Michigan 48202-2608*

Foreword

It is my pleasure to write the foreword for this text edited by my colleagues and friends Rinaldo Canalis and Paul Lambert. Having dedicated my career to otology, it is a great pleasure to see the development of a book which lives up to its title, *The Ear: Comprehensive Otology.*

The editors have assembled a group of recognized authorities in the field to write chapters on every aspect of the specialty. Topics from basic science through evaluation and then medical and surgical treatment of diseases from the external to the inner ear are discussed.

Otology and neurotology are rapidly developing fields. This book will provide an update on the latest developments in our exciting specialty.

Development of a text such as this requires tremendous effort not only on the part of the editors but of the many authors. People in training will be grateful to them for the basics that this book provides. Practitioners will thank them for conveying all of the latest information to them.

Congratulations Rinaldo and Paul for the development of this comprehensive text!

Derald E. Brackmann
House Ear Clinic, Inc.

Preface

The second half of our century has witnessed an explosive growth of knowledge and technical advancement in every medical discipline. Otology has been a full participant in this dynamic process in great part because of the efforts of a generation of men and women of exceptional intelligence, clear vision, and resolute dedication to the field. These efforts and otology's leadership on many scientific fronts, such as the development of microsurgery and sensory prostheses to name the most salient, have propelled it to a position of ever-increasing influence and have redefined its scope.

This enormous growth of knowledge has produced a corresponding expansion in the specialized literature. The large number of journals dedicated to otolaryngology and allied fields—many of recent appearance—along with the proliferation of electronic vehicles of communication have resulted in such a flood of information that it is a daunting task to integrate it and stay current within the context of otology.

We have felt for some time, and a careful survey of leaders in the field support this impression, that a book offering a comprehensive view of current otology could serve as an integrated teaching tool and point of reference within the specialty's literature. Therefore, the purpose of *The Ear: Comprehensive Otology* is to provide as complete coverage of the field of clinical otology as demanded by current knowledge in an authoritative, precise, and discriminating way. The book is oriented to serve both the otolaryngology resident as a practical didactic tool and the practicing otolaryngologist as an up-to-date reference source of clinical and basic information. The book has not been structured as a surgical guide but it does incorporate sufficient commentary and illustration of operative technique to give the reader a broad overview of surgical management.

The book has been divided into 12 sections containing 54 chapters written by authorities in the field. In order to give a dynamic perspective of otology, it opens with a historical overview and closes with a look at the way current changes—technical and otherwise—may influence otology in the near future. The scientific basis of the specialty is emphasized early with the initial 5 chapters addressing development, gross and microscopic anatomy of the ear, and auditory and vestibular physiology. The clinical chapters are problem-oriented, and, to avoid redundancy, include anatomical and physiological facts only as needed for the understanding of specific clinical problems. In general, the sections have been organized along anatomical lines (e.g., external ear, middle ear, vestibular system, facial nerve). Subjects such as trauma and neoplasia, that tend to simultaneously involve various anatomical areas, are addressed in separate sections. All chapters include summary points to guide the reader to the fundamental information contained within. At the end of each section one or more chapters address rehabilitation as pertaining to the system covered. Due to its importance and distinct orientation, auditory rehabilitation has been included in a separate section addressing amplification, education, and surgery for deafness.

Special emphasis has been placed on assessment techniques. For example, we have dedicated eight chapters to audiology and two chapters to the evaluation of patients with balance disorders. The audiology chapters have been specifically geared to the practicing otolaryngologist. To this end the various peripheral and central auditory methods of evaluation are discussed, correlating in detail physiology and pathology with test results, but without emphasizing technical issues.

Illustrations have been selected to clarify basic and complex concepts described in the text. Every effort has been made to include the best available illustrations, therefore, a number were chosen from previous publications because it was concluded that they could not be improved. Many color photographs have been incorporated into a single section; black and white versions of each of these are included and referenced in pertinent chapters.

We hope that the organization and content of this volume will provide the reader with a clear understanding of current views in otology, present a balanced perspective on controversial issues, and facilitate decision making in complex clinical situations.

Rinaldo F. Canalis, M.D.
Paul R. Lambert, M.D.

Acknowledgments

It is not possible to convey fully our gratitude to the many friends and colleagues who have contributed to this text. The depth of their expertise in the various reaches of otology have made this work truly comprehensive.

It is also not possible to name all the individuals who have nurtured this book during its development, but we do owe a special debt of gratitude to Danette Knopp, senior editor at Lippincott Williams & Wilkins, whose clear intelligence, availability, and experience were the cornerstone of this project from its inception. Special thanks are also due to our secretaries, Catalina Carreon (Harbor-UCLA) and Helen Koury (UVA), for their dedication, patience, and generosity with their time in the typing and retyping of so many chapters and innumerable editorial changes. Similarly, we are very grateful to Stephanie Harris, developmental editor, whose organizational skills were invaluable in bringing this book to completion.

Our sincere thanks are also due to Christine Coleman, M.A., who provided valuable assistance in the early organization of this book and to Donald D. Dirks, Ph.D., who not only contributed several audiology chapters, but also undertook much of the editing of this section.

Dedication to Our Mentors

VICTOR GOODHILL, M.D., F.A.C.S.

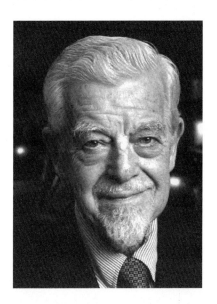

Dr. Victor Goodhill was born in Boston, Massachusetts in 1911. He received his medical degree in 1937 from the University of Southern California where he taught otology as clinical professor until joining the UCLA faculty in 1960. Dr. Goodhill was responsible for founding the hearing and speech clinic at Children's Hospital, Los Angeles County Hospital, and Cedars of Lebanon Hospital. He was also one of the founders of the John Tracy Clinic and created the Hope for Hearing Foundation. He was a member of Phi Beta Kappa and Alpha Omega Alpha. He was awarded the degree of Doctor of Humane Letters (*honoris causa*) by the University of Judaism-Jewish Theological Seminary in 1970. He received the Maimonides award of Wisconsin in 1974. He was the University of Southern California's Alumnus of the Year in 1972 and was honored with the Fifth Joseph Toynbee Memorial Lectureship at the Royal College of Surgeons (England) in 1976. Goodhill received the Sir William Wilde Discourse, Royal Society of Surgeons (Ireland) in 1983, and the distinguished Service Award from the California Speech, Language, Hearing Association in 1985.

Dr. Goodhill was fellow and former governor of the American College of Surgeons; fellow of the Acoustical Society; past chairman of the Section of Otorhinolaryngology of the American Medical Association; past president of the American Laryngological, Rhinological and Otological Society, the American Otological Society, and of the American Academy of Otolaryngology; and he held memberships in 19 other societies. He was an honorary member of the Otorhinolaryngological Societies of Japan, France, Australia, and England; former president of the Otosclerosis Study Group; and founding member of the Society of University Otolaryngologists.

Dr. Goodhill wrote the first textbook on stapes surgery in 1960 and an otology textbook entitled *Ear Diseases, Deafness and Dizziness* in 1979 which received the honorable mention award in the physician's category for the American Medical Writer's Association in 1980 and is the inspiration for this book. He wrote more than 150 journal articles and 25 chapters in medical textbooks. In 1983 he authored, in collaboration with the UCLA Office of Instructional Development, the award-winning video entitled "Beethoven: Triumph over Silence" which has been shown all over the world.

Dr. Goodhill was foremost a world-known otologic surgeon, a professor of surgery, an accomplished violinist, a talmudic scholar, and a physician of great wisdom in his interactions with patients. He was a teacher who had a profound influence on the young men and women who trained in the UCLA Division of Head and Neck Surgery and was often described as the sort of teacher who changes a student's life. Many of his former students are now department heads at universities throughout the world. The Victor Goodhill Ear Center was established in his honor at UCLA in 1984 to support research in hearing and balance disorders.

At his death at the age of 83 in 1994, Dr. Victor Goodhill was emeritus professor of otology at UCLA. To quote from Dean Goodhill, his son, "My father's favorite prayer was *LaDor VaDor*, which means 'from generation to generation.' It speaks to the continuity of life that binds us all to God and to those who have come before us. It links us inexorably to future men and women who will live with the legacy of whatever we leave behind."

This book, created by those he taught, is his legacy to the doctors and patients who meant so much to him.

Christine Coleman, M.A.
Executive Director
Hope for Hearing Foundation

HOWARD P. HOUSE, M.D.

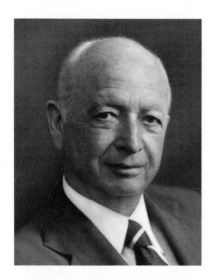

Few physicians have received more national and international recognition than Howard P. House, M.D. He has been president of almost all the major Otolaryngology-Head and Neck Surgery Societies and has received dozens of honorary degrees (in both medicine and law) and fellowships in international medical organizations. As an ear surgeon for over 55 years, his accomplishments in the field of otology are legendary. Particularly noteworthy are his pioneering role in otosclerosis surgery and his founding of the House Ear Institute and House Ear Clinic. These institutions have been a major force in otologic medicine and surgery in the latter half of the twentieth century, with significant contributions to hearing science and clinical research and with the education of hundreds of otolaryngologists in advanced ear surgery. On a personal note, all who have studied at Dr. House's side have marveled at the warmth, compassion, and empathy he shows his patients. I am grateful for his instruction not only in otologic surgery, but also in the finer points of the art of medicine.

WILLIAM F. HOUSE, M.D.

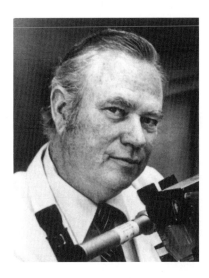

William F. House, M.D. is regarded as the father of neurotology. His contributions to the fields of acoustic tumor surgery, Meniere's disease, and the cochlear implant are the substance of that accolade. After completing his residency training in 1956, William House joined his brother Howard in practice and began his pioneering work on the inner ear. The legacies of this work are well known to all otolaryngologists; perhaps less well appreciated, however, are the implications these endeavors have had on microsurgery and on the collaborative efforts of otolaryngologists and neurosurgeons. In 1956, William and Howard House were among the first physicians in the United States to import a Zeiss microscope from Germany after hearing Professor Wullstein, head of the ENT department at the University of Würzburg, present his experience with microscopic middle ear surgery. The inaugural use of the operating microscope for intercranial surgery occurred two years later when William House performed a middle cranial fossa decompression of the internal auditory canal. Dr. House then refined this approach for acoustic tumors and introduced translabyrinthine surgery for resection of these lesions. These procedures became a major impetus for the integration of neurosurgical and otolaryngic skills in patient care. We as physicians, and our patients, are indebted to the wisdom and creativity of William House, and especially to his desire and ability to teach. Those of us who have sat at the microscope with him appreciate the singular educational experience we have had.

THE EAR
COMPREHENSIVE OTOLOGY

The Ear: Comprehensive Otology,
edited by R. F. Canalis and P.R. Lambert.
Lippincott Williams & Wilkins, Philadelphia © 2000.

CHAPTER 1

Otology—Unfolding of a Specialty

Dennis G. Pappas, Sr.

Modern otologists inherited from Hippocrates, the importance of etiology of diseases; from Eustachius, intricacies of the auditory tube; from a postmaster, how to sound the eustachian tube; from Valsalva, how to expel pus from the tympanum; from the father of Oscar Wilde, how to incise a mastoid; from the father of Arnold Toynbee, the importance of pathologic anatomy; from Politzer, the site of origin of otosclerosis being that of the cochlea; from a Nobel Prize laureate, caloric testing of the labyrinth; from a socialite Parisian physician, that the origin of dizziness was probably the labyrinth; and, from an Italian nobleman, the microscopic end structure of the auditory nerve.

Many of the great achievements in otology have passed the test of time and are as coveted today as when first introduced. Whether it's Lempert's fenestration, or Guyot's eustachian catheter, otology's legacy is perhaps one of the most stunning histories of medicine.

D. G. Pappas: Pappas Ear Clinic, Birmingham, Alabama 35233

In a chapter of this length only a sampling of personalities and events can be conveyed. Twentieth century contributions will undoubtedly be discussed by other authors in this text.

I feel that it is important that we realize the close relationship between otology and the history of medicine. With this in mind, it is important that we review an outline of Garrison's classification of the history of medicine (Table 1) (1).

ANCIENT MEDICINE TO THE RENAISSANCE

Perhaps the greatest accomplishment of the Egyptians was the practice of recording the voluminous data they assimilated. From the *Papyrus Ebers* we extract Egyptian knowledge of otologic remedies and prescriptions and from the *Papyrus Edwin Smith* we learn of deafness caused by injury.

TABLE 1. *Garrison's classification of the history of medicine*

I. Primitive Medicine
II. Egyptian Medicine
III. Greek Medicine
  1. Before Hippocrates
  2. The Classic Period (460–146 B.C.)
  3. The Greco-Roman Period (146 B.C.–A.D. 476)
IV. The Byzantine Period (A.D. 476–732)
V. The Mohammedan and Jewish Periods (A.D. 132–1096)
VI. The Medieval Period (1096–1438)
VII. The Period of the Renaissance. The Revival of Learning, and the Reformation (1438–1600)
VIII. The Seventeenth Century: The Age of Individual Scientific Endeavor
IX. The Eighteenth Century: The Age of Theories and Systems
X. The Nineteenth Century: The Beginnings of Organized Advancement of Science
XI. The Twentieth Century: The Beginnings of Organized Preventive Medicine

From Aesculapius (500 B.C.–A.D. 500) emerges a mixture of mythology and rational medicine (psychotherapy) (Fig. 1). Scientific medicine begins with Hippocrates, who developed the concept of individual diagnosis (principle of etiologic factors) and the doctrine of physis (the body itself tries to restore a disturbed equilibrium); then emerged the anatomic-physiologic work of Aristotle (382–322 B.C.). Galen (A.D. 121–199) advanced the anatomic work of Aristotle.

Prior to the Renaissance and especially before the era of the great Italian anatomists, knowledge of the structures of the ear was limited to those that were readily visible. Ear diseases were treated empirically, primarily with herbal elixirs, and otologic surgery was confined to trauma of the auricle and removal of foreign bodies from the external auditory canals.

During the Middle Ages, direct examination of the ear was seldom practiced; therefore, few otologic discoveries were made. Early in the fourteenth century, however, a few curious scientists began to lay a background for the innovative and daring studies of the ear done by the great Italian anatomists.

FORERUNNERS OF THE GREAT ITALIAN OTOANATOMISTS

Alessandro Achillini (1463–1512)

Achillini, a professor of anatomy at Bologna, has been mentioned by some as the first to describe the ossicles of the ear. According to J.H. Baas, Achillini reported this in *Annotations Anatomicae in Mundinum* (2), which was published posthumously in 1520. Adam Politzer, however, reported this not to be so. He had tracked down Achillini's rare text and found only a very scant description of the ear, perhaps including the tympanic membrane ("miringa"), but no mention of the ossicles in the manuscript. Politzer theorized that the assumption that Achillini discovered the ossicles probably resulted from the misinterpretation of a passage from Nicolaus Massa's 1536 report. (The malleoli [little hammers] were first mentioned in that work by Massa, however.) Politzer's contention was that Massa was simply referring to the

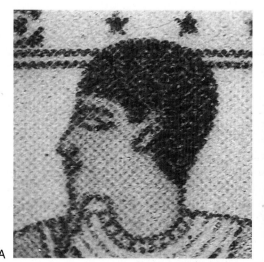
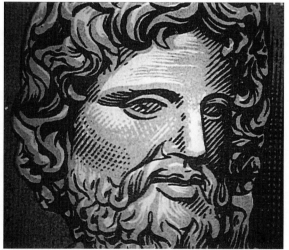

FIG. 1. A: Imhopteh, the first noted physician, was honored as a sage, a physician, an astronomer, and an architect. Imhopteh was deified, like Aesculapius of Greece, to full deity in 600 B.C. (From stamp, Egypt, 1928). **B:** Although Aesculapius (500 B.C.–A.D. 500) emerged as a mixture of mythology and rationality, the rational practice was a naturalistic point of view containing a degree of psychotherapy. Typically a patient came to the temple (Epidauras), mingled with other patients discussing symptoms, visited the magnificent outdoor theater and a stadium in which games were featured, received a potion to promote dreams, and was allowed to sleep in the abaton where Aesculapius or another physician applied medication to joints for arthritis, ointment for eye disease, etc. When fully awakened the patient was cured by prescribed drugs, diet, or other modes of treatment. (From stamp, Greece, 1960s.)

fact that the ossicles were discovered during the time of Achillini, and not that they were discovered by him (3).

Jacopo Berengario da Carpi (1470–1550)

da Carpi (1460–1530[?]) was one of the greatest physicians of his time. He was most often referred to as da Carpi, or Carpi, in recognition of the town in Modena where he was born. Carpi received his early instructions from his father, who was a surgeon, and his medical degree from Bologna. An accurate and patient investigator, he took pride in having dissected several hundred cadavers.

In his 1521 commentary on anatomy, entitled *Anatomi Carpi Isagogae...* (Bonon. 1514), Carpi successfully documented his knowledge of the two small ossicles, which he described as being adjacent to the tympanic membrane and within the tympanic cavity, which contained the "aer implantus." It was his theory that the vibrations of the ossicles that caused them to strike against each other were activated by movements in the outside air that reached them through the external auditory canal (4). He did not, however, name the malleus and incus; this was done later by Andreas Vesalius.

PERIOD OF THE RENAISSANCE

Andreas Vesalius (1514–1564)

Vesalius was born into a family of physicians in Brussels. He began his medical education at Montpelier and later went to Paris, eagerly looking forward to studying anatomy under the highly esteemed Sylvius. The disappointment he experienced would have disillusioned a young man of less spirit and courage to the point of abandoning his goals. The manner in which anatomy was taught there duplicated the Middle Ages method Mondino de Luzzi used in Bologna. Students were not allowed to dissect; they were required to sit in the audience while a barber surgeon followed directions from the script by Galen read by the professor. Vesalius reacted with such antagonistic determination to receive hands-on training that he was allowed to replace the barber surgeon on at least one occasion.

His persistence prompted him to move to Italy, where the socio-religious atmosphere was more lenient toward dissection. He went first to Venice and then to Padua, where he received his medical degree in 1537 and where he remained as a professor of surgery and anatomy.

The results of a dissection Vesalius performed in 1543 led to his first great contribution to anatomic knowledge in medical literature, which he completed in his late 20s. Frequently referred to as the *De fabrica,* this work contained the first significant medical illustrations (5). He has been reputed to have been the founder of modern anatomy, but it is obvious from the wood carvings in the

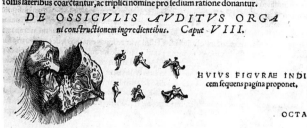

FIG. 2. First diagram of the ossicles. Vesalius came upon the ossicles in a perfunctory manner. Most startling was his omission of any mention of the stapes. Although he described the promontory of the middle ear, he made little mention of any other portion of the middle or internal ear. (From *De fabrica,* Reynold's Library, Birmingham, Alabama.)

De fabrica that, although his knowledge of many anatomic structures was impressive, his knowledge of otologic anatomy was lacking. They revealed a very poor conception of the shape of the ossicles and their attachment to each other (Fig. 2). Although Vesalius identified and named the malleus and incus, which he also referred to as the hammer and anvil, their articulation is misrepresented. He identified the tensor tympani, but did not recognize it as a muscle, and he described the anterior position of the oval window, which he compared to the more posterior position of the round window. Although he described the promontory position of the middle ear, he made little mention of any other portion of the middle or the internal ear. Most startling, however, is his omission of any mention of the stapes (6).

Vesalius was hot headed and stubborn, and he continued to fiercely oppose the manner in which anatomy was being taught (7). He apparently became exasperated with academic politics at Padua and exhausted by criticism of his pro-Galenic peers. Eventually he left to become court physician in Spain and later went to Jerusalem, but his heart remained in Padua and the memories of the work he had done there. When he was asked to return as successor to his student, Falloppio, who had died unexpectedly, his passage on an ill-fated ship became a victim of stormy seas. It wrecked on the Greek island of Zakynthos (Zante), in the Ionian Sea, and there his body was found and buried by a blacksmith (8).

In spite of his shortcomings in otologic anatomy, Vesalius initiated otologic studies that led to further investigations, and he startled the world with new anatomic discoveries.

Bartholomeus Eustachius (1510/1520–1574)

From the anatomy department of the University of Rome, Eustachius posed as a brash rival to the other anatomists in Italy. Although little is known of his personal life, his entire career seems to have been marked by a lack of dependence on other scientists. However, his close ties to the Catholic church, particularly to Pope Sixtus IV (1471 to 1484) to whom he was personal physician, may well have influenced his teachings and inhibited him from making public some of his findings and contradictions of Galen's theories.

Eustachius very openly positioned himself as the discoverer of the stapes and attempted to convince his colleagues of this. This issue remained divided among several possibilities until the credit ultimately was given to Giovanni Filippo Ingrassia (1510–1580) of Naples because of his clear and complete description of the structure.

Eustachius' anatomic skill and exact investigative policy were best indicated in his study of the most inaccessible anatomic structure in the body, the auditory tube. Scientists had shied away from exploring its function because of its perilous location at the base of the skull. Eustachius was the first to describe its bony and cartilaginous portion, its oval shape, and its course from the anterolateral skull base to the nasopharynx (Fig. 3). His description was so complete and thorough that the structure became known posthumously as the Eustachian tube (9), although the structure itself was known even to the ancients.

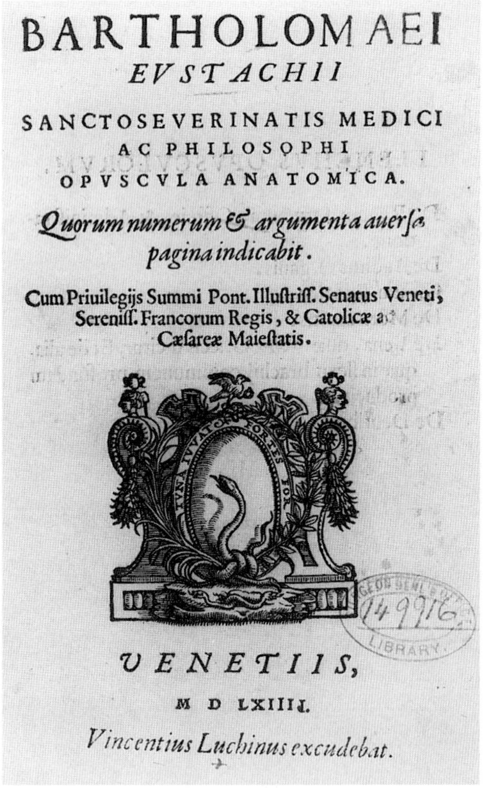
BARTHOLOMAEI
EVSTACHII
SANCTOSEVERINATIS MEDICI
AC PHILOSOPHI
OPVSCVLA ANATOMICA.
Quorum numerum & argumenta auersa pagina indicabit.
Cum Priuilegijs Summi Pont. Illuſtriſſ. Senatus Veneti, Sereniſſ. Francorum Regis, & Catolicæ ac Cæſareæ Maieſtatis.
VENETIIS,
M D LXIIII.
Vincentius Luchinus excudebat.

FIG. 3. Title page of Eustachius' *Opuscula Anatomica.* The text consisted of six chapters, one of which was devoted to the organ of hearing. This chapter probably represents the earliest written material dealing exclusively with the ear. (From the National Library of Medicine, Washington, D.C.)

Gabriele Falloppio (Fallopius) (1523–1562)

Falloppio was the son of a respected family in Modena and probably the greatest anatomist of his era. He studied under Vesalius and, in 1747, at the age of 24 he became professor of anatomy at Ferrara. One year later he became professor of anatomy at Pisa. In 1551, he succeeded Vesalius at Padua. Falloppio's contributions in anatomy, chemistry, botany, and surgery were made in a short academic lifetime (Fig. 4). He died of tuberculosis at the age of 39 (10).

Falloppio was an extremely careful observer who had the ability to make astute comparisons. It was he who gave the first clear description of the tympanic membrane and tympanic cavity. In addition, he described the facial canal that bears his name (aqueductus Fallopii) as resembling an aqueduct, and the chorda tympani; he recognized the separate origins of the VII and VIII cranial nerves; and he directed attention to the semicircular canals and sphenoid sinuses (11).

Other Renaissance Anatomists of Otologic Importance

Volcher Coiter (1534–1600) (Fig. 5) wrote the first treatise solely of the ear, *Extrenarum et Internarum Principalium Corpes Humani Partum Tabulae atque Anatomicae Exercititionis* (Noribergae: Theodorici Gerlatzeni, 1573), which contained *De auditus instrumento,* which was initially published as a separate work. Girolamo Fabrizzi (1533–1619) (Fig. 6) left a legacy of significant anatomic literature, including *De Visione, Voce, Auditu* (Venetiis: F. Balzetta, n.d.), which covered the eye and throat along with the ear. One of his students Guilio Casserio ([?]1561–1616) wrote the classic description of the voice and hearing organs, *De Vocis Audituso Organis* (Ferrariae: V. Baldinus, 1601), which contained the first complete anatomic study of the ear.

Concomitant Investigations by Others

While the most pivotal advances in otoanatomy took place in Italy during the Renaissance, the efforts of many scientists and physicians from a number of countries had a significant influence. A "post hoc: ergo propter hoc" philosophy of disease prevailed until the great anatomists began to shed light on the cause and effect of pathologic processes and in some countries even after. It should be kept in mind that even as late as the sixteenth century, little anatomy, especially of the ear, was known outside of Italy. As the need for surgical intervention developed, the important influence of keen anatomic awareness became apparent. This could account for the number of physi-

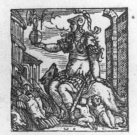

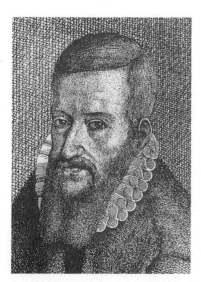

FIG. 4. A: *Gabriele Falloppio.* During his brief life, Falloppio produced one major written work, the *Observationes Anatomicae,* which was more of a narrative reflecting on the works of Vesalius than a classic textbook. Along with his correction of, and commentary on Vesalius' work, Falloppio reported some of his original work in this volume. Although a great deal of his attention was spent on the female reproductive organs, he gave a great deal of his attention to the anatomy of the ear. (From the author's collection.) **B:** Title page of *Observationes Anatomicae.* (From Reynold's Library, Birmingham, Alabama.)

FIG. 5. *Volcher Coiter.* Coiter (1534–1600) was born in The Netherlands and studied anatomy in Italy and Montpelier. He wrote two treatises that, taken together, form a compendium of all that was known concerning the ear in his day. Coiter discussed the anatomy and physiology of each part of the ear, particularly emphasizing the design and function of each. (From the author's collection.)

cians who converged to study under the noteworthy Italian anatomists and explain the coupling of operating skill and anatomic knowledge apparent in the renowned surgeons of this era (1400–1600). There were others, outside those in Italy, who became significant names in the history of medicine, such as Ambroïse Paré, the Huguenot son of a valet and one of the most outstanding surgeons in France; Paracelsus, of Switzerland; Platter of Basel, Switzerland; and, Hildanus, of Germany, all of whom made important otologic contributions.

Two very important clinical contributions during this period were those of Hieronymus Mercurialis (1530–1601), who introduced *De Compositione Medicamentorum* (12). In this treatise he addressed the medical treatment of diseases of the eye and ear; thus, this treatise is considered the first clinical otologic manual. The other otologic contribution of clinical significance was Girolamo Capivaccio's (1552–1589) discovery.

Capivaccio approached clinical evaluations with an attempt to ascribe the symptoms to a specific anatomic site. As edited by J.H. Baylo of Frankfurt in 1603, he related the origin of hearing losses to structures in the hearing pathway. If he was not the first to distinguish a conductive from a sensorineural hearing loss, he did intro-

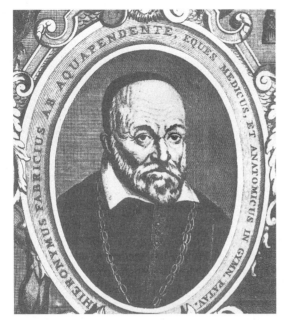

FIG. 6. *Fabricius ab Aquapendente (Girolamo Fabrizzi).* Fabricius was born in the town of Aquapendente, and, although his family was not wealthy, he received an education befitting a child of nobility. By his late teenage years his academic pursuits had taken him to the University of Padua, where he studied languages and philosophy and became an extern to Falloppio. After completing his medical studies (c. 1559), Fabricius set up medical practice and continued to follow his mentor's example of learning through dissections. He quickly became so recognized as an authority on dissection that by 1566 the Venetian Senate had appointed him chairman of surgery at his alma mater, the University of Padua. Fabricius left a legacy of significant anatomic literature including his description of the structures of the ear, yet he is best remembered as the mentor of William Harvey. (From Politzer's *Geschichte der Ohrenheilkunde, Volume I.*)

duce bone conduction testing to clinical otology. To determine the nature of a hearing loss, he had the patient grasp the end of an iron rod with the front teeth. The other end touched the strings of a zither. If sound was heard when the strings were plucked, he ascertained the hearing loss to be caused by a disease of the tympanic membrane (conductive). If no sound was heard, he concluded the hearing loss originated in the labyrinth (sensorineural) (13).

THE KINDLING OF OTOLOGY: NEW HORIZONS IN OTOLOGIC ANATOMY AND PHYSIOLOGY

Introduction of Inductive Science

Sir Francis Bacon (1561–1626) propounded the philosophy that new observations and experimental results should be melded with accepted facts to enable the discovery of the general physical principle behind a phenomenon (individual science).

Bacon had little regard for the disciples of Aristotle, saying that men should study the world around them instead of pouring over the works of antiquity. A Franciscan friar, he reasoned that if the world was God's handiwork, then studying it could be considered a form of piety (14).

Otology's First Clinical Primer: Duverney's Treatise

Guichard Joseph Duverney (1648–1730) was born the son of the village doctor in Feurs en Forez, France, on the banks of the Loire. At the age of 19 he received his medical degree from Avignon, and he moved to Paris to establish himself as an anatomist. There he matured into a handsome, personable, articulate, and extremely intelligent young scientist, with an insatiable desire to increase his knowledge and free it of misconceptions. He became a member of an elite group known as The Parisians, whose members discussed a variety of medical topics, such as respiration, hearing, smell, digestion, animals of Africa, muscles of dogs, and the comparative anatomy of various animals. While writing his *Traité de l'Organe de l'Ouie* (Paris: Estienne Michallet, 1683), he introduced the arrangement of diseases of the ear according to the anatomic structures affected. These he proceeded to discuss in a three-part format: (a) the anatomy of the ear, (b) the physiology of hearing, and (c) the pathology of the organ of hearing (15). Duverney's treatise (Fig. 7) exem-

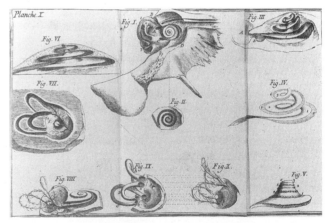

FIG. 7. Inner ear diagram from Duverney's treatise. *Guichard Joseph Duverney.* Duverney, for the first time, revealed that the osseous part of the external canal originated from the tympanic bone and that the tympanic ring is incomplete superiorly. With respect to the middle ear, Duverney presented the first detailed description of its structures, including the ossicles, and issued the first description of the communication between the tympanic cavity and the cells of the mastoid. In his description of the inner ear, Duverney divided the labyrinth into three parts: (a) the back portion, containing the three round canals; (b) the front portion, or cochlea; and (c) the vestibule, the area between the other two parts. He also included the first detailed description of the osseous labyrinth. One of the most outstanding sections of Duverney's book is that in which he thoroughly describes the embryologic anatomy of the ear in a fetus and compares it with the anatomy of the adult ear. In that comparison he found a number of dissimilarities. (From the author's collection.)

plified the desire of seventeenth century scientists, especially anatomists, to concentrate on specific organs and to pursue investigations and descriptions of their minute details. For example, he not only provided its length, direction, and structure, but he was the first to depict the arteries, veins, and nerve branches of the auricle.

Duverney's work was the first text relegated to the subject of the ear.

The First Comprehensive Account of the Minute Anatomy of the Ear

The late seventeenth and early eighteenth centuries also witnessed the results of the work of Antonio Mario Valsalva (1666–1723) (Fig. 8). A remarkable thread of genius can be found woven throughout the academic and professional life of this great anatomist, beginning with Malpighi, his mentor at the University of Bologna, and echoing through his devoted student, Giovanni (Joannis) Battista Morgagni (1682–1771), to Domenico Felice Antonio Cotugno (1736–1822) and Antonio Scarpa (1752–1832).

Valsalva's classic test on the anatomy of the ear was published in 1704. The six chapters of the book were considered an authoritative text for more than a century. His inner ear anatomy was especially exceptional. He described, in the book, finding ankylosis of the stapedial footplate secondary to ossification. In the first reported autopsy finding of otosclerosis he reported finding a bony hard annular ligament that contributed a continuous bone between the base of the stapes and the margin of the oval window, preventing all oscillation of the stapes (16).

Structural otologic anatomy was conveyed by Frederick Ruysch (1638–1731), Giovanni Santorini (1681–1737),

Johann Glaser (1629–1675), Claude Perrault (1613–1688), and Leopoldo Caldani (1725–1813) and his nephew Floriano Caldani. However, the newest insights in temporal bone anatomy were presented by Johann Cassebohn (1699/1700–1743), who had as his mentor Duverney's student Jakob Winslow. Cassebohn served as professor of anatomy at Frankfurt-on-Oder, Berlin, and in his native city of Halle. He introduced the present-day vernacular in describing the relationship of the location of the semicircular canals to that of the cochlea (Fig. 9) (17).

According to Cotugno (1736–1822), the older anatomists had failed to discover the labyrinthine fluid because they had worked on old cadavers.

Cotugno also boldly proceeded to introduce new concepts concerning the function of the duct and the fluid and hearing based on the conduction of the fluid. (Fig. 10). The source of the labyrinthine fluid, according to Cotugno, was an exhalation of blood vessels, and its function was to protect the nerve that might otherwise be injured by constant contact with the bony structures (18).

Cotugno's discovery of inner ear fluid was a great contribution at the time, but it was left to Antonio Scarpa to complete the description of the membranous portion of the inner ear. The failure of Cotugno to elaborate on the duct, which we know today as the vestibular aqueduct, allowed it to be rediscovered centuries later by otologists and anatomists in German-speaking universities.

After receiving his anatomy training under Morgagni at Padua and his surgical training in Bologna, Antonio Scarpa (1747–1832) became professor of anatomy and surgery at Modena. While there, he published his first

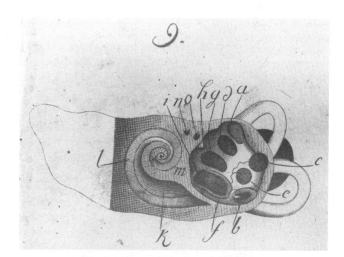

FIG. 9. *Johann Friedrich Cassebohn.* In the second of his two volumes, Cassebohn gave the most descriptive account of the labyrinth theretofore presented. In so doing he introduced the present-day vernacular in describing the relationship of the location of the semicircular canal to that of the cochlea, labyrinthine windows, and facial nerve (superior, inferior, and external). He took great pains to describe correctly the five openings of the semicircular canals. (From the author's collection.)

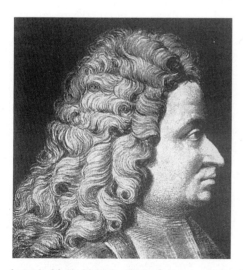

FIG. 8. *Antonio Mario Valsalva.* Valsalva was also a clinician and surgeon of note. He was the first physician to inspect the tympanic membrane in patients, and he felt that tears in this structure would heal easily and had no long-range adverse effect on hearing. (From the author's collection.)

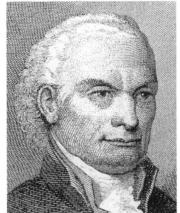
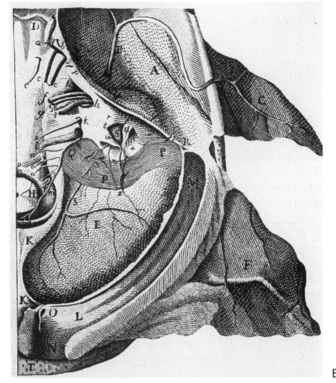

FIG. 10. A: *Domenico Felice Antonio Cotugno.* Cotugno was born into a very poor family in Ruvo, near Naples, on December 3, 1736. At the age of 24, while still a student of Morgagni, he wrote his famous dissertation on the fluid of the inner ear. By the time he was 30 years of age he was full professor of anatomy and surgery at the University of Naples. (From Politzer's *Geschichte der Ohrenheilkunde, Volume I.*) **B:** "Tab. 2." from Cotugno's anatomic dissertation. (From the author's collection.)

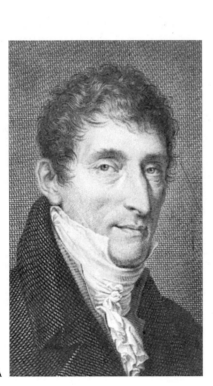
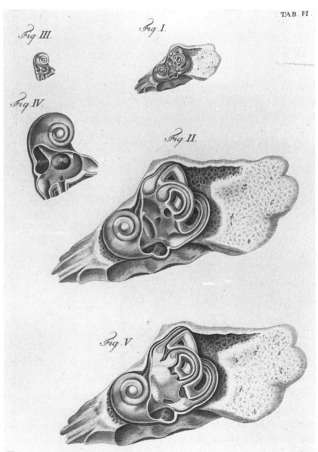

A
B

major work on the ear, in which he not only gave the first detailed anatomic description of the round window and the secondary drum, but also their embryologic development, along with extensive historic and anatomic investigations on the round window (19).

Scarpa's discovery of the membranous labyrinth was the ultimate evidence that the labyrinth contained fluid. In 1783 Scarpa became professor of anatomy in Pavia, and from that position he published the first edition of his description of the membranous labyrinth in 1789 (Fig. 11) (20). It was that work that eliminated once and for all the "aer implantus" theory of hearing.

CLINICAL APPLICATIONS

Seventeenth and eighteenth century identification of contemporary diagnoses included that of Thomas Willis (Paracusis of Willis, 1672) (21) and Carlos Mundini (cochlear dysplasia, 1791) (22).

Clinical Contributions of a Layman

Without doubt, the taproots of otology are found in the laboratories of the great anatomists, physiologists, and pathologists. Strangely, however, one of its most clinically significant aspects was germinated by a layman, the postmaster of Versailles, Edme-Gilles Guyot (1706–1786). His discovery perhaps could have been made earlier by any one of the scientists studying the hearing organ, based on the knowledge of the anatomy of the ear up to his time. Guyot had the incentive of a personal investment, however, for he was hard of hearing. Frustrated by the failure of the many physicians he had consulted, he ingeniously devised a pewter tube with a kneebend that he himself could insert behind the soft palate and into the eustachian tube—the first eustachian tube catheter. The external opening of the tube then was connected to a pump activated by two opposing cranks. The benefits of his invention were described in 1724 before the Académie Royale des Sciences in Paris (23).

The impetus provided for otology by the fundamental works of the great anatomists and the therapeutic achievements of the eighteenth and early nineteenth centuries was revitalized by three Frenchmen, Jean Marie Gaspard Itard (1755–1838), Antonine Saissy (1756–1822), and Nicholas Deleau (1799–1862). It was their supplementary works on eustachian tube catheterization, myringotomies, external otitis, and education of the deaf-mute that inaugurated otology as a clinical and surgical specialty.

Sir Astley Cooper: Paracentesis of the Tympanic Membrane

In 1801 Sir Astley Cooper was led to paracentesis (myringotomy) by a series of isolated historic cases that may have had nothing to do with the disease underlying the need for such surgery (24). There was also a vague report that paracentesis had been done in Paris around 1760 by a man named Eli, but who was Eli? There is scant information on him in the literature, and that which is available suggests that he was a charlatan in Paris who apparently had done this surgery to improve a patient's hearing. Antoine Portal and Raphael Bienveni Sabatier, both of whom were in Paris during the time of Eli, were unaware of any such surgery being done (25).

Institutions for the Deaf: Foundations of Otology in France

The two-volume treatise of Jean Marie Gaspard Itard on the maladies of the ear and hearing brought about a new phase in otology (26). Volume I dealt with the anatomy, physiology, and pathology of the ear, and Volume II with diseases of the ear. Itard took great care while examining his patients, and he meticulously presented, in Volume II, their histories together with an analysis of the appearance of the pathology he saw involving the external auditory canal and tympanic membrane. These two volumes, along with his famous two-part case report on

---

FIG. 11. A: *Antonio Scarpa.* Scarpa's profile as an individual was enigmatic. Born in Motta, Italy, in 1747, he became quite an influential faculty member at Pavia at the time when that institution was one of the most prominent of the European learning centers. It seems that he abused his leverage with tyranny and ruthlessness, however, shamelessly seeking to annihilate those whom he held in disfavor and imperiously promoting those whom he favored; and yet he was certainly held in the highest esteem as an anatomist and surgeon by his peers. He appeared to have used his exalted position to manipulate himself into the position of director of the medical faculty following his retirement so that he could retain his tyrannical control. The great wealth Scarpa acquired allowed him to collect an enviable number of paintings done by leading Italian masters, and his profuse and eclectic knowledge placed him in great demand as a speaker. All of these attributes doubtless provided him with abundant social opportunities that, as a bachelor, he pursued. His several romantic liaisons resulted in his fathering several sons, whom he sponsored in their chosen careers. (From the author's collection.) B: An accomplished artist, Scarpa provided the drawings from which the plates were made. Faustino Anderloni, whom Scarpa had actually trained to become the engraver of his illustrations, signed the above. Scarpa's drawings, along with those of Samuel Thomas Sömmerring (1755–1830), were considered among the best of those of all the great anatomists. (From the author's collection.)

the wild boy of Aveyron (27), developed for Itard an international reputation and a lucrative private practice. He became deeply concerned about the predicament of deaf-mutes, however, and eventually relinquished his private patients, some of whom were of nobility, to become resident physician at the Royal Institute for the Deaf and Dumb.

Itard's work was preceded by that of Jean Antoine Saissy (1756–1822), which was originally reported in an article (1819) in the *Dictionnaire des Sciences Medicales*. In 1827, Saissy's work was published as essays on diseases of the internal ear. This concise work exposes his knowledge of the anatomic studies of the ear carried out by his predecessors, as well as his contemporaries Astley Cooper, Marie Joseph Alard, and Itard. Because he was unable to find a previous report in the medical literature of a formed polyp on the tympanic membrane, Saissy claimed to be the first to observe this lesion (28). Clinically, he had strict prerequisites for paracentesis, especially in cases of eustachian tube obstruction.

The contributions Saissy made to otology, which greatly increased its prestige as a specialty, are remarkable, considering that his practice in the field covered only 12 years. Prior to that he served as a general surgeon on the Barbary Coast for 3 years and, after marrying the daughter of an obstetrician, had practiced obstetrics for a while. His publications on the effects of inoculation on smallpox and croup, on the phenomena exhibited by hibernating animals, and on other philosophical and chemical topics were recognized as well by the Academies of Science.

Nicholas Deleau (1797–1862), the third in the trio of French scientists, may have been the most talented clinically. Deleau had a great deal of experience in eustachian tube catheterization, which was the topic of his notable treatise. Using René Laennec's stethoscope, he attempted to diagnose ear diseases by the variation in sounds made when air was introduced into the ear through a eustachian tube catheter. He discarded Saissy's and Itard's method of irrigating the ear with water through the catheter, and he reintroduced the air douche for this purpose. In certain cases he would use medicated vapors instead of air, a practice that later became established throughout Europe (29).

A Physician to be Emulated: Sir William Wilde (1815–1876)

Wilde (Fig. 12) developed an otologic practice in the midst of the development of that new science. As a clinician he played a role as significant in advancing otology as did Toynbee as a pathoanatomist. His many contributions included his being the first to identify the cone of light in the anteroinferior portion of the tympanic membrane, which he found on physical examination, and his

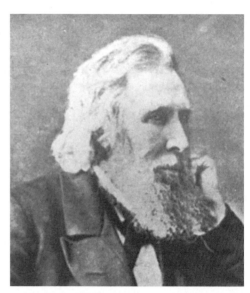

FIG. 12. *Sir William Wilde.* Wilde developed an extensive practice in both otology and ophthalmology in Dublin. He established St. Mark's Hospital (1841), which began as a small dispensary housed in an abandoned stable. During this period he was appointed medical commissioner of the Irish census, and it was for this service that he was knighted. As a result of his varied interests and his own fame, Wilde's social life was enriched by friends in science and literature. Undoubtedly making her contribution to his social circle was Wilde's wife, the Irish poetess Speranza. Although not particularly well known at the time of their marriage, her reputation among literary poets became quite respected over the years. Her works included poems and writings dealing with the ancient legends, charms, and superstitions of Ireland. Their son was the famous Oscar. (From the author's collection.)

invention of new instruments such as probes, a speculum, an aural snare, and aural dressing forceps. It is thought that angulation of the shaft of these instruments was his invention as well. His book on aural surgery (30) brought him acclaim by the time he was internationally known and was responsible for training physicians from America as well as Europe. He also was responsible for Wilde's incision for draining a periosteal extension of a mastoid abscess.

GERMAN APPLICATION OF ANATOMY

Sömmerring's Atlas: A Work of Art

Samuel Thomas von Sömmerring's anatomic atlas of 1806 was doubtless the most prominent influence on anatomy in Germany during the nineteenth century (31).

Sömmerring (1755–1830) insisted on presenting the ear in its natural state, undisturbed by disease or injury. He selected only the most perfect specimen among many, and he strove to represent the connections between different parts just as they occur in nature, and not to portray anything distorted in any way. The anatomy was not copied from existing descriptions, but was based on observations he had personally made (32). Sömmerring presented many of his investigations in a well-organized fashion. Although his text was quite credible, the most outstanding features were the drawings that he produced with the aid of Köck, a stucco worker and draftsman trained by Sömmerring to produce anatomic models and illustrations (Fig. 13). These remarkable illustrations were so accurate that they could very well be used today.

Knowledge of the gross anatomy of the ear culminated for the most part with the work of Scarpa; thereafter, anatomists and other researchers began to investigate the intricacies of individual structures and their components. Four of the important nineteenth century pioneers in otoanatomy who became associated with specific structures are Friedrich Christian Rosenthal (1780–1829), Emil Huschke (1797–1858), Friedrich Arnold (1803–1890), and Joseph Hyrtl (1810–1894).

Emil Huschke, professor of anatomy at Jena, revised Sömmerring's textbook. In 1824 he observed parallel rows of tall cells, which he considered to be basilar papilla and the excitatory structure of the cochlea. He referred to these tall cells with nuclei buried in the connective tissue of the limbus as "auditory teeth" (the auditory teeth of Huschke) (33,34). Two decades later Alfonso Corti was able to perceive and describe these cells and structures more clearly with the aid of the stronger compound microscope, and the structures became known as the organ of Corti (35).

SPECIAL SCIENTISTS, SPECIAL CONTRIBUTIONS

In addition to the German anatomists, anatomists of other countries, such as Gilbert Breschet (1784–1845) (Fig. 14) of Clermont-Gerrand, France, contributed to the foundation of otology. Breschet became head of the anatomy department at the Paris School of Medicine in 1818. He significantly advanced the knowledge of the

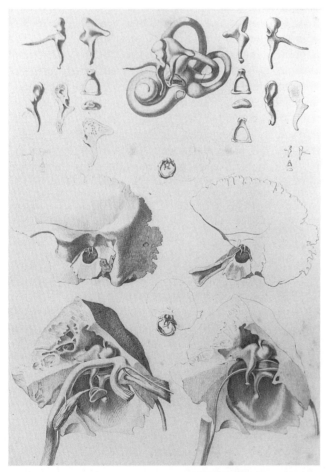

FIG. 13. From Sömmerring's *Abbildungen des menschlichen Höroganes. Samuel Thomas von Sömmerring.* Sömmerring, the son of a physician, was born in the East Prussian town of Thorn, the same city in which Copernicus had first seen the light of day some 300 years earlier. Although his father wished him to study to become a general practitioner, he obviously supported his son in his fervent study of anatomy. Sömmerring's medical education and training were acquired at Göttingen, where he studied with the great anatomist Heinrich August Wrisberg (1739–1808). (From the author's collection.)

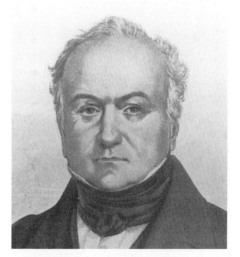

FIG. 14. *Gilbert Breschet.* Although he may generally have been more noted for his work on veins, he significantly advanced the knowledge of the morphology of the membranous labyrinth. Breschet particularly studied the labyrinthine fluid, and he differentiated the perilymph in the osseous labyrinth from the endolymph in the membranous labyrinth. His embryologic studies revealed that the two aqueducts were larger in fetuses and newborns than in adults. (From the author's collection.)

morphology of the membranous labyrinth, accurately describing the saccule and the utricle (the otocondria), and identifying the helicotrema (36).

Prosper Meniere (1799–1862)

Prior to the nineteenth century, balance disturbances were thought to be of central nervous system origin as advanced by Purkinje (1787–1869) and Flourens (1794–1867). Episodes of sudden severe vertigo were collectively categorized as "apoplectiform cerebral congestion." A Parisian physician who also had training in pathology, Prosper Meniere (Fig. 15) emphasized the role of the inner ear in producing vertiginous attacks. Meniere was called late one night by a colleague whose daughter had just fallen from the top of a stagecoach. This girl apparently became suddenly vertiginous, vomited, and complained of deafness. Despite Meniere's efforts, she died 5 days later. Meniere was granted autopsy permission. When he carefully inspected the brain, no focal abnormalities or evidence of congestion was noted. He also examined the inner ears, and on one side he found a blood-tinged exudate, prompting his hypothesis that this was the site of pathology. Intrigued by this initial finding, Meniere began to examine temporal bones of other patients who had dizziness, many of whom did have the disease process that now bears his name. Frequently, he found an inner ear abnormality. In 1861, 1 year prior to his death, he published these findings and forever turned our attention from the brain to the inner ear as the site of pathology for the symptom complex of episodic vertigo, hearing loss, and tinnitus (37). Parenthetically, on subsequent review of the child who fell from the stagecoach, it was determined that leukemia was the cause of dizziness and death and that there was no primary inner ear abnormality.

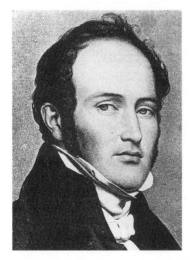

FIG. 15. *Prosper Meniere.* Meniere emphasized the role of the inner ear in producing vertiginous attacks.

STUDY OF TEMPORAL BONE PATHOLOGY: THE BEGINNING

Founder of Scientific Otology: Joseph Toynbee

In his classic book entitled *Diseases of the Ear,* the London physician Toynbee (1815–1866) (Fig. 16) stated that not one dissection of a diseased ear had been done prior to 1800, although thousands of dissections had been done on most other organs of the body (38). He proceeded to remedy this situation by dissecting more than two thousand temporal bones and thus was able to correlate the gross and microscopic pathology with the patient's symptoms. Of course, histochemical procedures were not available for close study of the cochlea, but Toynbee did describe cases of molluscous tumors (later recognized as cholesteatomas), ten cases of osteoid tumors, and ankylosis of the stapes to the oval window. The latter condition he referred to as "catarrhal sclerosis" decades later was recognized as otosclerosis.

James Hinton (1822–1875) was Toynbee's life-long and close friend. He possessed a remarkable memory that, no doubt, facilitated his studies of languages, history, and medicine, among other subjects. His insatiable quest for knowledge, which often led him to study late into the night, resulted in his securing a universal education. He was particularly well versed in philosophy, and his philosophical writings demonstrated his intellectual

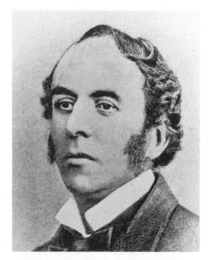

FIG. 16. *Joseph Toynbee.* Toynbee was born in Lincolnshire, England, in 1815. Following his early training in anatomy he became recognized for his investigative research. In a technical sense he could probably be considered an otopathologist, although he maintained a large and prosperous clinical practice. By the age of 26 he had the honor of being admitted to the Royal Society. To the literally inclined outside the field of medicine, the name Arnold Toynbee may be more familiar than that of his father, Joseph. Although the younger Toynbee died at the age of 26, he was a well-known sociologist, and it was for him that Toynbee Hall in the university settlement at White Chapel was named. (From Politzer's *Geschichte der Ohrenheilkunde, Volume II.*)

acumen; possibly the best known of these are *The Mystery of Pain* (Boston: Dewolfe, Fiske, 1866), *Man and His Dwelling Place* (New York: Redfield, 1859), and *Life in Nature* (London: Smith, Elder, 1862).

As an otologist, Hinton showed enormous technical knowledge. Some of his original observations are still meaningful today: the red sagging of the posterosuperior canal wall indicates acute mastoiditis; "molluscous tumors" (cholesteatomas) may cause death by eroding the tegmen of the mastoid and extending into the brain; and aural polyps must be considered a disease process of the middle ear or mastoid and not of the external canal. It was Hinton who first recommended early myringotomy in acute otitis media, as "it relieves pain, preserves hearing, and diminishes risk" (39).

The brilliant application of microscopic techniques exhibited by these nineteenth century scientists was followed by that of Magnus Gustaf (Gustave) Retzius (1842–1919), who left a mark in anatomic investigations of the labyrinth. A keen observer with a superior grasp of anatomic details, Retzius mastered the art of microdissection (40).

The precursor of today's head mirror was introduced in 1841 by Friedrich Hoffmann, Jr., a government public health surgeon of Burgsteinfurt, Germany. This handheld instrument had a handle attached to a concave mirror with a central perforation like that found on modern head mirrors. It was used predominantly for examining the ear, but it also was used to inspect the aural cavity and nose. Because he was a general practitioner, Hoffman also used it for rectal and gynecologic examinations. This original device is on exhibit in the Ear, Nose and Throat Clinic of Würzburg University. Hoffmann's mirror was introduced and popularized by Anton von Tröltsch, who typically is credited for inventing this device.

THE HONING OF OTOLOGY

Otology in Vienna

As far back as the Roman Empire, Vienna's location in the region along the Danube river ("Donauraum") predisposed it to be a borderland, strategic in trade and war, and a hub for migrating tribes. By the nineteenth century, it had become the churn in which central Europe was homogenized. It was in this eclectic city that the most remarkable facilities for medical education on the Eurasian continent developed. As the university clinics were being formed with the recognition that otology was emerging as a scientific specialty, Adam Politzer was being groomed to become one of its foremost teachers and one of the greatest of all otologists.

Adam Politzer (1835–1920): Quintessential Mentor

In 1861 Politzer (Fig. 17) began teaching his first course on diseases of the auditory organ before an audi-

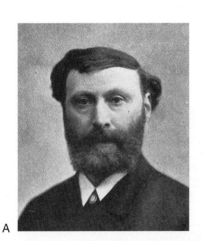
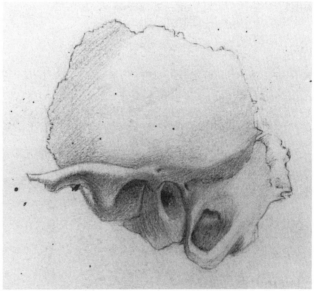

FIG. 17. A: *Adam Politzer.* An interest in art as well as personal artistic talent led Politzer to fraternize with some of the great masters of art in the Europe of his day and to assemble an enviable art collection as well. The waiting room in his office formed a gallery of fine paintings, and it is said that he never tired of recounting the incidents and stories associated with their acquisition. Politzer eventually donated his extensive library to the University of Vienna, and many of his paintings to the archives of the Institute of Medical History. His home in Alberti was designated as a shrine, but was subsequently adapted for office space under the Communist regime. It was later transformed into a movie house before its reclamation during the 1970s as a historical site by the Otolaryngological Society of Hungary. (Gift of Joseph B. Touma, M.D., Huntington, West Virginia.) **B:** A drawing for teaching purposes done by Politzer. (From the collection of the Academy of Otolaryngology-Head and Neck Surgery.)

ence of four students at the school of medicine in Vienna. His intense interest in his subject, his passion for scrupulous study and research, and his zealous lectures soon attracted students from around the world.

During the mid 1800s, the administration at the medical school in Vienna realized that no logical approach to the study of ear diseases was being offered on the European continent; little or no attempt was being made to investigate hearing systematically or to correlate aural disease with necropsy findings. Certainly, disorders that modern physicians would automatically consider complications of ear disease were present, but the ear often was overlooked in evaluations. (One reason for this may have been the lack of appropriate instruments.) Aware of the progressive moves in otology taking place in England, the faculty realized they needed someone with a primary interest in the auditory system if the medical school was to be contemporary.

Politzer had earned the admiration of his mentors and predecessors on the faculty, and many of them strongly advocated enlisting him to fill such a position. With these considerations in mind, Oppolzer, who had taken particular notice of Politzer, set him out on a program of training under outstanding tutors (Ludwig, Helmoltz, Kölliker, Bernard, Toynbee).

Politzer thought it imperative that his students recognize diagnostically significant changes in the tympanic membrane. The importance he attached to these manifestations was evidenced in two of his books, *The Membrana Tympani in Health and Disease* and *Atlas of Illustrations of the Healthy and Diseased Tympanic Membrane* (*Atlas der Beleuchtungsbilder des Trommelfells im gesunden und kranken Zustande für praktische Ärtze und Studierende,* Wien: Wilhelm Braumüller, 1896). The first of these must be considered one of the greatest contibutions to medical literature during that era. At the time of

its publication, inspection of the tympanic membrane was a new diagnostic concept endorsed by Politzer. Politzer's primary intent was that this book be used as a teaching tool for general practitioners, a reference source to be used in diagnosing ear disease. It contained instructions for inspecting the tympanic membrane for anomalies, opacities (such as the calcereous deposits in tympanosclerosis), and other signs of pathology. In addition, there were dissertations on perforations and tears, treatment of purulent catarrh of the middle ear, detachment of the membrane to the stapes, effects of disease on the convexity of the membrane, and the mobility of the membrane.

The contributions Politzer made to the literature on ear diseases were exceptional. He published more than 100 works, one of which was the most outstanding textbook of the last half of the nineteenth century. The first edition (1878) of his *Lehrbuch der Ohrenheilkunde* was translated into English and edited (1883) by a former student of Politzer, James Patterson Cassells, aural surgeon and lecturer at the Glasgow Hospital (41). Politzer continually revised and updated his text to accommodate the expanding knowledge of ear pathology and the rapid progress being made in the medical and surgical treatment of ear diseases. By 1908, it had undergone five editions and had been translated into English, French, and Spanish. The translated sixth edition (1926) amplified otologic literature considerably with a number of discussions on the labyrinth (42).

It was estimated that 7,000 students, many of whom referred to him affectionately as father, had attended his lectures by the end of his 46-year tenure (43). The esteem and affection of his students was demonstrated at celebrations such as that held in honor of the 25th anniversary of his teaching. During those ceremonies, they bestowed accolades upon him and presented him with a portrait by

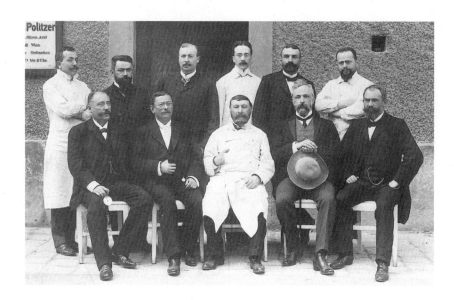

FIG. 18. Group photograph at Politzer Clinic c. 1903. Politzer, front row center. Second row, left to right: Heinrich Neumann, multifaceted otologic surgeon; Paul Manase, who made his reputation in the anatomic and pathologic histology a study of diseases of the ear; unknown; Frey; Victor Hinsberg, known for his surgical procedure for labyrinthitis; and Gustav Alexander (inner ear anatomy research). (From the Institute für Geschichte der Medizin der Universitat, Wien, Austria.)

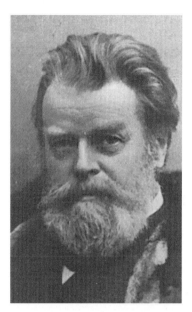

FIG. 19. *Friedrich von Bezold.* Bezold was a native of Rothenburg ob der Tauter. He never achieved the prestigious rank in otology as did Politzer, but Bezold was without question a quintessential scientist and teacher. His career can be followed if divided in specific areas as deaf education (recognition of residual hearing), clinical treatment (introduction of the remedy—boric acid—to a draining ear), clinical observation (Bezold's abscess), investigator (continuous tone series of tests to evaluate hearing), and academician (many of Bezold's students, such as Siebenmann, Denker, and Scheibe, became professors). (From the author's collection.)

the master artist Gustav Klemt (1864–1918). The appreciation of his students was displayed again, in 1909, when an affidavit, signed by 366 of them representing 21 countries, was presented to him during the festivities honoring him at his retirement.

Although his primary work was done on the hearing mechanism itself, there is no aspect of the anatomy, pathoanatomy, and physiology of the ear that Politzer did not influence during his nearly one-half century of scientific and teaching activities. As the works of other contributors in the field of otology are considered, the profound influence he had on time is revealed (Fig. 18).

It is quite probably that no other physician contributed as much to a specialty as did Adam Politzer.

The late nineteenth century conjured pioneers such as Von Tröltsch and Schwartze (reintroduction mastoidectomy), Stacke (meatoplasty), Lucae (inventions, new instruments), Jansen (neurotology), Trautmann (critical landmarks in mastoidectomy), Passow (fenestration), Katz (temporal bone findings in otosclerosis), Stenger (testing the hearing malingerer), Körner (Körner's septum), Scheibe (dysplasia), Wittmaack (research), Zaufal (mastoidectomy), and Bezold (mastoid tip abscess) (Fig. 19). A revolution in the practice of otology was brought about by these German-speaking pioneers (Fig. 20). This period started in Vienna with Politzer and ended in Vienna with the ousting of Heinrich Neumann by the Nazis following the Anschluss of Austria in 1938.

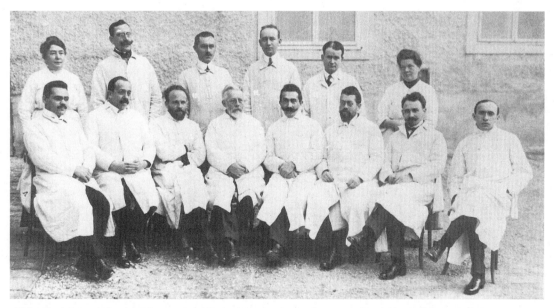

FIG. 20. Victor Urbantschitsch and his assistants in the General Hospital of Vienna. Seated first row, left to right: Oskar Beck, Heinrich Neumann, Robert Bárány, Victor Urbantschitsch, Gustav Bondy, Ernst Urbantschitsch, Erich Ruttin, and Emil Fröschels. (From the Institute für Geschichte der Medizin der Universitat, Wien, Austria.)

CONCLUSION

Acceleration of Otologic Progress: A New Surgical Era—The Influence of Antibiotics

The introduction of antibiotics very nearly eliminated the surgeries introduced by Emanuel Zaufal, Albert Jansen, Victor Hinsberg, Henrich Neumann, and others for labyrinthitis, cerebellar and cerebral abscesses, and similar conditions. Antibiotic therapy, along with immunizations and technically advanced diagnostic and surgical tools and procedures, produced stunning repercussions in otology during the first half of the twentieth century. As a result, the primary focus of that specialty was transformed from ablative procedures to reconstructive and preventive procedures.

The development of the fenestration operation (Julius Lempert), stapedectomy (John Shea), and tympanoplasty operations (Friz Zöllner and Horst Wullstein) were the most significant and dramatic advances during the first half of the twentieth century. The 1950s also were a crucial time in the history of otology, when the specialty was revolutionized by establishing new otoneurologic procedures (William House).

REFERENCES

1. Garrison FH. *An introduction to the history of medicine.* Philadelphia: WB Sanders, 1914:15.
2. Bass JH. *Outlines of the history of medicine and the medical profession.* Huntington, NY: RE Krieger, 1971:297. Handerson HE, translator.
3. Politzer A. *Geschichte der Ohrenheilkunde.* Stuttgart: Ferdinand Enke, 1907:73–77.
4. Politzer A. *Geschichte der Ohrenheilkunde.* Stuttgart: Ferdinand Enke, 1907:73–77.
5. Castiglioni A. *A history of medicine.* New York: AA Knopf, 1941:422. Bertrand J, translator.
6. Vesalius A. *De humani corporis fabrica libri septem.* Basileae: Joann. Oporini, 1543:32–33.
7. Robinson V. *The story of medicine.* New York: A & C Boni, 1931:253.
8. Ball JM. *Andreas Vesalius the reformer of anatomy.* St. Louis: Medical Scientific Press, 1910:123.
9. Eustachius B. *Opuscula anatomica.* Venetiis: V. Luchinus, 1564:148–164.
10. Ball JM. *Andreas Vesalius the reformer of anatomy.* St. Louis: Medical Scientific Press, 1910:123.
11. Falloppio G. *Observations anatomica.* Venetiis: M.A. Ulmum, 1561:10–222.
12. Mercurialis H. *De compositione medicamentorum.* Venetiis: Iuntas, 1601.
13. Capivaccio G. *De laeso auditu, in Opera omnia.* Venetiis: Iuntas, 1606:511.
14. Fremantle A. *Great ages of man: age of faith.* New York: Time, Inc., 1965:150.
15. Duverney GJ. *A treatise of the organ of hearing.* London: S. Baker, 1741:1–89. Marshall J, translator.
16. Valsalva AM. *De aure humana tractatus.* Bononiae: C. Pisarii, 1704:31.
17. Cassebohn JF. *Tractatus quatour anatomici de aure humana.* Halae, Magdeburgi: Orphotrophei, 1734; and *Tractatus quintus anatimicus de aure humana, cui accedit tacatus sextus de aura monstri humani.* Halae, Magdeburgi: Orphanotrophei, 1735, 45 of quintus section.
18. Cotungno D. *De aquaeductibus auris humanae internae anatomica dissertation.* Naepoli et Bononiae: Thomae Aquinatis, 1775.
19. Scarpa A. *De structura fenestrae rotundae auris, et de tympano secundario anatomicae observationes.* Mutinae: Apud Soc Typog, 1772:23–131.
20. Scarpa A. *Anatomicae disquisitiones de auditu et olfactu.* Tricini: Petri Galeatii, 1789:44–51.
21. Willis T. *De anima brutorum quae hominis...* Oxonii: Impensis R. Davis, 1672:76.
22. Mundini C. *Anatomia surdi nedi sectio, de Bononiensi scientiarum et artium institute atque academia commentarii 7.* 1791;28:419.
23. *Historie de l'Academie Royale des Sciences.* 1724:37.
24. Cooper A. Observations on the effects which take place from the destruction of the membrana tympani of the ear, in a letter to Everard Home, Esq. F.R.S., by whom some remarks are added. In: *Phil Trans Roy Soc SO* 1800:435–450.
25. St. John Roosa B. *A practical treatise on the diseases of the ear, including the anatomy of the organ,* 4th ed. New York: William Wood, 1878:321.
26. Itard JMG. *Traité des maladies de l'oreille et de l'audition.* Paris: Chez Meguignon-Marvis Libraire, 1821.
27. Lane H. *The wild boy of Aveyron.* Cambridge: Harvard Uinversity Press, 1979.
28. Saissy JA. *An essay on the diseases of the internal ear.* Baltimore: Hatch and Dunning, 1829:133. Smith NR, translator.
29. Deleau N. *Traité du cathétérisme de la trompe d'Eustachi.* Paris: Germer-Baillière, 1838.
30. Wilde WR. *Practical observations in aural surgery and the nature and treatment of diseases of the ear.* Philadelphia: Blanchard & Lea, 1853.
31. Von Sömmerring ST. *Abbildungen des menschlichen Hörorganes.* Frankfurt am Main: Varrentrapp und Wenner, 1806.
32. Bast T. The life and work of Samuel Thomas von Sömmerring. *Ann Med Hist* 1924;6:371.
33. Huschke E. *Lehre von den Eingeweiden und Sinnesorgan des menschlichen Körpers.* Leipzig:Voss, 1844.
34. Huschke E. Bermerkungen zur Anatmoie der Kinndaden Tod, XI. *Oken's Isis* 1825;18:1101.
35. Corti A. Recherches sur l'organe de l'ouïe des mammiféres. *Z Wiss Zool* 1851;3:109–169.
36. Breschet G. *Recherches anatomiques et physiologiques sur l'ouie et sur l'audition, dans l'homme et les animaux vertébrés.* Paris: JB Baillière, 1836:5–265.
37. Ménière P. Memoire sur das lesions de l'oreille interne donnant lier a das symptomes de congestion cerebral apoplectiforme. *Gaz Mad Paris* 1861;16:597–601.
38. Toynbee J. *The diseases of the ear: their nature, diagnosis, and treatment.* Philadelphia: Blanchard & Lea, 1860.
39. Toynbee J. *The diseases of the ear: their nature, diagnosis, and treatment, with a supplement of James Hinton, M.R.C.S.* London: H.K. Lewis, 1868:453.
40. Retzius MG. *Das Gehörorgan der Wirbelthiere.* Stockholm: Samson and Mallin, 1881–1884.
41. Politzer A. *A text-book of the diseases of the ear.* Philadelphia: HC Lea's Son, 1883. Cassells JP, translator and editor.
42. Politzer A. *Politzer's text-book of the ear,* 6th ed. Revised and largely rewritten by M.J. Ballin. Philadelphia: Lea & Febiger, 1926.
43. Lederer FL. A tribute to Adam Politzer. *Arch Otolaryngol* 1961;74:130–133.

The Ear: Comprehensive Otology,
edited by R. F. Canalis and P. R. Lambert.
Lippincott Williams & Wilkins, Philadelphia © 2000.

CHAPTER 2

Anatomy and Embryology of the Auditory and Vestibular Systems

Paul R. Lambert and Rinaldo F. Canalis

This chapter addresses the basic anatomic features of the ear and temporal bone and their development. It should be used as a general point of reference. Throughout this book, additional, often more detailed, anatomic descriptions are included in most chapters to clarify the discussion of specific clinical problems. Those aspects of anatomy that are particularly important from a clinical perspective are presented as summary points at the end of the chapter.

EMBRYOLOGY OF THE HUMAN EAR

Valsalva (1), in his classic treatise printed in Bologna in 1704, first divided the auditory organ into three parts: external, middle, and inner ear. Developmentally, the three primitive germ layers contribute in different ways to the various structures contained within these parts (Fig. 1). *Ectoderm* contributes to the formation of the auricular, meatal, and tympanic membrane (outer epithelial portion) components of the external ear and to the membranous labyrinth of the inner ear. *Mesoderm* gives rise to the auricular cartilages and muscles of the external and middle ear, the tympanic cleft, the ossicles, the middle (fibrous) layer of the tympanic membrane, and the periotic labyrinth and otic capsule of the inner ear. *Entoderm* contributes only to middle ear development, giving rise to the tubotympanic air cell system from the eustachian tube orifice to the most distant mastoid air cell and to the inner (mucosal) layer of the tympanic membrane.

Developmental Interrelations

Throughout their development, the three divisions of the human ear maintain several important interrelations. At the end of the third week of gestation, the *auditory placode* appears as an ectodermal thickening adjacent to

P. R. Lambert: Department of Otolaryngology–Head and Neck Surgery, University of Virginia Health Sciences Center, Charlottesville, Virginia 22908-2040

R. F. Canalis: Department of Surgery, University of California, Los Angeles, School of Medicine, Los Angeles, California 90095-1624

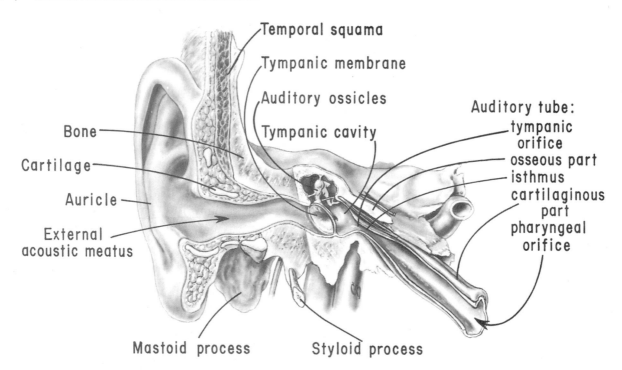

FIG. 1. Adult anatomy. (From Anson-Donaldson J, Duckert LG, Lambert PR, Rubel EW, eds. *Surgical anatomy of the temporal bone.* New York: Raven Press, 1992:61, with permission.)

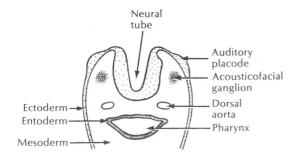

FIG. 2. Auditory placode stage in development of the ear. (Adapted from Pearson AA. *The development of the ear: a manual.* Rochester, MN: American Academy of Ophthalmology and Otolaryngology, 1967.)

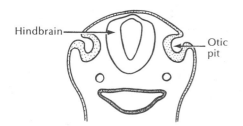

FIG. 3. Otic pit stage in development of the ear. (Adapted from Pearson AA. *The development of the ear: a manual.* Rochester, MN: American Academy of Ophthalmology and Otolaryngology, 1967.)

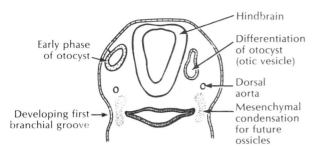

FIG. 4. Otocyst-otic vesicle development. (Adapted from Pearson AA. *The development of the ear: a manual.* Rochester, MN: American Academy of Ophthalmology and Otolaryngology, 1967.)

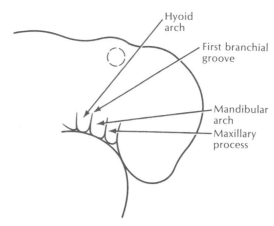

FIG. 5. Primitive branchial arch relations in development of the ear. (From Honrubia V, Goodhill V. Clinical anatomy and physiology of the peripheral ear. In: Goodhill V, ed. *Ear: diseases, deafness and dizziness.* Hagerstown, MD: Harper & Row, 1979:6, with permission.)

the neural tube and lateral to the acousticofacial ganglion (Fig. 2). At this point the auditory placode, which will contribute to the formation of the inner ear, and the primitive gut entoderm, which will form the middle ear cavity, are growing simultaneously.

The auditory placode invaginates, forming the *otic pit* (Fig. 3). It soon closes to form the *otocyst* (otic vesicle) (Fig. 4). Simultaneously, the *first branchial groove* begins to develop, with condensation of mesenchyme between the groove and the *entodermal pouch*. This mesenchymal condensation represents the anlage of future middle ear components, including the ossicles.

The *first branchial arch* (*mandibular*), the *second branchial arch* (*hyoid*), and the maxillary processes

develop (Fig. 5) at the same time that the otocyst and acousticofacial ganglion initiate the formation of the components of the membranous labyrinth (Fig. 6).

By the sixth week the *hillock formations* (Fig. 7) destined for the development of the auricle have appeared. The first branchial groove accompanied by first and second branchial arch derivatives will form the external auditory meatus.

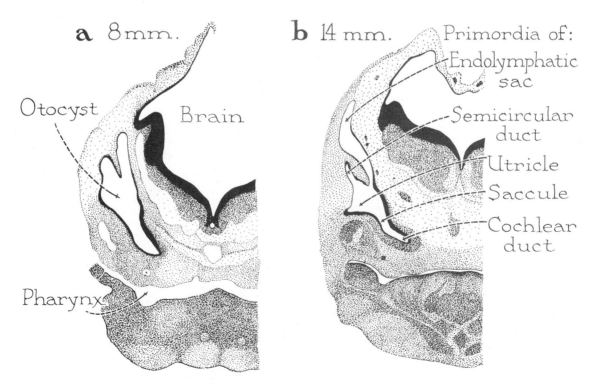

FIG. 6. Development of the otocyst from week 5 **(A)** to week 7 **(B)**. Parts of the membranous labyrinth are recognizable by the sixth to seventh week of gestation. (From Anson-Donaldson J, Duckert LG, Lambert PR, Rubel EW, eds. *Surgical anatomy of the temporal bone.* New York: Raven Press, 1992:93, with permission.)

(text continues on page 22)

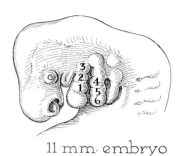

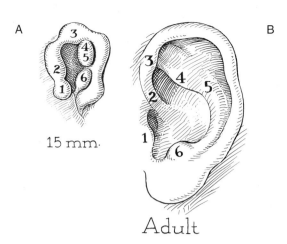

11 mm embryo

15 mm

Adult

A

B

FIG. 7. Hillock formations in an 11-mm embryo. (From Anson-Donaldson J, Duckert LG, Lambert PR, Rubel EW, eds. *Surgical anatomy of the temporal bone.* New York: Raven Press, 1992:56, with permission.)

FIG. 8. Progress of embryonic fusion of the hillocks to form the adult auricle. **A:** Six weeks of gestation. **B:** Adult auricle with corresponding numbers on the derived part. (From Anson-Donaldson J, Duckert LG, Lambert PR, Rubel EW, eds. *Surgical anatomy of the temporal bone.* New York: Raven Press, 1992:56, with permission.)

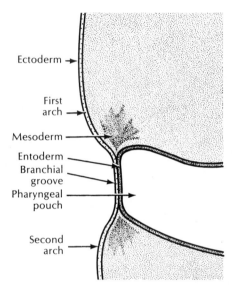

Ectoderm

First arch

Mesoderm

Entoderm
Branchial groove
Pharyngeal pouch

Second arch

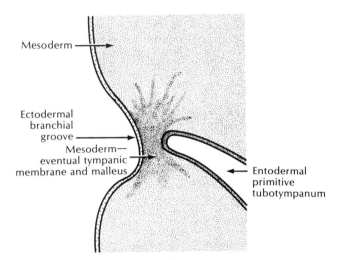

Mesoderm

Ectodermal branchial groove

Mesoderm— eventual tympanic membrane and malleus

Entodermal primitive tubotympanum

FIG. 9. Brief ectodermal-entodermal apposition. (From Honrubia V, Goodhill V. Clinical anatomy and physiology of the peripheral ear. In: Goodhill V, ed. *Ear: diseases, deafness and dizziness.* Hagerstown, MD: Harper & Row, 1979:7, with permission.)

FIG. 10. Mesodermal anlages of ossicles encroach on apposition area. (From Honrubia V, Goodhill V. Clinical anatomy and physiology of the peripheral ear. In: Goodhill V, ed. *Ear: diseases, deafness and dizziness.* Hagerstown, MD: Harper & Row, 1979:7, with permission.)

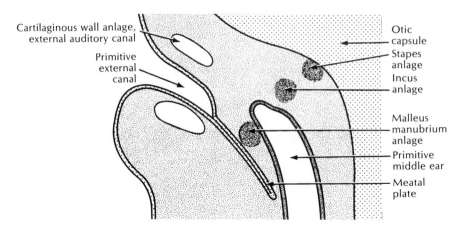

Cartilaginous wall anlage, external auditory canal

Primitive external canal

Otic capsule

Stapes anlage

Incus anlage

Malleus manubrium anlage

Primitive middle ear

Meatal plate

FIG. 11. Primitive external auditory canal, meatal plate, and middle ear. (From Honrubia V, Goodhill V. Clinical anatomy and physiology of the peripheral ear. In: Goodhill V, ed. *Ear: diseases, deafness and dizziness.* Hagerstown, MD: Harper & Row, 1979:7, with permission.)

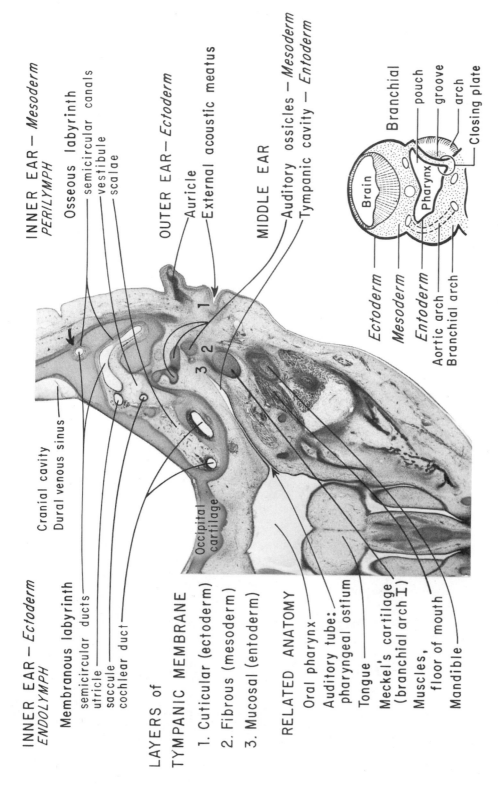

INNER EAR — *Mesoderm*
PERILYMPH

Osseous labyrinth
  semicircular canals
  vestibule
  scalae

OUTER EAR — *Ectoderm*

Auricle
External acoustic meatus

MIDDLE EAR

Auditory ossicles — *Mesoderm*
Tympanic cavity — *Entoderm*

Cranial cavity
Dural venous sinus

INNER EAR — *Ectoderm*
ENDOLYMPH

Membranous labyrinth
  semicircular ducts
  utricle
  saccule
  cochlear duct

LAYERS of
TYMPANIC MEMBRANE

1. Cuticular (ectoderm)
2. Fibrous (mesoderm)
3. Mucosal (entoderm)

RELATED ANATOMY

Oral pharynx
Auditory tube:
  pharyngeal ostium
Tongue
Meckel's cartilage
  (branchial arch I)
Muscles,
  floor of mouth
Mandible

Occipital
cartilage

Brain
Pharynx

Branchial
  pouch
  groove
  arch
Closing plate

Ectoderm
Mesoderm
Entoderm
Aortic arch
Branchial arch

FIG. 12. Transverse section through a 9-week-old fetus (40 mm). (From Anson-Donaldson J, Duckert LG, Lambert PR, Rubel EW, eds. *Surgical anatomy of the temporal bone.* New York: Raven Press, 1992:45, with permission.)

Development of the External Ear

The auricle develops around the first branchial grove from the *six hillocks of Hiss*. These hillocks are derived from the coalescence of the mandibular and hyoid arch anlages occurring during the third fetal month. The tragus develops from the first (mandibular) arch and the rest of the auricle from the remaining five hillocks, which are of second (hyoid) arch origin (Fig. 8). The branchial groove invaginates (Fig. 9) to meet the primitive entodermal pharyngeal pouch, but this ectodermal-entodermal apposition is encroached by superior and inferior mesodermal elements that rapidly separate this union (Fig. 10). These mesodermal anlages will form ossicular components as the pouch begins to form the primitive tubotympanum.

Mesodermal elements will form dorsal and ventral cartilaginous wall anlages around the primitive cartilaginous external auditory meatus and lateral external auditory canal. A solid core of epithelial cells, termed the *meatal plate*, grows toward the entodermal pharyngeal tube anlage (Fig. 11). Fetal development at 9 weeks is shown in Fig. 12.

Medial mesodermal elements begin to ossify during the fourth to fifth month to form the *tympanic ring* (annulus) for tympanic membrane support. However, it is not until the fifth to sixth fetal month that the solid ectodermal *epithelial core* (tympanic plate) begins dividing to form the lateral tympanic membrane epithelium and the skin of the bony external auditory canal, which arise simultaneously from the tympanic ring (Fig. 13).

In the fifth fetal month, the tympanic ring consists of several small centers of ossification. Osseous growth of the ring continues into the first postnatal year. As the ring develops, it actually encloses two spaces, the larger superior one being the external auditory canal and the smaller inferior one the foramen of Huschke. Continued growth of bone postnatally closes this latter foramen. After development, a defect in the tympanic ring persists in its superior portion, the tympanic incisure (notch of Rivinus). In addition to formation of the bony annulus, growth of the tympanic ring inferiorly increases the length of the meatus (Figs. 14 and 15).

Malformations of the auricle are due to failure in differentiation of the first and second branchial arches and may include anotia, microtia, and various auricular cartilage malformations, as well as malposition of the auricle. Failure of first branchial groove development is responsible for congenital atresia of the external canal, which usually is associated with an absent tympanic membrane, small middle ear space, and deformed ossicular chain (see Chapter 21).

Development of the Middle Ear

As the first (ectodermal) branchial groove invaginates to approach the primitive entodermal tubotympanic recess, mesodermal aggregations appear above and below to separate the primitive junction. Tympanic membrane and middle ear structures will develop from them, including ossicles, muscles, and tendons. The first pharyngeal pouch, which is lined by entoderm, expands to form the eustachian tube and middle ear cavity. As noted earlier, each of the three germ layers contributes to formation of the tympanic membrane.

The origin of the ossicles is complex (Fig. 16). It is thought that the superior portion of incus and malleus (forming the incudomalleal joint) arise from the first

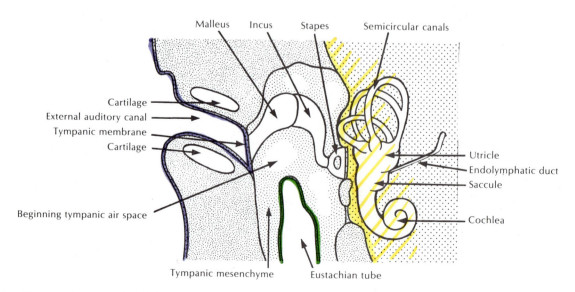

FIG. 13. Development of definite external, middle, and inner ear structures by seventh fetal month. (From Honrubia V, Goodhill V. Clinical anatomy and physiology of the peripheral ear. In: Goodhill V, ed. *Ear: diseases, deafness and dizziness.* Hagerstown, MD: Harper & Row, 1979:8, with permission.)

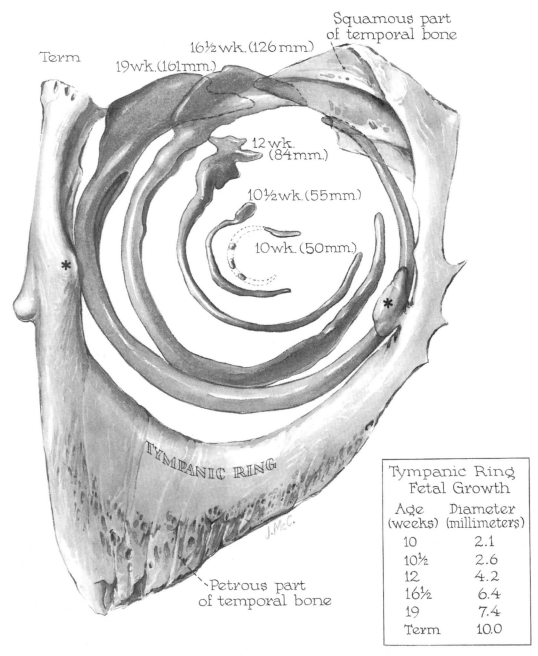

Tympanic Ring Fetal Growth	
Age (weeks)	Diameter (millimeters)
10	2.1
10½	2.6
12	4.2
16½	6.4
19	7.4
Term	10.0

FIG. 14. Developmental anatomy of the tympanic ring from week 10 to term. (From Anson-Donaldson J, Duckert LG, Lambert PR, Rubel EW, eds. *Surgical anatomy of the temporal bone.* New York: Raven Press, 1992:67, with permission.)

(mandibular) arch (*Meckel's cartilage*). The lower aspects of the incus and malleus and the arch of the stapes arise from the second (hyoid) arch (*Reichert's cartilage*). Initially the stapes is annular in appearance (chondral annulet), but by the fourth fetal month it is assuming a more stirruplike form. The stapes footplate has a dual origin, with the lateral (tympanic) portion arising from the hyoid arch and the medial (vestibular) portion from the otic capsule. At approximately the fourth fetal month, the ossicles begin to ossify. Branchial arch contributions to the ossicles and other head and neck structures are shown in Fig. 17.

As the ossicles develop and assume their positions within the mesotympanum, the eustachian tube remains an air-filled space, whereas tympanic mesenchyme still occupies the region of the future middle ear. Occasionally, mesenchyme may persist in the infant middle ear.

The entodermal primordium of the eustachian tube provides the ciliated epithelial lining for the tympanic cavity, attic, auntrum, and entire mastoid air cell system.

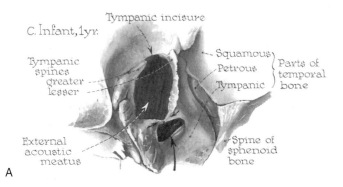

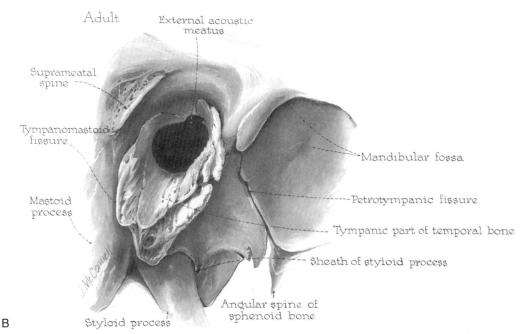

FIG. 15. A: At 1 year of age, the foramen of Huschke (*solid arrow*) is relatively large. **B:** Adult temporal bone showing full growth (meatal extension) of tympanic ring. (From Anson-Donaldson J, Duckert LG, Lambert PR, Rubel EW, eds. *Surgical anatomy of the temporal bone.* New York: Raven Press, 1992:68, with permission.)

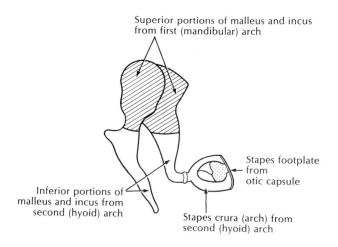

FIG. 16. Multiple origins for the three ossicles. (From Honrubia V, Goodhill V. Clinical anatomy and physiology of the peripheral ear. In: Goodhill V, ed. *Ear: diseases, deafness and dizziness.* Hagerstown, MD: Harper & Row, 1979:8, with permission.)

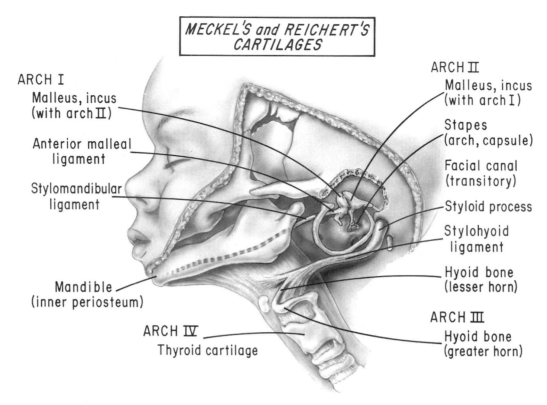

FIG. 17. Derivatives of the branchial arch system. (From Anson-Donaldson J, Duckert LG, Lambert PR, Rubel EW, eds. *Surgical anatomy of the temporal bone.* New York: Raven Press, 1992:51, with permission.)

Errors in first pharyngeal pouch differentiation may be responsible for maldevelopments of the eustachian tube, middle ear, and mastoid.

Development of the Inner Ear

The inner ear begins to develop 3 weeks after conception with the appearance of the *auditory placode*, an ectodermal thickening on either side of the rhombencephalon. The auditory placode rapidly invaginates to form a pit, which closes off at the surface to form the otocyst or *otic (auditory) vesicle*. Invaginations within the vesicular wall divide it into vestibular and cochlear components.

The primitive otocyst develops into the *vestibular duct* from which an anterior inferior *cochlear diverticulum* appears (Fig. 18). The vestibular duct differentiates into the three semicircular canals as the cochlear duct begins to develop from its saccular (inferior) portion (Fig. 19). By 7 to 8 weeks (20-mm stage) the semicircular canals are well formed, the cochlea is one turn in size, and the saccule and utricle are recognizable. By 9 to 10 weeks (30-mm stage) all of the mature components of the inner ear can be easily distinguished and the cochlea has grown to two full turns. At 25 weeks, the cochlear duct has two and one-half turns and appears adultlike.

Very early in the development of the inner ear (on the twelfth postfertilization day), *neuroepithelium* in the otocyst has progressed to form microvilli. By the tenth to twelfth week of gestation, sensory cells and supporting cells of the maculae of the saccule and utricle can be distinguished. At this time, the gelatinous otolithic membrane secreted by the supporting cells is apparent. Development of the three cristae proceeds along a similar time course.

The organ of Corti is represented by stratified epithelium during the first 2 fetal months. By the fifth month,

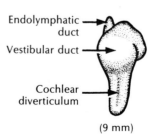

FIG. 18. Cochlear diverticulum appears from otic vesicle. (From Honrubia V, Goodhill V. Clinical anatomy and physiology of the peripheral ear. In: Goodhill V, ed. *Ear: diseases, deafness and dizziness.* Hagerstown, MD: Harper & Row, 1979:9, with permission.)

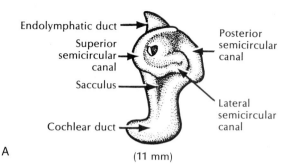

A

(11 mm)

FIG. 19. A: Semicircular canal and cochlear primordia. **B:** Canals, utricle, and saccule are developed. Cochlea still is primitive. **C:** At the 30-mm stage, full cochlear development is present. (From Honrubia V, Goodhill V. Clinical anatomy and physiology of the peripheral ear. In: Goodhill V, ed. *Ear: diseases, deafness and dizziness.* Hagerstown, MD: Harper & Row, 1979:9, with permission.)

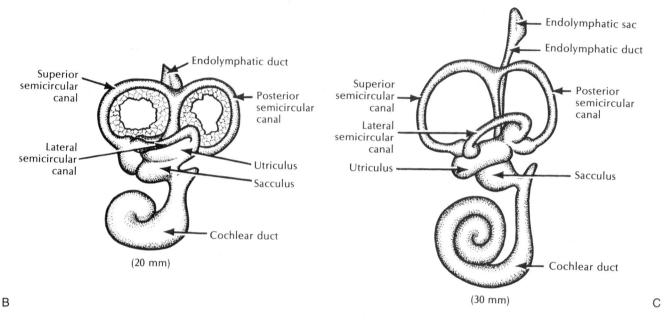

B

(20 mm)

(30 mm)

C

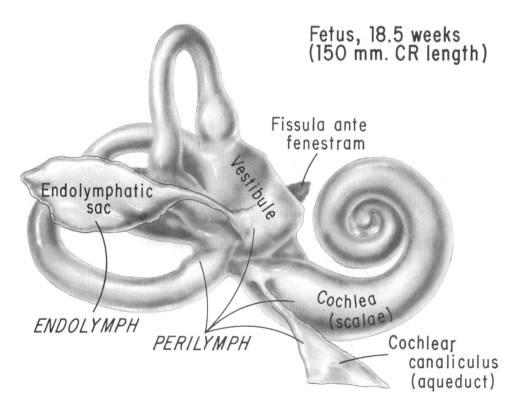

FIG. 20. Inner ear development. Note relatively straight course of endolymphatic duct early in fetal life. (From Anson-Donaldson J, Duckert LG, Lambert PR, Rubel EW, eds. *Surgical anatomy of the temporal bone.* New York: Raven Press, 1992:95, with permission.)

TABLE 1. *Time table of major events in human inner, middle, and external ear development*

Fetal week	Inner ear	Middle ear	External ear
3rd	Auditory placode; auditory pit	Tubotympanic recess begins to develop	
4th	Auditory vesicle (otocyst); vestibular-cochlear division		Tissue thickenings begin to form
5th			Primary auditory meatus begins
6th	Utricle and saccule present; semicircular canals begin		Six hillocks evident; cartilage begins to form
7th	One cochlear coil present; sensory cells in utricle and saccule		Auricle moves dorsolaterally
8th	Ductus reuniens present; sensory cells in semicircular canals	Incus and malleus present in cartilage; lower half of tympanic cavity formed	Outer cartilaginous third of external canal formed
9th		Three tissue layers at tympanic membrane are present	
11th	Two and one-half cochlear coils present; VIII nerve attaches to cochlear duct		
12th	Sensory cells in cochlea; membranous labyrinth complete; otic capsule begins to ossify		
15th		Cartilaginous stapes formed	
16th		Ossification of malleus and incus begins	
18th		Stapes begins to ossify	
20th	Maturation of internal ear; internal ear adult size		Auricle is adult shape, but continues to grow until age 9
21st		Meatal plug disintegrates, exposing tympanic membrane	
30th		Pneumatization of tympanum	External auditory canal continues to mature until age 7
32nd		Malleus and incus complete ossification	
34th		Mastoid air cells develop	
35th		Antrum is pneumatized	
37th		Epitympanum is pneumatized; stapes continues to develop until adulthood; tympanic membrane changes relative position during first 2 years of life	

From Northern, JL, Downs MP. *Hearing in children.* Baltimore: Williams and Wilkins, 1974.

the epithelium of the organ of Corti has differentiated and begun to assume adult characteristics. Development proceeds from the basal turn apically. By 25 weeks of gestation, the cochlear duct is probably functional, at least in the more basal regions. The appearance of the inner ear at approximately 20 weeks of gestation (150-mm stage) is shown in Fig. 20.

Concurrent with the development of the auditory placode, the *statoacoustic facial ganglion* forms from the neural crest at the end of the third week. The statoacoustic facial ganglion divides into a superior portion, which sends fibers to the utricle and to the superior and lateral ampullae, and into an inferior portion, from which fibers go to the saccule and posterior ampulla. The remainder of

the acoustic ganglion becomes the cochlear spiral ganglion. Facial nerve differentiation from the *facial ganglion* occurs simultaneously.

The primitive mesodermal anlage of the otic capsule, which forms the framework of the membranous labyrinth, relates laterally to the middle ear by the formation of the oval window and stapedial footplate and ligament, which seal the scala vestibuli. Similarly, the round window niche develops from the mesoderm, and its membrane becomes a mobile seal for the scala tympani.

Medial inner ear development relates to *vestibular* and *cochlear aqueduct* connections to the dura and subarachnoid space. Ectodermal otocyst components that form the neural elements of the inner ear interact with mesodermal

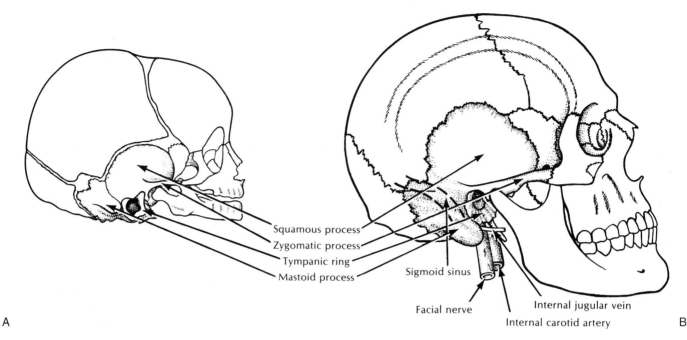

Squamous process
Zygomatic process
Tympanic ring
Mastoid process

Sigmoid sinus

Facial nerve

Internal jugular vein
Internal carotid artery

A   B

FIG. 21. A: Fetal skull. **B:** Adult skull. (From Honrubia V, Goodhill V. Clinical anatomy and physiology of the peripheral ear. In: Goodhill V, ed. *Ear: diseases, deafness and dizziness.* Hagerstown, MD: Harper & Row, 1979:11, with permission.)

plates to form these aqueducts. The "blind" end of the closed vestibular duct and sac in contact with the dura contrasts with the open communication of the cochlear aqueduct, providing hydraulic continuity between the perilymph of the scala tympani and the cerebral spinal fluid of the subarachnoid space.

The vestibular (endolymphatic) aqueduct extends from the junction of the utricular and saccular ducts as they exit the vestibule. In early fetal life, the duct is relatively straight, just medial to and paralleling the common crus of the superior and posterior semicircular canals. Later in fetal life, the vestibular duct turns downward at an angle of 30 to 60 degrees, which is the mature form. The duct terminates in an expanded portion termed the endolymphatic sac. An enlarged vestibular aqueduct is one of the most common congenital temporal bone anomalies. It usually is associated with progressive hearing loss (enlarged vestibular aqueduct syndrome) and may be unilateral or bilateral (see Chapter 29).

Because the membranous labyrinth derives from the ectodermal otocyst independently from the rest of the ear, which is primarily a branchial system apparatus, combined malformations of the inner ear and external and middle ear are infrequent. A summary of the time table of external, middle, and inner ear development is shown in Table 1).

Development of the Temporal Bone

The temporal bone develops in three parts, with the *petrous* portion deriving from cartilage and the *squa-*

mous and *tympanic* portions from membranous bone. The otic capsule around the labyrinth develops primarily from a cartilage model, although there are several areas of membranous bone that are involved in the ossification process. Distinct temporal bone development is recognizable by 8 to 12 weeks. The squama with its zygomatic process, the tympanic ring, and the primitive mastoid process are all present by the end of the fourth month (Fig. 21).

The primitive tympanic air space will lead first to the formation of the antrum and eventually to that of the entire mastoid air cell system. This system is created by a process in which a primitive connective tissue (embryonic mesenchyme) disappears with the invasion of mucosal epithelium from the first branchial pouch (via the eustachian tube anlage). As the mesenchyme disappears, many of its cells contribute to the epithelization of the various components of the tympanomastoid air space. The mucosa lining the mastoid is derived partly from mesenchyme and partly from first pharyngeal pouch gut entoderm.

ANATOMY OF THE TEMPORAL BONE

The temporal bone forms a large part of the lateral aspect of the skull and a significant portion of its base, integrating with the surrounding bones by tight articulations (synostoses) (Fig. 22). It consists of four parts: squamous, tympanic, mastoid, and petrous (Fig. 23). The large superior *squamous part* articulates with the

(text continues on page 33)

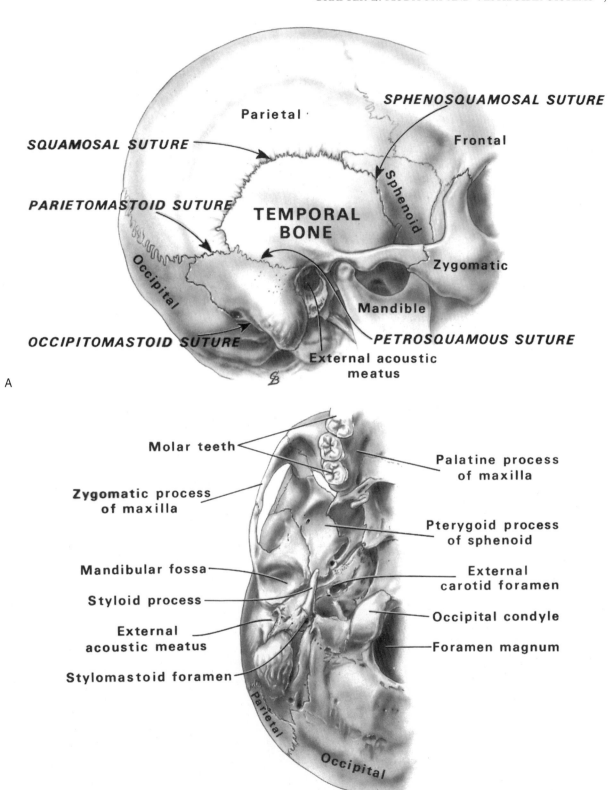

FIG. 22. A: The sutures of the squamous, mastoid, and tympanic parts of a right temporal bone. **B:** The relations of a right temporal bone to the sphenoid, frontal, parietal, and occipital bones. (From Anson-Donaldson J, Duckert LG, Lambert PR, Rubel EW, eds. *Surgical anatomy of the temporal bone.* New York: Raven Press, 1992:15, with permission.)

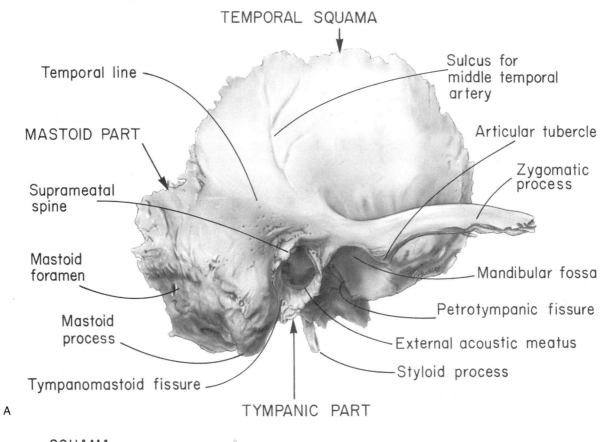

TEMPORAL SQUAMA

Temporal line

MASTOID PART

Suprameatal spine

Mastoid foramen

Mastoid process

Tympanomastoid fissure

Sulcus for middle temporal artery

Articular tubercle

Zygomatic process

Mandibular fossa

Petrotympanic fissure

External acoustic meatus

Styloid process

TYMPANIC PART

A

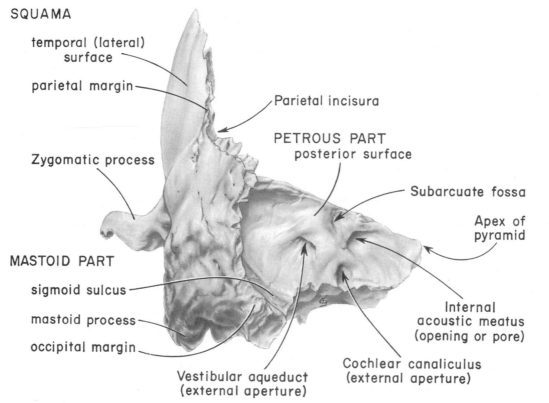

SQUAMA

temporal (lateral) surface

parietal margin

Zygomatic process

MASTOID PART

sigmoid sulcus

mastoid process

occipital margin

Parietal incisura

PETROUS PART
posterior surface

Subarcuate fossa

Apex of pyramid

Internal acoustic meatus (opening or pore)

Cochlear canaliculus (external aperture)

Vestibular aqueduct (external aperture)

B

FIG. 23. A: Lateral view of a right temporal bone. **B:** Posterolateral view of a left temporal bone. (From Anson-Donaldson J, Duckert LG, Lambert PR, Rubel EW, eds. *Surgical anatomy of the temporal bone.* New York: Raven Press, 1992:7, with permission.)

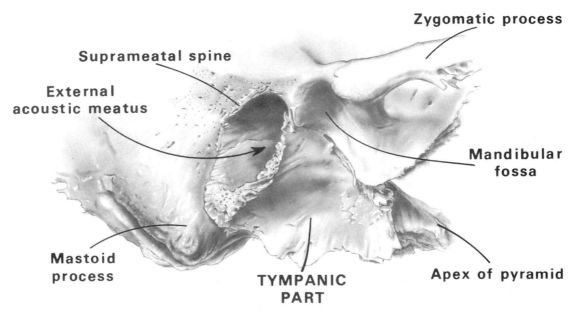

FIG. 24. Right temporomandibular fossa formed from zygomatic process of squamous part of temporal bone. (From Anson-Donaldson J, Duckert LG, Lambert PR, Rubel EW, eds. *Surgical anatomy of the temporal bone.* New York: Raven Press, 1992:13, with permission.)

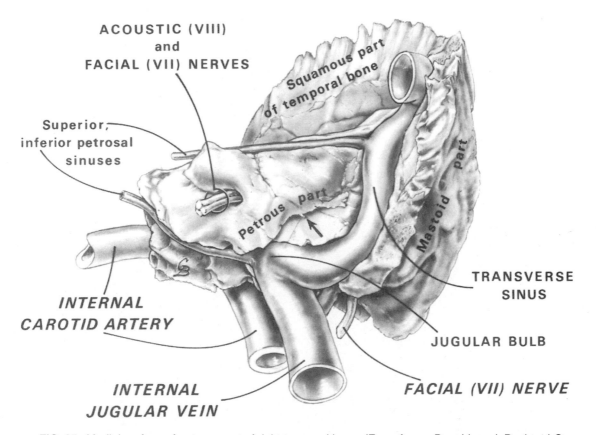

FIG. 25. Medial surface of petrous part of right temporal bone. (From Anson-Donaldson J, Duckert LG, Lambert PR, Rubel EW, eds. *Surgical anatomy of the temporal bone.* New York: Raven Press, 1992:334, with permission.)

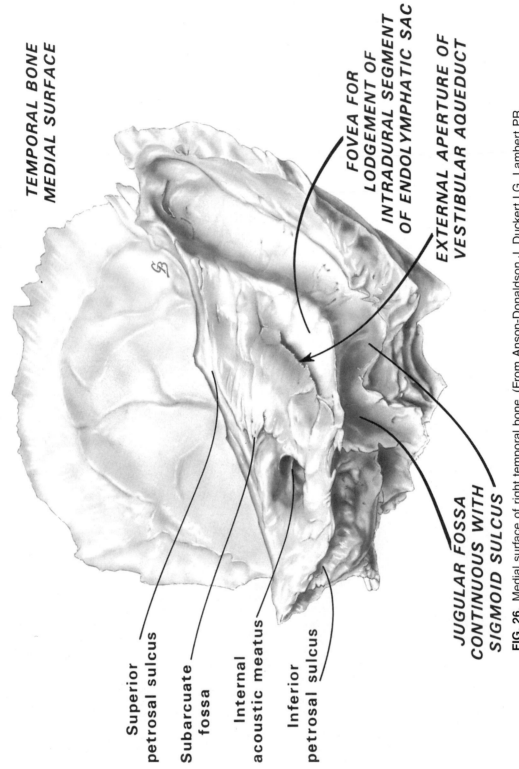

TEMPORAL BONE
MEDIAL SURFACE

FOVEA FOR
LODGEMENT OF
INTRADURAL SEGMENT
OF ENDOLYMPHATIC SAC

EXTERNAL APERTURE OF
VESTIBULAR AQUEDUCT

JUGULAR FOSSA
CONTINUOUS WITH
SIGMOID SULCUS

Superior
petrosal sulcus

Subarcuate
fossa

Internal
acoustic meatus

Inferior
petrosal sulcus

FIG. 26. Medial surface of right temporal bone. (From Anson-Donaldson J, Duckert LG, Lambert PR, Rubel EW, eds. *Surgical anatomy of the temporal bone.* New York: Raven Press, 1992:441, with permission.)

occipital, parietal, and sphenoid bones. It forms part of the lateral wall of the middle cranial fossa. Its anterior zygomatic portion (process) articulates with the zygoma and forms the roof of the temporomandibular fossa (Fig. 24). The small lateral *tympanic part* forms the external auditory canal. The posterior *mastoid part* articulates laterally with the parietal and occipital bones and houses a major portion of the mastoid air cell system, which communicates with the nasopharynx through the middle ear and eustachian tube. Medially, this system also is in continuity with the air cells of the petrous pyramid. The medial *petrous part* relates to the internal carotid artery, the sigmoid sinus, and the facial nerve. It contains the labyrinth with its neural aperture, the internal auditory canal (Fig. 25).

Medially, the anterior surface of the temporal bone contributes to the floor of the middle cranial fossa (Fig. 26). The posterior surface contributes to the floor of the posterior fossa and is almost at right angles to the anterior surface; the superior petrosal sulcus containing the superior petrosal sinus lies at the junction or apex of the posterior and anterior surfaces. The posterior surface landmarks include the depression for the sigmoid (lateral) sinus, the vestibular and cochlear aqueduct fossulae, the internal auditory meatus, and the jugular foramen.

The *internal auditory meatus* (Fig. 27) is the access route for the seventh and eighth cranial nerves from the cerebellopontine angle. The meatus is divided into superior and inferior portions by a transverse bony crest. The inferior portion serves as conduit for the cochlear division of the eighth nerve anteriorly and for the inferior vestibular nerve posteriorly. The latter also contains the foramen singulare, which transmits the saccular nerve to the posterior semicircular canal. The superior portion is divided by a *vertical crest (Bill's bar)* into an anterior channel for the seventh nerve and a posterior channel for the superior vestibular nerve, which supplies the superior and lateral semicircular canals and the utricle.

The seventh and eighth nerves in the cerebellopontine angle are in a superomedial relation with the fifth nerve; inferomedially they are relatively close to the ninth, tenth, and eleventh nerves and the jugular foramen (Fig. 28).

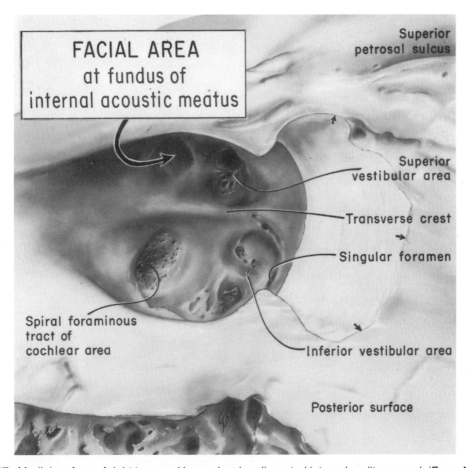

FIG. 27. Medial surface of right temporal bone showing dissected internal auditory canal. (From Anson-Donaldson J, Duckert LG, Lambert PR, Rubel EW, eds. *Surgical anatomy of the temporal bone.* New York: Raven Press, 1992:463, with permission.)

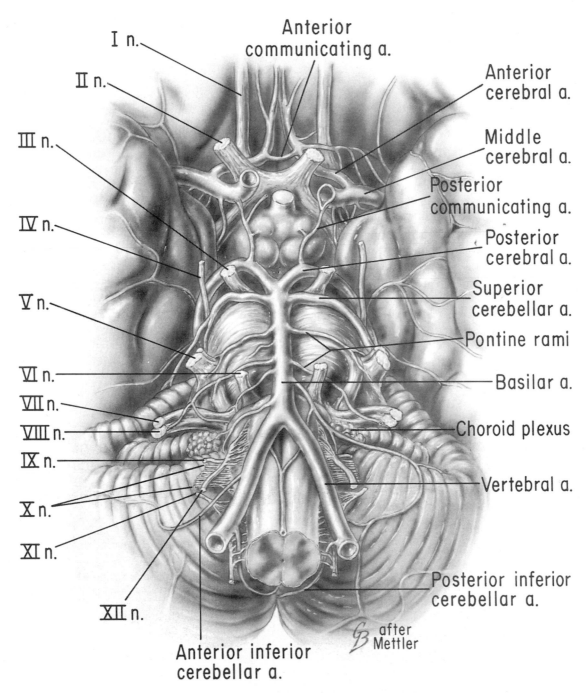

FIG. 28. Cranial nerves and arteries at the base of the brain. (From Anson-Donaldson J, Duckert LG, Lambert PR, Rubel EW, eds. *Surgical anatomy of the temporal bone.* New York: Raven Press, 1992:486, with permission.)

The *mastoid process* is the posterior part of the temporal bone visible as a bony protuberance behind the auricle. Clinically, the term mastoid refers not only to the mastoid process but to the entire interconnecting system of air cells contained within it. The *petrous apex*, which is at the base of the skull, has an air cell system that is in continuity with that of the mastoid. The petrous air cells remain open and aerated in only 30% of adult temporal bones. In the majority of adults the petrous tip consists of marrow and cortical bone. Therefore, petrous apicitis is often an osteitic or osteomyelitic process rather than one characterized by the coalescence of infected air cells.

The *periantral triangle* within the mastoid has boundaries defined by the posterior fossa plate and sigmoid sinus plate posteromedially, the middle fossa plate (tegmen) superiorly, and the posterior bony canal wall anteriorly. Normally, cellular pneumatization occurs throughout the temporal bone and may extend into the parietal, occipital, and zygomatic bones. The mucosa of the mastoid air cell system is in continuity with that of the middle ear, the eustachian tube, and the nasopharynx.

The mastoid air cell system contains the posterior genu and vertical portions of the facial (VII) nerve, the chorda tympani and stapedial nerves, a portion of the bony labyrinthine capsule (semicircular canals), and the sigmoid sinus (Fig. 29). The internal carotid artery is in anterior relation to the middle ear and to the eustachian tube and petrous apex.

Infant Anatomy

Although all major components are present in the infant's temporal bone, it differs from the adult in several important ways. The bony portion of the external canal consists only of the tympanic ring; thus, the external auditory canal of the infant is almost entirely cartilaginous. The petromastoid portion of the infant temporal bone contains at least one major air cell, the *mastoid antrum*, a primordium for development of the rest of the mastoid air cell system. The lateral bony margin of this antral cell is formed at birth by the squama. Because the mastoid tip is yet to develop, the infant stylomastoid foramen is very superficial; thus, the facial nerve may be traumatized during forceps delivery and other types of external trauma, including surgery.

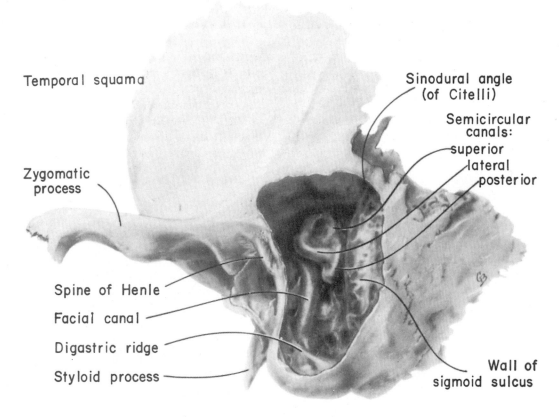

Temporal squama

Sinodural angle
(of Citelli)

Semicircular
canals:
superior
lateral
posterior

Zygomatic
process

Spine of Henle

Facial canal

Digastric ridge

Styloid process

Wall of
sigmoid sulcus

FIG. 29. Dissected mastoid cavity in a left temporal bone. (From Anson-Donaldson J, Duckert LG, Lambert PR, Rubel EW, eds. *Surgical anatomy of the temporal bone.* New York: Raven Press, 1992:254, with permission.)

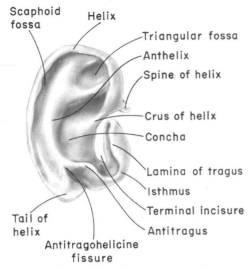

FIG. 30. The auricular framework. (From Anson-Donaldson J, Duckert LG, Lambert PR, Rubel EW, eds. *Surgical anatomy of the temporal bone.* New York: Raven Press, 1992:181, with permission.)

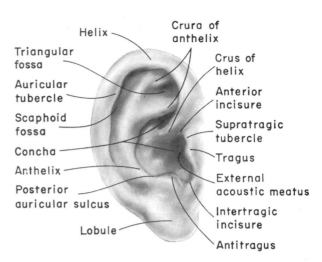

FIG. 31. The normal auricle. (From Anson-Donaldson J, Duckert LG, Lambert PR, Rubel EW, eds. *Surgical anatomy of the temporal bone.* New York: Raven Press, 1992:181, with permission.)

ANATOMY OF THE AURICLE

The auricular framework is a complex cartilaginous structure (Fig. 30). In the infant and young child it is soft, elastic, and shallow. The lateral superior margin of the auricle is the *helix*, which bounds (from posterior to anterior) the *scapha, antihelix, triangular fossa, antitragus,* and *concha* and is apposed anteriorly to the external auditory meatus by the *tragus* (Fig. 31). The *lobule* (noncartilaginous) is the inferior appendage of the auricle. The *intertragal notch* separates the antitragus from the tragus. The auricle has three extrinsic muscles—the anterior, superior, and posterior auricular—and six intrinsic muscles (Fig. 32). Further anatomic features of the pinna, including its special innervation and blood supply, are described in Chapter 19.

ANATOMY OF THE EXTERNAL EAR CANAL

The external auditory canal is approximately 25 mm in length posterosuperiorly and, because of the obliquity of the tympanic membrane, 30 mm long anteroinferiorly. It assumes a slight "s" configuration as it courses medially. The lateral aspect of the external auditory canal is constituted by cartilage covered by a thick epithelium (Fig. 33). The subepithelial stroma contains a very rich blood supply, hair follicles, and many ceruminal glands (Fig. 34). There are significant variations

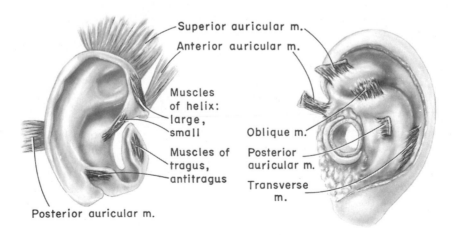

FIG. 32. The intrinsic and extrinsic auricular muscles. (From Anson-Donaldson J, Duckert LG, Lambert PR, Rubel EW, eds. *Surgical anatomy of the temporal bone.* New York: Raven Press, 1992:181, with permission.)

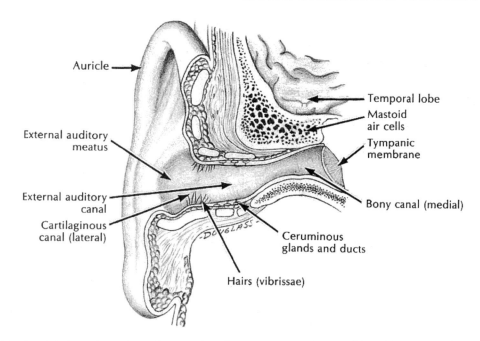

FIG. 33. Frontal view of auricle and external auditory meatus and canal. (From Honrubia V, Goodhill V. Clinical anatomy and physiology of the peripheral ear. In: Goodhill V, ed. *Ear: diseases, deafness and dizziness.* Hagerstown, MD: Harper & Row, 1979:18, with permission.)

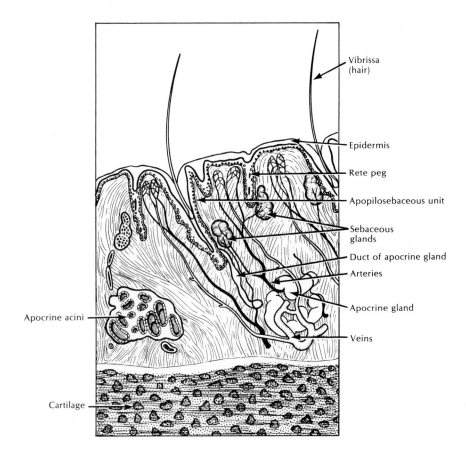

FIG. 34. Cartilaginous external canal skin with apocrine and sebaceous glands, pilosebaceous units, and vibrissas (hairs). (Adapted from Senturia BH. *Diseases of the external ear.* Springfield, IL: Charles C. Thomas Publisher, 1957:25.)

in diameter and shape of the infant and adult cartilaginous canals, and in the distribution and density of hairs and ceruminal glands. Additional details of external canal anatomy are included in Chapter 20. The medial aspect of the external canal is formed by the *tympanic bone*. This osseous portion comprises slightly more than half of the canal's length. It is lined by thin skin intimately attached to the periosteum and, in contrast with the cartilaginous canal, is extremely sensitive to touch. It lacks hairs and glands. The epithelium of the external canal is in continuity with the epidermal (squamous) layer of the tympanic membrane.

ANATOMY OF THE MIDDLE EAR

Tympanic Membrane

The *tympanic membrane* (eardrum) is a multilayered, cone-shaped structure measuring approximately 9 mm in diameter, with radii varying from 4 to 5 mm. It is anchored to the bony tympanic ring, and it separates the external and middle ear. The tympanic membrane is attached to the malleus handle (manubrium) between the short (lateral) process and umbo of that ossicle. The umbo is the medial apex of the tympanic membrane (Fig. 35).

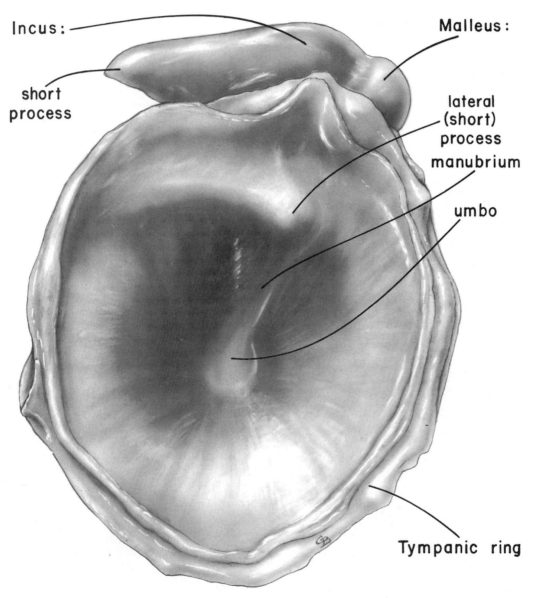

FIG. 35. The tympanic ring and tympanic membrane. (From Anson-Donaldson J, Duckert LG, Lambert PR, Rubel EW, eds. *Surgical anatomy of the temporal bone.* New York: Raven Press, 1992:184, with permission.)

The major portion of the tympanic membrane is the *pars tensa*, which is separated from the superior portion known as *pars flaccida* (Shrapnell's membrane) by the anterior and posterior malleal plicae (folds), which extend from the malleal short process to the annular rim. Medial to the pars flaccida is Prussak's space, a common area for primary cholesteatoma extension. The pars tensa is normally translucent, occasionally permitting visualization of the long process of the incus and the incudostapedial joint in its posterosuperior quadrant.

The tympanic membrane is approximately 0.1 mm thick and is constituted by a lateral (squamous), a middle (fibrous), and a medial (mucosal) layer. In the pars tensa the collagenous fibers of the middle layer are plentiful and organized both radially and circumferentially, whereas the fibers in the pars flaccida are less abundant and poorly organized. A thickening of the fibers at the limits of the pars tensa constitutes the *fibrous annulus,* an element lacking in the pars flaccida. These structural differences are responsible for the characteristic tightness of the pars tensa and the drapelike quality of the pars flaccida.

The Ossicles

The *malleus* (weight ±23 mg) consists of a head, neck, and three processes: the manubrium into which the tympanic membrane is inserted (Fig. 36A), the anterior process (usually vestigial), and the lateral (short) process. The malleal head, which occupies a major portion of the epitympanum (attic), is supported by a complex system of ligaments.

The *incus* (weight ±27 mg) consists of a body with a long and a short process (Fig. 36A). The body articulates with the head of the malleus, forming the incudomalleal joint. The short process projects into the posteroinferior portion of the epitympanic recess. In this position it can be seen from a mastoid view as a landmark in mastoidectomy. The long process descends in a posterior direction parallel to the malleal manubrium and, turning medially, ends at the lenticular process, which articulates with the head (capitulum) of the stapes to form the incudostapedial joint.

The *stapes* (weight ±2.5 mg) is the smallest bone in the body. It consists of a head (capitulum), which articulates with the incus at the incudostapedial joint, a neck, two crura or legs, and the footplate (Fig. 36A). The head, neck, and crura form the stapedial arch, which is attached to the footplate. The head and neck consist of marrow bone, whereas the crura consist of partly hollowed, semicylindrical shells of cortical bone. The crura form the boundaries of the obturator (stapedial) artery, which occupies this space in fetal life. Rarely, it may persist into adulthood, producing conductive hearing loss and tinnitus.

The *tensor tympani muscle* attaches to the proximal manubrium (or neck) of the malleus and maintains a variable tension on the tympanic membrane. In addition, there are superior, anterior, posterior, and mediolateral suspensory ligaments attaching to the malleus and incus. The *stapedius muscle* attaches to the head of the stapes (Fig. 36B).

The relations of the three intact ossicles *in situ* are shown in Fig. 37.

The Middle Ear Cleft

The *middle ear* (tympanum, tympanic cavity) is an air-containing space, contiguous anteroinferiorly with the eustachian tube and nasopharynx and posteriorly with the air cell system of the mastoid and petrous portions of the temporal bone. The middle ear is lined with a mucous membrane that is best described as modified respiratory mucosa. Cell types include ciliated cells, nonciliated cells with and without secretory granules, and goblet cells. Ciliated columnar epithelium predominate in the hypotympanum, near the eustachian tube orifice, and in the eustachian tube proper.

The middle ear cleft is formed by four walls, a roof, and a floor. The tegmen tympani forms the roof and the

AUDITORY OSSICLES – Normal Anatomy

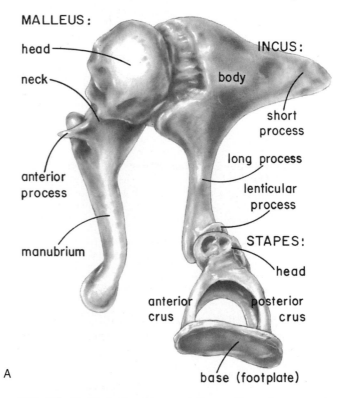

FIG. 36. A: Normal anatomy of the malleus, incus, and stapes. *Continued.*

AUDITORY OSSICLES – Ligaments and Muscles

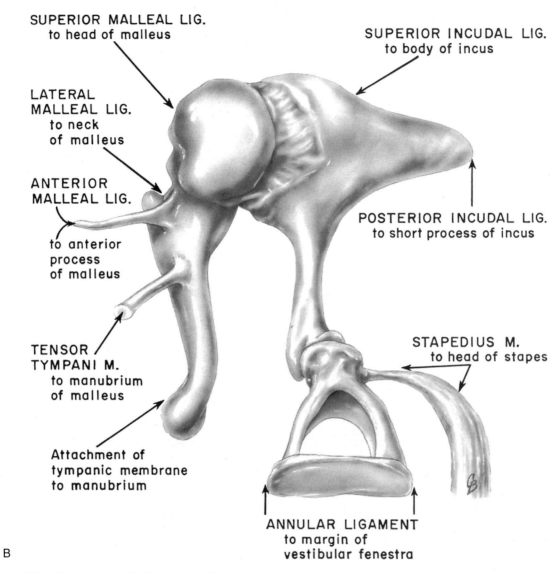

SUPERIOR MALLEAL LIG.
to head of malleus

SUPERIOR INCUDAL LIG.
to body of incus

LATERAL
MALLEAL LIG.
to neck
of malleus

ANTERIOR
MALLEAL LIG.

to anterior
process
of malleus

POSTERIOR INCUDAL LIG.
to short process of incus

TENSOR
TYMPANI M.
to manubrium
of malleus

STAPEDIUS M.
to head of stapes

Attachment of
tympanic membrane
to manubrium

ANNULAR LIGAMENT
to margin of
vestibular fenestra

B

FIG. 36. *Continued.* **B:** Muscles and ligaments that attach to the ossicles. (From Anson-Donaldson J, Duckert LG, Lambert PR, Rubel EW, eds. *Surgical anatomy of the temporal bone.* New York: Raven Press, 1992:224, 243, with permission.)

jugular bulb the floor. The posterior wall of the middle ear contains a number of anatomic structures including the pyramidal eminence, facial recess, and sinus tympani. Anteriorly, the major landmarks are the semicanal for the tensor tympani muscle, the wall of the internal carotid artery, and the eustachian tube orifice. The predominant structure of the medial wall of the middle ear is the basal turn of the cochlea (promontory); other important anatomic features include the oval and round windows, the fallopian canal for the horizontal segment of the facial nerve, and the cochleariform process from which the tensor tympani tendon emerges. The tympanic membrane forms the lateral wall of the middle ear

cleft. The middle ear also can be divided topographically into the epitympanum, mesotympanum, and hypotympanum.

The *epitympanum* (attic) houses the incudomalleal joint, the head of the malleus, and the body of the incus with their suspensory ligaments (Fig. 38). The epitympanic air space is in direct continuity anteriorly with the zygomatic air cell system and is bounded superiorly by the tegmen tympani, a thin bony plate separating the middle ear from the middle cranial fossa. Of particular note is the *anterior epitympanic recess (supratubal recess)*. This pneumatized area lies anterior to the head of the malleus. The ossicular heads partially obscure

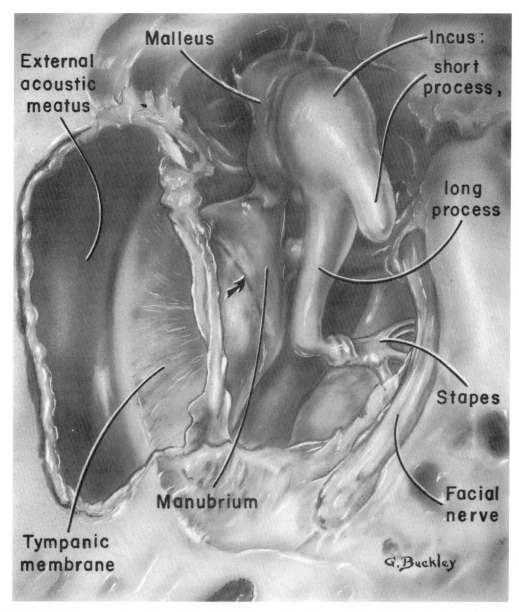

FIG. 37. Middle ear cavity with ossicles. (From Anson-Donaldson J, Duckert LG, Lambert PR, Rubel EW, eds. *Surgical anatomy of the temporal bone.* New York: Raven Press, 1992:182, with permission.)

this recess from inspection during surgical procedures, and for this reason complete removal of disease, particularly cholesteatoma, may be problematic (Fig. 39). The epitympanic air space communicates posteriorly through the aditus with the antrum, the primary cell of the mastoid air cell system. The medial wall of the epitympanum contains the anterior portions of the superior and lateral semicircular canals, and the horizontal segment of the facial canal. Laterally, it is bounded by the pars flaccida and the posterosuperior edge of the ear canal, or scutum.

The *mesotympanum* is the largest part of the middle ear. It is bound laterally by the pars tensa and contains the neck and manubrium of the malleus, the long process of the incus, the stapes and oval window, and the round window niche. The horizontal portion of the facial canal forms its superomedial boundary (Fig. 40). The oval window niche is occupied by the stapedial footplate (1.75 × 3.75 mm) and its annular ligament, providing a sealed but mobile communication between the middle ear and the vestibule. The cochlear promontory of the otic capsule is a rounded, smooth, bony surface forming one-third of the medial wall of the mesotympanum. It separates the oval window from the round window niche. The inferior portion of the promontory is the lower limit of the mesotympanum. The anterior portion of the meso-

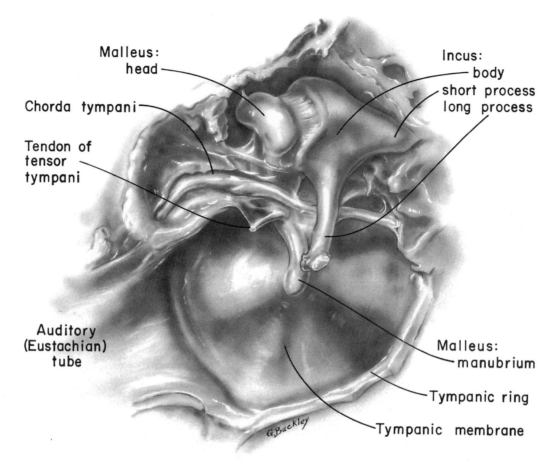

FIG. 38. Medial to lateral view of middle ear, emphasizing epitympanic space. (From Anson-Donaldson J, Duckert LG, Lambert PR, Rubel EW, eds. *Surgical anatomy of the temporal bone.* New York: Raven Press, 1992:189, with permission.)

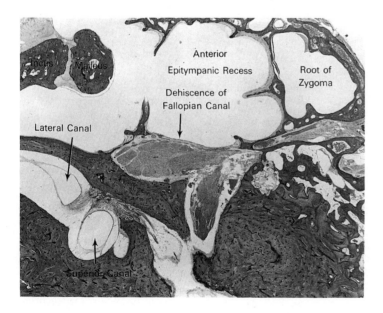

FIG. 39. Histologic section, emphasizing epitympanic recess anterior to head of malleus. (From Schuknecht HF. *Pathology of the ear,* 2nd ed. Philadelphia: Lea & Febiger, 1993:37, with permission.)

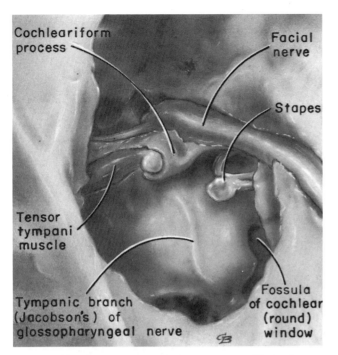

FIG. 40. Medial wall of the middle ear space. (From Anson-Donaldson J, Duckert LG, Lambert PR, Rubel EW, eds. *Surgical anatomy of the temporal bone.* New York: Raven Press, 1992:190, with permission.)

tympanum joins with the anterior epitympanum to form the protympanum (bony eustachian tube opening), which communicates with the cartilaginous eustachian tube (Fig. 41)

Along the posterior wall of the mesotympanum is the *sinus tympani*, a pneumatized recess that is bounded laterally by the mastoid segment of the facial nerve (Figs. 42

and 43). This recess is of varying size and is of clinical significance in surgery for chronic otitis media and cholesteatoma because of the difficulty in removing disease from its depths. Lateral to the mastoid segment of the facial nerve is another pneumatized space, the *facial recess*. This space is important surgically, as it provides an access route from the mastoid into the mesotympanum. The facial recess is bounded laterally by the chorda tympani nerve and superiorly by the fossa incudis (Figs. 44 and 45).

The *hypotympanum* is the lowest level of the middle ear space, and its floor is the dome of the jugular bulb. It communicates with the hypotympanic and retrofacial air cells anteriorly and posteriorly. The round window niche is a depression located inferoposterior to the promontory. The round window membrane, despite its name, is slightly elliptical in shape, measuring about 2 mm vertically and 1.7 mm horizontally. It inserts in the anterosuperior portion of the niche. It is in medial contact with the scala tympani and in close proximity to the labyrinthine opening of the cochlear aqueduct.

Structures within the Middle Ear

The *facial nerve* is derived from the second branchial arch. It contains efferent fibers that innervate the facial muscles, the stylohyoid muscle, the posterior belly of the digastric muscle, and the stapedius muscle. It also contains preganglionic parasympathetic fibers that innervate the lacrimal gland, seromucous glands of the nasal cavity, and the submandibular and sublingual glands. Taste from the anterior two-thirds of the tongue is carried via afferent fibers within the facial nerve.

The facial nerve exits the pons, crosses the cerebellopontine angle, and enters the internal auditory canal with

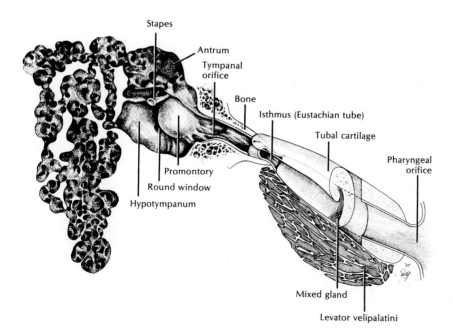

FIG. 41. Artist's view of middle ear, mastoid and eustachian tube, demonstrating anatomic landmarks. (From Lim DJ. Functional morphology of the lining membrane of the middle ear and eustachian tube. *Ann Otol Rhinol Laryngol* 1974;83[Suppl 11]:6, with permission.)

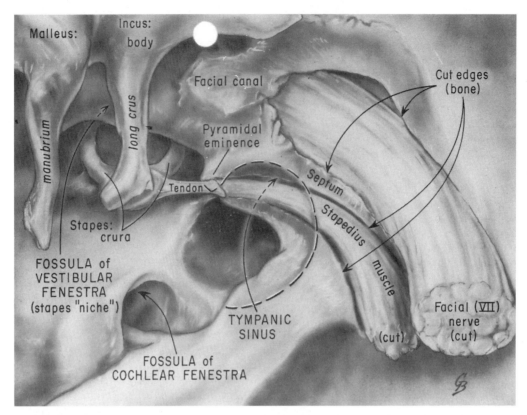

FIG. 42. The sinus tympani in the posterior medial wall of the middle ear. (From Anson-Donaldson J, Duckert LG, Lambert PR, Rubel EW, eds. *Surgical anatomy of the temporal bone.* New York: Raven Press, 1992:216, with permission.)

the vestibulocochlear nerve. The *labyrinthine segment* of the facial nerve is located between the lateral end of the internal auditory canal and the *geniculate ganglion.* At the geniculate ganglion, the nerve turns posteriorly (first or anterior genu) and enters the upper mesotympanum.

This *horizontal* or *tympanic segment* courses just superior to the oval window and then turns inferiorly near the horizontal semicircular canal. This second bend is termed the posterior or second genu. At this bend, the nerve enters the mastoid air cell system and is termed the *vertical* or

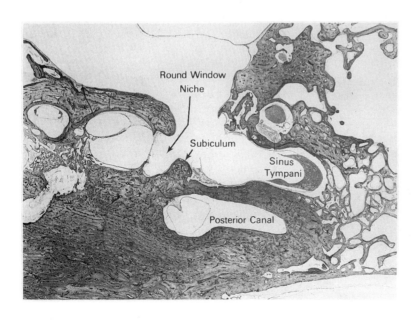

FIG. 43. Histologic section showing a large sinus tympani extending medial to facial nerve. (From Schuknecht HF. *Pathology of the ear,* 2nd ed. Philadelphia: Lea & Febiger, 1993:34, with permission.)

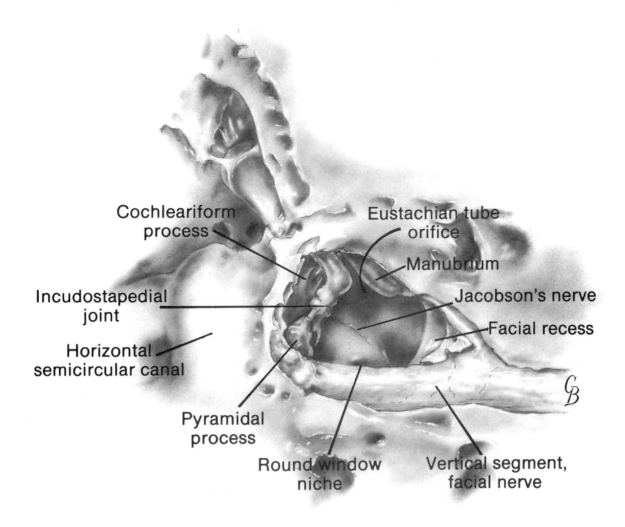

FIG. 44. Exposure of the middle ear through the facial recess. (From Anson-Donaldson J, Duckert LG, Lambert PR, Rubel EW, eds. *Surgical anatomy of the temporal bone.* New York: Raven Press, 1992:204, with permission.)

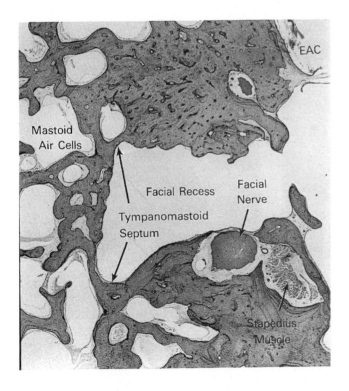

FIG. 45. Histologic section showing large facial recess lateral to the facial nerve. (From Schuknecht HF. *Pathology of the ear,* 2nd ed. Philadelphia: Lea & Febiger, 1993:35, with permission.)

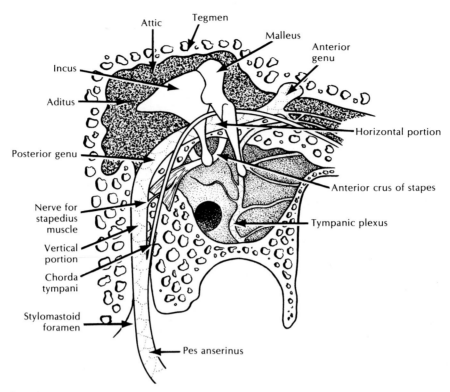

FIG. 46. Course of facial (VII) nerve through middle ear and mastoid. (From Honrubia V, Goodhill V. Clinical anatomy and physiology of the peripheral ear. In: Goodhill V, ed. *Ear: diseases, deafness and dizziness.* Hagerstown, MD: Harper & Row, 1979:31, with permission.)

mastoid segment. The nerve finally emerges into the parotid space through the stylomastoid foramen. From the lateral end (fundus) of the internal auditory canal to the stylomastoid foramen, the nerve is encased within the bony fallopian canal (Fig. 46). The anatomy of the facial nerve is described in detail in Chapter 44.

The mesotympanum contains two muscles. The *stapedius muscle* arises from the pyramidal eminence located just inferior to the lateral genu of the facial nerve and from a portion of the proximal mastoid segment of the fallopian canal. It attaches to the neck of the stapes and is innervated by the facial nerve. Contraction of this muscle limits movement of the stapes and is the basis for acoustic reflex testing. The *tensor tympani muscle* is approximately 2 cm in length and arises in part from the cartilaginous portion of the eustachian tube and in part from a semicanal parallel to the eustachian tube (Fig. 47). It courses posteriorly to a bony eminence, the cochleariform process, which overlies the tympanic portion of the fallopian canal. At this point, its tendon makes a right angle turn laterally to insert on the base of the manubrium of the malleus near its neck. The tensor tympani muscle is innervated by the mandibular branch of the trigeminal nerve. Contraction of this muscle causes the manubrium to move medially, tightening the tympanic membrane.

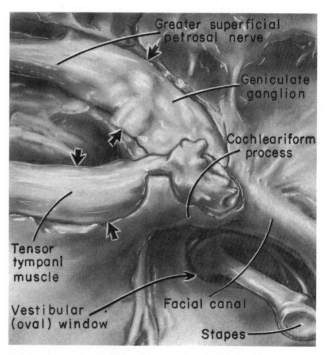

FIG. 47. The tensor tympani muscle. (From Anson-Donaldson J, Duckert LG, Lambert PR, Rubel EW, eds. *Surgical anatomy of the temporal bone.* New York: Raven Press, 1992:247, with permission.)

The *eustachian tube* is a 3.5-cm-long, part bony and part cartilaginous, tube that connects the nasopharynx with the middle ear (Fig. 41). Its upper (tympanic) orifice lies within the mesotympanum in a spacious bony channel, the protympanum, arising high on the anteromedial wall of the tympanic cavity. The tympanic portion of the eustachian tube is bony and measures approximately 10 mm in length and is shaped like a cone pointing inferolaterally. At the apex of the cone is the isthmus of the eustachian tube, its most narrow portion. Close to the cartilaginous portion the eustachian tube is oval in shape and approximately 3 mm high and 1.5 mm wide. Inferior to its isthmus the cartilaginous portion is approximately 2.5 mm in length and slitlike. Medially, it opens onto the lateral wall of the pharynx, near the lateral pharyngeal recess (fossa of Rosenmüller). Superomedially, it is surrounded by a C-shaped cartilage, to which are attached two muscles, the *tensor palatini*, laterally, and the *levator palatini*, medially. Unlike the osseus portion of the eustachian tube, which remains open, the cartilaginous portion usually is closed because of the incomplete cartilage ring. On swallowing, the eustachian tube opens, primarily by action of the levator palatini muscle.

Medial to the osseous portion of the eustachian tube is the *carotid canal*. The carotid canal forms the anterior boundary of the tympanic cavity and often is associated with air cells. Through this canal traverses the internal carotid artery and associated venous and neural plexuses.

Vascular Supply to the External and Middle Ears

The external auditory canal is supplied primarily by the posterior auricular and superficial temporal arteries, which are branches of the external carotid artery. The internal maxillary artery supplies blood to the tympanic membrane through its auricular branch (external surface) and its anterior tympanic branch (mucosal surface). The middle ear cavity, including the ossicles, are supplied by a number of arteries arising from the internal maxillary, middle meningeal, ascending pharyngeal, posterior auricular, and internal carotid arteries. Named vessels include the anterior, inferior, posterior, and superior tympanic arteries; stylomastoid artery; the caroticotympanic artery (from the internal carotid artery); and the superficial petrosal artery (Figs. 48 and 49). The veins of the middle ear run parallel to the arteries and drain into the pterygoid plexus and petrosal sinuses.

Sensory Innervation to the External and Middle Ears

Sensory innervation to the ear is supplied by cranial nerves V, VII, IX, and X, and the second and third cervical nerves. Innervation to the auricle is somewhat complex, with overlapping zones. The specific nerves involved include the auriculotemporal branch of the trigeminal nerve, the tympanic branch (Jacobson's nerve) of the glossopharyngeal nerve, the auricular branch (Arnold's nerve) of the vagus nerve, the lesser occipital nerve from C2, and the greater auricular nerve from C2 and C3 (Fig. 50).

The auriculotemporal nerve supplies the tragus and adjacent anterior one-third of the pinna above the meatus. The greater auricular nerve innervates the remainder of the lateral aspect of the pinna (except for the concavity of the concha) and most of the posterior surface of the pinna. The conchal area is innervated by cranial nerves VII, IX, and X. Skin overlying the mastoid is supplied by the lesser occipital nerve.

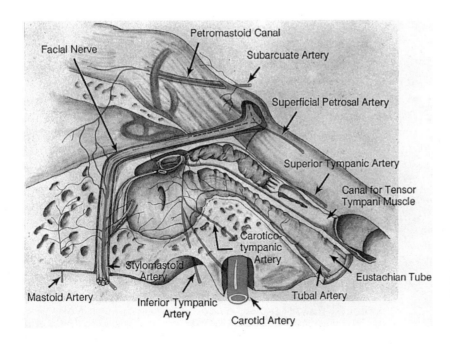

FIG. 48. Arterial supply of middle ear and mastoid exclusive of anterior tympanic artery. (From Schuknecht HF. *Pathology of the ear*, 2nd ed. Philadelphia: Lea & Febiger, 1993:38, with permission.)

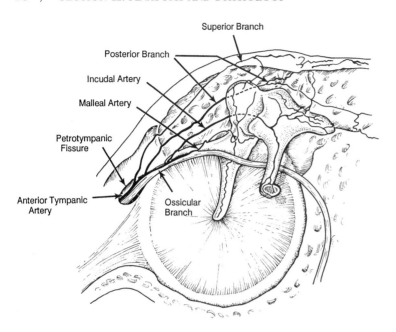

FIG. 49. Distribution of anterior tympanic artery. (From Schuknecht HF. *Pathology of the Ear,* 2nd ed. Philadelphia: Lea & Febiger, 1993:38, with permission.)

The anterior and superior external canal walls and the corresponding surface of the tympanic membrane are supplied by the auriculotemporal nerve. The posterior and inferior canal walls adjacent to the tympanic membrane are innervated by the auricular branch of the vagus nerve, probably with contribution from the glossopharyngeal and facial nerves. The medial surface of the tympanic membrane as well as the mucosa of the middle ear cavity are innervated by the tympanic plexus. The sensory portion of this plexus derives from the tympanic branch of the glossopharyngeal nerve. The plexus also contains preganglionic parasympathetic fibers from the glossopharyngeal nerve.

Anatomy of Specific Nerves

Although the *chorda tympani nerve* does not provide innervation to the middle ear structures, it traverses the middle ear cavity. The nerve contains sensory (taste) and preganglionic parasympathetic fibers. The cell bodies for the sensory fibers are in the geniculate ganglion and those for the secretory fibers are in the superior salivatory nucleus of the brainstem. The preganglionic fibers synapse in the submandibular ganglion and innervate the submandibular, sublingual, and minor salivary glands of the oral cavity.

The chorda tympani nerve can arise from various locations along the mastoid segment of the facial nerve, with the average takeoff being 5 mm proximal to the stylomastoid foramen. The nerve then enters the middle ear cavity through its posterior wall and courses anteriorly, passing just lateral to the long process of the incus and medial to the manubrium of the malleus. It exits the middle ear through the petrotympanic fissure and joins the lingual nerve for distribution to the anterior two-thirds of the tongue and the submandibular ganglion.

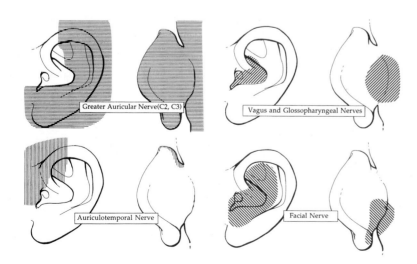

FIG. 50. Sensory innervation of lateral and posterior aspects of the ear. (From Lambert PR. Referred otalgia. In: Britton BH, ed. *Common problems in otology.* St. Louis, Mosby-Year Book, 1991:331, with permission.)

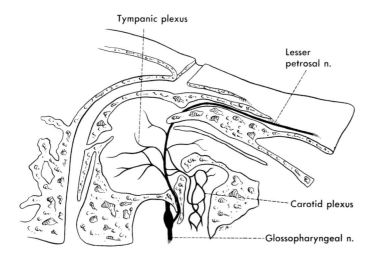

FIG. 51. The tympanic plexus. (From Hollinshead WH. *Anatomy for surgeons: The head and neck.* Hagerstown, MD: Harper & Row, 1982:200, with permission.)

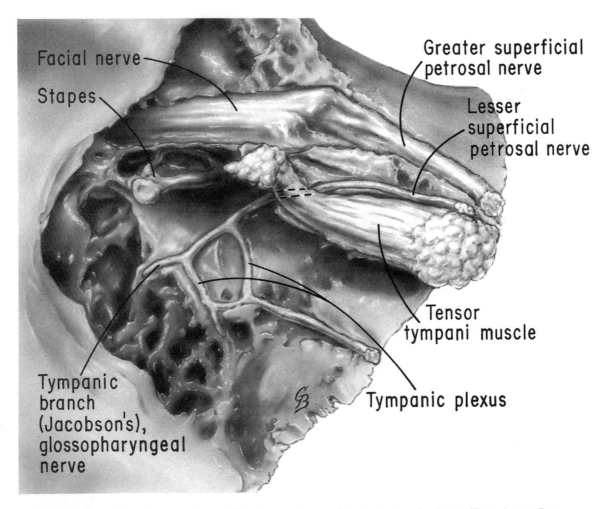

FIG. 52. Formation of the lesser superficial petrosal nerve from the tympanic plexus. (From Anson-Donaldson J, Duckert LG, Lambert PR, Rubel EW, eds. *Surgical anatomy of the temporal bone.* New York: Raven Press, 1992:245, with permission.)

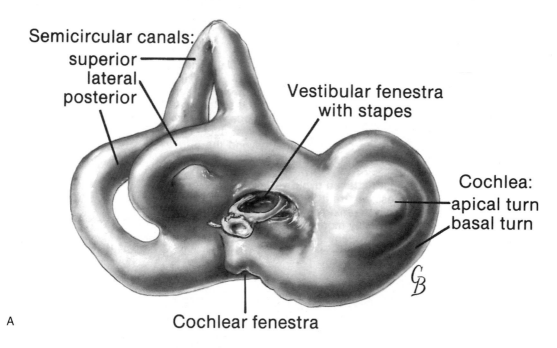

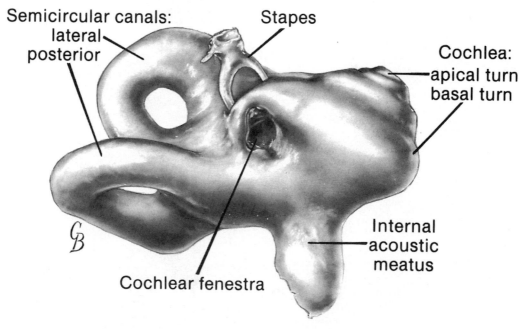

FIG. 53. Lateral **(A)** and inferior **(B)** view of osseous labyrinth. (From Anson-Donaldson J, Duckert LG, Lambert PR, Rubel EW, eds. *Surgical anatomy of the temporal bone.* New York: Raven Press, 1992:272–273, with permission.)

Jacobson's nerve (the tympanic branch of the glossopharyngeal nerve) contains both sensory fibers for the middle ear mucosa, including the eustachian tube, and preganglionic parasympathetic fibers destined for the parotid gland via the otic ganglion. Jacobson's nerve originates from the inferior (petrosal) ganglion of the glossopharyngeal nerve, just after that nerve has exited the skull base. The nerve then turns superiorly to enter the hypotympanum through the inferior tympanic canaliculus, located between the carotid canal and jugular foramen. As the nerve ascends in the middle ear, it lies in a groove or canal on the promontory wall. It is joined by caroticotympanic nerves (from the sympathetic plexus of the internal carotid artery) to form the *tympanic plexus* (Fig. 51). Near the cochleariform process, the tympanic plexus reunites and forms the *lesser superficial petrosal* nerve, which passes beneath the tensor tympani muscle and into the middle cranial fossa (Fig. 52).

Arnold's nerve is a composite structure, formed predominantly by the auricular branch of the vagus nerve with lesser contributions from the glossopharyngeal and facial nerves. The auricular branch of the vagus nerve enters the temporal bone through a small foramen in the jugular fossa, then passes posteriorly to exit the skull through the tympanomastoid fissure or stylomastoid foramen. With contributions from the facial and glossopharyngeal nerves, it provides sensation to the posterior portion of the external canal. The cutaneous vesicles from a herpes zoster infection (Ramsey Hunt syndrome) are thought to result from involvement of the facial nerve fibers in Arnold's nerve.

ANATOMY OF THE INNER EAR

Osseous Labyrinth

The inner ear is a neuromembranous structure contained within the otic capsule in the petrous portion of the temporal bone. The term *labyrinth* refers anatomically to the entire inner ear mechanism and includes two principal portions, the vestibule and semicircular canals superoposteriorly, and the cochlea inferoanteriorly. It is common in clinical practice, however, to use the term "labyrinth" to refer to the vestibular portion of the inner ear.

The bony labyrinth is a complex of interconnected bony cavities filled with *perilymph* and contained within the otic capsule (Fig. 53). Its central opening is the *vestibule*, an ovoid chamber approximately 4 mm in diameter, which connects with the three *semicircular canals* superiorly and posteriorly and the cochlea anteriorly. Along the medial walls of the vestibule are the elliptical recess for the utricle and the spherical recess for the saccule. In the lateral wall of the vestibule is the oval window containing the stapes footplate.

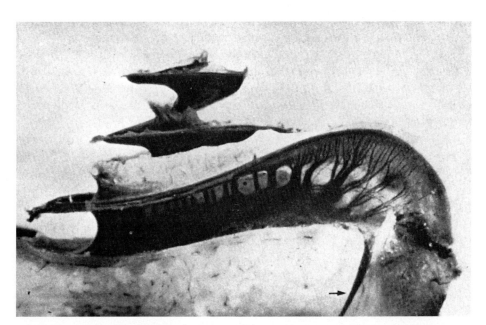

FIG. 54. Adult human cochlea showing modiolus with osseous spiral lamina and myelinated nerve bundles. The bony capsule, spiral ligament, and Reissner's membrane have been removed. The basal end of osseous spiral lamina is set **right**, and the lower basal coil extends to the **left**. Above it, the middle and apical coils are exposed. The cochlear aqueduct is shown lying opened (original magnification × 13). (From Bredberg G. *Acta Otolaryngol* 1968;[Suppl 236]:36, with permission.)

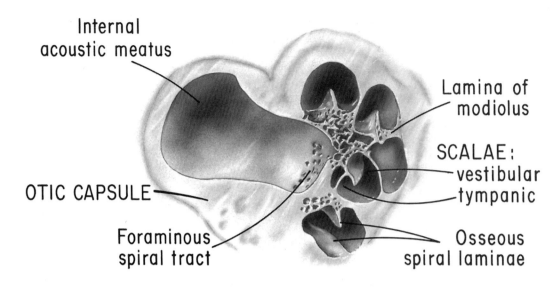

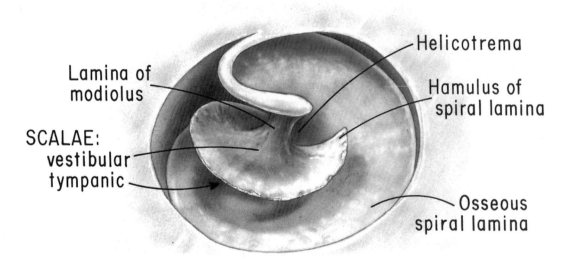

FIG. 55. Schematic diagram of the osseous spiral lamina of the cochlea. (From Anson-Donaldson J, Duckert LG, Lambert PR, Rubel EW, eds. *Surgical anatomy of the temporal bone.* New York: Raven Press, 1992:298, with permission.)

The hollow semicircular canals are arranged in three mutually perpendicular planes: horizontal (lateral), anterior vertical (superior), and posterior vertical (posterior). The lateral semicircular canal makes a 30-degree angle with the horizontal plane. The other two canals, in a position vertical to the horizontal, are orthogonal to each other. The superior canal in one ear is positioned in a plane parallel to the posterior canal contralaterally. These planes of orientation are fundamental to sensing angular acceleration (see Chapter 5). Each canal measures approximately 1 mm in diameter and resembles a semicircular arc with a diameter of about 6.5 mm. The horizontal canal joins the vestibule at each terminal end. The posterior limbs of the two vertical canals join to

form a common duct, the *crus commune*; their anterior limbs have separate openings into the vestibule. Thus, instead of six vestibular communications for the three canals, there are five. Each canal has one sensory organ, the *crista*, in its enlarged vestibular end, termed the *ampulla*.

The superior semicircular canal forms a ridge (*arcuate eminence*) on the floor of the middle cranial fossa. This bony landmark is important when identifying the internal auditory canal through a middle cranial fossa approach. The horizontal semicircular canal projects into the medial wall of the mastoid antrum and is an important landmark in performing most mastoid operations.

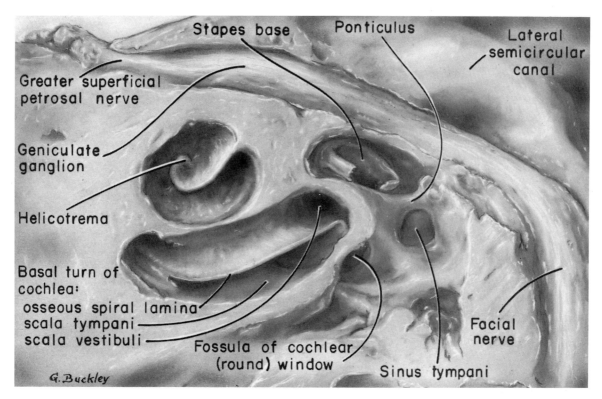

FIG. 56. The osseous spiral lamina in a dissected left temporal bone. (From Anson-Donaldson J, Duckert LG, Lambert PR, Rubel EW, eds. *Surgical anatomy of the temporal bone.* New York: Raven Press, 1992:364, with permission.)

Anteriorly, the vestibule connects with the cochlea. The first (basal) portion of the cochlea, known as the "hook," begins immediately inferior to the vestibule and transverses anteriorly and superiorly. The cochlea is about 31 to 33 mm in length and is rolled into a three-dimensional ascending spiral of 2.5 to 2.75 turns, around the central *modiolus.* These turns become smaller toward the apex, as the cochlear spiral points in an anterolateral direction (Fig. 54). Projecting out from the modious like the threads on a screw is the *osseus spiral lamina.* This thin bony plate partially divides the cochlea into a superior compartment (scala vestibuli) and an inferior compartment (scala tympani) (Figs. 55 and 56).

Membranous Labyrinth

Enclosed within the perilymphatic space of the osseus labyrinth is the endolymphatic system, or membranous labyrinth (Fig. 57), which consists of three main portions: the utricle and semicircular canals, the saccule and cochlear duct, and the endolymphatic duct and sac. Areas of sensory differentiation corresponding to the receptor organs are present in specific locations: the organ of Corti within the cochlear duct, the maculae of the utricle and saccule, and the three cristae of the semicircular canals.

MORPHOLOGY OF THE COCHLEA

A cross section of the cochlea shows that there are three compartments: the superior compartment is the *scala vestibuli,* the inferior is the *scala tympani,* and at the center there is a triangular-shaped cavity, the *cochlear duct,* or *scala media* (Fig. 58). The scala vestibuli tapers as it proceeds from the vestibule at the level of the oval window toward the apex. At the apex, it communicates through the *helicotrema* with the lower channel, the scala tympani, whose other end is at the round window (Fig. 59). Near the round window, the *cochlear aqueduct* connects the scala tympani (perilymphatic fluid) with the subarachnoid space (cerebral spinal fluid). This narrow bony channel averages 10 mm in length, with an internal (cochlear) aperture of 0.1 mm and an external aperture of 0.8 mm. The aqueduct contains a loose network of fibrous or periotic tissue that is continuous with arachnoid tissue from the posterior cranial fossa.

The scala media (Fig. 60) is separated from the scala vestibuli by the thin, obliquely lying, two-cell-layered

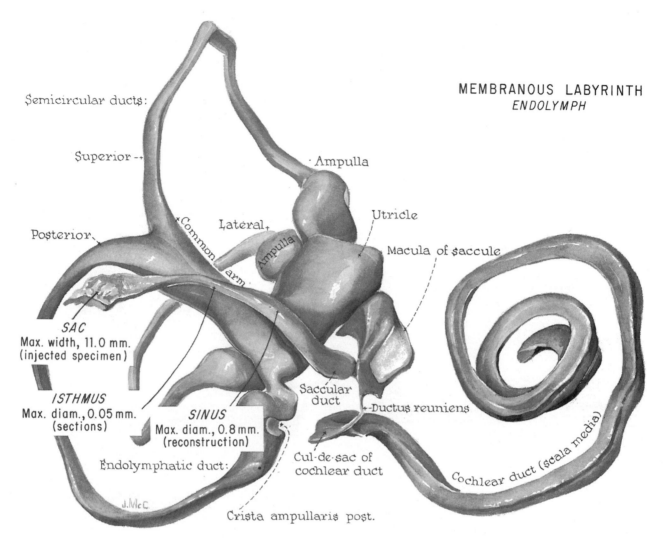

MEMBRANOUS LABYRINTH
ENDOLYMPH

Semicircular ducts:

Superior

Ampulla

Posterior

Lateral

Utricle

Common arm

Ampulla

Macula of saccule

SAC
Max. width, 11.0 mm.
(injected specimen)

ISTHMUS
Max. diam., 0.05 mm.
(sections)

SINUS
Max. diam., 0.8 mm.
(reconstruction)

Saccular
duct

Ductus reuniens

Cul-de-sac of
cochlear duct

Cochlear duct (scala media)

Endolymphatic duct:

J.McC.

Crista ampullaris post.

FIG. 57. The membranous labyrinth, viewed from medial to lateral. (From Anson-Donaldson J, Duckert LG, Lambert PR, Rubel EW, eds. *Surgical anatomy of the temporal bone.* New York: Raven Press, 1992:271, with permission.)

Reissner's membrane. Reissner's membrane extends from the spiral ligament on the external wall of the cochlear duct to the spiral limbus on the osseus spiral lamina. The *basilar membrane* that separates the scala media from the scala tympani is located between a crest in the inner side of the cochlear wall, the osseous spiral lamina, and the crest of the spiral ligament. The inner surface of the spiral ligament is covered by the *stria vascularis*, a three-layer membrane with secretory cells and a rich vascular bed. The basilar membrane averages 31 to 33 mm in length and varies in width from 0.1 mm at the base to 0.5 mm at the apex; it is also thinner at the apex.

The *organ of Corti* contains both sensory cells (inner and outer hair cells) and supporting cells. The approximate 15,500 hair cells are aligned in rows four or five cells deep (Fig. 61). The inner row of 3,500 cells is

anatomically different from the outer rows. A globular type of cell (type I hair cell) characterizes the inner hair cell group; it is separated from the outer hair cell group by a spiral space, Corti's tunnel. The outer hair cells (12,000) are cylindrical (type II cells) and placed in rows of three to four cells each. Several types of supporting cells complete the structure of the organ of Corti, including Deiters' cells, Hensen's cells, pillar cells, and inner and outer sulcus cells (Fig. 62). Hairs or stereocilia (approximately 50 to 150 per outer hair cell and 120 per inner hair cell) protrude from the cuticular plate at the top of each hair cell. A gelatinous *tectorial membrane* rests over the organ of Corti, supported medially at the limbus and laterally to the outer edge of the organ of Corti.

The bipolar *spiral ganglion* cells of the afferent auditory nerve fibers are located in the modiolus in its spiral

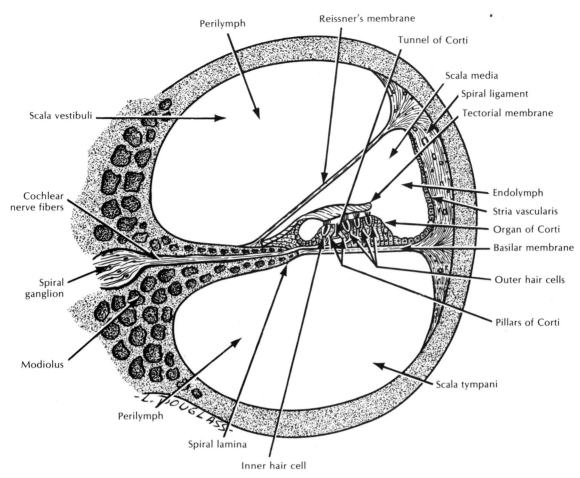

FIG. 58. The three cochlear compartments. (From Honrubia V, Goodhill V. Clinical anatomy and physiology of the peripheral ear. In: Goodhill V, ed. *Ear: diseases, deafness and dizziness.* Hagerstown, MD: Harper & Row, 1979:42, with permission.)

course. The terminal dendrite of each cell enters the cochlea through the habenular opening after traveling in a straight course through Rosenthal's canal (osseus spiral lamina). Next to the spiral ganglion is a group of nerve fibers belonging to the efferent system (*olivocochlear bundle*). These nerves originate in the superior olivary complex of the brainstem and terminate on the hair cells, predominately the outer ones. The afferent and efferent innervation patterns relate to the function of inner and outer hair cells as discussed in Chapter 4.

The cochlear duct ends at the apex in a cul-de-sac, the cupular cecum, and at the base (at the level of the vestibule) in another narrow cul-de-sac, the vestibular cecum. Here there is a communication with the saccule through the narrow, short *ductus reuniens*, thereby establishing continuity between the endolymphatic spaces of the auditory and vestibular systems.

MORPHOLOGY OF THE MEMBRANOUS VESTIBULAR LABYRINTH

The membranous vestibular labyrinth includes two globular cavities within the vestibule, the utricle and the saccule. The *saccule* lies in the medial wall in a spherical recess inferior to the utricle, with which it is in contact but without communication. The saccule communicates with the endolymphatic duct via the saccular duct and with the cochlear duct via the ductus reuniens. The sensory area, macula, contains both type I and type II hair cells and supporting cells. It is hook shaped and lies in a predominantly vertical position. The surface of the macula is covered by the *otolithic membrane*, a structure consisting of a mesh of fibers embedded in a gel made of acid mucopolysaccharides. Contained within this membrane are crystalline deposits called *otoconia*. Oto-

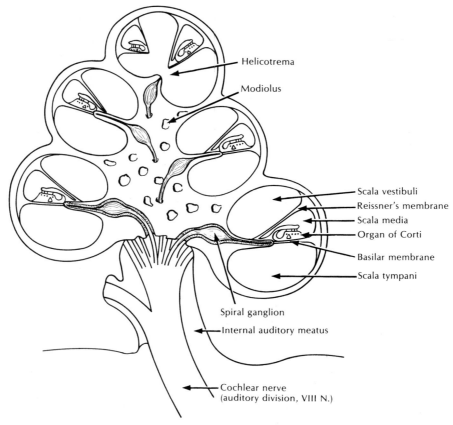

Helicotrema

Modiolus

Scala vestibuli
Reissner's membrane
Scala media
Organ of Corti
Basilar membrane
Scala tympani

Spiral ganglion
Internal auditory meatus

Cochlear nerve
(auditory division, VIII N.)

FIG. 59. Schematic midmodiolar section of the cochlea. (From Honrubia V, Goodhill V. Clinical anatomy and physiology of the peripheral ear. In: Goodhill V, ed. *Ear: diseases, deafness and dizziness.* Hagerstown, MD: Harper & Row, 1979:41, with permission.)

conia range in size from 0.5 to 30 μm, have a density more than twice that of water, and are composed of calcium carbonate.

The *utricle* lies superior to the saccule in the elliptical recess of the vestibule. It is oval in shape and communicates with the membranous semicircular canals via five openings. The macula of the utricle is located next to the anterior opening of the horizontal semicircular canal and lies in a horizontal position. Like the saccular macula, its type I and type II hair cells are embedded in an otoconial membrane. The utricular cavity communicates through the utricular duct with the sinus of the endolymphatic duct.

The *membranous semicircular canals* are three thin tubes (0.4-mm cross-sectional diameter) contained within the bony canals. They occupy eccentric positions within the bony semicircular canals, from which they are restrained by strands of connective tissue. The cavity outside the membranous tube is filled with perilymph whereas the inside contains endolymph, which is continuous with that of the utricle. Next to the anterior opening

of the horizontal and superior canals and to the inferior opening of the posterior canal, each tube enlarges to form an ampulla (Fig. 63). A crestlike septum, the crista, crosses the ampulla in a perpendicular direction to the longitudinal axis of the canal. It rests on the bone of the canal wall and consists of sensory epithelium resting on a mound of connective tissue, traversed by blood vessels and nerve fibers. On the surface of the crista are located the hair cells (type I and type II) with their cilia protruding into the endolymphatic space. A gelatinous mass, the *cupula*, of the same composition as the otolithic membrane, extends from the ceiling of the ampulla to the surface of the crista, making what appears to be a watertight seal (Fig. 64).

MORPHOLOGY OF THE ENDOLYMPHATIC DUCT AND SAC

The endolymphatic duct lies within a bony canal, the *vestibular aqueduct*. The utricular duct from the utricle and the saccular duct from the saccule combine in the

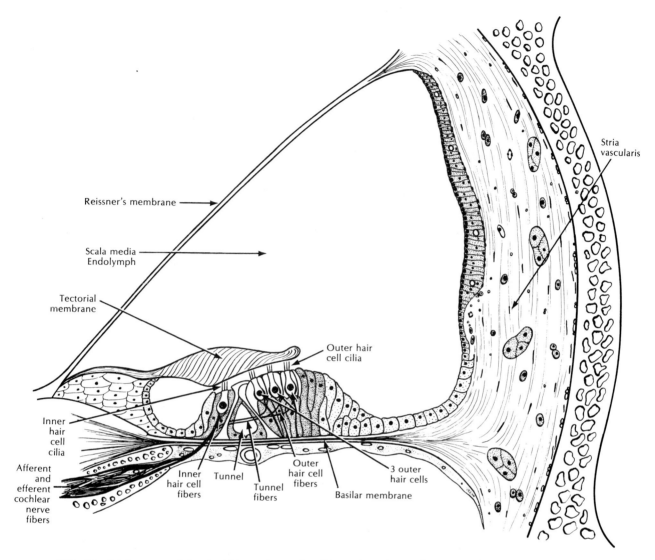

Reissner's membrane

Scala media
Endolymph

Tectorial
membrane

Stria
vascularis

Outer hair
cell cilia

Inner
hair
cell
cilia

Afferent
and
efferent
cochlear
nerve
fibers

Inner
hair cell
fibers

Tunnel

Tunnel
fibers

Outer
hair cell
fibers

3 outer
hair cells

Basilar membrane

FIG. 60. Adult organ of Corti within scala media. (From Honrubia V, Goodhill V. Clinical anatomy and physiology of the peripheral ear. In: Goodhill V, ed. *Ear: diseases, deafness and dizziness.* Hagerstown, MD: Harper & Row, 1979:43, with permission.)

vestibule to form the proximal portion of the endo-lymphatic duct (Fig. 65). The duct parallels and lies medial to the common crus, then makes a 30- to 60-degree turn posteriorly and inferiorly as it courses to the posterior surface of the petrous bone (Fig. 66). This proximal portion of the duct is somewhat expanded and is termed the sinus. As the vestibular aqueduct turns inferiorly, it narrows into an isthmus. The duct once again widens into its terminal enlargement called the *endolymphatic sac*. The proximal part of the sac lies within the bone, whereas the more distal portion is located within layers of the dura. The mid portion of the sac appears to be the most highly differentiated part, characterized by an irregular lumen with a series of interconnected channels. The endolymphatic sac is a

macroscopic structure of varying size, but it may have a width of up to 1 cm.

BLOOD SUPPLY OF THE INNER EAR

The vascularization of the inner ear is independent from that of the otic capsule and tympanic cavity. The *labyrinthine artery*, which supplies the membranous labyrinth and nerve structures, originates intracranially from the anterior inferior cerebellar artery, and in some cases from the basilar artery. As it enters the internal auditory meatus, it begins to branch out, supplying the ganglion cells, nerves, dura, and arachnoidal membranes. Shortly after entering the canal, the labyrinthine artery divides into two main branches: the *common cochlear*

(text continues on page 62)

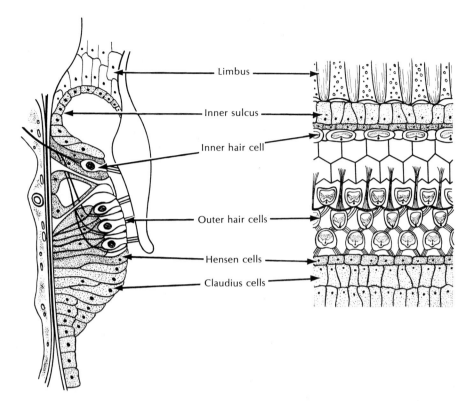

FIG. 61. Schematic correlation between light and transmission electron microscopic details of the organ of Corti. (From Honrubia V, Goodhill V. Clinical anatomy and physiology of the peripheral ear. In: Goodhill V, ed. *Ear: diseases, deafness and dizziness.* Hagerstown, MD: Harper & Row, 1979:44, with permission.)

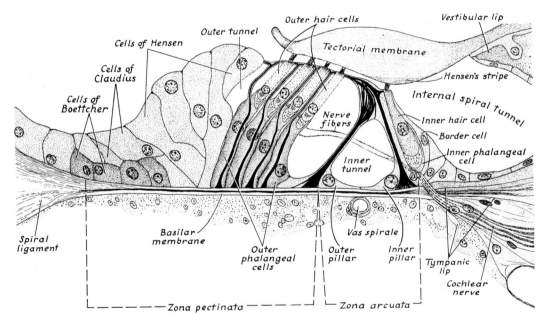

FIG. 62. The organ of Corti. (From Anson-Donaldson J, Duckert LG, Lambert PR, Rubel EW, eds. *Surgical anatomy of the temporal bone.* New York: Raven Press, 1992:300, with permission.)

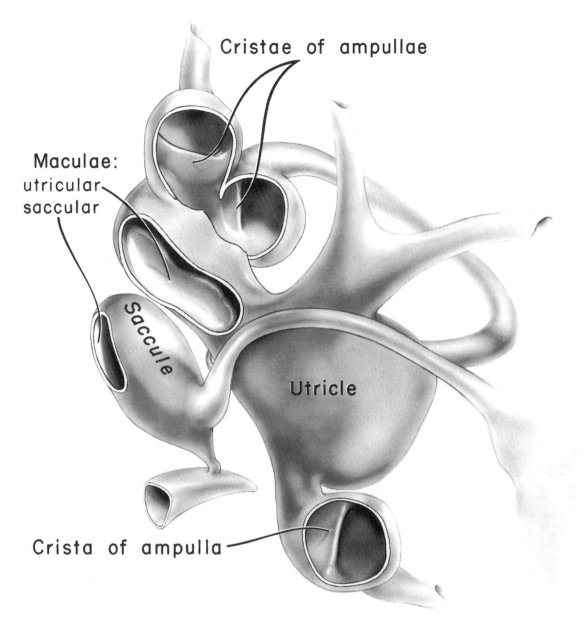

Cristae of ampullae

Maculae:
utricular
saccular

Saccule

Utricle

Crista of ampulla

FIG. 63. Ampullae of the semicircular canals. (From Anson-Donaldson J, Duckert LG, Lambert PR, Rubel EW, eds. *Surgical anatomy of the temporal bone.* New York: Raven Press, 1992:312, with permission.)

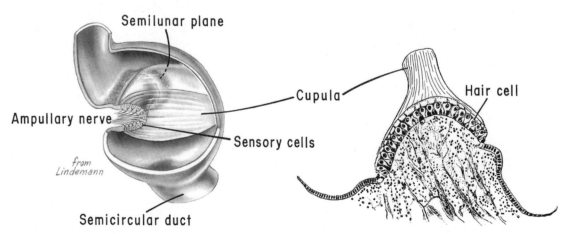

Semilunar plane

Cupula

Hair cell

Ampullary nerve

Sensory cells

from Lindemann

Semicircular duct

FIG. 64. Ampulla with contained crista and cupula. (From Anson-Donaldson J, Duckert LG, Lambert PR, Rubel EW, eds. *Surgical anatomy of the temporal bone.* New York: Raven Press, 1992:312, with permission.)

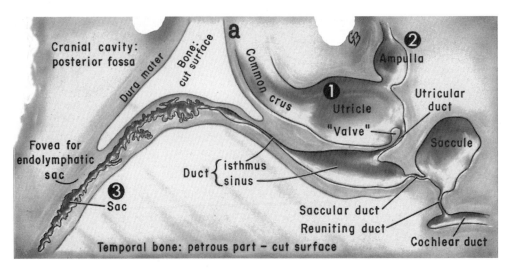

FIG. 65. Utricular and saccular ducts combining to form the endolymphatic duct. (From Anson-Donaldson J, Duckert LG, Lambert PR, Rubel EW, eds. *Surgical anatomy of the temporal bone.* New York: Raven Press, 1992:264, with permission.)

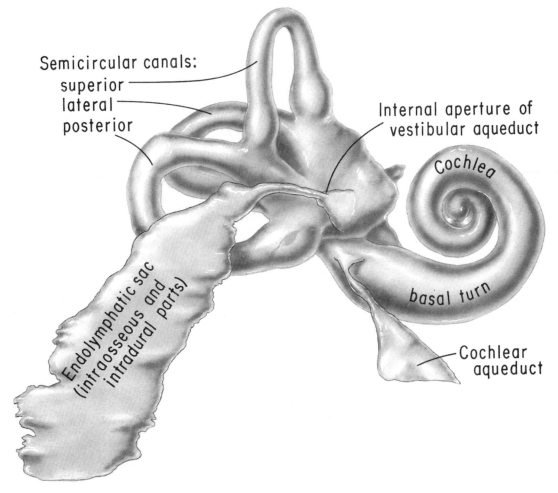

FIG. 66. Endolymphatic duct and sac in an adult. (From Anson-Donaldson J, Duckert LG, Lambert PR, Rubel EW, eds. *Surgical anatomy of the temporal bone.* New York: Raven Press, 1992:96, with permission.)

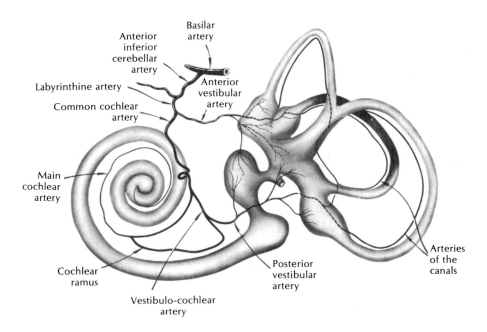

FIG. 67. Diagram of arterial system of mammalian membranous labyrinth. (From Schuknecht HF. *Pathology of the ear.* Cambridge: Harvard University Press, 1974:62, with permission.)

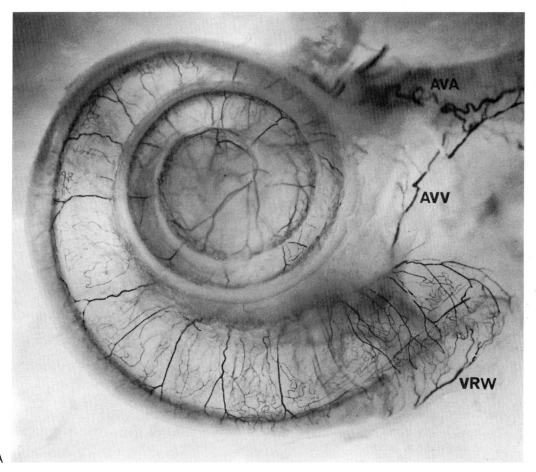

A

FIG. 68. A: Vascular pattern in scala vestibuli showing radiating arterioles from the anterior vestibular artery (AVA). AVV, anterior vestibular vein; VRW, vein of round window. *Continued.*

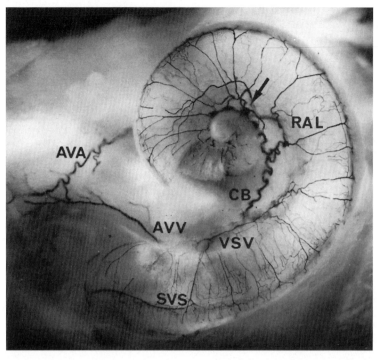

FIG. 68. *Continued.* **B:** Arterial supply to basal turn of cochlea from the main cochlear branch (CB) and spiral modiolar artery *(arrow).* RAL, radiating arterioles; SVS, vessels of stria vascularis; VSV, vein of scala vestibuli. (From Anson-Donaldson J, Duckert LG, Lambert PR, Rubel EW, eds. *Surgical anatomy of the temporal bone.* New York: Raven Press, 1992:497, with permission.)

artery and the *anterior vestibular artery* (Fig. 67). These arteries course independently within the canal. Therefore, it is possible for arteriolar occlusions to produce ischemic damage to segmental portions of the inner ear.

The common cochlear artery divides into two branches, the main cochlear artery and the vestibulocochlear artery. The main cochlear branch enters the central canal of the modiolus and gives off radiating arterioles, forming several plexuses supplying approximately 80% of the cochlea, including the spiral ganglion, the structures of the basilar membrane, and the stria vascularis (Fig. 68). The vestibulocochlear branch supplies the basal 20% of the cochlea (via the cochlear ramus) and gives rise to the posterior vestibular artery. The capillaries in the stria vascularis constitute a serpentine meshwork of interconnected vessels. The posterior vestibular artery supplies the macula of the saccule and the crista of the posterior semicircular canal. The anterior vestibular artery provides circulation to the macula of the utricle and to the cristae of the superior and horizontal semicircular canals.

Blood from the cochlea drains through the *common modiolar vein*. The anterior vestibular vein drains blood from the cristae of the superior and horizontal canals and from the utricle. The posterior vestibular vein drains blood from the saccule and crista of the posterior canal (and from a small portion of the cochlea). These two vestibular veins join to become the vestibulocochlear vein, which then combines with the common modiolar vein to form the *vein in the cochlear aqueduct,* which

drains into the *inferior petrosal sinus.* Blood from the semicircular canals also passes toward the vestibular aqueduct in a vein that accompanies the endolymphatic duct and drains into the lateral venous sinus (Fig. 69).

INNERVATION OF THE INNER EAR

The cochlea and vestibular organs are provided with afferent and efferent innervation. An autonomic system associated with the inner ear vasculature is also recognized.

Auditory System

Afferent innervation of the cochlear receptors is provided by bipolar cells from the *spiral ganglion of Corti.* There are approximately 32,000 to 35,000 spiral ganglion cells, and two types have been identified. The type I neurons comprise 95% of the total population and innervate inner hair cells. Type II spiral ganglion cells synapse with the outer hair cells and constitute about 5% of the total number of cochlear neurons. Each inner ear hair cell is innervated by 10 to 20 type I neurons, whereas ten outer hairs cells receive a single fiber from a type II spiral ganglion cell (Fig. 70).

To some degree, the tonotopic map of the cochlea and the spatial arrangement of the spiral ganglion cells are maintained in the auditory nerve and cochlear nucleus of the brainstem. The afferent fibers from the base of the cochlea, encoding high-frequency sounds, are located peripherally within the nerve trunk, whereas apical fibers

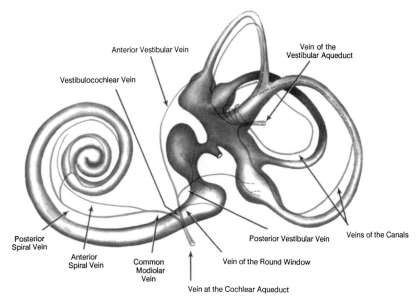

FIG. 69. Veins of the inner ear. (From Schuknecht HF. *Pathology of the ear,* 2nd ed. Philadelphia: Lea & Febiger, 1993:65, with permission.)

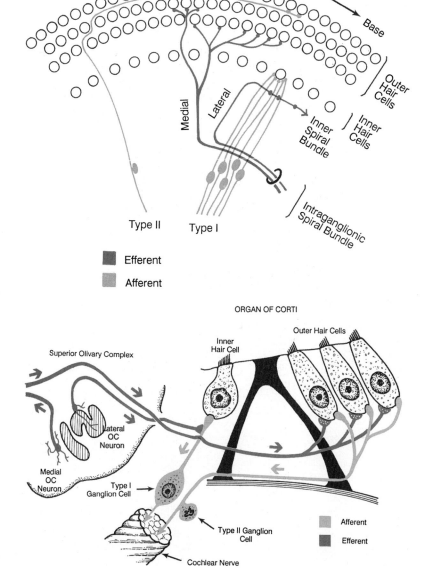

FIG. 70. Afferent and efferent innervation of the organ of Corti. (From Schuknecht HF. *Pathology of the ear,* 2nd ed. Philadelphia: Lea & Febiger, 1993:67, with permission.)

encoding low-frequency sounds are located in the central region. The major projection of the afferent nerve fibers is to the ventral cochlear nucleus (2).

In addition to afferent innervation, the hair cells of the cochlea also receive the *olivocochlear bundle* (3). This bundle originates in the superior olivary complex of the brainstem and contains approximately 500 to 600 fibers. As the olivocochlear bundle exits the brainstem beneath the cochlear nucleus, it travels with the inferior division of the vestibular nerve. Within the internal auditory canal, this bundle leaves the vestibular nerve and crosses to the cochlear nerve via the *vestibulo-cochlear anastomosis* (bundle of Oort) (Fig. 71). Most of these efferent nerve fibers terminate on the outer hair cells. Some do terminate on afferent nerve fibers of inner hair cells, but none on the body of the inner hair cell. The original group of efferent fibers ramify extensively, increasing their number many-fold. There is an average of three to four efferent nerve endings per outer hair cell (4).

Vestibular System

Afferent innervation of the vestibular organ is provided by bipolar ganglion cells (*Scarpa's ganglion*) located in the lateral end of the internal auditory canal. The superior cell group (superior division of the vestibular nerve) innervates the cristae of the superior and lateral canals and the macula of the utricle. The macula of the saccule and the crista of the posterior canal are supplied by the inferior cell group comprising the inferior vestibular nerve. (The singular nerve is the branch from the inferior vestibular nerve innervating the posterior canal). There are approximately 20,000 vestibular ganglion cells, which give rise to both large and small nerve fibers. The fibers with the largest diameter are found predominantly at the crest or center of the cristae and on the macular striola innervating type I hair cells with large chalicetype endings. The small-diameter fibers make contact with type II hair cells (5,6).

There is also an *efferent vestibular system* composed of 200 to 300 fibers that course together with efferents for the cochlear system in the internal auditory canal. All of the cristae and maculae receive efferent innervation, with boutontype synapses on hair cells and afferent nerve fibers. The efferent fibers originate from neurons located ventromedial to the lateral vestibular nuclei; each labyrinth receives equal efferent input from both sides of the brainstem (7).

On entering the brainstem with the cochlear nerve at the level of the cerebellopontine angle, the vestibular nerve divides into ascending and descending branches that make synaptic contacts with neurons of the various vestibular nuclei. Some of the fibers also send terminals to the cerebellum. No synaptic contact from primary vestibular fibers have been described with the neurons of the reticular substance or with the vestibular nuclei of the opposite side. The central projections of both the auditory and vestibular systems are discussed in Chapter 6.

Autonomic Innervation

Although the presence of an integral autonomic nerve supply to the auditory and vestibular organs is assumed, only the *sympathetic* (adrenergic) system has been demonstrated to date (8). Two types of adrenergic innervation have been found in the cochlea. The first (perivas-

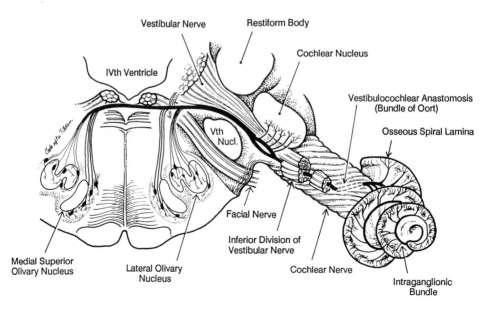

FIG. 71. The olivocochlear bundle (efferent auditory nerve fibers). (From Schuknecht HF. *Pathology of the ear,* 2nd ed. Philadelphia: Lea & Febiger, 1993:70, with permission.)

cular plexus) originates from the stellate ganglion and follows the plexus surrounding the anterior cerebellar and labyrinthine arteries into the greater modiolar artery but not beyond the osseous spiral lamina and the membranous labyrinth. The second (independent plexus) originates from the superior cervical ganglion and travels within the peripheral zone of the osseous spiral lamina. These adrenergic fibers are present in all turns of the cochlea, but apparently they are absent in the spiral ligament and stria vascularis.

A similar dual system is present in the vestibular organ, with adrenergic fibers following the blood vessels or independently reaching the undersurface of the sensory epithelium. They appear to have the same origin as the cochlear system and, similarly, their functional role is yet to be clarified (9).

SUMMARY POINTS

- By 25 weeks of development, the cochlea has grown to two and one-half turns and appears adultlike. The cochlea duct is probably functional, at least in the basal regions, as sensory development proceeds from the basal turn apically.
- The vestibular aqueduct is a bony canal containing the endolymphatic duct, which courses from the utricle and saccule to the endolymphatic sac located within layers of the posterior fossa dura. An enlarged vestibular aqueduct is a common congenital temporal bone anomaly associated with hearing loss.
- The petrous apex air cell system remains open and aerated in only 30% of adult temporal bones. As a consequence, infection in this area often presents as osteomyelitis rather than coalescence of infected air cells, as typically seen in the mastoid.
- At birth the mastoid tip is poorly developed and the stylomastoid foramen is very superficial. This predisposes the facial nerve to trauma during forceps delivery and must be considered during otologic surgery on an infant.
- The anterior epitympanic recess is a consistent, pneumatized space anterior to the head of the malleus. With the malleus present, this recess is difficult to inspect during surgical procedures and, therefore, may hide the presence of cholesteatoma.
- Cholesteatoma may be difficult to remove from the sinus tympani, a variably pneumatized recess located in the posterior wall of the mesotympanum. This recess is bounded laterally by the mastoid segment of the facial nerve.
- The carotid canal forms the anterior boundary of the tympanic cavity. It lies just anterior to the cochlea and medial to the osseous portion of the eustachian tube.
- Arnold's nerve is formed predominantly by the auricular branch of the vagus nerve, with lesser contributions from the glossopharyngeal and facial nerves. It provides sensation to the posterior portion of the external canal. The cutaneous vesicles from a herpes zoster infection are thought to result from involvement of the facial nerve fibers in Arnold's nerve.
- The superior semicircular canal forms a ridge (arcuate eminence) on the floor of the middle cranial fossa surgery. The horizontal semicircular canal projects into the mastoid antrum and is an important landmark in mastoid surgery.
- The labyrinthine artery provides the blood supply to the vestibular and cochlear portions of the inner ear. This artery usually originates intracranially from the anterior inferior cerebellar artery, but in some cases can arise directly from the basilar artery. Within the internal auditory canal the artery divides into a cochlear and vestibular branch; therefore, it is possible for an arteriolar occlusion to produce ischemic damage to segmental portions of the inner ear.

REFERENCES

1. Canalis RF. Valsalva's contribution to otology. *Am J Otolaryngol* 1990;11:420–427.
2. Lorente de No R. The sensory endings in the cochlea. *Laryngoscope* 1937;47:373–377.
3. Rasmussen G. Anatomic relationships of the ascending and descending auditory systems. In: Fields W, Alford B, eds. *Neurological aspects of auditory and vestibular disorders.* Springfield, IL: Charles C. Thomas Publishers, 1964:5–19.
4. Galambos R. Suppression of auditory nerve activity by stimulation of efferent fibers to the cochlea. *J Neurophysiol* 1956;19:424–437.
5. Gacek R. The innervation of the vestibular labyrinth. *Ann Otol Rhinol Laryngol* 1968;77:676–685.
6. Lorente de No R. Etudes sur l'anatomie et la physiologie du labyrinth del'oreille et du VIII nerf deuxieme partie. Quelques donnees au sujet de l'anatomie des organes sensoriels du labyrinth. *Trav Lab Rech Biol Univ Madrid* 1926;24:53.
7. Gacek R. Efferent component of the vestibular nerve. In: Rasmussen G, Windle W, eds. *Neural mechanisms of the auditory and vestibular systems.* Springfield, IL: Charles C. Thomas Publishers, 1960.
8. Spoendlin H, Lichtenstein W. The adrenergic innervation of the labyrinth. *Acta Otolaryngol (Stockh)* 1966;6:423–434.
9. Spoendlin H, Lichtenstein W. The sympathetic nerve supply of the inner ear. *Arch Klin Exp Ohr Nas Hehlk Heilk* 1967;189:246–266.

The Ear: Comprehensive Otology,
edited by R. F. Canalis and P. R. Lambert.
Lippincott Williams & Wilkins, Philadelphia © 2000.

CHAPTER 3

Temporal Bone Histology and Histopathology

A. Julianna Gulya

The purpose of this chapter is to provide a foundation of knowledge in the histology and histopathology of the temporal bone. Fascinating as such topics are in and of themselves, their relevance to the otologist lies in their ability to facilitate the understanding of diseases and disorders of, as well as surgical approaches to, the temporal bone.

Clearly, it is beyond the purview of these few pages to catalog exhaustively each and every feature of the normal and abnormal temporal bone, and only cameos of critical features are addressed in this chapter. For in-depth pursuit of particular topics of anatomic interest the reader is referred to *Anatomy of the Temporal Bone with Surgical Implications* (1) or *Surgical Anatomy of the Temporal Bone* (2). Pathology of the temporal bone is reviewed in *Pathology of the Ear* (3), *An Atlas of the Micropathology of the Temporal Bone* (4), and *Pathology of the Ear and Temporal Bone* (5).

HISTORY

Histopathologic examination of the temporal bone, characterized by light microscopic evaluation of serially

sectioned specimens, has been possible for well in excess of 100 years and has a recognized importance in improving our understanding of diseases and disorders of the temporal bone. The first temporal bone collections were established in Germany by Manasse and Wittmaak and in Switzerland by Nager (3). In the United States, initial collections were created by Guild in Baltimore, Lindsay in Chicago, and Anson and Bast, also in Chicago (3). In 1960, The Deafness Research Foundation developed the National Temporal Bone Banks program to encourage temporal bone donation and research (6); however, by the 1980s a number of factors contributed to an apparent waning of interest in such endeavors. To some extent, perhaps, the utility of the light microscopic examination had been exhausted, and even though electron microscopic examination enabled more detailed temporal bone study, the rigorous requirements of early postmortem harvesting and preparation rendered this modality impractical for routine use. More likely, though, the expense of the labor-intensive preparation process, coupled with the cost of storage, dominated in diminished enthusiasm. The number of active laboratories decreased and valuable collections were in danger of being lost forever.

In 1992 (7), to combat this trend, the National Institute on Deafness and Other Communication Disorders joined

A. J. Gulya: Department of Surgery (Otolaryngology–Head and Neck Surgery), The George Washington University, Washington DC 20037.

with the Deafness Research Foundation to establish the National Temporal Bone Hearing and Balance Pathology Resource Registry ("the Registry"). The Registry is an extension of the National Temporal Bone Banks Program, the founding mission of which was temporal bone donor enrollment and specimen acquisition, with the additional features of data bases allowing data access to the greater research community and a mechanism for saving "at risk" collections.

Concomitant with the Registry effort is a resurgence of the utility of temporal bone analysis. The human immunodeficiency virus epidemic carries with it a need to better understand, through histopathologic correlation, the effects of the virus on the structures of the ear. Even more exciting, though, is the development of procedures whereby archival temporal bones can be "recycled" for study with molecular biologic and molecular genetic probes (8), as well as with improved electron microscopic techniques (9,10). The development of these procedures has enhanced the value of, and interest in, temporal bone study. Now we are on the threshold to the future, where we have the ability to enhance our understanding of the etiopathogenesis of such disorders as Bell's palsy, otosclerosis, and sudden sensorineural hearing loss.

TEMPORAL BONE HARVESTING AND PREPARATION

As part of its mandate, the Registry has developed a series of instructional materials, including a recent review article (10) and a video tape, to educate individuals unacquainted with the steps involved in temporal bone harvesting. Temporal bone harvesting is only done with appropriate and specific patient and family consent. A prime consideration in the successful acquisition of temporal bone specimens useful for study is careful coordination and planning with the family, primary care physician, otolaryngologist, pathologist and diener, and funeral home director and staff (10).

For light microscopic, histopathologic evaluation, temporal bones should be harvested within 24 hours post mortem; whole-body refrigeration with fixative injection into the external auditory canal and middle ear, or, depending on available facilities, even into the inner ear, can act as temporizing measures if an unavoidable delay in temporal bone harvesting is anticipated. The window of opportunity for harvesting a specimen useful for electron microscopic study is even more restricted.

A variety of techniques can be used to actually remove the temporal bone. The selection depends on expertise, the anticipated temporal bone pathology, equipment available, and family member wishes (11). An oscillating saw with a plug cutter attachment expedites the preferred intracranial approach to temporal bone removal, which also allows for concomitant extraction of associated central nervous system structures. If the area of anticipated pathologic interest is beyond the perimeter of the plug cutter, for example, in a patient with a cochlear implant, then the "block method," in which a trapezoidal block encompassing the temporal bone is outlined with an oscillating saw, should be used.

An extracranial approach to temporal bone removal is used when a head autopsy will not be performed. Following a postauricular incision, the external auditory canal is transected; the temporal bone plug cutter then isolates the temporal bone specimen for removal (11).

Regardless of the approach used, the temporal bone specimen, once extracted, should be immersed immediately into fixative, preferably 10% neutral buffered formalin (11).

Preparation of the temporal bone for standard light microscopic analysis is a lengthy process, requiring several months for completion. For details, the reader should consult *Pathology of the Ear* (3), as only a capsule summary of the process is presented here.

Initial fixation of the temporal bone specimen begins with immersion in fixative solution, either formalin (10% to 20%, neutral, buffered) or Heidenhain-Susa, immediately after harvesting. Formalin is the preferred fixative if both light and electron microscopic study are contemplated, although Heidenhain-Susa tends to provide superior cytologic detail (3).

Decalcification with either trichloracetic acid or disodium ethylenediaminetetraacetate follows and, depending on the solution used, can require up to 6 to 9 months for completion. After neutralization (for the acid process) the temporal bone specimen undergoes dehydration by successive immersions in increasingly concentrated (50% to 100%) alcohol solutions, ending with an ether alcohol solution nearly 2 weeks later.

Over the ensuing 12 weeks, the specimen is embedded in celloidin and then undergoes hardening, an approximately 1-month process. Actual slicing of the temporal bone follows blocking, or positioning on a microtome so that sectioning is done in the appropriate plane—either horizontal or vertical. Sections are 20-μm thick. By convention, every tenth section is stained with hematoxylin and eosin and mounted on standard glass slides. Uniformity of section mounting, facilitated by means of a template, expedites subsequent light microscopic study.

After the finishing steps of coverslipping and labeling, the slides are finally ready for review, nearly 1 year after harvesting.

HORIZONTAL SERIAL SECTIONS

Serial horizontal sections, that is, those that are obtained when the temporal bone is sectioned in a horizontal plane that parallels the cochlear modiolus, are most commonly utilized in ordinary temporal bone analysis, for very practical reasons. With 20-μm sections, some 500 slices are generated from the average human specimen. Staining and mounting every tenth section yields a study set of some 50 slides, which provides a sufficient overview of the external, middle, and inner ear structures for histopathologic study; however, as the plane of sectioning parallels the basal and tegmental aspects of the temporal bone, these areas are not adequately assessed with horizontal sections.

The following series of a horizontally sectioned, right temporal bone proceeds from superior to inferior, and each section is oriented so that the lateral surface of the specimen is at the top of the figure, anterior is on the left, posterior is on the right, and the posterior cranial fossa surface is inferior.

Figure 1 is a section through the superior semicircular canal, the ampullated end of which is located lateral to the smaller, nonampullated end; the dense bone surrounding the inner ear organs is evident. The ampullated end of the lateral (or horizontal) semicircular canal is posterior to the ampullated end of the superior canal, and the bulge of the lateral canal constricts the passageway (the aditus ad antrum) from the epitympanum anteriorly to the antrum and mastoid posteriorly. The head of the malleus and the body of the incus figure prominently in the epitympanum. Anterior to the ossicles is the anterior

epitympanic recess, which at this level of sectioning appears separate from the epitympanum. The anterior epitympanic recess is an important consideration in surgery for chronic otitis media and cholesteatoma, as disease can remain concealed and escape extirpation; the head of the malleus and the body of the incus must be removed to visualize this area adequately. The superior aspect of the geniculate ganglion of the facial nerve is anteriorly located and is dehiscent in the floor of the middle cranial fossa; in the course of middle cranial fossa approaches to the internal auditory canal, dural elevation should proceed from posterior to anterior to avoid injury to the potentially exposed geniculate ganglion and the associated greater superficial petrosal nerve.

Figure 2 is approximately 3 mm inferior, with the internal auditory canal and its nerve bundle visible medially and the external auditory canal seen laterally. The cochlea is emerging from the dense petrous bone anteriorly, with its basal and middle turns apparent. The macula of the utricle is seen in the vestibule, posterior to the internal auditory canal. The posterior semicircular canal, paralleling the posterior cranial fossa surface of the temporal bone, is paralleled by the nonampullated end of the lateral semicircular canal.

The facial nerve is seen in its horizontal segment, crossing the surgical floor of the middle ear, accompa-

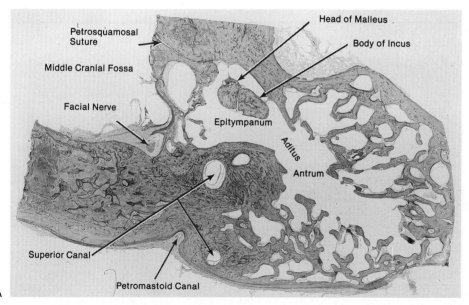

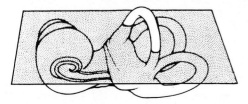

FIG. 1. A: Right temporal bone. Horizontal section at the level of the superior semicircular canal. (From Schuknecht HF. *Pathology of the ear.* Cambridge, MA: Harvard University Press, 1974, with permission.) **B:** Schematic diagram of bony labyrinth showing approximate level of sectioning. (From Gulya AJ, Schuknecht HF. *Anatomy of the temporal bone with surgical implications,* 2nd ed. Pearl River, NY: Parthenon Publishing, 1995, with permission.)

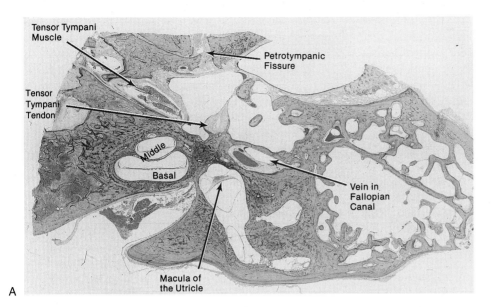

Tensor Tympani Muscle

Tensor Tympani Tendon

Middle

Basal

Petrotympanic Fissure

Vein in Fallopian Canal

Macula of the Utricle

A

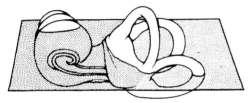

B

FIG. 2. A: Horizontal section inferior to Fig. 1A. (From Schuknecht HF. *Pathology of the ear.* Cambridge, MA: Harvard University Press, 1974, with permission.) **B:** Plane of sectioning. (From Gulya AJ, Schuknecht HF. *Anatomy of the temporal bone with surgical implications,* 2nd ed. Pearl River, NY: Parthenon Publishing, 1995, with permission.)

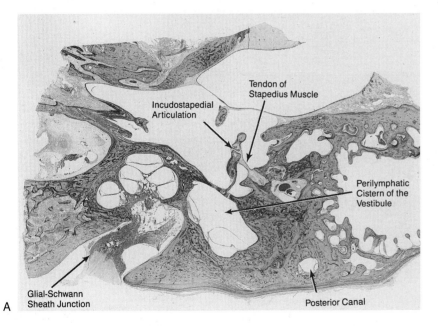

Incudostapedial Articulation

Tendon of Stapedius Muscle

Perilymphatic Cistern of the Vestibule

Glial-Schwann Sheath Junction

Posterior Canal

A

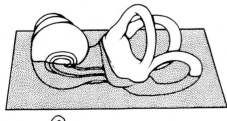

B

FIG. 3. A: Midmodiolar horizontal section. (*From Schuknecht HF. Pathology of the ear.* Cambridge, MA: Harvard University Press, 1974, with permission.) **B:** Plane of sectioning. (From Gulya AJ, Schuknecht HF. *Anatomy of the temporal bone with surgical implications,* 2nd ed. Pearl River, NY: Parthenon Publishing, 1995, with permission.)

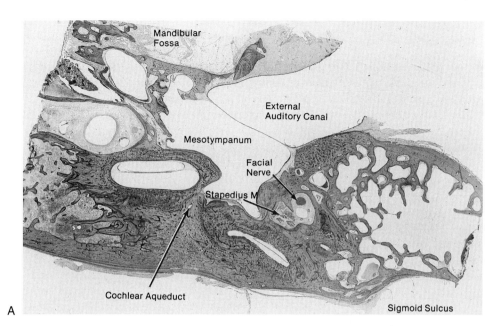

A

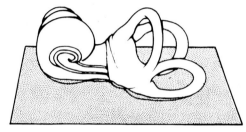

B

FIG. 4. **A:** Horizontal section through the inferior portion of the basal turn of the cochlea. (From Schuknecht HF. *Pathology of the ear.* Cambridge, MA: Harvard University Press, 1974, with permission.) **B:** Plane of sectioning. (From Gulya AJ, Schuknecht HF. *Anatomy of the temporal bone with surgical implications,* 2nd ed. Pearl River, NY: Parthenon Publishing, 1995, with permission.)

nied by a large vein. Just anterior to the facial nerve, the tensor tympani tendon swings around the cochleariform process to attach to the malleus; the chorda tympani nerve is suspended in middle ear mucosa as it passes medial to the malleus and lateral to the long process of the incus. The tympanic membrane is distinguishable at the medial aspect of the external auditory canal. The mastoid is divided into two compartments—a lateral squamous and a medial petrous—by Koerner's septum.

Figure 3 is a midmodiolar section, approximately 1.6 mm inferior to Fig. 2. The cochlear (anterior) and the inferior vestibular (posterior) nerves in the internal auditory canal both demonstrate the staining differential of the glial and Schwann sheaths. The cochlear nerve penetrates the cochlear modiolus to reach the primary auditory neurons in Rosenthal's spiral canal (compare to Fig. 13), whereas the saccular nerve fibers pass through the cribrose area of bone to reach the sensory neuroepithelium of the macula of the saccule. The stapes, with its footplate sealing the vestibule laterally, is tethered by the stapedius tendon emerging from the pyramidal eminence. Posteriorly, the facial nerve is seen in its vertical segment; the air space lateral to the facial nerve and anterior to the mastoid is the facial recess. Anterolateral to the cochlea is the carotid canal, with the internal

carotid artery and its pericarotid sympathetic and venous plexuses. The protympanum opens into the eustachian tube lateral to the internal carotid artery. The angle with which the anterior tympanic membrane meets the external auditory canal (the anterior tympanomeatal angle) is acute; fibrous obliteration (blunting) of this angle with anterior tympanoplasty can cause a conductive hearing loss after an otherwise successful procedure.

Figure 4 is a section through the basal turn of the cochlea, the bulge of which (the promontory) protrudes into the mesotympanum. The inferior aspect of the posterior semicircular canal is medial and posterior, whereas the facial nerve and stapedius muscle are lateral; the tongue of mesotympanum extending between these two structures is the sinus tympani. The sinus tympani demonstrates considerable interindividual variability and, in this case, remains relatively shallow. Its importance lies in its ability to shield cholesteatoma from the surgeon's view, an ability somewhat diminished by modern endoscopes. The mandibular fossa is anterior to the external auditory canal; in anterior canaloplasty, overzealous bone removal can lead to prolapse of the mandibular condyle into the external auditory canal.

VERTICAL SERIAL SECTIONS

Vertical sections, cut parallel to the plane of the cochlear modiolus and perpendicular to the long axis of the petrous pyramid, furnish the capacity to assess both the tegmental and the basal aspects of the temporal bone as well as the remaining structures of the ear; however, vertical sections are not used routinely in preparing human specimens for analysis. With vertical sectioning, the typical human temporal bone yields 800, 20-μm-thick sections. Staining and mounting every tenth section results in an 80-slide study set. Clearly, this endeavor is more laborious and hence more costly than the production of a horizontally sectioned study set. Nonetheless, for basal lesions such as glomus jugulare tumors or in the setting of tegmental disruption, as with cholesteatoma, vertical sectioning is preferable despite the expense.

Figures 5–8 are photomicrographs of a vertically sectioned, right temporal bone. The sections are arranged so that the series proceeds from posterolateral to anteromedial. Each section is oriented so that the tegmen is at the top of the figure, inferior is at the bottom, the posterior fossa surface is on the left, and the lateral aspect is on the right.

In Fig. 5, the most posterolateral of the series, the facial nerve is visualized ascending in its vertical seg-ment from the stylomastoid foramen to the external genu, just inferior to the lateral semicircular canal. Lateral to the facial nerve is an air cell of the facial recess, and even more laterally is the chorda tympani nerve near its posterior iter. The short process of the incus, which is the superior limit of the facial recess, is seen in the epitympanum. The posterior semicircular canal lies medial to the lateral semicircular canal and is bisected by the plane of sectioning, with the ampullated end located inferiorly. Extending the plane of the lateral semicircular canal through the posterior canal leads to the operculum and the intraosseous part of the endolymphatic sac; this relationship describes a landmark used in endolymphatic sac surgery known as Donaldson's line.

Figure 6 is 4.5 mm anteromedial to Fig. 5. The facial nerve is superior and medial to the cochleariform process and the tensor tympani tendon. This anatomic relationship is surgically important, especially in revision chronic ear cases in which alternative landmarks for locating the facial nerve are obscured by disease or eliminated by previous surgery. Jacobson's nerve, the tympanic branch of the glossopharyngeal nerve, is seen ascending the promontory. The horizontal orientation of the utricular macula in the vestibule can be appreciated, as can the origin of the endolymphatic duct from the medial aspect of the vestibule.

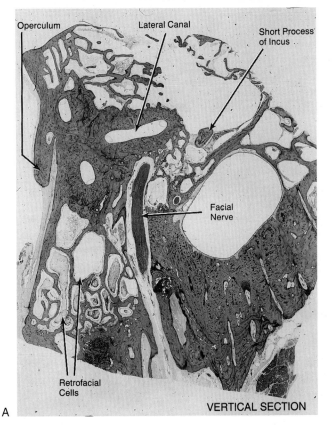

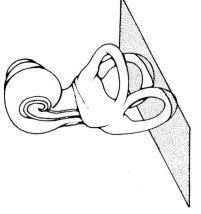

FIG. 5. A: Right temporal bone. Vertical section at the level of the vertical segment of the fallopian canal. B: Schematic diagram of the plane of sectioning. (From Gulya AJ, Schuknecht HF. *Anatomy of the temporal bone with surgical implications,* 2nd ed. Pearl River, NY: Parthenon Publishing, 1995, with permission.)

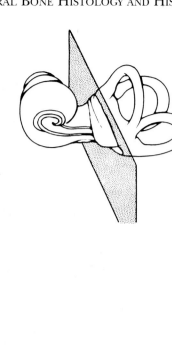

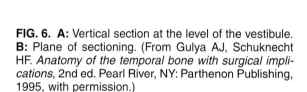

FIG. 6. A: Vertical section at the level of the vestibule. **B:** Plane of sectioning. (From Gulya AJ, Schuknecht HF. *Anatomy of the temporal bone with surgical implications,* 2nd ed. Pearl River, NY: Parthenon Publishing, 1995, with permission.)

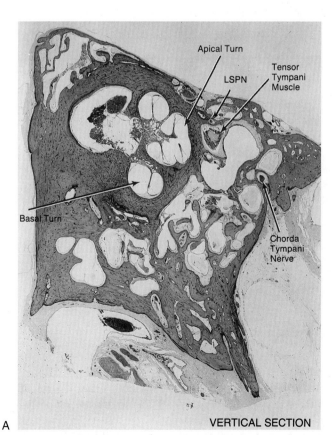

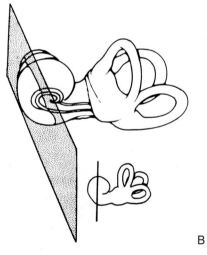

FIG. 7. A: Midmodiolar vertical section. **B:** Plane of sectioning. (From Gulya AJ, Schuknecht HF. *Anatomy of the temporal bone with surgical implications,* 2nd ed. Pearl River, NY: Parthenon Publishing, 1995, with permission.)

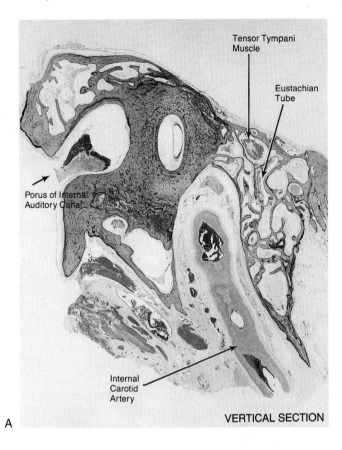

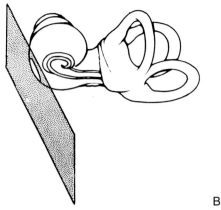

FIG. 8. A: Section at the anterior portion of the basal turn of the cochlea. **B:** Plane of sectioning. (From Gulya AJ, Schuknecht HF. *Anatomy of the temporal bone with surgical implications,* 2nd ed. Pearl River, NY: Parthenon Publishing, 1995, with permission.)

Figure 7 is a midmodiolar section and the helicotrema (the point of open communication between the perilymph of the scala tympani and the scala vestibuli) is seen in the apical turn of the cochlea. The jugular bulb emerges at the basal aspect of the temporal bone, surmounted by infralabyrinthine air cells. The protympanum has narrowed into the eustachian tube, bordered medially by the tensor tympani muscle in its semicanal. The chorda tympani nerve is in its anterior iter as it exits the temporal bone. Superior to the apical turn of the cochlea is the greater superficial petrosal nerve, which has just left the anterior aspect of the geniculate ganglion.

Figure 8 is the most anteromedial figure of the series. Only the basal turn of the cochlea remains in the plane of sectioning. The relationship of the internal carotid artery to both the cochlea and the eustachian tube is particularly well demonstrated in this section. Cochlear "drillout" procedures for electrode implantation are limited anteriorly by the proximity of the internal carotid artery to the basal turn of the cochlea.

CLINICALLY SIGNIFICANT ANATOMIC VARIANTS

There are a number of anatomic variants encountered in the human temporal bone that are generally asymptomatic but which may complicate surgical management of concomitant disease or may predispose to the development of disease.

Facial Nerve

Of all the recognized temporal bone anatomic variants, those involving the facial nerve are among the most relevant to the otologist. As already discussed, dehiscences or gaps in the fallopian canal render the facial nerve vulnerable to inadvertent injury by the unwary surgeon. The fallopian canal is most likely to be dehiscent in the region of the oval window (12–15), although the canal also may be dehiscent at the tensor tympani tendon, in the facial recess, in the floor of the middle cranial fossa, and in the medial aspect of the anterior epitympanic recess (1). The facial nerve may even herniate out through the dehiscence (Fig. 9), mimicking a tumor; such masses should not be biopsied, as facial paralysis will result.

Round Window Niche

The round window niche is prone to anatomic variation. As reported by Nomura (16), 70% of temporal bones studied had some sort of membrane covering the round window niche; the majority of membranes were perforated, but complete membranous closure (Fig. 10) was encountered in a substantial proportion of bones studied.

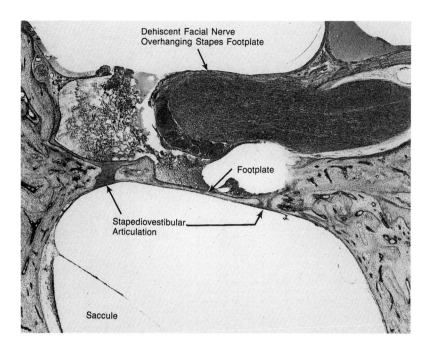

Dehiscent Facial Nerve
Overhanging Stapes Footplate

Footplate

Stapediovestibular
Articulation

Saccule

FIG. 9. Right temporal bone, horizontal section. A dehiscent facial nerve overhangs the stapes footplate. (From Gulya AJ, Schuknecht HF. *Anatomy of the temporal bone with surgical implications,* 2nd ed. Pearl River, NY: Parthenon Publishing, 1995, with permission.)

In exploratory tympanotomy for suspected perilymph fistula at the round window, it is of paramount importance that the operating surgeon confirm identification of the round window membrane, for example, by means of the round window reflex, to avoid "repairing" a perforate membrane overlying the true round window membrane.

Hyrtl's Fissure

Hyrtl's fissure (the tympanomeningeal hiatus) follows a course parallel to the cochlear aqueduct; in the course of normal embryonic development, the hiatus is obliterated, but on occasion it may persist as a result of incomplete ossification to serve as a passage for spontaneous

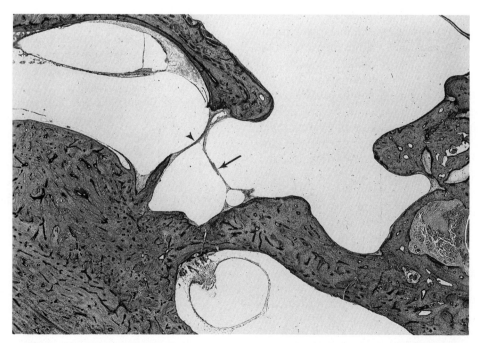

FIG. 10. Right temporal bone, horizontal section. A membranous fold (*arrow*) cloaks the true round window membrane (*arrowhead*). (From Gulya AJ, Schuknecht HF. *Anatomy of the temporal bone with surgical implications,* 2nd ed. Pearl River, NY: Parthenon Publishing, 1995, with permission.)

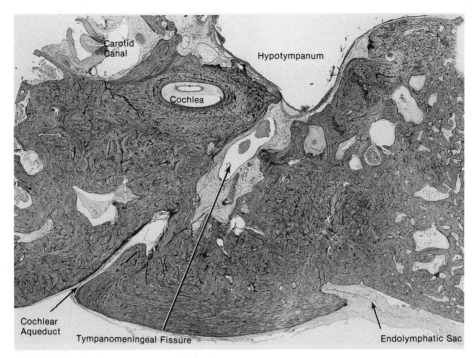

FIG. 11. Right temporal bone, horizontal section. The cochlear aqueduct is paralleled by the persistent tympanomeningeal hiatus. (From Gulya AJ, Schuknecht HF. *Anatomy of the temporal bone with surgical implications,* 2nd ed. Pearl River, NY: Parthenon Publishing, 1995, with permission.)

cerebrospinal fluid leakage from the depths of the round window niche (Fig. 11) (17).

Perilymph Oozers

The cochlear aqueduct extends from the scala tympani of the basal turn of the cochlea to the medial aspect of the jugular fossa. The widely patent cochlear aqueduct, as seen on temporal bone histologic examination (Fig. 12), is thought to be the anatomic basis for the so-called perilymph oozer occasionally encountered in stapedotomy (18). High-resolution temporal bone computerized tomographic scanning is unable to detect all but the most widely patent cochlear aqueducts (larger than 2-mm diameter width throughout) (19).

Perilymph Gusher

The perilymph gusher (18) describes the dramatic outflow of predominantly cerebrospinal fluid (with a few lambda of perilymph) that occasionally occurs with stapedotomy. The histopathologic correlate to this phenomenon is a developmental failure of the formation of the cochlear modiolus (Fig. 13), which results in a wide communication between the subarachnoid space of the internal auditory canal and the scala vestibuli of the basal turn of the cochlea; disruption of the footplate seal over the vestibule allows for the free flow of fluid (18).

Pacchionian Bodies

Arachnoid granulations (Fig. 14), better known as pacchionian bodies (1), comprise multiple arachnoid villi projecting intradurally into the major venous sinuses of the brain. Loose arachnoid tissue, which is a continuation of the subarachnoid space, makes up the core of the villi, thought to resorb cerebrospinal fluid into the intracranial venous system. Where the arachnoid granulations protrude through dura adjacent to bone, including the middle and posterior cranial fossa surfaces of the temporal bone, they create depressions, or foveae granulares. Surgical exposure of such granulations usually does not precipitate a cerebrospinal fluid leak, but those granulations that have eroded bone to enter the mastoid air cell system have been linked to spontaneous, adult-onset fluid (i.e., cerebrospinal fluid) in the tympanomastoid compartment (20). The bony and dural defects associated with arachnoid granulations typically are multiple and can be found at both the posterior and middle cranial fossa surfaces of the human temporal bone.

Jugular Bulb

The jugular bulb normally rests at the basal aspect of the temporal bone, inferior to the infralabyrinthine air cells (Fig. 7). Variants of jugular bulb anatomy exist and

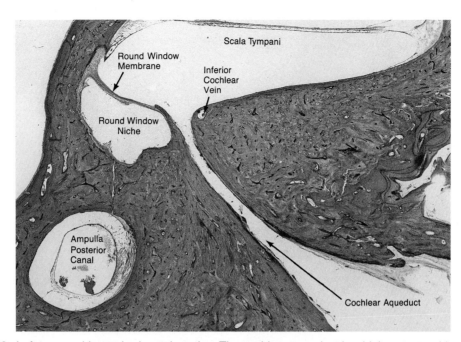

FIG. 12. Left temporal bone, horizontal section. The cochlear aqueduct is widely patent, a histopathologic finding thought to correlate to the "perilymph oozer." There also is a microfissure between the round window niche and the posterior semicircular canal ampulla. This microfissure is uniformly observed in temporal bones from individuals over the age of 6 years and is of no clinical importance. (From Schuknecht HF, Seifi AE. Experimental observations on the fluid physiology of the inner ear. *Ann Otol Rhinol Laryngol* 1963;72:687.)

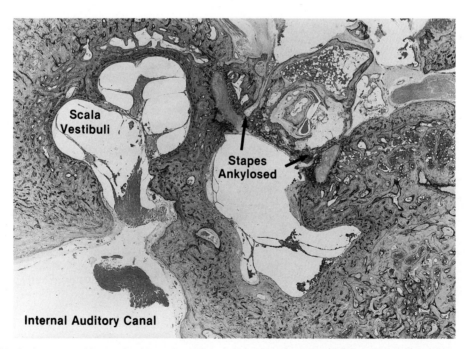

FIG. 13. Left temporal bone, horizontal section. Incomplete formation of the cochlear modiolus allows for wide communication between the basal cochlear turn and the internal auditory canal subarachnoid space. There is congenital stapes fixation as well. (From Shi S-R. Temporal bone findings in a case of otopalatodigital syndrome. *Arch Otolaryngol* 1985;111:120, with permission.)

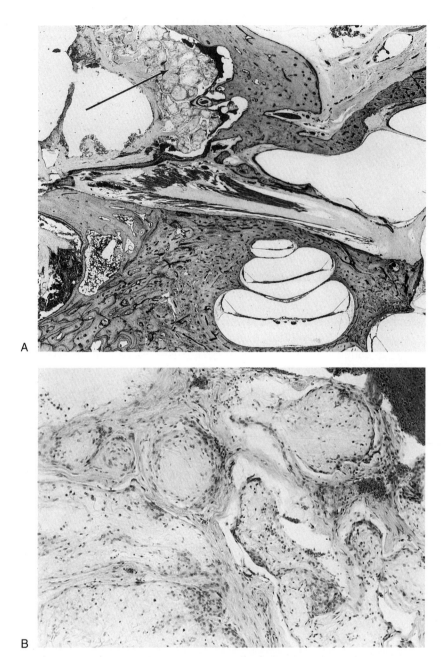

FIG. 14. A: Right temporal bone, horizontal section. Arachnoid granulations at the middle cranial fossa surface (*arrow*). **B:** At higher magnification, the architecture of the arachnoid granulations is evident and consists of a loose arachnoid tissue core surrounded by arachnoid cells and fibrous tissue. (From Gulya AJ, Schuknecht HF. *Anatomy of the temporal bone with surgical implications,* 2nd ed. Pearl River, NY: Parthenon Publishing, 1995, with permission.)

include the high-riding jugular bulb (Fig. 15), the dehiscent jugular bulb, the jugular bulb diverticulum, and the jugular "megabulb" (21). The anomalous jugular bulb in most cases is asymptomatic but may, depending on its size and location, give rise to pulsatile tinnitus (21), conductive hearing loss, and the symptoms of Meniere's disease (22). The high-riding jugular bulb may be confused with a glomus tumor and may complicate tym-

panostomy as well as internal auditory canal tumor removal.

Vascular Loops

An anomaly located within the internal auditory canal is the presence of a vascular loop (Fig. 16), most commonly the anterior inferior cerebellar artery (23); although

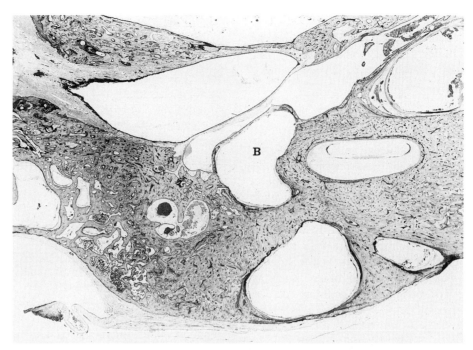

FIG. 15. Left temporal bone, horizontal section. There is a high-riding jugular bulb (*B*) with areas of dehiscence in its bony shell. (From Gulya AJ, Schuknecht HF. *Anatomy of the temporal bone with surgical implications,* 2nd ed. Pearl River, NY: Parthenon Publishing, 1995, with permission.)

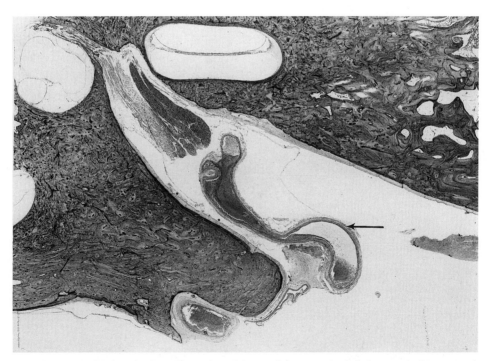

FIG. 16. Left temporal bone, horizontal section. A loop of the anterior inferior cerebellar artery (*arrow*) abuts and enters the internal auditory canal. (From Gulya AJ, Schuknecht HF. *Anatomy of the temporal bone with surgical implications,* 2nd ed. Pearl River, NY: Parthenon Publishing, 1995, with permission.)

nearly 40% of specimens studied (23) had a vessel loop within the internal auditory canal, the precipitation of symptoms such as tinnitus, sensorineural hearing loss, and vertigo by such loops appears to be an exceedingly unusual occurrence (24).

HISTOPATHOLOGIC ENTITIES

Systematic study of the normal temporal bone allows for the development of criteria to distinguish normal anatomic variants from those structural and functional alterations caused by disease processes. The following histopathologic entities have been selected for presentation because of their relevance to the practicing otologist, as well as the ability of the photomicrograph to capture their essence. Accordingly, entities such as exostoses and vestibular schwannomas are illustrated, whereas others, such as depletion of hair cells or spiral ganglion cells, are not.

Exostoses

Exostoses of the external auditory canal (Fig. 17) are bilaterally symmetric, (usually) multiple, bony protuberances. They are believed to result from repetitive refrigeration periostitis, as with, for example, habitually swimming or surfing in cold water. Histopathologically, exostoses have an unique appearance, consisting of lamellae of bone. In contrast, osteomas of the external auditory canal are solitary, unilateral lesions that consist of bony trabeculae with interspersed fibrous tissue.

Tympanic Membrane Perforations

Tympanic membrane perforations (Fig. 18) are readily identified by a loss of continuity of the membrane and medial growth of squamous epithelium. With chronic perforations, there may be medialization of the manubrium as the pull of the tensor tympani tendon overcomes the lateral pull of the tympanic membrane remnant. The resultant middle ear space is contracted, and tympanoplasty in such cases is facilitated by forcible lateralization of the manubrium and, if necessary, sectioning of the tensor tympani tendon.

Chronic Otitis Media

Chronic suppurative otitis media and mastoiditis comprise episodic or incessant purulent otorrhea through a perforated tympanic membrane. Accompanying the malodorous discharge can be conductive hearing loss, sensorineural hearing loss, vertigo, and facial nerve dysfunction, depending on the location and extent of disease.

The pathologic correlates to the clinical manifestations of active chronic otitis media include purulent debris in the tympanomastoid compartment, thickening and polypoid degeneration of the middle ear mucosa, resorptive osteitis of the ossicles, labyrinthine fistulization, cholesteatoma, and cholesterol granuloma (3) within the temporal bone. Central nervous system complications stemming from extratemporal spread of chronic otitis media encompass meningitis, abscess formation, and otitic hydrocephalus.

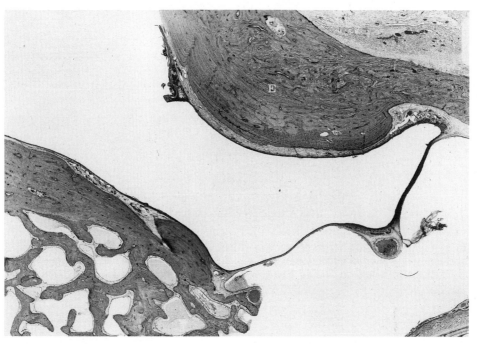

FIG. 17. Left temporal bone, horizontal section. There is a broad-based, anterior canal wall exostosis (*E*). (From Schuknecht HF. *Pathology of the ear.* Cambridge, MA: Harvard University Press, 1974, with permission.)

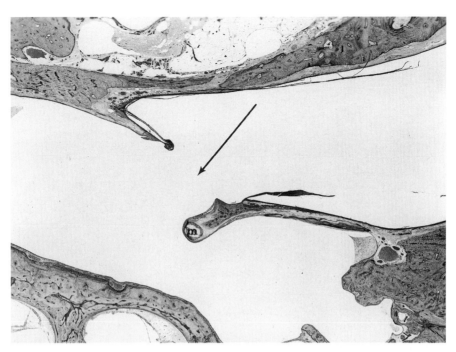

FIG. 18. Right temporal bone, horizontal section. There is an anterior, central tympanic membrane perforation (*arrow*). The manubrium (*m*) is medially displaced.

The sequelae of "chronic healed otitis media and mastoiditis" (3), i.e., spontaneously resolved infection, are less commonly detailed and include such entities as tympanic membrane retraction pockets, dormant middle ear polyps, epidermization, fibrocystic sclerosis, and new bone formation (Fig. 19).

Otosclerosis

Otosclerosis is a disorder of human labyrinthine bone that manifests in the prime clinical manifestation of conductive hearing loss owing to its predilection for occurrence at the anteromedial aspect of the oval window with consequent stapes immobilization (Fig. 20). With early otosclerosis, the predominantly fibrous fixation of the stapes causes a mild, low-frequency conductive hearing loss. With maturation of the otosclerotic focus, the osseous ankylosis firmly fixes the stapes, resulting in a maximal conductive loss. Rarely, with additional extreme involvement of the cochlea, sensorineural hearing loss may be seen as well.

On histopathologic examination, the first sign of a developing otosclerotic focus is an area of perivascular bony resorption (3). Subsequently, immature bone is

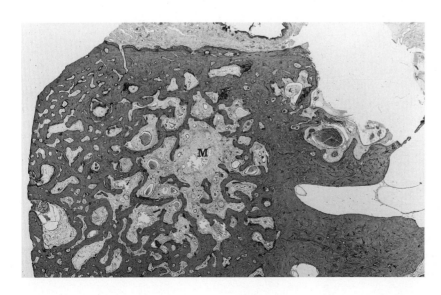

FIG. 19. Left temporal bone, horizontal section. The mastoid (*M*) is obliterated by a combination of osseous and fibrous tissue. (From Schuknecht HF. *Pathology of the ear.* Cambridge, MA: Harvard University Press, 1974, with permission.)

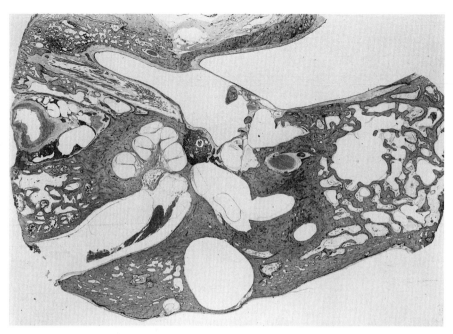

FIG. 20. Right temporal bone, horizontal section. There is an otosclerotic focus (*O*) at the anterior oval window, which has fixed the stapes.

deposited, which has a dearth of collagen, but an abundance of ground substance. The bone undergoes resorption and remodeling—at variable rates and variable degrees within the focus. Eventually, mature bone, collagen-rich and poor in ground substance, is deposited (3).

Current surgical management of the conductive hearing loss of otosclerosis is centered on stapedotomy or partial stapedotomy facilitated by a variety of lasers, and placement of a prosthesis (Fig. 21). In skilled hands, stapes surgery is very effective in eliminating the conductive component of the hearing loss and complications, such as tympanic membrane perforation, anacusis, and prolonged vertigo, are uncommon.

Vestibular Schwannomas

Vestibular schwannomas, also known as acoustic neuromas, are benign tumors of Schwann cell origin that precipitate sensorineural hearing loss, tinnitus, dysequilibrium, as well as other neurologic manifestations, by

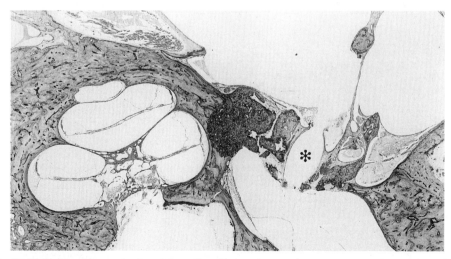

FIG. 21. Right temporal bone, horizontal section. The patient underwent a stapedotomy, but there was no subsequent hearing improvement. The deeply placed piston prosthesis (silhouette at *) has disrupted the saccular wall. (From Schuknecht HF, Mendoza AM. Cochlear pathology after stapedectomy. *Am J Otolaryngol* 1981;2:182.)

both direct and indirect tumor effects (Fig. 22). Direct tumor effects (Fig. 22) include neural compression, frank destruction of nerve fibers, and intralabyrinthine extension (3). It is also hypothesized, but not proven, that partial vascular obstruction by the intracanalicular component of the tumor results in end organ ischemic degeneration (25).

By altering the biochemical homeostasis of the inner ear, vestibular schwannomas may provoke symptomatology related to end organ dysfunction. The eosinophilic staining of inner ear fluids (Fig. 22) associated with vestibular schwannomas is a manifestation of their increased protein content (26). Johnsson and colleagues (27) suggested that it is the consequent increase in viscosity that alters cochlear hydrodynamics to result in sensorineural hearing loss, whereas Schuknecht (3) theorized that the biochemical changes in and of themselves were at least partly etiologic.

The treatment of choice for vestibular schwannomas continues to be complete surgical excision, where possible. The surgeon now aspires not only to preserve facial nerve function but, increasingly, to preserve hearing as well. There are two histopathologic observations that may argue against uniform success in attaining the goal of complete tumor excision with hearing preservation—the infiltrative quality of vestibular schwannoma growth and the microanatomy of cochlear and vestibular nerve union.

First, as shown by studies of the nerve–tumor interface in small vestibular schwannomas of superior vestibular nerve origin (28), the tumor remains distinct from the cochlear nerve. The same is not true for small tumors of inferior vestibular nerve origin; however, in such tumors the cochlear nerve was found to become incorporated into the substance of the tumor as evaluation encompassed the lateral extent of the tumor. The delineation of a discrete tumor–nerve interface defies even immunohistochemical analysis (29,30).

Second, as reported by Silverstein (31), in 25% of normal eighth nerves, the vestibular and cochlear nerves blend imperceptibly in the cerebellopontine angle. Clearly, it would be an exercise in futility to attempt to excise a tumor arising in such an anatomic milieu while leaving the cochlear nerve intact.

Temporal Bone Metastases

Metastatic tumors also may implant in the internal auditory canal (Fig. 23), precipitating symptomatology reminiscent of vestibular schwannomas, but generally within a more compressed time frame (32). Additionally, the presence of facial nerve paralysis or significant paresis, uncommon with vestibular schwannomas, suggests malignant disease. More common than internal auditory canal involvement are metastatic tumor deposits in the marrow of the petrous apex, the sinusoidal capillaries of which, with their slow flow, provide the ideal environment for hematogenous tumor cell deposition (33).

Petrous Apex Lesions

The petrous apex is not only a favored site for metastatic tumor deposition, but also, and more commonly, is the

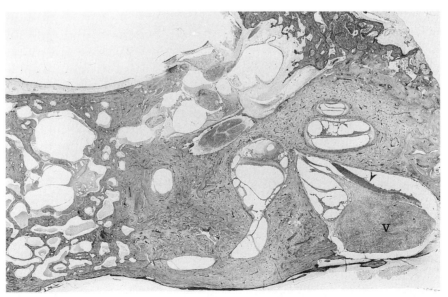

FIG. 22. Left temporal bone, horizontal section. The intracanalicular vestibular schwannoma (*V*) has compressed the facial nerve (*arrowhead*). Preparation artifact causes disproportionate shrinkage of the soft tissues in comparison to bone. (From Schuknecht HF, Shinozaki-Hori N. Patterns of degeneration of the facial nerve. *Am J Otol* 1985;[Suppl 6]:47–54, with permission.)

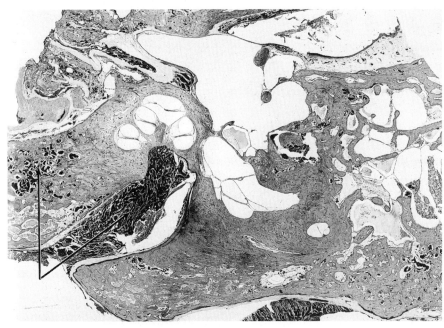

FIG. 23. Right temporal bone, horizontal section. Metastatic breast carcinoma occupies both the internal auditory canal and the petrous apex (*arrows*). Clinical manifestations included a sudden-onset, right facial paralysis, sensorineural hearing loss, and vertigo. (From Schuknecht HF. *Pathology of the ear.* Cambridge, MA: Harvard University Press, 1974, with permission.)

site of occurrence of a variety of benign primary lesions, such as cholesteatomas and cholesterol granulomas. Tumors may invade the petrous apex by direct extension as well. If impinging on the internal auditory canal, the petrous apex lesion can provoke sensorineural hearing loss and vertigo, whereas compression of the eustachian tube and the internal auditory canal (Fig. 24) can cause unilateral serous otitis media and even hemiparesis (32).

Fallopian Canal Lesions

The fallopian canal may be impacted by direct tumor extension, for example, by paragangliomas (34), or by primary tumor development, as with facial neuromas or ossifying hemangiomas, to result in a (generally) progressive facial paralysis. Facial paralysis of sudden onset is ordinarily ascribed to Bell's palsy, but it is important to

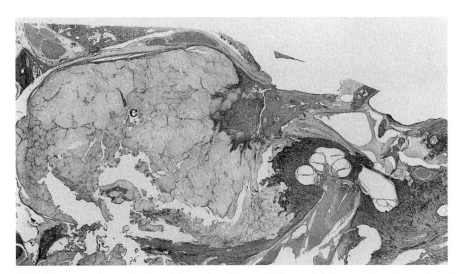

FIG. 24. Right temporal bone, horizontal section. The anterior petrous apex has been invaded by a chondromyxosarcoma (*C*), which has occluded both the eustachian tube and the internal carotid artery. Clinical manifestations included right serous otitis media and left hemiparesis. (From Schuknecht HF. *Pathology of the ear.* Cambridge, MA: Harvard University Press, 1974, with permission.)

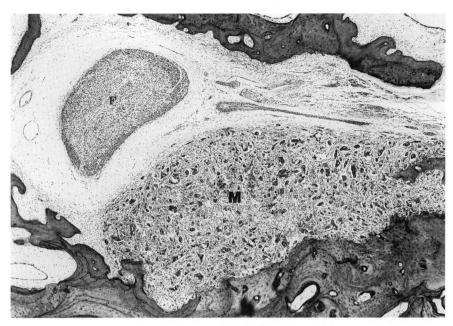

FIG. 25. Left temporal bone, horizontal section. The facial nerve (*F*) is compressed by a nodule of metastatic undifferentiated lung carcinoma (*M*). The patient experienced a rapidly progressive, left facial paralysis. (From Schuknecht HF, Shinozaki-Hori N. Patterns of degeneration of the facial nerve. *Am J Otol* 1985;[Suppl 6]:47–54, with permission.)

consider the possibility of tumor metastasis to the fallopian canal (Fig. 25) (35).

Internal Carotid Artery Disorders

The internal carotid artery, coursing in the anterior petrous apex, is potentially involved in the primary and secondary disorders of the petrous apex, as noted previously. In addition, the internal carotid artery has inherent pathologic disorders, which may manifest within the confines of the temporal bone. With aging, there may be atrophy of the carotid artery wall, leaving only intima and the temporal bone constraining blood flow (Fig. 26). Blind probing in the protympanum or eustachian tube, as in the course of extirpation of cholesteatoma and chronic otitis media (36) or extended temporal bone dissection, may disrupt this thin barrier, resulting in profuse hemorrhage. Alternatively, the internal carotid artery may develop atherosclerotic changes (Fig. 27) precipitating thromboembolic central nervous system dysfunction, either spontaneously or with surgical manipulation.

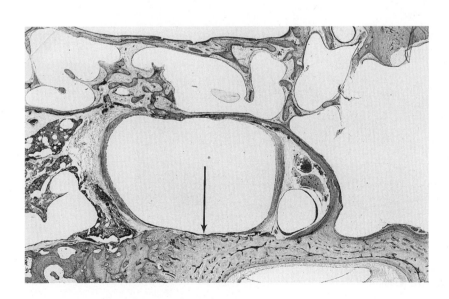

FIG. 26. Right temporal bone, horizontal section. Extreme thinning of the internal carotid artery wall (*arrow*) in a 72-year-old woman. (From Schuknecht HF. *Pathology of the ear.* Cambridge, MA: Harvard University Press, 1974, with permission.)

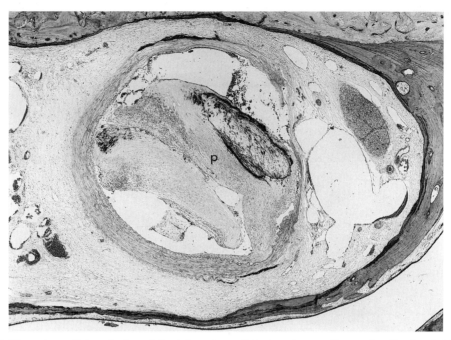

FIG. 27. There is partial occlusion of the internal carotid artery by an atherosclerotic plug (*p*) in a 70-year-old man. (From Schuknecht HF. *Pathology of the ear.* Cambridge, MA: Harvard University Press, 1974, with permission.)

Labyrinthitis Ossificans

Osteoneogenesis that obliterates the fluid spaces of the labyrinth, better known as labyrinthitis ossificans (Fig. 28), can develop as a consequence of inner ear trauma, infection, or vascular insult (37). Labyrinthitis ossificans also can be a feature of far-advanced otosclerosis and autoimmune inner ear disease, as well as other less common disorders of the inner ear (38). Although the pattern of cochlear involvement with labyrinthitis ossificans varies somewhat according to etiology (38), the basal scala tympani is most commonly

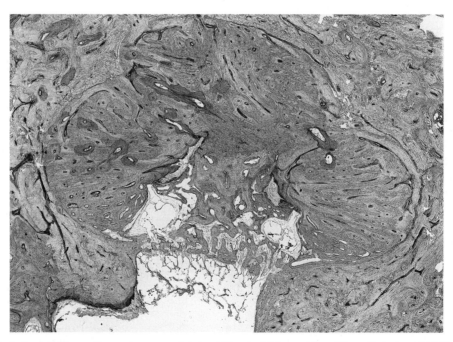

FIG. 28. Labyrinthitis ossificans has completely obliterated this cochlea. (From Schuknecht HF. *Pathology of the ear.* Cambridge, MA: Harvard University Press, 1974, with permission.)

and usually most extensively involved. Moreover, at least with postmeningitic labyrinthitis ossificans, new bone formation can begin as soon as 4 weeks after the acute phase (39).

The presence of labyrinthitis ossificans impacts both on the surgery for cochlear implantation and the success of the implant, once positioned. As the majority of today's devices utilize the scala tympani as the insertion route, extensive obliteration of this chamber by labyrinthitis ossificans requires consideration of alternative procedures for implantation—either cochlear drillout (40) or, where possible, insertion via the scala vestibuli (41). The extent of labyrinthitis ossificans also has an effect on the surviving spiral ganglion cell population. Although even in severe cases a substantial population of surviving spiral ganglion cells remains (42), concern exists nonetheless regarding the adequacy of the remaining population to provide sufficient stimulus transmission from the implant for efficacy.

SUMMARY POINTS

- The anterior epitympanic recess can serve as a hiding place for cholesteatoma. Adequate visualization of this space requires removal of the body of the incus and the head of the malleus.
- The sinus tympani, a recess of considerable interindividual variability in extent of development, can shield cholesteatoma from surgical visualization. Endoscopes can be helpful in assessing this region of the mesotympanum.
- A surgically important anatomic relationship is the superior and medial position of the facial nerve with respect to the cochleariform process.
- The most common location for a dehiscence of the fallopian canal is at the oval window.
- In the vast majority of cases, there is some sort of membrane covering the round window niche.
- With long-standing tympanic membrane perforations the manubrium may assume a more medial position than normal ("medialization of the malleus") due to the unopposed pull of the tensor tympani muscle.
- Vestibular schwannomas can precipitate a broad spectrum of neurotologic symptoms by both direct and indirect mechanisms.
- Hematogenous metastases to the temporal bone have a predilection for the marrow of the petrous apex.
- The internal carotid artery may be injured in the course of surgical manipulations in the protympanum and eustachian tube.

REFERENCES

1. Gulya AJ, Schuknecht HF. *Anatomy of the temporal bone with surgical implications,* 2nd ed. Pearl River, NY: Parthenon Publishing, 1995.
2. Donaldson JA, Duckert LG, Lambert PM, Rubel EW. *Anson-Donaldson: surgical anatomy of the temporal bone,* 4th ed. Philadelphia: Lippincott-Raven Publishers, 1992.
3. Schuknecht HF. *Pathology of the ear,* 2nd ed. Philadelphia: Lea & Febiger, 1993.
4. Linthicum FH Jr, Schwartzman JA. *An atlas of the micropathology of the temporal bone.* San Diego: Singular Publishing, 1994.
5. Nager GT, Hyams VJ. *Pathology of the ear and temporal bone.* Baltimore: Williams & Wilkins, 1994.
6. Schuknecht HF. Temporal bone collections in Europe and the United States: observations on a productive laboratory, pathologic findings of clinical relevance, and recommendations. *Ann Otol Rhinol Laryngol* 1987;96[Suppl 130]:3–19.
7. Merchant SN, Schuknecht HF, Rauch SD, et al. The National Temporal Bone, Hearing, and Balance Pathology Resource Registry. *Arch Otolaryngol Head Neck Surg* 1993;119:846–853.
8. Wackym PA, Simpson TA, Gantz BJ, Smith RJH. Polymerase chain reaction amplification of DNA from archival celloidin-embedded human temporal bone sections. *Laryngoscope* 1993;103:583–588.
9. Portmann D, Fayad J, Wackym PA, Shiroishi H, Linthicum FH Jr, Rask-Andersen H. A technique for reembedding celloidin sections for electron microscopy. *Laryngoscope* 1990;100:195–199.
10. Wackym PA, Micevych PE, Ward PH. Immunoelectron microscopy of the human inner ear. *Laryngoscope* 1990;100:447–454.
11. Nadol JB Jr. Scientific Advisory Council of the National Institute on Deafness and other Communication Disorders National Temporal Bone, Hearing and Balance Pathology Resource Registry. Techniques for human temporal bone removal: information for the scientific community. *Otolaryngol Head Neck Surg* 1996;115:298–305.
12. Baxter A. Dehiscence of the fallopian canal. An anatomical study. *J Laryngol Otol* 1971;85:587–594.
13. Takahashi H, Sando I. Facial canal dehiscence: histologic study and computer reconstruction. *Ann Otol Rhinol Laryngol* 1992;101:925–930.
14. Moreano EH, Paparella MM, Zelterman D, Goycoolea MV. Prevalence of facial canal dehiscence and of persistent stapedial artery in the human middle ear: a report of 1000 temporal bones. *Laryngoscope* 1994;104:309–320.
15. Li D, Cao Y. Facial canal dehiscence: a report of 1,465 stapes operations. *Ann Otol Rhinol Laryngol* 1996;105:467–471.
16. Nomura Y. Otological significance of the round window. *Adv Otorhinolaryngol* 1984;33:1–159.
17. Gacek RR, Leipzig B. Congenital cerebrospinal fluid otorrhea. *Ann Otol Rhinol Laryngol* 1979;88:358–365.
18. Schuknecht HF, Reisser C. The morphologic basis for perilymphatic gushers and oozers. *Adv Otorhinolaryngol* 1988;39:1–12.
19. Jackler RK, Hwang PH. Enlargement of the cochlear aqueduct: fact or fiction? *Otolaryngol Head Neck Surg* 1993;109:14–25.
20. Gacek RR. Arachnoid granulation cerebrospinal fluid otorrhea. *Ann Otol Rhinol Laryngol* 1990;99:854–862.
21. Buckwalter JA, Sasaki CT, Virapongse C, Kier EL, Bauman N. Pulsatile tinnitus arising from jugular megabulb deformity: a treatment rationale. *Laryngoscope* 1983;93:1534–1539.
22. Jahrsdoerfer RA, Cail WS, Cantrell RW. Endolymphatic duct obstruction from a jugular bulb diverticulum. *Ann Otol Rhinol Laryngol* 1981;90:619–623.
23. Mazzoni A. Internal auditory canal arterial relations at the porus acusticus. *Ann Otol Rhinol Laryngol* 1969;78:797–814.
24. Reisser C, Schuknecht HF. The anterior inferior cerebellar artery in the internal auditory canal. *Laryngoscope* 1991;101:761–766.
25. Suga F, Lindsay JR. Inner ear degeneration in acoustic neuroma. *Ann Otol Rhinol Laryngol* 1976;85:343–358.
26. Silverstein H. Inner ear fluid proteins in acoustic neuroma, Meniere's disease, and otosclerosis. *Ann Otol Rhinol Laryngol* 1971;80:27–35.
27. Johnsson L-G, Hawkins JE Jr, Rouse RC. Sensorineural and vascular changes in an ear with acoustic neurinoma. *Am J Otolaryngol* 1984;5:49–59.
28. Neely JG, Hough JVD. Histologic findings in two very small intracanalicular solitary schwannomas of the eighth nerve. *Ann Otol Rhinol Laryngol* 1986;95:460–465.

29. Hebbar GK, McKenna MJ, Linthicum FH Jr. Immunohistochemical localization of vimentin and S-100 antigen in small acoustic tumors and adjacent cochlear nerves. *Am J Otol* 1990;11:310–313.

30. Marquet JFE, Forton GEJ, Offeciers FE, Moeneclaey LLM. The solitary schwannoma of the eighth cranial nerve. An immunohistochemical study of cochlear nerve tumor interface. *Arch Otolaryngol Head Neck Surg* 1990;116:1023–1025.

31. Silverstein H. Cochlear and vestibular gross and histologic anatomy (as seen from postauricular approach). *Otolaryngol Head Neck Surg* 1984;92:207–211.

32. Schuknecht HF. *Pathology of the ear.* Cambridge, MA: Harvard University Press, 1974.

33. Nelson EG, Hinojosa R. Histopathology of metastatic temporal bone tumors. *Arch Otolaryngol Head Neck Surg* 1991;117:189–193.

34. Makek M, Franklin DJ, Zhao J-C, Fisch U. Neural infiltration of glomus temporale tumors. *Am J Otol* 1990;11:1–5.

35. Schuknecht HF, Shinozaki-Hori N. Patterns of degeneration of the facial nerve. *Am J Otol* 1985;[Suppl 6]:47–54.

36. Welling DB, Glasscock ME III, Tarasidis N. Management of carotid artery hemorrhage in middle ear surgery. *Otolaryngol Head Neck Surg* 1993;109:996–999.

37. Suga F, Lindsay JR. Labyrinthitis ossificans. *Ann Otol Rhinol Laryngol* 1977;86:17–29.

38. Green JD Jr, Marion MS, Hinojosa R. Labyrinthitis ossificans: histopathologic consideration for cochlear implantation. *Otolaryngol Head Neck Surg* 1991;104:320–326.

39. Novak MA, Fifer RC, Barkmeier JC, Firszt JB. Labyrinthine ossification after meningitis: its implications for cochlear implantation. *Otolaryngol Head Neck Surg* 1990;103:351–356.

40. Gantz BJ, McCabe BF, Tyler RS. Use of multichannel cochlear implants in obstructed and obliterated cochleas. *Otolaryngol Head Neck Surg* 1988;98:72–81.

41. Gulya AJ, Steenerson RL. The scala vestibuli for cochlear implantation: an anatomic study. *Arch Otolaryngol Head Neck Surg* 1996;122:130–132.

42. Nadol JB Jr, Hsu W. Histopathologic correlation of spiral ganglion cell count and new bone formation in the cochlea following meningogenic labyrinthitis and deafness. *Ann Otol Rhinol Laryngol* 1991;100:712–716.

The Ear: Comprehensive Otology,
edited by R. F. Canalis and P. R. Lambert.
Lippincott Williams & Wilkins, Philadelphia © 2000.

CHAPTER 4

Physiologic Acoustics—The Auditory Periphery

John D. Durrant and John A. Ferraro

Sound is created when an object, such as a tuning fork, is set into vibration within a medium, such as air. As the tongs of the tuning fork vibrate back and forth, the molecules of air expand and compress accordingly to create local alterations of the static pressure. The healthy human ear is capable of detecting sound pressure changes equal to steady air pressures as small as 0.00000001 (or 10^{-8}) atm. Even sound pressures capable of causing pain correspond to steady pressures of merely 0.1 (10^{-1}) atm. This illustrates both the exquisite sensitivity and enormous dynamic range of the auditory system [i.e., $10^{7}:1$ in sound pressure or $(10^{7})^{2}:1 = 10^{14}:1$ in acoustic intensity, that is, "sound power"].

PHYSICS OF SOUND AND LIMITS OF HUMAN HEARING

Quantifying sound actually involves two measures: magnitude and frequency. Magnitude (i.e., amplitude, for

J.D. Durrant: Departments of Communication Science and Disorders and Otolaryngology, University of Pittsburgh, Pittsburgh, Pennsylvania 15260; and Department of Otorhinolaryngology, Université Claude Bernard (Lyon 1), Hôpital Edouard Herriot, Lyon 69003, France

J.A. Ferraro: Department of Hearing and Speech, University of Kansas Medical Center, Kansas City, Kansas 66160-7605

pure tones, and related measures are measured in units of sound pressure called pascals, where 1 Pa = 1 N/m²). The minimal detectable sound in a healthy ear is approximately 20 μPa, but sounds on the order of 2,000 μPa or higher are common in our environment. Given the dynamic range of human hearing and the range of sound pressures to which the ear is commonly exposed, a more convenient (and conventional) unit of sound pressure is the decibel (dB). Decibels are logarithmic numbers based on the ratio of a measured sound pressure to that of a reference pressure (i.e., 20 μPa). Transforming the magnitude of sound pressure to dB yields the sound pressure level (SPL); the dynamic range of human hearing spans from approximately 0 to 140 dB SPL. Except near the limits of hearing, humans generally are capable of discriminating 1-dB steps in SPL, which, in turn, is proportional to the acoustic intensity, or power, of the sound (1). The "physical" quantities have corresponding "psychological" quantities. The percept of loudness thus corresponds to intensity, but loudness is not directly scaled by such measures as μPa or dB SPL, although the latter is more representative of the loudness scale than the former [see Durrant and Lovrinic (2) for an overview of concepts of physical/acoustic measures and the psychological attributes of sound discussed in this section].

Frequency, however, is a measure of the rate of vibration of the sound source (also a physical measure) and is the primary determinant of pitch (a psychologic attribute). The unit of measure for frequency is cycles per second and has been given the name hertz (Hz). The perceptible range of frequencies for the human ear extends from approximately 20 to 20,000 Hz. The limits of frequency discrimination are a bit more complicated to characterize than intensity discrimination. Suffice it to say here that for simple tones presented sequentially, changes of a few hertz or less are readily detectable at suprathreshold levels (3).

Considering again the example of the tuning fork, it is important to realize that the sound produced by this device is relatively simple, reflecting oscillations at a single frequency. Most sounds in nature, however, are considerably more complex, typically comprising several frequencies or more that vary in amplitude among frequency components and over time. Despite this, these sounds can be analyzed according to their "spectrum," that is to say, measuring the magnitude of each frequency component. Sounds of particular interest to humans—speech, music, and environmental noise—have complex spectra that tend to change rapidly over time. Thus, for sound to be heard and understood, the auditory system must be able to perform some form of spectral analysis at relatively high rates and continuously update the analysis. In addition to loudness and pitch, the spectrum of the sound also determines the perceived qualities of timbre, volume, and density. The auditory system's ability to analyze these features allows us to distinguish between, for example, the sound of a piano versus a trumpet, even though they are playing the same note (i.e., sounds of equal pitch).

Although not directly corresponding to perceptual units, as alluded to previously, it is often more convenient, or even desirable, to characterize auditory capabilities by the physical measures of the stimuli that elicit them. The basic measures of sound, for example, can be used to map the human auditory response area (Fig. 1). This is a two-dimensional space, with axes of frequency (in Hz) and sound pressure (in SPL), again defining the dynamic range of hearing (4–7). As noted previously, the sensitivity of hearing is exquisite and is characterized by the lower boundary of the auditory response—the minimum audibility curve. It has been speculated that further improvement of hearing sensitivity in humans would be of little practical value, because such sensitivity would approach levels at which the molecular motion of the medium could be detected but the threshold of hearing is significantly above this limit (8). The upper limit of the auditory response area is defined by the physiologic tolerance of the system and cross-modal stimulation. Sounds approaching 140-dB SPL are extremely loud and typically uncomfortable (7), if not painful, and definitely are harmful to the ear. Prolonged exposures to sounds as low as 90-dB SPL (A-scale weighted), if not lower, can cause permanent damage to the organ of hearing. This particular level has been stipulated by the National Institute of Occupational Safety and Health as the maximal limit of noise to which workers can be exposed for 8 hours/day on a daily basis without being required to wear ear protection (9). Maximum allowable exposure times decrease as the level of workplace noise increases. Even brief exposures to very intense sounds, such as explosive noises, may cause immediate and permanent damage to the hearing organ, a condition referred to as acoustic trauma.

Examining again the lower limit of the auditory response area (Fig. 1), this curve represents specifically the thresholds of sound detection by a group of otologically normal young subjects, as a function of frequency. This

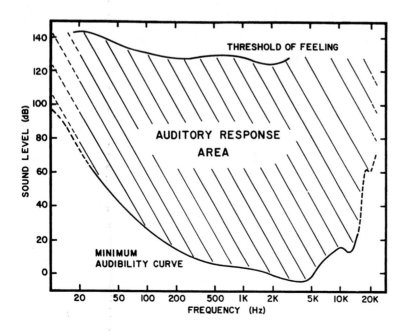

FIG. 1. The auditory response area, defined by the minimum audibility curve [based on data of Robinson and Dadson (5) and, for the extreme low- and high-frequency portions of the curve (*broken line*), data of Yeowart and Evans (6) and Corso (4), respectively], and the threshold-of-feeling curve [based on data of Wegel (7)]. (From Durrant JD, Lovrinic JH. *Bases of hearing science,* 3rd ed. Baltimore: Williams and Wilkins, 1995;259, with permission.)

function, the minimum audibility curve, serves as the basis by which to detect diminished hearing sensitivity, i.e., one of the most common manifestations of diseases/disorders of the ear and auditory system. The clinical chart of hearing sensitivity—the audiogram—represents the norms of hearing as a straight line (i.e., 0-dB hearing [threshold] level; see Chapter 10), but clearly, the threshold of hearing is not constant across frequency when measured in SPL. For example, less SPL is needed for humans to hear a 2,000-Hz tone than a 100-Hz tone. The frequency range of hearing and the shape of the minimum audibility curve tend to be species dependent. The frequencies to which a dog is most sensitive are higher than humans, but lower than the mouse. For humans, the usable frequency range is centered around the speech spectrum; telephones, for example, are engineered to reproduce a range of only about 300 to 3,000 Hz. The range of human hearing (again, from approximately 20 and 20,000 Hz) clearly extends well beyond the frequencies needed for speech recognition/understanding. However, much lower and higher frequencies are capable of exciting the human auditory (4,6), but sounds beyond the nominal limits of hearing must be presented at rather high SPLs to be detected, tend to sound distorted (9), and may be devoid of pitch (4,10).

The most sensitive hearing, nevertheless, coincides with the speech frequency range. As will be shown in the following section, this is the range of most efficient function of the combined outer and middle ear systems. The overall role of the outer and middle ears in hearing is relatively straightforward—they collect sound energy and route it to the inner ear, housing the organ of hearing. This particular physical task and its formative influence on hearing, however, cannot be fully appreciated without considering the basic underlying acoustic and mechanical principles involved. At first glance, the outer ear in humans seems expendable, and there is no doubt that the middle ear contributes considerably more to our auditory capabilities. It thus is fitting to begin our discussion of physiologic acoustics at this level of the auditory system.

FUNCTION OF THE MIDDLE EAR

Middle Ear Transformer

The need of the middle ear for efficient hearing can be appreciated by considering the problem of transmitting sound energy through different media. For example, consider what happens when acoustic energy traveling through air encounters water. Under the best circumstances, only a fraction (approximately 0.1%) of the energy will be transmitted below the surface of the water, whereas the majority of it (i.e., 99.9%) will be reflected (11). This loss from air to water represents approximately 30 dB. Applying this analogy to the auditory system, our hearing would be compromised by approximately 30 dB if sound waves were transferred directly from our air-filled environment to the

fluids of the inner ear. The role of the middle ear, consequently, is to compensate for this situation.

It is well known from physics that the primary determinant of how much power is transmitted from one medium to another is the ratio of impedances between these media (11). Impedance is a form of opposition to the transfer of power and is determined by the combined physical characteristics of the medium (i.e., its mass or density, stiffness [elasticity], and friction). The best transfer occurs when the impedance ratio between media is unity (i.e., when the impedances are matched to each other). For example, the output impedance of a stereo sound system must be matched to the input impedance of the loud speakers to achieve the greatest frequency response and best overall efficiency. If, per chance, the impedances are "mismatched," a transformer can be used to correct the situation. Transformers are commonly used for electrical applications when transferring electrical power from one source to another. Likewise, transformers can be applied in acoustic and mechanical systems. The middle ear mechanism likewise serves as a transformer to match the impedance of air to that the cochlea.

The classic model of the middle ear treats it as a system of pistons and levers, as illustrated in Fig. 2. This

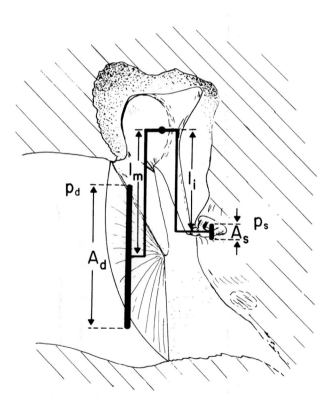

FIG. 2. Components of the middle ear transformer modeled as a system of two pistons connected by a folded lever. A, area; l, length; p, sound pressure. Subscripts: d, eardrum; i, long crus of the incus; m, manubrium of the malleus; s, stapes footplate. [Drawing of piston model after Zwislocki (13), from Durrant JD, Lovrinic JH. *Bases of hearing science,* 3rd ed. Baltimore: Williams and Wilkins, 1995;163, with permission.]

description has received considerable attention in the literature (2,12–14) and is presented only conceptually here. The component of the transformation performed by this system that has the largest effect and most obvious physically is the areal ratio between the TM or tympanic membrane (d) and the stapes footplate or oval window (s). Although this ratio is approximately 20:1, not all of the surface of the ear drum is free to vibrate. The effective ratio is closer to 14:1. Sound waves exert pressure on surface area d and thus create an input force: $Force_d = Pressure_d \times Area_d$. Likewise, transmission of mechanical energy through the middle ear produces a force at s, the output of the system. This force (F_s), in turn, is equal to the product of pressure and area at s. If we assume for now that $F_d = F_s$ (i.e., that the middle ear is a lossless system), then $P_d \times A_d = P_s \times A_s$. Inserting the effective d and s areas into this equation, $P_d \times 14 = P_s$ (Note: $P_s \times 1 = P_s$). Thus, $d{:}s$, the areal ratio, allows for a 14-fold increase in pressure as energy is funneled through this system. An additional, but small, amplification of force is achieved through the lever system formed by the ossicular chain. In this system, the lever is folded and may be treated as a class II lever. As such, the input force is applied at one end of the lever arm, the fulcrum is at the other end, and the force to be moved (i.e., the output force) is in between. The manubrium of the malleus represents the lever arm that receives the input force from the TM, the fulcrum is the malleoincudal joint, and the long crus of the incus represents that portion of the lever arm between the fulcrum and the output force (i.e., via the stapes in the oval window). Class II levers always operate at a mechanical advantage. This means that the force coming into the system will be amplified by the time it comes out. The amount of force amplification is determined by the ratio of the lengths of the lever arms. For humans, the length of the malleus:incus is approximately 1.3:1. Thus, the output force of the ossicular lever system is 1.3 times greater than the input force. When the pressure amplification factor due to $d{:}s$ (14) is combined with the force amplification factor of the ossicular chain lever system (1.3), the total amplification factor becomes $14 \times 1.3 \approx 18$. This corresponds to a sound pressure gain of approximately 25 dB.

Worth of the Middle Ear and Other Considerations

The sound pressure gain computed in this manner is attractive as an estimate of the "worth" of the middle ear because it clearly approximates the 30-dB air-water mismatch noted earlier. This amount of sound pressure amplification is also seen experimentally, in animals like the cat (Fig. 3A, 500- to 5,000-Hz range) (15), wherein it is possible to compare directly the sound pressure at the tympanic membrane and the pressure gradient across the cochlear partition (CP), the effective stimulus of the organ of Corti (see following). However, the more critical analysis pre-

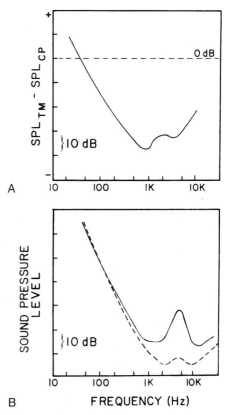

FIG. 3. Comparison of **(A)** sound pressure gradient across the cochlear partition and **(B)** behavioral thresholds (minimal audibility curve) in the cat with (*solid line*) and without (*dashed line*) correction for effects of ear canal resonance. CP, cochlear partition; SPL, sound pressure level; TM, tympanic membrane. In **B** the middle ear cavity was open; hence, the slightly different low-frequency slopes. [Based on data of **(A)** Nedzelnitsky (15) and **(B)** an adaptation of graph by Dallos (12). From ref. Durrant JD, Lovrinic JH. *Bases of hearing science,* 3rd ed. Baltimore: Williams and Wilkins, 1995;167, with permission.]

cludes this as the final solution on various points. Two of the most salient are that the cochlear input impedance must differ significantly from that of water, and that full use of the sound pressure gain presumes the cochlea to be a pure pressure transducer. That the cochlear impedance is different, i.e., less than that of water, is dictated by the simple logic that sound energy must find a path into the inner ear. Because the body is largely water in composition, it is clear that specific effects of sound on the cochlea would be difficult were the input impedance not uniquely different. It also is well known that the stapes must move in the oval window to excite the cochlear mechanical events essential to hearing (see following) (12,14). Additionally, the input impedance to the cochlea does not effectively approach infinity (13,16) (as required for pure pressure detection); thus, significant power transfer to the cochlear must occur. The complete analysis of the worth of the middle ear, consequently, requires consideration of the volume velocity of the stapes, not just sound pressure, and, more generally, the impedance transform ratio—the comparison of input impedance of the cochlea to that of the middle ear. The impedance transform ratio calculated on the basis of the classic piston-lever model and related measurements, however, yields rather pessimistic estimates of the worth of the middle ear (e.g., approximately 14 dB) (2,12). It is beyond our scope here to delve further into this still-unresolved issue in the literature, although considerable strides have been made in analysis of the middle ear acousticomechanical circuit, input impedance to the ear/middle ear, and related issues, including how the system is altered by pathology and surgical treatment (16–19). One century-old-plus mystery is whether or not there is a significant transformation performed by the curvature of the eardrum itself, as it is clear that the tympanic membrane vibrating like a rigid piston is unrealistic (20).

Therefore, as well as the general principals of middle ear function are established (12,14,21,22), there remains less than a completely satisfying account of its dB value in hearing. Still, there is no doubt of its significance for overall hearing sensitivity. This is demonstrated by the effects of middle ear effusion and other pathologies that cause conductive hearing loss (see Chapter 10). More fundamentally, because the efficiency of the middle ear transformer is not constant across frequency, it is primarily responsible for the shape of the minimum audibility curve (12,15,21) (compare curves in Figs. 3A and B; note also the minimum audibility curve in Fig. 1). The middle ear (together with the outer ear [see following]) thus imposes a filter function on the frequency response of the auditory system (see Fig. 5A). Another contribution is so-called protection of the round window. As noted previously, the effective input signal for the organ of Corti (i.e., for generating the cochlear hydromechanical waves of the cochlea excited by the vibration of the stapes footplate [see following]) is the sound pressure differential generated subsequently across the CP. Because the two windows see opposite sides of the partition, the problem with sound waves striking the two windows is self-evident. Therefore, the middle ear mechanism, by providing a particularly efficient path for sound to the oval window—a path of least "resistance"—effectively protects the round window from efficient transmission of sound energy. Not only is the air-to-cochlea mismatch encountered by sound arriving at the round window, there is the additional mismatch created by the eardrum and middle ear cavity beforehand. More critical consideration of this factor, however, reveals that direct exposure of both windows to sound waves cannot lead to complete sound cancellation in the first place because the two windows do not lie in the same plane. Consequently, some phase difference is inevitable (22). In any practical consideration (e.g., an ossicular chain disarticulated at the stapes), there also is the reality that the two windows are covered in remarkably different ways—the round window by a membrane and the oval window by the stapes footplate

and annular ligament. The middle-inner ear package thus is well designed for maintaining a sound pressure differential across the CP at all odds. This is fortunate, because pathology such as middle ear effusion may compromise the "protection" of the round window. Yet, such conditions do not cause profound deafness (see Chapter 10).

Other remarkable anatomic features of the middle ear include not only the somewhat elaborate system of cavities, but also the auditory (eustachian) tube connecting the middle ear space to the nasopharynx. The normal functioning of the middle ear requires a balance of air pressure on the two sides of the tympanic membrane, which is accomplished by opening of the auditory tube. Manipulating air pressure differentially across the eardrum also is a useful way of testing the middle ear system (i.e., tympanometry). The topics of eustachian tube functioning and tympanometry are considered elsewhere in this book (see Chapters 12 and 23).

Acoustic Reflex

Still other remarkable features are the middle ear muscles—tensor tympani and stapedius. The auditory system itself has the ability to alter the impedance (or admittance) of the middle ear to some extent and, thereby, alter the transmission of sound through the middle ear (12,21,23). This is made possible by the musculature of the middle ear, primarily through the action of the stapedius muscle. The stapedius muscle reacts reflexively to sound. Consequently, this response of the auditory system is called the acoustic or stapedius reflex. As shown in Fig. 4, the magnitude of the response increases with increasing intensity of the stimulus, although it ultimately saturates at very high levels of sound (23) (around 120-dB SPL). The reflex is bilateral; a sound stimulus delivered via an earphone to one ear will elicit the reflex in both ears. The threshold of the reflex response is seen to be approximately 80-dB SPL for individuals with normal hearing or relatively minor hearing loss (that is, as measured with clinical immittance equipment and no response averaging). However, the sensitivity of the acoustic reflex can be substantially enhanced by the occurrence of a preceding sound (24).

The role of the acoustic reflex is often described in terms of protection of the cochlea (21). However, the protection provided by the acoustic reflex is limited because, again, the transmission of sound is affected only below frequencies of about 1,200 kHz. Higher-frequency sounds generally have been viewed as potentially more hazardous to hearing, and yet it is in this range of frequencies that the reflex offers little or no attenuation. Another problem with the protection theory is that the reflex is not instantaneous; rather, a certain minimal time is required for it to be activated (10 ms or more to develop full contractile force, depending on the intensity of the sound stimulus). The acoustic reflex thus can afford little

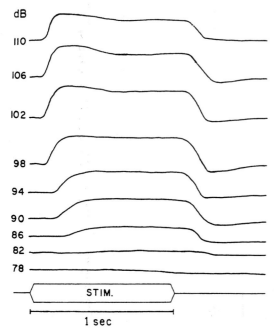

FIG. 4. Input-output function of the acoustic reflex (i.e., response magnitude in relative units of stiffness versus sound pressure level of the stimulus (STIM.) indicated in sound pressure level (dB). (From Durrant JD, Lovrinic JH. *Bases of hearing science,* 3rd ed. Baltimore: Williams and Wilkins, 1995;172, with permission.)

protection from impulsive sounds, such as gunshots, unless the reflex is coincidentally "primed" via the sensitization effect discussed above. However, the protection theory also has its problems from an evolutionary perspective, because it is difficult to imagine the impetus in nature.

The regulatory role of the acoustic reflex is similarly limited, i.e., limited dynamic range of influence, frequency range of effect, and speed of response. By comparison, the effects of the pupillary reflex are dramatic. Yet, it perhaps is the more subtle influence of the middle ear muscles that is important. Even without activation, like all skeletal muscles, these muscles still have tonus. Their mere presence has a damping effect so as to smooth the frequency response of the middle ear mechanism. Otherwise, there would be sharp dips and peaks at various frequencies (resonances and antiresonances, respectively) (25). Interestingly, the muscles also are activated before and during vocalization (26). Consequently, the intensity of one's own voice reaching the cochlea is attenuated. Finally, it is noteworthy that the acoustic reflex is not entirely controlled by events in the periphery. It can be modified by the organism's state of attention to the sound stimulus (27), and it is mediated by a reflex arc or "circuit" involving lower centers of the brain (21). The acoustic reflex, however, is only one of two mechanisms by which the central system can exercise come control over the input to the system at the periphery (28) (see otoacoustic emissions following). Some of the most

recent thinking suggests such mechanisms to be important in helping to maintain the most favorable signal-to-noise ratio for processing of the input signals by the central system (29). Consequently, even if the contribution of the middle ear muscles and the acoustic reflex is not as dramatic as the pupil and the pupillary reflex in vision, they appear to significantly influence auditory function.

FUNCTION OF THE OUTER EAR

Ear Canal Resonance (Outer Ear Transformer)

Sound energy must first pass through another system—the outer ear. Up to this point, the acoustic contribution of the outer ear has been ignored. However, in a detailed comparison between the minimum audibility curve and the response characteristics of the middle ear, differences are evident that are attributable, in part, to the contribution of the outer ear (see Figs. 3b and 5) (12,30, 31). Sensitivity of hearing is actually improved by the presence of the external meatus, particularly at frequencies above 1,000 Hz. Acoustically, the external meatus resembles a pipe with one end open (laterally) and the other end closed (medially, by the tympanic membrane). Therefore, standing waves form at odd-integer multiples of the frequency whose wavelength is four times the length of the ear canal. In humans, the length of the external canal is approximately 2.5 cm, yielding a fundamental mode at ≈ 3,400 Hz, as confirmed experimentally (32). At modal frequencies (i.e., higher, odd-integer multiple frequencies), a pressure node occurs at the entrance of the canal with an antinode at the tympanic membrane. Thus, there is sound pressure amplification at the closed end of the "pipe." More fundamentally, the ear canal acts

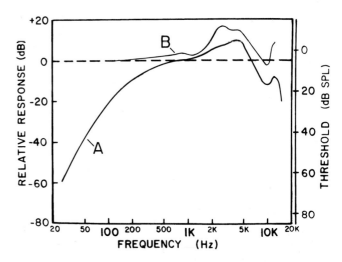

FIG. 5. Frequency response of the auditory system, estimated from the minimum audibility curve **(A)** and contribution of the head-baffle and ear-canal resonance effects **(B).** [As adapted from Shaw (31) by Durrant (30). From Durrant JD, Lovrinic JH. *Bases of hearing science,* 3rd ed. Baltimore: Williams and Wilkins, 1995;177, with permission.]

as another impedance matching transformer (i.e., air to middle ear). The exact frequencies of the resonance peaks, especially the higher modes, and the amount of gain from ear canal resonance differ somewhat from those calculated for a simple hard-walled tube. The real ear canal, of course, bends somewhat and is lined with skin (an absorptive material; absorption limits resonance peaks). Nevertheless, the ear canal provides some 12–15 dB gain near the first mode (31,32). This peak, however, is shifted down somewhat in frequency (2,700 Hz) and broadened overall by the combined acoustic effects of the concha and the pinna- (auricle-) and head-baffle effects.

Head-/Pinna-baffle versus Diffraction Effects— Bases of Sound Localization

Even if it were located on the surface of the head, the SPL appearing at the eardrum would not necessarily equal the SPL measured in the sound field in the absence of the head (11). In effect, sound gets to the eardrum through a hole in a wall. The "hole" is the entrance to the external auditory meatus, whereas the combination of the auricle and head forms the wall or baffle, in acoustic terms. Hearing laboratories and clinics, more often than not, work on one side or the other of this spherical baffle and/or largely obviate some of the head and pinna effects by using earphones to evaluate one-eared hearing. The majority of information presented earlier was based on experiments involving monaural listening paradigms. This is a great simplification of real-life listening. The real world is a binaural world, and binaural hearing offers substantive advantages over monaural. The binaural absolute threshold, for example, is better than the monaural absolute threshold; this advantage may be worth as much as 3 dB (33). Sounds also sound louder when heard binaurally. These are examples of binaural summation (34). There are yet other binaural effects that could be described, but certainly none appears as compelling as binaural hearing in the location of sounds in space. However, there is more to the sound localization story than simply "two ears are better than one," and at the heart of this story are outer ear and head-baffle diffraction effects.

Time versus Intensity Cues for Localization

Spectral disparities resulting from differences in the intensity and/or arrival time of sound at the two ears arise from diffraction and baffle effects of the head (35–37) The general scheme of events is summarized in Fig. 6. For sounds with relatively long wavelengths, the head has little effect on the SPL at the eardrum, regardless of which way the head is turned. An idea of the frequencies at which diffraction can be expected to occur is obtained simply by solving for f in the equation for wavelength, $\lambda = c/f$, given $\lambda = 0.18$ m (the approximate diameter of the average adult head). The frequency of 2,000 Hz has a

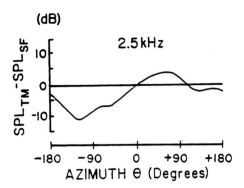

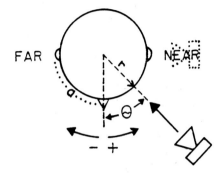

FIG. 6. Bases of intensity and time cues for sound localization. **Top:** Changes in sound pressure level versus azimuth (angle theta) of sound at relatively high frequencies, i.e., as the source is moved about the head in the horizontal plane, as illustrated at the bottom. [Based on data of **(top)** Shaw (31).] **Bottom:** At relatively low frequencies, head shadow/baffle is minimal due to diffraction, but there remain time differences in arrival of sound at the two ears. The greatest interaural difference occurs with the source located at +90-degree azimuth (indicated by *dotted outline* of loudspeaker), wherein the sound must travel a total distance of r (radius of the head) plus a (one-fourth circumference of the head).

wavelength of about 0.18 m, so for the human, no diffraction is anticipated above 2,000 Hz. With decreasing frequency, total diffraction is approached around 150 Hz for real heads; so, little or no sound pressure buildup occurs at relatively low frequencies. Again, for real human heads, diffraction actually begins to diminish appreciably above 500 Hz. At higher frequencies, then, the SPL at the tympanic membrane for a given ear will vary systematically as a function of azimuth of the head (Fig. 6) (31). The range of change is defined by the extremes of optimal head baffle (or maximal sound buildup), wherein the sound source is directed at the ear, and maximal head shadow, wherein the sound source is on the opposite side of the head. A well-known problem among hearing-impaired listeners with substantial unilateral or asymmetric high-frequency hearing loss is the increased difficulty understanding a speaker located on the side of the "bad" ear.

That low frequency sounds essentially wrap around the head does not mean that nothing interesting is going on here; this is a time-consuming process (35,36). Other than the case in which the two ears are located at equal distances from the sound source (i.e., head on), a time disparity occurs between the arrival of sound at the two ears. The maximal time difference occurs when one ear is pointing directly toward the sound source (90-degree azimuth). As illustrated in Fig. 6, the total distance of travel of the sound wave from the "near" ear to the "far" ear will involve two distances, r (the "line of sight" travel) and a (the distance of the curved portion of the path around the part of the head out of "line of sight"). The former is equal to the radius of the head, approximately 0.09 m. The latter is equal to one-fourth the circumference of the head: $1/4 \times 2\pi r = 0.25 \times 2 \times 3.14 \times 0.09 \approx 0.14$ m. The total distance d then is $r + a = 0.09 + 0.14 = 0.23$ m. Assuming the speed of sound c to be 343 m/s, the maximal time difference possible is $\Delta t = d/c = 0.23/343 \approx 6.71 \times 10^{-4} \approx 0.67$ ms. For other azimuths the time disparities will be less than 0.67 ms. Time disparities also introduce phase differences, i.e., in ongoing sounds. It is interesting in this regard that the estimated 0.67-ms upper limit for (natural) time disparities corresponds to the period of 1,500 Hz ($T = 1/f = 1/1500 \approx 0.00067$ s = 0.67 ms). At higher frequencies, interaural phase disparities become ambiguous (i.e., >360 degrees). Of course, as noted previously, diffraction is nil at frequencies approaching 2,000 Hz and above.

The notion that binaural sound localization, and the related effect under earphone call lateralization, is dependent on time and intensity disparities at low and high frequencies, respectively, is the principal tenant of what is called the duplex theory, attributed to the acoustician Lord Rayleigh. The duplex theory accounts well for the sound localization of simple sounds, but it does not appear to account so well for the localization of complex sounds that, in turn, depends more on temporal cues, even for sounds of predominantly high-frequency sound energy (37). Temporal cues at high frequencies are possible by virtue of interaural differences in the amplitude envelopes of these sounds.

Sound Localization Ability and Other Considerations

The multiple factors influencing binaural localization make it difficult to specify a single index to fully characterize this capability of the auditory system. Perhaps the most direct index, and one characterizing the sensitivity of the system, is the minimum audible angle (36). This is a measure of the ability of a listener to determine whether two successive sounds were at different azimuths. The data are complicated by changes in sensitivity as the source moves around the head, but the minimum audible angle is on the order of 2 degrees (determined near 0-degree azimuth). At other azimuths, spatial resolution diminishes, and the minimum audible angle increases as a function of frequency, becoming indeterminately large in the vicinity of 1,500 Hz as the sound approaches the

90-degree azimuth. This means that the most precise directional hearing (for all frequencies) is realized when the listener is essentially facing the sound source.

Unfortunately, unambiguous interaural differences occur only in the horizontal plane; in the real world, sounds also come from different elevations. For such vertical localization, the auricle becomes the crucial part of the outer ear. Its convoluted surface creates variations in the sound spectrum as the head is tilted up and down (38); front-to-back discrimination also depends on the auditory system's ability to interpret such cues. However, the pinna baffle is small, so its contribution is limited to fairly short-wavelength sounds, i.e., high frequencies, over 4,000 Hz. Consequently, for the most accurate judgment of sound elevation, the spectrum of the sound must contain energy at frequencies above 4,000 Hz (39). Furthermore, to create the sensation of three-dimensional sound space via earphones, it is necessary to compensate the response of the earphones to include these subtle spectral cues, namely, according to what are called head-related transfer functions (40).

The total story of sound localization cannot be told without consideration of the central auditory system (see Chapter 6). Nevertheless, it should be clear from the foregoing that the outer ear, and subsequently the middle ear, contributes significantly to auditory processing, although by largely passive acousticomechanical mechanisms. It is a general characteristic of sensory systems that there is a functional component dedicated to the efficient coupling of the energy of the stimulus to the transduction mechanism proper. In the auditory system, this obviously complex function is further elaborated via mechanisms within the inner ear.

COCHLEAR FUNCTION

The auditory part of the inner ear is the cochlea. The cochlea's job is to couple the vibratory energy at the oval window to the receptor cells of the hearing organ—the hair cells of the organ of Corti. The cochlea represents a unique and intriguing hydrodynamic (fluid-mechanical) system that must be considered at multiple levels of function to be fully appreciated. This includes, before considering any of the mechanisms of transduction and encoding of the auditory stimulus, the general physiology of the cochlear system.

Cochlear Fluid Systems

The fluids of the inner ear create specific environments for the sensory cells, which have ramification for both hydromechanical and electrochemical processes, as will be described. That there are two types of fluid in the inner ear (41,42)—the endolymph filling the membranous labyrinth and perilymph surrounding it—suggests two of the more interesting issues in auditory physiology: (a) how the two fluids are produced, and (b) how fluid pressure is regulated within the cochlea. Perilymph is the more abundant fluid and is characterized by a concentration of sodium (Na⁺) about 30 times that of potassium (K⁺) (Fig. 7). Perilymph thus resembles interstitial fluid. There are basically two theories concerning the origin of perilymph. One is that it is a filtrate of blood serum that is produced by capillaries in the spiral ligament. The other theory is that it is merely cerebrospinal fluid (CSF), on the assumption that CSF can enter the cochlea via the cochlear aqueduct. The bone of contention is whether this duct is functionally patent, especially in adults (42–44). The consensus is that a free exchange of fluid between the subarachnoid space and scala tympany is unlikely; perilymph has not been found to be identical in composition to CSF (42,45).

Endolymph is far more curious, particularly as an extracellular fluid; the Na⁺-K⁺ mix is opposite to that of perilymph (Fig. 7), thus making endolymph much like intracellular fluid. The specific mechanisms of endolymph production remain to be described completely, and such details are beyond the scope of coverage here. The most salient and well-established fact is that cochlear production of endolymph directly involves the stria vascularis. Current thinking on the matter suggests the existence of K⁺-Na⁺ exchange "pumps" in the stria wherein ions are moved across Reissner's membrane. The chemical balance between endolymph and perilymph appears to be maintained by local ion exchange circuits all along the cochlear duct (42,45,46).

The cochlear fluid system appears to have a mechanism for regulating the overall fluid pressure within the inner ear (Fig. 7) (42,47). Even in the absence of free flow of CSF through the cochlear aqueduct, it seems

likely that there is sufficient fluid movement to provide a mechanism of static pressure control for perilymph. Similarly, endolymph appears to be slowly absorbed by the endolymphatic sac. This sac is located in a subdural space and communicates with the remainder of the membranous labyrinth via the endolymphatic duct. This makes for a hydraulic circuit between the two cochlear fluids and between the cochlear fluids and the CSF without their active intermingling. Overall, cochlear fluid pressure can influence cochlear perfusion or blood flow (analogous to the effects of CSF pressure on cerebral perfusion), so the fluid balance of the inner ear is an integral part of its own homeostasis.

Underlying this system is a rich vascular supply (see also Chapter 3). The common cochlear artery and common modiolar vein branch to form intricate beds of minute vessels—arterioles and venules—which supply and drain, respectively, capillary beds in the cochlea (48,49). The stria vascularis, spiral limbus, and spiral ligament are major areas of concentration of vessels. A limited number of vessels also run beneath the organ of Corti on the scala tympani side of the basilar membrane (BM). The vascular network of the stria vascularis reflects the high level of metabolic activity believed to be primarily associated with the maintenance of the ionic composition of endolymph in scala media, as well as an associated electrical potential or voltage—the endocochlear potential. However, the stria does not appear to provide life support, as such, to the organ of Corti. It appears that nutrients and oxygen are supplied to the cells of the organ of Corti by perilymph that, in turn, appears to flow freely into the spaces of the organ of Corti (50).

Generic Hair Cell Mechanoreceptor

The most basic aspect of the cochlea's job (although by no means basic in detailed analysis) is the function of the receptor cells of the organ of Corti. Although representing the final path in the transduction of sound, it will be useful to consider first how these cells work fundamentally. At this juncture, we are particularly interested in what it takes to stimulate the sensory receptor cells that we call hair cells. Hair cells are a type of mechanoreceptor cell not entirely unique to the ear. Much of the earlier work pursued in quest of an understanding of cochlear hair cells was based on a combination of theory, observations from extracellular recordings of cochlear electrical potentials in animals, and extracellular and intracellular recordings from lateral line organs in fish and frogs and other amphibia (51). Findings from the latter were supplemented by observations from their vestibular organs (52). Both auditory and vestibular sensory organs of fish and amphibia have hair cells with a single kinocilium and several stereocilia. As illustrated in Fig. 8A the kinocilium represents a morphologic signpost that indicates the preferred direction of deflection of the sensory hairs nec-

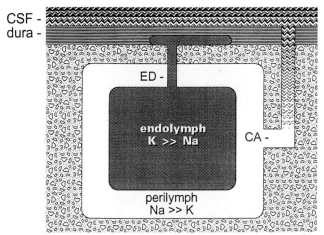

FIG. 7. Pressure balance and relative concentration of sodium and potassium in the cochlear fluids. CA, cochlear aqueduct; CSF, cerebrospinal fluid; ED, endocochlear duct and sac system. (From Durrant JD, Lovrinic JH. *Bases of hearing science,* 3rd ed. Baltimore: Williams and Wilkins, 1995;132, with permission.)

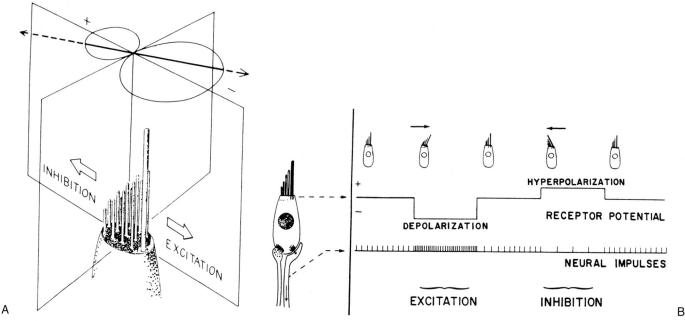

FIG. 8. A: Directional sensitivity of the hair cell. **B:** Relation of discharge rate of action potentials in the afferent neuron as the hair cell responds to different directions of shearing of the hairs. [Adapted from Flock (51). From Durrant JD, Lovrinic JH. *Bases of hearing science,* 3rd ed. Baltimore: Williams and Wilkins, 1995;144, with permission.]

essary to stimulate/inhibit the sensory cell. Back-and-forth deflection of the hair bundle along the axis defined by the kinocilium results in alternating depolarization and hyperpolarization of the cell, whereas displacement at right angles to this axis is ineffective. Depolarization/hyperpolarization of the sensory cell, in turn, leads to the excitation/inhibition of the nerve fibers that innervate the cell.

The model for the conversion of hydromechanical to electrical energy at the level of the hair cell that has guided research in the area for over 30 years is that of the late Hallowell Davis (53). Davis postulated that the bending of the sensory cilia alters membrane resistance. That is, deflection in one direction decreases this resistance and leads to depolarization of the cell, whereas bending in opposite direction increases resistance and causes hyperpolarization. The hair cell also appears to be "leaky" in that a small amount of ionic current constantly flows across its membrane. This leakage current is presumably the stimulus for the spontaneous and random discharges seen in the nerve fibers that innervate the cell. When the sensory cilia are deflected in an excitatory direction, current flow through the cell increases. This leads to an increased release of excitatory transmitter substance at the base of the hair cell where it is in synaptic contact with a nerve fiber. The nerve fiber, in turn, responds by increasing the rate and organizing the pattern of spike action potentials subsequently excited in the axon of the primary auditory neuron (51,54). Figure 8B illustrates this process. Although a considerably greater

understanding of the underlying membrane biophysics has been achieved in the past decade or so, much of the knowledge gained in this area supports the tenet of the original Davis model (12,55,56).

An important component of the Davis model, which dealt specifically with cochlear hair cells, was the suggested role of the resting potential of the fluid of the scala media, i.e., the endolymphatic potential (57), as noted previously. Generated, again, by the stria vascularis, the endolymphatic potential is thought to provide an extra pressure for driving current through the hair cell (53). The endolymphatic potential and membrane resting potential of the hair cell are analogous to two batteries that are wired in series, thus essentially doubling the transmembrane potential of the hair cell. As the cochlear potentials (discussed in the following) are readily modified by changes in the endolymphatic potential, a normal endolymphatic potential is essential for a truly normally functioning hearing organ (12,58).

Cochlear Hair Cell

Cochlear hair cells in humans and other mammals are notably different in morphology than the "generic" hair cell described previously, starting with the fact that they have no kinocilia. However, considerable anatomic and electrophysiologic evidence indicates that the stereocilia atop cochlear hair cells also are directionally sensitive, and there are morphologic indicators (59). One is the organization of the stereocilia of outer hair cells (OHCs).

A characteristic W-shaped pattern is formed by these hairs, which are present is several rows that vary in height, i.e., from short to tall moving radially away from the cochlear modiolus and with the tallest row at the base of the "W," also away from the modiolus. Maximal excitation of the hair cell occurs when displacement of the stereocilia is in the direction of their tallest row, toward the base of the "W." Optimal displacement thus occurs when the stereocila are deflected in a radial direction (Fig. 9) (59,60).

The recent discovery of fine linkages between the stereocilia called "cross links" and "tip links" provides yet another compelling morphologic signpost of the direction of depolarizing deflection of the hairs (61,62). The cross links are horizontally oriented (with respect to the hair-bearing surface of the cell) and are believed to subserve stiffening of the hair bundle. Tip links, however, are oriented almost vertically near the upper end of the hairs and are thought to play a significant role in the transduction process. Specifically, tip links may act as molecular gates to regulate the flow of current into and out of the hair cell via ion channels in the stereocilia themselves. The tip links are aligned radially in a manner that connects each stereocilium in a shorter row of hairs to one in the next taller row.

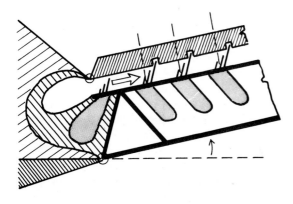

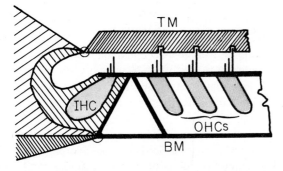

FIG. 9. Mode of shearing displacements (radially) of the stereocilia in response to displacements ("vertically") of the basilar membrane (BM). IHC, inner hair cell; OHC, outer hair cell; TM, tectorial membrane. [Adapted from Ryan and Dallos (60). From Durrant JD, Lovrinic JH. *Bases of hearing science,* 3rd ed. Baltimore: Williams and Wilkins, 1995;149, with permission.]

Given the ciliary properties, a crucial problem in stimulating cochlear sensory cells is how to cause radial deflection of the hairs via the up-and-down vibratory motion of the CP. A plausible solution to this puzzle involves the structural relation between the tectorial membrane (TM) and BM, which constitute the upper and lower boundaries, respectively, of the CP. As illustrated in Fig. 9, the tectorial membrane (TM) pivots effectively at the lip of the internal sulcus, whereas the BM, on which the organ of Corti sits, effectively pivots at or near its attachment to the osseous spiral lamina. The net effect is that up-and-down vibration of the CP creates a radial shear between the units. Also, as shown in Fig. 9, the stereocilia are normally stiff (63), and the tallest row of OHC hairs are attached to the undersurface of the TM (64). Thus, the radial, shearing movement created by the up-and-down displacement of the CP leads to the appropriate deflection of the OHC stereocilia (remembering that the hairs are linked to each other).

The mode of displacement of the inner hair cell (IHC) stereocilia is less obvious than that of the OHCs, primarily because the IHC hairs are, at best, only lightly coupled to the TM. However, it should be remembered that this is a fluid-filled system, and fluids have the property of viscosity. Displacement of the CP sets this fluid into motion at a certain velocity (related to the frequency of displacement). The viscous drag of the fluid moving across the top of the IHCs, in turn, displaces their stereocilia (60). Consequently, the response of the OHCs reflects the displacement of the CP, whereas the velocity at which this displacement occurs is the effective input of the IHCs (65). Actually, both velocity and displacement responses have been observed electrophysiologically for IHCs (66). However, the latter is small at best, given the lack of tight coupling between the IHC stereocilia and the TM. This particular characteristic (i.e., the degree of coupling between the stereocilia and the TM) represents one of the several anatomic features clearly pointing to different roles for IHCs versus OHCs.

Macromechanics to Micromechanics Interface

As described previously, the essential mechanical event for exciting cochlear hair cells is the back-and-forth bending of their cilia, which results (again) from the up-and-down vibration of the CP. The basis of this motion, revealed by the classic experiments of Georg von Bekesy (67), is illustrated in Fig. 10A. The input to the cochlea is represented by the oval window, which communicates with the scala vestibuli. The round window, which seals the scala tympani, serves as the outlet for pressure changes introduced to the system at its input. Although the helicotrema represents an opening through which pressure changes in cochlear fluid between the scalae vestibuli and tympani can be accommodated, this only occurs in humans at very low frequencies (68). In other

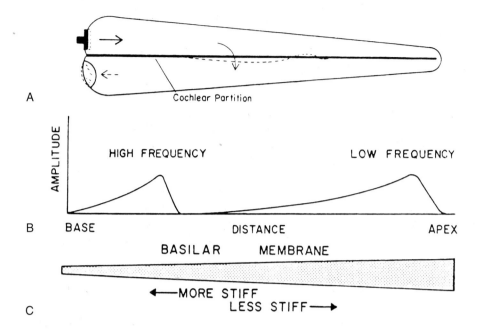

FIG. 10. A: Mode of displacement of the basilar membrane, actually the entire cochlear partition, in response to stapes displacement. **B:** Envelopes of overall peak magnitudes displacements of the cochlear partition due to the formation of traveling waves at different frequencies. **C:** Change of basilar membrane width, and consequently stiffness, from base to apex. [Adaptation of drawings by Durrant and Lovrinic (2), based on drawings and data of Bekesy (67) and data of Rhode (72). From Durrant JD. Physical and physiologic bases of hearing. In: Bluestone CD, Stool SE, Kenna MA, eds. *Pediatric otolaryngology, volume 1,* 3rd ed. Philadelphia: WB Saunders, 1996:127–149, with permission.]

words, throughout most of the audible frequency range, the helicotrema remains functionally closed. Rather, inward movement of the stapes footplate creates a positive pressure in the fluid of the scala vestibuli. This pressure from above displaces the flexible CP downward, which pushes the fluid of the scala tympani and causes the membranous round window to bulge outward into the middle ear space. Outward movement of the footplate creates the opposite effect, resulting in upward displacement of the CP and inward movement of the round window. Thus, inward-outward movement of the footplate at the oval window sets the CP into "sympathetic" vibration with the stapes.

In Fig. 10A, the cochlea is uncoiled for illustrative purposes, and the CP is represented as a single membrane separating the two perilymphatic scalae. Displacement of the CP produced by the inward-outward movement of the stapes is not uniform along its entire length. Rather, a traveling wave is initiated at its basal end that continues to grow as it moves apically until it reaches a crest, whereupon it decays very rapidly (67). The site where the traveling wave crests, in turn, is uniquely related to the frequency of vibration of the stapes. It is important to note that the mechanics of the CP responsible for this phenomena are determined extensively by the physical properties of the BM. As shown in Fig. 10B, high-frequency stimulation produces a traveling wave that peaks in the base of the cochlea, whereas maximum displacement of the traveling wave for low-frequency stimuli occurs in the apex. It is in this way that frequency is transformed into place of excitation. The ability of the central auditory system to utilize this transformation is addressed elsewhere in this book (see Chapter 6).

Although a description of how traveling waves occur is a matter too involved to delve into here, the primary para-

meter that governs their behavior is simple to describe. As shown in Fig. 10C, the width of the BM increases toward the apex of the cochlea. However, the crucial parameter associated with this characteristic is an accompanying stiffness gradient of the BM (67,69). Because the BM is approximately ten times wider at the apex of the cochlea than it is at the base, it is nearly 100 times more flexible. This dramatic decrease in the stiffness of the BM as it extends from base to apex provides the basis for a unique mechanical system that efficiently handles a broad range of frequencies. Of course, there are several other aspects of the CP in addition to the stiffness gradient of the BM that contributes to the detailed mechanical events of the cochlea. These include such microstructural features as the change in number, length, and stiffness of the stereocilia, the angle of orientation of the W pattern, and/or the TM-stereocilia interface from base to apex (59,70).

Conclusion—Cochlear Mechanics Are Active (or The Outer Hair Cells Are Special)

Although it is widely accepted that BM displacement is the effective stimulus of the hearing organs, this notion is not without historical controversy. Earlier estimates had suggested that the degree displacement of the BM needed to stimulate hair cells at just detectable levels of sound must be on the order of the diameter of a hydrogen atom, or even less! It was difficult to conceive of such minute displacements, let alone how they would be sufficient to lead to significant movement of the stereocilia. These estimates, however, were based on the assumption that the system behaves linearly. It is now well accepted that the motion of the BM is nonlinear, and that the system is compressive (i.e., displays a saturating input-output relationship; Fig. 11) (59,71–73). It was recognized only rela-

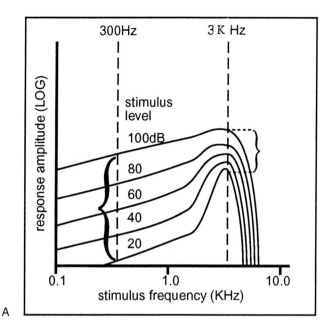

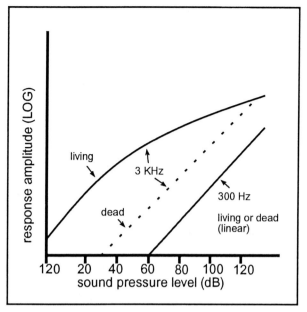

FIG. 11. A: Relative displacement of the basilar membrane in the live cochlea at a given point of observation—in this illustration, "place" of characteristic frequency (CF) = 3 kHz. **B:** Displacement input-output functions under indicated conditions, contrasting displacement at CF in the live versus dead cochlea and between CF and a much lower frequency. [Courtesy of J. Siegel, Northwestern University, Evanston, Illinois. From Durrant JD, Lovrinic JH. *Bases of hearing science,* 3rd ed. Baltimore: Williams and Wilkins, 1995;158 with permission.]

tively recently that nonlinearity not only occurs during sound transduction by the hearing organ, but it is an essential aspect of the hair cell transduction process (74).

Even with this knowledge at hand, it still is difficult to explain how the ear detects the minute stimulus intensities represented by normal hearing thresholds (i.e., perhaps involving no more than 0.3 nM [or 3×10^{-10} M] deflection at the tips of the stereocilia) (59). Our understanding of this process has been facilitated during the last decade or so by research involving the role of the OHCs. It is now clear that the OHCs are crucial to the remarkable sensitivity of the ear—not so much as receptors, but as effectors! The OHCs have a "dual personality" (i.e., sensory and motor), dominated perhaps by their motoric function. The presence of contractile proteins in the stereocilia and other parts of the hair cell provide anatomic evidence for this phenomenon. For example, actin is present in the fiberlike structure of the stereocilia, whereas myosin is abundant in the cuticular plate. Actin and myosin interact to cause contractions in muscle tissue. Although the configuration of these proteins in the structure of hair cells is nothing like that of muscle cells, their presence in hair cells suggests the prospect of contractile movements of the hairs or the hair cell itself (75). One of the most exciting of recent findings in hearing science is that the lengths of isolated OHCs change in reaction to an applied electrical field (76,77). Thus, the cell presumably can change its length *in situ* in response to

stimulation by virtue of its own receptor potential. Given the tight degree of coupling between OHC stereocilia and the TM, changes in the length of the hair cell would be expected to alter the mechanical properties of the CP, whether or not transduction leads to significant movement of the partition (78). Thus it is apparent that the OHCs do not just passively "go along for the ride" during the transduction process. They play an "active" role that accounts for the wide dynamic range, exquisite sensitivity, and precise frequency discrimination associated with human hearing (74).

PERIPHERAL NEURAL ENCODING OF SOUND AND BASIC AUDITORY INFORMATION PROCESSING

Frequency

The hair cells and central nervous system are connected via the primary auditory neurons that richly innervate the organ of Corti. The response area of an individual neuron, in turn, can be examined using microelectrodes (79). The SPL for a criterion increase in spike discharge rate (above the spontaneous rate) is plotted as a function of stimulus frequency. Figure 12A displays such a function, which is somewhat analogous to a minimum audibility curve. The resultant plot is referred to a "tuning curve." As shown in Fig. 12a, the tuning curve of an individual auditory neuron

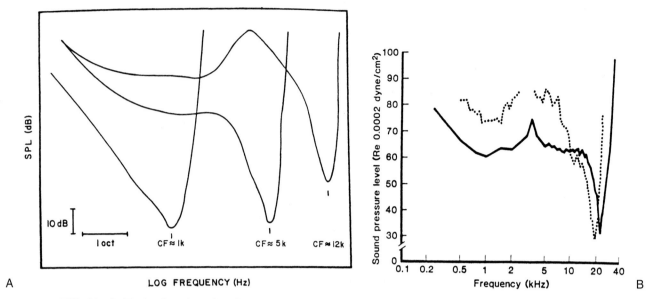

FIG. 12. A: Tuning functions (in effect, "audiograms") of single primary auditory neurons (cat)—sound pressure level (SPL in dB) for criterion spike discharge rates as a function of frequency. [Based on data of Kiang and Moxon (80), as presented by Zwicker (83)]. **B:** Comparison of tuning functions for the response of the basilar membrane (*solid line,* SPL as function of frequency required for 3 × 108 cm basilar membrane displacement in base of cat cochlea) versus that a single-unit tuning function [Khanna and Leonard (81) (*dotted line graph,* data from different animal and laboratory, courtesy of M. C. Liberman)]. [Adapted from Durrant and Lovrinic (2). From Durrant JD. Physical and physiologic bases of hearing. In: Bluestone CD, Stool SE, Kenna MA, eds. *Pediatric otolaryngology, volume 1,* 3rd ed. Philadelphia: WB Saunders, 1996:127–149, with permission.]

has a sharp minimum or peak of sensitivity at one characteristic frequency (CF). The value of the CF depends on the site of origin of the neuron along the BM. Consequently, neurons with high CFs innervate the basal regions of the cochlea, whereas low-frequency neurons innervate apical hair cells. It also is evident from Fig. 12A that, although primary neurons are selective in their sensitivity to a particular CF, they are not insensitive to other frequencies. However, the rolloff in sensitivity is much steeper for frequencies above versus those below the CF, particularly once the SPL has been increased by approximately 40 dB above the level needed for the CF to evoke a discharge (80).

The question that has baffled researchers for years is what accounts for the observed pattern of the tuning function, especially the degree of frequency sensitivity represented by the tip region around the CF. Is this extraordinary selectivity attributable to the cochlear hydromechanical events described earlier, or is there an additional (i.e., second) "filter" between the receptor and nerve cells? The answer is now known to be the former. As illustrated in Fig. 12B, the peripheral mechanical events provide all the selectivity necessary to account for the precise tuning of auditory neurons (81,82). Psychoacoustic tuning curves (83), involving the entire auditory pathway, show little increase in selectivity over the tuning functions of single primary auditory neurons; therefore, it appears that cochlear mechanics essentially account for the frequency

discrimination ability of the auditory system. As discussed later, however, some central processing is essential for pitch perception, particularly for complex sounds such as speech. This is because the spectral elements of such sounds create complex patterns of BM motion due to overlapping traveling waves (84). It is even possible, through tedious and meticulous electrophysiologic experiments, to reconstruct the overall pattern of BM motion from activity recorded from nerve fibers throughout the acoustic nerve (85). However, the resultant "perception" of such sounds requires interpretation of these events at the level of the central nervous system.

As described previously, auditory neurons leave the hearing organ in an orderly fashion with respect to their CF. Given the tuning of each neuron, due in turn to the tuning of each place along the BM, the hearing organ behaves as a bank or array of bandpass filters, each connected to the central nervous system via a primary auditory neuron (Fig. 13A). The resulting frequency-to-place scheme is known as "tonotopic organization" (Fig. 13B). This scheme is well maintained centrally with tonotopic/cochleotopic organization being demonstrated for all major nuclei of the central pathways and, finally, the primary auditory cortex (86–88).

The pervasiveness of tonotopicity throughout the central auditory system bespeaks the importance of the place code in the encoding and processing of frequency information. However, place of excitation, again, is not

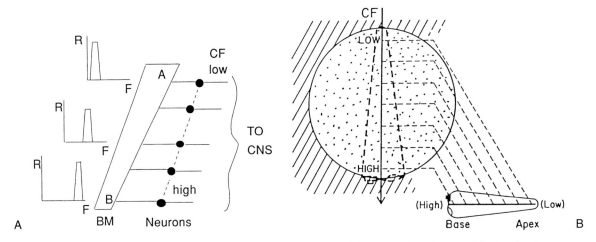

FIG. 13. A: Concept of bank of cochlear filters (only three of the more than 30 possible for simultaneous/broadband stimulation) created effectively by the frequency-to-place transformation of the traveling waves. **B:** Concept of tonotopical organization; by virtue of the orderly "wiring" of the cochlea to the brain stem, via neurons in **A**, a tonal map of the cochlea is projected onto an auditory nucleus. An electrode traversing the nucleus in the appropriate direction encounters neurons with systematically progressing characteristic frequencies (CF), reflecting the "places" of the first-order neurons peripherally. (Based on drawings from Durrant JD, Lovrinic JH. *Bases of hearing science,* 3rd ed. Baltimore: Williams and Wilkins, 1995;221.)

the only cue for frequency perception. Auditory neurons also show considerable ability to encode temporal features of the stimulus. It once was thought that auditory neurons used a simple volley mechanism to do this, because their maximum firing rate renders them incapable of following each cycle of the stimulus except at relatively low frequencies, i.e., on the order of a few hundred hertz at most (89). As illustrated in Fig. 14, a more statistical concept is now used to describe how the temporal pattern of discharges is used for interpreting

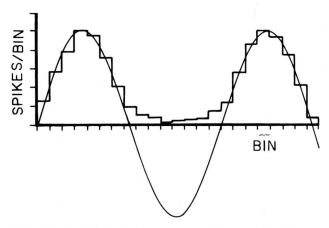

FIG. 14. Periodicity in the pattern of neural discharges reflected by a histogram of the spikes occurring in each time bin over the period observed. [Based on Brugge et al. (90). From Durrant JD. Physical and physiologic bases of hearing. In: Bluestone CD, Stool SE, Kenna MA, eds. *Pediatric oto-laryngology, volume 1,* 3rd ed. WB Philadelphia: Saunders, 1996:127–149, with permission.]

frequency information. Here, it is shown that, although individual discharges are are not locked to a particular phase of the time history or waveform of the stimulus, their probability of occurrence at any time does reflect the stimulus waveform (90,91). It is in this way that auditory neurons appear to be capable of representing the periodicity of the stimulus, at least for frequencies up to 5,000 Hz. This information then is extracted by the central system to provide a sense of fundamental pitch as well as other temporal discriminations needed for the encoding and processing of complex sounds. Thus, the auditory system functions, in part, as a high-speed temporal processor and not solely as a high-speed or (virtually) real-time spectrum analyzer.

Intensity

In addition to frequency, the intensity of sound must be encoded for neural transmission to, and processing by, the central auditory system. At the first level of encoding, the auditory system, like most sensory systems, translates intensity into spike discharge rate (Fig. 15A) (92). Thus, the more intense the stimulus, the higher the rate of discharge of the auditory neuron. There are limits to this, however. First, the stimulus must be strong enough to cause a significant increase in discharges above the background (spontaneous) rate. A possible exception to this is that the temporal pattern of discharges, with or without a net increase in firing rate, may serve as a code for intensity, at least at relatively low frequencies (91). The second limitation is that the discharge rate ultimately saturates. At CF, saturation of firing rate typically occurs at only 20 to 30

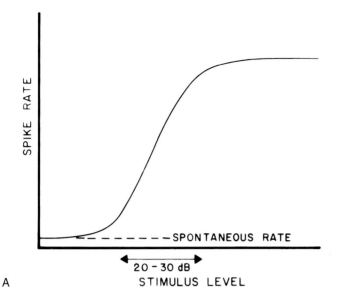

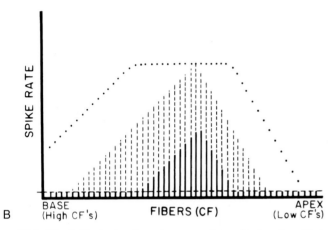

FIG. 15. A: Typical spike rate versus intensity function (first-order neuron) monitored at the characteristic frequency. [Based on data from the cat from Kiang (92).] **B:** Hypothetical histogram type of plot of the spike rate of an array of fibers and limit imposed by saturation of spike rates (*dotted line*). [Modified after Whitfield (95). From Durrant JD, Lovrinic JH. *Bases of hearing science,* 3rd ed. Baltimore: Williams and Wilkins, 1995;226, with permission.]

dB. Off CF, saturation may occur some 40 dB or more beyond the intensity needed to cause a significant increase in discharges over the spontaneous rate (93,94).

The saturation effect described raises an interesting question regarding dynamic ranges at different levels or for different functions of the auditory system. Namely, if the dynamic range of a single neuron near CF is only 20 to 40 dB, how is it that the dynamic range measured behaviorally is 140 dB (refer back to Fig. 1)? A plausible, but not infallible, answer to this puzzling question involves the number of neurons firing at any time (as opposed to the number of firings per neuron). Although primary neurons are finely tuned, they still respond to

frequencies other than their CF if the stimulus in intense enough. This is because the traveling wave represents a pattern or region of displacement, not a discrete point of vibration. Thus, as stimulus intensity increases, spread of excitation occurs (Fig. 15B). The central auditory system, in turn, sees the total density of neural discharges resulting from increased levels of stimulation, even after the individual neurons tuned to the stimulus have saturated (95,96). The role of "off-frequency" listening remains controversial (97), but spread of excitation is unquestionably a factor in the growth of compound nerve potentials that can be evoked by sound stimuli and recorded by electrophysiologic methods (see following). Neural responses, however, are only one of several sound-evoked responses that may be recorded and that, in turn, provide objective indicators of the activation of the auditory periphery.

INNERVATION OF THE HEARING ORGAN–FUNCTIONAL IMPLICATIONS AND POSSIBLE CONSEQUENCES

The auditory periphery uses both afferent and efferent neurons and, thus, bidirectional communication with the central auditory system. Only the OHCs, however, receive direct efferent innervation (i.e., with nerve endings directly terminating on the hair cell). Efferent endings in the vicinity of IHCs tend to terminate on associated afferent nerve endings (Fig. 16) (98–100). Various afferent and efferent transmitter substances have been identified in the body and, in turn, suggested as cochlear transmitters. The afferent transmitter released by hair cells still is debated, but glutamate or a similar substance is the strongest candidate. The efferent transmitter appears to be acetylcholine (101).

There is a descending pathway that more or less parallels the ascending pathway(s) (see Chapter 6), although it is less well established in neuroanatomic detail or function (102). The best known part of the efferent system on both counts is the olivocochlear system (Fig. 16), which is the part of the pathway that provides the efferent endings just described (99). The olivocochlear fibers course from the superior olivary complex through the internal auditory meatus to the organ of Corti as bundles bilaterally within the vestibular part of the eighth cranial nerves. There are crossed and uncrossed fibers in the olivocochlear bundles (OCBs), constituting two distinct subsystems—the medial and lateral olivocochlear bundles. The fibers in the medial olivocochlear bundles project from areas in the vicinity of the medial superior olives, are relatively large in diameter and myelinated, innervate the OHCs, and follow both crossed and uncrossed paths. The fibers of the lateral olivocochlear bundles, however, originate from areas near the lateral superior olive, are small in diameter and unmyelinated, and make synapses on the afferents from the IHCs.

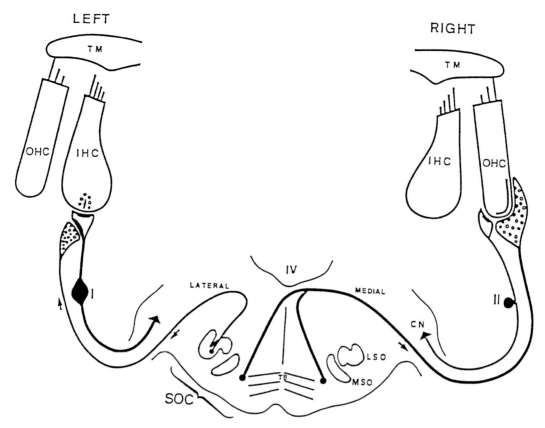

FIG. 16. Schematic diagram of lateral and crossed and uncrossed medial olivocochlear fibers and their termination on outer hair cells (OHC) or neurons (afferent, type I, bipolar) innervating inner hair cells (IHC). CN, cochlear nucleus: type II, pseudomonopolar neuron; IV, fourth ventricle; LSO, lateral superior olive; MSO, medial superior olive; SOC, superior olivary complex; TM, tectorial membrane. (Adapted from Eybalin M. Neurotransmitters and neuromodulators of the mammalian cochlea. *Physiol Rev* 1993;73:309–373.)

This interesting dichotomy of innervation further underscores the special characteristics of the OHCs, yet it seems entirely consistent with the presumption of a motoric function of the OHCs, as does the pattern of afferent innervation of the hair cells. Here, of course, the IHCs are dominant, receiving the vast majority of nerve endings and representing the vast majority of nerve fibers in general (i.e., approximately 95%) (103, 104). Numerous afferent fibers innervate individual IHCs. These neurons are largely bipolar, type I, neurons that have relatively large-diameter axons that are myelinated. The more numerous OHCs thus must share a small minority of the afferent neurons. Consequently, one afferent neuron branches to many OHCs, and these tend to be pseudomonopolar or type II neurons that, in turn, have relatively small-diameter unmyelinated axons. The complete innervation scheme is dichotomous and bespeaks a mode of operation in which the IHCs essentially do all the listening. The question is whether there are significant effects of activation of the efferents.

That the olivocochlear fibers have the potential to act directly on the periphery has been clearly demonstrated experimentally. For example, electrical stimulation via electrodes placed in the floor of the fourth ventricle leads to changes in the cochlear potentials and suppression of the whole-nerve action potentials (105). The olivocochlear bundle fibers have been found to be spontaneously active in awake animals and have been shown to respond to sound stimuli. Research has revealed afferentlike tuning properties in the auditory efferents (106,107). What is unclear, however, is the extent to which the olivocochlear bundles influence the periphery under natural, real-world/real-time operation. The seeming paradox is that there are relatively few efferent fibers compared to the number of afferent fibers. These several-hundred-plus fibers clearly are much less numerous than OHCs; consequently, the innervation pattern is divergent (100), as also is the case for afferent innervation of these cells. Each efferent neuron gives rise to tens of nerve endings. At first glance, then, this scheme does not seem to offer fine control. However, because the majority of efferent endings terminate on OHCs and the OHCs contribute significantly to the sensitivity and frequency resolution of the hearing organ, efferent activation has the potential to substantially influence the cochlear analysis of sound, perhaps in a frequency-specific manner. Yet, complete sectioning of the efferents, as most likely occurs in cases of vestibular neurotomy in the treatment of intractable dizziness, appears to cause little change in hearing ability (108).

Definitive effects of efferent activation by natural/sound stimulation have been demonstrated in animals (109,110), although results have not been as compelling as those realized with direct electrical stimulation. The measurement of otoacoustic emissions (OAEs) during contralateral stimulation has provided a research tool particularly applicable to humans (111,112). OAEs are sound-evoked acoustic responses of the hearing organ, attributed to OHC motility (see following). Thus, the OAEs excited in one ear have been shown to be depressed. The effect is greatly reduced or eliminated in cases of vestibular neurotomy (113). The reduction in OAEs observed, however, is typically only a few decibels or less (depending on the method of measurement/analysis), but this may be more significant if the role of the efferents is to enhance signal-to-noise ratio in the system, as has been proposed (114,115). Whereas this and various other issues remain to be resolved, it seems clear that the efferent and acoustic (middle ear) reflexes together provide some amount of feedback to the auditory periphery (Fig. 17). It is attractive to suppose that the two reflexes work symbiotically to enhance signal-to-noise ratio (28,29). This notion, however, only raises more questions [e.g., can these systems function quickly enough for real-time speech processing (116)?], so this area can be expected to continue to be one of active research, fervent debate, and growing clinical interests.

SOUND-EVOKED RESPONSES OF THE COCHEAR HAIR CELLS AND THE AUDITORY NERVE AND APPLICATIONS

Much of the information presented in this chapter was derived from experiments involving single unit recordings in animals (other than humans). Such approaches allow investigators to measure the electrical responses of single cells with microelectrodes near or even within these cells. However, there are numerous gross or compound potentials that also can be recorded from the auditory system with electrodes placed on the surface of the skin (e.g., on the scalp, or in the ear canal) or via minimally invasive methods, in general. Evoked responses represent inherently the activity of many cells (receptor, neural, or other) but have provided valuable electrophysiologic indices for use in basic and applied research of auditory function. Most also are recordable in humans and have emerged as important clinical tools. A brief description of the most clinically useful responses is provided here.

Electrocochleography

Electrocochleography is a technique for recording the stimulus-related potentials of the cochlea and auditory nerve (see also Chapter 13). The resultant waveform is referred to as an electrocochleogram. Three potentials (two receptor and one neural) comprise the electrocochleogram; the receptor potentials in question are the cochlear microphonic and summating potential (12). Figure 18 displays cochlear microphonic and summating potential waveforms in response to a tone burst stimulus (bottom tracing). An electrode placed within the cochlea or on the round window or promontory will pick up these potentials simultaneously. With the application of signal processing, the electrode can be placed at more remote (and noninvasive) sites, such as the eardrum or ear canal. The waveform of the

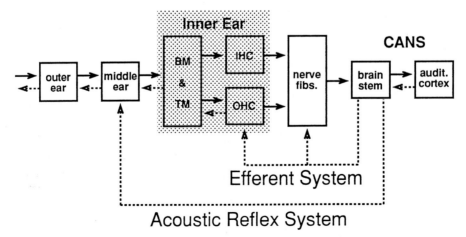

FIG. 17. Block diagram of the feedback control circuit of the auditory periphery. BM, basilar membrane; CANS, central auditory nervous system; IHC, inner hair cell; OHC, outer hair cell; nerve fibs., primary, afferent auditory nerve fibers; TM, tectorial membrane. [After Dallos (28). From Durrant JD, Lovrinic JH. *Bases of hearing science,* 3rd ed. Baltimore: Williams and Wilkins, 1995;243, with permission.]

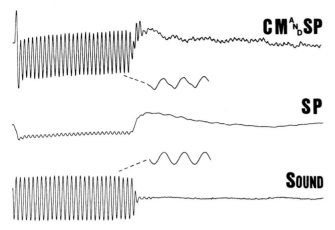

FIG. 18. Cochlear microphonic (CM) and summating potential (SP), obtained via intracochlear recording in guinea pig, in response to a tone burst (Sound). **Insets** provide detailed comparison of CM and Sound, suggesting some distortion in the CM (in this case due to cochlear distortion). (From Durrant JD. Auditory physiology and an auditory physiologist's view of tinnitus. *J Laryngol Otol* 1981; [Suppl 4]: 21–28, with permission.)

cochlear microphonic mimics the electrical waveform of the acoustic stimulus. Thus, as shown in Fig. 18, if the stimulus is a tone burst, the cochlear microphonic will appear as a sinusoidal pulse. However, as also shown in Fig. 18 (top tracing), the cochlear microphonic will often appear to be offset (i.e., the zero axis is shifted above or

below the baseline of the recording). This direct-current shift represents the summating potential, which can be seen more clearly if the cochlear microphonic is filtered (via low-pass filtering) or averaged (via phase cancellation) out (Fig. 18, middle tracing). For the most part, the cochlear microphonic and summating potential are products of the mechanoelectric transduction processes of the hair cells. In a normal cochlea, the electrical responses of the OHCs dominate these grossly recorded potentials (12), but as recorded outside of the cochlea, presumably by conduction through the round window, the summating potential appears to reflect contributions from both types of hair cells (117). In any event, both the summating potential and cochlear microphonic can provide useful indices of hydromechanical events in the cochlea and reflect the integrity of the hair cells (12,117–119).

The other component potential of the electrocochleogram is the whole-nerve action potential, i.e., of the auditory nerve. The action potential, as typically recorded, represents the summed discharges of thousands of auditory nerve fibers. As shown in Fig. 19, this generally occurs at the onset and offset of a sound stimulus, at which time the primary neurons are responding most vigorously and in a synchronized manner (119). Although each individual neural discharge is an all-or-none phenomenon, the magnitude of the whole-nerve action potential varies in proportion to the number of neurons firing (120). In general, the most robust action potentials tend to be obtained in

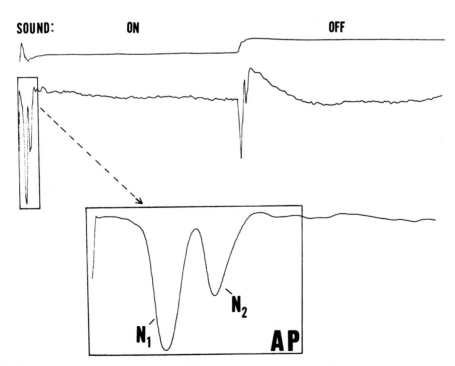

FIG. 19. The whole-nerve action potential (AP and components N1 and N2; time base expanded in **inset**), obtained via intracochlear recording in guinea pig. Precise timing of sound activation of the organ of Corti was demarked in this recording by concurrent measurement of the summating potential. Note occurrence of onset and offset APs, although the onset response is more robust. (From Durrant JD. Auditory physiology and an auditory physiologist's view of tinnitus. *J Laryngol Otol* 1981;[Suppl 4]: 21–28, with permission.)

response to a broadband transient stimulus such as the acoustic "click," created by applying a brief (100-μs) direct-current pulse to an earphone. This is because the click has an abrupt onset and offset and broad spectrum that simultaneously excites numerous neurons. However, because synchronization of neural firing is best for neurons originating in the base of the cochlea (i.e., high-frequency fibers), due to the high velocity of the traveling wave there, the action potential response to a click tends to be biased toward the basal end of the cochlea (121). Still apical-ward activity can be elicited and registered with the use of more frequency-specific stimuli and other techniques. Like the cochlear microphonic and summating potential, the action potential also can be recorded from inside or outside the cochlea, including the earlobe.

Recording at extracochlear sites is not without costs. Sensitivity, in particular, decreases systematically as the distance between the recording electrode and response generators increases. Thus, the magnitude of a response recorded with an electrode at the promontory will be considerably larger than the magnitude of recordings from the ear canal or eardrum, and the potentials continue to decrease systematically as the recording electrode is moved laterally along the canal (122). Measurements from the promontory and more distant extracochlear sites require appropriate methods of recording and signal processing–computer-based signal averaging (123,124). Although maximum sensitivity is achieved with transtympanic approaches (123), extratympanic electrocochleography, especially via an electrode on the eardrum (125), has been shown to have a variety of useful clinical applications (124,126). Nevertheless, for limited purposes, the action potential component is accessible strictly via surface

recording techniques (e.g., one electrode at the vertex and the other on the earlobe or mastoid).

As shown in Fig. 20, the action potential constitutes the first wave of the sequence of short-latency components, the so-called brainstem auditory evoked response (i.e., auditory evoked potentials with peaks occurring 10 ms or less after the stimulus; see Chapter 13). Still, as seen in Fig. 20, electrocochleography via ear canal or "deeper" recording techniques is useful for enhancing brainstem recordings, allowing for better definition of the first wave (i.e., the action potential) (127). This is especially useful in cases of significant peripheral hearing loss and is important in differential diagnosis (see Chapter 13).

Measurement of Otoacoustic Emissions

von Bekesy (67), approximately a half century ago, found that he could not fully account for distortion observed in the ear canal from results of distortion analysis of the stimulus transducer. In a similar time frame, a scientist by the name of Gold proposed an active model of hair cell transduction implying the feedback of some sound energy that, in turn, must be emitted from the cochlea, back into the external ear canal. However, it is only relatively recently that the presence of such "cochlear echoes"—now known as OAEs—has been confirmed by delicate sound recordings in humans (128). Some two decades after its discovery, the OAE has become one of the most extensively studied phenomena in physiologic acoustics (129). Although not an electrophysiologic response *per se*, their measurement is accomplished by similar instrumentation and analyses, and OAEs provide clear signs of the reaction of the hearing organ to sound. Most intriguing, they appear

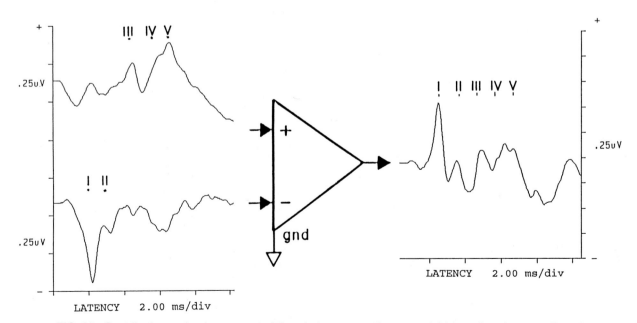

FIG. 20. Contribution and enhancement of the whole-nerve action potential (wave I) to the recording of the "auditory brainstem response" (waves I to V) via combined electrocochleography (electrode on tympanic membrane) and scalp-electrode recordings in a human subject. A click stimulus was presented via a tubal insert earphone (11.1/s at 90-dB normal hearing level).

to reflect uniquely (at least under certain stimulus conditions) the active micromechanical process of OHC transduction, i.e., hair cell motility.

OAEs are recorded from the ear canal via a very sensitive miniature microphone and small efficient transducers for sound generation, packaged essentially in an earplug-sized probe assembly (130). Computer signal processing techniques are used, similar to methods used for extratympanic electrocochleography and other evoked potential measurements. Figure 21 illustrates a click-evoked OAE, one of several OAE measures available. Confirmation that OAEs originate from the interior of the cochlea is based on several factors: (a) the acoustic response has a latency and persists beyond a mere reflection (i.e. echo) off of the eardrum; (b) OAEs are highly vulnerable to adverse metabolic conditions; (c) they are absent in cases of partial or complete cochlear deafness (and in dummy/test cavities simulating the volume of the ear canal); and (d) they grow nonlinearly with stimulus level or manifest other nonlinearities (128–132). In addition to clicks, which tend to be the most popular stimulus for clinical/screening paradigms, OAEs can be elicited by brief tones and continuous sounds (129). Many normal-hearing adults and most newborns produce emissions in the absence of external stimulation. These spontaneous OAEs may appear at one to five or more frequencies (129,133). Finally, distortion products in the OAE, as suggested by von Bekesy's observations and as implied previously, also can be recorded. These include the cubic distortion product $2f_1 - f_2$, which is of primary interest for research and clinical applications (134).

OAE and other evoked response testing and their clinical applications are discussed in more detail elsewhere in this book (see Chapter 14). This summary is intended merely as an introduction, but demonstrates the robust signals available to clinicians and researchers alike to determine, monitor, or quantify the activation of the auditory periphery. The workings of the peripheral system thus are more accessible than ever, and in rather intimate ways. As noted, the advent of OAE measurement has opened the door to still other aspects of auditory function activation of the auditory efferents, which again interface most extensively with the OHCs. Accessibility of this system in humans is particularly exciting as the descending pathways and their contribution to audition have been elusive. Evoked response technology thus may be expected to provide useful information and tools for years to come.

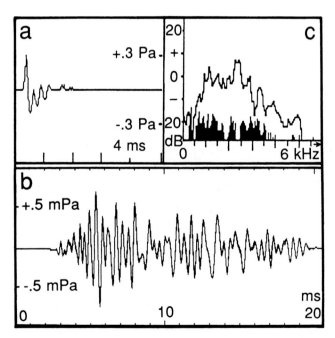

FIG. 21. Recording of the transient (click-evoked) otoacoustic emission (OAE). **A:** Click stimulus. **B:** Amplified and windowed recording to emphasize the OAE itself (i.e., effectively removing the stimulus waveform). **C:** Spectra of the OAE (*white*) and noise floor of the recording (*black*). (From Durrant JD. Physical and physiologic bases of hearing. In: Bluestone CD, Stool SE, Kenna MA, eds. *Pediatric otolaryngology, volume 1,* 3rd ed. Philadelphia: WB Saunders, 1996:127–149, with permission.)

SUMMARY POINTS

- The auditory periphery represents the front end of an exquisitely sensitive system, capable of very fine discriminations among sounds. As such, it must accomplish the transduction of the energy in the sound and encode it into a signal of neural discharges destined for the brain.
- The most peripheral components of the system function as acousticomechanical transformers to enhance efficiency of the transduction process. In so doing, the outer and middle ears shape the sensitivity per frequency of the system.
- The outer ear provides the bases for monaural (vertical plane) and binaural (horizontal plane) localization of sound.
- The middle ear system also includes one of the two feedback mechanisms by which the central auditory system may exercise some control over the periphery (i.e., via the acoustic reflex).
- The coupling of energy to the hair cells, the sensory-specific transducer cells of the organ of Corti, involves some of the finest structures found in the inner ear. In this process, frequency-to-place and timing codes are set up across the array of afferent neurons innervating the hair cells.
- The great dynamic range of operation of the auditory system is accomplished via nonlinear compression of the input signal (i.e., sound). Additional feedback control of the periphery derives from descending pathways, with the most direct influence being expressed through innervation of the OHC.
- The OHCs appear to play an active, rather than passive, role in the transduction of sound energy.

REFERENCES

1. Jesteadt W, Wier CC, Green DM. Intensity discrimination as a function of frequency and sensation level. *J Acoust Soc Am* 1977;61:169–177.
2. Durrant JD, Lovrinic JH. *Bases of hearing science,* 3rd ed. Baltimore: Williams and Wilkins, 1995.
3. Wier CC, Jesteadt W, Green DM. Frequency discrimination as a function of frequency and sensation level. *J Acoust Soc Am* 1977;61:178–184.
4. Corso JF. *The experimental psychology of sensory behavior.* New York: Holt, Rinehart and Winston, 1967.
5. Robinson DW, Dadson RS. A redetermination of the equal loudness relations for pure tones. *Br J Appl Phys* 1956;7:166–181.
6. Yeowart NS, Evans MJ. Thresholds of audibility for very low-frequency pure tones. *J Acoust Soc Am* 1974;55:814–818.
7. Wegel RL. Physical data and physiology of excitation of the auditory nerve. *Ann Otol Rhinol Laryngol* 1932;41:740–779.
8. Green DM. *An introduction to hearing.* Hillsdale, NJ: Lawrence Erlbaum Associates, 1976.
9. Sutter AH. Hearing conservation. In: Berger EH, Ward WD, Morrill JC, eds. *Noise and hearing conservation manual.* Akron, OH: American Industrial Hygiene Association, 1986;1–18.
10. Wever EG, Bray CM. The perception of low tones and the resonance volley theory. *J Psychol* 1937;3:101–114.
11. Kinsler LE, Frey AR. *Fundamentals of acoustics.* New York: John Wiley and Sons, 1962.
12. Dallos P. *The auditory periphery: biophysics and physiology.* New York: Academic Press, 1973.
13. Zwislocki J. Analysis of some auditory characteristics. In: Luce R, Bush R, Galenter E, eds. *Handbook of mathematical psychology, volume 3.* New York: John Wiley and Sons, 1965:197.
14. Zwislocki J. The role of the external and middle ear in sound transmission. In Eagles EL, ed. *The nervous system, volume 3. Human communication and its disorders.* New York, Raven Press, 1975;45–55.
15. Nedzelnitsky V. Measurement of sound pressure in the cochleae of anesthetized cats. In: Zwicker E, Terhardt E, eds. *Facts and models in hearing.* New York: Springer-Verlag, 1974:45–53.
16. Merchant SN, Ravicz ME, Rosowski JJ. Acoustic input impedance of the stapes and cochlea in human temporal bones. *Hear Res* 1996;97:30–45.
17. Rosowski JJ, Merchant SN, Ravicz ME. Middle ear mechanics of type IV and type V tympanoplasty: I. Model analysis and predictions. *Am J Otol* 1995;16:555–564.
18. Keefe DH, Ling R, Bulen JC. Method to measure acoustic impedance and reflection coefficient. *J Acoust Soc Am* 1992;91:470–485.
19. Keefe DH, Levi E. Maturation of the middle and external ears: acoustic power-based responses and reflectance tympanometry. *Ear Hear* 1996;17:361–373.
20. Tonndorf J, Khanna SM. The role of the tympanic membrane in middle ear transmission. *Ann Otolaryngol* 1970;79:743–753.
21. Moller AR. *Auditory physiology.* New York: Academic Press, 1983.
22. Merchant SN, Ravicz ME, Puria S, et al. Analysis of middle ear mechanics and application to diseased and reconstructed ears. *Am J Otol* 1997;18:139–154.
23. Sprague BH, Wiley TL, Block MG. Dynamics of acoustic reflex growth. *Audiology* 1981;20:15–40.
24. Cacace AT, Margolis RH, Relkin, EM. Short-term poststimulatory response characteristics of the human acoustic stapedius reflex: monotic and dichotic stimulation. *J Acoust Soc Am* 1992;91:203–214.
25. Guinan JJ, Peake WT. Middle-ear characteristics of anesthetized cats. *J Acoust Soc Am* 1967;41:1237–1261.
26. Borg E, Zakrisson, JE. The activity of the stapedius muscle in man during vocalization. *Acta Otolaryngol* 1975;79:325–333.
27. Durrant JD, Shallop JK. Effects of differing states of attention on acoustic reflex activity and temporary threshold shift. *J Acoust Soc Am.* 1969;46:907–913.
28. Dallos P. Cochlear neurobiology: revolutionary developments. *ASHA* 1988;30:50–56.
29. Liberman MC, Guinan JJ Jr. Feedback control of the auditory periphery: anti-masking effects of middle ear vs. olivocochlear efferents. *J Commun Disord* 1998;31(6):471–482.
30. Durrant JD. Fundamentals of sound generation. In: Moore EJ, ed. *Bases of auditory brain stem evoked responses.* New York: Grune & Stratton, 1983;15–49.
31. Shaw EAG. The external ear. In: Keidel WD, Neff WD, eds. *Handbook of sensory physiology, volume V/1. Auditory system: anatomy, physiology (ear).* New York: Springer-Verlag, 1974:455–490.
32. Wiener FM, Ross DA. The pressure distribution in the auditory canal in a progressive sound field. *J Acoust Soc Am* 1946;18:401–408.
33. Diercks KF, Jeffress LA. Interaural phase and the absolute threshold for tone. *J Acoust Soc Am* 1962;34:981–984.
34. Durlach NI, Colburn, HS. Binaural phenomena. In: Carterette EC, Friedman MP, eds. *Handbook of perception, volume 4. Hearing.* New York: Academic Press, 1978:365–466.
35. Middlebrooks JC, Green DM. Sound localization by human listeners. *Annu Rev Psychol* 1991;42:135–159.
36. Mills AW. Auditory localization. In: Tobias JV, ed. *Foundations of modern auditory theory, volume 1.* New York: Academic Press, 1972:303–348.
37. Yost WA, Gourevitch G, eds. *Directional hearing.* New York: Springer-Verlag, 1987.
38. Kuhn GF. Physical acoustics and measurements pertaining to directional hearing. In: Yost WA, Gourevitch G, eds. *Directional hearing.* New York: Springer-Verlag, 1987:3–25.
39. Butler RA, Helwig CC. The spatial attributes of stimulus frequency in the median sagittal plane and their role in sound localization. *Am J Otolaryngol* 1983;4:165–173.
40. Wightman FL, Kistler DJ, et al. A new approach to the study of human sound localization. In: Yost WA, Gourevitch G, eds. *Directional hearing.* New York: Springer-Verlag, 1987:26–48.
41. Naftalin L, Harrison MS. Circulation of labyrinthine fluids. *J Laryngol Otol* 1958;72:118–136
42. Salt AN, Thalmann R. Cochlear fluid dynamics. In: Jahn AF, Santos-Sachi J, eds. *Physiology of the ear.* New York: Raven Press, 1988:341–357.
43. Palva T, Raunio V, Karma P, Ylikoski J. Fluid pathways in temporal bones. *Acta Otolaryngol* 1979;87:310–317.
44. Ritter FN, Lawrence M. A histological and experimental study of the cochlear aqueduct patency in the adult human. *Laryngoscope* 1965;75:1224–1233.
45. Wangemann P, Schacht J. Homeostatic mechanisms in the cochlea. In: Dallos P, Popper AN, Fay RR, eds. *The cochlea.* New York: Springer, 1996:130–185.
46. Offner FF, Dallos P, Cheatham MA. Positive endocochlear potential: mechanism of production by marginal cells of stria vascularis. *Hear Res* 1987;29:117–124.
47. Marchbanks RJ, Reid A. Cochlear and cerebrospinal fluid pressure: their inter-relationship and control mechanisms. *Br J Audiol* 1990;24:179–187.
48. Axelsson A. The blood supply of the inner ear in mammals. In: Keidel WD, Neff WD, eds. *Handbook of sensory physiology, volume V/1. Auditory system: anatomy, physiology (ear).* New York: Springer-Verlag, 1974:213–260.
49. Smith CA. Vascular patterns of the membranous labyrinth. In: deLorenzo ADJ, ed. *Vascular disorders and hearing defects.* Baltimore: University Park Press, 1973:1–21.
50. Nadol JB. Synaptic morphology of inner and outer hair cells of the human organ of corti. *J Electron Microsc Tech* 1990;15:187–196.
51. Flock A. Transducing mechanisms in the lateral line canal organ receptors. *Cold Spring Harbor Symp Quant Biol* 1965;30:133–144.
52. Duvall AJ, Flock A, Wersall J. The ultrastructure of the sensory hairs and associated organelles of the cochlear inner hair cell with reference to directional sensitivity. *J Cell Biol* 1966;29:497–505.
53. Davis H. A model for transducer action in the cochlea. *Cold Spring Harbor Symp Quant Biol* 1965;30:181–189.
54. Flock A, Jorgensen M, Russell I. The physiology of individual hair cells and their synapses. In: Moller AR, ed. *Basic mechanisms in hearing.* New York: Academic Press, 1973:273–302.
55. Dallos P. Cochlear physiology. *Annu Rev Psychol* 1981;32:153–190.
56. Tonndorf J. Davis 1961 revisited: signal transmission in the cochlear hair cell-nerve junction. *Arch Otolaryngol* 1975;101:528–535.
57. Tasaki I, Spyropoulos CS. Stria vascularis as source of endocochlear potential. *J Neurophysiol* 1959;22:149–155.
58. Honrubia V, Ward PH. Dependence of the cochlear microphonics and the summating potential on the endocochlear potential. *J Acoust Soc Am* 1969;46:388–392.
59. Dallos P. Overview: cochlear neurobiology. In: Dallos P, Popper AN, Fay RR, eds. *The cochlea.* New York: Springer, 1996:1–43.
60. Ryan A, Dallos P. Physiology of the cochlea. In: Northern JL, ed. *Hearing disorders,* 2nd ed. Boston: Little, Brown and Company, 1984:253–266.

61. Pickles JO, Corey DP. Mechanoelectrical transduction by hair cells. *Trends Neurosci* 1992;15:254–259.

62. Pickles JO, Comis SD, Osborne MP. Cross-links between stereocilia in the guinea pig organ of corti and their possible relation to sensory transduction. *Hear Res* 1984;15:103–112.

63. Flock A, Cheung HC. Actin filaments in sensory hairs of inner ear receptor cells. *J Cell Biol* 1977;75:339–343.

64. Hunter-Duvar IM. Electron microscopic assessment of the cochlea. *Acta Otolaryngol Suppl* 1978;351:3–23.

65. Dallos P, Billone MC, Durrant JD, Wang CY, Raynor S. Cochlear inner and outer hair cells: functional differences. *Science* 1972;177:356–358.

66. Zwislocki JJ, Sokolich WG. Velocity and displacement in auditory-nerve fibers. *Science* 1973;182:64–66.

67. von Bekesy G. *Experiments in hearing*, New York: McGraw-Hill, 1960. Wever EG, translator and editor.

68. Dallos P. Low-frequency auditory characteristics: species dependence. *J Acoust Soc Am* 1970;48:489–499.

69. Tonndorf J. The hydrodynamic origin of aural harmonics in the cochlea. *Ann Otol Rhinol Laryngol* 1958;67:754–774

70. Lim DJ. Cochlear micromechanics in understanding otoacoustic emission. *Scand Audiol Suppl* 1986;25:17–25.

71. Johnstone BM, Patuzzi R, Yates GK. Basilar membrane measurements and the travelling wave. *Hearing Res* 1986;22:147–153.

72. Rhode WS. An investigation of post-mortem cochlear mechanics using the Mossbauer effect. In: Moller AR, ed. *Basic mechanisms in hearing*. New York: Academic Press, 1973:39–63.

73. Rhode WS. Basilar membrane motion: results of mossbauer measurements. *Scand Audiol Suppl* 1986;25:7–15.

74. Dallos P. The active cochlea. *J Neurosci* 1992;12:4575–4585.

75. Tilney LG, Derosier DJ, Mulroy MJ. The organization of actin filaments in the stereocilia of cochlear hair cells. *J Cell Biol* 1980;86:244–259.

76. Brownell WE, Bader CR, Bertrand D, de Ribaupierre Y. Evoked mechanical responses of isolated cochlear outer hair cells. *Science* 1985;227:194–196.

77. Dallos P, Evans BN, Hallworth R. Nature of the motor element in electrokinetic shape changes of cochlear outer hair cells. *Nature* 1991;350:155–157.

78. Geisler CD. A cochlear model using feedback from motile outer hair cells. *Hear Res* 1991;54:105–117.

79. Kiang NYS. *Discharge patterns of single fibers in the cat's auditory nerve*. Cambridge, MA: MIT Press, 1965.

80. Kiang NYS, Moxon EC. Tails of tuning curves of auditory-nerve fibers. *J Acoust Soc Am* 1974;55:620–630.

81. Khanna SM, Leonard DGB. Basilar membrane tuning in the cat cochlea. *Science* 1982;215:305–306.

82. Russell IJ, Sellick PM. Tuning properties of cochlear hair cells. *Nature* 1977;267:858–860.

83. Zwicker E. On a psychoacoustical equivalent of tuning curves. In: Zwicker E, Terhardt E, eds. *Facts and models in hearing*. New York: Springer-Verlag, 1974:132–141.

84. Keidel WE. Neurophysiological requirements for implanted cochlear prostheses. *Audiology* 1980;19:105–127.

85. Pfeiffer RR, Kim DO. Cochlear nerve fiber responses: distribution along the cochlear partition. *J Acoust Soc Am* 1975;58:867–869.

86. Brugge JF, Geisler CD. Auditory mechanisms of the lower brainstem. *Ann Rev Neurosci* 1978;1:363–394.

87. Merzenich MM, Knight PL, Roth GL. Representation of cochlea within primary auditory cortex in the cat. *J Neurophysiol* 1975;38:231–249.

88. Walzl EM. Representation of the cochlea in the cerebral cortex. *Laryngoscope* 1947;57:778–787.

89. Wever EG. *Theory of fearing*. New York: Dover Publications, 1949.

90. Brugge JF, Anderson DJ, Hind JE, Rose JE. Time structure of discharges in single auditory nerve fibers of the squirrel monkey in response to complex periodic sounds. *J Neurophysiol* 1969;32:386–401.

91. Rose JE, Brugge JF, Anderson DJ, Hind JE. Phase-locked response to low-frequency tones in single auditory nerve fibers of the squirrel monkey. *J Neurophysiol* 1967;30:769–793.

92. Kiang NYS. A survey of recent developments in the study of auditory physiology. *Ann Otol* 1968;77:656–675.

93. Sachs MB, Abbas PJ. Rate versus level functions for auditory-nerve fibers in cats: tone-burst stimuli. *J Acoust Soc Am* 1974;56:1835–1847.

94. Sachs MB, Young ED. Encoding of steady-state vowels in the auditory nerve: representation in terms of discharge rate. *J Acoust Soc Am* 1979;66:470–479.

95. Whitfield IC. Electrophysiology of the central auditory pathway. *Br Med Bull* 1956;12:105–109.

96. Whitfield IC. Coding in the auditory nervous system. *Nature* 1967;213:756–760.

97. Viemeister NF. Auditory intensity discrimination at high frequencies in the presence of noise. *Science* 1983;221:1206–1208.

98. Eybalin M. Neurotransmitters and neuromodulators of the mammalian cochlea. *Physiol Rev* 1993;73:309–373.

99. Guinan JJ. Physiology of olivocochlear efferents. In: Dallos P, Popper AN, Fay RR, eds. *The cochlea*. New York: Springer, 1996:435–501.

100. Warr WB, Guinan JJ. Efferent innervation of the organ of corti: two separate systems. *Brain Res* 1979;173:152–155.

101. Sewell WF. Neurotransmitters and synaptic transmission. In: Dallos P, Popper AN, Fay RR, eds. *The cochlea*. New York: Springer, 1996:501–533.

102. Galambos R. Neural mechanisms in audition. *Laryngoscope* 1958;68:388–401.

103. Spoendlin H. Neural connections of the outer hair cell system. *Acta Otolaryngol* 1976;87:381–387.

104. Spoendlin H. Neural anatomy of the inner ear. In: Jahn AF, Santos-Sachi J, eds. *Physiology of the ear*. New York: Raven Press, 1988:201–219.

105. Klinke R, Galley N. Efferent innervation of vestibular and auditory receptors. *Physiol Rev* 1974;54:316–357.

106. Cody AR, Johnstone BM. Acoustically evoked activity of single efferent neurons in the guinea pig cochlea. *J Acoust Soc Am* 1982;72:280–282.

107. Liberman MC. Physiology of cochlear efferent and afferent neurons: direct comparisons in the same animal. *Hearing Res* 1988;34:179–191.

108. Scharf B, Magnan J, Chays A. On the role of the olivocochlear bundle in hearing: 16 case studies. *Hear Res* 1997;103:101–122.

109. Liberman MC. Rapid assessment of sound-evoked olivocochlear feedback: suppressions on compound action potentials by contralateral sound. *Hear Res* 1989;38:47–56.

110. Puria S, Guinan JJ, Liberman MC. Olivocochlear reflex assays: effects of contralateral sound on compound action potentials versus ear-canal distortion products. *J Acoust Soc Am* 1996;99:500–507.

111. Collet L, Kemp DT, Veuillet E, Duclaux R, Moulin A, Morgon A. Effect of contralateral auditory stimuli on active cochlear micromechanical properties in human subjects. *Hear Res* 1990;43:251–262.

112. Moulin A, Collet L, Duclaux R. Contralateral auditory stimulation alters acoustic distortion products in humans. *Hear Res* 1993;65:193–210.

113. Giraud AL, Collet L, Chery-Croze S, Magnan J, Chays A. Evidence of a medial olivocochlear involvement in contralateal suppression of otoacoustic emissions in humans. *Brain Res* 1995;705:15–23.

114. Comis SD. Detection of signals in noisy backgrounds: a role for centrifugal fibres. *J Laryngol Otol* 1973;87:529–534.

115. Kawase T, Liberman MC. Antimasking effects of the olivocochlear reflex. I. Enhancement of compound action potentials to masked tones. *J Neurophysiol* 1993;70:2519–2532.

116. Durrant JD. Contralateral suppression of otoacoustic emissions—delay of effect? *J Commun Disord* 1998;31(6):485–488.

117. Durrant JD, Wang J, Ding DL, Salvi RJ. Are inner or outer hair cells the source of summating potentials recorded from the round window? *J Acoust Soc Am* 1998;104:370–377.

118. Durrant JD. Comments on the effects of overstimulation on microphonic sensitivity. *J Acoust Soc Am* 1979;66:597–598.

119. Durrant JD. Auditory physiology and an auditory physiologist's view of tinnitus. *J Laryngol Otol* 1981; [Suppl 4]: 21–28.

120. Katz B. *Nerve, muscle, and synapse*. New York: McGraw-Hill, 1966.

121. Kiang NYS. Stimulus representation in the discharge patterns of auditory neurons. In: Eagles EL, ed. *The nervous system, volume 3. Human communication and its disorders*. New York: Raven Press, 1975:81–96.

122. Coats AC. On electrocochleographic electrode design. *J Acoust Soc Am* 1974;56:708–711.

123. Aran JM, Portmann M, Portmann M. Electrocochleography in adults and children. Electrophysiological study of the peripheral receptor. *Audiology* 1972;11:77–89.

124. Ferraro JA, Ruth RA. Electrocochleography. In: Jacobson JT, ed. *Principles and applications in auditory evoked potentials*. Boston: Allyn & Bacon, 1994:101–122.

125. Stypulkowski PH, Staller SJ. Clinical evaluation of a new ECocG recording electrode. *Ear Hear* 1987;8:304–310.

126. Coats AC. The summating potential and Meniere's disease. I. Summating potential amplitude in Meniere and non-Meniere ears. *Arch Otolaryngol* 1981;107:199–208.

127. Durrant JD. Combined EcochGABR versus conventional ABR recordings. *Semin Hear* 1986;7:289–305.
128. Kemp DT. Stimulated acoustic emissions from within the human auditory system. *J Acoust Soc Am* 1978;64:1386–1391.
129. Probst R. Otoacoustic emissions: an overview. In: Pfaltz CR, ed. *New aspects of cochlear mechanics and inner ear pathophysiology*. Basel: Karger, 1990:1–91.
130. Kemp DT. Developments in cochlear mechanics and techniques for noninvasive evaluation. *Adv Audiol* 1988;5:27–45.
131. Kim DO, Paparello J, Jung MD, Smurzynski J, Sun X. Distortion product otoacoustic emission test of sensorineural heraring lsos: performance regarding sensitivity, specificity and receiver operating characteristics. *Acta Otolaryngol* 1996;116:3–11.
132. Probst R, Lonsbury-Martin BL, Martin GK, Coats AC. Otoacoustic emissions in ears with hearing loss. *Am J Otolaryngol* 1987;8: 73–81.
133. Zurek PM. Spontaneous narrowband acoustic signals emitted by human ears. *J Acoust Soc* Am 1981;69:514–523.
134. Lonsbury-Martin BL, Whitehead ML, Martin GK. Clinical applications of otoacoustic emissions. *J Speech Hear Res* 1991;34:964–981.

The Ear: Comprehensive Otology,
edited by R. F. Canalis and P. R. Lambert.
Lippincott Williams & Wilkins, Philadelphia © 2000.

CHAPTER 5

Applied Physiology of the Vestibular System

Kamran Barin and John D. Durrant

<table>
<tr><td>

Overview of Vestibular Function
  Vestibulospinal Reflex
  Vestibuloocular Reflex
  Effects of Vestibular Receptors on the Autonomic
    System
  Adaptation of Vestibular Responses
  Implications for Clinical Evaluation of the Vestibular
    Function
Structure of the Vestibular System
  Hair Cell Structure
  Functional Significance of Structure of Semicircular
    Canals
  Structure of Otolith Organs
  Vestibular Nerve and Its Central Connections

</td><td>

Functional Organization of Vestibular
  Responses
  Stimulation of the Semicircular Canals: Responses to
    Head Rotation
  Vestibular Nystagmus
  Stimulation of the Semicircular Canals: Responses to
    Temperature Gradients
  Stimulation of the Otolith Organs
  Adaptation of Vestibular Responses
Effects of Peripheral Vestibular Lesions
  Effects of Unilateral Vestibular Lesions
  Vestibular Compensation after a Unilateral Vestibular
    Lesion
  Effects of Bilateral Vestibular Lesion

</td></tr>
</table>

OVERVIEW OF VESTIBULAR FUNCTION

The human vestibular system participates in two important reflexes that are essential to our normal daily activities—the vestibulospinal reflex (VSR) and the vestibuloocular reflex (VOR) (1). These reflexes are intended to operate quickly and efficiently with the overall objective of keeping one's body, head, and eyes oriented in space at all times. The vestibular system contributes to orientation during routine tasks such as standing upright or walking, as well as more complex motor tasks such as running or walking while turning the head. The somewhat independent movement of the eyes adds yet another demand on the nervous system for information processing and control, namely, the need to maintain clear vision. Before describing the mechanisms of the vestibular system and their physiologic bases, it will

be worthwhile to more completely characterize these two motor reflexes, as well as other functions reflecting the considerable degree to which information from vestibular sensors is integrated to control or influence a diverse array of bodily and nervous system functions. The vestibular system and its pathways are summarized schematically in Fig. 1.

Vestibulospinal Reflex

The vestibular receptors participate in maintaining upright postural stability and generating purposeful movements by providing the central nervous system (CNS) with sensory information about the movements and orientation of the head. The VSR, which generates compensatory body movements, includes the peripheral vestibular end organs, central vestibular pathways, and motor centers such as the spinal cord (2).

In addition to vestibular input, the VSR receives information from other sensory modalities, namely, the visual and proprioceptive systems. Although there is some overlap among the sensory inputs, the frequency range for optimal operation of each sensor is somewhat distinct. For example, the visual system operates best for slow,

K. Barin: Department of Otolaryngology, The Ohio State University, Columbus, Ohio 43210

J.D. Durrant: Departments of Communication Science and Disorders and Otolaryngology, University of Pittsburgh, Pittsburgh, Pennsylvania 15260; and Department of Otorhinolaryngology, Université Claude Bernard (Lyon 1), Hôpital Edouard Herriot, Lyon 69003, France

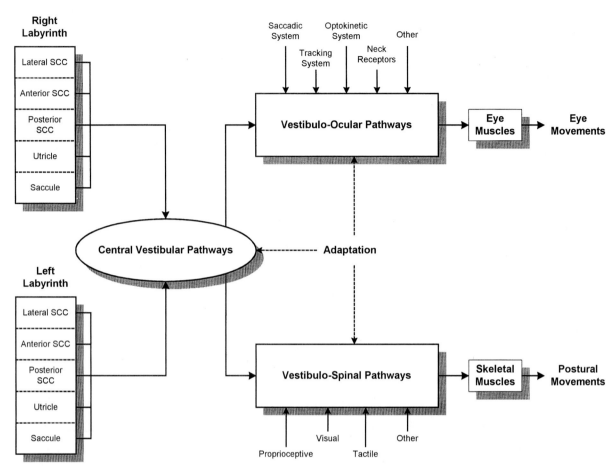

FIG. 1. Overview of the vestibular pathways and their interactions with other sensory mechanisms. SCC, semicircular canal.

low-frequency movements, whereas the proprioceptive system is best suited for fast, high-frequency activities (3). The frequency range of the vestibular receptors, approximately 0.1 to 3 Hz, falls somewhere between the operational frequencies of visual and proprioceptive inputs and corresponds well with the natural frequency of head movements.

The input from the vestibular system differs from those of the other systems in one other significant way. The orientation information from the visual and proprioceptive receptors are generally relative to a reference frame that itself may vary with respect to an absolute frame of reference, such as that of gravity (4). These inputs must be converted to absolute orientation information to be useful in maintaining upright posture. The takeoff phase of a plane provides an example of the distinction between the sensory receptors. Because the visual system provides information relative to the external environment, it cannot provide accurate orientation information unless one can look out the window and first detect the orientation of the plane with respect to ground.

Similarly, the proprioceptive system provides information about the orientation of one body segment with respect to another body segment. For upright stability, this information can be used to derive absolute orientation information only if the orientation of the support surface is known. If the support surface is moving or compliant, the proprioceptive cues are not likely to be an accurate representation of absolute orientation.

In contrast, the vestibular system during locomotion on earth provides absolute information regarding the orientation of the head with respect to gravity. Because the direction of gravity is not variable, the vestibular cues are not as easily affected as those from other sensors. For this reason, as well as its frequency range, the vestibular system seems to operate as the final arbitrator in the hierarchical control of posture (5). That is, if a discrepancy among the sensory inputs develops with regard to the orientation of posture, the VSR relies on vestibular signals to determine the appropriate strategy for preserving balance.

Vestibuloocular Reflex

The other important function in which the vestibular system participates is the task of providing clear vision during head movements. This task is accomplished through the VOR, which maintains a steady retinal image by generating compensatory eye movements in response to head motion (6). In addition to the vestibular pathways, other sensorimotor mechanisms participate in the stabilization of gaze. These mechanisms both extend the operational frequency range of the VOR and provide the necessary redundancy to make the overall system more fault tolerant.

The visual equivalent of the vestibular system that contributes to generating compensatory eye movements during low-frequency head motion is the optokinetic system (7). The optokinetic and vestibular reflexes are integrated to generate eye movement signals that can precisely counteract the head movements under a variety of conditions. The hallmark of optokinetic activation is the sensation of self-motion. The most compelling demonstration of this effect occurs when one car waiting at a traffic light starts to move. The driver of the adjacent vehicle, observing the motion in the peripheral vision, often perceives that it is his or her own car that actually is moving and reflexively pushes harder on the brake pedal, thus attempting to prevent the apparent movement.

In humans, two other visual subsystems contribute to the control of eye movements: the saccadic system and the smooth pursuit system. The saccadic system is responsible for generating fast eye movements that redirect the attention from one target to another, by quickly placing the image of the new target on the fovea (8). Because both the vestibular and optokinetic mechanisms cause the eyes to move away from center gaze, the saccadic system ensures that the eyes do not remain deviated to one side by quickly resetting the eyes toward the center gaze (9).

The smooth pursuit or tracking system is designed to keep the image of a moving target on the fovea (10). Smooth pursuit and optokinetic eye movements often are misidentified due to their close association. However, they have significant differences and clearly originate from different sensory modalities. For example, the smooth pursuit eye movements are voluntary, whereas the optokinetic eye movements are reflexive. The stimulus for the optokinetic system is the full visual field motion, whereas the smooth pursuit system is mainly activated by motion of small targets whose images fit within the fovea. Finally, the sensation of self-motion is an exclusive property of the optokinetic system activation. The interaction of the smooth pursuit with the vestibular system initially was thought to be inhibitory in nature; the smooth pursuit eye movements are used to suppress vestibular responses in conditions where they are deemed to be inappropriate for gaze stabilization (11). Although this view has proved to be somewhat of an oversimplification, it nonetheless highlights the overall goal of visual-vestibular interaction, which is to provide clear vision during a wide range of conditions.

In addition to the visual system, the proprioceptive mechanisms contribute to gaze stabilization through the neck receptors and the cervicoocular reflex (12). The contribution of the cervicoocular reflex in many tasks is often overshadowed in the presence of a normal functioning vestibular system. However, eye movements purely generated by the cervicoocular reflex can be seen in patients with bilateral loss of vestibular function as well as during movements of the torso relative to the stationary head.

Effects of Vestibular Receptors on the Autonomic System

Although the main function of the vestibular system is related to maintaining balance and coordination, motion-induced anomalies, such as emesis, are well-known consequences associated with vestibular responses (13). Autonomic nervous symptoms in such cases are not limited to nausea and vomiting, but include circulatory and respiratory responses as well (14). These symptoms seem to occur when the CNS receives conflicting information from different sensory mechanisms. More accurately, the deviation of vestibular, visual, and other sensory inputs from their expected behavior leads to the development of motion sickness (15). The most well-known example of such a sensory conflict occurs when one is placed inside a moving vehicle without allowing visual contact with the environment outside the vehicle. In this case, the motion of the vehicle is sensed by the vestibular system but the visual system does not provide a matching input. This type of visual-vestibular conflict causes motion sickness in susceptible individuals.

A number of animal studies have established the direct role of the vestibular system in generating motion-induced autonomic symptoms (16,17). In these studies, animals produced emesis responses after prolonged or excessive vestibular stimulation. When the vestibular apparatus was destroyed in some animals by labyrinthectomy or deafferentation of the vestibular nerve, those animals no longer exhibited the emesis response after vestibular stimulation. On the other hand, the control animals with the intact vestibular system continued to suffer from the autonomic symptoms.

In recent years, the neural pathways that link the vestibular responses with the centers that control autonomic responses have begun to be identified (18). However, the functional basis for such connections is not yet fully established. Some have speculated that autonomic responses such as nausea and vomiting serve as a protective mechanism. The stimuli that trigger such responses usually are generated by movements that are intense and well beyond normal daily activities. It is also clear that the cardiovascular system faces significant challenges during standing or lying down due to changes in the height of the orthostatic column. Therefore, motion-induced changes in the autonomic responses seem to provide the necessary regulation during such activities.

Adaptation of Vestibular Responses

The vestibular pathways are highly adaptive. Such plasticity is essential to overcome the effects of changes due to disease and trauma as well as environmental and developmental changes, such as aging (19). When the changes are due to dysfunction of the vestibular system, the adaptive process usually is referred to as *vestibular compensation* (20) (see Chapter 42). However, regardless of whether the changes are due to natural or disease processes, the adaptive strategies appear to be similar. Such strategies may include readjusting the properties of the vestibular response (magnitude, timing) or substituting alternative sensory mechanisms.

The adaptive mechanisms appear to be activated when the vestibular responses are not within the anticipated behavior of the system. For example, most of our normal daily activities generate vestibular activities that are usually short in duration. When the responses do not subside quickly, as may be the case after a labyrinthine lesion or during an extended flight, a recalibration of the vestibular reflexes becomes necessary. It is important to recognize that the adaptive behavior of the vestibular receptors is not yet fully understood. There also are significant individual differences in the extent and type of adaptive mechanisms used. Understanding these differences is important in the rehabilitation of vestibular disorders.

Implications for Clinical Evaluation of the Vestibular Function

This brief overview of vestibular system function highlights two issues that are highly relevant to the clinical assessment and management of the vestibular disorders. First, in laboratory evaluation of the human vestibular function, there is no direct access to the activities of the vestibular end organ. One must rely on secondary responses, such as eye or postural movements, to evaluate the vestibular system. Because many other sensory mechanisms participate in the control of eye and postural movements, it should not come as a surprise that vestibular tests often yield nonspecific and nonlocalizing findings.

Second, the plasticity of the neural pathways, although essential for optimal functioning of the VOR and VSR, poses a challenge in testing the vestibular system. Because the nature and timing of vestibular lesions can affect the outcome of function tests, the correct interpretation of the results depends on understanding the vestibular compensation process. In addition, the recent advances in the rehabilitation of patients with vestibular disorders are critically dependent on the design and implementation of physical therapy routines that activate the proper adaptive mechanisms.

STRUCTURE OF THE VESTIBULAR SYSTEM

The vestibular receptors are embedded within the membranous labyrinth. The membranous labyrinth is enclosed within the bony labyrinth, a series of hollow channels in the petrous portion of the temporal bone that also houses the auditory sensory receptors (see figure 1, Chapter 2). The space for the bony labyrinth is divided into three distinct parts: a cochlear part, a vestibular part, and a central chamber called the vestibule. The vestibular portion is represented by three semicircular canals with their openings converging at the vestibule. The bony labyrinth is filled with perilymphatic fluid, the chemical composition of which is similar to that of the extracellular fluid with a higher ratio of sodium to potassium concentration (21). Although the electrolyte composition of perilymph is similar to that of the cerebrospinal fluid, the difference in the protein contents provides compelling evidence against a direct connection between the two. It is possible, however, that a small portion of the perilymph is produced by the filtration of the cerebrospinal fluid. The main source for perilymph production is considered to be the filtration of blood from the vessels within the perilymphatic space.

The membranous labyrinth is suspended within the bony labyrinth through a group of connective tissues. The membranous labyrinth is filled with endolymph, a fluid that has a different composition than that of the perilymph. The chemical composition of endolymphatic fluid resembles that of intracellular fluid, with a higher ratio of potassium to sodium concentration (22). In an intact vestibular structure, there is no contact between the endolymphatic and perilymphatic fluids. The cochlear endolymph is most likely produced by the secretory cells within the stria vascularis (see Chapter 4). The dark cells within the vestibular labyrinth share many characteristics with the cells of the stria vascularis (23). The dark cells are the most likely source of vestibular endolymph production. The absorption of endolymph is believed to occur in the endolymphatic sac (24).

The vestibular sensory cells are concentrated in different areas within the membranous labyrinth (Fig. 2). Three of these areas are located in the enlarged portion (ampulla) of each semicircular canal where the neuroepithelia, called the cristae ampullaris, reside. The macula of the utricle and saccule within the cavities of the vestibule also are packed with sensory cells. The arrangement and spatial orientation of the sensory receptors within each area are unique, allowing for differential sensitivity to different types of head movement.

The membranous labyrinth receives its blood supply through the labyrinthine artery. The basilar artery is the supplier to the labyrinthine artery either directly, or more commonly through the anterior inferior cerebellar branch

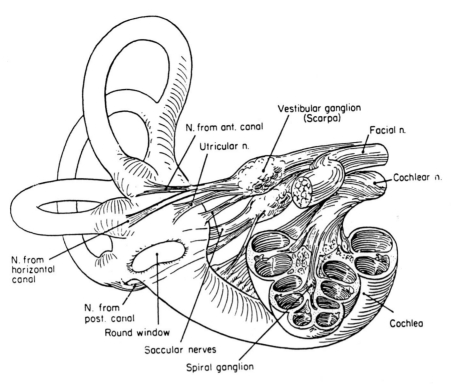

FIG. 2. Vestibular receptors within the membranous labyrinth. (From Baloh RW, Honrubia V. *Clinical neurophysiology of the vestibular system.* Philadelphia: F.A. Davis, 1990;10, with permission.)

(25,26). The vestibular portion of the labyrinthine artery has an anterior branch and a posterior branch, each supplying blood to various parts of the labyrinth. The posterior vestibular artery is a branch of the vestibulocochlear artery. The vestibular apparatus is susceptible to ischemic events because labyrinthine arteries lack collateral anastomotic connections with other major arterial branches (27). A short 15-second interruption of blood circulation can cause impairment of the sensory receptors (28). The impairment may become irreversible after a prolonged ischemia. Such events can damage one area of the labyrinth without affecting others, because the arterial branches take independent paths within the labyrinth (29).

Hair Cell Structure

The vestibular sensory receptors are members of a group of specialized cells that transduce mechanical energy to neural activities. These cells, referred to as *hair cells* due to their unique structure, are similar to those found in the organ of Corti. The general principles of hair cell function are described in Chapter 4. Suffice it to say here that, in the vestibular system, the energy of the stimulus is hydromechanical and generated in association with the forces that are produced either by head movements or by gravity. Microscopic displacement of the hair cells subsequent to the applied force causes the chemical reaction that releases neurotransmitter substance and changes the neural firing rate of the primary vestibular neurons (30).

Figure 3 shows the general structure of a hair cell. Three major parts can be identified: the cilia, the cell body, and the nerve endings. The cilia, or *hairs*, are the distinctive feature of these sensory cells. In the vestibular apparatus, the cilia of the sensory cells consist of approximately 70 short hairs called *stereocilia* and a single, thicker, longer hair called a *kinocilium*. The stereocilia do

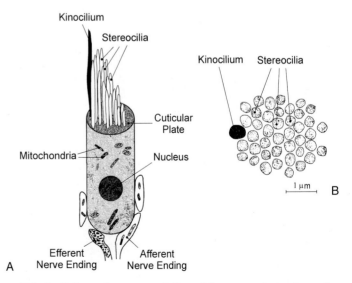

FIG. 3. Schematic representation of the general structure of a hair cell. **A:** Side view. **B:** Top view. (Based on drawings from Baloh RW, Honrubia V. *Clinical neurophysiology of the vestibular system.* Philadelphia: F.A. Davis, 1990.)

not surround the kinocilium, nor do they line up in a plane. Instead, they form a bundle atop the cell body with the kinocilium on one side. This is a relatively rigid bundle as the applied force is easily transmitted from one hair to the other (31). The length of the stereocilia for each hair cell increases as they get closer to the kinocilium. However, the relative length of stereocilia is variable for hair cells in different receptor organs and even for hair cells in different locations within the same organ.

Two types of vestibular hair cells have been identified in mammals (Fig. 4). The main morphologic differences between the two types are in the shape of the cell body and the connection of the nerve endings to the cell body. *Type I* hair cells have a cell body that is narrower at the apex and wider at the base, much like a flask. These cells are distinguished by the presence of a large afferent nerve ending termed the chalice or *calyx*. In type I cells, the calyx almost completely surrounds the cell body. The efferent nerve ending is attached to the calyx and does not directly contact the body of a type I cell. *Type II* hair cells have a cylindrical cell body with multiple afferent nerve connections. The efferent nerve terminal in type II cells lies directly on the cell body.

The relative distribution of the two hair cell types differs from one receptor area to another and from one species to another (32). For example, in primates, the crista ampullares are predominantly comprised of type I cells, whereas the maculae consist of both type I and type II cells. On the other hand, in lower animals such as rodents, the ratio of type I to type II cells is closer to one.

In recent years, differences in the functional properties of the two hair cell types have begun to emerge. A detailed review of these differences is beyond the scope of this text, but it should be noted that the differences in the afferent and efferent nerve endings may have a profound effect on the adaptive responses of the two cell types (29).

Despite the differences, type I and type II hair cells both have two important characteristics. First, the majority of them generate spontaneous neural firing at rest (Fig. 5A). The steady release of neurotransmitters across the junction of the hair cell and its afferent neurons appears to be the mechanism that provokes this tonic neural activity in the absence of any external stimulus (33). The magnitude of spontaneous firing varies among species. In mammals, the average spontaneous firing rate of each afferent nerve fiber is about 70 to 90 spikes per second (34). Because there are more than 20,000 fibers in each vestibular nerve, the tonic activity transmitted to the central pathways is on the order of an astonishing 1.5 million spikes per second!

The second common characteristic of the hair cells, as discussed in Chapter 4, is their directional polarization (35). When the stereocilia bundle is bent toward the kinocilium, the firing rate of the afferent nerve fiber connected to that cell increases (Fig. 5B). Bending of the stereocilia away from the kinocilium causes a decrease in the firing rate (Fig. 5C). In general, the change in the firing rate of the afferent neuron is proportional to the displacement of the stereocilia. However, there is an inherent asymmetry between the excitatory and inhibitory responses. The firing rate of neurons can increase from the tonic level to approximately 400 spikes per second during the excitatory phase. However, the inhibitory responses are limited to cessation of the neural activity and therefore cannot exceed the spontaneous firing rate.

The most effective stimulus to hair cells is a force applied in a plane that passes through the kinocilium and divides the stereocilia bundle in half (Fig. 5) (36). Forces applied in the planes that are perpendicular to the described plane are not effective in activating the hair cell (37). The displacement of hair cells is proportional to the applied force and consequently to the acceleration of the motion, in the plane of hair cell activation. Most of our normal daily activities do not induce asymmetric behavior from the hair cells.

The hair cells within the labyrinthine neuroepithelia are surrounded by supporting cells. Supporting cells lie just below the cuticle, where the kinocilium and stereocilia attach to the cell body, and extend to the base of the membrane. The support cells form a ring around the body of the hair cells. The tight binding between the two cell types separates the endolymph that surrounds the stereocilia and kinocilium from the perilymph that covers the base of the membrane.

Functional Significance of the Structure of the Semicircular Canals

It is neither trivial nor a matter of redundancy that there are three semicircular canals within each labyrinth—*lateral* (or *horizontal*), *anterior* (or *supe-*

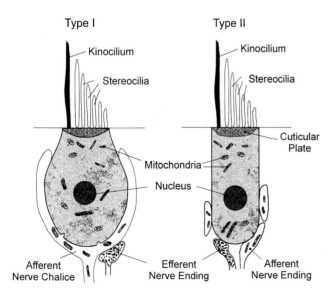

FIG. 4. Schematic drawings of type I and type II hair cells. (Adapted from Baloh RW, Honrubia V. *Clinical neurophysiology of the vestibular system.* Philadelphia: F.A. Davis, 1990.)

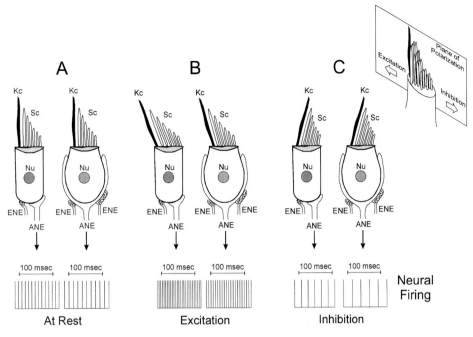

FIG. 5. Modulation of the firing rate of the primary afferent nerve fibers as a function of the stereocilia displacement. **A:** At rest. **B:** Depolarization as a result of bending toward the kinocilium (excitatory response). **C:** Hyperpolarization as a result of bending away from the kinocilium (inhibitory response). ANE, afferent nerve ending; ENE, efferent nerve ending; Kc, kinocilium; Nu, nucleus; Sc, stereocilia. (Based on Baloh RW. *Dizziness, hearing loss, and tinnitus: the essentials of neurotology.* Philadelphia: F.A. Davis, 1984.)

rior[1]), and *posterior.* These canals are organized in three nearly orthogonal (i.e., mutually perpendicular) planes (Fig. 6). The lateral canal resides in a plane that makes a 30-degree upward angle with the horizontal plane when the head is in a natural upright position. The other two canals are roughly vertical, each oriented at an approximately 45-degree angle with respect to the sagittal plane that bisects the head (38). Each semicircular canal in the right ear is synergistically paired with a canal in the left ear such that they reside in approximately parallel planes. The three pairs consist of two lateral canals, right anterior and left posterior canals, and right posterior and left anterior canals. Because the semicircular canals are not perfectly perpendicular and because the canal pairs are not exactly parallel, most natural head movements stimulate all of the semicircular canals simultaneously.

Each semicircular canal forms a closed ring with an opening to a shared cavity in the utricular sac of the vestibule (Fig. 7). The canal is filled with endolymphatic fluid. Near its junction with the utricular sac, the semicircular duct enlarges to form the *ampulla.* The crista ampullaris, the neuroepithelium packed with sensory hair

cells, extends across the floor of the ampulla. A gelatinous mass called the *cupula* protrudes from the surface of the crista and completely seals the ampullar cavity (39). This fluid-tight plug partitions the semicircular canal duct into two chambers.

The cilia rise from the cell bodies on the crista and become embedded in the cupula. The nerve endings from the hair cells join to form a bundle that constitutes the primary afferent nerve fiber for each semicircular canal. An important characteristic of the hair cells in the crista ampullaris is their identical polarization direction. That is, in each crista, the hair cells are oriented with their kinocilia pointing in the same direction. Therefore, any movement of the cupula causes excitation or inhibition of all of the hair cells simultaneously. The orientation of hair cells in the lateral canal is the opposite of the orientation in the vertical canals. In the anterior and posterior canals the kinocilia are aligned toward the canal side of the ampulla. Thus, the deflection of the cupula away from the utricular sac (utriculofugal or ampullofugal) results in excitatory responses in the vertical canals. On the other hand, the kinocilia in the horizontal canals are polarized such that the deflection of the cupula toward the utricular sac (utriculopedal or ampullopedal) causes an increase in the neural firing rate.

The response characteristic of the semicircular canals to head movements is dependent on the fluid dynamics of the

---

[1]The use of the term *anterior* instead of *superior* is common in describing the orientation of the semicircular canals. This terminology can be misleading, because it implies that the anterior and posterior canals reside in parallel planes. In this text, the term *anterior* is used mainly to be consistent with other texts on the subject.

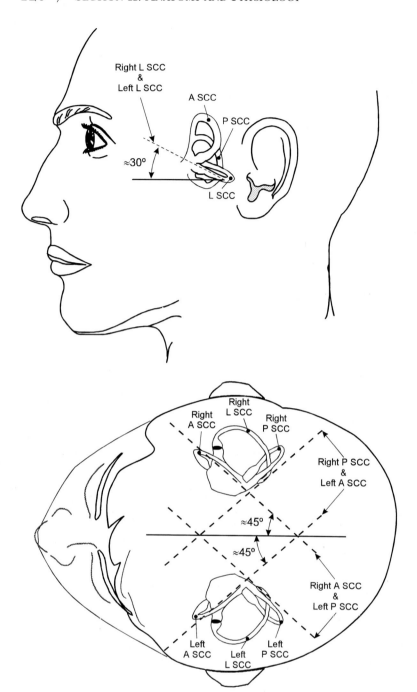

FIG. 6. Spatial orientation of the semicircular canals. A SCC, anterior semicircular canal; L SCC, lateral semicircular canal; P SCC, posterior semicircular canal. (Based on drawings from Blanks RHI, Curthoys IS, Markham CH. Planar relationships of semicircular canals in man. *Acta Otolaryngol* 1975;80:185–196 and Barber HO, Stockwell CW. *Manual of electronystagmography.* St. Louis: Mosby, 1980.)

system (Fig. 7). The cupula and the endolymph have identical densities (specific gravity of approximately 1.0) (40). When the head is motionless, the cupula floats in the endolymph, keeping the hairs in their resting positions. The density of neural firing is equal to the sum of tonic inputs from individual nerve fibers. If the head is rotated in the plane of the canal, the canal walls follow the movement of the head; however, the viscosity of the endolymph causes a lag in the motion of the fluid, thus creating a relative motion of the endolymph with respect to the canal wall. Because the cupula completely blocks the flow of endolymph, the fluid motion generates a force across the cupula and bends it in the direction of endolymph flow. If the head

rotation continues for an extended period of time at a constant velocity, the cupula eventually returns to its resting position as the fluid motion catches up with the motion of the canal wall. In humans, it takes about 15 to 20 seconds for the cupula to return to its resting position after a sudden change in the head velocity (34). If the head now is brought to a sudden stop, the relative motion of the endolymph to canal wall will be reversed and the cupula will be bent in the opposite direction. The pattern of neural firing in this case, as well as the sensation experienced by the subject, is the same as if the subject was rotated in the opposite direction of the initial head rotation, given again that the response of the hair cell is bidirectional.

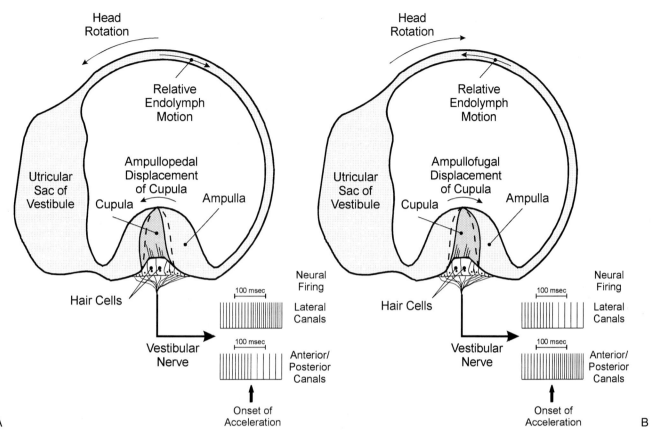

FIG. 7. Schematic drawing of the structure and fluid dynamics of semicircular canals. Neural firing rate of the afferent nerve fibers in response to counter-clockwise **(A)** and clockwise **(B)** rotation of the head in the plane of the semicircular canal. (From Melvill Jones G. Organization of neural control in the vestibulo-ocular reflex arc. In: Bach-Y-Rita P, Collins CC, Hyde JE, eds. *The control of eye movements,* New York: Academic Press, 1971:497–518.)

It is clear from this discussion that the stimulus to the semicircular canals is the change in the angular velocity of the head, i.e., in essence, the acceleration of the head along a circular path. The semicircular canals are mostly unresponsive to motion in a straight line. However, the semicircular canals are by no means perfect *angular accelerometers*. As shown in Fig. 8A, the afferent neural firing pattern is a damped version of the head acceleration and does not exactly match it. The damping effect is due to the combination of inertia and friction posed by the endolymph-cupula dynamics (i.e., due to properties such as mass and viscosity). The neural firing rate nearly perfectly mirrors the head velocity for head movements that consist of brief acceleration and deceleration, with almost no period of constant velocity rotation (Fig. 8B). For these head movements, which are representative of natural head movements, the semicircular canals act as velocity meters. Another source of deviation from being an ideal accelerometer is the response asymmetry of individual canals for clockwise versus counterclockwise rotations, although asymmetries become apparent only for large-amplitude rotations and are not encountered in our normal daily activities.

The asymmetry is due to the differences in the saturation level of excitatory and inhibitory responses of the hair cells (41). As will be discussed later, fortunately the synergetic pairing of the canals effectively neutralizes the effects of this asymmetry.

As noted briefly earlier, linear motion of the head is not an effective stimulus for the semicircular canal system. Because the cupula and endolymph have the same density, linear accelerations, including gravity, generate little displacement of the cupula. Consequently, the neural activity of the canals produced by linear acceleration of the head is negligible.

Structure of Otolith Organs

In addition to the crista ampullaris, vestibular sensory cells are found in two other areas: the macula of the saccule and the macula of the utricle. The vestibular receptors formed by these two areas are known collectively as the *otolith organs*. They respond to an entirely different class of stimuli when compared to the semicircular canals.

The utricle and saccule are two cavities within the vestibule. They are filled with endolymph and each con-

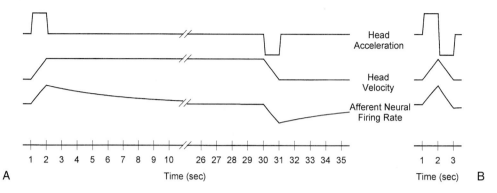

FIG. 8. Response of the primary afferent nerve fiber of a semicircular canal to head rotation in the plane of the canal. **A:** Prolonged rotation. **B:** Brief rotation. (Adapted from Barber HO, Stockwell CW. *Manual of electronystagmography.* St. Louis: Mosby, 1980.)

tains a sensory neuroepithelium, called the *macula.* The macula of the utricle is an oval-shaped structure, with its average plane roughly parallel to that of the lateral semicircular canals (Fig. 9) (42). The macula of the saccule is also a curved structure, with its average plane roughly parallel to the vertical plane (more accurately, parallel to the sagittal plane bisecting the head).

The macula is analogous to the crista in the semicircular canal. It is packed with hair cells and supporting structures necessary for transducing mechanical forces to neural firings (Fig. 10). The cilia from the hair cells in each macula protrude into its own *otolithic membrane.* The otolithic membrane is analogous to the cupula of the canals. It consists of a gelatinous lower surface topped by crystal

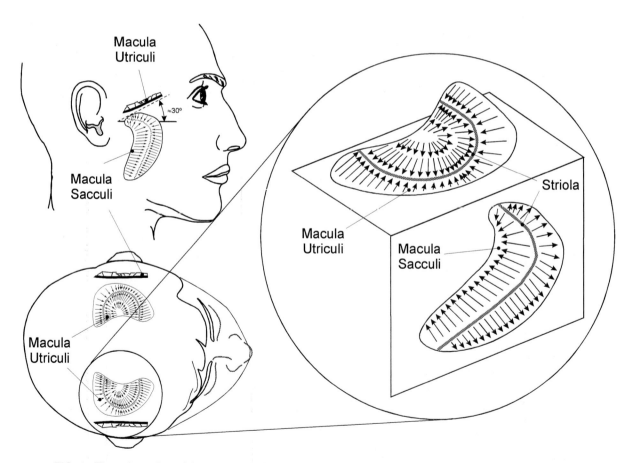

FIG. 9. The orientation of the maculae of the utricle and the saccule. The *arrows* indicate the direction for the excitatory responses of the hair cells. (Based on drawings from Barber HO, Stockwell CW. *Manual of electronystagmography.* St. Louis: Mosby, 1980 and Howard IP. *Human visual orientation.* New York: John Wiley & Sons, 1982.)

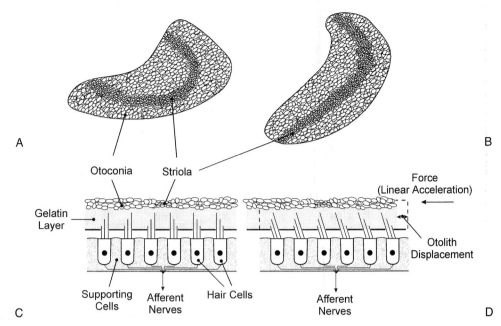

FIG. 10. Structure of the macula and its mechanism of stimulation. **A:** Macula of utricle. **B:** Macula of saccule. Orientation of the otoconia and hair cells at rest **(C)** and in response to linear acceleration of the head **(D)**. (Adapted from Baloh RW, Honrubia V. Physiology of the vestibular system. In: Cummings CW, Fredrickson JM, Harker LA, Krause CJ, Schuller DE, eds. *Otolaryngology—head and neck surgery*, 2nd ed. St. Louis: Mosby, 1995:2604–2642.)

deposits called *otoconia* or *otoliths* (43). The otoconia are composed of calcium carbonate or calcite deposits of varying size (usually 5 to 7 μm) (44). Unlike the cupula, the specific gravity of the otolithic membrane is roughly three times higher than the specific gravity of the endolymph (40). Both maculae have a thin stripe through the middle of their otolithic membranes called the *striola*. The otoconia in this area are very small, and the thickness of the otolithic membrane is different compared to the adjacent tissue. In the utricle, the striola is thinner, whereas in the saccule, it is thicker than the surrounding membrane. The striola clearly divides the macula into regions in which the underlying hair cells have different patterns of polarization. Unlike the crista, the hair cells in the macula are not all polarized in the same direction. In the utricle, the hair cells are arranged with their kinocilia pointing toward the striola. In the saccule, the hair cells are aligned with the kinocilia pointing away from the striola (Fig. 9). Because both maculae are nonplanar and both striolae are curved, the hair cell activation patterns are complex.

The mechanism of stimulation for the otolith organs is any force that displaces the otolithic membrane with respect to the macula. Any arbitrary force applied to the head has two components, one that is parallel, and the other that is perpendicular, to the plane of the macula. The perpendicular component is a compressive force to the hair cells of that macula and therefore does not affect the firing rate of the corresponding afferent neurons. The parallel component, on the other hand, is a shear force that can displace the hair cells and generate neural activ-

ity. Because the maculae of the utricle and saccule lie roughly in perpendicular planes, any force component that is compressive to the hair cells in one macula will act as a shear force to the hair cells in the other macula. Therefore, the direction and the magnitude of any force can be decoded by its relative effect on the two maculae.

Because the applied force is proportional to the linear acceleration of the head, the otolith organs are assumed to be *linear accelerometers*. This assumption is somewhat misleading however, because the induced neural activities are complex and not proportional to the linear acceleration of the head. It is more accurate to think of the otoliths as systems that are stimulated by linear acceleration of the head but with highly nonlinear response patterns that are yet to be fully characterized.

On earth, the most prominent force of linear acceleration is gravity (45). Because of the specific configuration of the otoliths, they are intimately involved in detecting the direction of the gravitational vector.[2] This is an important function that allows the vestibular receptors to provide absolute orientation information and distinguishes them from other sensory mechanisms. Clearly, the otolith receptors are capable of sensing dynamic changes of the head velocity, i.e., acceleration. Because of their sensitivity to gravity, they also are capable of detecting static head tilts. This function is related to the fact that the relative distribution of

---

[2]Force, velocity, acceleration, and related physical quantities are characterized as having both magnitude and direction; such quantities constitute vectors in mathematical and graphical analyses.

the gravity vector on the two maculae changes depending on the direction and the magnitude of the head tilt.

Vestibular Nerve and Its Central Connections

The afferent nerve fibers from the semicircular canals and the otolith organs merge to form the vestibular nerve. The vestibular nerve and the auditory nerve are two branches of the eighth (vestibulocochlear) cranial nerve. The eighth and seventh (facial) nerves form a bundle that travels through the internal auditory canal and enters the brainstem lateral to the cerebellopontine angle (42).

Vestibular nerve fibers are bipolar neurons with their cell bodies in Scarpa's (vestibular) ganglion, their peripheral synapses on the hair cells, and their central synapses on the central vestibular structures. Scarpa's ganglion consists of two portions, a superior portion and an inferior portion (Fig. 2). The latter comprises the nerve fibers from the crista of the posterior canal and the macula of the saccule. The nerve fibers from the remaining three vestibular receptors (cristae of the lateral and anterior canals and macula of the utricle) as well as a branch of the saccular nerve converge on the superior portion of the Scarpa's ganglion. The vestibular nerve maintains two branches as it leaves the superior and inferior ganglia (1).

The primary destination of the vestibular nerve fibers is the vestibular nuclei, although some fibers innervate the cerebellum directly (Fig. 11) (46). The vestibular

nuclei are a group of neurons located mainly in the pons and extending into the medulla. Two sets of nuclei exist, one on the right side and the other on the left side. Each side consists of more than ten distinct groups of neurons (47). Four of them, the superior, medial, lateral, and descending nuclei, are considered the most prominent ones. Contrary to what is implied by the name, direct vestibular connections constitute only a fraction of the nerve fibers that innervate the vestibular nuclei. Other sources that supply afferent nerve fibers to the vestibular nuclei include the cerebellum, the reticular formation, the spinal cord, and the cervical area. There are also a considerable number of interconnecting fibers between the vestibular nuclei on the right and left sides. The efferent nerve fibers from the vestibular nuclei project to the same parts that supply afferent neurons to them.

As the vestibular neurons enter the brainstem, they take two separate pathways. The ascending pathway terminates either in the superior vestibular nucleus or in the cerebellum, while the descending branch terminates in one of the other three main vestibular nuclei (46). The vestibular nuclei are the main processors of the vestibular signal where the initial integration of the sensory inputs takes place. The role of the cerebellum is to monitor the vestibular responses and provide adaptive changes as necessitated by the changes in the environmental factors or the properties of the vestibular pathways (48).

The structures of the central vestibular pathways are an order of magnitude more complex than the peripheral structures. Significant gaps remain in our understanding of these pathways. Nonetheless, a brief discussion of the VOR and VSR is valuable for clinical assessment and management of vestibular disorders. Figure 12 shows a simplified view of the VOR and VSR pathways. The VOR pathways make two distinct connections between the vestibular nuclei and oculomotor neurons: a direct one using the nerve fibers in the medial longitudinal fasciculus and an indirect one mediated through the reticular formation (49). The precise control of vestibular-driven eye movements requires coordinated activities of both pathways. The signals from the vestibular nuclei, regardless of their pathway, project to the oculomotor nuclear complex: the third (oculomotor), the fourth (trochlear), and the sixth (abducens) nucleus. Each nucleus is composed of a pair of cell groups, one on each side of the brain midline. Excitatory responses from one side usually are coupled with inhibitory responses from the opposite side to generate conjugate eye movements. The motor neurons from the oculomotor nuclei drive three pairs of extraocular muscles in each eye. The muscle pairs are arranged to move the eye in planes that roughly coincide with the planes of the semicircular canals. This arrangement simplifies the task of generating compensatory eye movements in response to head motion by enabling one pair of canals to drive only one pair of extraocular muscles. A functional description of the VOR pathways is provided in the next section.

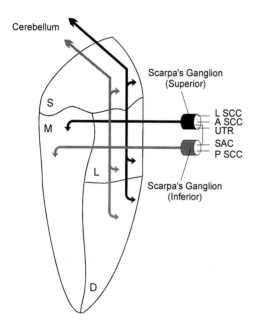

FIG. 11. Innervation of afferent nerve fibers from the vestibular receptors within the vestibular nuclei. A SCC, anterior semicircular canal; D, descending nucleus; L, lateral nucleus; L SCC, lateral semicircular canal; M, medial nucleus; P SCC, posterior semicircular canal; S, superior nucleus; SAC, saccule; UTR, utricle. (Modified from Baloh RW, Honrubia V. *Clinical neurophysiology of the vestibular system.* Philadelphia: F.A. Davis, 1990.)

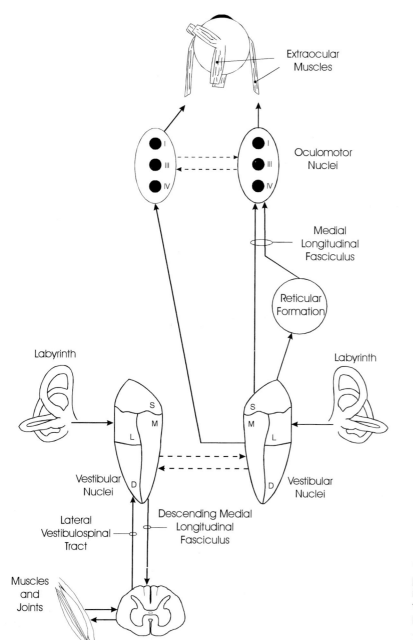

FIG. 12. Vestibuloocular and vestibulospinal pathways. Abbreviations for vestibular nuclei as in Fig. 11. (Modified from Brodal A. Anatomy of the vestibular nuclei and their connections. In: Kornhuber HH, ed. *Handbook of sensory physiology: the vestibular system.* Berlin: Springer-Verlag, 1974:239–352.)

The VSR pathways are far more complex than those of the VOR. This is not surprising considering that the task of postural control requires regulation of the activities of many more muscles and joints and integration of more complex sensory signals. The VSR is not a single reflex as is the VOR, but rather it is composed of a series of context-sensitive reflexes that are initiated on the basis of the available sensory inputs and the required motor task. The anterior horn cells of the spinal cord are the motor neurons that control the activities of the skeletal muscles. These motor neurons are connected to the vestibular nuclei via three primary pathways: the lateral vestibulospinal tract, the medial vestibulospinal tract, and the reticulospinal tract. The first two tracts (shown in Fig. 12) project directly from the sec-

ondary vestibular neurons, whereas the third tract projects indirectly from the reticular formation that receives input from the vestibular nuclei. All three tracts are highly influenced by the cerebellum. For a comprehensive description of the VSR, see Brooks (2).

FUNCTIONAL ORGANIZATION OF VESTIBULAR RESPONSES

The microstructure and mechanism of stimulation for individual vestibular receptors were considered in the previous section. In this section, the functional organization of the peripheral and central vestibular pathways and their responses to various stimuli are described. Much of our current knowledge about the function of the vestibular system is based on the study of eye movements. Therefore, this section concentrates primarily on the responses from the VOR pathways.

Stimulation of the Semicircular Canals: Responses to Head Rotation

As noted before, an important function of the vestibular system is to participate in generating compensatory eye movements to maintain clear vision during head movements. The primary role of the semicircular canals is to detect rotational acceleration of the head. When the head undergoes an angular acceleration in the plane of one of the canals, the firing rate of the afferent nerve fibers changes accordingly. The characteristics of vestibular responses to rotation is highly influenced by synergistic pairing of the canals. Any head motion that generates an excitatory response in one canal also generates an equal inhibitory response from the paired canal in the opposite labyrinth. This type of arrangement is referred to as a *push-pull* organization in the engineering literature.

There are a number of advantages to the push-pull organization of the canal responses (45). First, it improves the resolution of the system by supplying the CNS with a signal that is twice as large as that produced by a single canal. Second, it desensitizes the system to changes in the afferent neural firing that are not produced by head motion. For example, changes in the body temperature or the chemical composition of the inner ear fluids alter the tonic activity of the vestibular neurons from a single canal. However, because these changes affect both labyrinths simultaneously, they are not falsely perceived as signals generated by head motion. Third, the push-pull arrangement of the canals provides a level of redundancy such that a failure of one labyrinth does not completely impair the vestibular function. Finally, this arrangement effectively neutralizes the inherent asymmetry between the excitatory and inhibitory responses of a single canal. High acceleration stimuli in one direction that saturate the inhibitory response of one canal will induce a similar saturation in the output of the paired canal for rotation in the opposite direction. Thus, the net input to the central vestibular pathways is the same regardless of the direction.

The process for generating compensatory eye movements in response to head rotation can be best illustrated by considering rotations in the plane of the lateral canals (30). Figure 13 shows the changes in the afferent neural firing of the two labyrinths in response to a counterclockwise acceleration of the head. The arrangement of the hair cells in the lateral canals is such that the neural firing from the leading ear (the left ear, in this case) increases, whereas the firing rate from the opposite side decreases from its tonic level. For most normal daily activities, the magnitude of

the asymmetry between the responses from the two sides is proportional to the head velocity. This asymmetry is a signal to the central vestibular pathways to drive the eyes in the opposite direction of the motion with an amplitude that matches the head velocity.

To understand how neural activities from the peripheral vestibular system are converted to compensatory eye movements, one must become familiar with the way oculomotor pathways generate eye movements in general. Figure 14 shows a highly simplified and somewhat speculative sequence of events that are necessary to move the eyes rapidly from the center gaze to a new position right of the center (50). The neural command to the ipsilateral paramedian pontine reticular formation (PPRF) is a short-duration sudden surge in the firing rate (excitation *pulse*). The contralateral PPRF simultaneously receives a sudden decrease in the firing rate of the input neurons (inhibitory *inverse pulse*). Three pairs of muscles in each eye are used to move the eye in three different planes. The lateral rectus muscle and the medial rectus muscle move the eyes in the horizontal plane. For movements in any direction, one muscle contracts to pull the eye in the direction of movement (agonist muscle) while the paired muscle relaxes to allow movement in the opposite direction (antagonist muscle). For a rightward eye movement, the right lateral rectus and left medial rectus muscles act as agonists and the right medial and left lateral rectus muscles act as antagonists. The excitatory pulse and inhibitory inverse pulse to the PPRF are transformed as they travel through the medial longitudinal fasciculus and oculomotor nuclei before supplying the muscles via the motor neurons. The agonist muscles receive a sudden increase in the neural firing rate followed by a drop to a new level that is slightly higher than the initial firing rate of the neurons (*pulse-step*). The pulse provides the muscle contraction to move the eyes quickly to the new position and the step allows the increased level of contraction required to keep the eyes in the new position. Similarly, the antagonist muscles receive an *inverse pulse-step* to provide the necessary muscle relaxation for initiating the eye movement and maintaining the new eye position.

The responses of the oculomotor system to other stimuli can be inferred from the eye movements generated by the pulse command to the PPRF. The table in Fig. 14 lists the type of command, the resulting eye movement, and the possible origin of such a command for a number of different stimuli. Of particular interest are the stimuli generated by the secondary vestibular neurons from the vestibular nuclei. As noted in Fig. 13, the afferent vestibular signal in response to an angular acceleration of the head is an increase in the firing rate of neurons from the leading ear and a decrease of firing rate from the opposite ear. For natural head movements, the excitatory neural firing rate is approximately a triangular waveform resembling the head velocity. Unlike the pulse

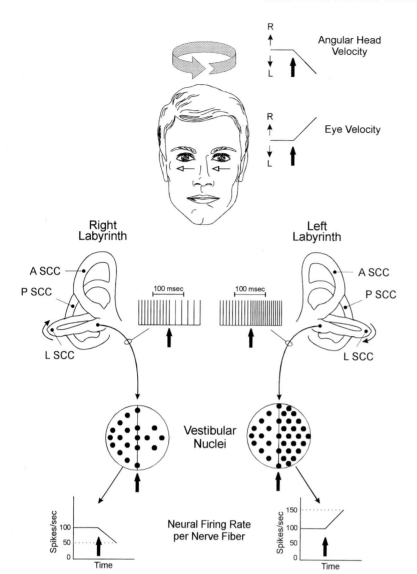

FIG. 13. The changes in the afferent neural firing of the labyrinths and the resulting compensatory eye movements (direction identified by *hollow arrowheads*) immediately after the onset of a counterclockwise head rotation (identified by *solid arrows*). The density of *dots* represents the level of neural firing. Abbreviations for semicircular canals as in Fig. 6. (Adapted from Baloh RW. *Dizziness, hearing loss, and tinnitus: the essentials of neurotology.* Philadelphia: F.A. Davis, 1984.)

that, when applied to the PPRF, causes a quick change in the eye position, the triangular waveform results in a slow drift of the eye from one position to another (51,52). The speed of the eye movement is proportional to the rate of the increase in neural firing and, consequently, to the velocity of the head. The signals from the vestibular nuclei cross the midbrain and connect to the contralateral PPRF. Thus, the response to a brief head rotation is a movement of the eyes in the opposite direction of head motion. Because the eye velocity matches the head velocity, the eyes will remain virtually stationary in space.

When the head rotation is sustained, the asymmetry in the firing rate of the right-left vestibular neurons persists for a much longer time. If there were no other intervention, the eyes would drift slowly in the opposite direction, reach their orbital limits, and remain in that position until the neural asymmetry subsided. Because such a response is not desirable for maintaining a stationary image on the

retina, a pulse is applied to the PPRF to move the eyes back toward the midline. The drift and the subsequent resetting of the eyes continue as long as the neural asymmetry persists. The source of the pulse is most likely the pulse generator in the saccadic system, which is responsible for moving the eyes quickly from one target to another (9). Intuitively, one might assume that eyes must reach the limit of the orbit before the pulse resets them to the center. This is the case for afoveate animals such as rabbits. In humans, however, the occurrence of the pulse appears to depend on the position and velocity of the eyes and can occur well in advance of the eyes reaching their limit. In other words, the pulse generator is triggered by an anticipatory process that keeps the eyes near the midline at all times (53). The specific to-and-fro pattern of eye movements generated by vestibular stimulation belongs to the class of eye movements known as *nystagmus*. Vestibular nystagmus will be discussed in detail in the next section.

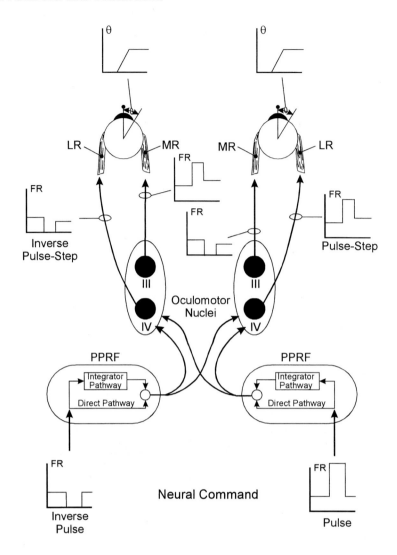

Neural Command		Source	Eye Movement	Comments
Pulse	⊓	Saccadic System (Pulse Generator)	Saccades	Redirects attention from one target to another.
Sinusoidal	∿	Tracking System (Sinusoidal Target Motion)	Sinusoidal Pursuit	For tracking slow-moving small targets.
Triangular	⋀	Vestibular System (Brief Head Rotation)	Slow Compensatory Eye Movement	Eye velocity matches head velocity in the opposite direction.
Exponential	⌒‿	Vestibular System (Sustained Head Rotation)	Nystagmus	Pulse generator resets the eyes as they approach the orbital limit.

FIG. 14. Simplified diagram for generating eye movements in response to an excitation pulse. Eye movement responses to other stimuli are summarized in the *table.* θ, eye position; FR, neural firing rate; LR, lateral rectus muscle; MR, medial rectus muscle; PPRF, paramedian pontine reticular formation. (Based on drawings from Barber HO, Stockwell CW. *Manual of electronystagmography.* St. Louis: Mosby, 1980.)

The studies of oculomotor responses mediated by the vertical semicircular canals have been limited because of the complexity of the instruments needed to generate vertical stimuli as well as technical difficulties in recording vertical eye movements. Yet it is clear that the rotation of the head in the plane of the vertical semicircular canals does generate compensatory eye movements in that plane.

The neural process, however, is complicated because the orientation of the planes of the semicircular canals and eye muscles is somewhat different. Therefore, the spatial information from the canals must be mapped on the coordinates of the eye muscles through a transformation. Such a transformation occurs as the semicircular canal output travels through the vestibular and oculomotor nuclei (42).

Vestibular Nystagmus

Nystagmus is a rhythmic to-and-fro eye movement typically identified by a slow drift of the eyes in one direction followed by a fast reset in the opposite direction. In case of vestibular nystagmus, the slow component is generated by the VOR while the fast component is generated by the pulse generator of the saccadic system. Because the firing rate of the vestibular neurons does not change significantly during each nystagmus beat (approximately 1 second or less), the slow phase of vestibular nystagmus is linear. That is, the slow-phase velocity is relatively constant during each nystagmus beat. Nystagmus is characterized by its fast phases. Thus, right-beating nystagmus indicates slow leftward eye movements followed by fast rightward phases. When nystagmus is provoked by head motion, the nystagmus typically beats in the direction of the acceleration. For instance, in Fig. 13, acceleration toward the left ear (counterclockwise rotation) causes left-beating nystagmus. Note that if the subject is brought to a sudden stop after prolonged constant-velocity counterclockwise rotation, the resulting nystagmus will be right-beating because deceleration of the head is equivalent to accelerating the head in the opposite direction of the initial rotation.

In addition to the acceleration of the head, two other conditions are necessary to observe vestibular nystagmus. First, the type of eye movements described in Fig. 13 can be observed only in the absence of vision (eyes closed or in darkness). With vision present, other visual mechanisms, namely, the optokinetic and tracking systems, interact with the vestibular responses in generating compensatory eye movements (52). In the example in which the subject is suddenly stopped after a prolonged rotation, vestibular nystagmus can be observed in darkness. However, when vision is permitted, vestibular nystagmus is quickly suppressed. This is functionally reasonable because, in the absence of head motion, such compensatory eye movements are not required. The second condition for the formation of vestibular nystagmus is the mental alertness of the subject (54). Alertness appears to be necessary only for generating the fast phase of the nystagmus. It has been demonstrated that vestibular stimulation in comatose individuals does produce the slow drift of the eyes (55). However, once the eyes reach the periphery of the orbit, they remain deviated to one side.

An important property of the VOR pathways is revealed by examining eye movement responses during a prolonged constant-velocity rotation. As described earlier, the canal response consists of a sudden change in the firing rate of the peripheral neurons, which returns to its baseline exponentially as the cupula returns to its resting position. The intensity of the resulting vestibular nystagmus (slow-phase velocity) also undergoes a similar pattern, rising immediately after the initiation of motion and dissipating exponentially over time. However, there is a significant difference between the time course of the two events. Whereas the canal responses disappear after 15 to 20 seconds, the nystagmus persists almost three times longer (Fig. 15A) (56). The prolongation of the nystagmus is due to a neural integrator aptly named the *velocity storage mechanism.* The integrator acts as a storage tank in which an outflow valve can control the flow of neural activity so that it is not as rapid as the inflow. Consequently, there is a buildup of the neural activity that continues even after the input signal has ceased. The overall effect of the velocity storage mechanism is to extend the frequency response of the VOR pathways to lower frequencies. This effect is demonstrated in Fig. 15B. The gain (ratio of slow-phase eye velocity to head velocity) and phase (temporal difference of slow-phase eye velocity to head velocity) are shown for different frequencies of sinusoidal head movements. For ideal compensatory eye movements, the slow-phase eye velocity will be exactly the same amplitude as the head velocity but in the opposite direction. The frequency responses in Fig. 15B show the deviation of the resulting eye movements from ideal ones for different frequencies. When the gain is equal to one and the phase is equal to zero, the eye movements are completely compensatory. Without the velocity storage mechanism, the ideal responses are limited to the frequency range from 0.3 to 10 Hz. For frequencies lower than 0.3 Hz, the slow-phase eye velocity is less than the head velocity (gain less than one), and there is a time difference between the two (phase greater than zero). With the addition of the velocity storage mechanism, the effective range of the canal-ocular responses is extended to 0.1 to 10 Hz.

Stimulation of the Semicircular Canals: Responses to Temperature Gradients

The natural mode of stimulation for vestibular receptors is head motion; however, nonphysiologic stimuli are common in clinical testing of the vestibular system. In particular, the caloric test is still one of the most effective means of assessing vestibular function because it permits stimulation of each labyrinth independently. The caloric testing is administered with the subject in a supine position with the head bent forward by 30 degrees (Fig. 16). With the head in this position, the lateral semicircular canals are placed in the vertical plane. If a significant temperature gradient develops between the endolymphatic fluid on one side of the canal with respect to the fluid on the opposite side, the endolymph will begin to move, thus displacing the cupula (57). Such a temperature gradient can be induced by irrigating the external auditory canal with a medium (air or water) that has a significantly different temperature when compared to the body temperature.

The underlying mechanism for the movement of the endolymph during caloric irrigations is the temperature-induced change in the density of the endolymph. For example, a warm stimulus causes the fluid closest to the auditory canal to become lighter than the rest of the endolymph and rise due to the effect of gravity (Fig. 16). This causes an ampullopedal flow of the endolymph and leads to an excitatory response of the afferent neurons

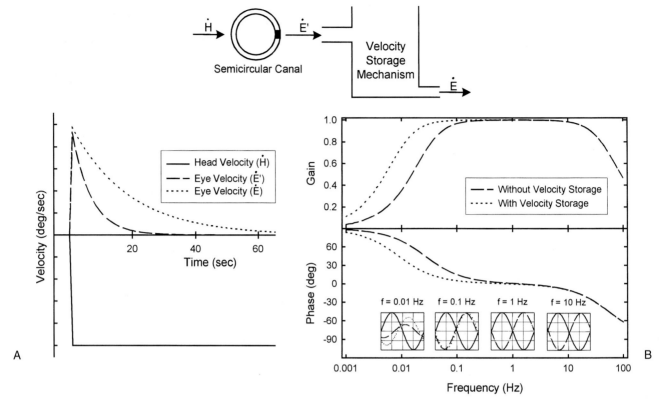

FIG. 15. The role of the velocity storage mechanism. **A:** Responses to a sudden change in head velocity. **B:** Frequency responses (gain and phase) to sinusoidal head rotations. Eye movement responses to various head rotation frequencies are shown in the **bottom** of the figure. (Adapted from Baloh RW, Honrubia V. *Clinical neurophysiology of the vestibular system.* Philadelphia: F.A. Davis, 1990.)

from the irrigated ear. The asymmetry between the neural firing rates from the two labyrinths is identical to that produced by the horizontal angular acceleration of the head toward the irrigated ear. Similarly, the resulting vestibular nystagmus has the same characteristics as those described earlier. A cold irrigation of the ear results in the flow of the endolymph in the opposite direction and decreases the neural firing rate of the irrigated ear. An acronym, COWS (cold opposite, warm same), is used to quickly identify the direction of the nystagmus generated by different irrigations. For example, cool irrigation of the left ear causes right-beating nystagmus exactly the same way as if the patient was being accelerated toward the right ear.

It is clear from this discussion that gravity is essential to explain the theory for generation of caloric responses. However, experiments in the space shuttle in the early 1980s cast doubt on the validity of this assumption when caloric responses were apparently produced in the absence of gravity. Yet compelling evidence remains to support the explanation. Figure 17 shows the direction of the endolymph flow if the subject is placed in a prone position with the head tilted forward by 30 degrees. Warm irrigation of the external auditory canal in this head position generates ampullofugal flow and decreases the neural firing rate from the irrigated side (58). The change in the direction of the nystagmus when the subject

moves from supine to prone or from prone to supine positions can be interpreted only by considering the effect of reversing the gravity vector. Today, the general consensus is that gravity is primarily responsible for generating caloric responses, although small changes in the firing rate of the neurons can be attributed to the direct effect of the temperature on the afferent nerve fibers (59).

Caloric responses are mediated primarily by the lateral semicircular canals. Theoretically, it also is possible to generate caloric responses from vertical canals if they are placed in the plane of gravity. However, the anatomic organization of the labyrinths is such that the vertical semicircular canals are distant from the external auditory canal. As a result, it is not possible to create the temperature gradient necessary to generate adequate vestibular stimulation for the vertical canals.

Stimulation of the Otolith Organs

The maculae of the utricle and saccule transduce forces applied to the head into neural signals. In contrast to the semicircular canals, the otolith organs respond to dynamic changes in linear velocity as well as static changes in the orientation of the head. The sensitivity of the otoliths to head tilts is due to presence of the gravitational field, which imposes a constant linear acceleration. Although only two

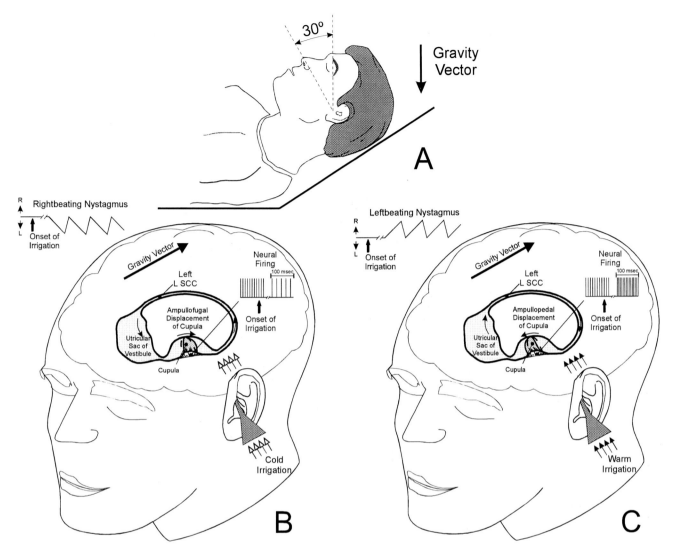

FIG. 16. Principle of caloric stimulation. **A:** Standard caloric test position with the lateral semicircular canals placed in the vertical plane. Modulation of neural firing rates and eye movement responses to cold **(B)** and warm **(C)** irrigations. (Inspired by drawings from Baloh RW. *Dizziness, hearing loss, and tinnitus: the essentials of neurotology.* Philadelphia: F.A. Davis, 1984.)

sensory receptors are available for linear motion, the distinct arrangement of the macular hair cells allows the otoliths to sense motion in all three dimensions. This same arrangement also is responsible for creating synergistic pairing of the otoliths that is much more complex than that of the canals (37). In otoliths, the push-pull arrangement might be confined to only one area of the macula on each side instead of involving the entire sensory organ.

As is the case for the semicircular canals, stimulation of the otoliths also is expected to produce compensatory eye movements. Electrical stimulation of the utricular and saccular nerve fibers, as well as direct stimulation of macular regions, produce steady eye deviations (60). The direction of the eye deviations depends on the polarization of the hair cells in each region. Nystagmus eye movements have been reported, but it is not clear whether

nystagmus responses were the result of inadvertent stimulation of semicircular canal nerve fibers (61).

When otolith stimulation is generated by head tilts, the resulting eye movements can be either torsional (rotation of the eyes in the orbit about the visual axis) or rotational (similar to horizontal eye movements but may include a vertical component). The type of response is different among species and depends on the orientation of eyes and the direction of tilt (42). In humans, lateral head tilts generate torsional eye movements known as *ocular counter-rolling* (62). Although these eye movements are compensatory, they are not efficient in counteracting the effect of head tilts. The amplitude of eye torsion even for large tilts is only around 10% of the amplitude of the head tilt. Head tilts in the pitch plane generate vertical movements of the eyes. However, the effect of the vertical semicircular

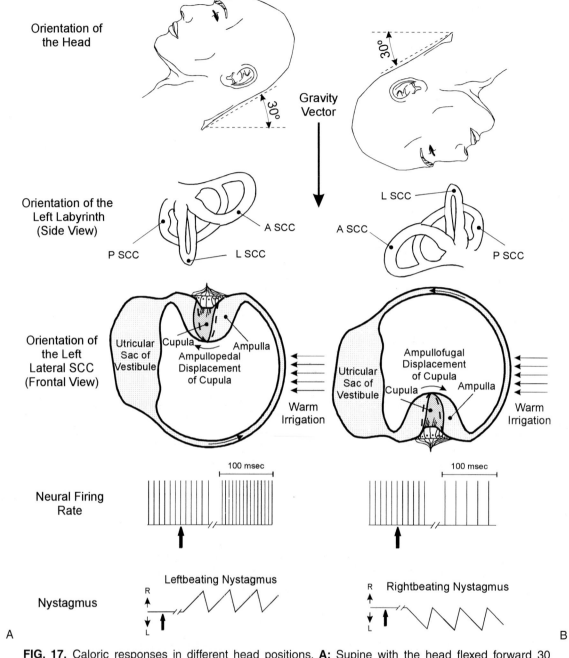

FIG. 17. Caloric responses in different head positions. **A:** Supine with the head flexed forward 30 degrees (standard caloric test position). **B:** Prone with the head flexed forward 30 degrees. Abbreviations for semicircular canals as in Fig. 6.

canals in generating such eye movements during the acceleration phase of the tilt should not be overlooked.

The effect of linear head acceleration in generating compensatory eye movements is more controversial. If the otoliths are viewed as sensors that respond to the combination of all forces applied to the head, then compensatory eye movements for linear acceleration in the lateral plane (along the interaural axis) will be ocular counterrolling similar to those generated by lateral head tilts. Instead, experiments using such an acceleration have

produced horizontal nystagmus (61). Similarly, linear accelerations in the pitch plane (along the occipitonasal axis) have failed to produce vertical eye movements as expected. These observations indicate that the otolith-ocular pathways do not respond the same way to other linear accelerations as they do to gravity. This is logical, because the role of the vestibular receptors is to complement the visual system. This can be best accomplished if gravity is treated differently than other linear accelerations that induce motion.

Overall, otolith-induced eye movements are not studied as extensively as those produced by the semicircular canals. Significant gaps remain in our understanding of the organization and the exact function of the otolith-ocular pathways.

Adaptation of Vestibular Responses

A discussion of vestibular function is incomplete without consideration of the role of adaptation. Adaptation is the process of making adjustments to the vestibular pathways to improve their performance under a variety of conditions. The cerebellum is thought to be the origin of the adaptive control mechanisms. These mechanisms are part of a more global compensation system that is responsible for recovering from a vestibular lesion. Whereas compensation can take many different forms (see the next section), adaptation primarily involves changing the sensitivity (gain) of the vestibular pathways (19). It should be noted, however, that because the VOR is a dynamic system, changing the gain means more than simply changing the intensity of the eye movements. Other response characteristics, such as timing and direction of eye movements, also may be affected.

As noted before, normal vestibular responses usually are short in duration, often lasting only a few seconds. When the asymmetry from right-left afferent nerve fibers persists for longer than the anticipated time, the sensitivity of the VOR, and consequently the intensity of the nystagmus, is reduced (42). This adjustment can take place in a relatively short period of time. For example, if caloric stimulation is applied for an extended period of time, the adaptive changes can begin within a few minutes (4). Similarly, repeated stimulation of the vestibular system can activate the adaptive mechanisms. For example, the intensity of induced nystagmus declines after repeated exposure to rotation. A more drastic example of adaptation occurs during space flights (63). Removal of the gravitational vector causes a change in the firing pattern of the otolith neurons. Whereas a change in the gain of the VOR may be helpful in the short term to alleviate motion sickness symptoms, a more intricate change in the organization of the otolith pathways is needed to deal with the long-term consequences of space flight on the vestibular system. Once the astronauts return to earth, a similar reorganization must take place to adapt to gravity.

EFFECTS OF PERIPHERAL VESTIBULAR LESIONS

Peripheral vestibular disorders are the major cause of dizziness and balance disorders in humans. Understanding the underlying process of vestibular pathologies and central compensation mechanisms can provide a significant insight into the assessment and management of dizzy patients. The scope of peripheral vestibular disorders can be best appreciated by an abstract analysis of the problem. The vestibular system consists of ten receptors, five per labyrinth. If one assumes each receptor can develop a lesion independently, there will be more than 1,000 combinations of ways that the vestibular receptors may become dysfunctional. This simple analysis does not include damage to the surrounding support structures and many other aspects of lesions, such as complete versus partial, transient versus permanent, or sudden versus gradual. Also not considered is the differentiation of the type of lesion that impairs receptor function from the type of lesion that distorts function.[3] Therefore, one should not be surprised by the myriad of the symptoms reported by patients with diseases of the labyrinths and the vestibular nerve. It is humbling to consider that our assessment methods can only evaluate a handful of peripheral vestibular anomalies.

Effects of Unilateral Vestibular Lesions

Figure 18 shows the effect of a peripheral vestibular lesion that reduces or obliterates the tonic activity of the vestibular nerve from one labyrinth (60). Such a lesion can be caused by a disease process that destroys the hair cells in the labyrinth or directly affects the peripheral nerve function. The unilateral decrease in the tonic neural activity results in an asymmetry identical to that produced by head rotation. The patient perceives the head rotating toward the intact ear. This illusion of motion is called *vertigo*. In this case, because there is a conflict between the information from the vestibular system and those from other sensory modalities, the patient will likely experience vegetative symptoms associated with such a sensory conflict, such as nausea and vomiting. Additionally, the patient will have vestibular nystagmus, which has similar characteristics to those produced in response to physiologic stimuli and described in the previous section. This pathologic nystagmus is often referred to as *spontaneous nystagmus* to highlight that it is present in the absence of head motion. However, in this chapter, this often misused terminology is avoided because the same term also is used to describe *any* pathologic nystagmus regardless of its origin or characteristics.

The sudden unilateral loss of labyrinthine function produces vestibular nystagmus that is predominantly horizontal but sometimes also has a torsional component. The horizontal component of the nystagmus is caused by the loss of tonic activity from the afferent neurons of the lateral canal on the damaged side (20). The slow phase of this nystagmus will be directed toward the damaged side because the CNS perceives the head rotation being toward the intact ear. It should be noted, however, that the direction of nystagmus can change because of vestibular compensation and is not always a reliable indicator of the side of lesion (see following). Pathologic vestibular nystagmus does not

---

[3]An example of the type of lesion that causes impairment is labyrinthitis, which causes loss of hair cell function and reduction of tonic neural activity. An example of the type of lesion that causes distortion is benign paroxysmal positional vertigo, which makes the posterior semicircular canals sensitive to certain head movements.

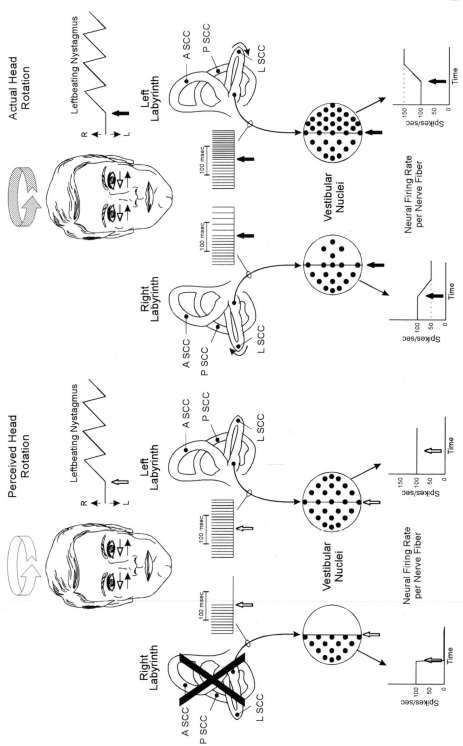

FIG. 18. A: Changes in neural firing rates and the resulting eye movements immediately after a unilateral vestibular lesion (identified by *hollow arrows*). **B:** Changes in neural firing rates and the resulting eye movements immediately after a counterclockwise head rotation (identified by *solid arrows*). The directions of nystagmus fast and slow phases are as in Fig. 6. The density of *dots* represents the level of neural firing. (Modified from Baloh RW. *Dizziness, hearing loss, and tinnitus: the essentials of neurotology.* Philadelphia: F.A. Davis, 1984.)

have a vertical component. Vertical eye movements that are generated by the vertical semicircular canals from one ear are in the opposite direction. The net result is the cancellation of the vertical component because the anterior and posterior canals from the intact side have no functioning match in the damaged side. These canals produce torsional eye movements that are in the same direction, thus explaining the torsional component of the nystagmus (64).

Acute unilateral vestibular loss also causes other postural abnormalities, including head tilt toward the side of lesion and disequilibrium (20). Many of these effects are temporary and recover quickly after compensation. One manifestation of unilateral vestibular loss, which seems to persist permanently, is a static torsion of the eyes toward the side of lesion. This *ocular tilt reaction* is likely caused by the unilateral loss of otolithic function.

Vestibular Compensation after a Unilateral Vestibular Lesion

The persistent asymmetry in the firing rate of vestibular neurons triggers the vestibular compensation mechanisms (19). In this case, vestibular compensation consists of two distinct processes. First, the static balance in the tonic neural activities of the two labyrinths is restored. Second, the characteristics of the vestibular pathways (e.g., sensitivity or gain) are modified to accommodate dynamic changes due to the loss of motion-induced neural activities from one labyrinth.

Figure 19 shows various steps during the static compensation process that lead to the restoration of tonic neural activities (42). This is used as a simplified and functional illustration of a complex process and does not necessarily match the exact physiologic events. Figure 19A shows the neural activity for a stationary head followed a counterclockwise head acceleration, when both labyrinths are intact. The asymmetry in the neural firing rates immediately after a sudden unilateral vestibular loss (Fig. 19B) is reduced by "clamping" the neural activity of the intact labyrinth (Fig. 19C). This step can begin within days, if not hours, after the initial damage to the labyrinth. The decrease in the asymmetry of neural activities reduces the intensity of the symptoms. The effect is similar to that of the antivertiginous medications that suppress the vestibular activity at the brainstem level. Within 1 week after the onset of the lesion, neural activity appears in the vestibular nuclei at the site innervated by the afferent nerve fibers from the damaged side (Fig. 19D). This neural activity originates not from the labyrinth, but from other sources within the CNS. At the same time, the activity from the intact side begins to increase as the clamping of the vestibular input is eased. After a few weeks, the static compensation is completed when the tonic neural firing from the intact side returns to its prelesion level and the neural activity is restored at the vestibular nuclei of the damaged side (Fig. 19E). The static compensation process occurs regardless of whether the unilateral vestibular loss is sudden or gradual. In case of a gradual loss, the entire compensation process takes place repeatedly in small increments. As a result, a patient with such a loss may not experience the kind of severe symptoms associated with a sudden unilateral lesion (60).

After a unilateral vestibular loss, the inherent asymmetry between the excitatory and inhibitory neural firings from one semicircular canal is no longer offset by the responses from the paired canal. Therefore, it is expected that the responses for clockwise and counterclockwise rotations will be asymmetric after a unilateral lesion. In practice, this type of asymmetry is seen only in the early stage of static compensation during the period when the responses from the intact ear are suppressed (Figs. 19C and D). In this stage, rotation away from the side of lesion will quickly saturate the response as the neural firing rate is reduced to zero. The rotation toward the intact side will be unaffected as the excitatory responses can increase significantly more. After the completion of static compensation, the response asymmetries can be seen only for high-acceleration stimuli.

The process of static compensation is most effective when the lesion is stable. Fluctuations in the status of the labyrinth disrupt the compensation process and cause symptoms that usually are more troublesome to the patient than those caused by a stable lesion, even when the lesion is permanent. If function is restored to the damaged labyrinth during the compensation steps for which the neural activity of the intact side is suppressed (Fig. 19C or D), the asymmetry in the neural activity of right-left labyrinths will be reversed. This reversal leads to eye movements known as *recovery nystagmus* (64). The slow phase of the recovery nystagmus is in the opposite direction of the slow phase of the nystagmus seen immediately after an acute vestibular lesion. Otherwise, the two types of nystagmus have identical characteristics and cannot be differentiated. Therefore, one cannot rely solely on the direction of the nystagmus as an indicator of side of lesion.

Figure 19F shows the neural activity after a counterclockwise head acceleration, after the completion of static compensation. It is clear that head rotation once again will generate the neural asymmetry necessary for detecting the direction of rotation. However, the magnitude of the asymmetry is half of that generated by two functioning labyrinths for the same head acceleration. During the dynamic phase of compensation, the vestibular pathways are recalibrated such that the new pattern of the head velocity to neural firing rates is transformed into compensatory eye movements with appropriate intensities (19). Intuitively, the gain of the VOR pathways must be doubled to generate the same amplitude of eye movements as those generated before the lesion. However, because the VOR is a dynamic system, a change in the gain of the pathway could affect other characteristics, including its frequency response. Recall the analogy used

(text continues on page 138)

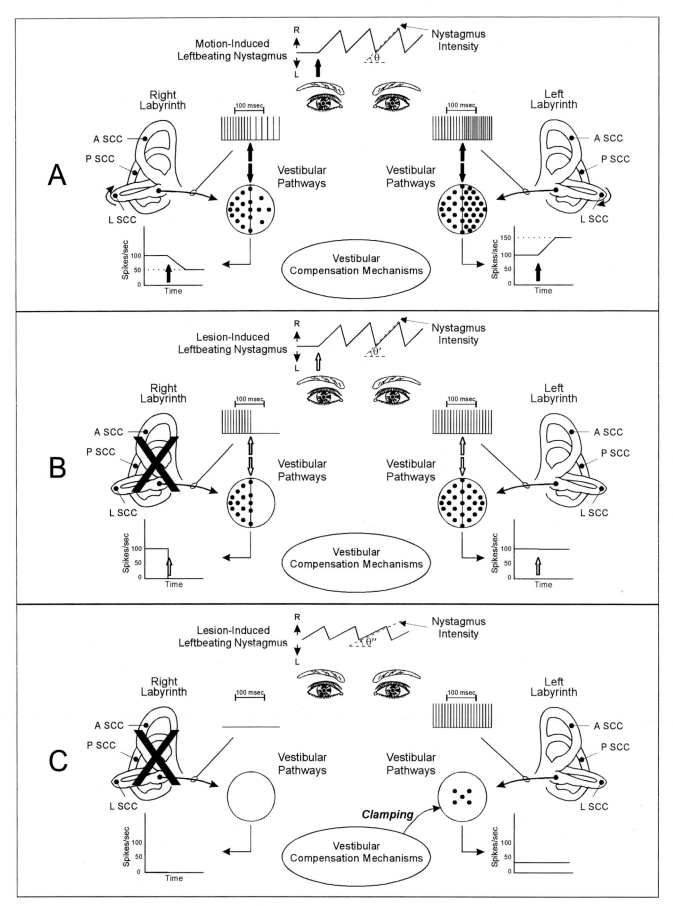

FIG. 19. A simplified illustration of the vestibular compensation process after a unilateral vestibular lesion. (Inspired by Barber HO, Stockwell CW. *Manual of electronystagmography.* St. Louis: Mosby, 1980.) *Solid arrows* identify the onset of the head acceleration. *Hollow arrows* identify the onset of the lesion. The density of *dots* represents the level of neural firing. θ, θ′, and θ″ represent slow-phase nystagmus intensities. Abbreviations for semicircular canals as in Fig. 6. See text for a description of compensation steps.

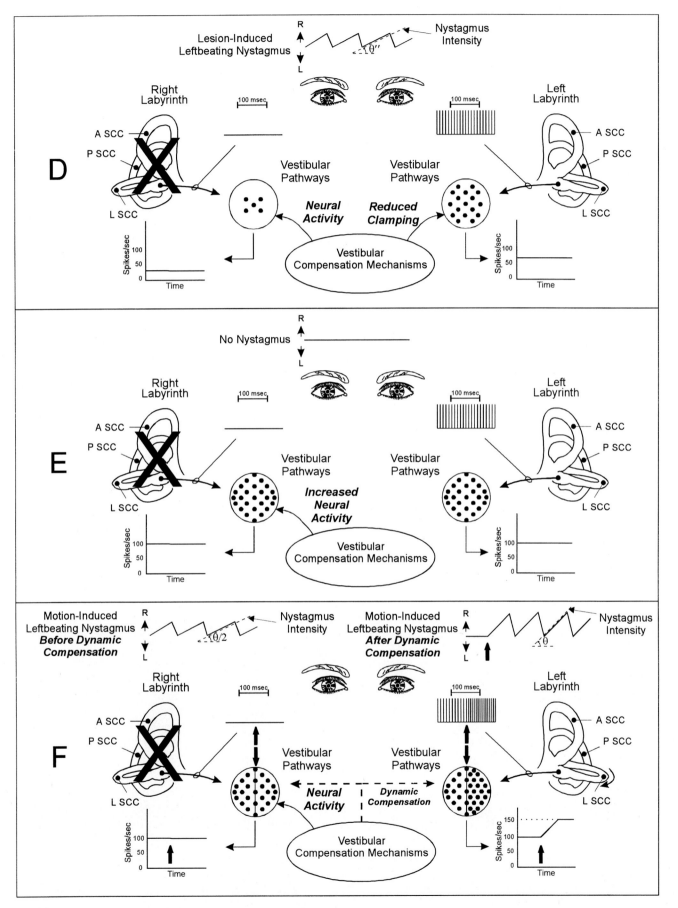

FIG. 19. *Continued.*

for the velocity storage mechanism. One way to increase the sensitivity is to increase the gain of the integrator in the VOR pathway. This is analogous to increasing the outflow of the velocity storage mechanism. Although this action increases the sensitivity, it also diminishes the storage capacity of the integrator. Consequently, the low-frequency performance of the system will be degraded. This can be best appreciated by revisiting Fig. 15. If the effectiveness of the velocity storage mechanism is gradually decreased, the frequency response of the VOR in Fig. 15B will move from the configuration represented by the dotted line to that represented by the dashed line.

Degradation of low-frequency VOR performance is associated with unilateral loss of vestibular function (65). Rotational tests in patients with such lesions show that the ratio of the slow-phase eye velocity to head velocity decreases and the phase difference between them increases for low frequencies. However, the process of dynamic compensation is more complex than simply increasing the gain of the VOR. Most likely, a remapping of the vestibular signals is necessary to ensure precise integration of the information from all sensory mechanisms.

Effects of Bilateral Vestibular Lesion

Bilateral vestibular lesions are far less common than unilateral ones. Although the long-term functional consequences of bilateral lesions are considerably more serious, ironically, the symptoms are not as severe as those after a sudden unilateral lesion. Because there is no asymmetry between the right-left neural firing rates, patients with bilateral lesions do not experience vertigo, nystagmus, or vegetative symptoms. The main complaints of these patients are disequilibrium and oscillopsia. Oscillopsia is the illusion that stationary objects are moving during head motion (66). This symptom is caused by the impairment of the VOR after loss of both labyrinths. Because vestibular-driven compensatory eye movements are no longer possible, the images of the objects are not stationary long enough to have clear vision during head motion.

Bilateral vestibular lesions can be complete or partial (42). The loss of function for partial lesions is confined to low-frequency head movements, whereas the high-frequency responses are preserved until the loss is complete. In the case of a complete vestibular loss, there is no vestibular-mediated mechanism to restore function. Instead, the central compensation mechanisms utilize other sensorimotor inputs to substitute for the labyrinthine function (19). The visual and neck receptors are the most appropriate alternatives for both postural and visual stabilization. The compensation methods for bilateral lesions are not nearly as effective as the methods described for unilateral lesions. Patients with complete and permanent bilateral lesions are not as likely to regain their prelesion functional status as well as patients with a unilateral loss.

SUMMARY POINTS

- The vestibular receptors are responsible for sensing the three-dimensional orientation and movements of the head.
- The information from the vestibular system is used by the VSR and VOR to maintain a stable upright posture and to provide a clear vision during head movements.
- Three semicircular canals in each labyrinth respond to rotational movements of the head and generate an afferent neural firing pattern that is a damped version of the head acceleration. For natural head movements, the neural firing rate is proportional to the head velocity.
- When the head undergoes an angular acceleration in the plane of one of the semicircular canals, the firing rate of the afferent nerve fibers from the leading ear increases, whereas the firing rate from the opposite side decreases from its tonic level.
- The asymmetry in the firing rate of the right-left vestibular neurons generates compensatory eye movements known as nystagmus. When nystagmus is provoked by head rotation, its slow phase is in the opposite direction of the head acceleration.
- The role of otolith organs, the maculae of utricle and saccule, is to sense linear accelerations of the head. Because of their sensitivity to gravity, the otoliths also are responsible for detecting the static orientation of the head.
- Caloric stimulation of the labyrinth in the standard caloric position (head tilted forward 30 degrees from the supine position) causes movement of the endolymph and changes the neural firing rate from the irrigated ear. A cold irrigation of the ear decreases the firing rate, whereas a warm irrigation increases it.
- An acronym, COWS (cold opposite, warm same), is used to identify the fast phase of the nystagmus generated by different irrigations in the standard caloric position.
- The unilateral loss or reduction of labyrinthine function produces vertigo and vestibular nystagmus. For acute lesions, the perceived head rotation is toward the intact ear and the slow phase of the nystagmus is directed toward the damaged side.
- The persistent asymmetry in the firing rate of vestibular neurons after a unilateral vestibular loss triggers vestibular compensation mechanisms. These mechanisms restore the balance in the tonic neural activities (static compensation) and modify the vestibular pathways to accommodate for the loss of motion-induced neural activities from one labyrinth (dynamic compensation).

ACKNOWLEDGMENTS

The authors thank Lois J. Barin and Vinita Brinda for their assistance in preparation of this chapter. The figures in this chapter were produced using CorelDraw 4.

REFERENCES

1. Wilson VJ, Melvill Jones, G. *Mammalian vestibular physiology.* New York: Plenum Press, 1979.
2. Brooks VB. *The neural basis of motor control.* New York: Oxford University Press, 1986.
3. Shepard NT, Telian SA. *Practical management of the balance disorder patient.* San Diego: Singular Publishing, 1996.
4. Howard IP. *Human visual orientation.* New York: John Wiley & Sons, 1982.
5. Nashner LM, McCollum G. The organization of human postural movements: a formal basis and experimental synthesis. *Behav Brain Sci* 1985;8:135–172.
6. Leigh RJ, Zee DS. *The neurology of eye movement.* Philadelphia: F.A. Davis, 1983.
7. van Die G, Collewijn H. Optokinetic nystagmus in man: role of central and peripheral retina and occurrence of asymmetries. *Hum Neurobiol* 1982;1:111–119.
8. Westheimer G. Mechanism of saccadic eye movements. *AMA Arch Ophthalmol* 1954;52:710–724.
9. Cohen B, Henn V. The origin of quick phases of nystagmus in the horizontal plane. *Bibl Ophthalmol* 1972;82:36–55.
10. Pola J, Wyatt HJ. Target position and velocity: the stimuli for smooth pursuit eye movements. *Vision Res* 1980;20:523–534.
11. Waespe W, Henn V. Gaze stabilization in the primate: the interaction of the vestibuloocular reflex, optokinetic nystagmus, and smooth pursuit. *Rev Physiol Biochem Pharmacol* 1987;106:37–125.
12. Barlow D, Freedman W. Cervico-ocular reflex in the normal adult. *Acta Otolaryngol* 1980;89:487–496.
13. Reason JT, Brand JJ. *Motion sickness.* New York: Academic Press, 1975.
14. Yates BJ, Miller AD. Overview of vestibular autonomic regulation. In: Yates BJ, Miller AD, eds. *Vestibular autonomic regulation.* Boca Raton: CRC Press, 1996:1–3.
15. Money KE. Motion sickness. *Physiol Rev* 1970;50:1–39.
16. Wang SC, Chinn HI. Experimental motion sickness in dogs: importance of labyrinth and vestibular cerebellum. *Am J Physiol* 1956;185:617–623.
17. Brizzee KR, Igarashi M. Effect of macular ablation on frequency and latency of motion-induced emesis in the squirrel monkey. *Aviat Space Environ Med* 1986;57:1066–1170.
18. Furman JM, Jacob RG, Redfern MS. Clinical evidence that the vestibular system participates in autonomic control. *J Vestib Res* 1998;8:27–34.
19. Zee DS. Vestibular adaptation. In: Herdman SJ, ed. *Vestibular rehabilitation.* Philadelphia: F.A. Davis, 1994:68–79.
20. Halmagyi GM, Curthoys IS. Clinical changes in vestibular function over time after lesions: the consequences of unilateral vestibular deafferentation. In: Herdman SJ, ed. *Vestibular rehabilitation.* Philadelphia: F.A. Davis, 1994:90–109.
21. Sterkers O, Ferrary E, Amiel C. Production of inner ear fluids. *Physiol Rev* 1988;68:1083–1128.
22. Salt AN, Konishi T. The cochlear fluids: perilymph and endolymph. In: Altschuler RA, Hoffman DW, Bobbin RP, eds. *Neurobiology of hearing: the cochlea.* New York: Raven Press, 1986:109–122.
23. Kimura RS. Distribution, structure, and function of dark cells in the vestibular labyrinth. *Ann Otol Rhinol Laryngol* 1969;78:542–561.
24. Lysakowski A, McCrea RA, Tomlinson RD. Anatomy of vestibular end organs and neural pathways. In: Cummings, et al., eds. *Otolaryngology—head and neck surgery,* 2nd ed. St. Louis: Mosby, 1995:2525–2547.
25. Wende S, Nakayama N, Schwerdtfeger P. The internal auditory artery: embryology, anatomy, angiography, pathology. *J Neurol* 1975;210:21–31.
26. Schucknecht HF. *Pathology of the ear.* Cambridge: Harvard University Press, 1974.
27. Perlman HB, Kimura RS, Fernandez C. Experiments on temporary obstruction of the internal auditory artery. *Laryngoscope* 1959;69:591–613.
28. Konishi T, Butler RA, Fernandez C. Effect of anoxia on cochlear potentials. *J Acoust Soc Amer* 1961;33:349–356.
29. Durrant JD, Freeman AR. Concepts in vestibular physiology. In: Finestone AJ, ed. *Evaluation and clinical management of dizziness and vertigo.* Boston: John Wright, 1982:13–43.
30. Baloh RW, Honrubia V. Physiology of the vestibular system. In: Cummings, et al., eds. *Otolaryngology—head and neck surgery,* 2nd ed. St. Louis: Mosby, 1995:2604–2642.
31. Flock A, Orman S. Micromechanical properties of sensory hairs on receptor cells of the inner ear. *Hear Res* 1983;11:249–260.
32. Goldberg JM, Lysakowski A, Fernandez C. Structure and function of vestibular nerve fibers in the chinchilla and squirrel monkey. In: Cohen B, Tomko DL, Guedry F, eds. Sensing and controlling motion: vestibular and sensorimotor function. *Proc N Y Acad Sci* 1992;656:92–107.
33. Honrubia V, Hoffman LF. Practical anatomy and physiology of the vestibular pathways. In: Jacobson GP, Newman CW, Kartush JM, eds. *Handbook of balance function testing,* St. Louis: Mosby-Year Book, 1993:9–47.
34. Goldberg JM, Fernandez C. Physiology of peripheral neurons innervating semicircular canals of the squirrel monkey. I. Resting discharge and response to constant angular accelerations. *J Neurophysiol* 1971;34:635–660.
35. Flock A, Jorgensen M, Russell I. The physiology of individual hair cells and their synapses. In: Moller AR, ed. *Basic mechanisms in hearing.* New York: Academic Press, 1973;273–306.
36. Hudspeth AJ. Mechanoelectrical transduction by hair cells in the acousticolateralis sensory system. *Annu Rev Neurosci* 1983;6:187–215.
37. Fernandez C, Goldberg JM. Physiology of peripheral neurons innervating otolith organs of the squirrel monkey. II. Directional selectivity and force-response relations. *J Neurophysiol* 1976;39:985–995.
38. Blanks RHI, Curthoys IS, Markham CH. Planar relationships of semicircular canals in man. *Acta Otolaryngol* 1975;80:185–196.
39. Dohlmann GF. The attachment of the cupulae, otolith, and tectorial membranes to the sensory cell areas. *Acta Otolaryngol* 1971;71:89–105.
40. Money KE, Bonen L, Beatty JD, Kuehn LA, Sokoloff M, Weaver RS. Physical properties of fluids and structures of vestibular apparatus of the pigeon. *Am J Physiol* 1971;220:140–147.
41. Fernandez C, Goldberg JM. Physiology of peripheral neurons innervating semicircular canals of the squirrel monkey. II. Response to sinusoidal stimulation and dynamics of peripheral vestibular system. *J Neurophysiol* 1971;34:661–675.
42. Baloh RW, Honrubia V. *Clinical neurophysiology of the vestibular system.* Philadelphia: F.A. Davis, 1990.
43. Lim DJ. The development and structure of the otoconia. In: Friedman I, Ballantyne J, eds. *Ultrastructural atlas of the inner ear.* London: Butterworths, 1984:245–269.
44. Lindeman HH. Studies on the morphology of the sensory regions of the vestibular apparatus with 45 figures. *Ergeb Anat EntwicklungsGesch* 1969;42:1–113.
45. Hain TC, Hillman MA. Anatomy and physiology of the normal vestibular system. In: Herdman SJ, ed. *Vestibular rehabilitation.* Philadelphia: F.A. Davis, 1994:3–21.
46. Brodal A. Anatomy of the vestibular nuclei and their connections. In: Kornhuber HH, ed. *Handbook of sensory physiology: the vestibular system.* Berlin: Springer-Verlag, 1974:239–352.
47. Precht W. Labyrinthine influences on the vestibular nuclei. *Prog Brain Res* 1979;50:369–381.
48. Robinson DA. Adaptive gain control of the vestibulo-ocular reflex by the cerebellum. *J Neurophysiol* 1976;39:954–969.
49. Cohen B. The vestibulo-ocular reflex arc. In: Kornhuber HH, ed. *Handbook of sensory physiology: the vestibular system,* Berlin: Springer-Verlag, 1974:477–540.
50. Barber HO, Stockwell CW. *Manual of electronystagmography.* St. Louis: Mosby, 1980.
51. Maeda M, Shimazu H, Shinoda Y. Nature of synaptic events in cat abducens motoneurons at slow and quick phase of vestibular nystagmus. *J Neurophysiol* 1972;35:279–296.
52. Robinson DA. Control of eye movements. In: Brooks VB, ed. *Handbook of physiology: the nervous system.* Washington, DC: American Physiological Society, 1981:1275–1313.
53. Honrubia V, Baloh RW, Lau CG, Sills AW. The patterns of eye movements during physiologic vestibular nystagmus in man. *Trans Am Acad Ophthalmol Otolaryngol* 1977;84:339–347.
54. Collins WE. Manipulation of arousal and its effects upon human

vestibular nystagmus induced by caloric irrigation and angular accelerations. *Aerospace Med* 1963;34:124–129.

55. Leigh RJ, Hanley DF, Munschauer FE 3d, Lasker AG. Eye movements induced by head rotation in unresponsive patients. *Ann Neurol* 1984;15:465–473.

56. Raphan T, Matsuo V, Cohen B. Velocity storage in the vestibulo-ocular reflex arc. *Exp Brain Res* 1979;35:229–248.

57. O'Neill G. The caloric stimulus. Temperature generation within the temporal bone. *Acta Otolaryngol* 1987;103:266–272.

58. Coats AC, Smith SY. Body position and the intensity of caloric nystagmus. *Acta Otolaryngol* 1967;63:515–532.

59. Paige G. Caloric responses after canal inactivation. *Acta Otolaryngol* 1985;100:321–327.

60. Baloh RW. *Dizziness, hearing loss, and tinnitus: the essentials of neurotology.* Philadelphia: F.A. Davis, 1984.

61. Niven JI, Hixson WC, Correia, MJ. Elicitation of horizontal nystagmus by periodic linear acceleration. *Acta Otolaryngol* 1966;62:429–441.

62. Miller EF. Counterrolling of the human eye produced by head tilt with respect to gravity. *Acta Otolaryngol* 1962;54:479–501.

63. Oman CM, Lichtenberg BK, Money KE, McCoy RK. MIT/Canadian vestibular experiments on the Spacelab-1 mission: 4. Space motion sickness: symptoms, stimuli, and predictability. *Exp Brain Res* 1986; 64:316–334.

64. Furman JM, Cass SP. *Balance disorders: a case-study approach.* Philadelphia: F.A. Davis, 1996.

65. Wolfe JW, Engelken EJ, Olson JE. Low-frequency harmonic acceleration in evaluation of patients with peripheral labyrinthine disorders. In: Honrubia V, Brazier MAB, eds. *Nystagmus and vertigo: clinical approaches to the patient with dizziness.* New York: Academic Press, 1982:95–105.

66. Bender MB. Oscillopsia. *Arch Neurol* 1965;13:203–213.

67. Melvill Jones G. Organization of neural control in the vestibulo-ocular reflex arc. In: Bach-Y-Rita P, Cullins CC, Hyde JE, eds. *The control of eye movements,* New York: Academic Press, 1971;497–518.

The Ear: Comprehensive Otology,
edited by R. F. Canalis and P. R. Lambert.
Lippincott Williams & Wilkins, Philadelphia © 2000.

CHAPTER 6

Central Representation of the Eighth Cranial Nerve

Anita N. Newman, Ian S. Storper, and Phillip A. Wackym

The foundation of our understanding of the central nervous system (CNS) anatomy of the auditory and vestibular system has been provided by the meticulous, painstaking work of anatomists such as the late professor Rafael Lorente de Nó. In addition to his many contributions regarding the organization of the receptors of the cochlear and vestibular labyrinth, Lorente de Nó, using Golgi preparations or nerve degeneration techniques, described the central projections of the cochlear and vestibular nerves (1), the cytoarchitecture of the cochlear nucleus (2), the anatomy of the vestibuloocular reflex arc (3), and the role of interneurons in vestibular reflex function (4). The advent of computer-assisted representation and specific labeling techniques such as immunocytochemistry and immunoelectron microscopy has markedly improved our understanding of the central projections of the eighth cranial nerve. In contrast to other biosensory systems, the projections of the vestibular and auditory nerves are extremely complex, and many details remain unknown. More is known about the

auditory than the vestibular system. Although many of the gross vestibular projections are understood, details about the precise anatomic connections between cells, the distributions of neurotransmitters, neuromodulators, and receptors, and the types of neurotransmission, whether excitatory or inhibitory, remain to be elucidated.

In this chapter we summarize the information currently available about the CNS projections of the auditory and vestibular divisions of the eighth cranial nerve. This information is intended to complement Chapters 2–5, which describe the peripheral organization of these nerves at the level of the receptor end organs. It also is intended to be used in conjunction with the clinical information available elsewhere in this book.

AUDITORY PROJECTIONS

The cochlear nerve is a bipolar sensory nerve. Its cell bodies lie within the spiral ganglion, located in the modiolus, within Rosenthal's canal. Peripherally, the dendrites of 95% of the neurons of the cochlear nerve innervate the inner hair cells of the cochlea. Only 5% of the neurons innervate the outer hair cells of the cochlea (Fig. 1). There is evidence that the central processes of the ganglion cells project directly to the rhombencephalon (hindbrain including the pons and medulla). Through secondary and possibly tertiary fibers, the mesencephalon (midbrain) and prosencephalon (forebrain) also are supplied (Fig. 2). The

A. N. Newman: Department of Head and Neck Surgery, University of Southern California School of Medicine, Los Angeles, California 90020

I. S. Storper: Department of Otolaryngology, College of Physicians and Surgeons, Columbia University, New York, New York 10032

P. A. Wackym: Department of Otolaryngology and Communication Sciences, Medical College of Wisconsin, Milwaukee, Wisconsin 53226

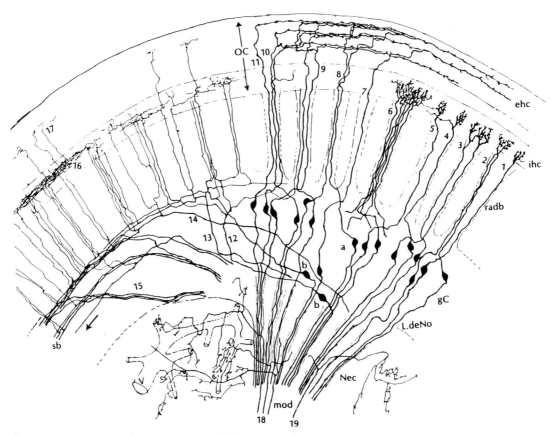

FIG. 1. Except for fibers 18 and 19, which innervate blood vessels, drawing shows nerve cells and fibers in a single section passing through the basal spiral turn of the cochlea. Eight-day-old mouse (Golgi's rapid method). *gC,* Ganglion of Corti; *Nec,* cochlear nerve; *mod,* modiolus; *OC,* organ of Corti. Ganglion cells (*a*) give rise to specific radial fibers (*1–6*) for internal (inner) hair cells (*ihc*) and to external spiral fibers (*7–11*) for external (outer) hair cells (*ehc*). Ganglion cells (*b*) give rise to unspecific radial fibers for internal hair cells (ramified fibers *12, 13,* and *14* are shown); *radb,* radial bundles; *sb,* spiral bundles (*arrow* points toward apex of cochlea); *15,* bundle of fibers joining the spiral system; *16* and *17,* bundles of fibers probably belonging to Rasmussen's efferent system.

cochlear nerve, composed of approximately 35,000 cells, travels with the vestibular nerves in the vicinity of the porus acusticus internus (5) to form the eighth cranial nerve. At approximately the level of the porus acusticus, the nerve reaches the Obersteiner-Redlich zone, where the transition from Schwann sheathing to glial sheathing cells occurs (6). As the nerve progresses centrally, it forms one structure, which again becomes separated into two roots by the inferior cerebellar peduncle at the pontomedullary junction. The cochlear root is located superior to the inferior cerebellar peduncle.

Afferent First-order Neurons

The auditory nerve enters the brainstem posteriorly and laterally at the pontomedullary junction, where all cells terminate within a protuberance comprised of the cochlear nuclei (Figs. 3–5). With Nissl's staining method, three cell groups have been found within this complex: the anteroventral cochlear nucleus (AVCN), the posteroventral cochlear nucleus (PVCN), and the dorsal cochlear nucleus

(DCN). The AVCN and PVCN form the ventral cochlear nucleus (VCN); the DCN also is called the *tuberculum acusticum.* Lorente de Nó, using Golgi's stain, identified 50 different cell types in the cochlear nuclei (7); Osen identified nine distinct cell classes in cat cochlear nuclei (8). Other investigators have classified numerous distinct cell types in these nuclei in various species, including *Homo sapiens* (9). Among other cell types, commonly accepted ones include octopus, fusiform, corn, stellate, bushy, granular, and multipolar (Figs. 6–8).

The individual cochlear nerve fibers enter the brainstem and immediately bifurcate into the ascending (ventral or anterior) branch to the AVCN and the descending (dorsal or posterior) branch to the PVCN and DCN. Each cochlear fiber projects to the DCN, the AVCN, and the PVCN. The VCN also projects to the DCN. The first synapse of cells of the auditory nerve occurs within the cochlear nuclei, both with second-order neurons and with cells confined to the cochlear nuclei (7). Organization is tonotopic or cochleotopic with high-frequency neurons (originating from the basal cochlea) that project dorsally

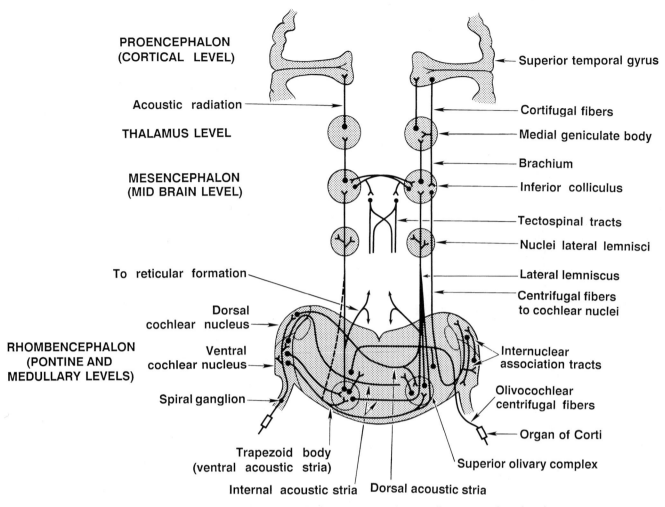

PROENCEPHALON (CORTICAL LEVEL)

Acoustic radiation

THALAMUS LEVEL

MESENCEPHALON (MID BRAIN LEVEL)

To reticular formation

Dorsal cochlear nucleus

RHOMBENCEPHALON (PONTINE AND MEDULLARY LEVELS)

Ventral cochlear nucleus

Spiral ganglion

Trapezoid body (ventral acoustic stria)

Internal acoustic stria   Dorsal acoustic stria

Superior temporal gyrus

Cortifugal fibers

Medial geniculate body

Brachium

Inferior colliculus

Tectospinal tracts

Nuclei lateral lemnisci

Lateral lemniscus

Centrifugal fibers to cochlear nuclei

Internuclear association tracts

Olivocochlear centrifugal fibers

Organ of Corti

Superior olivary complex

FIG. 2. Block diagram of acoustic system. *Left,* Only uncrossed ascending or centripetal pathways are presented. *Right,* In addition to crossed centripetal pathways, there are descending or centrifugal pathways. *Dashed line,* Probable supply of fibers from trapezoid body to homolateral lemniscus.

and low-frequency neurons (originating from the apical cochlea) that project ventrally (10). As a result of this organization, individual neurons have specific excitatory frequency ranges. The frequency with the lowest threshold for excitation is known as the characteristic frequency of that neuron (11). Individual cochlear fibers innervate the cochlea with characteristic types of nerve endings. For example, there are calcine endings in the ascending pathways, and boutons *terminaux* or boutons *en passant* in the descending pathways (12). Numerous interneurons and afferent neurons from other regions of the auditory brainstem also innervate cells of the descending pathways. The main excitatory neurotransmitter in the auditory system remains unknown; Wickesberg and Oertel suggested that it may be an excitatory amino acid (13).

Afferent Second-order Neurons

The second-order neurons ascend from the cochlear nuclei through three fiber bundles that project both ipsilat-

erally and contralaterally (see Fig. 2). The dorsal acoustic stria, also known as the bundle of Monakow, is a contralateral pathway that originates from the DCN, decussates in the floor of the fourth ventricle, and traveling through the contralateral lateral lemniscus synapses on the nuclei of the lateral lemniscus and the central nucleus of the inferior colliculus (14,15). The intermediate acoustic stria, also known as the tract of Held, originates primarily in the PVCN. Some fibers project bilaterally to the preolivary nuclei; some bypass these nuclei and ascend to the contralateral lateral lemniscus; some send projections to the nucleus of the lateral lemniscus (NLL); the rest of the neurons project to the inferior colliculus (16,17). The ventral acoustic stria, also known as the trapezoid body, arising from cells in the AVCN and PVCN courses in the ventromedial direction. Ipsilateral fibers project to the medial superior olivary nucleus (MSO) and lateral superior olivary nucleus (LSO). Many contralateral fibers cross the brainstem to terminate in the contralateral medial trapezoid body or MSO. In other words, each MSO receives input bilaterally from each

(text continues on page 147)

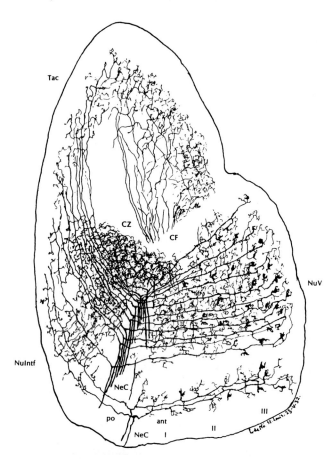

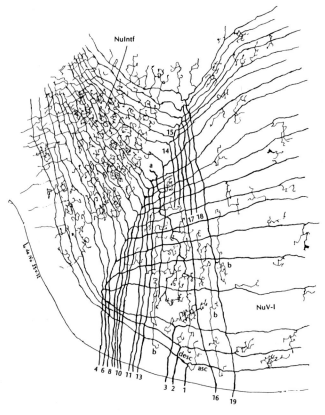

FIG. 3. Parasagittal section through primary acoustic nuclei of 4-day-old cat. Root fibers of the cochlear nerve (*NeC*) bifurcate to yield anterior (*ant*) and posterior (*po*) branches. The anterior branches cross through the three subdivisions (*I, II, III*) of the ventral nucleus (*NuV* [VCN in text]). The posterior branches cross through interfascicular nucleus (*NuIntf*) to reach acoustic tubercle (*Tac* [DCN in text]); *CF,* bundle of centrifugal fibers ending in cortex of dorsal cochlear nucleus; *CZ,* confluence zone of anterior and posterior lateral nuclei (Golgi's rapid method). (From Lorente de Nó R. *Laryngoscope* 1937;47:373–377, with permission.)

FIG. 4. Parasagittal section through cochlear root and neighboring parts of (*NuV* [VCN in text]) and interfascicular nucleus (*NuIntf*). The endogenous fiber (*a*) forms an extensive ramification in caudal part of *NuV-1* (VCN in text). The cochlear root fibers (*1–19*) display a very regular arrangement of their points of division into anterior and posterior branches. Fiber *1* is supposed to belong to the apical end, and fiber *19* to the basal end, of the ganglion of Corti. A number of root fibers give off collateral branches (*b*) at variable distances from their points of division. Cat a few days of age (Golgi's rapid method). (asc, ascending; desc, descending.) (From Lorento de Nó R. Anatomy of the eighth nerve: the central projection of the nerve endings of the internal ear. *Laryngoscope* 1933;43:1–38, with permission.)

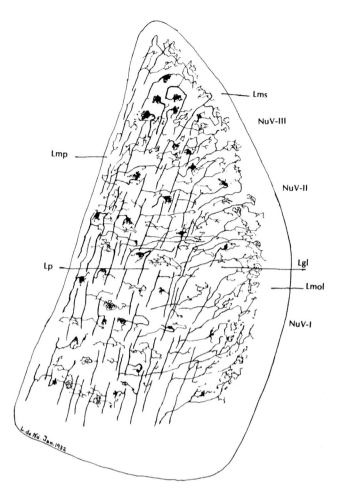

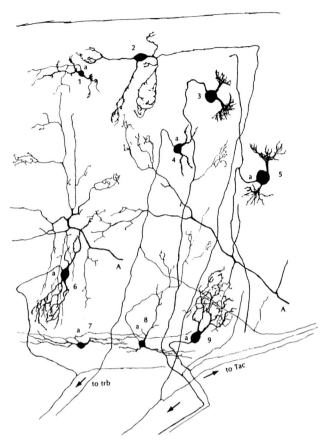

FIG. 5. Oblique frontal section through the *NuV* (VCN in text) shows the three streams of anterior cochlear branches present in each elementary lamella (a thin layer of the nucleus that receives fibers from a narrow zone of the ganglion of Corti). Cat several days old (Golgi's rapid method). *NuV-I, NuV-II, NuV-III,* subdivisions of the ventral cochlear nucleus (VCN); *Lms,* superficial marginal layer; *Lmp,* deep marginal layer; *Lp,* principal layer; *Lgl,* glomerular layer; *Lmol,* molecular layer.

FIG. 6. Frontal section through NuV-II (second subdivision of the ventral cochlear nucleus) immediately adjacent to caudal end of NuV-III (third subdivision of the ventral cochlear nucleus) containing cells with long or efferent axons of two different types—brush cells (*3, 5*) and multipolar or basket cells (*2, 4, 6, 9*)—and cells with short axons (*1, 7, 8*). *A,* end arborizations of short axons. Only the initial parts of the dendrites of cell *4* have been reproduced. *Arrows* at bottom indicate that the efferent axons divide into two branches going in different directions, toward trapezoid body (*to trb*) and toward Tac (DCN in text) (*to Tac*). Cat a few days old (Golgi's rapid method).

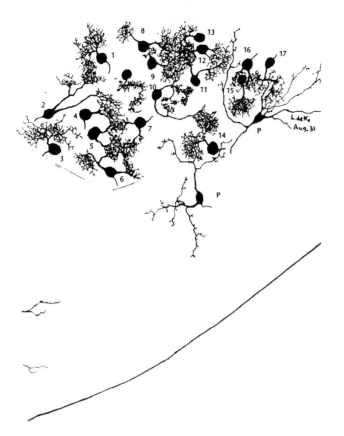

FIG. 7. Longitudinal section through the part of NuV-III (third subdivision of ventral cochlear nucleus) that belongs to central part of Corti's ganglion. All cells (*1–17*) are brush cells. *P,* Polygonal neurons, presumably with efferent axons. Adult cat (Golgi-Cox method).

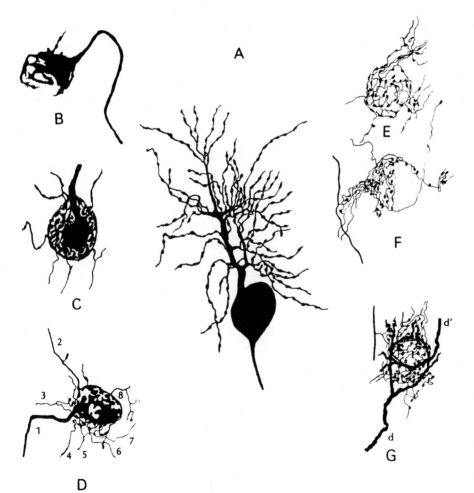

FIG. 8. Spheroidal brush cell of Nuv-II (second subdivision of ventral cochlear nerve) **(A)**. Arborization of the single dendrite has been reproduced as accurately as possible. Held chalice **(B, C)** or two articulated Held bulbs (**D**: *1, 2*) cannot cover more than one hemisphere of the cell body or that synaptic boutons formed by other fibers (**D**: *3–8*) are present in the "holes" of the Held endings. The other hemisphere of the synaptic shell is formed by synaptic boutons of ordinary sizes. *d, d',* Terminal dendritic branches of a basket cell surrounding the synaptic shell of a brush cell. Adult cat (Golgi-Cox method) **(A)**. Synaptic shell from cats a few days old (Golgi's rapid method) **(B–G)**.

AVCN and PVCN. Each LSO receives ipsilateral input from the ipsilateral VCN and contralateral input from the ipsilateral medial trapezoid body (18).

Superior Olivary Complex

The superior olivary complex contains a number of nuclei in the ventrolateral portion of the pons. These cells receive copious input from the VCN, and after numerous local circuits are completed relay information to the midbrain through the lateral lemniscus (19). In most mammalian species, four nuclei are easily recognized with Nissl's staining. The largest of these is the S-shaped LSO, which consists of multipolar cells with flat, two-dimensional dendritic fields that travel rostrocaudally. Its innervation is bilateral. Ipsilateral innervation is through the trapezoid body from the AVCN. This portion is nearly exclusively excitatory and is highly tonotopically organized. Contralateral innervation is through globular bushy cells in the caudal AVCN and the rostral PVCN and reaches the LSO through inhibitory neurons located in the medial nucleus of the trapezoid body. These connections are believed to be glycine mediated (20). The LSO appears to be most sensitive to stimuli higher than 5 kHz in frequency (21).

Next to the LSO is the MSO, also known as the accessory olivary nucleus. It is predominantly sensitive to low-frequency stimuli. The MSO receives input from direct projections from bushy cells of the contralateral and the ipsilateral AVCN. Incoming axons branch within the flat layers between MSO neurons. Most cells in this region are probably excited by auditory stimulation to either ear; the likely neurotransmitter is an excitatory amino acid. This nucleus is highly tonotopically organized, and the output resembles that of the rostral AVCN, which is the likely source of input (22,23). The medial nucleus of the trapezoid body (MNTB) lies within the trapezoid body. The fourth group of cells, the preolivary nuclei, curve around the MSO and LSO. There are the medial and lateral preolivary nuclei (MPO and LPO). For each one of these, the principal sources of input are the AVCN and the PVCN. The LPO is activated by ipsilateral acoustic stimulation; the MPO is activated by stimulation of either ear and also receives descending input from the inferior colliculus and the NLL (24,25).

Other groups of cells around this area are the periolivary nuclei. They compose up to six groups of cells that receive afferent input from the PVCN and the DCN over all three acoustic striae (26,27). Tracer studies from this area indicate that many of these neurons project back to the cochlea as two separate systems, medial and lateral, to the areas beneath the inner and outer hair cells (28,29). Some of these neurons send axons to the cochlear nuclei to provide central mechanisms for peripheral sensory coding. It is believed that the bilateral convergence onto the superior olivary complex from the VCN results in performance of the first binaural interaction operations at this level, including sound localization through temporal and intensity differences in bilateral auditory input (17,30,31).

Lateral Lemniscus

Each lateral lemniscus and its nuclei are rhombencephalic structures located rostral to the superior olivary complex. The lateral lemniscus is a pathway that travels rostrally to connect second- and third-order contralateral and ipsilateral neurons of the superior olivary complex and cochlear nuclei with the inferior colliculus, a mesencephalic structure (32). The ventral nucleus of the lateral lemniscus (VNLL) receives input from the contralateral VCN and lesser input from the superior olivary complex. Most of the cells in the VNLL are affected by contralateral acoustic stimulation. The intermediate nucleus of the lateral lemniscus (INLL) receives bilateral innervation from each VCN and LSO. The dorsal nucleus of the lateral lemniscus (DNLL) receives contralateral input from the VCN and bilateral input from each LSO and MSO. The commissure of Probst connects both DNLLs reciprocally. Most of the neurons in this nucleus are affected by acoustic stimulation of either ear (17,33). All of the nuclei of the lateral lemnisci are tonotopically organized. Cells that respond best to low frequencies are located dorsally; cells that respond best to higher frequencies are located ventrally (18).

Inferior Colliculus

The inferior colliculus is part of the corpora quadrigemina of the midbrain and forms a portion of the tectum. These structures receive all or nearly all of the input ascending from the hindbrain. Each inferior colliculus may be divided into three nuclei: the central or main nucleus (ICC), the external nucleus (ICX), and the pericentral nucleus (ICP) (34). The ICC has two cell types: stellate neurons with branched, spherical dendritic fields and neurons with disc-shaped dendritic fields. It may be subdivided into dorsomedial and ventrolateral portions (35). The dorsomedial portion contains multipolar, large cells and receives neurons from the lateral lemniscus, contralateral inferior colliculus, and the auditory cortex (through layer V pyramidal cells) (16). The ventrolateral portion comprises small- and medium-sized neurons and receives ascending neurons from the NLL, the superior olivary complex, and the cochlear nucleus. These cells have disc-shaped dendritic fields and a laminar appearance. The dorsal acoustic stria from the contralateral side projects fibers directly from the cochlear nucleus. The VCN projects through the ipsilateral and contralateral superior olivary complex. Each LSO projects bilaterally to this portion; MSO projections are ipsilateral. There is evidence of tonotopic organization; high-frequency fibers are located ventromedially and low-frequency fibers are located dorsolaterally. The commissure of the inferior colliculus connects the dorsomedial portions bilaterally.

The ICX receives fibers from ascending projections from the central nucleus. ICP and ICX neurons have very broad response areas. In the ICX there appear to be cells activated by both auditory and somatosensory input; this implies that the function of this area may be to integrate auditory input with other sensory modalities (36). Fibers that project to the forebrain do so through the brachium of the inferior colliculus, an ipsilateral pathway that runs to the medial geniculate body of the thalamus (MGB), giving off projections to the ICX, the interstitial nucleus of the inferior colliculus, and the parabrachial region of the tegmentum. The MGB receives bilateral projections and is highly tonotopically organized (37).

Superior Colliculus

The superior colliculus is a component of the tectum of the midbrain that has visual input to the superficial layers and multimodal sensory input to the deeper layers. Auditory input arises from the inferior colliculus and its brachium, the auditory cortex, the VNLL, and the periolivary nuclei. Output from this region mediates eye, head, neck, and ear movement. Neurons in this region respond to tones delivered monaurally or binaurally (38,39).

Medial Geniculate Body

The MGB is the main auditory relay station of the thalamus. All ascending auditory projections to the cortex pass through this region. There are three main divisions: ventral, dorsal, and medial. The ventral division receives massive ipsilateral afferent input from the ventrolateral nucleus of the inferior colliculus and projects to the auditory cortex. It is subdivided into a pars ovoidea and a pars lateralis. There arc only two types of ncurons: gcniculocortical and Golgi type II (40). There is tonotopic organization in this region; high frequencies are represented laterally, and lower frequencies are represented medially (41). The dorsal division receives mainly corticogeniculate input and has complex synaptic organization of four neuron types. The medial division of the MGB receives input from the inferior colliculus and is broadly tuned with respect to frequency. Somatosensory and vibratory stimuli also are represented here. It is part of a pulvinar-posterior complex that includes the pulvinar, nucleus posterior, and nucleus lateralis posterior. In this complex, neurons are narrowly tuned with respect to frequency (42).

Cortical Projections

Afferent fibers project from the lateral surface of the thalamus as part of the internal capsule and project to the auditory cortex. The primary auditory area is located in the temporal lobe of each hemisphere of the brain. The afferent points project to synaptic points on the anterior and posterior temporal gyri, which comprise part of the floor of the sylvian fissure and span the superior tempo-ral gyrus. This area is called A1 and considered the primary auditory core surrounded by other auditory regions (43). The core is believed to receive projections from the ventral nucleus of the MGB, and the surrounding belt is believed to receive input from all of the MGB. The auditory cortex is tonotopically organized, but the organization differs with location (44). There may be intensity mapping, but evidence is not strong. Through the corpus callosum, the auditory and association areas of each side of the brain are interconnected.

In addition to the afferent, ascending pathways, there are efferent, descending pathways. Corticofugal fibers parallel the ascending system. There are projections to the MGB and inferior colliculus, and from these regions there are projections to the preolivary and periolivary areas (17,31,32,40). The crossed and uncrossed olivocochlear bundles then project to the cochlea (28,29). The cell bodies of this bundle are located within the superior olivary complex, and this bundle may be divided into crossed and uncrossed components or medial and lateral components (28). The medial division contains myelinated neurons originating from large cells in the medial superior olivary complex. Just below the floor of the fourth ventricle, axons cross to the other side of the brainstem, joining ipsilateral fibers. These fibers travel peripherally with the vestibular nerve and join the cochlear nerve through Oort's anastomosis. After they enter the modiolus, these fibers form the intraganglionic bundle in Rosenthal's canal. The fibers then become unmyelinated and pass through the habenula perforata into the organ of Corti; they then travel across the tunnel of Corti and synapse on the bases of the outer hair cells. The lateral division is unmyelinated and originates from small cells in the lateral superior olivary complex. These fibers course within the medial division to the organ of Corti. In the organ of Corti they travel beneath the inner hair cells and are known as the inner spiral bundle. They then terminate on dendrites of cochlear nerve fibers beneath the inner hair cells. The medial olivocochlear bundle may be able to modify the response of the outer hair cells to sound, and the modification affects cochlear mechanics; the lateral olivocochlear bundle possibly influences activity of the auditory nerve (31).

VESTIBULAR PROJECTIONS

The ability of the brain to integrate head and body motion in space requires interaction of almost every sensory modality, including the vestibular end organs, the visual system, and the somatosensory system. These pathways are therefore more complex than the auditory pathways and consequently less well known. The vestibular nuclei receive their primary afferent projections through the vestibular nerve from the vestibular end organs. This nerve contains approximately 18,000 myelinated afferents of bipolar ganglion cells. Two percent of vestibular nerve axons are efferent fibers (45).

Afferent Vestibular System

The vestibular neuroepithelium is innervated by bipolar ganglion cells the cell bodies of which are located in the vestibular (Scarpa's) ganglion. Centrally, these ganglion cells innervate the vestibular nuclei and part of the cerebellum (Fig. 9). Scarpa's ganglion has superior and inferior divisions. The inferior division contains cell bodies of neurons that innervate the posterior canal cristae and most of the the macula of the saccule. The superior division contains cell bodies of neurons that innervate the horizontal and superior semicircular canal cristae, the macula of the utricle, and a small portion of the macula of the saccule (46,47). Large-diameter fibers are located centrally in the nerve; small-diameter fibers are located peripherally. This organization persists into the nerve roots.

The vestibular nuclei are located in the dorsolateral region of the rostral medulla and in the caudal pons. There are four major nuclei: superior (SVN, nucleus of Bekhterev, angular nucleus), medial (MVN, principal nucleus, triangular nucleus, Schwalbe's nucleus), lateral (LVN, Deiters' nucleus), and inferior (IVN, spinal nucleus, or descending nucleus). Other related cell groups include groups x, y, and z of Brodal cells, the interstitial nucleus of the vestibular nerve, and the supravestibular nucleus (48). Group p has been identified in some animals (49,50).

The fibers from the vestibular nerve penetrate the brainstem immediately caudad to the point of the facial nerve entrance. Once inside the brainstem, the fibers travel in a dorsomedial direction in a sigmoid trajectory. In their course, the fibers surround the column of cells that form the interstitial nucleus—the first and most lateral of the vestibular nuclei to be innervated. As the fibers travel medially, they divide into several fascicles before reaching the main vestibular areas. Near the nuclear area the fibers split into ascending and descending secondary branches that form the vestibular tract. Tertiary collaterals of the vestibular tract project to the major and minor vestibular nuclei and to the cerebellum.

Classic anatomic studies showed that the CNS receives fibers from the five labyrinthine receptors in different parts of the vestibular nuclei, but the precise pattern of innervation from each receptor has been determined only recently. Newer tract-tracing techniques with substances such as horseradish peroxidase to label the vestibular afferent fibers have enabled visualization of the fiber projections from individual receptors in the CNS.

In the nerve root, fibers segregate according to the receptor of origin (46,51,52); fibers from the semicircular canals occupy the rostrodorsal part of the root, and those from the maculae occupy the caudoventral area. In the vestibular tract segregation of fibers according to the receptor of origin has been identified (52).

All the end organ receptors project fibers to all the major and minor vestibular nuclei except group y, which is innervated only by the sacculus. Projection areas of the tertiary branches of various end organs exhibit considerable overlap within the major vestibular nuclei. However, differences in projection pattern can be identified. In the superior nucleus, fibers from the posterior semicircular canal project medially, and the horizontal semicircular canal and superior semicircular canal project centrally and laterally (46,47,50,53). In some mammals (54), the saccule and utricle have been found to have a large number of projections to the superior nucleus, whereas few or no projections have been found in others (46,47,53,55). It has been considered that the superior nucleus is a principal relay center for the ocular reflexes mediated by the semicircular canals (56) because of heavy input from the semicircular canals and efferent innervation to the motor nuclei of the extrinsic eye muscles (57). Prominent projections from the otoliths to the superior nucleus suggest that these organs might play a more important role in the vestibulooocular reflexes.

The projections to the lateral nucleus are concentrated in its ventral part; there are few or no dorsal projections (46,47,50,53,58–61). The rostroventral portion of the lateral nucleus receives afferent fibers primarily from the utricle (46,55) and from the saccule (46,53). The projections from the cristae are believed to be limited (46) or absent (47,53,55). Unlike the afferent fibers from vestibular end organs, primary and secondary spinal afferent fibers (59,62–64) and fibers from the cerebellum (59,61) are known to project to the dorsocaudal lateral nucleus.

Some studies have found that in the medial nucleus, primary afferent fibers project predominantly in the rostral areas (47,50,58,65). Others studies have found a relatively uniform pattern of projection throughout the nucleus (55,61). Various patterns of location of the terminals in the medial rectus from individual receptors have been described (46,47,53,55). Semicircular canal projections have been found in the central to dorsal part of the rostral medial nucleus (47). Projection areas of the utricular and saccular maculae have been found in the middle of the medial nucleus (46,55).

Projections from vestibular end organs in the descending nucleus are abundant in its rostral part and progressively decrease caudally. The projection of individual receptors is specific in this nucleus. The superior canal and horizontal canal project ventrolaterally and centrally; the posterior canal projects most medially; the utricle projects in the central and lateral region; and the saccule projects in the dorsolateral region. The superior canal and the horizontal canal project primarily in the rostral part of the descending nucleus, and the projection areas of the utricle and saccule extend more caudally (47,54,61).

Among minor vestibular nuclei, the interstitial nucleus, groups p, 1, and y receive primary afferent vestibular projections. The interstitial nucleus is the most richly innervated of all the vestibular nuclei. Fibers from the vestibular root send an enormous number of short branches that terminate throughout the nucleus. Some authors report that only ampullar fibers project to the

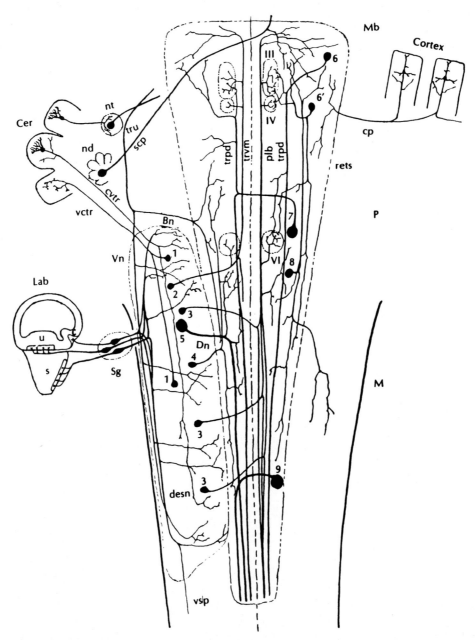

FIG. 9. Diagram of main connections of vestibular nerve. *M,* Medulla; *P,* pons; *Mb,* midbrain; *Lab,* labyrinth; *Cer,* cerebellum; *Cortex,* cerebral cortex; *Sg,* Scarpa's ganglion; *rets,* reticular substance. Vestibular nerve innervates cristae of semicircular canals (*c*), utricular macula (*u*), and saccular macula (*s*). It ends in the primary vestibular nuclei, the main divisions of which are Bekhterev's nucleus (*Bn* [SVN in text]), Deiters' nucleus (*Dn* [LVN in text]), and the descending nucleus (*desn* [DVN in text]); *1–5,* cells of vestibular nuclei (*Vn*). *1,* With axon reaching cerebellar cortex through vestibulocerebellar tracts (*vctr*); *2,* with axon joining tractus vestibulomesencephalicus (*trvm*); *3,* with axon joining posterior longitudinal bundle (*plb*); *4,* with axon ending in reticular substance; *5,* with axon joining tractus deiterospinalis; *vsp,* thin branches of vestibular nerve reaching cervical segments of spinal cord. Part of reticular substance (*rets*) with vestibular connections contains various types of cells (*6, 7, 8,* and *9*), axons of which form either short pathways (*6, 8*) or join the tractus predorsalis (*trpd*) and descend to spinal cord (*6', 7, 8, 9*). The reticular formation receives many vestibular fibers and sends branches to vestibular nuclei. Cerebellum establishes connections with vestibular nuclei by means of axons of Purkinje's cells (*cvtr*) and by means of axons of cells of nucleus tecti (*nt*), which form tractus uncinatus (*tru*). This tract also has connections with reticular substance. The superior cerebellar peduncle (*scp*), which arises from the nucleus dentatus (*nd*), gives branches to the reticular formation in the oral portion of the midbrain (*Mb*). The cerebral cortex establishes connections with the reticular formation by means of descending cortical paths (*cp*). The motor nuclei of the eye muscles (*III, IV,* and *VI*) receive branches from the vestibular and reticular tracts. (From Lorente de Nó R, Berens C. Nystagmus. In: Piersol, ed. *The cyclopedia of medicine.* Philadelphia: FA Davis, 1938:684–706, with permission.)

interstitial nucleus (46,55). Others suggest that fibers from the maculae also innervate this nucleus (47). Some authors consider the interstitial nucleus to be a displaced part of the lateral nucleus (66). The function of the interstitial nucleus is unclear. It is believed that this nucleus projects to the cerebellum and to the spinal cord (62,64) and may be the source of commissural fibers (67).

Group p has been described in guinea pig (49), chinchillas (50), and squirrel monkeys (68). It receives afferent innervation primarily from the otolith organs. Group l has been considered to be a special part of the lateral nucleus because of its neighboring location, and the similarity in their efferent projections to the cord (62). Group y is known to receive primary projections from the saccule (46,53,54). The function of group y is considered to be related to vertical eye movement (69,70). Groups x and f receive primary afferent vestibular fibers (46,47,58, 59,61). These nuclei receive fibers from the spinal cord (59,62–64) and receive fibers from and project fibers to the cerebellum (66,71).

The vestibular nuclei have numerous secondary projections to various portions of the CNS. These include projections to the flocculus, nodulus, uvula, and fastigial nucleus of the cerebellum; projections to the reticular formation; projections to the oculomotor, trochlear, and abducens nuclei; projections to all levels of the spinal cord; and projections to contralateral vestibular nuclei. These second-order projections tend to mediate bilateral interactions and are considered to be efferent from the nuclei (45).

Efferent Vestibular System

Much effort has been directed at understanding the afferent mechanisms of transducing the forces associated with head acceleration and gravity into a biologic signal. The role of the efferent vestibular system in modulating this afferent input to the CNS is of fundamental importance in understanding general sensory processing of the vestibular system. There is little information regarding the anatomic organization of the efferent vestibular neurons, particularly in humans. The best studied feature of the organization of efferent vestibular neurons is the location of their somata within the brainstems of rats, gerbils, cats, and squirrel monkeys (72,73). Early studies entailed classic techniques of identifying efferent vestibular neurons and fibers after transection of the vestibular nerve or with acetylcholinesterase histochemical analysis in which the vestibular efferent bundle was followed into the nerve and end organs. More recent studies have entailed retrograde tract-tracing techniques with horseradish peroxidase, fluorescent labels, or tritiated amino acids to identify efferent vestibular neurons. Efferent vestibular neuron somata have been found in two groups bordering the facial nerve genu in most species (group E neurons) and in the caudal pontine reticular nucleus (72,73) (Fig. 10). Cells from each group project ipsilaterally and contralaterally, although the detailed innervation patterns are not known.

The detailed neurotransmitter and receptor anatomy of the efferent neurons innervating the afferent vestibular receptors is unknown; however, efferent vestibular neurons are described as cholinergic. Perachio and Kevetter (74) reported that the vestibular efferent neurons of gerbils contain both calcitonin gene-related peptide (CGRP) and choline acetyltransferase (ChAT), implying the presence of acetylcholine. Ohno et al. (75) reported that more than 90% of retrograde-labeled efferent vestibular neurons of rat contained ChAT immunoreactivity. They also reported that approximately 55% of ChAT immunoreactive efferent vestibular neurons contained CGRP immunoreactivity (CGRPi). The regulation of these individual transmitters in efferent vestibular neurons may be important in the modulation of synaptic activity in the vestibular system (72,73).

Experiments in our laboratories indicate that all neurons in group E and scattered neurons throughout the caudal pontine reticular regions expressed αCGRP messenger RNA (mRNA) and translated the message to CGRP (see Fig. 10). αCGRP mRNA is not found in the primary vestibular afferent cell bodies in Scarpa's ganglion or in the intratemporal bone efferent fibers. The absence of CGRPi and αCGRP mRNA within somata of the primary afferent Scarpa's ganglion indicates that the CGRPi terminals within the vestibular end organs are of efferent origin (73). We found that in the vestibular pathways expression of αCGRP mRNA occurs only in areas associated with brainstem efferent somata; therefore the CGRPi fibers that innervate the vestibular neurosensory epithelium are exclusively efferent. In summary, the distribution of αCGRP mRNA and CGRPi in the vestibular efferent system suggests a role for this neuroactive peptide in the regulation of afferent signaling in the vestibular system. The uniform distribution of CGRP-containing neurons within all regions of group E and the caudal pontine reticular nucleus suggests that CGRP has a more important role in efferent vestibular function than proposed by other investigators.

Vestibular efferent (second-order) connections to the cerebellum appear to originate in the ventrolateral IVN, the ventral MVN, and cell group x. These connections have been shown to relay both labyrinthine and spinal information. The fibers terminate in the vestibulocerebellum—that is, the nodulus, flocculus, ventral paraflocculus, and uvula—as mossy fibers (48). In frogs, the flocculus projects Purkinje's cells back to the vestibular nuclei, providing feedback control.

Vestibulospinal Connections

The vestibulospinal tracts convey vestibular information to the spinal cord for maintenance of posture and balance (76). There are two such pathways: the lateral vestibulospinal tract and the medial vestibulospinal tract. The lateral vestibulospinal tract is a complex pathway that begins mainly in Deiters' nucleus and extends ipsi-

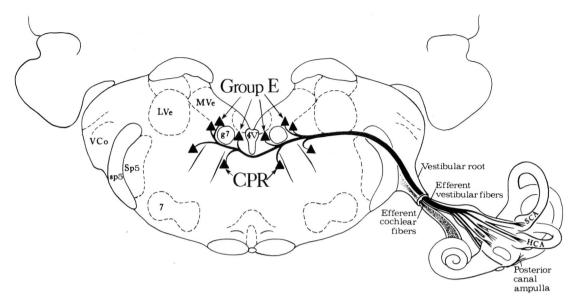

FIG. 10. A single rat brainstem. *Triangles,* calcitonin gene-related peptide immunoreactivity (CGRPi) and αCGRP messenger RNA colocalization in adjacent sections in individual cell bodies. Cell bodies in both the dorsolateral and medial group E cells and the caudal pontine reticular nucleus (*CPR*) colocalize CGRPi and αCGRP mRNA. CGRPi axons originating from the efferent vestibular neuron somata containing CGRPi and αCGRP mRNA, group E and CPR, which project contralaterally beneath the ependyma of the fourth ventricle (*4V*) out through the root of the vestibular nerve and Scarpa's ganglion to the individual vestibular end organs. CPR somata are localized on either side of the ascending facial nerve. *4v,* Fourth ventricle; *g7,* genu of the facial nerve; *7,* facial nucleus; *HCA,* horizontal canal ampulla; *LVe,* lateral vestibular nucleus; *MVe,* medial vestibular nucleus; *SCA,* superior canal ampulla; *Sp5,* spinal nucleus of the fifth nerve; *sp5,* spinal tract of the fifth nerve; *VCo,* ventral cochlear nucleus. (Copyright © 1991 P. A. Wackym, published with permission.)

laterally to the lumbosacral region of the spinal cord in the ventral funiculus. Some fibers are short and terminate in the upper or lower cervical region. In cats most fibers are longer and reach the lumbosacral region of the spinal cord. This tract contains a wide variety of fiber diameters; conduction velocities range from 20 to 140 m/s (77). The final effect is on limb α-motoneurons, axial α-motoneurons, or interneurons (78,79). In the limbs of cats, ipsilateral extensor activation and flexor inhibition occur when this tract is stimulated. Excitation can be monosynaptic (quadriceps, soleus muscles) or polysynaptic (quadriceps, biceps, soleus, plantaris muscles). Inhibition is disynaptic, through γ-motoneurons. Most connections are polysynaptic (80).

The medial vestibulospinal tract originates from the MVN, IVN, and Deiters' nucleus. Its fibers descend bilaterally in the spinal cord. Most neurons extend no more caudally than the upper cervical region. According to Wilson and Jones (80) and Shinoda et al. (81), in cats the medial vestibulospinal tract has a close relation with the cervical muscles. This tract contains inhibitory and excitatory fibers that exert effects on upper cervical and thoracic motoneurons but not on limb motoneurons (82). Many connections to motoneurons are monosynaptic, but

not enough information has been elucidated to determine whether all connections are monosynaptic.

Oculomotor Connections

The connections of the vestibular nuclei to the motor nuclei of the extraocular muscles have been carefully studied (Fig. 11) (83,84). The close relation between eye movement and head movement implies a highly organized set of connections for this reflex. The fibers in the median longitudinal fasciculus originate from all four vestibular nuclei, cell group x, and the interstitial nucleus of the vestibular nerve. The fibers originating from the SVN travel ipsilaterally; the fibers originating from the remaining nuclei travel bilaterally. The median longitudinal fasciculus innervates the oculomotor, trochlear, and abducens nuclei, the interstitial nucleus of Cajal, the red nucleus, and the thalamus. The vestibuloocular reflex is the output of a three-neuron arc. This reflex excites agonists and inhibits antagonists to compensatory eye motions. Excitatory activity is carried by the contralateral median longitudinal fasciculus, and inhibitory activity is carried by the ipsilateral median longitudinal fasciculus. The SVN inhibits oculomotor neurons in all nuclei on the

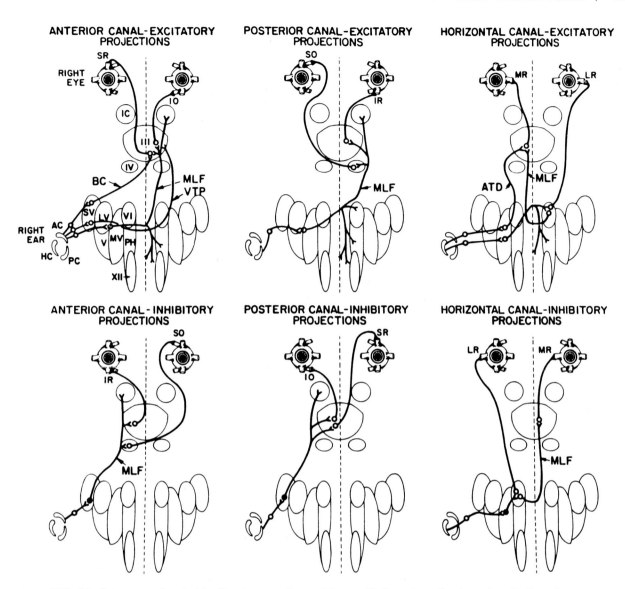

FIG. 11. Summary of probable direct connections of the vestibuloocular reflex based on findings from a number of species. Excitatory neurons are indicated by *open circles,* inhibitory neurons by *closed circles. III,* Oculomotor nuclear complex; *IV,* trochlear nucleus; *VI,* abducens nucleus; *XII,* hypoglossal nucleus; *AC,* anterior semicircular canal; *ATD,* ascending tract of Deiters; *BC,* brachium conjunctivum; *HC,* horizontal or lateral semicircular canal; *IC,* interstitial nucleus of Cajal; *IO,* inferior oblique muscle; *IR,* inferior rectus muscle; *LR,* lateral rectus muscle; *LV,* lateral vestibular nucleus; *MLF,* medial longitudinal fasciculus; *MR,* medial rectus muscle; *MV,* medial vestibular nucleus; *PC,* posterior semicircular canal; *PH,* prepositus nucleus; *SV,* superior vestibular nucleus; *SO,* superior oblique muscle; *SR,* superior rectus muscle; *V,* inferior vestibular nucleus; *VTP,* ventral tegmental pathway. (From Leigh RJ, Zee DS. *The neurology of eye movements,* 2nd ed. Philadelphia: FA Davis, 1991, with permission.)

same side and in the motor nucleus of the medial rectus muscle of the opposite side. The rostral two thirds of the MVN contains neurons that make excitatory synaptic connections to all contralateral subnuclei except the medial rectus nucleus, which is excited ipsilaterally.

Unfortunately, the exact vestibulothalamic projections that ultimately project to the vestibular cortex have not been clearly demonstrated. Some evidence exists for

existence of fibers projecting to the hypothalamus, the thalamic nuclei, the Darkshevich's nucleus, and the interstitial nucleus of Cajal (45).

Cortical Vestibular Projections

There is disagreement about the exact location of the vestibular cortex and whether it is ipsilateral, contralateral, or bilateral. The vestibular cortex is located in the postcentral gyrus between the first and second somatosensory cortices (85,86). Braun (87) proposed the existence of two vestibulocortical areas: area 1 in the anterior suprasylvian and anterior ectosylvian gyri and area 2 in the middle and posterior ectosylvian gyri (45,87). The cortical response can be elicited with stimulation of the vestibular end organs and nuclei, the cerebellum, the thalamus, and the reticular formation.

All four vestibular nuclei project to the medial two thirds of the pontomedullary reticular formation, although in unequal proportions (88). Connections can be ipsilateral, bilateral, or contralateral. These connections are related to the vestibuloocular and vestibulospinal reflexes (89). There is an extensive network of commissural connections between the vestibular nuclei.

Vestibular efferent fibers allow the CNS to influence the end organs (90). The vestibular efferent fibers originate in caudal areas in the vestibular nuclear region lateral to the nucleus of the sixth nerve. These neurons enter the vestibular roots in the brainstem, where they join efferent cochlear fibers. These fibers have extensive terminal branching. The exact function of this system is not well understood.

In addition to the fibers that project from the vestibular nuclei, there exist numerous afferent connections from multiple sensory modalities. The main source of afferent fibers to the vestibular system is the cerebellum (91). There are two sources of cerebellar input: the fastigial nucleus and the cerebellar cortex (vermis, especially anterior lobe and flocculus). The main areas of termination of these fibers are the LVN and certain areas of other nuclei. The fibers from the fastigial nucleus originate from the rostral portion and travel ipsilaterally. They supply the dorsal portion of the LVN, MVN, and SVN. The caudal third of the fastigial nucleus generates a crossed tract and ends in the ventrolateral MVN and IVN, the ventral LVN, and the peripheral SVN.

There exist a substantial number of spinovestibular neurons that project from the spinal cord to the vestibular nuclei. These neurons originate from the lumbosacral region of the cord; these connections are exclusively ipsilateral. These tracts travel in the dorsal half of the lateral funiculus, terminating in the caudal MVN and IVN, cell groups x and z, and the dorsocaudal LVN. These tracts are believed to mediate extralabyrinthine proprioception (66).

Descending neurons to the vestibular nuclei originate from parts of the cortex that have not yet been completely defined and travel in the median longitudinal fasciculus. They are found in the interstitial nucleus of Cajal. The area of termination of these fibers is the ipsilateral dorsal and caudal MVN (62). Other projections to the vestibular nuclei are known to exist but are poorly understood. These include projections from the inferior olive, the olivocerebellar fibers, the nucleus gracilis, the mandibu-

lar nerve, the glossopharyngeal nerve, the nucleus prepositus, and the nucleus reticularis gigantocellularis (16).

SUMMARY POINTS

- Spiral ganglion dendrites of 95% of the neurons of the cochlear nerve innervate the inner hair cells of the cochlea; only 5% of the neurons innervate the outer hair cells.
- Approximately 35,000 neurons make up each cochlear nerve.
- Approximately 18,000 neurons make up each vestibular nerve.
- Broad understanding of the central auditory and vestibular systems is necessary to understand both diagnostic tests and the pathophysiologic processes of disorders that affect these systems.

REFERENCES

1. Lorente de Nó R. Anatomy of the eighth nerve: the central projection of the nerve endings of the internal ear. *Laryngoscope* 1933;43:1–39.
2. Lorente de Nó R. Anatomy of the eighth nerve, III: general plan of structure of the primary cochlear nuclei. *Laryngoscope* 1933;43:327.
3. Lorente de Nó R. Vestibulo-ocular reflex arc. *Arch Neurol Psych* 1933;30:245.
4. Lorente de Nó R. Analysis of the activity of the chains of internuncial neurons. *J Neurophysiol* 1938:207.
5. Rasmussen GL. Efferent fibers of the cochlear nerve and cochlear nucleus. In: Rasmussen GL, Windle WF, eds. *Neuromechanisms of the auditory and vestibular systems.* Springfield, Ill.: Charles C Thomas, 1960.
6. Bebin J. Pathophysiology of acoustic tumors. In: House WF, Leutje CM, eds. *Acoustic tumors.* Baltimore: University Park Press, 1979.
7. Lorente de Nó R. *The primary acoustic nuclei.* New York: Raven Press, 1981.
8. Osen KK. Cytoarchitecture of the cochlear nuclei in the cat. *J Comp Neurol* 1969;136:453.
9. Moore JK, Osen KK. The cochlear nuclei in man. *Am J Anat* 1970; 154:393.
10. Osen KK. Course and termination of the primary afferents in the cochlear nuclei of the cat: an experimental anatomical study. *Arch Ital Biol* 1970;108:21.
11. Liberman MC. The cochlea frequency map for the cat: labeling auditory nerve fibers of known characteristic frequency. *J Acoust Soc Am* 1982;72:1441.
12. Brawer JR, Morest DK. Relations between auditory nerve endings and cell types in the cat's anteroventral cochlear nucleus seen with the Golgi method and Nomarski optics. *J Comp Neurol* 1975;160:491.
13. Wickesberg RE, Oertel D. Auditory nerve neurotransmitter acts on a kainate receptor: evidence from intracellular recordings in brain slices from mice. *Brain Res* 1989;486:39.
14. Fernandez C, Karapas F. The course and terminations of the striae of Monakow and Held in the cat. *J Comp Neurol* 1967;131:171.
15. Osen KK. Projection of the cochlear nuclei on the inferior colliculus in the cat. *J Comp Neurol* 1972;144:355.
16. Brugge JF. Neurophysiology of the central auditory and vestibular systems. In: Paparella MM, Shumrick DA, Gluckman JL, Meyerhoff WL, eds. *Otolaryngology,* 3rd ed. Philadelphia: Saunders, 1991:280–314.
17. Thompson G. Structure and function of the central auditory system. In: Northern GL, ed. *Seminars in hearing.* New York: Thieme-Stratton, 1983.
18. Neely JG, Dennis JM, Lippe WR. Anatomy of the auditory end organ and neural pathways. In: Cummings CW, Fredrickson JM, Harker LA,

Krause CJ, Schuller DE, eds. *Otolaryngology–head and neck surgery.* St. Louis: Mosby, 1986:2571–2607.

19. Irvine DRF. The auditory brainstem: a review of the structure and function of auditory brainstem processing mechanisms. In: Ottoson D, ed. *Progress in sensory physiology 7.* Berlin: Springer-Verlag, 1976.

20. Caspary DM, Findlayson PG. Superior olivary complex: functional neuropharmacology of the principal cell types. In: Altschuler RA, Hoffman DW, Bobbin RP, eds. *Neurobiology of hearing: the central auditory system.* New York: Raven Press, 1990.

21. Tolbert LP, Morest DK, Yurgelun-Todd DA. The neuronal architecture of the anteroventral cochlear nucleus of the cat in the region of the cochlear nerve root: horseradish peroxidase labelling of identified cell types. *Neuroscience* 1982;7:303.

22. Goldberg JM, Brown PB. Response of binaural neurons of dog superior olivary complex to dichotic tonal stimuli: some physiological mechanisms of sound localization. *J Neurophysiol* 1969;32:613.

23. Guinan JJ Jr, Guinan SS, Norris BE. Single auditory units in the superior olivary complex, I: responses to sounds and classification based on physiological properties. *Int J Neurosci* 1972;4:101.

24. Rasmussen GL. Anatomic relationships of the ascending and descending auditory systems. In: Field WS, Alford BR, eds. *Neural mechanisms of auditory and vestibular disorders.* Springfield, Ill.: Charles C Thomas, 1964.

25. Moore RY, Goldberg JM. Projections of the inferior colliculus in the monkey. *Exp Neurol* 1966;14:429.

26. Warr RB. Fiber degeneration following lesions in the posterioventral cochlear nucleus of the cat. *Exp Neurol* 1969;23:140.

27. Morest DK. Auditory neurons of the brain stem. *Adv Otorhinolaryngol* 1973;20:337.

28. Warr WB. Olivocochlear and vestibular efferent neurons of the feline brain stem: their location, morphology, and number determined by retrograde axonal transport and acetylcholinesterase histochemistry. *J Comp Neurol* 1975;161:159.

29. Guinan JJ Jr, Warr WB, Norris BE. Differential olivocochlear projections from lateral versus medial zones of the superior olivary complex. *J Comp Neurol* 1983;221:358.

30. Masterton B, et al. Neuroanatomical basis for binaural phase-difference analysis for sound localization: a comparative study. *J Comp Physiol Psychol* 1975;89:379.

31. Pickles JO. *An introduction to the physiology of hearing.* New York: Academic Press, 1982.

32. Möhler AR. *Auditory physiology.* New York: Academic Press, 1983.

33. Goldberg JM. Physiological studies of the auditory nuclei of the pons. In: Wolff D, Keidel WD, Neff WD, eds. *Handbook of sensory physiology: auditory system, physiology (CNS) behavioral studies psychoacoustics.* New York: Springer-Verlag, 1975.

34. vanNoort J. *The structure and connection of the inferior colliculus.* Assen: The Netherlands, 1969.

35. Rockel AJ, Jones EG. Observation and fine structure of the central nucleus of the inferior colliculus of the cat. *J Comp Neurol* 1973;149:301.

36. Wright CG, Barnes CD. Audio-spinal reflex responses in decerebrate and chloralose anesthetized cats. *Brain Res* 1972;36:307.

37. Anderson RA, Roth GL, Aitkin LM, Merzenich MM. The efferent projections of the central nucleus and the pericentral nucleus of the inferior colliculus in the cat. *J Comp Neurol* 1980;194:649.

38. Wise LZ, Irvine DRF. Interaural intensity sensitivity based on facilitatory binaural interaction in cat superior colliculus. *Hear Res* 1984;16:181.

39. Hirsch JA, Chan JCK, Yin CT. Responses of neurons in the cat's superior colliculus to acoustic stimuli, I: monaural and binaural response properties. *J Neurophysiol* 1985;53:726.

40. Morest DK. Synaptic relations of Golgi type II cells in the medial geniculate body in the cat. *J Comp Neurol* 1975;162:157.

41. Imig TJ, Morel A. Tonotopic organization in ventral nucleus of medial geniculate body in the cat. *J Neurophysiol* 1985;53:309.

42. Aitkin LM. Medial geniculate body of the cat: responses to tonal stimuli of neurons in medial division. *J Neurophysiol* 1973;36:275.

43. Neff WD, Diamond IT, Casseday JH. Behavioral studies of auditory discrimination: central nervous system. In: Keidel WD, Neff WD, eds. *Handbook of sensory physiology.* New York: Springer-Verlag, 1975.

44. Reale RA, Imig TJ. Tonotopic organization of the auditory cortex of the cat. *J Comp Neurol* 1980;192:265.

45. Ryu JH. Anatomy of the vestibular end organ and neural pathways. In: Cummings CW, Fredrickson JM, Harker LA, Krause CJ, Schuller DE, eds. *Otolaryngology–head and neck surgery.* St. Louis: Mosby, 1986: 2609–2631.

46. Gacek RR. The course and central termination of first order neurons supplying vestibular end organs in the cat. *Acta Otolaryngol Suppl (Stockh)* 1969;254:5.

47. Stein BM, Carpenter MB. Central projections of portions of the vestibular ganglia innervating specific parts of the labyrinth in the rhesus monkey. *Am J Anat* 1967;120:281.

48. Brodal A, Pompeiano O, Walberg F. *The vestibular nuclei and their connections: anatomy functional correlations.* London: Oliver & Boyd, 1962.

49. Gstoettner W, Burian M. Vestibular nuclear complex in the guinea pig: a cytoarchitectronic study and map in three planes. *J Comp Neurol* 1987;257:176.

50. Suarez C, Honrubia V, Gomez J, Lee WS, Newman A. Primary vestibular projections in the chinchilla. *Arch Otorhinolaryngol* 1989;246:242.

51. Sando I, Black FO, Hemensway WG. Spatial distribution of vestibular nerve in the internal auditory canal. *Ann Otol Rhinol Laryngol* 1972; 81:305.

52. Lee WS, Newman AN, Honrubia V. Afferent innervation of the vestibular nuclei in the chinchilla, I: methods for labeling the individual vestibular receptors with horseradish peroxidase. *Brain Res* 1992;597:269.

53. Kevetter GA, Perachio AA. Central projections of first order vestibular neurons innervating the sacculus and posterior canal in the gerbil. *Prog Clin Biol Res* 1985;176:279.

54. Newman AN, Suarez C, Lee W, Honrubia V. Afferent innervation of the vestibular nuclei in the chinchilla, II: description of the vestibular nerve and nuclei. *Brain Res* 1992;597:278.

55. Siegborn J, Grant G. Brainstem projections of different branches of the vestibular nerve: an experimental study by transganglionic transport of horseradish peroxidase in the cat, I: the horizontal ampullar and utricular nerves. *Arch Ital Biol* 1983;121:237.

56. Baloh RW, Honrubia V. The central vestibular system. *Contemp Neurol Ser* 1979;18:47.

57. Mitsacos A, Reisine H, Highstein SM. The superior vestibular nucleus: an intracellular HRP study in the cat, I: vestibulo-ocular neurons. *J Comp Neurol* 1983;215:78.

58. Walberg F, Bowsher D, Brodal A. The termination of primary vestibular fibers in the vestibular nuclei in the cat: an experimental study with silver methods. *J Comp Neurol* 1958;110:391.

59. Henkel CK, Martin GF. The vestibular complex of the American opossum *Didelphis virginiana,* II: afferent and efferent connections. *J Comp Neurol* 1977;172:321.

60. Sugawara T. The cytoarchitecture of the vestibular nuclei and central projections of primary vestibular fibers in the rabbit. *Med J Osaka Univ* 1978;28:245.

61. Carleton SC, Carpenter MB. Distribution of primary vestibular fibers in the brainstem and cerebellum of the monkey. *Brain Res* 1984;294:281.

62. Pompeiano O, Walberg F. Descending connections to the vestibular nuclei: An experimental study in the cat. *J Comp Neurol* 1957;108:465.

63. Brodal A, Angaut P. The termination of spinovestibular fibers in the cat. *Brain Res* 1967;5:494.

64. Rubertone JA, Haines DE. Secondary vestibulocerebellar projections to the flocculonodular lobe in a prosimian primate, *Galagno senegalensis. J Comp Neurol* 1981;200:255.

65. Sato F, Sasaki H, Ishizuka N, Sasaki S, Mannen H. Morphology of single primary afferents originating from the horizontal semicircular canal in the cat. *J Comp Neurol* 1989;290:423.

66. Brodal A, Angaut P. The termination of spinovestibular fibers in the cat. *Brain Res* 1967;5:494.

67. Pompeiano O, Mergner T, Corvaja N. Commissural, perihypoglossal, and reticular afferent projections to the vestibular nuclei in the cat: an experimental anatomical study with the method of horseradish peroxidase. *Arch Ital Biol* 1978;116:130.

68. Naito Y, Newman AN, Lee WS, Beykirch K. Projections of the individual vestibular end organs on the brainstem of the squirrel monkey. *Brain Res* (in press).

69. Fluur E. The interaction between the utricle and the saccule. *Acta Otolaryngol (Stockh)* 1970;69:17.

70. Chubb MC, Fuchs AF. The role of the dentate nucleus and y-group in the generation of vertical smooth eye movement. *Ann N Y Acad Sci* 1981;374:446.

71. Kotchabhakdi N, Walberg F. Cerebellar afferent projections from the vestibular nuclei in the cat: an experimental study with the method of

retrograde axonal transport of horseradish peroxidase. *Exp Brain Res* 1978;31:591.

72. Wackym PA, Popper P, Ward PH, Micevych PE. Cell and molecular anatomy of nicotinic acetylcholine receptor subunits and calcitonin gene-related peptide in the rat vestibular system. *Otolaryngol Head Neck Surg* 1991;105:493.

73. Wackym PA. Ultrastructural organization of calcitonin gene-related peptide immunoreactive efferent axons and terminals in the rat vestibular periphery. *Am J Otol* 1993;14:41.

74. Perachio AA, Kevetter GA. Coexistence of choline acetyltransferase and calcitonin gene-related peptide in vestibular efferents of the gerbil. *Neurosci Abstr* 1989;15:518.

75. Ohno K, Takeda N, Yamano M, Matsunaga T, Tohyama M. Coexistence of acetylcholine and calcitonin gene-related peptide in the vestibular efferent neurons in the rat. *Brain Res* 1991;566:103.

76. Storper IS, Honrubia V. Is human triceps surae electromyogram a vestibulospinal reflex response? *Otolaryngol Head Neck Surg* 1992; 107:527.

77. Ito M, Hongo T, Yoshida M, Okada Y, Obata K. Antidromic and trans-synaptic activation of Deiter's neurones induced from the spinal cord. *Jpn J Physiol* 1964;14:638.

78. Marchand AR, Amblard B, Cremieux J. Visual and vestibular control of locomotion in early and late sensory-deprived cats. *Prog Brain Res* 1988;76:229–238.

79. Petras JM. Cortical, tectal, and tegmental fiber connections in the spinal cord of the cat. *Brain Res* 1967;6:275.

80. Wilson VJ, Jones GM. *Mammalian vestibular physiology.* New York: Plenum Press, 1970:185–248.

81. Shinoda Y, Ohgaki T, Futami T, Sugiuchi Y. Vestibular projections to the spinal cord: the morphology of single vestibulospinal axons. *Prog Brain Res* 1988;76:17.

82. Akaike T, Fanardjian VV, Ito M, Ohno T. Electrophysiological analysis of the vestibulospinal reflex pathway of rabbit, II: synaptic actions upon spinal neurones. *Exp Brain Res* 1973;17:497.

83. McMasters RE, Weiss AH, Carpenter MB. Vestibular projections to the nuclei of the extraocular muscles: degeneration resulting from discrete partial lesions of the vestibular nuclei in the monkey. *Am J Anat* 1966; 118:163.

84. Tarlov E. Organization of the vestibulo-oculomotor projection in the cat. *Brain Res* 1970;20:159.

85. Walzl E, Mountcastle VB. Projection of the vestibular nerve to cerebral cortex of the cat. *Am J Physiol* 1949;159:595.

86. Fredrickson JM. Vestibular nerve projections to the cerebral cortex of the rhesus monkey. *Exp Brain Res* 1966;2:318.

87. Braun GV. Averaged evoked cortical response to vestibular stimulation in the cat [master's thesis]. Iowa City: University of Iowa, 1971.

88. Ladpli R, Brodal A. Experimental studies of commissural and reticular formation projection from the vestibular nuclei in the cat. *Brain Res* 1968;8:65.

89. McCabe BF. The quick component of nystagmus. *Laryngoscope* 1965; 75:1619.

90. Gacek RR, Lyon M. Localization of vestibular effector neurons in the kitten with horseradish peroxidase. *Acta Otolaryngol (Stockh)* 1974;72:92.

91. Brodal A. Anatomy of the vestibular nuclei and their connections. In: Kornhuber HH, ed. *Handbook of sensory physiology.* New York: Springer-Verlag, 1974.

The Ear: Comprehensive Otology,
edited by R. F. Canalis and P. R. Lambert.
Lippincott Williams & Wilkins, Philadelphia © 2000.

CHAPTER 7

Otologic History and Physical Examination of the Ear

Barry Strasnick and David S. Haynes

The history and physical examination are the most important components of the evaluation of a patient with a hearing or balance disorder. They enable the clinician to develop a differential diagnosis before audiologic or vestibular testing and provide the basis for treatment planning. This chapter addresses the basic otologic history and physical examination and some aspects of the regional neurologic evaluation that are important in the complete assessment of ear disease.

HISTORY

General

As with any other medical disorder, the history is the essential component in evaluating a patient for ear disease. The physical examination is important, but when

  B. Strasnick: Department of Otolaryngology, Eastern Virginia Medical School, Norfolk, Virginia 23507 and DePaul Medical Center, Norfolk, Virginia 23505
  D. S. Haynes: Department of Otolaryngology, Vanderbilt University Medical Center, Nashville, Tennessee 37232; St. Thomas Hospital, Nashville, Tennessee 37205

compared with other anatomic areas, the ear often lends itself to relatively limited exploration. Therefore the examiner must be thorough and precise. A complete, systematic evaluation can be facilitated by a use of questionnaire (1,2) (Fig. 1).

Use of the standard principles of patient care makes an otologic examination efficient, functional, and effective. The patient history should not be limited to symptoms related to the ear. A full clinical account including a review of the patient's past and current illnesses is essential. The possibility of associated systemic disorders that may contribute to hearing loss, such as diabetes, heart disease, thyroid dysfunction, viral and bacterial infection, and rheumatologic disease, should always be explored in detail. A history of mild or severe environmental or pharmacologic allergies and symptoms of hay fever or asthma should be carefully investigated. Past surgical procedures, head trauma, and occupational, recreational, and military noise exposure should be recorded in the history (2–5). A review of the patient's medications is important. A list of ototoxic medications is provided in Table 1. Many of these drugs, such as furosemide, salicylates, and

MC 4920 (2/97)

Vanderbilt University Medical Center

OTOLARYNGOLOGY
Nashville, TN 37232-5555
(615) 322-6180

OTOLOGY/NEUROTOLOGY
ASSESSMENT FORM

Patient Name: Date:

DOB: AGE:

MR #

Referring Physician:

Dictation: Y   N

Chief Complaint:

HPI:

HEARING	Right	Left	VERTIGO
Duration			Onset
Prog.			Frequency
Tinnitus			Duration
Fullness			Spinning
Otitis			Unsteadiness
Bet. Ear			Nausea
Fluctuation			Positional
Hearing Aid			MRI

Current Medications: Allergies:

Trauma:

Family History

Noise Exposure:

Physical Exam:

Right		Left		Neurotology Exam
	Normal			Romberg
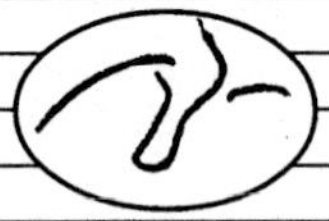	Perf w/ chol			Cerebellar
	Perf w/o chol			Cranial Nerve
	Serous OM			Nystagmus
	Acute OM			Dix Hallpike

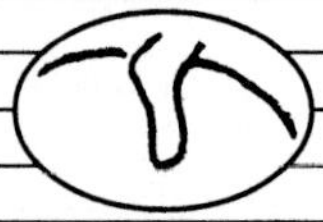

AC>BC ; BC>AC   (W)   AC>BC ; BC>AC

HEENT: Bruits:

IMPRESSION:

EVALUATION:

Imaging:	Lab Work	Vestibular Testing	TREATMENT
CT	FTA	ENG	
Temporal Bone	ESR	ECoG	
Coronal Sinus	ANA	Rotary Chair	
MRI head w/GAD	RF	Posturography	
w/o GAD	Chol	Vestibular Rehab.	
	SMA-20		

Follow up	
Audiogram	

FIG. 1. Otologic and neurotologic assessment form.

TABLE 1. *Ototoxic medications*

Quinine
Salicylates
Diuretics
    Furosemide
    Ethacrynic acid
Antibiotics
    Vancomycin
    Erythromycin
    Gentamicin
    Neomycin
    Streptomycin
    Kanamycin
    Amikacin
    Tobramycin
    Dihydrostreptomycin
Chemotherapeutic agents
    Cisplatin
    Nitrogen mustard

quinine, are commonly used and may cause tinnitus and hearing loss. Others may cause otologic symptoms without being directly ototoxic. For example, some antihypertensive agents, especially β-blockers, can lead to a sense of imbalance for some patients. Somnolence is common with many medications and can exacerbate symptoms of imbalance, especially among elderly patients (6). Cochlear and vestibular ototoxicity is discussed in Chapter 35.

Auditory System

Information important in the evaluation of hearing loss includes age at onset, duration, rate of progression (sudden or gradual over weeks or years), and whether the impairment is unilateral, bilateral, or fluctuating. Associated symptoms such as high fever, upper respiratory infection, tinnitus, or vertigo should be explored. Prior use of amplification should be recorded (7).

Evaluation of a child for hearing loss requires a detailed interview with the parents. Gestational, perinatal, postnatal, and family histories are necessary components of the historical inventory. The gestational history helps identify factors that may have adversely affected the auditory system during fetal development. Environmental teratogens, including maternal infections, use of drugs, and metabolic and nutritional disturbances, should be identified. Maternal infections that influence fetal development include rubella, cytomegalovirus infection, syphilis, toxoplasmosis, and herpes. Drug ingestion during pregnancy can lead to irreparable damage to the developing neuroepithelium of the inner ear. Morphologic and functional defects of the external and inner ear have been associated with exposure to streptomycin, quinine, chloroquine, and thalidomide. Maternal alcoholism has also been demonstrated to be teratogenic to the developing auditory system.

Perinatal events, including placental insufficiency, prematurity, birth trauma, neonatal jaundice, and neonatal infection, may be associated with hearing loss among children. Postnatal infections, including measles, mumps, encephalitis, varicella, and tick-borne diseases, should be recorded. Bacterial meningitis may lead to unilateral or bilateral sensorineural hearing loss. The patient should be questioned regarding the presence of otorrhea and its characteristics, such as profuse or scant, purulent, clear, mucoid, bloody, or foul smelling (8).

Many patients have undergone multiple ear operations. It is critical to obtain information regarding the type and approximate date of the procedures. The patient should always be asked which ear is the better-hearing ear regardless of what the physical examination, tuning fork test, or audiogram reveals.

Otalgia is uncommon among patients with hearing loss not associated with infection of the external canal or middle ear. If otalgia is present, is it severe or mild? Is it relieved by otorrhea, drops, or antibiotics? Are there any exacerbating features, such as pain with chewing as occurs in temporomandibular joint dysfunction? Has there been recent dental work? Do dentures fit properly? Otalgia may be referred from neoplastic processes in the oropharynx, hypopharynx, or larynx, which have to be excluded with a complete head and neck examination.

Eustachian tube dysfunction may be a cause of otalgia, but it is generally described as ear fullness or pressure sometimes alleviated with a Valsalva maneuver. A history of autophony (ability to hear one's own voice) or hearing one's own breathing in the affected ear suggests a patulous eustachian tube and can help to differentiate this problem from inadequate eustachian tube function.

Tinnitus is defined as any abnormal noise perceived when no external acoustic stimulus exists. It is generally divided into two categories, objective and subjective. Objective tinnitus is infrequent and refers to internal noise that may be audible to the examiner. Subjective tinnitus is much more common than objective tinnitus and is not audible to the examiner (see Chapter 34).

Objective tinnitus may be caused by vascular, neurologic, or eustachian tube disorders. Vascular disorders may cause pulsatile tinnitus by generating turbulent flow in vessels in the vicinity of the temporal bone. They include arterial bruits, venous hums, arteriovenous malformations and shunts, aneurysms, vascular neoplasms, and aberrant vessels.

Neurologic disorders that cause objective tinnitus include palatomyoclonus and idiopathic stapedial and tensor tympani muscle spasms. Palatomyoclonus is characterized by an irregular, rapid, clicking sound in the ear. The sound is generated when the mucosa of the eustachian tube snaps together as the palatal muscles undergo myoclonic contraction. Patients may report aural fullness, hearing loss, or sound distortion. Middle ear muscle spasms produce a rough, crackling noise in the ear. External sounds may accentuate these spasms.

Subjective tinnitus is far more common than objective tinnitus and is generally associated with high-frequency sensorineural hearing loss usually caused by noise exposure or aging. Other causes are idiopathic, metabolic, cardiologic, neurologic, pharmacologic, dental, psychologic, and otologic factors. Tinnitus associated with symmetric sensorineural hearing loss may not necessitate evaluation beyond a complete audiologic and head and neck examination. Unilateral or pulsatile tinnitus and tinnitus associated with asymmetric sensorineural hearing loss or conductive hearing loss generally necessitates additional investigation by means of imaging or neurophysiologic testing.

Vestibular System

Imbalance is an extremely complex symptom referable to several organ systems besides the labyrinth (9–11). The clinician should establish the duration, severity, and progression of disequilibrium (12). Onset, whether sudden and violent or slow and insidious, may help to determine the diagnosis. Is it vertigo, imbalance, or unsteadiness? Have the symptoms progressed? Are they related to position? Is the vertigo constant or episodic? If episodic, what is the duration of the episodes? Are there symptoms between episodes? Are the vestibular symptoms associated with hearing loss or tinnitus, focal neurologic signs, migraine, severe nausea and vomiting? Is there a history of physical or barometric trauma? Is there a history of chronic ear disease with or without drainage (13,14)? Chapters 8 and 9 discuss dizziness in detail.

PHYSICAL EXAMINATION

Patients with hearing loss, tinnitus, or vestibular dysfunction should undergo a thorough otologic and neurotologic examination. As with any medical disorder, there is no substitute for a complete physical examination, and there is no excuse for an overlooked physical finding as a result of an examination done in haste. The physical examination includes a general examination of the head and neck, ear, nose, and throat and a specific otologic and neurotologic examination.

OTOLOGIC EXAMINATION

Auricle

An otologic examination begins with inspection of the auricle to find evidence of prior surgery, trauma, infection, or neoplasia. The size, shape, and position of the pinna are recorded, as is evidence of abnormal embryonic development, which may suggest deformation of underlying structures. Preauricular pits or skin tags may be present and indicate faulty fusion of the auricular hillocks. Movement of the auricle often causes pain when external otitis is present.

External Auditory Canal

The examiner can visualize the external auditory canal by drawing the tragus anteriorly while pulling the auricle superiorly. This maneuver is particularly helpful in examinations of children, who may be apprehensive about the use of an ear speculum. This preliminary maneuver assists in determining the correct size ear speculum to use. The largest speculum that can comfortably be inserted into the ear canal typically is chosen. Care is taken to insert the speculum only into the cartilaginous canal because deeper penetration into the bony canal can be painful. The patient's head must be properly positioned to compensate for the normal inclination of the ear canal.

Although a hand-held otoscope is useful as a screening tool (Fig. 2), its use is limited by the absence of binocular vision. An operating microscope is used when there is any question regarding the status of the ear. Careful cleaning of the external auditory canal is a prerequisite for otologic diagnosis. Cerumen, desquamated skin, and purulent debris must be completely removed with loops, alligator forceps, curettes, or suction. Video otoscopic examination (Fig. 3) can be performed easily in the office and assists greatly in photodocumentation and patient counseling. With video monitors in direct patient view, patient can better appreciate any pathologic process because they can see for themselves the ear and external canal. Video otoscopic examination can be performed with the 0-degree sinus scopes found commonly in the

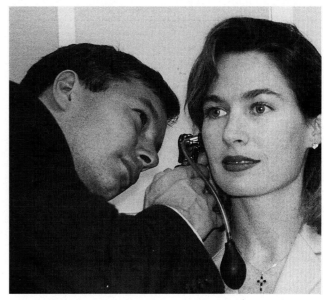

FIG. 2. Otoscopic examination with a hand-held otoscope.

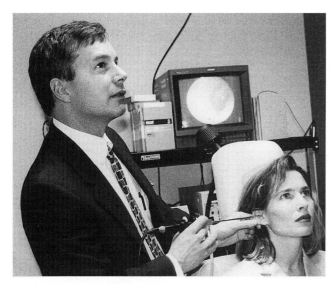

FIG. 3. Otologic examination with endoscopes and video monitoring. This technique is useful for patient education.

otolaryngologist's office (see Fig. 3) or with easier to use shorter otoscopes designed for otoscopic examination.

The external auditory canal is inspected for furuncles, cysts, dermatitis, exposed bone, and neoplastic changes. The presence of granulation tissue is assessed. Bony osteoma or exostosis is confirmed by means of direct palpation. Aural polyps are manipulated to determine their site of origin. It is important to differentiate polyps arising from the external ear canal from those that arise from the middle ear or tympanic membrane. Polypoid disease emanating from the tympanic membrane often suggests chronic middle ear disease or cholesteatoma. It is unwise to attempt removal of aural polyps in the office, because these lesions may be intimately involved with vital structures such as the ossicular chain and facial nerve (15,16).

Tympanic Membrane

After careful inspection of the external canal, thorough inspection of the tympanic membrane is conducted. In addition to the usual inspection for eardrum retraction, perforation, effusion, or cholesteatoma, mobility of the tympanic membrane is assessed to determine the status of the eustachian tube. The position of the tympanic membrane is evaluated to rule out lateralization or blunting, which may contribute to hearing loss. A monomeric area of the tympanic membrane must be differentiated from true perforation. Vascular lesions such as a dehiscent jugular bulb or glomus tumor are seen as a blue or red mass behind the eardrum. A white mass behind or within the tympanic membrane may represent cholesteatoma, tympanosclerosis, osteoma or, rarely, adenoma or neuroma.

In examinations of patients who have undergone surgical procedures, careful inspection is necessary to rule out

osteitis, recurrent cholesteatoma, and poor wound healing. In canal wall down mastoid cavities assessment of meatal size and height of the facial ridge is necessary. Evidence of granulation tissue, dural herniation, or leakage of cerebrospinal fluid is recorded (16,17).

Disorders associated with atelectasis and atrophy of the tympanic membrane can be difficult to diagnose. Retraction of the tympanic membrane is important to identify occult cholesteatoma. Severe retraction without cholesteatoma formation may lead to ossicular discontinuity and conductive hearing loss. Pneumotoscopy can be useful to diagnose disorders associated with retraction pockets. A standard otoscope with a pneumatic bulb or a Siegle's otoscope (Fig. 4) assists in evaluating retraction pockets and small perforations of the tympanic membrane that are not easily visualized. Pneumatic otoscopy can be useful to differentiate tympanosclerotic plaques on the surface of the tympanic membrane and cholesteatoma. It also can be useful to differentiate cholesteatoma from severe retraction of the tympanic membrane onto the promontory (18–20).

Eustachian Tube

The functional status of the eustachian tube should be evaluated when a patient has otologic symptoms. A satisfactory view of the eustachian tube orifice can be obtained by use of a small mirror or nasopharyngoscope. Any mass that impinges on the eustachian tube orifice must be fully investigated to rule out a neoplasm. The presence of hypertrophic adenoidal tissue may cause recurrent episodes of otitis media or chronic otorrhea. Acute or chronic nasopharyngitis or scarring of the eustachian tube orifice is evaluated. Mucosal or submu-

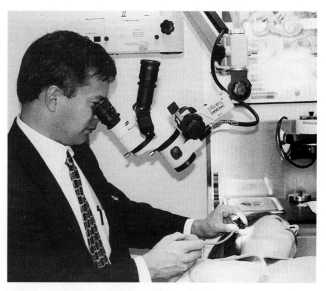

FIG. 4. Otoscopic examination with a microscope and Siegle's otoscope.

cosal clefting of the soft palate impairs eustachian tube function by means of deficient activity of the levator muscles of the palate. An abnormally patulous eustachian tube is rare but can often be confused with abnormal occlusion. Patients often describe disagreeable resounding of their own voice in their ear (autophony) or the ability to hear their own breathing.

HEAD AND NECK EXAMINATION

A complete head and neck examination is performed on all patients with otologic symptoms. Particular attention is paid to the parotid, parapharyngeal, and neck regions to find evidence of neoplasia. Auscultation of the head and neck is mandatory for all patients with pulsatile tinnitus. Although most tinnitus is subjective (heard only by the patient), objective tinnitus (heard by examiner) occasionally is present. The presence of pulsatile tinnitus may imply a vascular anomaly or tumor (21,22). Bruits are appreciable when turbulent blood flow is present. Otalgia may be caused by referred pain from simultaneously innervated structures within the head and neck. Common sources of referred otalgia include temporomandibular joint disorders and diseases of the larynx and/or hypopharynx.

Auscultation of the ear canal may be performed with a Toynbee otoscope or other modified electronic stethoscope. In the neck, the carotid arteries are auscultated with the patient's head in the midline. Auscultation of the head is necessary, including the orbits, mastoid region, and temporal area. A Valsalva maneuver is used to increase subtle vascular flow abnormalities (8).

TESTS OF NEUROLOGIC FUNCTION

Cranial nerve dysfunction frequently is associated with neurotologic disease. Therefore a comprehensive cranial nerve examination is part of the general otologic evaluation (23).

Cranial Nerve I: Olfactory

Disturbance in the sense of smell may be caused by transport loss, sensory loss, neural loss, or a central nervous system lesion. Several different types of tests are available to test olfaction. The most widely used office test is the three-bottle test. In the test, the patient is asked to smell three bottles, one containing coffee, one containing ammonia, and one that is empty. If the patient identifies all bottles correctly, smell is probably normal. If the patient is unable to smell the coffee bottle but is able to correctly identify the ammonia container, smell may be abnormal. However, if the patient denies smelling anything, the problem is likely functional, because ammonia stimulates the fifth nerve and is perceived even in the absence of olfaction. More definitive tests of olfaction extend the examiner's ability to detect loss of olfaction. One example is the University of Pennsylvania Smell Identification Test.

Cranial Nerve II: Optic

Optic nerve function can be rapidly assessed by means of examining visual acuity, visual fields, and pupillary reflex. Visual acuity is tested with a Snellen card. A person with 20/20 corrected vision likely has a normally functioning optic nerve. Visual fields are assessed in all four quadrants to find evidence of field deficits. A visual field deficit may imply a defect along the optic tract to the visual cortex. The pupillary reflex is assessed by means of alternating a light into each eye and searching for pupillary constriction. The sensory pathway of the pupillary reflex is through the optic nerve, and the motor response is through the third cranial nerve. If light does not produce constriction in either eye, there is an optic nerve problem in that eye. Lack of constriction on the stimulated side alone indicates a third nerve deficit on that side. In addition to evaluation of acuity, pupillary response and visual fields, funduscopic examination can be extremely helpful in the neurotologic assessment. Papilledema suggests elevation in intracranial pressure, which may be caused by cavernous sinus disease, sigmoid sinus thrombosis, a space-occupying lesion, or benign intracranial hypertension.

Cranial Nerves III, IV, and VI: Oculomotor, Trochlear, Abducens

Cranial nerves III (oculomotor), IV (trochlear), and VI (abducens) serve the extraocular muscles. Loss of third-nerve function leads to paralysis of the levator palpebra so the eye remains closed. The pupil is dilated and nonreactive because of involvement of the parasympathetic fibers that travel with the third nerve. Extraocular motility is affected except for eye movements served by the lateral rectus (cranial nerve IV) and superior oblique (cranial nerve VI). Loss of fourth-nerve function leads to paralysis of the ipsilateral superior oblique muscle and an inability to perform intorsion. Affected patients often report vertical diplopia. Loss of sixth-nerve function leads to an inability to laterally deviate the affected eye, a movement directed by the lateral rectus muscle. Horner's syndrome, characterized by unilateral ptosis, miosis, and anhidrosis of the ipsilateral face may be caused by a tumor of the cranial base or a lesion within the cavernous sinus. This syndrome is caused by interruption of postganglionic sympathetic fibers that arise from the superior cervical ganglion.

Cranial Nerve V: Trigeminal

The fifth cranial nerve consists of both a motor and sensory division. The three sensory divisions (ophthalmic, maxillary, and mandibular) provide sensation to the face. Loss of facial sensation may be tested by means of applying light touch, temperature changes, or pin pricks to the ipsilateral face. An important test of fifth-nerve sensory function is the corneal reflex. Touching the cornea with a wisp of cotton should produce blinking of both eyes. If the cornea is stimulated and neither eye blinks, the patient has a sensory deficit on the side tested. If only the opposite eye blinks, there is a seventh-nerve deficit on the tested side.

The motor division of the fifth nerve supplies the temporalis and masseter muscles with jaw opening. A fifth-nerve motor deficit typically leads to deviation of the jaw toward the side of the lesion because of the action of the relatively stronger muscles on the contralateral side. Fifth-nerve dysfunction may be seen with tumors of the cerebellopontine angle, middle cranial fossa, or paranasal sinuses.

Cranial Nerve VII: Facial

Facial nerve motor function is assessed in the three main areas of muscle innervation: frontal, periorbital, and perioral. Strength of voluntary muscle contraction is compared with that on the contralateral side. Asymmetry in movement of facial musculature implies weakness or paralysis of the involved side. A six-part grading system has been developed by the American Academy of Otolaryngology–Head and Neck Surgery to assist in uniform reporting of facial nerve injury and recovery.

In addition to motor function, the facial nerve possesses parasympathetic and sensory components that can be assessed for competence. Tearing, a function controlled by the parasympathetic division of the seventh nerve, can be tested with the Schirmer test. Submandibular salivary gland secretion represents another parasympathetic function of the facial nerve, although it is rarely tested clinically. Sensory fibers of the facial nerve travel with the chorda tympani nerve to supply taste to the anterior two thirds of the ipsilateral tongue. Taste can be tested to a variety of stimulants such as sugar, salt, and vinegar. A decrease in taste capabilities on the stimulated side implies a deficit of sensory innervation (24).

Cranial Nerves IX and X: Glossopharyngeal, Vagus

In its normal state, the palate is symmetric with the uvula in the midline. Voluntary elevation of the palate should be symmetric, and the uvula should remain in the midline. Deviation of the palate to one side implies dysfunction of the ninth and tenth cranial nerves on the side that does not elevate well. The uvula deviates to the nonparalyzed side. A diminished gag reflex also indicates ninth and tenth nerve dysfunction on the stimulated side. Tenth-nerve function can readily be assessed by means of laryngeal evaluation. Loss of tenth-nerve function causes

immobility of the ipsilateral vocal cord due to involvement of the recurrent laryngeal nerve. Swallowing may be affected if the lesion is proximal to the pharyngeal and superior laryngeal components of the tenth nerve.

Cranial Nerve XI: Spinal Accessory

The eleventh cranial nerve is tested by means of determining the strength of the sternocleidomastoid and trapezius muscles. A weak shoulder shrug indicates eleventh-nerve involvement, as does winging of the ipsilateral scapula. Notable reduction in voluntary head turning against resistance implies reduced innervation of the sternocleidomastoid muscle on the side contralateral to the resistance.

Cranial Nerve XII: Hypoglossal

The twelfth cranial nerve supplies the tongue muscles. Peripheral twelfth-nerve paralysis causes the tongue to deviate toward the side of the lesion because of the unopposed action of the contralateral tongue muscles. Fasciculation may be seen with twelfth-nerve lesions.

Hallpike Examination

The physical examination of a patient with vertigo includes the otologic and neurotologic examinations and an abbreviated neuroophthalmologic examination. The eyes are evaluated for nystagmus in all directions of gaze. Nystagmus may be present in both peripheral and central causes of vertigo. Nystagmus usually is horizontal but may be vertical or horizontal-rotary. Nystagmus may be spontaneous, present only during lateral gaze, or present with certain head positions, such as the Dix-Hallpike maneuver (25,26).

A Hallpike examination (Fig. 5) is performed on any patient with a history that suggests positional vertigo, that is, patients who describe brief, self-limiting, vertigo while looking up, lying down, or turning over in bed (27). As are all aspects of the physical examination, this test and why it is being performed are explained to the patient before the test is performed. When the examination begins the patient is sitting. The patient then is gently placed in a lying position with the head turned and slightly hanging to the right. The patient is asked to report any subjective vertigo while the examiner documents any nystagmus. The nystagmus that develops is characteristic: it is generally horizontal-rotary, delayed in onset, builds in intensity, peaks, and slowly resolves. The test is repeated with the head turned to the left. The affected ear is identified as the ear eliciting vertigo or nystagmus when turned down (28–30).

Cerebellar Function

Cerebellar disease may be manifest as asynergia and dysmetria. In cerebellar disorders, muscle movements

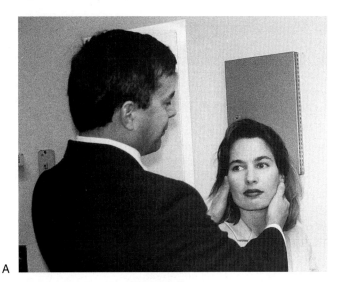

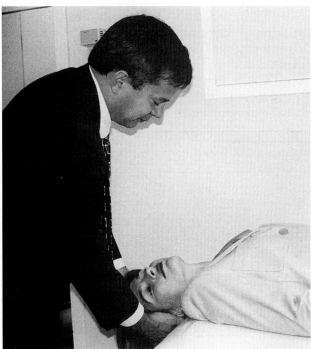

FIG. 5. A: Starting position for Dix-Hallpike maneuver (right ear). **B:** Ending position in Dix-Hallpike maneuver (right ear).

may be irregular, uncoordinated, or dissociated. Dysmetria implies inability to control the range of motion, so targets are overshot or undershot. Tests of cerebellar function typically involve repetitive movements such as finger-to-finger, toe-to-finger, and heel-to-shin. Rebound is the inability to control movement of an extremity after it is released from forceful restraint or displacement. The presence of rebound implies a loss of control of muscle coordination typically related to cerebellar dysfunction. Romberg testing is a test of static posture control. The patient is asked to stand still with the eyes open and then with the eyes closed. Romberg testing and gait assessment are measures of both central and peripheral input to

the limb and spinal muscles. The presence of ataxia generally implies cerebellar dysfunction. Not all abnormalities may be identified with these postural tests. For example, a patient with a severe labyrinthine deficit may have both a normal gait and a normal Romberg examination if the deficit is well compensated.

Motor and Sensory Function

Concise assessment of a patient's gross and fine motor movements includes evaluation of strength, bulk, and tone. Absent, diminished, or hyperactive reflexes may imply an upper or lower motor neuron lesion. Sensory responses to light touch, pin prick, and vibration are particularly helpful in the evaluation of balance dysfunction.

Tuning Fork Tests

A tuning fork examination is an important part of a bedside examination and a critical part of an office examination. A tuning fork examination can help to confirm the audiometric findings for any patient, especially those who are difficult to examine. Instructions are best given to the patient before the test and not during the test to avoid confusion. Although most patients with otologic symptoms are likely to undergo formal audiometric testing, a tuning fork test is a mandatory component of an office evaluation.

In Weber's test (Fig. 6) a vibrating tuning fork is placed on the glabella, nasal dorsum, central incisors of the maxilla, or mandibular symphysis. These solid midline structures conduct the sound energy of the tuning fork to the cochlear end organ. A patient who hears the tuning fork more clearly in one ear is said to have *lateralized* to that ear. Patients with a unilateral conductive hearing loss are

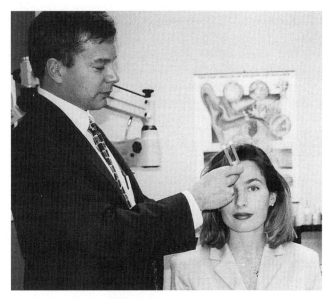

FIG. 6. Weber's test.

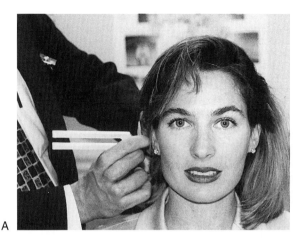
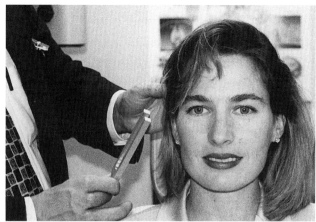

A   B

FIG. 7. A Rinne test.

sometimes tentative to respond to hearing a tone better in the "bad" ear. It may be useful to explain this fact to the patient during the examination if this is apparent. Tuning fork tests typically use 512 Hz vibratory stimuli, although useful information can be obtained with 1,024 Hz and 2,048 Hz tuning forks. As a rule, sound energy that lateralizes to one ear implies either an ipsilateral conductive loss (typically 15 to 25 dB with a 512 Hz fork) in the better hearing ear or a sensorineural loss in the contralateral ear.

A Rinne test (Fig. 7) further defines the Weber's test response. As with Weber's test, the test is briefly explained to the patient before it is begun. The examiner performs a Rinne test by first placing the vibrating tuning fork firmly against the mastoid process (bone conduction) and comparing its loudness with that of the tuning fork placed just outside the canal (air conduction). If the patient perceives the sound as being louder at the ear canal, air conduction is said to be greater than bone conduction. This implies either normal hearing or sensorineural hearing loss. If the sound is louder when the tuning fork is placed on the mastoid tip, bone conduction is said to be greater than air conduction. This implies conductive hearing loss. An approximately 20 dB conductive hearing loss is required before bone conduction becomes greater than air conduction. The importance of the tuning fork test as both a bedside and an office examination cannot be overemphasized. The tuning fork examination can confirm or refute audiometric test results, making these tests critical in otologic diagnosis (31,32).

SUMMARY POINTS

- The otologic history and physical examination are the cornerstones of the evaluation of a patient with hearing loss, vertigo, tinnitus, or other otologic symptoms.

- A complete neurotologic examination comprises otologic examination, evaluation of the head and neck, neurologic examination, vestibular examination, and office hearing testing.
- The need for further investigation, including vestibular tests, audiologic tests, blood tests, or imaging studies, is guided by the information obtained in the initial interview.
- The otologic history and physical examination should be performed efficiently, systematically, and accurately.

REFERENCES

1. Glasscock ME, Shambaugh GE. *Surgery of the ear,* 4th ed. Philadelphia: WB Saunders, 1991.
2. House JW. Otologic and neurotologic history and physical examination. In: Cummings CA, et al., eds. *Otolaryngology–head and neck surgery,* 2nd ed. St. Louis: Mosby–Year Book, 1993:2643–2651.
3. Rybak L. Metabolic disorders of the vestibular system. *Otolaryngol Head Neck Surg* 1995;112:128–132.
4. Goebel JA. Vertigo. In: Gates GA, ed. *Current therapy in otolaryngology–head and neck surgery.* St. Louis: Mosby Year Book, 1994:66–72.
5. Glasscock ME, Haynes DS, Storper IS, Bohrer P, Swazzu . Otology and neurotology. In: Adkins RB, Scott HW, eds. *Surgical care of the elderly,* 2nd ed. Philadelphia: Lippincott–Raven, 1998:193–200.
6. Hart CW. Clinical evaluation of the dizzy patient. In: Hughes GB, Pensak ML, eds. *Clinical otology* New York: Thieme, 1997:169–174.
7. Asher VA, Kveton JF. Clinical evaluation of hearing loss. In: Hughes GB, Pensak ML, eds. *Clinical otology.* New York: Thieme, 1997: 159–168, 215–232.
8. Bluestone CD, Klein JO. Methods of examination: clinical examination. In: Bluestone CD, Stool SE, Kenna MA, eds *Pediatric otolaryngology,* 3rd ed. Philadelphia: WB Saunders, 1996:150–164.
9. Kumar A, Applebaum EL. Evaluation of the vestibular system. In: Schuknecht HF, Nadol JB, eds. *Surgery of the ear and temporal bone.* New York: Raven Press, 1993:57–70.
10. Stockwell CW. Vestibular function tests. In: Paparella MM, et al., eds. *Otolaryngology.* Philadelphia: WB Saunders, 1991:921–948.
11. Cyr DG, Harker LA. Vestibular function tests. In: Cummings CA, et al., eds. *Otolaryngology–head and neck surgery,* 2nd ed. St. Louis: Mosby–Year Book, 1993:2652–2682.
12. DeWeese DD. Differential diagnosis of dizziness and vertigo. In: Paparella MM, et al., eds. *Otolaryngology.* Philadelphia: WB Saunders, 1991:1683–1687.

13. Schuknecht HF, Brackman DE, Glasscock ME, Jenkins H. Difficult decisions: Meniere's disease. *Operative Techniques Otolaryngol Head Neck Surg* 1991;2:47–53.

14. Singleton GT. Evaluation of the dizzy patient. In: Bailey BJ, Pillsbury HC, eds. *Head and neck surgery–otolaryngology.* Philadelphia: JB Lippincott, 1993:1870–1876.

15. Novick NL. Fundamentals of dermatologic diagnosis and therapy. In: Lucente FE, Lawsom W, Novick NL, eds. *The external ear.* Philadelphia: WB Saunders, 1995:25–39.

16. Lucente FE. Techniques of examination. In: Lucente FE, Lawson W, Novick NL, eds. *The external ear.* Philadelphia: WB Saunders, 1995:18–24.

17. Glasscock ME, Haynes DS, Storper IS, Bohrer PS. Surgery for chronic ear disease. In: Hughes GB, Pensak ML, eds. *Clinical otology.* New York: Thieme, 1997:215–232.

18. Paparella MM, Morris MS. Otologic diagnosis. In: Paparella MM, et al., eds. *Otolaryngology.* Philadelphia: WB Saunders, 1991:885–903.

19. Meyerhoff WL, Roland PS. Physical examination of the ear. In: Paparella MM, et al., eds. *Otolaryngology.* Philadelphia: WB Saunders, 1991:905–909.

20. Schuknecht HF. Office examination of the ear. In: Schuknecht HF, Nadol JB, eds. *Surgery of the ear and temporal bone.* New York: Raven Press, 1993:1–10.

21. Dickens JRE, Graham SS. Differential diagnosis of tumors of the cranial base. In Jackson CG, ed. *Surgery of skull base tumors.* New York: Churchill Livingstone, 1991:11–18.

22. Pillsbury HC, Woods CI. Clinical, neurophysiologic, and radiologic diagnosis of skull base lesions. In Jackson CG, ed. *Surgery of skull base tumors.* New York: Churchill Livingstone, 1991:19–48.

23. Burton MJ, Niparko JK. Evaluation of the cranial nerves. In: Hughes GB, Pensak ML, eds. *Clinical otology.* New York: Thieme, 1997:131–146.

24. Kumar A, Applebaum EL. Evaluation of the facial nerve. In: Schuknecht HF, Nadol JB, eds. *Surgery of the ear and temporal bone.* New York: Raven Press, 1993:71–77.

25. Zee DS, Leigh RJ. Evaluation of eye movements in the diagnosis of disease of the vestibular system. In: Cummings CA, et al., eds. *Otolaryngology–head and neck surgery, 2nd ed.* St. Louis: Mosby–Year Book 1993;2683–2697.

26. Leigh RJ, Zee DS. *The neurology of eye movement,* 2nd ed. Philadelphia: FA Davis, 1991.

27. Dix MR, Hallpike CS. The pathology, symptomatology and diagnosis of certain common disorders of the vestibular system. *Ann Otol Rhinol Laryngol* 1952;61:987–1016.

28. Herdman SJ, Tusa RJ, Zee DS, et al. Single treatment approaches to benign paroxysmal positional vertigo. *Arch Otolaryngol Head Neck Surg* 1993;101:523–528.

29. Brandt TRB. Physical therapy for benign paroxysmal positional vertigo. *Arch Otolaryngol* 1980;106:484–485.

30. Semont A, Freyss G, Vitte E. Curing the BPPV with a liberatory maneuver. *Adv Otorhinolaryngol* 1988;42:290–293.

31. Capper JW, Slack RW, Maw AR. Tuning fork tests in children. *J Laryngol Otol* 1987;101:780–783.

32. Sheehy JL, Gardner G Jr, Hambley WM. Tuning fork tests in modern otology. *Arch Otolaryngol* 1971;94:132–138.

The Ear: Comprehensive Otology,
edited by R. F. Canalis and P. R. Lambert.
Lippincott Williams & Wilkins, Philadelphia © 2000.

CHAPTER 8

History and Physical Examination of a Patient with Dizziness

Paul R. Lambert

Disequilibrium is a common disability that affects all age groups, especially the elderly. The myriad factors that can underlie this symptom contribute to the frustration and perplexity that often attend both patient and physician. To facilitate the approach to care of a patient with dizziness, it is important to focus on the following objectives:

1. To identify serious pathologic conditions, such as central nervous system lesions, brainstem ischemia, or cardiac arrhythmia
2. To recognize diseases that can be treated medically or surgically, such as endocrine abnormality, middle ear infection, Meniere's disease, or drug reaction
3. To provide reassurance or rehabilitation to patients excluded from the first two objectives

The purpose of this chapter is to outline a systematic approach to the evaluation of patients with dizziness that meets the three objectives in an efficient and comprehensive manner.

P.R. Lambert: Department of Otolaryngology–Head and Neck Surgery, University of Virginia Health Sciences Center, Charlottesville, Virginia 22908-0430

ANATOMY AND PHYSIOLOGY

The clinical evaluation of any disease or symptom complex must be based on a solid understanding of the pertinent anatomic and physiologic features. This precept is especially germane to the symptom of dizziness, which usually involves one or more of the following systems: peripheral vestibular, central vestibular, visual, and somatosensory. Only a superficial discussion of anatomy and physiology is considered here; this information is presented in detail in Chapters 2 through 6.

The cristae of the semicircular canals sense angular acceleration, and the maculae of the utricle and saccule sense linear acceleration and gravitational force. The hair cells of these vestibular organs are innervated by bipolar neurons (approximately 20,000), which constitute the superior and inferior vestibular nerves. The cell bodies of these neurons compose Scarpa's ganglion, which is located within the internal auditory canal. These first-order vestibular neurons project primarily to the four vestibular nuclei (superior, lateral, medial, and descending) in the brainstem; a small percentage of fibers synapse directly in the cerebellum.

The anatomic organization of the vestibular nuclei and their connections with the central and peripheral nervous systems are complex. Briefly, the vestibular nuclei receive afferent fibers, in addition to those from the vestibular nuclei, from the cerebellum, reticular formation, contralateral vestibular nuclei, spinal cord, and cortex. Of these additional sources of input, the afferent fibers from the cerebellum provide the largest number. Efferent fibers from the vestibular nuclei project to the cerebellum, spinal cord (vestibulospinal track), reticular formation of the midbrain, oculomotor nuclei through the medial longitudinal fasciculus, and temporal lobe cortex.

The vestibular nerve fibers have a constant, resting discharge rate. Physiologic stimulation that produces endolymph flow within the semicircular canals changes this baseline activity to produce an increase in firing from the semicircular canals on one side and a corresponding decrease from the contralateral side. This equal but opposite change in neural activity is interpreted centrally as head movement of a certain speed in a certain plane. Activation of the oculomotor nuclei provides compensatory eye movements so that the field of last gaze is maintained (vestibuloocular reflex). Muscle tone and muscle reflexes are adjusted by cerebellar and vestibulospinal inputs to maintain posture and balance.

From this brief overview of physiology, the consequences of a disease such as Meniere's disease or labyrinthitis that alters baseline neural activity from one labyrinth can be understood. Disparity in peripheral vestibular inputs can be interpreted, on the basis of experience, as head motion, even though the patient is stationary. This constant illusion of motion defines vertigo. The misinformation is relayed to the ocular muscles, which make compensatory movements for the supposed head motion, causing nystagmus. Misinformation directed at the cerebellum and vestibulospinal system produces inappropriate adjustment of muscle tone and reflexes and causes incoordination and ataxia. Stimulation of the vagus nerve causes nausea and vomiting. The central nervous system is able to compensate over time for most vestibular insults.

HISTORY

The most important aspect of the evaluation of a patient with dizziness is the history. Physical examination is all too often unrevealing; it is the information provided by the patient that directs further objective testing and treatment. Although some patients can provide a succinct and precise account of their dizziness, the highly subjective, often emotional, perception of this symptom and its functional impact frequently result in a history that is disjointed and long. This fact, combined with the many causes of dizziness that must be considered in the differential diagnosis, makes it imperative that the history be clinician directed and structured. One way to accomplish this is with a dizziness questionnaire. This approach can expedite the interview and provide both a structure and recall mechanism for the patient's comments. Whether or not a questionnaire is used, a complete history includes the following components:

Description of the dizziness
Severity
Temporal pattern
Precipitating and exacerbating factors
Associated symptoms
Circumstances of the initial event
Medications and toxins
Other disease processes

Description

A precise description of the dizziness by the patient is the initial point elicited. The patient must differentiate a variety of possible descriptors: vertigo, light-headedness, blurred vision, incoordination, loss of motor function or consciousness, disorientation, and vague sensations, such as poor concentration, floating, and heavy- or fuzzy-headedness. If patients have difficulty articulating their symptoms, they can focus on the first episode of dizziness, because it may have been the most frightening and still the most vivid in their memory.

Vertigo implies an actual sensation of motion (the patient or the environment). It is usually rotary but may have a vertical or even pulsive component. A description of vertigo strongly suggests a peripheral or occasionally a central vestibular lesion.

Oscillopsia is the perception that a stationary object is in motion. It most frequently results from a bilateral peripheral vestibular pathologic process. Without vestibular input to the ocular muscles (vestibuloocular reflex), a stable retinal image cannot be maintained with head or body motion. Stationary objects in the visual field appear blurred or bobbing (e.g., difficulty reading signs while walking or riding in a car). Oscillopsia is not experienced if the person is stationary.

Light-headedness directs the clinician to the vascular system, particularly if it is associated with posture change (e.g., postural hypotension) or exercise (e.g., cardiac dysfunction). Vasovagal attacks, metabolic disorders (especially glucose abnormalities), and anxiety with hyperventilation also can produce light-headedness.

Blurred vision does not specifically implicate one system as the underlying problem. Unilateral vestibular lesions that cause nystagmus usually are perceived as vertigo; however, very fine nystagmus may cause blurring of the vision. Blurred vision with head movement (oscillopsia) suggests bilateral vestibular loss. Refractive errors, ocular motor abnormalities, or optic nerve lesions (e.g., demyelination) also cause this symptom.

Incoordination is a nonspecific symptom caused by a variety of pathologic conditions such as central lesions (including acoustic tumors), proprioceptive deficits, and middle ear infection (serous labyrinthitis).

Loss of motor function or consciousness points toward a structural or vascular lesion of the central nervous system.

Disorientation, poor concentration, floating, and fuzzy-headedness are not characteristic of most peripheral vestibular disorders. Patients in this category frequently relay a long history (months to years) of constant symptoms. This history further mitigates against a peripheral vestibular cause. Metabolic disorders, psychogenic causes, and, rarely, central lesions must be considered.

Side effects of medications and ingested or inhaled toxins (e.g., hydrocarbon fumes) rarely cause vertigo but are considered in the differential diagnosis of the other dizziness descriptors.

Severity

Determining the severity of dizziness, especially in terms of its functional impact on daily activities, further refines the symptom. Specific questions include the following:

1. Are you able to function during the dizziness? Can you walk, work, drive an automobile? Do you have to sit or lie down a great deal?
2. What leisure or daily activities, if any, have you stopped because of the dizziness?
3. If you have undergone electronystagmography (ENG), how do you compare the dizziness in severity and quality with the vertigo experienced with the caloric examination?

During the episode of dizziness, the severity may change. The dizziness typically is most severe initially and subsides with time; this is true for benign paroxysmal positional vertigo (BPPV), Meniere's disease, and viral labyrinthitis. Dizziness that is continuous in intensity over months to years usually is not vestibular in origin. With any vestibular lesion, including complete unilateral loss of peripheral vestibular function, compensatory mechanisms in the central nervous system are expected to ameliorate the symptom within days to weeks. An exception is an unstable vestibular lesion, that is, one in which vestibular function fluctuates. In this circumstance, adaptive central nervous system mechanisms are compromised because of varying vestibular inputs.

Temporal Pattern

The temporal pattern of dizziness often is diagnostic of a specific disorder. Although intermittent dizzy spells may vary in *duration,* the patient should be able to classify the typical episode as lasting seconds, minutes, hours, days or as constant (weeks to months). Examples of diseases that correspond to these time frames are listed in Table 1.

TABLE 1. *Differential diagnosis of dizziness on the basis of temporal pattern*

Seconds	Benign paroxysmal positional vertigo, postural hypotension
Minutes	Transient ischemic attacks
Hours	Meniere's disease
Days	Viral labyrinthitis
Constant	Metabolic, psychogenic, or toxic disorder or drug side effect (unlikely to be vestibular)

The *frequency* of attacks is determined. In a number of disorders the episodes are random with no set frequency pattern. In general, however, it is possible to differentiate attacks that occur daily, weekly, monthly, or yearly and to quantify the average number of episodes within those time frames. In addition to having diagnostic significance, this information is important in assessing response to various therapies. The patient is asked to specify the longest time between attacks.

Precipitating and Exacerbating Factors

A number of factors can precipitate dizziness, and eliciting this information often can point to an underlying pathologic process. Specific events to be explored in this context include food ingestion, sudden head movement, turning over in bed, coughing or sneezing, loud noise, postural change, and exercise. Ingestion of large amounts of sodium can precipitate an attack of Meniere's disease for some patients; others with this disease can experience dizziness after eating certain foods, as though the attack were an allergic reaction.

Vertigo of short duration (less than 1 minute) precipitated by sudden head movement or turning over in bed strongly suggests BPPV. However, any type of sudden head or body movement places considerable demands on the vestibular system. Such movements, therefore, can exacerbate vertigo from a variety of vestibular lesions.

Dizziness caused by coughing or sneezing could be caused by a perilymph fistula or central nervous system disorder that causes increased intracranial pressure. Fibrosis within the vestibule caused by Meniere's disease or syphilis can produce dizziness in response to loud sounds (Tullio phenomenon) as stapes displacement exerts traction on the saccule or utricle. Dizziness precipitated by a change in posture or by exercise suggests a cardiovascular problem such as postural hypotension or cardiac disease.

Associated Symptoms

Vestibular disorders that cause vertigo frequently are accompanied by diaphoresis, nausea, and vomiting. A history of such autonomic symptoms strongly points to the inner ear as the source of dizziness. Other symptoms that implicate the peripheral labyrinth include hearing loss, tinnitus, aural fullness or pressure, and otorrhea. Episodes of vertigo with fluctuating hearing loss, low-pitch tinnitus, and aural pressure are pathognomonic for Meniere's disease. Vertigo in the presence of otorrhea suggests serous or suppurative labyrinthitis.

Dizziness associated with diplopia, dysarthria, weakness, or paresthesia suggests a central vascular abnormality such as transient ischemic attacks or stroke, depending on the time course of the neurologic deficit. Multiple sclerosis can cause a similar complex of neurologic symptoms. Visual changes (e.g., scotoma, tunnel vision, flashing lights) with headache and dizziness point to migraine. Dizziness associated with shortness of breath, palpitations, or chest discomfort suggests cardiac disease.

Although paresthesia can be associated with several neurologic disorders, circumoral numbness and tingling of the fingers suggest hyperventilation and possible underlying anxiety as the cause of dizziness. Falling is a rather nonspecific symptom, but drop attacks are indicative of a more specific abnormality such as vertebral-basilar insufficiency, seizure disorder, crisis of Tumarkin (a variant of Meniere's disease), cardiac disease, or vaso-vagal syncope.

Initial Event

Having patients recall the initial episode of dizziness can often assist them in describing their symptoms more precisely. The events precipitating or surrounding the initial episode may provide insight into the causation. For example, did the dizziness occur spontaneously and suddenly, or did it develop after physical straining or barotrauma from scuba diving or air flight? The latter circumstances would be consistent with an inner ear fistula, whereas the former would be consistent with Meniere's disease, viral labyrinthitis, or a vascular lesion. Dizziness after blunt trauma to the head or cervical region also suggests inner ear disease or possible damage to the central vestibular pathways. The patient is questioned about any travel, exposure to toxins, or substantial emotional stress near the time the dizziness began. It is also important to ascertain the current character of the dizziness in terms of severity, frequency, and associated symptoms compared with the initial episode.

Medications and Toxins

The patient's current medications and those used in the recent past, including during hospitalizations, especially intravenous antibiotics such as aminoglycosides, are reviewed. In a study involving patients seeking evaluation in an emergency department because of dizziness, medications were found to be the cause 10% of the time.

Among patients older than 60 years, the incidence was 20% (1). Drugs may cause orthostatic hypotension (e.g., antihypertensives), central vestibular dysfunction resulting in nonspecific disequilibrium (e.g., antidepressants, sedatives, antihistamines), and direct damage to vestibular sensory cells (e.g., aminoglycoside antibiotics). Exposure to toxins such as mercury, lead, and organic solvents can cause damage to the cerebellum and other central vestibular structures (2,3).

Other Diseases

Because spatial equilibrium depends on visual and somatosensory input in addition to that from the vestibular system, diseases that affect the eyes or proprioception may cause or contribute to the symptoms. Recent changes in *visual acuity,* such as refraction errors, macular damage, cataract surgery, or new glasses, can precipitate disequilibrium, particularly among persons who may have preexisting vestibular deficits but have compensated in part with greater reliance on visual input. This circumstance often is encountered among the elderly. Diseases that cause *peripheral neuropathy,* such as diabetes, alcoholism, and vitamin B_{12} deficiency, can affect proprioception.

A common manifestation of *cardiac disease* is dizziness or light-headedness. Abnormalities of conduction, valvular disease, and congestive failure all must be considered in the evaluation of a patient with dizziness.

One of the most common factors underlying the general feeling of dizziness as opposed to the more specific symptom of vertigo is a *psychogenic disorder,* such as stress, acute or chronic anxiety, or depression. This problem may be the entire basis for the patient's dizziness or it may contribute by intensifying other disease processes or impairing physiologic compensation. Although psychogenic disorders are frequently encountered, it is essential that the patient's dizziness be attributed to this diagnosis only after a thorough history and physical examination have excluded other potential causes.

One is alerted to the possibility of psychogenic dizziness when patients describe multiple somatic problems, such as tension headaches, backache, or chronic fatigue. Panic attacks, which can be characterized by a variety of symptoms including dizziness, trembling, palpitations, shortness of breath, weakness, paresthesia, sweating, and chest tightness, are a specific type of acute anxiety. As a method of introducing this aspect of the evaluation process, examiners can ask patients to quantify on a scale of 1 to 10 their level of stress, anxiety, or depression.

PHYSICAL EXAMINATION

The multiplicity of potential causes of dizziness requires a thorough physical examination of several systems, including the ear and peripheral vestibular system and the vascular and neurologic systems. A neurologic examination includes the cranial nerves, cerebellar testing, Romberg testing, eye movements, gait, and general motor and sensory testing. Hyperventilation testing can be performed if the history suggests a psychogenic origin of the dizziness. This test is considered positive if 1 minute of forceful and rapid breathing reproduces the symptoms. Because nystagmus is the only objective sign of vertigo, the examination initially focuses on the presence or absence of this abnormality.

Nystagmus

Nystagmus is involuntary, repetitive oscillation of the eyes. If present, nystagmus is defined with the following parameters: direction, plane, intensity, and evoking maneuvers. One examines for nystagmus occurring spontaneously or in response to changes in eye position or head movement. This examination includes the use of Frenzel glasses, which prevent visual fixation (Figs. 1, 2). This testing condition is important because visual fixation can suppress nystagmus, especially that caused by peripheral labyrinthine dysfunction. Preventing visual fixation can assist in the diagnosis of a recent labyrinthine lesion that has undergone compensation and no longer exhibits spontaneous nystagmus. Frenzel glasses consist of +20 diopter lenses in a frame that has a light source. These glasses magnify and illuminate the eyes for the examiner and prevent the patient from visually fixating. Loss of visual fixation often can uncover nystagmus that has persisted many months after the initial vestibular insult.

Direction

Vestibular dysfunction causes asymmetric oscillation of the eyes with a slow drift in one direction and fast compensatory movement in the opposite. By convention, the direction of the fast phase is used to specify the type

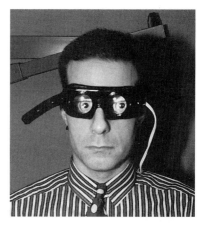

FIG. 2. Frenzel glasses help uncover nystagmus by preventing visual fixation. The eyes are illuminated by the light source and magnified with high-diopter lenses.

of nystagmus (e.g., right beating or left beating). The direction of the slow phase, however, usually points toward the diseased labyrinth.

Nystagmus can be further characterized as direction fixed or direction changing. Direction-changing nystagmus suggests a central lesion, whereas most acute, unilateral peripheral vestibular disorders cause direction-fixed nystagmus that beats away the affected labyrinth. Interruption of the resting discharges from a diseased labyrinth causes relative hyperactivity from the normal side. Because this disparate information is processed centrally, it is interpreted, on the basis of experience, as head rotation away from the diseased labyrinth (i.e., rotation of the head to the left with right labyrinthine dysfunction). The result of this illusion of constant head motion is vertigo. Nystagmus develops as the vestibular imbalance directs the ocular muscles to compensate for this supposed head movement. Slow deviation of the eyes toward the diseased labyrinth occurs in an attempt to maintain the field of last gaze. As the eyes reach the extreme of lateral gaze, compensatory rapid eye movement returns them toward the midline (i.e., rapid eye movement toward the intact labyrinth). This condition is simulated during the caloric examination with irrigation of an ear canal with cold water, which temporarily reduces activity from that labyrinth.

Plane

Nystagmus can be horizontal, rotary, or vertical. Peripheral vestibular disorders characteristically produce horizontal or horizontal-rotary nystagmus. Lesions of the peripheral vestibular system rarely involve just one semicircular canal but affect the entire labyrinth or vestibular nerve on one side. As a result, the disparate inputs from the two vertical semicircular canals (i.e., right posterior and left superior and vice versa) largely cancel out, allowing the asymmetric input from the right and left horizontal

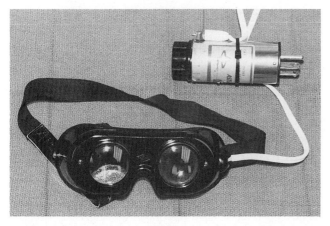

FIG. 1. Frenzel glasses used to examine for nystagmus.

canals to predominate. Central vestibular disorders can cause nystagmus in any plane, but vertical nystagmus (upbeat or downbeat) strongly suggests a central pathologic condition.

Intensity

If spontaneous nystagmus is observed (with or without Frenzel glasses), intensity is graded as first, second, or third degree. This classification is based on the effect of direction of gaze on nystagmus. Nystagmus present only when gaze is in the direction of the fast phase is first degree; this is the least intense nystagmus. Nystagmus present when the eyes are also midline is second degree. The strongest nystagmus, third degree, occurs even when gaze is in the direction of the slow phase. Third-degree nystagmus is seen in all eye positions. Regression in the degree of nystagmus over time (e.g., from third to second or second to first) can be used as an objective indicator of the clinical course of the labyrinthine injury. The intensity of nystagmus may be affected by direction of gaze. Looking in the direction of the fast phase increases the amplitude of nystagmus secondary to a peripheral vestibular abnormality but usually has no effect on nystagmus of central origin. This observation is known as Alexander's law (4).

Evoking Maneuvers

Several provocative stimuli are used to induce nystagmus. These include gaze testing (asking the patient to follow the examiner's finger across the field of vision) and *Hallpike testing* (rapidly changing the patient's head position). Healthy persons can have nystagmus if eye deviation is more than 40 degrees from the middle position (end point nystagmus).

A specific type of gaze nystagmus indicative of a central lesion is *gaze paretic nystagmus.* Gaze paretic nystagmus is characterized by an inability to maintain lateral gaze. As the patient attempts to look toward the right or left, the eyes slowly return to midline (slow phase) and make a rapid corrective movement (fast phase) back toward the periphery. On right lateral gaze a right beating nystagmus is present, and on left lateral gaze a left beating nystagmus is present. The most common causes of this type of nystagmus are ingestion of drugs such as alcohol or anticonvulsants and specific central nervous system lesions, including multiple sclerosis, myasthenia gravis, and cerebellar atrophy (5–8). Gaze paretic nystagmus frequently occurs among patients awakening from general anesthesia and therefore must be differentiated from pathologic nystagmus caused by otologic or neurotologic surgery.

The Hallpike test is performed in examinations for paroxysmal positional nystagmus, which if classic in presentation indicates BPPV, a specific peripheral vestibular disorder. This test is performed by rapidly changing the patient from a seated position to a supine one with the head hanging right or left (Figs. 3, 4). Nystagmus (and vertigo) that has a 2 to 10 second latency before onset, is predominately rotary, and lasts 10 to 30 seconds is characteristic of BPPV. This diagnosis is further substantiated if the nystagmus is fatigable; that is, repeated positioning of the patient causes the nystagmus to be less intense and then finally not occur. Nystagmus is present usually in only one head-hanging position. This observation allows identification of the diseased labyrinth, because the nystagmus typically occurs when the abnormal ear is on the bottom (9–11). Paroxysmal positional nystagmus that appears without latency, lasts more than 30 seconds (often as long as the head position is maintained), is not fatigable with repeated testing, and can be direction changing depending on the head position is indicative of a central vestibular lesion (9,12,13).

Central versus Peripheral Nystagmus

It often is not possible to differentiate nystagmus of peripheral origin (labyrinth, eighth nerve) from nystagmus caused by a central lesion (brainstem, cerebellum, or cortex). Certain characteristics of eye movement, how-

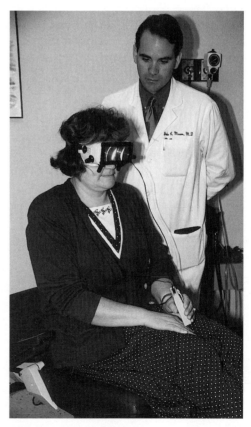

FIG. 3. Hallpike testing begins with the patient seated in an examination chair with the back fully reclined. Frenzel glasses can be used.

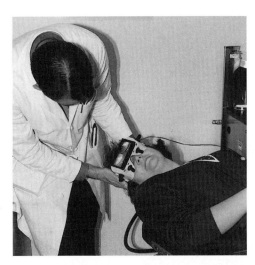

FIG. 4. The patient is quickly placed in a head hanging position (right or left) and kept there for 15 to 20 seconds while the examiner looks for nystagmus or subjective symptoms of dizziness. If the test is negative, the patient is returned to the seated position, then quickly placed supine with the head turned to the opposite side.

ever, suggest peripheral as opposed to central abnormality. Those characteristics are summarized in Table 2.

Otologic Examination

Otoscopy is performed to look for pathologic conditions of the middle ear, such as otitis media or cholesteatoma, that can cause dizziness. In the setting of acute otitis media, toxins can diffuse across the round window membrane and cause serous labyrinthitis. Infection associated with cholesteatoma can produce similar pathologic features. A cholesteatoma can directly erode the labyrinthine bone (most frequently the horizontal semicircular canal) and cause serous or purulent labyrinthitis.

A fistula test is performed at otoscopy using a pneumatic otoscope with a tight fitting speculum or, ideally, a Siegle otoscope (Fig. 5). The Siegle otoscope is designed to be used with a microscope (3). The shape of the Siegle specula helps assure a tight seal, and the pneumatic bulb allows insufflation of a large volume of air. Frenzel glasses are worn by the patient. A positive test is defined as a burst of nystagmus in response to positive or negative pressure on the tympanic membrane. The subjective symptom of dizziness without nystagmus is interpreted as equivocal. A positive fistula test can occur in the setting of a break in the oval window or round window membrane, as from barotrauma, erosion into the labyrinth, as from cholesteatoma, or adhesions in the vestibule connecting the medial surface of the stapes footplate with the saccule. The last condition can be caused by Meniere's disease or syphilis.

Vascular System Examination

Altered vascular flow to the peripheral or central vestibular systems is a common cause of dizziness and disequilibrium. Hypoperfusion can occur acutely (postural hypotension, cardiac arrhythmia, vertebral basilar insufficiency) or chronically (atherosclerosis, impaired cardiac muscle function). The physical examination cannot investigate all causes of hypoperfusion, but postural blood pressure measurements should be documented, and auscultation of the neck and chest should be performed to rule out bruits, murmurs, and irregularities in cardiac rhythm.

Neurologic Examination

The neurologic examination is performed to evaluate the cranial nerves, cerebellar function, and various components of the peripheral and central vestibular systems (vestibuloocular and vestibulospinal reflexes, vestibuloocular control, and proprioception). Gross motor and sensory function is assessed. Muscular abnormalities such as weakness or spasticity can contribute to imbalance, and sensory loss, particularly in a stocking or glove pattern, is indicative of peripheral neuropathy with possible impairment of proprioceptive input.

TABLE 2. *Peripheral versus central nystagmus*

Characteristic	Peripheral	Central
Spontaneous Nystagmus		
Direction	Horizontal–rotary	Any direction, including vertical
	Direction fixed	Direction fixed or changing
Intensity	Diminished by visual fixation	No change with visual fixation
	Increased by gaze in direction of fast phase (Alexander's law)	Gaze has little or no effect
Evoked Nystagmus (Hallpike)		
Latency	2–10 seconds	Immediate onset
Direction	Predominantly rotary	Any direction, including vertical
Duration	<30 seconds	>45 seconds
Fatigability	Yes	No

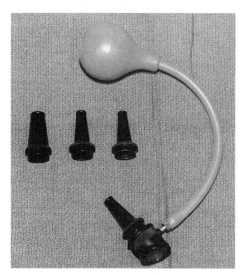

FIG. 5. The Siegle otoscope with an assortment of specula.

Cranial Nerves

Cranial nerves II through XII are examined with particular focus on visual acuity (cranial nerve II), extraocular muscles (cranial nerves III, IV, VI), facial and corneal sensation (cranial nerve V), facial muscle function (cranial nerve VII), and auditory and vestibular function (cranial nerve VIII). Uncorrected refraction errors can contribute to or occasionally cause dizziness. Use of the Snellen chart or a near-vision card can provide an approximation of visual acuity. Assessment of visual fields is included. The extraocular muscles are assessed by having a patient look in all directions of gaze. The presence of muscle weakness (the patient usually describes diplopia), nystagmus, or drooping of the eyelid (ptosis) is documented.

Trigeminal nerve function is assessed by having the patient compare, side to side, the light touch of cotton on the forehead, cheek, and chin. The corneal reflex is examined by touching the lateral (temporal) corneal edge of each eye with a tightly wound wisp of cotton. The patient gazes toward the contralateral side, so that the cotton wisp or examiner's hand does not enter the visual field. Touching the lateral sclera can be used as a control, because this stimulus does not elicit a reflex blink. Decreased facial or corneal sensation can occur with vestibular schwannoma (acoustic tumor) and petrous apex lesions.

The facial muscles are examined for hyperactivity (hemifacial spasm) or hypoactivity (paresis). Various temporal bone and central nervous system tumors (vestibular or facial schwannomas, petrous apex cholesteatoma, or cholesterol granuloma) can produce facial nerve dysfunction and disequilibrium. Paresis or paralysis of the mid and lower face with sparing of frontalis and orbicularis oculi function points toward a cortical (supranuclear) lesion.

Hearing is qualitatively assessed with a 512 Hz tuning fork. Weber's and Rinne tests can be used to differentiate conductive from sensorineural hearing loss. The vestibuloocular reflex can be assessed with the *head shaking test* and the *dynamic visual acuity test* (Fig. 6). With Frenzel glasses in place, the patient quickly shakes his or her head back and forth (horizontal plane) 15 to 20 times. The presence of nystagmus after head shaking suggests an imbalance in the vestibuloocular pathway (14). The dynamic visual acuity test is used to assess visual acuity with the head at rest and in motion. The patient first reads a Snellen chart with the head stationary and then with the head randomly rotated about the visual axis by the examiner. A drop in acuity of two lines or more indicates an abnormality, usually bilateral, within the vestibuloocular reflex (15). A patient with a positive test typically describes oscillopsia, that is, instability of the visual surround with motion such as walking or riding in a vehicle. More objective information about auditory and peripheral dysfunction is provided by audiometric testing and ENG.

Cerebellar Testing

Midline or vermis lesions of the cerebellum can cause ataxia, especially truncal ataxia, and intention tremor, whereas hemispheric lesions affect fine motor control and cause clumsiness in performing finger to nose and rapid alternating hand movements. Ataxia is assessed by having the patient walk heel to toe (tandem gait). Testing of fine motor control involves the patient's touching his or her nose and with an outstretched arm the examiner's finger, which is moved to different positions for each trial. Incoordination of arm and hand movement (undershooting or overshooting) is termed *dysmetria*. Rapidly moving the hands from a pronated to supinated position

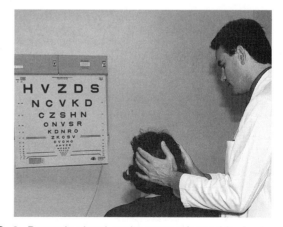

FIG. 6. Dynamic visual acuity test performed by having the patient read a Snellen chart with the head at rest and during random head movements produced when the examiner moves the patient's head about the visual axis.

also tests fine motor control; impaired ability to perform this task is termed *dysdiadochokinesia.*

Visual-Ocular Testing

The visual-ocular control system involves *saccadic* and *smooth-pursuit eye movements.* Abnormalities in this system are indicative of a central lesion. Saccadic and smooth-pursuit testing is a routine part of ENG. At physical examination, saccadic eye movement is assessed by having the patient look back and forth between the examiner's finger as it is quickly moved from approximately 30 degrees right of center to 30 degrees left of center. Abnormal saccadic movement is characterized by overshooting or undershooting. Smooth pursuit is tested as the patient follows the slow back and forth motion of the examiner's finger across the visual field. The eyes should show a smooth, pendular motion without saccadic or other erratic eye movements.

Vestibulospinal Testing

The vestibulospinal system involves complex reflexes that act on many joints, adjusting muscle tension to maintain body stability with respect to gravity. *Romberg testing* and gait provide qualitative information on the integrity of this system (Figs. 7, 8). Romberg testing is

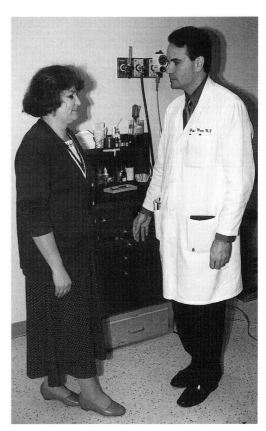

FIG. 8. Sharpened Romberg test with feet in tandem and eyes opened or closed.

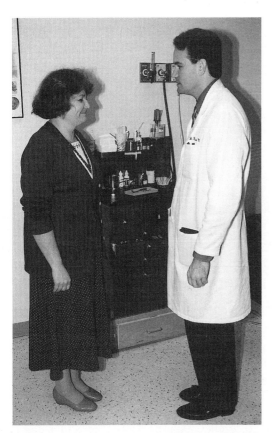

FIG. 7. Romberg testing with feet together and eyes opened or closed.

first performed with the patient standing erect with feet together. If this task is performed without difficulty, the patient is asked to close their eyes. Consistent falling to one side is considered a positive test result. The sharpened Romberg test, a more sensitive indicator of a pathologic condition, is performed by having the patient stand with feet aligned (in tandem). Gait is evaluated by having the patient walk back and forth in a straight path with rapid 180-degree turns. An alternative is trying to maintain balance while walking in a tight figure of eight.

Vestibulospinal reflexes depend on proprioceptive, visual, and vestibular input. Romberg testing with eyes closed eliminates the visual input and isolates the vestibular and proprioceptive systems. Proprioceptive input can be largely negated by having patients stand on a 6-inch (15-cm) foam mat during the Romberg test.

DISEASES AND DISORDERS

To properly focus the evaluation, it is important to have a broad differential diagnosis of dizziness in mind. To that end, the following diseases and disorders are discussed, and salient features of the history and physical examination are highlighted.

Benign Paroxysmal Positional Vertigo

Pathophysiology

BPPV is one of the most common abnormalities of the peripheral labyrinth. It is thought to result from the presence of particles of inner ear debris (possibly degenerated otoconia from the utricular macula) in the posterior semicircular canal. These particles may attach to the cupula of the posterior semicircular canal and make it sensitive to gravity (16). Another explanation is that the particles, which have a higher specific gravity than the surrounding endolymph, may remain free floating and produce abnormal cupular deflection with certain head movements (17). A history of head trauma or viral labyrinthitis may be elicited from some patients, but most patients have no obvious predisposing factors.

Evaluation

The history usually allows the clinician to make the diagnosis of BPPV. The typical patient describes sudden, fleeting (less than 30 seconds) episodes of intense vertigo precipitated by certain head or body movements (turning over in bed, looking upward, bending down). Although the vertigo is transient, a feeling of nausea or unsteadiness may linger for several minutes. Hallpike testing usually confirms positional nystagmus (rotatory) with either the right ear or left ear on the bottom; the ear on the bottom is the abnormal one. A presumptive diagnosis of BPPV can be made from the history without a positive Hallpike test.

Meniere's Disease

Pathophysiology

The cause of Meniere's disease is uncertain. For more than a half century, the histologic correlate of this disorder has been known (18). Temporal bone studies show dilatation, distortion, and membrane ruptures within the membranous labyrinth, especially the scala media and saccule. These changes are caused by an increased volume of endolymph thought to result from underabsorption rather than overproduction of this fluid. The endolymphatic sac has been implicated in a variety of ways, such as resorption site or immunologic abnormality, in the pathogenesis of Meniere's disease (19,20).

Evaluation

Although the symptoms of Meniere's disease can vary greatly from one patient to another, and even temporally within the same patient, the history is sufficiently distinct to make the definitive diagnosis in most instances. Sudden episodes of vertigo lasting 20 minutes to 12 hours (usually 2 to 8 hours) associated with diminished hearing, roaring tinnitus, and pressure or fullness in one ear are classic for Meniere's disease. Early in the course of the disease, there may be little or no hearing loss and minimal tinnitus. With time, the full symptom complex develops. Physical examination may reveal unilateral sensorineural hearing loss at tuning fork testing. During an acute attack of vertigo, nystagmus is evident.

Labyrinthitis

Pathophysiology

Bacteria and viruses can cause an inflammatory response within the labyrinth. Serous or purulent labyrinthitis develops as bacteria or their toxins diffuse across the round window membrane (e.g., from acute otitis media), enter through a bony fistula (e.g., erosion of the horizontal semicircular canal by cholesteatoma), or traverse the cochlear aqueduct or internal auditory canal (e.g., from meningitis). More common than bacterial labyrinthitis is the clinical condition called *vestibular neuritis* or *viral labyrinthitis*. Although a viral cause has not been demonstrated unequivocally, there are good epidemiologic and histopathologic data implicating a viral infection of the inner ear in this disorder (21).

Evaluation

Patients with viral labyrinthitis describe sudden onset of intense vertigo that lasts several days to a week and necessitates bed rest. Unilateral hearing loss may occur. The dizziness gradually resolves over several weeks, although mild unsteadiness or transient vertigo with sudden movement may persist for several months, particularly among elderly patients. If seen immediately, the patient demonstrates nystagmus that beats away from the side of the lesion. Otologic examination otherwise is normal. In the case of bacterial labyrinthitis, physical examination of the ear may reveal acute otitis media or a cholesteatoma. Vertigo may be sudden and severe in these conditions, although it may be preceded by several days of less intense unsteadiness.

Vestibular Schwannoma (Acoustic Tumor)

Pathophysiology

Vestibular schwannoma is a benign Schwann cell tumor that originates from the vestibular division of the eighth cranial nerve. As the tumor enlarges, it compresses the eighth nerve within the internal auditory canal, and the compression causes hearing loss, tinnitus, and possibly mild disequilibrium. With further growth into the cerebellopontine angle, the tumor compresses the cerebellum and brainstem.

Evaluation

The primary symptom of an acoustic tumor is likely to be tinnitus and slowly progressive unilateral hearing loss rather than dizziness. Vertigo is rare, but mild unsteadiness or clumsiness may be acknowledged. With larger tumors, paresthesia of the ipsilateral face may be noticed. Sensorineural hearing loss can be documented with tuning fork testing. Decreased corneal sensation usually is present if the tumor extends to the brainstem. Facial weakness is uncommon. With increasing compression of the cerebellum and brainstem, ataxia and gaze paretic nystagmus occur.

Vertebral Basilar Insufficiency

Pathophysiology

Vertebral basilar insufficiency usually is caused by atherosclerosis involving the subclavian, vertebral, or basilar arteries.

Evaluation

Vertebral basilar insufficiency typically occurs among patients older than 50 years. Vertigo or disequilibrium is a common initial symptom of this disorder and usually lasts several minutes. The key to diagnosis is finding associated symptoms of posterior circulation ischemia, such as visual changes (field defects, diplopia), weakness, paresthesia, and drop attacks. The physical examination usually is normal.

Presyncopal Light-headedness

Pathophysiology

Decreased cerebral perfusion on a global rather than focal basis can cause light-headedness or dizziness. Common disorders that precipitate central ischemia include postural hypotension, cardiac disease, vasovagal attacks, hyperventilation, and autonomic dysfunction.

Evaluation

Patients with postural hypertension describe light-headedness with quick standing. The history often reveals a contributing factor such as use of antihypertensive medications, hypovolemia, or diabetes and secondary autonomic dysfunction. Confirmation of this diagnosis is made by measuring blood pressure and pulse in the supine and standing positions. Most patients with light-headedness from cardiac disease have a history of heart problems. One must be alert, however, to the possibility of dizziness as a presenting symptom of arrhythmia or other cardiac abnormality, especially among the elderly. The physical examination may show an irregular pulse or heart murmur. A history of fear or acute or chronic anxiety usually can be elicited from patients experiencing light-headedness that has a psychogenic basis (22). Symptoms associated with hyperventilation include circumoral numbness and paresthesia of the fingers, air hunger, and chest tightness. This diagnosis can be confirmed during the physical examination if hyperventilation reproduces dizziness.

Perilymph Fistula

Pathophysiology

A leak of perilymph fluid from the inner ear into the middle ear or mastoid can result from surgery, trauma, infection, or sudden change in cerebral spinal fluid pressure. Less commonly, it can occur spontaneously, usually from developmental abnormalities of the inner ear, such as Mondini dysplasia. Trauma includes both penetrating injuries to the labyrinth and atmospheric pressure changes (barotrauma), which cause rupture of the oval window or round window membrane. Cholesteatoma and other middle ear or mastoid infectious processes can erode into the horizontal semicircular canal or cochlea. A sudden increase in cerebrospinal fluid pressure, as with severe straining, lifting, or sneezing, can be transmitted to the perilymph and rupture the round window membrane.

[handwritten marginal note: true. Mondini doesn't give CSF fistula]

Evaluation

The sudden onset of vertigo or dizziness after penetrating injury to the ear or after flying, scuba diving, or severe straining suggests an inner ear fistula. A patient with a cholesteatoma and dizziness is assumed to have a fistula of the horizontal semicircular canal. The vestibular symptoms experienced by a patient with a fistula can vary from vertigo to unsteadiness. Coughing, sneezing, or straining often exacerbates the dizziness. Tinnitus and hearing loss may be present. The onset of the hearing loss usually is coincident with the dizziness, but it may fluctuate in severity. A positive fistula test (nystagmus with pneumatic otoscopy) strongly suggests the presence of a perilymph fistula.

Ototoxicity

Pathophysiology

Ototoxins can damage the peripheral vestibular organs (e.g., aminoglycosides) or central vestibular system (e.g., hydrocarbons, mercury, and possibly lead). Aminoglycoside ototoxicity causes death of hair cells in the cochlea, cristae of the semicircular canals, and maculae of the utricle and saccule. The cristae are more vulnerable to damage than are the otolithic organs. The mechanisms by which organic solvents cause balance dysfunction are incompletely understood, but loss of neurons within the cerebellum has been seen in experiments and in post-mortem studies of humans (23).

Evaluation

Patients with vague descriptions of dizziness or ataxia are asked about exposure to industrial solvents during work or in recreational activities. Mercury intoxication, which can occur after eating contaminated fish, is considered if paresthesias in the extremities or constriction of visual fields is present. Actual vertigo is uncommon after parenteral aminoglycoside toxicity because vestibular organs are affected bilaterally. Marked unsteadiness or oscillopsia can occur. Patients with ototoxic exposure may show unsteadiness with gait, a positive Romberg test result, and a positive dynamic visual acuity test result. Sensorineural hearing loss and tinnitus may be present.

Trauma

Pathophysiology

Trauma to the vestibular system includes penetrating injuries, blunt skull trauma with temporal bone fracture or concussive damage to the inner ear, and barotrauma (oval window or round window membrane break). Depending on the injury, disruption of the membranous labyrinth with damage to the sensory epithelium by physical or chemical (perilymph and endolymph mixing) means can occur. The result is partial or total loss of vestibular function on the affected side. Temporal bone trauma can dislodge particulate matter, which becomes free floating within the endolymph and causes positional vertigo.

Evaluation

Injury to the vestibular labyrinth is suspected in a patient with dizziness after barotrauma or direct injury to the ear or skull. Depending on the extent of trauma, one or more of the following may be found during the physical examination: sensorineural hearing loss, nystagmus, ataxia, positive Hallpike test result, and a positive fistula test result.

Disequilibrium of Aging

Pathophysiology

Changes in the peripheral and central vestibular system that occur with aging include loss of sensory epithelium, neuronal atrophy or loss, neurofiber degeneration, and accumulation of lipofuscin and other inclusion bodies (24). It has been demonstrated in patients older than 70 years that a 40% loss of hair cells occurs in the cristae and a 20% loss in the maculae (25). These diffuse changes can alter input (visual, proprioceptive, and vestibular), central processing, and the motor response.

Evaluation

Disequilibrium of aging is suggested when an older patient experiences slowly progressive disequilibrium or ataxia. Because peripheral vestibular changes with aging may be compensated in large part by visual input, patients often notice more disequilibrium at night. A sudden change in vision may initiate the symptoms for the same reason. Physical examination shows changes in gait and poor Romberg test results, especially with eyes closed or standing on foam. Cerebellar testing may be impaired. These abnormal test results usually show no localizing (right versus left) signs.

Central Nervous System Lesion

Dizziness can be the presenting symptom of a central nervous system lesion or, more commonly, can develop at some time during the course of the illness. Because these lesions may have serious health implications, it is imperative to maintain a high index of suspicion and perform the necessary diagnostic tests (usually magnetic resonance imaging) as appropriate. The following are examples of central nervous system diseases to be considered in the evaluation of dizziness.

Migraine

Dizziness may predate the onset of headaches, especially among younger patients. The dizziness may not be synchronous with the headache but can occur as an isolated event. A family history of migraine and the presence of other symptoms such as nausea and vomiting and an aura (visual or somatosensory) help confirm the diagnosis.

Multiple Sclerosis

Although dizziness is rarely an initial symptom of multiple sclerosis, it is a common symptom at some point in the illness. The diagnosis is suggested when a young adult has a history of various neurologic deficits characterized by remissions and exacerbations.

Communicating Hydrocephalus

Disequilibrium, ataxia, urinary frequency, and forgetfulness experienced by an elderly patient suggest communicating hydrocephalus. A shunt can improve the symptoms.

Arnold-Chiari Type I Malformation

Slowly progressive unsteadiness of gait, usually with nystagmus, especially down beating, suggests Arnold-Chiari type I malformation, a cranial vertebral abnormality.

Tumors

Tumors of the brainstem (glioma), cerebellum (medulloblastoma), posterior fossa (meningioma, arachnoid cyst), and temporal bone (epidermoid tumor) may cause dizziness, but typically the diagnosis is suggested by the presence of associated neurologic deficits.

Other

Other central nervous system lesions to be considered in the differential diagnosis of dizziness include Parkinson's disease, cerebellar degeneration, and familial ataxia.

SUMMARY POINTS

- The history is the most important aspect in the evaluation of a patient with dizziness.
- Dizziness should be more precisely defined as vertigo, which strongly suggests a vestibular lesion; light-headedness; incoordination; oscillopsia; or loss of motor function or consciousness.
- The temporal pattern of dizziness often is diagnostic for a specific disorder (e.g., seconds, BPPV; hours, Meniere's disease; days, labyrinthitis).
- Associated symptoms may provide important diagnostic information; for example, fluctuating hearing loss and tinnitus suggest Meniere's disease; diplopia, dysarthria, and paresthesias suggest central ischemia; and headaches, scotomata, and flashing lights suggest migraine).
- Dizziness, particularly among elderly patients, may be related to medications. Orthostatic hypotension, nonspecific central vestibular dysfunction, and direct peripheral vestibular end organ damage are possible side effects of a number of common medications.
- Nystagmus is the best objective sign of vertigo. Nystagmus that is latent (suppressed by visual fixation and other compensatory mechanisms) may be uncovered with use of Frenzel glasses or the head-shaking test.
- Vertical nystagmus (upbeat or downbeat) suggests a central pathologic condition.
- The classic response to Hallpike testing for BPPV is transient (less than 30 seconds) rotary nystagmus that has a several-second latency and is fatigable. The nystagmus usually is present in only one head-hanging position, and the ear on the bottom is the abnormal one.
- A neurologic examination includes cranial nerve assessment, cerebellar testing (tandem gait, fine motor control), saccadic and smooth-pursuit eye movements, and Romberg testing.
- To focus the history and physical examination of a patient with dizziness, a broad differential diagnosis of vestibular and nonvestibular causes of this symptom is essential.

REFERENCES

1. Skiendzielewski JJ, Martyak G. The weak and dizzy patient. *Ann Emerg Med* 1980;9:353–356.
2. Moller C, Odkvist LM, Thell J, et al. Otoneurological findings in psycho-organic syndrome caused by industrial solvent exposure. *Acta Otolaryngol (Stockh)* 1989;107:5–12.
3. Mizukoshi K, Nagaba M, Ohno Y, et al. Neurotological studies upon intoxication by organic mercury compounds. *ORL J Otorhinolaryngol Relat Spec* 1975;37:74–87.
4. Robinson DA, Zee DS, Hain TC, Holmes A, Rosenberg LF. Alexander's law: its behavior and origin in the human vestibulo-ocular reflex. *Ann Neurol* 1984;16:714–722.
5. Herishanu Y, Osimand A, Louzoun Z. Unidirectional gaze paretic nystagmus induced by phenytoin intoxication. *Am J Ophthalmol* 1982;94:122–123.
6. Kattah JC, Schilling R, Liu SJ, Cohan SL. Oculo-motor manifestations of acute alcohol intoxication. In: Smith JL, Katz RS, eds. *Neuro-ophthalmology enters the nineties*. Hialeah, FL: Duton Press, 1988:233–243.
7. Reulen JPH, Sanders EACM, Hogenhuis LAH. Eye movement disorders in multiple sclerosis and optic neuritis. *Brain* 1983;106:121–140.
8. Zee DS, Yee RD, Cogan DG, Robinson DA, Engel WK. Ocular motor abnormalities in hereditary cerebellar ataxia. *Brain* 1976;99:207–234.
9. Harrison MS, Ozahinoglu C. Positional vertigo. *Arch Otolaryngol* 1975;101:675–678.
10. Dix MR, Hallpike CS. The pathology, symptomatology, and diagnosis of certain disorders of the vestibular system. *Ann Otol Rhinol Laryngol* 1952;61:987–1016.
11. Cawthorne T. Positional nystagmus. *Ann Otol Rhinol Laryngol* 1954;63:481–490.
12. Cawthorn T, Hinchcliffe R. Positional nystagmus of the central type as evidence of subtentorial metastases. *Brain* 1961;84:415–426.
13. Hallpike CS. Vertigo of central origin. *Proc R Soc Med* 1962;55:364–370.
14. Hain TC, Fetter M, Zee DS. Head-shaking nystagmus in patients with unilateral peripheral vestibular lesions. *Am J Otolaryngol* 1987;8:36–47.
15. Longridge NS, Mallinson AI. A discussion of the dynamic illegible "E"-test: a new method of screening for aminoglycoside vestibulotoxicity. *Otolaryngol Head Neck Surg* 1984;92:671–677.
16. Schuknecht HD. Cupololithiasis. *Arch Otolaryngol* 1969;90:113–126.
17. Parnes LS, McClure JA. Free-floating endolymph particles: a new operative finding during posterior semicircular canal occlusion. *Laryngoscope* 1992;102:988–92.
18. Hallpike CS, Cairns H. Observations on the pathology of Meniere's syndrome. *J Laryngol Otol* 1938;53:625–655.
19. Kimura RS. Experimental blockage of the endolymphatic duct and sac and its effect on the inner ear of the guinea pig: a study on endolymphatic hydrops. *Ann Otol Rhinol Laryngol* 1967;76:644–687.
20. Wackym PA, Linthicum FH Jr, Ward PH, House WF, Micevych PE, Bagger-Sjoback D. Re-evaluation of the role of the human endolymphatic sac in Meniere's disease. *Otolaryngol Head Neck Surg* 1990;102:732–744.
21. Schuknecht HF, Kitamura K. Vestibular neuritis. *Ann Otol Rhinol Laryngol* 1981;90[Suppl 78]:1–19.
22. Katon W. Panic disorder and somatization. *Am J Med* 1984;77:101–106.
23. Odvist LM, Larsby B, Fredrickson JM, Liedgren SR, Tham R. Vestibular and oculomotor disturbances caused by industrial solvents. *J Otolaryngol* 1980;9:53–59.
24. Fujii M, Goto N, Kikuchi K. Nerve fiber analysis and the aging process of the vestibulocochlear nerve. *Ann Otol Rhinol Laryngol* 1990;99:863–870.
25. Rosenhall U, Rubin W. Degenerative changes in the human vestibular sensory epithelia. *Acta Otolaryngol (Stockh)* 1975;79:67–80.

The Ear: Comprehensive Otology,
edited by R. F. Canalis and P. R. Lambert.
Lippincott Williams & Wilkins, Philadelphia © 2000.

CHAPTER 9

Objective Evaluation of a Patient with Dizziness

Dennis I. Bojrab and Sanjay A. Bhansali

Electronystagmography	Rotary Chair Testing
Method of Electronystagmographic Testing	Head-shake Testing
Evaluation of Abnormal Eye Movements	**Posturography**
Evaluation of Vestibular-Oculomotor Function	Sensory Organization Test
Evaluation of Visual-Oculomotor Function	Motor Coordination Test
Clinical Application	Pressure Test
Rotation Tests	Clinical Significance

Objective evaluation of dizziness is undertaken after a thorough history and physical examination provide the information needed to formulate a diagnostic impression. Vestibular tests are used to confirm the clinical diagnostic impression. Too often objective vestibular tests are used with the hope of finding a diagnosis when they may lead to acquisition of erroneous or negative information. For instance, two common vestibular disorders characterized by dizziness are benign paroxysmal positional vertigo (BPPV) and Meniere's disease. In both conditions, results of objective vestibular tests may be normal during remission, but the patient's symptoms usually are consistent with the illness. Conversely, a patient may have a test result that suggests unilateral vestibular loss, but the presenting symptoms may be consistent with vascular syncope and unrelated to such a finding. In general, vestibular function tests should aid in determining whether a disorder is peripheral or central, localizing the side of lesion, supporting the clinical diagnosis, establishing treatment, and evaluating the patient's progress.

Vestibular function tests are clinical techniques used to examine and evaluate part of the human balance system. A brief review of vestibular anatomy and physiology is needed to understand vestibular function testing. The vestibular system is one of the oldest on the phylogenetic scale. It is generally divided into a peripheral part (the inner ear balance organs or labyrinth and the vestibular nerves) and a central part (the vestibular nuclei in the brainstem and its numerous connections to the cerebellum and higher centers) (1). The purpose of the vestibular portion of the inner ear is to provide the brain with information regarding orientation of the head in space. The labyrinth works by converting acceleration or gravity forces into a neural signal that responds to linear and angular movement. The paired vestibular end organs are dynamic structures that constantly discharge neural impulses to the brain even when at rest (2). Acceleration of the head produces a change in this signal pattern, which is what the brain interprets as motion. If both labyrinths are simultaneously stimulated or inhibited, they cancel each other, and no reaction occurs—the brain does not perceive any change. Natural head motion stimulates one side and inhibits the other side, causing a reaction and perception of motion. Caloric irrigation, heating or cooling the inner ear, stimulates one side at a time and causes a predictable reaction and perception of motion— vertigo. There are several ways in which the inner ear can be stimulated, including thermal, electrical (galvanic), gravitational (positional), and head motion (acceleration). Vestibular function tests are limited to thermal, gravitational, and head motion stimuli because effective electrical stimulation is painful.

Stimulation of the inner ear causes a specific eye movement called *nystagmus*. Nystagmus is a reflexive repetitive eye movement and is integral to the evaluation of the vestibular system. Nystagmus is produced by

   D. I. Bojrab: Department of Otolaryngology, Wayne State University, Michigan Ear Institute, Farmington Hills, Michigan 48334; Department of Otolaryngology–Head and Neck Surgery, Beaumont Hospital, Royal Oak, Michigan 48075

   S. A. Bhansali: Atlanta Ear, Nose, and Throat Associates, Atlanta, Georgia 30342-1703

means of vestibular stimulation or inhibition. It may be considered extrinsic, as in vestibular function testing, or intrinsic, as in inner ear disease. Electronystagmography (ENG) and rotation testing measure nystagmus to provide objective assessment of vestibular system function.

It is important to understand the interaction of the vestibular system with other organ systems that help maintain balance and posture. The brain acts as the central processor to produce motor reflexes that maintain posture and equilibrium and to stabilize gaze based on information it receives from the inner ear (vestibular), the eyes (visual), and muscle and joint receptors (proprioception). These systems are connected within the central nervous system (CNS), and reflex pathways provide continuous information not perceived by the person. The most important reflex pathways are the vestibuloocular reflex (VOR), which integrates information between the inner ear and the eyes (the extraocular muscles), and the vestibulospinal reflex, which integrates information from the skeletal system. One system may be more dominant and override the other in certain situations, but these interactions and their adaptive control are not completely understood (3).

The vestibular function tests in current use are ENG, rotary chair testing, and posturography. Most of this chapter is devoted to ENG because it is the most widely used, the most useful, and the most economical of the vestibular function tests.

ELECTRONYSTAGMOGRAPHY

ENG gets its name from the oldest method of recording nystagmus. In ENG periorbital skin surface electrodes are attached near the eye and detect the tiny electrical potential that naturally exists between the cornea and the retina, the corneoretinal potential. Eye movement causes deflection in the ENG recording that produces a characteristic tracing. Nystagmus has a fast phase and a slow phase. The velocity of the slow phase provides a sensitive and accurate measure of intensity. In the past, recordings were made with a polygraph tracer. During the 1980s, computerized ENG recording became available for clinical use. This provided the advantages of efficient storage and retrieval of actual eye movement tracings, eliminated cutting and pasting of strip chart records, and delivered automatic, rapid calculation and analysis of various parameters and formulas that are critical in ENG testing. Computerization also provided greater sophistication of analysis for saccade, tracking, and caloric tests and allowed automatic comparison of individual eye movement recordings with statistical norms at a variety of different frequencies. This would be too laborious, time consuming, and impractical to do manually. For these reasons, computerized ENG recording is now routinely used (4).

Although ENG refers to the electrical method of recording eye movements, ENG testing is a battery of vestibular tests performed and recorded with ENG. To avoid confusion some authors refer to the ENG method of recording eye movements as electrooculography and the testing battery as ENG testing. ENG recording has limitations, such as inability to record patients who have little or no corneoretinal potential (blind persons) and inability to record very small or pure torsional eye movements.

If ENG is analogous to electrocardiography, then visual observation of the patient's eyes is analogous to listening to heart sounds with a stethoscope. Direct visual observation, with or without Frenzel lenses, is an inexpensive and easily available method of assessing nystagmus, but there is no permanent record and the velocity of nystagmus is not assessed. Duration and frequency (beats per 10 seconds) can be measured by means of observation, but these parameters are not as sensitive or accurate as maximum slow-phase velocity (SPV) of nystagmus in describing the intensity of a vestibular reaction (5). Direct observation can, however, be a useful part of an office examination. Frenzel lenses (very high diopter, magnifying glasses) enlarge the view of a patient's eyes and inhibit visual fixation, often exposing occult spontaneous nystagmus.

Use of skin surface electrodes (ENG) remains the most popular clinical method of recording nystagmus because it is simple, noninvasive, inexpensive, and reliable. Other methods of recording eye movements are available, but cost factors and practical issues limit their use. The following is a brief description of these techniques. Infrared videography involves use of an infrared camera system that provides video monitoring of the eyes supplemented by computerized recording of nystagmus (6). Direct infrared oculography involves use of an array of tiny infrared lights reflected off the surface of the eye and uses the differential reflection between the iris and the sclera. This provides a clean, sensitive recording but requires testing with eyes open and technical expertise for accurate use (7,8). Scleral search coils are the most accurate devices for measuring eye movement. They are not practical for routine clinical use, however, because the patient must wear a difficult-to-adapt contact lens that contains an electrical coil. Scleral coils are used mostly as research tools.

METHOD OF ELECTRONYSTAGMOGRAPHIC TESTING

The ENG test battery consists of eight procedures that may be divided into three groups (3,9,10). The first group of tests looks for the *presence of abnormal eye movements* and whether the movements change with head position. The following are the tests in this group: (a) The *gaze test* is used to evaluate limitation of eye movements, gaze stability, ocular flutter, spontaneous nystagmus, and latent nystagmus. (b) *The Dix-Hallpike maneuver* is used to evaluate for BPPV. (c) The *positional test* determines whether various head positions cause or modify a nystagmus. The second group of tests investigates *vestibular-oculomotor function*: (d) The *bithermal caloric test* is the cornerstone of the ENG test battery and is used primarily to detect labyrinthine or vestibular nerve dysfunction and to localize the side of involvement. (e) The *head-shake test* involves use of an imprecise rotational stimulus to generate nystagmus. It is not part of the traditional ENG test battery, but it takes little time to perform and often verifies the presence of a peripheral vestibular disorder. The *third group of tests is used to evaluate visual-oculomotor function* or nonvestibular (tracking) eye movements: (f) The *saccade test* is used to detect disorders of the saccade eye movement control system. (g) The *tracking (smooth pursuit) test* and (h) the *optokinetic test* are used to detect disorders of the pursuit eye movement control system. A normal computerized ENG test result is shown in Fig. 1.

Evaluation of Abnormal Eye Movements

Gaze Test

The gaze test discloses nystagmus in the absence of vestibular stimulation. It may be the first step in identification of vestibular, central, or congenital disorders that present with nystagmus. The test is performed by recording the patient's eye movements first in the primary position (gazing straight ahead) and then while looking 30 to 40 degrees to the right, to the left, up, and down (11,12). Eye position should be held for at least 30 seconds. Vestibular *spontaneous nystagmus* occurs when there is an imbalance in the tonic input from the vestibular apparatuses. It is typically seen during and after unilateral vestibular dysfunction, and the nystagmus usually beats away from the side of the diseased labyrinth or nerve. Vestibular spontaneous nystagmus is seen at ENG as a horizontal nystagmus, but it may be horizontal-torsional. The intensity of spontaneous nystagmus may change with change in eye position, being stronger when gaze is directed toward the direction of the nystagmus (Alexander's law). Gaze deviation beyond 40 degrees may cause end-point nystagmus even among healthy persons. Spontaneous nystagmus that does not lessen or increases with visual fixation suggests a central lesion (failure of fixation suppression) (11).

Gaze-evoked nystagmus may be a side effect of various medications, including anticonvulsants, sedatives, and alcohol. It can also occur in such diverse conditions as myasthenia gravis, multiple sclerosis, and cerebellar atrophy. The most common type of disconjugate nystagmus (internuclear ophthalmoplegia) occurs with lesions of the medial longitudinal fasciculus (12,13).

Dix-Hallpike Maneuver

The Dix-Hallpike maneuver (sometimes called the Nylen-Barany maneuver) is used to diagnose the most commonly seen peripheral vestibular disorder, BPPV. Barany gave the first detailed clinical description of this condition in 1921 and Nylen further characterized it in

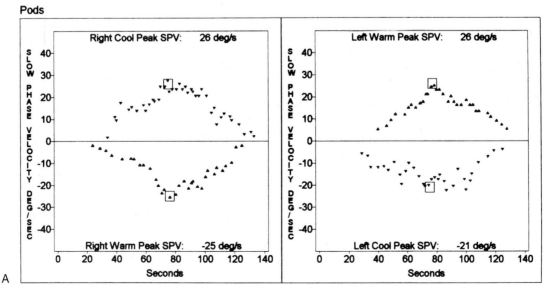

FIG. 1. Normal results of computerized electronystagmography. *Continued.*

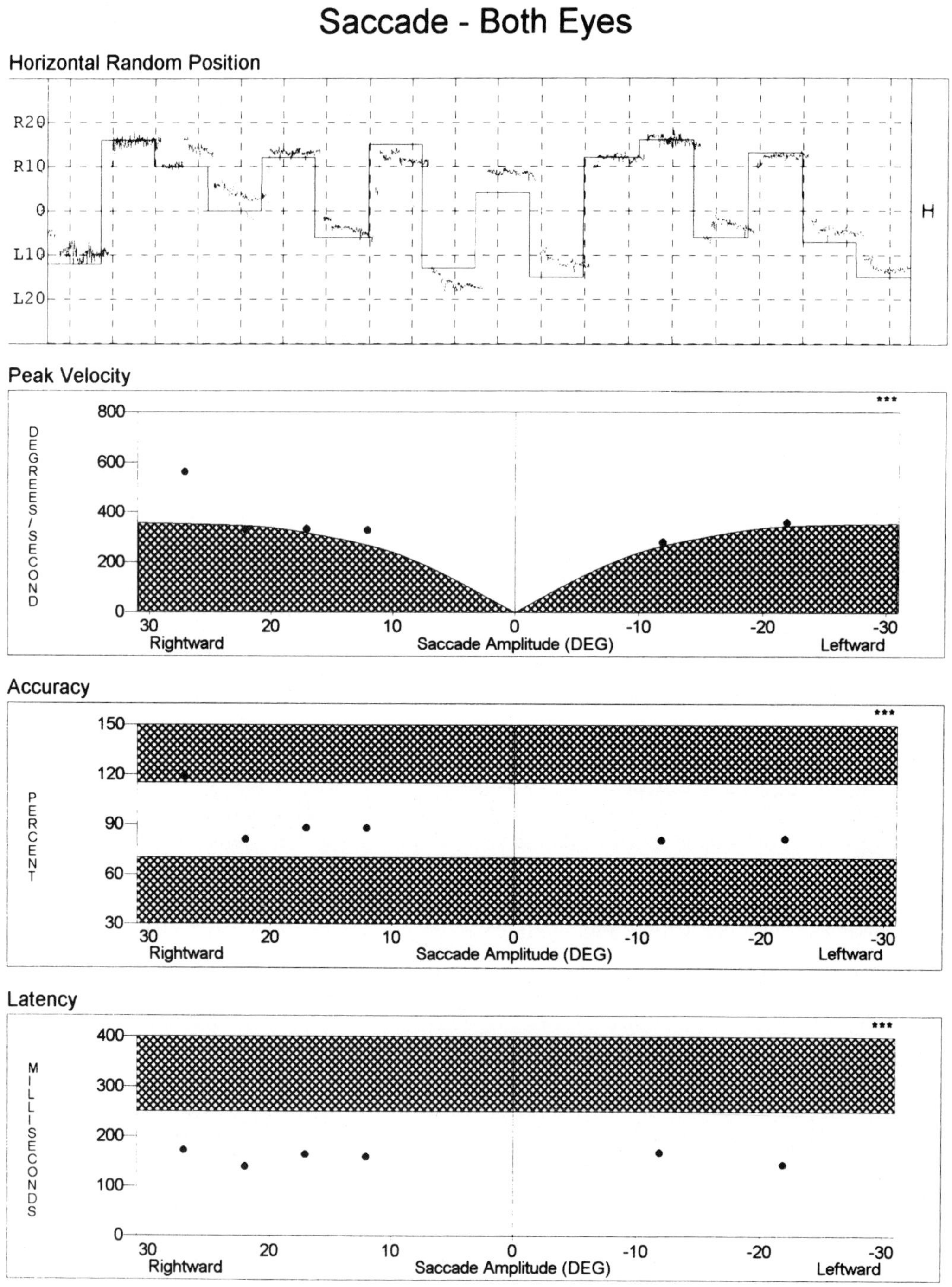

Saccade - Both Eyes

Horizontal Random Position

Peak Velocity

Accuracy

Latency

B

FIG. 1. *Continued.*

1952 (14,15). Dix and Hallpike provided histologic correlation to the inner ear in a patient with BPPV. Their report of 100 cases provided the impetus for common recognition of the disorder (16). Schuknecht found basophilic deposits on the cupula of the posterior semicircular canals of patients with BPPV, and he coined the term *cupulolithiasis* to describe the condition (17). Schuknecht presented evidence to support his theory that inner ear debris, perhaps from the otoconia of a degener-

ating utricular macula, settles in the posterior semicircular canal and displaces the cupula in the head-hanging lateral position. Evidence suggests that most patients with BPPV have free-floating particles in the endolymph of the posterior semicircular canal (canalithiasis) of the affected side that are mobilized by the force of quick head displacement (18).

The Dix-Hallpike maneuver is designed to stimulate the posterior semicircular canal on one side, thus it needs

Tracking - Both Eyes

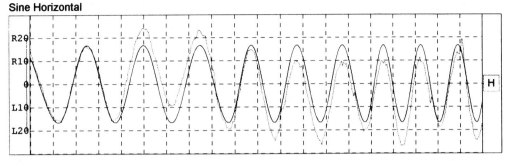

Sine Horizontal

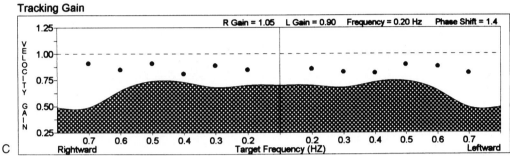

Tracking Gain

R Gain = 1.05   L Gain = 0.90   Frequency = 0.20 Hz   Phase Shift = 1.4

C

Caloric Weakness: 4% in the left ear
Directional Preponderance: 6% to the left

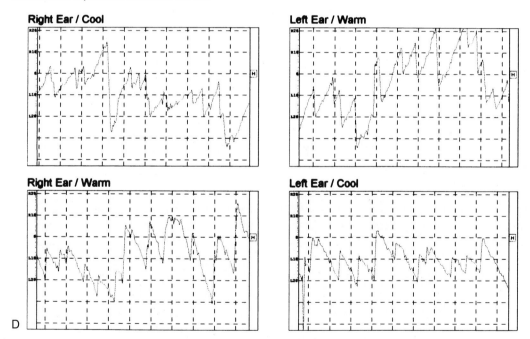

Right Ear / Cool   Left Ear / Warm

Right Ear / Warm   Left Ear / Cool

D

FIG. 1. *Continued.*

to be performed twice (once for each side). The maneuver involves quick movement from the sitting to reclining position with the head hanging slightly. The patient's head is first turned 45 degrees toward one side (the side being tested) and the patient is instructed to fall backward quickly. The examiner holds the patient's head, keeps it turned and hanging for at least 20 seconds, and monitors the eyes for nystagmus (use of Frenzel glasses is recommended, but the nystagmus response usually is strong and is not suppressed by fixation). The nystagmus usually intensifies to a crescendo and then dies away completely. The patient is returned to the sitting position with the head still turned, and the eyes are assessed for nystagmus, which now occurs in the opposite direction.

When the Dix-Hallpike maneuver induces nystagmus with the following six characteristics it is pathognomonic for posterior canal BPPV: (a) It has a latency, that is, onset is delayed by a few seconds. (b) It is paroxysmal, appearing for several seconds and disappearing completely. (c) It is accompanied by vertigo, which is usually intense and parallels the intensity of the nystagmus as it wanes. (d) It is geotropic rotatory, or beating toward the floor, or bottom ear. (Nystagmus may appear disconjugate depending on the eye position or gaze. When the gaze is away from the affected side, the nystagmus in the top eye is vertical, that is, toward the forehead.) (e) Its direction reverses when the person sits up. (f) It is usually fatigable (repeated maneuvers cause a decreasing response). When the nystagmus does not have these characteristics, the underlying disorder is not typical posterior canal BPPV, and the likelihood of a variant BPPV or central vestibular disorder increases. A possible exception is positioning nystagmus that lasts longer than 1 minute, which can be explained by cupulolithiasis, in which the cupula remains deflected as long as the position is held. Positioning nystagmus that lasts longer than 1 minute, nystagmus that does not fatigue with repeated positioning, actively beating positional nystagmus not associated with vertigo, ageotropic rotary nystagmus (beating toward the ceiling or the top ear), and conjugate vertical positioning nystagmus (down-beat or up-beat nystagmus) are signs of CNS disease (11,12). Typically, though, investigation for CNS disease infrequently yields positive findings, suggesting that some of these patients may have a type of peripheral vestibular disorder that has not yet been characterized.

In 1985, McClure (19) described a variant of BPPV that affects the horizontal or lateral semicircular canal. In this condition, which has been called horizontal canal BPPV, the positioning maneuver (done the same way as for posterior canal BPPV) results in horizontal nystagmus (as opposed to a rotary nystagmus) that displays some of the characteristics as that of posterior canal BPPV (paroxysmal, accompanied by vertigo). The nystagmus may be *geotropic* (toward the involved ear, which is on the bottom) or *ageotropic* (away from the involved ear) and may not fatigue with repeated positioning (20). The nystagmus also is elicited with positioning maneuvers other than the Dix-Hallpike, such as quick rotation of the head from facing the ceiling to facing the wall while supine.

Positional Tests

The purpose of positional testing is to determine whether different head positions, not head movements, induce or modify vestibular nystagmus. Nystagmus induced by positional testing is called *positional nystagmus* or *static positional nystagmus* to differentiate it from *paroxysmal* or *positioning nystagmus,* which is associated

with the Dix-Hallpike maneuver. Positional testing is performed by monitoring the eyes for nystagmus in at least four head positions: sitting, supine, right lateral, and left lateral. If nystagmus is seen or modified in either lateral head position, the patient is positioned in the lateral decubitus position on that side to evaluate the effect of neck rotation. If the nystagmus disappears, it was caused at least partly by neck rotation. This rarely occurs. The assumption with the positional test is that the nystagmus generated is caused by the orientation of the head with respect to gravity and not by head movement. Thus the patient's head is slowly moved into position rather than moved quickly, as in the Dix-Hallpike maneuver. Each head position is held for 20 seconds with eyes open and 20 seconds with eyes closed. It is more reliable to interpret the eyes-open test by preventing visual fixation with Frenzel glasses or performing it in the dark (21).

Positional nystagmus may be intermittent or persistent, unlike positioning nystagmus, which disappears if the head is still. Persistent positional nystagmus is sustained as long as the head position is held and may reflect the effect of changing otolithic influence. As with positioning nystagmus, the terms *geotropic* and *ageotropic* may be used to describe the direction of the nystagmus. The nystagmus may be *direction fixed* (beating in the same direction in different head positions) or *direction changing* (beating in a different direction in different head positions). Both of these types of nystagmus occur most commonly with peripheral vestibular disorders, but they may occur with central lesions. Peripheral vestibular nystagmus usually stops with visual fixation. Positional nystagmus has little localizing value but is a valuable indicator of vestibular system dysfunction. Other signs and clinical data must be used to localize the lesion. The most common abnormality seen with the positional test is spontaneous nystagmus. When persistent nystagmus is found, it is important to observe it for at least 2 minutes because certain types of direction-changing nystagmus reverse direction every 2 minutes (acquired periodic alternating nystagmus). This type of nystagmus usually is caused by a CNS lesion, but vestibular stimulation can reset the oscillation (22).

Evaluation of Vestibular-Oculomotor Function

Bithermal Caloric Test

The caloric test is the most difficult, the most time-consuming, and the most important test in the ENG test battery. No other test has proved as useful in lateralizing a vestibular lesion or identifying disorders of the labyrinth and vestibular nerve. It is an invaluable aid in the diagnosis of peripheral vestibular disorders, such as Meniere's disease, vestibular neuronitis, labyrinthitis, and ototoxicity. It is the only test that allows stimulation of each ear separately.

The theory of caloric stimulation was proposed by Robert Barany, who received the Nobel Prize for medicine in 1914 for his work on the vestibular system. Barany proposed that caloric irrigation induces endolymphatic flow in the lateral semicircular canal by producing a temperature gradient from one side of the canal to the other. The temperature change alters the density of endolymph on the lateral aspect of the canal (closest to the temperature source). Gravity causes the fluid to move, deflect the cupula, and stimulate or inhibit the vestibular nerve and the afferent pathway. Cold stimuli produce ampullofugal (away from the cupula) deviation, and warm stimuli cause in ampullopetal deviation. We now know that this theory is incomplete because caloric responses are seen (though diminished) in monkeys even after occlusion of the horizontal semicircular canal and in humans tested in microgravity (outer space) (23,24). Thus the mechanism of caloric stimulation probably involves endolymphatic convection and a direct effect of temperature change on the discharge rate of the superior vestibular nerve (cold temperature depresses the firing rate, and warm temperature elevates the firing rate).

A variety of caloric stimuli have been based predominantly on changes in the temperature and duration of the stimulus (water or air) applied to the eardrum (25). The current standard caloric test evolved from the bithermal caloric test introduced by Fitzgerald and Hallpike in 1942 (26). The primary reasons for using it are as follows (a) the labyrinth is tested serially (excited when warmed, inhibited when cooled); (b) each ear is tested separately; (c) the caloric stimulus is highly reproducible from one side to the other in almost all patients; and (d) the test is usually well tolerated.

The bithermal caloric test is performed with the patient supine with the head flexed 30 degrees so that the horizontal canal is in the vertical plane. Four irrigations are performed separately (two for each ear) with at least 5 minutes rest between irrigations to avoid additive effects. The temperatures of the standard caloric stimuli are equally above and below body temperature. Irrigation is done with 250 mL of water over 30 seconds at 30°C for the cool irrigation and at 44°C for the warm irrigation. Water caloric testing may be performed by means of direct irrigation, wetting the ear canal and eardrum, or a closed-loop system (usually a small latex balloon) through which the water circulates but does not wet the ear. Closed-loop and air irrigation systems are used to examine patients with perforated eardrums. Use of closed-loop systems carries risk for perforation of the eardrum if the balloon suddenly ruptures during irrigation. Air irrigation is performed with 8 L of air over 60 seconds at 24°C for the warm irrigation and 50°C for the cool irrigation. With these values water and air produce equivalent stimuli that can be reproduced reliably (27). Warm air irrigation sometimes can produce paradoxic cooling in the ear by means of evaporation when tympanic membrane perforation is present and the ear is wet. In such a situation the direction of the nystagmus produced is opposite that expected. The intensity of the stimulus increases when the eardrum is perforated or the ear has been surgically altered (canal-wall-down mastoidectomy); comparison of sides may not be possible when the anatomic features are markedly different.

If the nystagmus response is weak or absent, additional irrigation with ice water is warranted. The standard test consists of placing 2 mL of ice water in the ear canal for 30 seconds and dumping it out. The patient is immediately placed supine; nystagmus is recorded for 2 minutes. Ice water irrigation should be repeated in the prone position if a response is not obtained when the patient is supine, the reading is in doubt, or spontaneous nystagmus exists. When a cold stimulus is applied to the ear in the prone position, endolymph flow is ampullopetal (toward the ampulla), and according to Ewald's law, ampullopetal deviation of the cupula of the lateral semicircular canal evokes a stronger response than ampullofugal deviation (cold stimulus in the supine position). In cases of bilateral weakness, six or more caloric irrigations may be needed to obtain meaningful information.

The magnitude of the caloric response is highly dependent on the patient's level of mental alertness and on the degree of visual fixation allowed during the test. Low mental alertness results in a weak or poor response; therefore patients are always given enhancement tasks during the postirrigation phase, such as counting backward, multiplication, or naming lists. Visual fixation may be controlled in three ways: (a) eyes open and fixating, (b) eyes open but denied fixation (Frenzel glasses or total darkness), or (c) eyes closed. When fixation is allowed (eyes open), the VOR and the pursuit system interact, and the VOR is affected by fixation (3). Caloric testing is often conducted with eyes closed, but the least variation in response is found when patients are tested with eyes open and denied fixation with either Frenzel glasses or total darkness. Eye closure causes slight upward deviation of the eyes (Bell's phenomenon), which can lead to suppression of nystagmus (28).

The most commonly seen abnormal finding in caloric testing is unilateral weakness. Because the caloric stimulus delivered to each ear is the same, the assumption is that if the ears are normal, the responses should be about equal. Unilateral weakness is determined by using the Jongkees formula to compare the response strengths of the two sides (29):

$$\frac{(RW + RC) - (LW + LC)}{RW + RC + LW + LC} \times 100 = \%UW$$

where RW, RC, LW, and LC represent the peak SPV of the nystagmus response to right warm, right cool, left warm, and left cool irrigations, and UW is unilateral weakness. The accepted normal limits should be determined by each testing laboratory (3,27,29–35) (H. O. Barber, G. Wright,

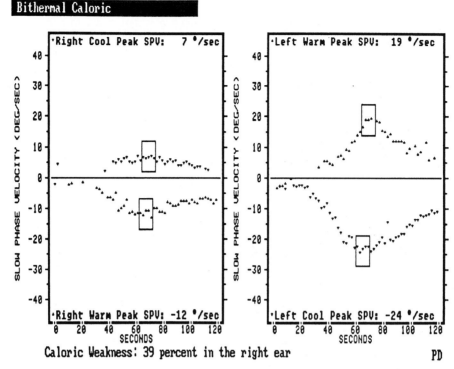

FIG. 2. Computerized electronystagmogram shows unilateral weakness.

unpublished data, 1979). If a UW value greater than the upper limit of normal is found, unilateral weakness is said to exist. This finding almost always signifies the presence of a peripheral vestibular lesion, but some central lesions affecting the vestibular nuclei may display unilateral weakness. Figure 2 shows a computerized ENG result showing unilateral weakness. Clinical history and examination findings, audiometric findings, and auditory brainstem response test results are integrated to further characterize the lesion and establish a diagnosis.

Sometimes, as in the case of an acute peripheral vestibular lesion, a patient has spontaneous nystagmus and unilateral weakness. The spontaneous nystagmus creates a new baseline for the caloric test equal to the SPV (including the direction) of the nystagmus. In such cases, it would be difficult to differentiate the effect of the spontaneous nystagmus from unilateral weakness on the basis of peak SPV if only one irrigation per ear were used in the caloric test. When two irrigations, warm and cool, are used, responses occur in opposite directions. When the sum of each peak response is used to characterize the degree of integrity of each ear, the effect of the spontaneous nystagmus is canceled and a valid interaural comparison is possible (11).

Bilateral vestibular weakness usually is defined as the sum of peak caloric responses (warm plus cool) of each ear that fall below 10°C/s, because the range of each caloric response can be as low as 5°C/s and still be within the 95% confidence interval for healthy persons (36).

This finding is most commonly seen with peripheral disorders such as ototoxicity and bilateral Meniere's disease (37). CNS disease also may produce bilateral vestibular weakness but is usually accompanied by other neurologic symptoms (11).

Head-shake Test

Some laboratories include a short head-shake test as part of the ENG battery when spontaneous nystagmus is not present. The test is performed with the patient in the seated position. The patient's head is rapidly rotated the in the horizontal (yaw) plane, as if signing "no". The rotation must be performed at approximately 1 Hz or faster for 20 to 30 cycles and abruptly stopped. The patient may shake his or her own head as directed (autorotation) or may be assisted by the examiner, who grasps the head firmly and rotates it side to side. Patients with peripheral vestibular dysfunction display a few beats of nystagmus, usually away from the affected side (38). Visual fixation is prevented with Frenzel lenses or darkness.

Evaluation of Visual-Oculomotor Function

Saccade Test

The saccade test is used to calibrate the ENG recording system and to look for defects of the saccadic eye system. The purpose of the saccadic system is to rapidly capture onto the fovea interesting visual targets in the periphery of the visual field. This action produces a quick eye movement, known as a *saccade,* and is the fastest type of eye movement, sometimes with peak velocities as high as 700 degrees/s. Saccades may be involuntary or voluntary. The fast phase of nystagmus and rapid eye movements that occur during sleep are examples of involuntary saccades. Normal voluntary saccadic eye movements are highly accurate in locking in on a target. Overshooting the target is rare for healthy persons, but undershooting by a small amount is frequent (10% of the amplitude of the saccade for unpredictable visual targets). Once the target is acquired, fixation is readily held (no postsaccadic drift or glissade) (12).

The saccade test may be performed with three dots placed on a wall parallel to the floor, spaced apart at a known distance requiring a 20-degree angle of visual excursion for the patient between the farthest dots. With computerized testing, target dots are generated on a screen or light bar in front of the patient and are moved through a computer-controlled series of jumps back and forth in an unpredictable sequence. The entire sequence may consist of 80 target jumps (40 to the right and 40 to the left) with varying amplitudes. The computer analyzes the eye movement recordings, calculates three values of interest for each saccade (peak velocity, accuracy, and latency), and plots these data graphically against standardized normative values.

Disorders of the saccadic system generally are categorized according to the three values of interest; thus there are disorders of velocity, accuracy, or latency. Abnormally slow saccades are seen with many degenerative and metabolic diseases of the CNS, including internuclear ophthalmoplegia, disturbances in the cerebral hemispheres, superior colliculus, or oculomotor neurons and disorders of the extraocular muscles, drug intoxication, drowsiness, or inattentiveness. Abnormally fast-appearing saccades may occur with orbital tumors and myasthenia gravis. Inaccurate saccades, or dysmetria, are classified as hypermetria (overshooting the target) or hypometria (undershooting). Saccadic hypermetria is the hallmark of cerebellar disease but also may be caused by brainstem lesions (12). Saccadic hypometria also occurs with various cerebellar and brainstem disorders. Disorders of saccadic latency, or initiation, occur with abnormal vision, Parkinson's disease, Huntington's disease, Alzheimer's disease, and focal hemispheric lesions. A thorough review of saccadic abnormalities has been made by Leigh and Zee (12).

Pursuit Tests (Tracking and Optokinetic)

Although saccadic eye movements capture an image of interest in the fovea, maintaining that image on a moving target requires pursuit function. The smooth-pursuit system generates smooth tracking movements of the eyes that closely match the speed of the target. This system is used to track targets at slower speeds and operates when the eyes move within the orbit and the head is still. At faster speeds and when the head moves, the VOR is brought into play. The pursuit eye function tests performed in the ENG examination are the smooth-pursuit or tracking test and the optokinetic test.

The neural pathways that serve the pursuit system are distributed in different areas of the brain. Smooth-pursuit function involves the fovea and several cortical and subcortical pathways. Optokinetic function is phylogenetically older and has been demonstrated in animals without well-developed fovea, unlike the smooth-pursuit system. The optokinetic pathways, for the most part, are subcortical, involving the accessory optic system. In humans there is an overlap of functions by neurons in the cortical and subcortical visual systems (3). The smooth-pursuit system dominates the operation of the overall pursuit system (5).

Although a tracking test can be performed with a pendulum swinging back and forth to produce a sinusoidally moving target, varying the velocity of the target to predetermined frequencies is difficult. This may be overcome with a computer-controlled light bar that provides precise control of a moving target over a series of velocities. The patient follows a lighted dot that moves back and forth in the horizontal plane in a sinusoidal waveform at frequencies from 0.2 to 0.8 Hz. The computer analyzes eye velocity with respect to target velocity in each direction and calculates the gain for each frequency in each direction while pursuit software analyzes the spectral purity of the sine wave generated by the eye movement. These data are plotted graphically against standardized normative values.

Patients with impaired smooth pursuit require frequent corrective saccades to keep up with the target; this produces a cogwheel pattern when plotted graphically, or saccadic pursuit. Abnormal smooth-pursuit function is of limited localizing value because it may occur with disorders throughout the CNS. Smooth-pursuit is especially impaired in the presence of cerebellar lesions; the result is failure of fixation suppression of vestibular responses such as the caloric response (39). Acute peripheral vestibular lesions may impair smooth pursuit contralateral to the affected side when the eyes are moving against the slow phase of spontaneous nystagmus. Inattentive or tired patients may display some saccades. Healthy elderly subjects show marked variability in tracking ability, therefore their pursuit testing results must be interpreted with caution (21).

The optokinetic test is a variation of the tracking test. The target consists of a moving, large-patterned surface, such as projected stripes, a striped drum, or projected dots randomly placed on a sphere or an electronic facsimile (electronically controlled light bar). The tracking motion of the eye is interrupted by short, quick opposite saccades that generate a characteristic pattern of nystagmus. Subjects follow a series of dots in one direction (the slow phase) and return with a quick eye movement (the fast phase) to the starting point. The head is kept still, and function is tested in both directions. As with tracking of pursuit movements, the velocity of the eye should match the velocity of the target. Abnormalities of the optokinetic slow phase generally mimic abnormalities of smooth pursuit, and abnormalities of the optokinetic fast phase correlate with abnormalities of voluntary saccades. Symmetrically decreased slow-phase velocity is caused by diffuse disease of the cortex, diencephalon, brainstem, and cerebellum (3). Impaired optokinetic nystagmus is seen in focal lateralized disease of the parietal occipital region, brainstem, and cerebellum when the target moves toward the damaged side.

Clinical Application

ENG testing has stood the test of time and has proved to be clinically invaluable in the evaluation of patients with dizziness (3,11). The battery of tests provides site-of-lesion information about peripheral vestibular lesions and objective data that support diagnoses of BPPV, vestibular neuronitis, Meniere's disease, labyrinthitis, ototoxicity, otosyphilis, and autoimmune inner ear disease. ENG testing is not used to diagnose acoustic neuroma, but ENG plays a role in evaluating some patients for degree of vestibular impairment before surgical treatment and in predicting to some extent the likelihood of vertigo and balance problems. If the response to caloric irrigation is normal, sacrifice of the superior vestibular nerve will likely produce intense nystagmus and vertigo. If the caloric response is diminished or absent, tumor removal will probably produce a minimal effect on balance.

Abnormalities in any of the components of the ENG test battery when the caloric and head-shake tests and the Hallpike maneuver are normal usually indicate a CNS disorder. CNS disorders often are test specific. Examples are internuclear ophthalmoplegia, which localizes a lesion to the medial longitudinal fasciculus in the brainstem between the third and sixth cranial nerve nuclei, and failure of fixation suppression, which is evidence of a cerebellar (floccular) lesion.

ROTATION TESTS

Rotation tests have been in use longer than any other and are based on use of head acceleration to stimulate the semicircular canals. Angular acceleration is delivered most efficiently and economically by means of rotation, which may be passive or active. Passive rotation involves whole-body rotation (as in a rotary chair). In active rotation the patient rotates his or her own head while the body remains still. In either test, rotation occurs around the vertical axis through the center of the body. Like ENG testing, rotary testing elicits the horizontal semicircular

canal ocular reflex because it is the easiest to stimulate and record. Unlike ENG testing, a rotational stimulus is independent of the physical features of the external auditory canal or temporal bone, so a more precise and physiologic stimulus and response are possible. In addition, multiple stepped stimuli can be delivered relatively quickly, and testing is well tolerated. However, because rotational stimuli affect both labyrinths simultaneously, identifying the diseased side is not always possible.

Rotary Chair Testing

Historically, three types of passive rotation stimuli have been used clinically: impulsive, constant, and sinusoidal oscillations. Barany (40) in 1907 used an impulsive rotation test in which the chair and patient were manually rotated 10 turns in 20 seconds and suddenly stopped. Response was measured on the basis of duration of visually monitored nystagmus after clockwise and counterclockwise rotation. Van Egmond et al. (41) modified this test by accelerating patients to different velocities and suddenly stopping the chair. They also used duration of nystagmus as a response measure and generated a "cupulogram" by plotting nystagmus duration versus the log of stimulus magnitude.

As ENG techniques became available for recording nystagmus, constant and sinusoidal rotation tests became popular. Montandon (42) introduced a constant acceleration test in which the patient was slowly brought to a constant angular velocity, and after a period of constant speed (3 minutes), the chair was slowly stopped. The nystagmus threshold (the rate of acceleration and deceleration at which nystagmus was first seen) was used as the response measure for a series of different constant accelerations. Threshold measurements, however, are not a pure reflection of the vestibular signal (3).

Early sinusoidal oscillation tests were called *torsion swing tests,* and they were popularized in France. In the torsion swing test a chair fitted with a spring was used to produce oscillations. Because the stimulus intensity depended on the weight of the patient and mass distribution, the stimulus intensity varied from patient to patient. The modern era of rotation testing began in the 1960s when methods became available for generating precise, repeatable rotational stimuli (motorized rotary chair) and for quantitative measurement of eye movements.

Method

Rotary chair testing is controlled and analyzed by computer. The patient sits on a servo-controlled, motorized chair that is enclosed in a light-proof circular booth. Patients keep their eyes open in total darkness. Patients are constantly asked questions to maintain mental alertness. Both impulsive and sinusoidal oscillation tests are performed.

In the typical *impulsive test,* the chair is rotated in a series of velocity steps to the right and to the left, each with an angular acceleration of 100 degrees/s for 1 second. The response measure, as in caloric testing, is the maximum SPV of the nystagmus. Three parameters are used to measure the nystagmus response: gain, time constant, and symmetry. *Gain* is the ratio of eye velocity (maximum SPV) to head (chair) velocity. *Time constant* is the time it takes, in seconds, for the response to decline to 37% of its peak value. *Symmetry* is the ratio of maximum SPV of the nystagmus to rightward and leftward steps.

In the *sinusoidal oscillation test,* the chair is rotated in a series of oscillations at frequencies from 0.01 Hz to 0.64 Hz at octave intervals (0.01, 0.02, 0.04, and so on) with peak angular chair velocities of 50 degrees/s at each frequency. Three parameters are used to measure the nystagmus response: gain, phase, and symmetry. *Gain* is the ratio of eye velocity (maximum SPV) to head (chair) velocity. *Phase* is a comparison of the time of the maximum head (chair) velocity to the time of maximum eye SPV. Among healthy subjects, the maximum eye SPV leads the maximum head (chair) velocity at low frequencies of sinusoidal rotation (phase lead). *Symmetry* is the ratio of maximum SPV of the nystagmus to rightward and leftward stimuli at each frequency. Figure 3 shows a report of a computerized rotary chair test for a healthy person.

Clinical Application

Unilateral Vestibular Loss

Although rotary chair testing is less able to localize vestibular disease than ENG testing, it is important because it provides a precise stimulus that can be administered quickly and at several grades of intensity.

In many instances, rotary chair testing can give more information about the vestibular system than can caloric testing. Patients who undergo the test soon after experiencing a sudden, unilateral loss of vestibular function show asymmetry on the impulsive tests; on the sinusoidal oscillation test they show abnormal phase leads and reduced gain at the lower test frequencies and asymmetry at the higher test frequencies (43–45). The asymmetry usually is toward the side of the peripheral vestibular lesion. It is believed to be partly caused by the following: (a) a dc bias resulting from spontaneous nystagmus and (b) the difference in response to ampullopetal and ampullofugal stimulation of the remaining intact labyrinth (46). Figures 4 and 5 demonstrate the results of testing of a patient with an acute right unilateral vestibular lesion and a patient with a chronic left vestibular lesion.

Patients with recent unilateral vestibular lesions show abnormal (decreased) function at the lower frequencies of sinusoidal oscillation testing. It is not surprising that such patients also show unilateral weakness at caloric testing, which is a lower-frequency stimulus than the lowest frequency tested with oscillation rotation tests. More severe vestibular insults, such as bilateral vestibular loss, also cause abnormal function at higher frequencies of sinusoidal oscillation testing (47).

Bilateral Vestibular Loss

The most important application of rotary chair testing is in evaluation of patients with bilateral vestibular loss. Patients who show artifactually decreased responses to caloric irrigation because of variant temporal bone anatomy (narrow or curved ear canal) show normal nystagmus responses to rotation testing. Patients with bilateral vestibular loss at caloric testing frequently show

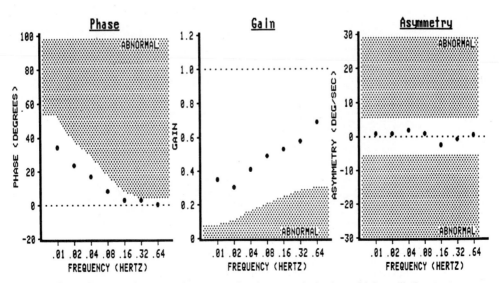

FIG. 3. Report of a normal computerized rotary chair sinusoidal oscillation test.

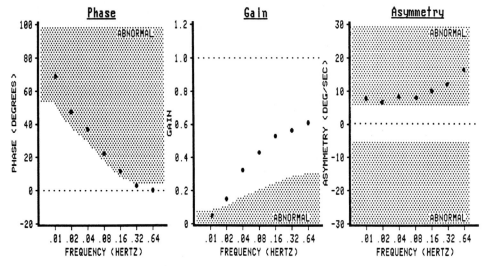

FIG. 4. Report of computerized rotary chair sinusoidal oscillation test of a patient with an acute right unilateral peripheral vestibular lesion.

deficits at lower frequencies and preserved function at the higher frequencies on sinusoidal oscillation testing (47) (Fig. 6). Absence of caloric response, even to ice water stimulation, does not mean complete loss of vestibular function. High-frequency sinusoidal oscillation testing, however, is not a sensitive measure of vestibular deficit. Patients with bilateral peripheral vestibular loss show a similar, but more pronounced, pattern of low-frequency gain and phase abnormalities at sinusoidal oscillation testing as patients with compensated unilateral peripheral vestibular weakness (48).

Compensation

Compensation is the neurophysiologic process by which the brain adapts to normalize balance function

after a peripheral vestibular insult. After compensation occurs, acute spontaneous nystagmus subsides, and gain asymmetry on rotary chair testing decreases but never entirely disappears. Phase asymmetry also decreases but never fully disappears (43).

Central Nervous System Lesions

Central vestibular lesions, like peripheral lesions, can show decreased gain or gain asymmetry at rotary chair testing. Lesions that involve the nerve root or vestibular nucleus may produce responses identical to those of a peripheral vestibular lesion. The variety of abnormal responses is greater with central vestibular lesions; nystagmus can appear disorganized or distorted in certain

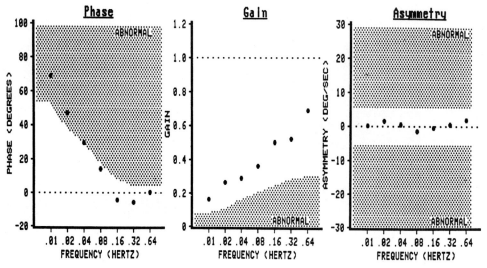

FIG. 5. Report of computerized rotary chair sinusoidal oscillation test of a patient with a chronic left unilateral peripheral lesion.

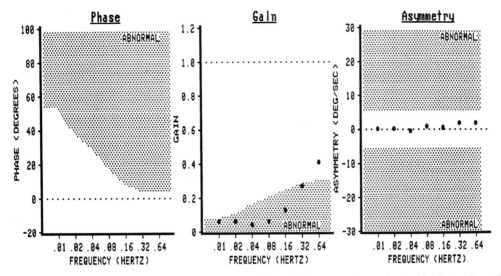

FIG. 6. Report of computerized rotary chair sinusoidal oscillation test of a patient with bilateral vestibular weakness.

conditions. Gain values may even be increased among some patients with cerebellar lesions (3).

Altered Temporal Bone Anatomy

Other uses of rotation testing are in evaluations of patients with a surgically altered temporal bone, such as after canal-wall-down mastoidectomy, and patients with a draining ear or congenital aural atresia. Caloric testing often is meaningless or contraindicated in such cases, but rotary chair testing can sometimes provide useful information about the vestibular system when chronic middle ear infection and inner ear disease coexist.

Head-shake Testing

Because passive rotation testing (rotary chair) requires expensive equipment and does not evaluate vestibular responses to quick head motions such as those encountered in daily activities, active rotation testing has been introduced into vestibular function testing. There are two types of active rotation testing—the head-shake test and the vestibular autorotation test. Both involve the patient's shaking his or her head back and forth with the ears level to each other and parallel to the ground.

The head-shake test entails a period of head shaking as the vestibular stimulus, and the nystagmus response is measured after the rotation is stopped. Although this is considered an active rotation test, it may be done passively; the examiner can shake the subject's head to ensure maintenance of a fast rotation frequency. Head shaking is done at a frequency of at least 1 Hz and for at least 20 cycles. The motion is abruptly stopped, and nystagmus is assessed either visually or with ENG monitoring (38,49,50). This test may be performed as part of an office examination after evaluation for spontaneous nystagmus or as part of ENG testing. Nystagmus usually beats away from the diseased ear.

The vestibular autorotation test also uses a head-shake stimulus, but rather than waiting to monitor nystagmus (as in the head-shake test), the examiner records eye movements during active head rotation. The patient wears a headband with a velocity sensor attached to it to monitor head motion with ENG. Thus head motion and eye motion are quantified. With these measurements, values for gain, phase, and symmetry can be calculated (51,52). Additional refinements include head shaking at the rhythm of a metronome to control the frequencies of head rotation and a vertical head-shake test. The clinical utility of vertical head-shake testing awaits further elucidation.

POSTUROGRAPHY

Postural sway has been recognized for many years as an important clinical indicator of balance function. It is used to measure changes in body position under conditions that challenge postural control mechanisms by interfering with somatosensory and visual feedback functions. It is used specifically to explore a subject's ability to maintain and regain balance under various sensory input situations.

Computerized dynamic platform posturography (CDDP) is based on a computerized testing device (Equitest) that consists of a force plate capable of rotating in the pitch plane about an axis collinear with the patient's ankles. The patient stands on the force plate capable of rotating about the same axis and faces a scene that subtends the patient's entire field of view. The device incorporates shifting, tilting, or perturbing the support surface or other methods of challenging the patient with unexpected movements. There also is a degree of isolation of visual and somatosensory contributions to balance so that these influences can be analyzed separately from vestibular influences. As the patient sways back and forth, the force plate measures the changes in the position of the body's center of pressure. These data are transferred to a computer, which calculates the angle of body sway in the pitch plane. Three tests can be performed with the Equitest device: sensory organization, movement coordination, and pressure.

Nashner (52a) analyzed postural control in the pitch plane with the patient standing on a firm surface in a lighted room. He showed that during quiet standing, either visual or proprioceptive cues are sufficient for maintaining postural stability and that the vestibular system is only secondary in this setting. To detect a vestibular deficit, the patient must be made to rely solely on vestibular cues, and the visual and proprioceptive systems must be excluded. The sensory organization test is based on this rationale (53). All the possible outcomes of the sensory organization test have not been specified, but it is clear that at least four types of abnormality exist: vestibular deficit, vestibular and visual deficit, vestibular and proprioceptive deficit, and severe vestibular deficit.

Sensory Organization Test

The sensory organization test places the patient in six different test conditions. Under conditions 1, 2, and 3 the supporting surface is fixed so the patient has correct proprioceptive cues, and visual cues are varied. Under conditions 4 through 6, the supporting service is rotated in proportion to the angle of the body sway, and the visual cues are varied as before. The six conditions are as follows:

Condition 1: Visual field is fixed so that visual cues are correct.
Condition 2: The patient closes the eyes to deny visual cues.
Condition 3: The visual scene is rotated in proportion to the angle of body sway (sway referenced) so that visual and proprioceptive cues are in conflict; the proprioceptive cues are erroneous, indicating that the subject is motionless.
Condition 4: The visual scene is fixed so that the visual and proprioceptive cues are again in conflict; the visual cues are correct, and the proprioceptive cues are erroneous, indicating that the subject is motionless.
Condition 5: The patient closes the eyes so that visual cues are denied and proprioceptive cues are erroneous, indicating that the subjective is motionless. Under this condition the only correct cue regarding the direction of gravity comes from the vestibular system.
Condition 6: The visual scene is rotated in proportion to the angle of body sway so that both visual and propri-

oceptive cues indicate that the patient is motionless. The only correct cue regarding the direction of gravity comes from the vestibular system.

The test is performed in three 20-second trials under each condition. Body sway data are used to calculate a performance index, which is measured on the basis of the peak-to-peak body sway that would be possible without actually falling.

Motor Coordination Test

In the motor coordination test the patient undergoes a series of translations of the supporting surface in the backward direction followed by a series of toes up rotations about an axis collinear with the ankle joints. This series is succeeded by an identical series of translations in the backward direction followed by a series of toes down rotations. Body sway responses are monitored with the force plate. The computer uses these data to calculate various response entities, including response latency, amplitude, and left or right symmetry. The ability of a patient to adapt to support surface rotation followed by repeated exposure to support surface translations (forward, backward or side to side) is calculated. The motor coordination test is intended primarily to evaluate disorders of movement coordination caused by head injury and metabolic and degenerative disorders of the brain and neuromuscular system. This test rarely yields abnormalities among patients with a primary symptom of vertigo or dizziness.

Pressure Test

The patient's eye movements during body sway are monitored while pressure changes are induced in the external ear canal. ENG is used to monitor eye movements with the eyes closed. With an impedance bridge, pressure in the external ear canal of the ear believed to be abnormal is increased rapidly to positive 200 mm of water and maintained at this level for 14 to 20 seconds, decreased rapidly to negative 400 mm of water and maintained at this level for 15 to 20 seconds, and finally atmospheric pressure is restored. The sequence is repeated several times. When the pressure test provokes nystagmus, the direction of nystagmus may be either toward or away from the involved ear, and there are generally both positive and negative pressure changes. Nystagmus and vertigo usually persist for as long as the pressure change is held. Symptoms induced with this test may persist for several minutes.

When body sway is recorded, the patient is asked to stand with eyes closed on the posturography platform with support surface sway reference, thus denying both visual and proprioceptive cues. With a computer-controlled impedance bridge, the pressure in the external ear canal of the ear believed to be abnormal is rapidly increased to positive 300 mm of water and returned to atmospheric pressure. Ten trials are performed. Body sway in both the anterior-posterior and lateral directions is monitored during each trial, and the computer calculates average body sway over the ten trials. This ten-trial sequence is repeated with pressure, decreased to negative 300 mm of water. Among healthy persons the procedure does not produce body sways that are time locked to the pressure changes. Among patients with disorders such as perilymphatic fistula, active Meniere's disease, or syphilis with inner ear disease the procedure does produce time-locked body sways.

Clinical Significance

CDDP fulfills most criteria for a reliable and valid test of postural stability (54,55) and has gained acceptance in some specific situations. It has been shown to enable differentiation between subjects with normal and abnormal vestibular function compared with the clinical standard of reference (56,57). Recovery of postural control after a unilateral vestibular lesion has been measured with CDDP (53,58), and it has been reported to be useful in assessing the progress of vestibular rehabilitation (59–62). Additional clinical and experimental work is needed to clearly establish the clinical significance of CDDP. Such an understanding is complex because vestibulospinal disorders are characterized mainly by subjective sensations difficult to measure with any testing modality.

SUMMARY POINTS

- Vestibular tests are used to confirm a clinical diagnosis formulated after a thorough history and physical examination.
- ENG testing remains the most useful tool for assessing abnormalities of the vestibular system. Caloric testing documents the site of a lesion; bithermal stimulation is important in the evaluation of spontaneous nystagmus.
- Visual oculomotor function is explored with the saccade and pursuit tests. Pursuit tests include the tracking and optokinetic tests. Impaired tracking ability produces a cogwheel pattern.
- Rotary chair testing can be useful in evaluating the entire spectrum of vestibular function. It provides a wider range of stimuli and a more physiologic stimulus than caloric testing.
- Low-frequency sinusoidal rotation is a sensitive indicator of vestibular disease. It is especially useful in evaluating patients with bilateral vestibular loss and those with abnormal temporal bone anatomy.

- Rotational tests do not reliably indicate the side of a lesion and do not help to differentiate between peripheral and central vestibular lesions. The results are best interpreted with findings of other vestibular function tests, such as ENG.
- Active rotation testing can be performed with a head-shake test or with an autorotation test. However, the results are imprecise and less quantifiable than rotary chair testing.
- Head-shake testing is used to evaluate the higher frequencies of vestibular function, which are not as sensitive to vestibular disease as the lower frequencies.
- Posturography may be used to monitor the progress of patients undergoing vestibular rehabilitation therapy, identify patients with symptoms of disequilibrium for whom conventional vestibular test results are negative, assess disability, and identify malingerers and patients at risk for falls.

REFERENCES

1. Lorente De Nò R. Anatomy of the eighth nerve: the central projection of the nerve endings of the internal ear. *Laryngoscope* 1933;43:1.
2. Ryu JH, McCabe BF, Funasaka S. Types of neuronal activity in the medial vestibular nucleus. *Acta Otolaryngol (Stockh)* 1971;72:288.
3. Baloh RW, Honrubia V. *Clinical neurophysiology of the vestibular system,* 2nd ed. Philadelphia: FA Davis, 1990.
4. Honrubia V. Contemporary vestibular function testing: accomplishments and future perspectives. *Otolaryngol Head Neck Surg* 1995; 112:64–77.
5. Baloh RW, Sills AW, Honrubia V. Caloric testing, III: patients with peripheral and central vestibular lesions. *Ann Otol Rhinol Laryngol* 1977;86[Suppl 43]:24.
6. Waldorf RA. Observations of eye movements related to vestibular and other neurological problems using the House infrared/video ENG system. In: Arenberg IK, ed. *Dizziness and balance disorders.* New York: Kugler, 1993:277–281.
7. Nykiel F, Torok N. A simplified nystagmograph. *Ann Otol Rhinol Laryngol* 1963;72:647.
8. Kumar A, Krol G. Binocular infrared oculography. *Laryngoscope* 1992;102:367–378.
9. von Gierke HE, Barber H, Cohen B, et al. Working group on evaluation of test for vestibular function (CHABA). *Aviat Space Environ Med* 1992;63[Suppl 2]:A1-A34.
10. Bhansali S, Honrubia V. The current status of electronystagmography testing. *Otolaryngol Head Neck Surg* 1999;120:419–426.
11. Barber HO, Stockwell CW. *Manual of electronystagmography.* St. Louis: Mosby, 1980.
12. Leigh RJ, Zee DS. *The neurology of eye movements,* 2nd ed. Philadelphia: FA Davis, 1991:393,416–418.
13. Highstein SM, Baker R. Excitatory termination of abducens internuclear neurons on medial rectus motoneurons: relationship to syndrome of internuclear ophthalmoplegia. *J Neurophysiol* 1978;41:1647–1661.
14. Barany R. Diagnose von Krankheitserschernungen in Bereiche des Otolithenapparates. *Acta Otolaryngol (Stockh)* 1921;2:434–37
15. Nylen CO. Positional nystagmus: a review and future prospects. *J Laryngol Otol* 1950;64:295–318.
16. Dix MR, Hallpike CS. Pathology, symptomatology and diagnosis of certain disorders of the vestibular system. *Proc R Soc Med* 1952;45: 341–354.
17. Schuknecht HF. Cupulolithiasis. *Arch Otolaryngol* 1969;90:765–778.
18. Hall SF, Ruby RF, McClure JA. The mechanics of benign paroxysmal vertigo. *J Otolaryngol* 1979;8:151–158.
19. McClure JA. Horizontal canal benign positional vertigo. *J Otolaryngol* 1985;14:30–35.

20. Pagnini P, Nuti D, Vannucchi P. Benign positional vertigo of the horizontal canal. *ORL J Otorhinolaryngol Relat Spec* 1989;51:161–170.

21. Stockwell CW, Bojrab DI. Vestibular function tests. In: Paparella MM, et al., eds. *Otolaryngology,* 3rd ed. Philadelphia: WB Saunders, 1991; 921–948.

22. Leigh RJ, Robinson DA, Zee DS. A hypothetical explanation for periodic alternating nystagmus: instability in the optokinetic-vestibular system. *Ann N Y Acad Sci* 1981;374:619–635.

23. Paige G. Caloric vestibular responses despite canal inactivation. *Invest Ophthalmol Vis Sci* 1984;25[Suppl]:229–232.

24. Scherer H, Brandt U, Clarke AH, et al. European vestibular experiments on the spacelab I mission, III: caloric nystagmus in microgravity. *Exp Brain Res* 1986;64:255.

25. Bhansali SA. Other caloric tests. In: Arenberg IK, ed. *Dizziness and balance disorders.* New York: Kugler, 1993:283–287.

26. Fitzgerald G, Hallpike CS. Studies in human vestibular function, I: observations on the directional preponderance of caloric nystagmus resulting from cerebral lesions. *Brain* 1942;65:115–137.

27. Ford CR, Stockwell CW. Reliabilities of air and water caloric responses. *Arch Otolaryngol* 1978;104:380.

28. Baloh RW, Solingen L, Sills AW, Honrubia V. Caloric testing, I: effect of different conditions of ocular fixation. *Ann Otol Rhinol Laryngol* 1977;86[Suppl 43]:1–6.

29. Jongkees LBW, Philipszoon AJ. Electronystagmography. *Acta Otolaryngol (Stockh)* 1964;[Suppl 189].

30. Custer DD, Black FO, Hemenway WG, Thorby JI. The sequential, bithermal caloric test, I: a statistical analysis of normal subject responses. *Ann Otol Rhinol Laryngol* 1973;83[Suppl 6]:3–9.

31. Hamersma H. The caloric test: a nystagmographical study [thesis]. Amsterdam: University of Amsterdam, 1957.

32. Mehra YG. Electronystagmography: a study of caloric tests in normal subjects. *J Laryngol Otol* 1964;78:520.

33. Henriksson NG. Speed of slow component and duration in caloric nystagmus. *Acta Otolaryngol (Stockh)* 1956;[Suppl 125].

34. Capps MJ, Preciado MC, Paparella M, Hoppe WE. Evaluation of air caloric tests as a routine examination procedure. *Laryngoscope* 1973; 83:1013.

35. Benitez JT, Bouchard KR, Choe YK. Air calorics: a technique and results. *Ann Otol Rhinol Laryngol* 1978;87:216.

36. Sills AW, Baloh RW, Honrubia V. Caloric testing, II: results in normal subjects. *Ann Otol Rhinol Laryngol* 1977;86[Suppl 43]:7.

37. Hess K, Baloh RW, Honrubia V, Yee RD. Rotational testing in patients with bilateral peripheral vestibular disease. *Laryngoscope* 1985;95: 85–88.

38. Hain TC, Fretter M, Zee DS. Head-shaking nystagmus in patients with unilateral peripheral vestibular lesions. *Am J Otolaryngol* 1987;8: 36–47.

39. Demanez JP. L'influence de la fixation oculaire sur le nystagmus postcalorique. *Acta Otolaryngol Belg* 1968;22:7.

40. Bàràny R. Physiologie and Pathologie des Bogengangsapparates beim Menschen. Vienna: Deuticke, 1907.

41. Van Egmond AAJ, Groen JJ, Jongkees LBW. The turning test with small regulable stimuli, I: method of examination—cupulometria. *J Laryngol Otol* 1948;2:63.

42. Montandon A. A new technique for vestibular investigation. *Acta Otolaryngol (Stockh)* 1954;39:594.

43. Jenkins HR, Honrubia V, Baloh RW. Evaluation of multiple frequency rotatory testing in patients with peripheral labyrinthine weakness. *Am J Otolaryngol* 1982;3:182.

44. Wolfe JW, Engelken EJ, Kos CM. Low-frequency harmonic acceleration as a test of labyrinthine function: basic methods and illustrative cases. *Trans Am Acad Ophthalmol Otolaryngol* 1978;86:130–142.

45. Baloh RW, Hess K, Honrubia V, Yee RD. Low and high frequency sinusoidal rotational testing in patients with peripheral vestibular lesions. *Acta Otolaryngol (Stockh)* 1984;406[Suppl]:189–193.

46. Honrubia V, Jenkins HA, Minser K, Baloh RW, Yee RD. Vestibulo-ocular reflexes in peripheral labyrinthine lesions, II: Caloric testing. *Am J Otolaryngol* 1984;5:93.

47. Bhansali SA, Stockwell CW, Bojrab DI. Oscillopsia in patients with loss of vestibular function. *Otolaryngol Head Neck Surg* 1993;109:120–125.

48. Baloh RW, Jacobson K, Honrubia V. Idiopathic bilateral vestibulopathy. *Neurology* 1989;39:272.

49. Takahashi S, Fetter M, Koenig E, et al. The clinical significance of head-shaking nystagmus in the dizzy patient. *Acta Otolaryngol (Stockh)* 1990;109:8–14.

50. Kamei T, Kornhuber HH. Spontaneous and head-shaking nystagmus in normals and in patients with central lesions. *Can J Otolaryngol* 1979;3:372–380.

51. O'Leary DP, Davis LL. Vestibular autorotation testing of Meniere's disease. *Otolaryngol Head Neck Surg* 1990;103:66–71.

52. Kitsigianis GA, O'Leary DP, Davis LL. Active head-movement analysis of cisplatin-induced vestibulotoxicity. *Otolaryngol Head Neck Surg* 1988;98:82–87.

52a. Nashner LM, Black FO, Wall C. Adaptation to altered support and visual conditions during stance: patients with vestibular deficits. *J Neurosci* 1982;2(5):536–544.

53. Black FO, Shupeert CL, Peterka RJ, Nashner LM. Effects of unilateral loss of vestibular function on the vestibulo-ocular reflex and postural control. *Ann Otol Rhinol Laryngol* 1989;98:884–889.

54. Ford-Smith CD, Wyman JF, Elswick LK, Fernandez T, Newton RA. Test-retest reliability of the sensory organization test in institutionalized older adults. *Arch Phys Med Rehabil* 1995;76:77–81.

55. Hamid MA, Hughes GB, Kinney SE. Specificity and sensitivity of dynamic posturography. *Acta Otolaryngol (Stockh)* 1991;[Suppl 481]: 596–600.

56. Goebel JA, Paige GD. Dynamic posturography and caloric test results in patients with and without vertigo. *Otolaryngol Head Neck Surg* 1989;100:553–558.

57. Vorhees RL. Dynamic posturography findings in central nervous system disorders. *Otolaryngol Head Neck Surg* 1990;103:96–101.

58. Cass SP, Kartush JM, Graham MD. Patterns of vestibular function following vestibular nerve section. *Laryngoscope* 1992;102:388–394.

59. Shepard NT, Telian SA, Smith-Weelock M, Raj A. Vestibular and balance rehabilitation therapy. *Ann Otol Rhinol Laryngol* 1993;102; 198–205.

60. Cevette MJ, Puetz B, Marion MS, Wertz ML, Muenter MD. A physiologic performance on dynamic posturography. Otolaryngol Head Neck Surg 1995;112:676–688.

61. Jacobson GP, Newman CW, Hunter L, Balzer GK. Balance function test correlates of the dizziness handicap inventory. *J Am Acad Audiol* 1991;2:253–260.

62. Monsel EM, Furman JM, Herdman SJ, Konrad HR, Shepard NT. Computerized dynamic platform posturography. Otolaryngol Head Neck Surg 1997;117:394–398.

The Ear: Comprehensive Otology,
edited by R. F. Canalis and P. R. Lambert.
Lippincott Williams & Wilkins, Philadelphia © 2000.

CHAPTER 10

Auditory Sensitivity: Air and Bone Conduction

Donald D. Dirks, Jayne B. Ahlstrom, and Donald E. Morgan

There are two primary reasons for administering hearing tests to patients. The first is to provide information that can assist in diagnosing the anatomic site of a lesion, from which inferences can be made concerning the disease or pathologic process. The second is to determine the receptive communication capabilities of the patient. Because reduced auditory sensitivity is common to most auditory disorders of peripheral origin, an estimate of the magnitude of the sensitivity loss forms the nucleus of auditory diagnostic testing. The purpose of this chapter is to describe normal auditory sensitivity and the clinical measurement of pure tone air conduction thresholds, which has become the standard behavioral procedure for determination of auditory sensitivity. The clinical use of bone conduction threshold measurements is discussed because the results combined with the air conduction thresholds are used to estimate the integrity of the sensorineural system and the magnitude of middle ear disorders.

UNITS OF MEASUREMENT

The normal human ear is remarkable in terms of its absolute sensitivity to sound and the dynamic range over which it can respond. The human ear is most sensitive in

the midfrequency region of audibility (2.0 to 3.0 kHz), and the dynamic range encompasses approximately 140 dB. This dynamic range corresponds to a power ratio of 10 million to 1. Because the normal human ear can hear over such a wide range, it is not practical to describe and measure sound intensities directly. Thus a logarithmic scale that expresses the ratio of two intensities is used. One intensity (I_0) is chosen as the reference, and the other intensity (I_1) is described relative to the reference. The measurement unit used to describe intensity is the bel, which corresponds to an intensity ratio of 10:1. The number of bels corresponding to a particular intensity ratio is calculated by taking the logarithm to the base 10 of the intensity ratio (number of bels = $\log_{10}(I_0/I_1)$). For more discrete resolution of the measured levels, the bel is divided into 10 decibels (dB). Thus the number of decibels that corresponds to a given ratio of acoustic intensity or power is formulated as number of dB = $10\log_{10}(I_0/I_1)$.

From the foregoing description, it is clear that the decibel represents an intensity or power ratio, not an absolute intensity. To specify the absolute intensity of a sound, it is necessary to refer the particular intensity to a standard reference level. The reference level most commonly used is the power of 10^{-16} watts per square centimeter (w/cm^2), which is equivalent to a pressure of 0.0002 dynes per square centimeter (dynes/cm^2). For most audiologic indices, measurements are made and described in decibels expressed as a ratio of pressure, that is, the amount of force acting on each unit area. Intensity or power is proportional to the square of pressure. Thus if a sound has an intensity (or power) of I_1, and an amplitude (or pressure) A_1, and a second sound

D. D. Dirks: Division of Head and Neck Surgery, University of California, Los Angeles, School of Medicine, Los Angeles, California 90095

J. B. Ahlstrom: Department of Otolaryngology and Communicative Sciences, Medical University of South Carolina, Charleston, South Carolina 29425

D. E. Morgan: Decibel Instruments, Inc., Fremont, California 94555

has an intensity of I_2 and an amplitude of A_2, the difference in level between them is

$$\text{Number of dB} = 10\log_{10}(I_1/I_2) = 10\log_{10}(A_1/A_2)^2 \text{ or}$$
$$20\log_{10}(A_1/A_2)$$

As a consequence, a tenfold increase in amplitude (pressure) corresponds to a 100-fold increase in intensity (power), or 20 dB.

The reference sound pressure level used to specify a sound is commonly referenced to 0.0002 dynes/cm². This reference level (0 dB) is now expressed in the International System of Units as 2×10^{-5} N/m² or 20 µPa (micropascals). A sound level described in terms of this reference is called sound pressure level (SPL).

For physical measurements of the output levels from earphones or loudspeakers, the levels are described in terms of SPL. For clinical and diagnostic purposes, however, it is desirable to compare the hearing sensitivity of a given patient to "normal" threshold values to determine the presence or absence of a hearing loss. For this purpose, the described level is referenced to normal hearing sensitivity, or the "threshold" as determined from a group of young listeners with normal hearing. Thus when hearing is tested with a clinical audiometer, the measured level is expressed in hearing level (HL). The SPL equivalents at 0 dB HL for various audiometric test frequencies are available in a standard document on the specification of audiometers from the American National Standards Institute (ANSI S3.6-1996) (1). The current standard on the specifications of audiometers contains recommendations for air conduction testing with several types of earphones and information on calibration for bone conduction testing with a vibrator and sound field measurements with a loudspeaker.

SENSITIVITY OF A NORMAL HUMAN EAR

Threshold of Audibility

Determination of the absolute threshold for listeners with normal hearing has been studied by a large number of investigators. Because the procedural methods and specification of the signals used has varied greatly among investigators, there are discrepancies in reported results. To establish the general configuration of the normal audibility curve, some investigators have presented tones in the sound field through a loudspeaker, and the measured thresholds are described in terms of the minimum audible field (MAF). Other experimenters have delivered the tonal stimuli through earphones and monitored the SPL in the ear canal that corresponds to those thresholds. This procedure yields a measure called the minimum audible pressure (MAP). The physical calibration of tonal SPL is different for each of these measurements. For the MAF thresholds, SPL is determined either in the ear canal or at the eardrum of the subject or

at a position occupied by the center of the head, the listener having been removed from the sound field. For the MAP procedure, SPL is measured by means of calibration of the earphones with an "artificial ear", or coupler, which approximates the volume under an earphone when the earphone is coupled to the ear of the average person. The artificial ear used for standard audiometric calibration of earphones consists of a condenser microphone and one of several standard couplers; the choice depends on the type of earphone.

Figure 1 provides a representative example of the normal hearing thresholds obtained from measurements obtained with MAP and MAF procedures. These average audibility curves were obtained from thresholds taken from a large number of otologically normal ears evaluated by Dadson and King in 1952 (2) for the MAP measurements and by Robinson and Dadson (3) in 1956 for the MAF measurements. MAF thresholds were measured in the sound field of an anechoic chamber with the loudspeaker located at 0° azimuth. Several results in Fig. 1 are noteworthy. First, the threshold of audibility is different for earphone and sound field measurements. Second, the normal human ear is most sensitive to sounds between 2.0 and 4.0 kHz. Third, absolute thresholds become progressively poorer above and below these frequencies.

Although it might be anticipated that the threshold would be the same whether or not the measurements were taken in the sound field or with earphones, the threshold of audibility is consistently found at higher SPLs for MAP than for MAF measurements. In the frequency region between 0.20 and 8.0 kHz, the difference between thresholds averages 6 dB. For this reason, Munson and Wiener (4) called the difference in MAP and MAF thresholds the missing 6 dB. The differences in the higher frequencies are caused by the effects of head diffraction

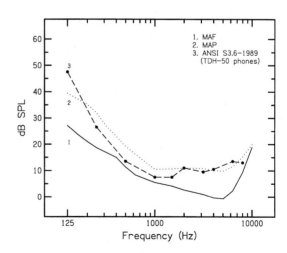

FIG. 1. Representative example of normal hearing thresholds obtained from minimum audible pressure (MAP) and minimum audible field (MAF) measurements. Also shown are recommended sound pressure levels for 0 dB HL for a TDH-50 earphone taken from ANSI S3.6-1989.

and ear canal and pinna resonances that influence MAF measurements. These effects contribute less to threshold determination when the ear is covered by an earphone (MAP) than when measured in the sound field with the ear uncovered (MAF). The larger differences in the low frequencies have received more extensive investigation. Rudmose (5,6), Villchur (7), and Shaw and Piercy (8) accounted for much of the difference in the low frequencies by demonstrating a large masking effect that occurs under earphone conditions because of increased physiologic noise in the ear canal. Anderson and Whittle (9) obtained masking levels of 11 dB because of physiologic noise at 0.125 kHz during MAP measurements. Thus low frequency MAP thresholds, up to 0.25 kHz, are essentially masked thresholds resulting from high physiologic noise levels generated under the earphone cushion. When the aforementioned low and high frequency effects are accounted for, the differences between thresholds for MAP and MAF are essentially absent. As Killion (10) suggested after review of the relevant literature, nothing is really missing.

The coupler pressure that corresponds to MAP threshold measurements depends on the particular earphone used with the audiometer. Michael and Bienvenue (11), for example, compared the results obtained with several clinically used earphones. In the standard used to specify the SPL for 0 dB HL, values differ somewhat depending on the type of earphone used. The TDH-50 earphone is widely used in clinical practice. This earphone is mounted in an earphone cushion (MX41/AR) the dimensions of which are standardized. In Fig. 1, the recommended SPLs for 0 dB HL with a TDH-50 earphone at major test frequencies are provided for comparison with MAF and MAP thresholds. The standard recommended thresholds agree, in general, with the MAP values reported by Dadson and King (2).

TDH-50 earphones are widely used both clinically and experimentally because of their uniform response across most of the important audible frequency range for humans. The MX41/AR cushions are supraaural in design, that is, they touch and press against the pinna, unlike circumaural earphone-cushion arrangements, which encircle the pinna. The NBS-9A coupler, which is used for standard calibration, accommodates only earphones encased in supraaural cushions.

A national standard (ANSI S3.7-1986) (12) describes the physical dimensions of the coupler used to calibrate earphones. The standard 6-cc coupler (NSB-9A) simulates the enclosed volume under an earphone for a human ear but does not replicate the impedance of the human ear. A coupler developed by Zwislocki (13,14) and usually referred to as an ear simulator, approximates closely the impedance of the human ear. However, because of the recent development and higher cost of the ear simulator, the 6-cc coupler continues to be used for calibrating earphones on clinical audiometers.

Insert earphones have been introduced as an alternative to air conduction earphones housed in circumaural or supraaural cushions. The revised standard for audiometers (ANSI S3.6-1996) describes the reference equivalent threshold SPL for two insert earphones, the Etymotic ER-3A and the EARtone 3A insert phones. These insert earphones provide certain real-ear coupling advantages over supraaural cushions. These advantages are detailed later. The insert earphones require either a HA-1 or HA-2 coupler or an occluded ear simulator for calibration, because the ear canal volume is smaller when these phones are coupled to the ear than when a TDH-50 supraaural phone is used, which simply covers the ear canal opening.

Temporal Duration

Numerous investigators (15,16) have reported that both absolute thresholds and loudness of sounds depend on the duration of the stimulus. The studies cited earlier concerning MAP and MAF measurements all were conducted with pure tone stimuli the duration of which generally exceeded 500 ms. Figure 2 shows a representative example of the average change in threshold for a pure tone at 1.0 kHz. In general, when the duration of a short tone burst is increased, the threshold of audibility decreases at the approximate rate of 3 dB per doubling of duration. This is true for normal-hearing listeners up to a duration of approximately 200 ms, at which point the change in threshold with duration asymptotes. For example, if a subject's threshold at a particular frequency is 15 dB for a 25-ms duration, then the threshold would be approximately 12 dB for a tone 50 ms in duration. Thus over a reasonable range of duration (10 to 500 ms), the ear appears to integrate the energy of the stimulus over time (temporal integration).

To avoid the intersubject variability associated with establishing threshold for short-duration tones and variations in temporal integration found in some ears with sensorineural hearing loss (17), it is usually recommended

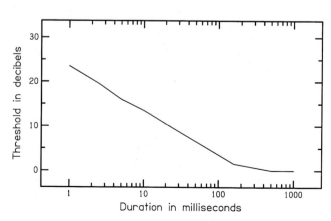

FIG. 2. Representative example of the average change in threshold for a 1,000-Hz tone as a function of duration.

that tonal signals used to measure clinical thresholds have a duration of at least 200 ms. Automatic audiometers, in which the tonal duration is not under manual control of the tester, typically provide a duration of at least 200 ms with an off period of 200 ms before the next tone burst is presented. For manual signal presentation, clinicians typically provide a signal of 200 to 750 ms duration when testing pure tone thresholds.

MEASUREMENT OF CLINICAL THRESHOLDS: AIR CONDUCTION

An estimate of sensitivity loss as a function of frequency is usually the initial measurement obtained during an auditory diagnostic examination. Pure tones at selected frequencies over the most sensitive auditory frequency region (0.25 to 8.0 kHz) are presented through an air conduction receiver (earphone, insert phone, or loudspeaker) or bone conduction vibrator, and threshold measurements are obtained. Before the advent of audiometers, measurements of auditory sensitivity were estimated with tuning forks. Tuning fork tests are discussed in Chapter 7 as part of the otologic examination.

Pure Tone Audiometry

Pure tone threshold audiometry has become the accepted behavioral procedure for quantifying auditory sensitivity. Audiometric threshold testing is conducted either by means of manual audiometry, in which the examiner controls the signal parameters, or automatic audiometry, in which the listener controls the signal intensity with an adjustment procedure as the test signals are presented at discrete or systematically changing frequencies. In most clinics, pure tone air and bone conduction threshold tests are performed by means of manual audiometry.

Another general methodologic consideration is whether to perform the threshold tests with earphones or in the sound field. Although most routine testing is conducted with earphones, a substantial amount of threshold testing is conducted in the sound field. Sound field testing is necessary for infants, young children, and difficult-to-test patients who cannot or will not tolerate earphones. In examinations of adults and children, sound field thresholds may be used to assess the real ear gain available from amplification systems

Although standards are available that specify the physical characteristics for audiometers and the SPL for normal thresholds with various earphones, no standards have been universally accepted for sound field testing. Neither have national standards been accepted for specifying the procedural methods to be used for determination of thresholds with earphones or in the sound field. Guidelines for pure tone manual audiometry (18), sound field testing (19), and the symbols used to record auditory

results (20) have been suggested by working committees on audiologic evaluation sponsored by the American Speech-Language-Hearing Association (ASHA) in an effort to standardize audiometric test procedures. Some of the more important issues cited in these guidelines have been incorporated into this chapter.

Earphone Measurements

Test Condition

The current standard (ANSI S3.6-1996) (1) for audiometers provides reference SPLs for normal hearing (0 dB HL) for several earphones encased in supraaural cushions. The current standard also provides reference threshold levels for an insert earphone (Etymotic ER-3A). Figure 3 shows a typical pair of insert earphones and a pair of supraaural earphones.

Insert earphones were developed to minimize common clinical problems associated with use of supraaural earphones, such as an occlusion effect and interaural attenuation between the ears, which often leads to problems when the nontest ear needs masking. These issues are discussed later. Insert earphones are placed in the external auditory meatus with foam eartips, which are supplied by the manufacturer. After the eartips are inserted in the canal, the foam expands to provide an acoustic seal. Insert earphones alleviate most of the acoustic leakage associated with use of supraaural earphones, especially notable at frequencies below 0.50 kHz. Although insertion depth in the ear canal is a variable with insert earphones, test-retest reliability between a shallow and a deep insertion is small, according to data summarized from several studies and reported by Wilbur et al. (21). For some patients, when an earphone with a supraaural cushion is applied to the pinna, the soft cartilaginous portion of the ear canal collapses and prevents complete transmission of the test signal to the eardrum. For ears in which there is a possibility that use of earphones with

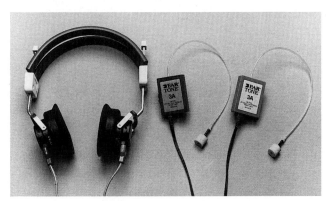

FIG. 3. A typical pair of insert earphones (*right*) together with a pair of supraaural earphones (*left*).

supraaural cushions will cause tragal occlusion of the external canal, insert earphones are a necessity. Insert earphones are more comfortable for most patients than traditional supraaural cushions, especially when the test period is prolonged.

Audiological testing is conducted in a room that is quiet enough to avoid masking by environmental noise, which exists in all rooms. Permissible ambient noise levels for earphone testing have been established and standardized (ANSI S3.1-1991) (22). Because the ear is unoccluded for bone conduction and sound field testing, additional permissible noise levels are recommended in the standard for testing with the ear uncovered. The latter permissible noise levels are more restrictive than for earphone testing, in which the earphone and cushion or insert tip provide some attenuation of ambient noise.

For practical purposes, the magnitude of hearing loss usually is measured at selected frequencies between 0.25 and 8.0 kHz. There is, however, increasing interest in testing thresholds at frequencies greater than 8.0 kHz, because the effects of aging and certain ototoxic drugs may first be evidenced at these high frequencies. Many clinical audiometers are not designed for testing at frequencies above 8.0 kHz; however, these options are available from some manufacturers. ANSI standard S3.6-1996 contains an appendix with recommended reference levels for test frequencies up to 16.0 kHz. Reference threshold SPLs for normal-hearing listeners at selected test frequencies from 8.0 to 20.0 kHz have been published (23,24).

Test Procedure

An important variable in determining pure tone thresholds is the particular psychophysical method used. The commonly used procedure in clinical pure tone audiometry incorporates elements of a manual procedure initially described by Hughson and Westlake in 1944 (25). This procedure received further theoretic and practical confirmation by Carhart and Jerger (26) and is essentially the same as the procedure recommended by the ASHA committee on audiologic evaluation (18). The basic procedure consists of two parts—familiarization with the signal and the threshold measurement itself. The patient is presented with the tone at a hearing level well above the assumed threshold. If no clear response is elicited, the tone can be presented at progressively higher levels until a response is obtained for each stimulus presentation. Once the patient is familiar with the tonal stimulus and the response task, measurement of the threshold begins. The tone is decreased in 10-dB steps until no response occurs. The tone then is increased in level in 5-dB steps until the patient responds. After the response, the level is decreased by 10 dB, and another ascending series begins in 5-dB steps. The threshold usually is defined as the lowest level at which responses occur in at least half of a series of ascending trials. A minimum of three responses is required at a signal presentation level. By convention this procedure leads to an intensity level that produces a 50% chance of detection. Because the step size used in clinical audiometry is large (5 dB), it is sometimes difficult to obtain the exact level for 50% detection. Clinical thresholds obtained with manual audiometry usually are higher than 50% detection.

Masking

In clinical air conduction testing, it is not uncommon that the two ears have different threshold levels. Results for such a patient are illustrated in Fig. 4. Although the difference in threshold between the ears is small (<40 dB) in the low frequencies, it exceeds 40 dB in the frequencies above 0.50 kHz. The validity of the thresholds in the left ear is questionable because the head does not sufficiently attenuate signals transcranially to ensure that all signals presented to the poorer left ear are not heard by the normal-hearing right ear. The difference (in decibels) between the level of the signal in the car canal of the test ear and the level in the opposite cochlea is called *interaural attenuation.* When standard supraaural earphones with cushions are used, interaural attenuation between the ears varies from 40 to 65 dB (27).

Two simultaneous pathways determine interaural attenuation during standard earphone testing: an *air conduction pathway* around the head and into the opposite ear canal and a *bone conduction pathway,* which extends from the air enclosed under the earphone, through the skin, into the bone of the skull, and finally to the opposite cochlea. In practice, this means that whenever the air conduction presentation level to the test ear exceeds the bone conduction threshold in the opposite ear by more than the most conservative estimated interaural attenuation (40 dB), it is necessary to apply a masking signal to the nontest ear to ensure that the nontest ear does not contribute to the results from the poorer ear (28). For the example in Fig. 4, the difference in thresholds (air conduction thresholds in the left ear minus bone conduction thresholds in the right ear) between the two ears at 0.25 and 0.50 kHz are less than 40 dB, thus masking would not be required in the right ear at those frequencies for testing of the left ear. However, at other test frequencies, masking would be necessary in the right ear to validate the thresholds of the poorer left ear. The goal of the masking procedure is to elevate the thresholds of the nontest ear and at the same time produce no influence on the threshold of the test ear. The details of the techniques used for masking are beyond the scope of this chapter, but the procedures have been discussed in numerous publications (29).

Two especially relevant factors should be recognized in regard to masking. First, as described by Fletcher (30) only a small portion of the masking energy around the test

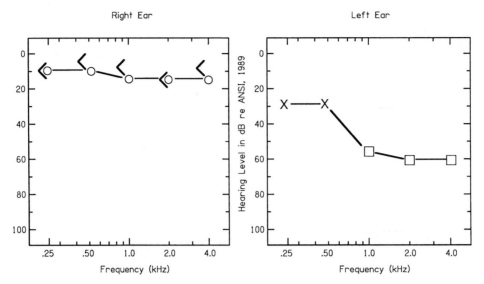

FIG. 4. Audiometric results from a patient with normal hearing according to air (O-O) and bone (<-<) conduction testing in the right ear and a hearing loss according to air conduction testing in the left ear. The air conduction thresholds in the left ear were measured without masking in the nontest ear (x-x) at 0.25 and 0.5 kHz. Thresholds at 1.0, 2.0, and 4.0 kHz were measured with masking applied to the non-test ear (□-□).

frequency provides the masking that elevates the threshold. Thus the most efficient masker is one that consists of a narrow band of noise centered on the test frequency. Masking energy above and below the test frequency contributes only to the overall level and loudness of the masker but not to the elevation of the threshold at the test frequency. Most modern audiometers have narrow bands of noise that change with frequency and are most often calibrated in terms of effective masking levels, that is, the hearing level to which the threshold is shifted, regardless of hearing loss, given a specified amount of noise.

A second interesting and clinically useful observation in regard to masking was made by Zwislocki in 1953 (27). While studying interaural attenuation, Zwislocki observed that attenuation between ears could be increased by reducing the area of the head that comes in contact with the masking transducer. By using insert earphones, he found that interaural attenuation was substantially increased and thus the likelihood of overmasking (masker level so high that it begins to crossover to mask the test ear) was reduced. Use of insert earphones, such as those shown in Fig. 3, would also reduce the need for masking during testing of air conduction thresholds, because of the increase in interaural attenuation between the ears. In summary, the use of narrow bands of noise and insert earphones has greatly reduced the confounding factors that occur with masking the nontest ear.

Sound Field Audiometry

Auditory measurements of sensitivity can be obtained in the sound field with a loudspeaker as the transducer

instead of an earphone. Sound field audiometry is used most often to test infants and young children and occasionally for difficult-to-test adult patients who do not tolerate earphones. Although sound field measurements for threshold and speech recognition are an integral part of many clinical assessments, there are no official standards for these measurements. Because sound field measurements are rarely conducted in an anechoic chamber (a test room with no reverberation), the test environment imposes several limitations on these measurements that are not usually encountered with earphone test conditions. These factors include reflections from the walls and objects in the room, background noise, movement of the head of the listener, and the physical characteristics of the loudspeaker. Each of these issues presents special problems not encountered when testing is conducted with earphones.

Ambient Noise Level

Low ambient noise levels in audiometric test rooms are essential for accurate measurement of thresholds. This is especially true for sound field conditions, in which the person undergoing testing is not provided the degree of attenuation of ambient noise available when the ears are covered during earphone test conditions.

The purpose of measuring the ambient noise in a room is to estimate the potential masking effect of that noise on threshold. In practice, the ambient noise of single-walled test chambers in relatively noisy, outside surroundings severely restricts measurement of hearing sensitivity for persons with normal hearing or mild hearing loss. Maximum permissible levels of ambient noise for both sound field and earphone testing have been published in ANSI S3.1-1991 (22). The permissible ambient noise levels are lower for sound field, open ear testing than for earphone testing. It is often necessary to administer auditory tests in rooms where the ambient noise level is higher than the recommended permissible levels, and this limits the potential for measuring normal or near normal thresholds. In most of these situations (e.g. medical settings for patients treated with potentially ototoxic drugs and hearing screening tests in schools), tests are conducted with earphones. Because the highest intensity of typical room noise is in the lower-frequency region, air conduction thresholds for 0.25 and 0.50 kHz are most affected. The problem can be minimized with use of insert earphones, which seal the auditory meatus and reduce the noise level within the ear canal. It is highly desirable to measure the noise level to calculate its effect. If it is not practical to measure the noise, a tester with normal hearing can measure his or her own thresholds in the room and estimate the magnitude of the effect on threshold measurements.

Loudspeakers

A loudspeaker used in clinical testing should have a wide bandwidth (100 to 10,000 Hz) that encompasses both the audible frequency range in humans and the important frequency regions for communication of speech. The frequency response of the loudspeaker also should be relatively consistent so that the spectrum of broadband stimuli, such as speech, does not differ greatly from that of the original recording. This requirement is difficult to achieve, especially for loudspeakers with diaphragms large enough to produce sufficient acoustic output for examinations of patients with moderate or severe hearing loss. Loudspeakers with high-level acoustic output and a relatively consistent frequency response characteristic can be found, but most are expensive.

The frequency response characteristics of the loudspeaker are modified in most test rooms because of interaction between the direct sound from the loudspeaker and the indirect sound created by reflections from the walls. Audiometric test chambers are constructed with a primary goal of reducing the level of sound from the outside environment, but most have large reflective surfaces such as glass windows. Many test rooms also contain reflective objects, such as speaker enclosures, tables, and chairs. As a result, the sound field from the loudspeaker often is modified by interaction between the direct sound from the loudspeaker and the indirect sound from the reflective surfaces and objects. This interaction produces a reverberant sound field and prolongs the original signal after it stops. The location of the listener's head and the location of the loudspeaker in the test room therefore must be carefully considered so that the effects of the reflections

are minimized. In most commercial test rooms, reverberation time is short, and the effects of the reflective surfaces are reduced by use of a rug on the floor and having only essential furniture in the room.

In general, loudspeakers are placed in the corner of the test room, and the listener is seated near the center of the room away from the reflective walls or other reflective surfaces. The location of the loudspeaker and the patient in the test room should not be determined arbitrarily. Guidelines for the physical measurements of room characteristics and their potential influences on the test environment have been published (31), and the ASHA committee on audiologic evaluation has developed a tutorial on sound field measurements (19).

Stimuli

Testing in the sound field involves presentation of frequency-specific or speech stimuli. For most test rooms, pure tones used in earphone audiometry are an inappropriate choice of stimulus for sound field measurements. When pure tones are introduced into the sound field, interaction between the direct and indirect sounds produces standing wave patterns that introduce variations in SPL at different locations. To minimize this problem and still maintain frequency-specific stimuli, it is recommended that signals broader than pure tones be used for testing. The most commonly preferred alternatives to pure tones include frequency-modulated (FM; warble) tones and narrow bands of noise. Both of these types of complex signals effectively overcome the effects of standing wave patterns because their bandwidths exceed the bandwidths of the nodes and antinodes caused by the physical characteristics of the room. Signal level variability in the room decreases as the stimulus bandwidth increases, effectively providing an average measure of SPL that minimizes the effect of the standing wave.

FM tones are characterized by their carrier frequency, modulation rate, and frequency deviation. The *carrier frequency* may be modulated by a square or a sine wave. It is not clear which resulting waveform is most advantageous for audiometric purposes. *Modulation rate* refers to the number of times per second the frequency is swept. *Frequency deviation* refers to percentage frequency change from the nominal frequency and is expressed in cycles per second (Hz). Frequency-specific narrow bands of noise are generated by passing a broadband noise through a band-pass filter. One-third octave bands of noise at various test frequencies are useful for sound field testing because they are sufficiently frequency specific.

The choice of stimuli, FM tones, or narrow bands of noise depends on the need for increased stimulus bandwidth to ensure uniformity of the sound field and the need for frequency specificity to obtain accurate representation of threshold sensitivity at discrete frequencies. Both types of complex signals produce similar thresholds if the physical characteristics in terms of bandwidth and rejection rate (how fast the signal intensity drops on either side of the signal band) are similar. Regardless of choice of stimulus, the bandwidth must be narrow and the rejection rate fast enough so that rapid changes in hearing sensitivity, such as precipitous high-frequency hearing losses, can be measured accurately. When the bandwidth is too wide or the rejection rate outside the band too slow, the actual slope of an audiogram cannot be measured accurately. Walker et al. (31) recommended specific bandwidths for sound field audiometry. For procedures in which sound field uniformity is critical (testing of infants or children), these investigators recommend stimulus bandwidths approximately one-third octave wide. More restrictive bandwidths are recommended when accuracy of the audiometric configuration is the critical criterion. Many commercially available audiometers contain narrow bands of noise or FM tones that approximate one-third octave bandwidths.

Physical Calibration of the Sound Field

The SPL of the test stimulus typically is measured at the point in the sound field where the listener's head is to be placed. This procedure is referred to as the *substitution method*. Although SPL measured in this manner does not reflect the precise level of the sound arriving at the listener's ear (with the listener present), it is an acceptable procedure that allows threshold comparisons between clinics and measurements of the stability of the sound source over time.

For frequency-specific stimuli (such as FM tones or narrow bands of noise), each test stimulus is measured in the sound field by means of the substitution method. Although no sound field standards exist for normal hearing sensitivity levels, several investigators (31–33) have recommended SPL levels for FM tonal thresholds obtained in the sound field.

Because speech is a complex stimulus that varies over time in both frequency and intensity, it usually is not possible to measure the SPL of this signal the way continuous tones or narrow bands of noise are measured. In ANSI S3.6-1996 (1), reference levels are recommended for speech delivered from loudspeakers located at 0-, 45-, and 90-degree locations relative to the center of the patient's head. The standard suggests use of a 1.0-kHz tone signal for the calibration measurement. However, because of problems associated with using pure tones in the sound field, some investigators have suggested (32,33) that a wide-band stimulus, such as speech-spectrum noise, be substituted for pure tones to determine the SPL measured at the test location in the room. The amplitude of the noise is adjusted to produce a volume unit meter deflection equivalent to the average peaks of the speech signal. These investigators provided recommendations for SPL levels that correspond to speech reception thresholds for normal-hearing listeners for various loudspeaker locations relative to the listener's head.

MEASUREMENT OF CLINICAL THRESHOLDS: BONE CONDUCTION

Before the advent of clinical immittance measurements, the primary audiologic tests used to differentiate conductive hearing loss from sensorineural hearing loss was comparative measurement of air and bone conduction thresholds. The psychophysical procedure for measuring bone conduction thresholds is similar to that for measuring air conduction thresholds, except that the signal is transduced with a vibrator, which usually is coupled to the mastoid process.

The diagnostic utility of the difference between air and bone conduction threshold measures is based on two principle assumptions. The first is that the air conduction threshold is a measure of the total auditory system; the second is that the threshold for bone conduction is primarily a measure of the integrity of the sensorineural auditory system. Thus the difference between these thresholds provides an estimate of the conductive component. If both thresholds are essentially the same, the result indicates that the hearing loss is sensorineural in origin. The second assumption implies that bone conduction sensitivity is independent of the state of the external or middle ear. There is sufficient documentation from both animal and human experiments that the second assumption cannot be completely accepted. Understanding the basic mechanism of bone conduction should clarify this issue.

Mechanism of Bone Conduction

Many of our currently held concepts regarding bone conduction evolved from early investigations by Herzog and Krainz (34), Bekesy (35), and Barany (36) and more recent comprehensive investigations by Tonndorf (37). Tonndorf's investigation emphasized the futility of attempting to account for all bone conduction phenomena with a single mechanism. Among the several factors that contribute to the total bone conduction response, three important factors were identified: (a) the reception of sound energy radiated into the external canal, (b) the inertial response of the middle ear ossicles and inner ear fluid, and (c) the compressional response of the inner ear spaces.

Tonndorf found that when the vibrating signal was applied to the skull, energy was produced by the walls of the external canal and transmitted to the tympanic membrane. The magnitude of this energy may be increased or decreased by unoccluding or occluding the external ear canal, changing the canal resonance, or changing the impedance at the tympanic membrane. Impairment of the middle ear may change the relative influence of this mode of transmission of energy.

The inertial response identified by Bekesy and Barany was cited by Tonndorf as a principle mechanism of conduction. The inertia of the ossicles during forced vibration of the skull sets up relative motion between the stapes and the oval window. This motion leads to cochlear stimulation similar to that produced by air conduction. Tonndorf emphasized that the inertial response is primarily caused by impedance of the middle ear ossicles and inertia of inner ear fluid. Tonndorf further demonstrated this point by reporting elevation of bone conduction responses in various species of animals after removal or immobilization of the ossicular chain. The frequency region of maximal loss in the bone conduction response was related to the ossicular resonant frequency characteristics of the particular animal species examined. In the human ear that frequency region is near 2.0 kHz. Reduction of middle ear participation in the total bone conduction threshold caused by otosclerosis appears to account for the notch in bone conduction thresholds, observed first by Carhart (38), at that frequency region.

An example of the Carhart notch is illustrated in Fig. 5, which shows the pre- and postoperative air and bone conduction thresholds of a patient with unilateral otosclerosis. The preoperative air conduction responses (see Fig. 5, *left*) demonstrate a hearing loss of 40 to 50 dB HL at most frequencies. The preoperative bone conduction threshold is normal except in the 2.0-kHz frequency region where threshold sensitivity is reduced. After successful stapes mobilization (see Fig. 5, *right*), the air conduction threshold level at 2.0 kHz is better than the preoperative bone conduction threshold. This overclosure of the preoperative bone gap was no doubt caused by the mechanical changes on the ossicular

chain system that occurred during the stapes mobilization operation. The preoperative reduction in bone conduction threshold reflects absence of the inertial effects that contribute to the total bone conduction threshold of a normal-hearing listener. The inertial component was reactivated after the successful stapes mobilization operation. The results for the patient described in Fig. 5 illustrate how a conductive disorder that affects the function of the middle ear structures can influence measurement of the bone conduction threshold. The example also demonstrates that for patients with middle ear disorders, the bone conduction threshold cannot be assumed to represent, in an absolute manner, cochlear reserve. Identification of an air-bone gap and prediction of postoperative air conduction threshold sensitivity must always be predicated on an understanding of the potential effects of preoperative middle ear mechanics on bone conduction measurements of threshold sensitivity.

The third important mechanism for bone conduction is the compressional response. This response, identified originally by Herzog and Krainz (34), is a product of distortional vibrations of the skull, which may be alternately compressed and expanded in response to bone conduction vibration. Because the stiffness of the oval window membrane is greater than that of the round window membrane, the cochlear fluid must yield under the influence of these opposite movements, and the basilar membrane is displaced. The total bone conduction response thus is a result of the complex interaction of several mechanisms, two of which (external ear canal radiated energy and middle ear inertia) may be influenced by conditions that affect outer or middle ear function.

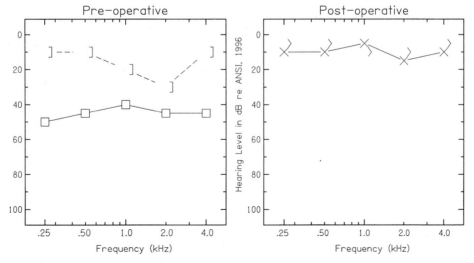

FIG. 5. Pre- and postoperative audiometric results for a patient with otosclerosis. Masked air (□-□) and masked bone (]-]) conduction thresholds are shown in the preoperative ear, and unmasked air conduction (x-x) and bone conduction (>->) thresholds are shown in the postoperative ear.

Considerations in Testing Clinical Bone Conduction

Because the mode of excitation of the auditory system is so different for bone conduction than for air conduction stimulation, a number of equipment and procedural issues vary.

The Bone Conduction Vibrator

In the early days of clinical bone conduction audiometry, bone vibrators were held by hand against the mastoid process. The housing of the vibrator was essentially isolated from the vibratory tip itself. These vibrators were cumbersome to use, and once hearing aid vibrators were developed, they were quickly adopted for use in clinical threshold measurement. The vibrators commonly used today are small in comparison with the old style and are coupled to the skull with a headband. Because the vibrators were developed originally as hearing aids, they generally produce a greater response in the middle frequencies, where speech cues are most important to the listener. The frequency response of the commonly used Radioear B-71 vibrator is shown in Fig. 6. The results were obtained with the bone vibrator coupled to an artificial mastoid with physical characteristics approximating the mechanical impedance of the skull. The artificial mastoid (artificial headbone) is used for calibrating bone vibrators for audiometric purposes. The recommended impedance values for its construction are contained in ANSI standard S3.13-1987 (39).

Threshold Measurements

To measure the magnitude of hearing loss, it is necessary to know the force level needed at a test frequency to produce the normal hearing threshold (0 db HL) for bone-conducted stimuli. After much investigative effort, such information has been accumulated, and standard

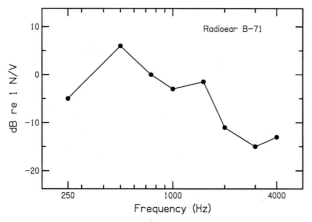

FIG. 6. Frequency response of the Radioear B-71 bone vibrator obtained on an artificial headbone conforming to ANSI S3.13-1987.

force levels necessary for normal thresholds of bone conduction have been recommended (ANSI S3.43-1992) (40). These reference levels are included in ANSI S3.6-1996 (1). The levels needed for normal thresholds are applicable to vibrators such as the Radioear B-71, which has a rounded vibrating tip of specific dimensions and is applied to the skull with a force of 5.4 ± 0.5 newtons. Although the vibrator mentioned previously (B-71), is one of several that conform to the standard in physical specifications, an application force of 5.4 newtons is seldom attained in clinical practice with commercially available headbands. The actual force level achieved with these headbands is determined by the tension of the headband and the size of the patient's skull. Because of these factors, some variability occurs in the force of vibrator application among individual patients.

The force level needed for normal threshold is also determined according to the location of the vibrator on the skull. The most sensitive thresholds are obtained when the vibrator is located on the mastoid process. There has been much interest in testing with the vibrator located on the forehead. This location results in less intersubject variability, but the thresholds are 6 to 15 dB less sensitive, depending on stimulus frequency, at the forehead than at the mastoid process. Thus most clinical tests of bone conduction thresholds are obtained with the vibrator located on the mastoid process.

Masking

During testing with standard supraaural earphones, the mass of the head provides an average interaural attenuation of 40 to 50 dB for air conduction measurements. For bone conduction, however, the interaural attenuation factor is negligible, because the entire skull vibrates regardless of the location of the vibrator on the head. As a consequence, it is generally necessary to use a masking noise in the nontest ear for testing by means of bone conduction. In the case of bilateral symmetric sensorineural hearing loss, however, in which the bone conduction thresholds are as poor as the air conduction thresholds, masking is not essential. Thus the presence of a sensorineural hearing loss in both ears can be documented without applying a masker as long as the magnitude of loss is approximately the same in both ears. The criteria for masking for bone conduction are stricter than those for air conduction. In general, whenever the bone conduction threshold in the test ear is 10 dB or more higher than the air conduction threshold in the same ear, masking must be applied to the contralateral ear.

A so-called masking dilemma occurs under any conditions in which it is not possible to effectively mask the nontest ear without risk for contralateral (test ear) interference from the masker. Such dilemmas are encountered clinically in examinations of patients with moderate to severe bilateral hearing loss when one or both ears have normal or near-normal bone conduction thresholds. The primary route of cross-cranial transmission from the test ear to the nontest cochlea is bone conduction for both air conduction and bone conduction testing. When testing is conducted with conventional supraaural earphones, two questions arise. First, are the air conduction thresholds an accurate reflection of the ear being tested, or do they represent cross-cranial transmission to the nontest ear? Second, can sufficient masking by air conduction be applied to the nontest ear to assure that the thresholds measured with bone conduction are from the cochlea of the ear being tested? When conventional earphones are used, the air conduction masking level needed to eliminate the nontest ear may be so high that the masking signal is transmitted to the opposite cochlea by means of cross-cranial conduction and increases the bone conduction threshold in the test ear. An example of a masking dilemma in bilateral asymmetric hearing loss is presented in Fig. 7.

When air conduction is tested, no dilemma exists. Air conduction thresholds in the left ear (see Fig. 7) are valid without masking because they do not exceed 40 dB HL, the conservative estimate of interaural attenuation for air conduction. Air and bone conduction thresholds from the right ear are valid because masking can be presented to the left ear without participation of the better, left ear and without risk that the masker will cross to the right cochlea. During testing of the air or bone conduction thresholds of the right ear, effective masking levels of 20 to 30 dB can safely be applied to the left ear before the masking stimulus crosses over to the right cochlea. An effective masking level of 30 dB indicates that the bone

conduction threshold in the test ear has been shifted 30 dB, sufficient to mask the nontest ear while the right ear thresholds are obtained.

The left ear bone conduction thresholds (see Fig. 7) reveal the masking dilemma. Questions arise concerning the validity of the unmasked bone conduction thresholds of the left ear. Are these thresholds valid, or do they simply reflect responses from the right ear? Unfortunately, the right ear air conduction threshold levels (~60 dB HL) preclude presentation of masking to the right ear without the masking stimulus crossing to the left cochlea and shifting the threshold of the cochlea being tested (left ear). In this example, the diagnostic dilemma is the unknown sensitivity of the left cochlea as estimated with the left ear bone conduction threshold. Other evaluation procedures, such as tympanometry and otologic examination, must be used to infer the condition of the left cochlea. More complicated masking dilemmas are encountered when there is bilateral symmetric air conduction hearing loss of greater magnitude than the example in Fig. 7.

The masking dilemma described in Fig. 7 may be reduced considerably with the use of insert earphones to deliver the masking stimulus. These earphones substantially increase the interaural attenuation for air conduction. Thus less sound is transmitted to the bones of the head, and transmission of the stimulus to the cochlea of either ear is reduced. When masking is insufficient for adequate decisions regarding the presence or degree of a conductive lesion in each ear, immittance measurements are of great diagnostic assistance in determining the presence or absence of a conductive lesion. These measurements are discussed in Chapter 12.

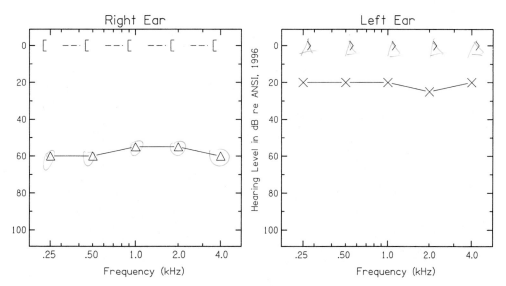

FIG. 7. Audiometric results for a patient with bilateral asymmetric hearing loss. *Right ear,* masked air conduction thresholds (Δ-Δ) and masked bone conduction thresholds ([-[). *Left ear,* unmasked air conduction thresholds (x-x) and unmasked bone conduction (>->) thresholds.

SUMMARY POINTS

- Pure tone air conduction audiometry is used to obtain an estimate of the magnitude of a hearing loss and forms the nucleus of auditory diagnostic testing.
- Thresholds of audibility are commonly measured at octave frequencies within the range of 0.25 kHz through 8.0 kHz. The sound pressure level (SPL) of the measured thresholds is expressed in hearing level (HL) and referenced at each test frequency to normal hearing sensitivity.
- The threshold of audibility usually is measured clinically with an earphone the output of which is calibrated in an artificial ear or coupler that approximates certain physical characteristics of an average ear.
- Air conduction thresholds may be measured in the sound field with a loudspeaker. Sound field testing often is used to obtain measurements in examinations of infants, young children, and difficult-to-test adults who cannot be fitted with or do not tolerate an earphone. Sound field thresholds are referenced to normal hearing sensitivity measured with a microphone located at the point in the sound field where the listener's head is to be positioned (substitution method).
- Whenever the air conduction presentation level to the test ear exceeds the bone conduction threshold in the opposite ear by more than approximately 40 dB, it is necessary to apply a masking signal to the nontest ear. The masking noise raises the threshold in the nontest ear and ensures that this ear does not contribute to the results for the test ear.
- Thresholds obtained by means of bone conduction provide an estimate of the integrity of the sensorineural auditory system. The difference between the thresholds of air and bone conduction indicates the magnitude of conductive hearing loss.
- Bone conduction thresholds are most often measured clinically with a vibrator located on the mastoid process. Bone-conducted stimuli are calibrated on an artificial mastoid the physical characteristics of which approximate the mechanical impedance of the skull.
- Masking of the nontest ear is routinely needed for measurement of bone conduction thresholds because the interaural attenuation for bone conduction is essentially 0 dB.

REFERENCES

1. American National Standards Institute. American national standard specifications for audiometers; ANSI-S3.6-1996. New York: ANSI, 1996.
2. Dadson R, King J. A determination of the normal threshold of hearing and its relation to the standardization of audiometers. *J Laryngol Otol* 1952;46:366–378.
3. Robinson D, Dadson R. A re-determination of the equal loudness relations for pure tones. *Br J Appl Physics* 1956;7:166–181.
4. Munson W, Weiner F. In search of the missing 6 dB. *J Acoust Soc Am* 1952;24:498–501.
5. Rudmose W. Pressure vs free-field thresholds at low frequencies. Proceedings of the 4th International Congress on Acoustics; Copenhagen 1962; paper H52.
6. Rudmose W. On the lack of agreement between earphone pressures and loudspeaker pressures for loudness balances at low frequencies. *J Acoust Soc Am* 1963;35:S1906(abst).
7. Villchur E. Free-field calibration of earphones. *J Acoust Soc Am* 1969; 46:1527–1534.
8. Shaw E, Piercy J. Audiometry and physiological noise. Proceedings of the 4th International Congress on Acoustics; Copenhagen 1962; paper H46.
9. Anderson C, Whittle L. Physiological noise and the missing 6 dB. *Acustica* 1971;24:261–272.
10. Killion M. Revised estimate of minimum audible pressure: where is the "missing 6 dB"? *J Acoust Soc Am* 1978;63:1501–1508.
11. Michael P, Bienvenue G. Real-ear threshold level comparisons between the telephonics TDH-39 earphone with a metal outer shell and the TDH-39, TDH-49, and TDH-50 earphones with plastic outer shells. *J Acoust Soc Am* 1977;61:1640–1642.
12. American National Standards Institute. American national standard for coupler calibration of earphones; ANSI S3.7-1986. New York: ANSI, 1986.
13. Zwislocki J. An acoustic coupler for earphone calibration: Rep-LSC-S-7. Syracuse, NY: Syracuse University Laboratory for Sensory Communication, 1970.
14. Zwislocki J. An acoustic coupler for earphone calibration: Rep-LSC-S-9. Syracuse, NY: Syracuse University Laboratory for Sensory Communication, 1971.
15. Zwislocki J. Theory of temporal auditory summation. *J Acoust Soc Am* 1960;32:1046–1060.
16. Watson C, Gengel R. Signal duration and signal frequency in relation to auditory sensitivity. *J Acoust Soc Am* 1969;46:989–998.
17. Olsen W, Rose D, Noffsinger PD. Brief-tone audiometry with normal, cochlear and eight nerve tumor patients. *Arch Otolaryngol* 1974;99: 185–191.
18. American Speech and Hearing Association. Guidelines for manual pure-tone threshold audiometry. *ASHA* 1978;20:297–305.
19. American Speech-Language-Hearing Association. Soundfield measurement tutorial. *ASHA* 1991;33[Suppl 3]:25–28.
20. American Speech-Language-Hearing Association. Guidelines for audiometric symbols. *ASHA* 1990;32[Suppl 2].
21. Wilbur L, Kruger B, Killion M. Reference thresholds for the ER-3A insert earphone. *J Acoust Soc Am* 1988;83:669–676.
22. American National Standards Institute. American national standard criteria for permissible ambient noise during audiometric testing; ANSI S3.1-1991. New York: ANSI, 1991.
23. Stelmachowicz PG, Beauchaine KA, Kalberer A, Jesteadt W. Normative thresholds in 8 to 20 kHz range as a function of age. *J Acoust Soc Am* 1989;86:1384–1391
24. Frank KT. High frequency hearing threshold in young adults using a commercially available audiometer. *Ear Hear* 1990;11:450.
25. Hughson W, Westlake H. Manual for program outline for rehabilitation of aural casualties both military and civilian. *Trans Am Acad Ophthalmol* 1944;[Otolaryngol Suppl]48:1–15.
26. Carhart R, Jerger J. Preferred method for clinical determination of pure-tone thresholds. *J Speech Hear Disord* 1959;24:330–345.
27. Zwislocki J. Acoustic attenuation between ears. *J Acoust Soc Am* 1953; 25:752–759.
28. Studebaker G. On masking in bone conduction testing. *J Speech Hear Res* 1962;5:215–227.
29. Studebaker G. Clinical masking. In: WF Rintelman, ed. *Hearing assessment.* Baltimore: University Park Press, 1979:51–100.

30. Fletcher H. Auditory patterns. *Rev Mod Physics* 1940;12:47–65.
31. Walker G, Dillon H, Bryne D. Sound field audiometry: recommended stimuli and procedures. *Ear Hear* 1984;5:13–21.
32. Morgan D, Dirks D, Bower D. Suggested threshold sound pressure levels for frequency modulated (warble) tones in the sound field. *J Speech Hear Disord* 1979;44:37–54.
33. Dirks D, Stream R, Wilson R. Speech audiometry: earphone and sound field. *J Speech Hear Dis* 1972;37:371–383.
34. Herzog H, Krainz W. Das Knochenleitungsproblem. Z Hals Usw Heilk 15 1926. Cited in Tonndorf J. Bone conduction. *Acta Otolaryngol* 1966; [Suppl 213].
35. Bekesy G. Zur theorie des horens bei der schallaufnahme durch knochenleitung. *Ann Physik* 1932;13:111–136.
36. Barany E. A contribution to the physiology of bone conduction. *Acta Otolaryngol* 1938;[Suppl 26]:1–223.
37. Tonndorf J. Bone conduction; studies in experimental animals. *Acta Otolaryngol* 1966;[Suppl 213]:1–65.
38. Carhart R. Effect of stapes fixation on bone conduction. In: Schuknecht HF, ed. *International Symposium on Otosclerosis.* Boston: Little, Brown, 1962.
39. American National Standards Institute. American national standard specification for mechanical coupler for measurement of bone vibrators; ANSI S3.13-1987. New York: ANSI, 1987.
40. American National Standards Institute. Standard reference zero for the calibration of pure-tone bone-conduction audiometers; ANSI S3.43-1992. New York: ANSI, 1992.

The Ear: Comprehensive Otology,
edited by R. F. Canalis and P. R. Lambert.
Lippincott Williams & Wilkins, Philadelphia © 2000.

CHAPTER 11

Measures of Auditory Function Using Speech Stimuli

Judy R. Dubno and Donald D. Dirks

The two principal purposes for conducting behavioral or electrophysiologic tests of the auditory system are to determine the type and location of auditory abnormalities and to evaluate receptive communication abilities. Measurement of pure tone air conduction and bone conduction thresholds provides important information about the function of the auditory system. However, these threshold measurements are obtained with frequency-specific stimuli (pure tones) and provide only limited information about a person's ability to hear more spectrally complex stimuli, such as speech, or to understand spoken syllables, words, or sentences. Because speech is the primary means by which people communicate, it is critical that evaluations of the auditory system include measurements of the ability to hear and understand speech. Audiometric

measurements with speech stimuli also are used to select and assess the benefit of amplification devices such as hearing aids; to determine candidacy, a suitable programming setting, or an appropriate signal-processing scheme for an electrical device such as a cochlear implant; and to measure benefit provided by an aural rehabilitation program. This chapter reviews traditional measures of auditory function with speech stimuli. These include the speech reception threshold (SRT), speech recognition (speech discrimination) score, and other measures, such as speech detection threshold, loudness discomfort level (LDL), and most comfortable listening level (MCL).

INSTRUMENTATION AND ELECTROACOUSTIC CALIBRATION OF SPEECH

Measures of auditory function with speech stimuli are conducted with an audiometer. In addition to generating, amplifying, and attenuating pure tone and other frequency-specific stimuli, an audiometer routes signals from a phonograph, audio tape player, compact disc

J. R. Dubno: Department of Otolaryngology and Communicative Sciences, Medical University of South Carolina, Charleston, South Carolina 29425

D. D. Dirks: Division of Head and Neck Surgery, University of California, Los Angeles, School of Medicine, Los Angeles, California 90095

player, digital audio tape player, or microphone; allows for monitoring of speech level with a volume unit (VU) meter; amplifies or attenuates speech signals; and delivers speech signals through earphones or loudspeakers. This equipment must conform to standards published by the American National Standards Institute (1). Specific procedures have been reviewed and explained by ASHA (2). Recommended procedures for calibration of signals through loudspeakers (i.e., in a soundfield) are discussed in Chapter 10.

Speech differs from pure tones in the temporal domain and in the frequency domain. Whereas a pure tone has most of its energy contained within a 1-Hz bandwidth, speech has energy across a wide frequency range. The frequency regions are not equal in intensity, primarily because of unique features of the human vocal tract and intensity differences of vowels and consonants. Thus speech level may be represented by a mathematical average of the waveforms of a large number of words or sentences recorded by many talkers. Intensity is computed within narrow frequency regions by means of Fourier analysis, and average intensity is plotted as a function of frequency. The result of this analysis is called a *long-term average speech spectrum*; an example is shown by the solid line in Fig. 1. In Fig. 1, the speech spectrum is defined in reference to auditory thresholds and is plotted on an audiogram. The shaded area indicates the dynamic range of speech energy (around 30 dB) from the least intense to the most intense speech sounds across frequency. For example, vowels are high-intensity, low to middle frequency sounds, whereas nasal sounds such as /m/ and /n/ are lower-intensity sounds with energy in the low to middle frequencies. Stop consonants, such as /b,d,g,p,t,k/, and fricative consonants, such as /f,v/, are low-intensity sounds with energy in the higher frequencies. The precise shape of the spectrum and the overall

level of the speech depend on several factors, including the number, sex, and vocal effort of the talkers, the type of speech items (syllables, words, sentences), and the length of silent periods included in the averaging. The shape of the long-term average speech spectrum is an important factor in interpreting the results of tests of auditory function using speech stimuli, especially for persons with elevated pure tone thresholds. This is discussed later.

AUDITORY THRESHOLDS FOR SPEECH STIMULI

Measurement of threshold for speech stimuli is traditionally considered part of the standard audiometric test battery. Like measurement of pure tone air conduction thresholds, it is an estimate of the magnitude of hearing loss for speech stimuli presented through an earphone. The rationale for incorporating a measurement of threshold for speech in an audiologic test battery often includes the following four points:

1. Because there is a strong association between thresholds for pure tones at certain frequencies and thresholds for speech, thresholds for speech may be used to verify the accuracy of pure tone thresholds.
2. Thresholds obtained with speech stimuli may be more valid indicators of a person's communication abilities than thresholds obtained with frequency-specific stimuli.
3. Thresholds for speech stimuli may be used to determine the sensation level (SL, or decibels relative to threshold) at which other speech materials are presented, such as the one-syllable words used to measure the speech recognition score.
4. For some patients, such as young children or persons with developmental disabilities, threshold measurements with speech stimuli may represent the only method available to obtain a reliable estimate of auditory sensitivity.

Although many terms have been used to describe the threshold for speech (speech recognition threshold, speech reception threshold, hearing loss for speech, and threshold of audibility), the term *speech reception threshold* (SRT) is used in this chapter.

Test Materials

Early audiometric tests with speech stimuli included lists of digits, nonsense syllables, and sentences and were often designed to obtain an articulation function, more commonly called a *performance-intensity function* (3,4). A performance-intensity function is analogous to a psychometric function in psychophysical experiments in which performance (e.g., proportion of total number of stimuli detected) is plotted as a function of one aspect of

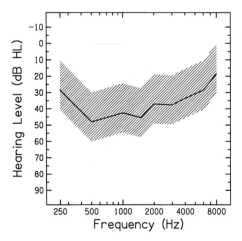

FIG. 1. Typical long-term average spectrum of speech (*solid line*). The *shaded area* indicates the range from the least intense to the most intense speech sounds across frequency.

the stimulus (e.g., intensity). That is, a psychometric function for speech plots the percentage of speech items correctly identified as a function of the intensity of the speech items. The intensity that corresponds to a specific point on the function (e.g., 50% correct) may be operationally defined as *threshold*. Under conditions in which the stimuli are very similar in familiarity, difficulty, and audibility, the percentage of words identified correctly should increase from 0% to 100% within a very narrow range of intensities, as is the case for a psychometric function for detection of a pure tone. However, differences in familiarity, difficulty, and audibility among the test items alter the shape and slope of the psychometric function and therefore the SRT estimated from that function. The rate at which speech recognition increases with intensity determines how precisely and rapidly the threshold may be determined.

In 1942, Hughson and Thompson (5) demonstrated that a relation existed between hearing loss for pure tones and the threshold of intelligibility for lists of sentences developed at the Bell Telephone Laboratories. This threshold for sentences was called the SRT. Later Carhart (6) determined that the threshold for the Bell Telephone sentences was similar to the threshold obtained for two-syllable words that have equal stress on each syllable (*spondaic words* or *spondees*). The term SRT has been used for the threshold obtained with spondees.

For the measurement of the SRT, Hudgins et al. (7), at the Psycho-Acoustics Laboratory at Harvard University, developed a list of 84 spondees and produced several test recordings. Words were selected according to their familiarity, to be homogeneous with respect to their thresholds, to provide a broad sample of English sounds, and to be phonetically distinct. These authors also suggested that thresholds correspond to the intensity at which 50% of the words are correctly identified. The psychometric function for the specific list of spondees should be relatively steep because, first, a fixed set of response choices is defined (closed set) rather than allowing listeners to respond with any word in their vocabulary (open set) and, second, two-syllable words composed of two one-syllable words (such as baseball and stairway) make it easy for listeners to guess correctly even if only part of the word is understood. As predicted, the slope of the psychometric function for the 84 spondees for normal-hearing listeners was steep, rising at a rate of 10%/dB. A typical psychometric function for spondees obtained from a group of normal-hearing individuals is shown in Fig. 2.

Some years later, researchers at the Central Institute for the Deaf (CID) in St. Louis (8) reported that the original list of 84 spondees contained some items that could be understood at substantially lower intensities than others. These authors also found that SRTs with the original list of test items had more intersubject variability than would be predicted from testing of subjects whose pure

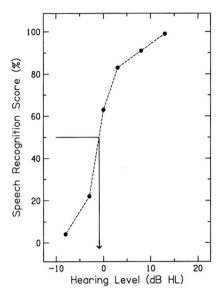

FIG. 2. Psychometric function for spondaic words obtained for normal-hearing listeners (*dashed line*). *Solid lines* and *arrow* indicate the speech level at which 50% performance is estimated (approximately 20 dB sound pressure level or 0 dB hearing level).

tone thresholds were nearly equivalent. In an effort to improve the homogeneity of the test materials, the list of words was shortened to 36 on the basis of additional tests of familiarity. The new list was recorded with each word following the carrier phrase "Say the word_____," and minor adjustments in intensity were made to equate intelligibility. With these recordings (known as CID Auditory Test W-1), mean SRT for normal-hearing listeners was approximately 20 dB sound pressure level (SPL). Performance increased from 0% to 100% over a 20-dB range, and the slope of the psychometric function was approximately 8%/dB.

The CID Auditory Test W-1 recording of 36 spondees has become standard for measurement of the SRT in most audiology clinics in the United States. Table 1 is an alphabetic list of the 36 words. To compare the SRT of a given

TABLE 1. *Alphabetic list of spondaic words used in Central Institute for the Deaf (CID) Auditory Test W-1*

airplane	eardrum	iceberg	railroad
armchair	farewell	inkwell	schoolboy
baseball	grandson	mousetrap	sidewalk
birthday	greyhound	mushroom	stairway
cowboy	hardware	northwest	sunset
daybreak	headlight	oatmeal	toothbrush
doormat	horseshoe	padlock	whitewash
drawbridge	hotdog	pancake	woodwork
duckpond	hothouse	playground	workshop

From Hirsh I, Davis H, Silverman S, Reynolds E, Eldert E, Benson R. Development of materials for speech audiometry. *J Speech Hear Disord* 1952;17:321–337, with permission.

person with normal results, the mean SRT for normal-hearing listeners (approximately 20 dB SPL) is equivalent to 0 dB hearing level (HL) for spondaic words when the SRT is measured through a specific type of earphone-cushion combination. The reference threshold corresponding to 0 dB HL for speech and reference levels for pure tones at frequencies ranging from 125 Hz to 8,000 Hz can be found in the American National Standards Institute standard S3.6-1996 (1).

Presentation of Test Materials

For threshold measurements, the initial presentation level for the test materials may be higher than the predicted SRT, each subsequent level decreasing to approach threshold. This is known as a *descending approach to threshold.* An ascending approach also may be chosen whereby a relatively low initial presentation level is selected, or a combination of approaches may be used (bracketing). Early investigations of the SRT (7,8) support the descending approach except in cases in which the patient's threshold may be exaggerated. Bracketing procedures tend to be less systematic than other approaches and therefore are not widely recommended for this purpose. Bracketing methods based on well-established psychophysical procedures, such as simple, up-down or forced-choice adaptive procedures, often are used in laboratory settings for the measurement of recognition thresholds for speech stimuli.

Although the preferred method for presenting speech items is by means of a standardized recording, it may be necessary for the audiologist to present each item to the patient through a microphone connected to the audiometer while monitoring the peak level of each item with the VU meter on the audiometer. This method, known as monitored live voice, introduces additional talker, level, and calibration differences that may affect the accuracy of the SRT. Under certain situations, however, including testing of young children, presentation of speech stimuli by means of monitored live voice provides the flexibility and speed that may be required.

Procedure for Determining Threshold

The most accurate procedure for determining threshold is to construct a psychometric function and identify the intensity corresponding to 50% performance. However, this is a time-consuming process and usually is not feasible in a clinical setting. The procedure adopted by ASHA in its Guidelines for Determining Threshold Level for Speech (9) has five steps: instructions, familiarization, determination of starting level, test phase, and calculation of the SRT. After instructions are given and the test words are reviewed, a descending technique is used to determine the starting level. During the test phase, two spondees are presented (one at a time) at the starting level and responses (correct or incorrect) are recorded on a worksheet. The presentation level is decreased by 2 dB, two more spondees are presented, and the patient's responses are recorded. This process is continued until the patient responds incorrectly to five of six words. Threshold is computed by means of subtracting the total number of correct responses from the starting level and adding a correction factor of 1. The procedure also accommodates a 5-dB step size; five test words are presented at each level, and a correction factor of 2 is added in the SRT computation.

Relation between Speech Reception Thresholds and Pure Tone Thresholds

SRT is an estimate of magnitude of hearing loss for speech stimuli presented through an earphone. Because pure tone air conduction thresholds also are measures of magnitude of hearing loss, it is reasonable to assume that pure tone thresholds and the SRT are highly correlated and that the SRT may be accurately predicted from pure tone thresholds.

The average of the three pure tone air conduction thresholds at 500, 1,000, and 2,000 Hz has been shown to provide a reasonably accurate estimate of the SRT and is equivalent to the predictive accuracy of more complex regression formulas and weighting strategies (6). However, for patients with large threshold differences at 500, 1,000, and 2,000 Hz, the three-frequency pure tone average (PTA) may lead to an overestimate of the SRT. For example, when pure tone thresholds at 500, 1,000, and 2,000 Hz are 15 dB HL, 15 dB HL, and 60 dB HL (PTA, 30 dB), an SRT of 30 dB HL is predicted. However, it would not be unreasonable for the SRT to be substantially lower than 30 dB HL and possibly closer to 15 to 20 dB HL. This is because of the combined effects of the near-normal auditory thresholds at 500 and 1,000 Hz and the long-term average spectrum for spondaic words, which is characterized by a peak in the lower-frequency region (similar to Fig. 1). In this case, a more accurate prediction of the SRT may be obtained from the average of the two better (lower) thresholds, referred to as the *Fletcher average* (10). The SRT may be considerably better than the three-frequency PTA in cases of suspected pseudohypacusis. The SRT may be worse than predicted from the PTA among patients with central auditory system abnormalities, cognitive or language disorders, or other nonauditory disorders that affect ability to repeat simple words. Despite the relatively high correlation between the three-frequency PTA and the SRT for spondees, spectral information contained in frequency regions below 500 Hz and above 2,000 Hz is important for speech recognition of other speech materials. Thus the SRT is necessarily restricted to assessment of a person's ability to understand highly redundant, easy-to-understand two-syllable words.

Summary

Although the SRT is well established in the audiologic testing battery, it is useful to review the purpose of this measurement and evaluate its contribution to the test battery. Wilson and Margolis (4) provided a detailed critique of each of the four points of the rationale for measuring the SRT. Although the SRT is considered a more appropriate indicator of communication ability than pure tone thresholds, the use of thresholds for easy-to-understand, two-syllable words measured with earphones for predicting performance in realistic listening conditions has questionable validity. These authors also suggest that the use of the SRT as a reference level for the measurement of speech recognition (speech discrimination) scores is somewhat arbitrary because the SRT is not a detection threshold. Moreover, SRTs are typically measured with two-syllable spondees, whereas speech recognition scores are commonly measured with one-syllable words. Nevertheless, the rationale for using the SRT as a reference level is traditionally based on empirical data identifying the level (decibels relative to the SRT) at which normal-hearing listeners obtain maximum speech recognition scores for specific speech materials. The SRT does, however, contribute important information in the evaluation of auditory function of patients whose pure tone thresholds are difficult to obtain or are highly unreliable (as may be the case for young children or patients who show evidence of pseudohypacusis).

MEASUREMENT OF SUPRATHRESHOLD SPEECH RECOGNITION (SPEECH DISCRIMINATION)

The second traditional measure of auditory function with speech stimuli is the speech recognition score. Although the SRT is a measure of magnitude of hearing loss for speech stimuli, the SRT does not provide evidence of a patient's ability to differentiate the sounds of speech at conversational levels. Rather than a threshold (in decibels), the speech recognition score is conventionally measured as the percentage of items correctly recognized by a listener at a suprathreshold level. Although many terms have been used to describe this measurement (most commonly speech discrimination score), the preferred term is *speech recognition score* because it is a more accurate description of the process and is consistent with accepted psychophysical terminology.

A speech recognition score ideally is obtained at several speech sensation levels (dB SL) or hearing levels for speech (dB HL). There are two principal reasons for measuring the speech recognition score—as a diagnostic tool to determine the site of auditory abnormality and as an indication of communication ability. In either case, it is important to determine a patient's maximum speech recognition performance rather than to obtain one score at an arbitrary speech level.

Test Materials and Procedures

During the 1940s, interest in speech recognition testing increased dramatically because of the need to evaluate telephone and other communication equipment. Early pioneers working at the Psycho-Acoustic Laboratory developed 50-item lists of commonly used monosyllabic words (11). Because the relative proportions of speech sounds in each list were approximately equivalent to their occurrences in English, the lists were considered to be phonetically balanced (PB) and therefore appropriate for measuring receptive communication ability. These lists were later adapted to evaluate speech recognition of persons with hearing losses. Hirsh et al. at CID (8) made additional modifications because these lists contained many unfamiliar words and did not completely meet the criterion of phonetic balance. The resulting test, known as CID Auditory Test W-22, consists of four 50-word PB lists recorded with the carrier phrase "You will say _____." The slope of the psychometric function for these materials (approximately 5.5%/dB) is less steep than for spondees, and the threshold is higher. This is because of differences in the homogeneity and size of the stimulus sets and difficulty of the test items. Typical psychometric functions for normal-hearing listeners for spondaic and monosyllabic words are shown in Fig. 3 (functions 1 and 2).

Lehiste and Peterson (12) developed lists of words of the consonant–nucleus (vowel)–consonant type using word familiarity and phonemic balance as the criteria for word selection. Investigators at Northwestern University (13,14) later reduced the number of consonant-nucleus-consonant items to improve phonemic balance and recorded four 50-word lists that have become known as

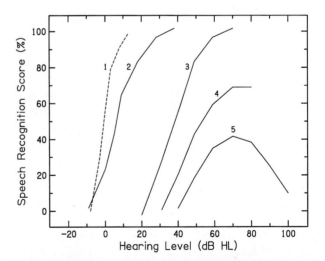

FIG. 3. Psychometric functions for spondaic words (*1*) and monosyllabic words (*2*) for normal-hearing listeners. Other psychometric functions are for monosyllabic words for a patient with conductive hearing loss (*3*), a patient with sensorineural hearing loss of cochlear origin (*4*), and a patient with an eighth-nerve lesion (*5*).

Northwestern University Test No. 6, or NU-6. CID Auditory Test W-22, NU-6 recordings, and an Auditec recording of the NU-6 lists are the most commonly used speech materials for measurement of the speech recognition score. Because of variations among different recordings of the same word lists, a speech recognition test is not the printed list of words but is the *recording* of the list.

Other test materials developed for determining the speech recognition score include closed-set nonsense syllable and monosyllabic word tests and sentence tests (15–17). A noteworthy example is the Speech Perception in Noise test, or SPIN (18). This test consists of lists of short, natural, English sentences. The listener is instructed to repeat the final word of the sentence. In half the sentences, contextual cues in the sentence provide information about the final word (for example, Stir your coffee with a *spoon*). The other half of the sentences includes the same set of final words without contextual information (for example, Bob could have known about the *spoon*). The sentences are presented in a background of speech-like noise (or babble), a recording of 12 people talking simultaneously. Because its spectral and temporal characteristics are similar to speech, babble provides a more realistic masker than white or other noise. Differences in final-word recognition for the two types of sentences suggest how well a listener is able to benefit from acoustic-phonetic cues and from linguistic-semantic (contextual) information.

Procedure for Determining the Speech Recognition Score

In the measurement of the speech recognition score, patients are presented 50 recorded monosyllabic words each in a carrier phrase. Traditionally each test word is scored as correct or incorrect regardless of the number of elements (consonants and vowels) that are repeated correctly. Thus the speech recognition score is the percentage of words correctly identified. By far the most important variable in the measurement of the speech recognition score is the intensity at which the test items are presented. Because the speech recognition score is intended to indicate a person's maximum performance, the preferred method is to obtain scores at several speech levels, plot the psychometric function, and find the maximum score (PB_{max}).

Unfortunately, measurement of the psychometric function for speech often is not practical in clinical settings because of time constraints. The most common clinical practice is to measure the speech recognition score at a single intensity. A relatively moderate intensity (30 to 40 dB above SRT) is chosen to increase the probability that the speech recognition score obtained is a reasonable estimate of PB_{max}. If test words are presented at only a single intensity, the speech recognition score should be interpreted not as a general assessment of receptive communication ability in everyday listening situations but as an indication of speech recognition ability under one particular condition. The question remains, for diagnostic purposes, whether a speech recognition score obtained at a single suprathreshold intensity can be used reliably to differentiate conductive and sensorineural hearing loss, hearing loss associated with cochlear and retrocochlear pathologic conditions, and cochlear abnormalities (see later).

Assessing the Diagnostic Value of Speech Recognition Scores

Measurement of speech recognition scores has traditionally been included as part of the standard audiometric testing battery for differential diagnosis of the site of an auditory abnormality. For test results to be used for this purpose, they must allow reliable and accurate assignment of diagnostic category (e.g., normal, conductive, cochlear, retrocochlear) or associate a particular pattern of results with a specific causation (e.g., Meniere's disease, presbycusis, ototoxicity). There is compelling evidence that a speech recognition score obtained at a single suprathreshold level selected to estimate PB_{max} is of limited diagnostic value because of the wide range of scores obtained within diagnostic or etiologic categories (16,19,20). For example, most patients with conductive hearing loss have near-normal speech recognition scores at high speech levels. However, at high speech levels many persons with sensorineural hearing loss of cochlear origin can also achieve relatively high speech recognition scores. For another example, whereas it is assumed that maximum speech recognition scores for patients with retrocochlear disease are disproportionately poor in relation to the magnitude of their pure tone hearing loss, persons with certain cochlear abnormalities also may have markedly reduced speech recognition. Some patients with eighth-nerve lesions may even have normal pure tone thresholds and speech recognition scores. In two studies involving large numbers of patients with retrocochlear abnormalities, PB_{max} for nearly half the patients was more than 60% (21), and no one had a score less than 30% (22). Thus PB_{max} ranges for persons with normal hearing, conductive hearing loss, and sensorineural hearing loss can overlap substantially. For differential diagnosis of auditory abnormalities, measurement of a speech recognition score at a single suprathreshold level may not confirm a diagnosis.

For diagnostic purposes, the preferred method is to obtain speech recognition scores at several speech levels and plot the psychometric function. Jerger and Jerger (23) observed distinguishing characteristics of the shapes of psychometric functions for various diagnostic categories of patients. They suggested that sensorineural hearing loss of cochlear and retrocochlear origin may be differentiated on the basis of a change in speech recognition scores with increasing intensities. Representative psychometric functions obtained for monosyllabic words for persons with hearing losses are shown in Fig. 3 (functions 3 through 5). In the presence of conductive hearing loss (function 3), the function is parallel to the function obtained for a normal-hearing listener (function 2) but is shifted to the right because of the magnitude of the hearing loss. That is, scores equivalent to normal are obtained when speech levels are increased by approximately 30 dB. For the patient with cochlear hearing loss (function 4), PB_{max} is reduced (70%) at higher speech levels, and scores remain constant with further increases in speech level. In contrast, the function for a patient with a retrocochlear lesion (function 5) shows reduced PB_{max} (40%) with further increases in speech level that cause marked decreases in scores, often called *rollover*.

The *rollover index* is a normalized ratio of differences between PB_{max} and the minimum score (PB_{min}) obtained at an intensity higher than that yielding PB_{max}. When PB_{max} and PB_{min} are determined with small-intensity step sizes, the rollover index has been shown to aid categorization of patients with cochlear and retrocochlear lesions (24). Because of differences in test materials and procedures among clinics, a criterion rollover index for differentiating cochlear and retrocochlear abnormalities should be determined by individual clinics (24).

Because measurement of a psychometric function is time consuming and other objective differential diagnostic measures are routine (including otoacoustic emissions, acoustic reflex measures, and auditory brainstem responses), the use of speech recognition scores for differentiating conductive and sensorineural hearing loss and disorders of the cochlea and eighth nerve has diminished in importance in recent years. Nevertheless, diagnostic measurements with speech stimuli remain an important component of the battery of tests used in the evaluation of the central auditory nervous system (see Chapter 15).

Assessing the Variability of Speech Recognition Scores

Measures of auditory function with speech stimuli are often used to assess and monitor benefit derived from rehabilitation or other treatment programs and to differentiate listening conditions. For example, the success of medical or surgical intervention may be evaluated with comparisons of speech recognition scores before and after treatment. If the criterion for benefit or success provided by a treatment is defined by improvement in speech recognition, it is necessary to compute the change in speech recognition score that is considered statistically significant. That is, a significant change in performance must be a result of the change in condition (i.e., surgery, hearing aid, rehabilitation) and not simply the normal variation in scores expected with a particular test. To determine this critical difference, it is important to understand the factors that determine the variability associated with speech recognition scores.

In 1978, Thornton and Raffin (25) proposed a simple model to describe the variability associated with speech recognition scores. Using an approximation of the binomial model, they computed 95% critical differences for each percentage score for commonly used numbers of test items (100, 50, 25, and 10 items). Critical differences for 50-, 25-, and 10-item lists are shown in Table 2. Once a score is obtained with a particular test list, values in the table may be used to determine the score that must be achieved in a second administration of the test to be considered statistically significantly different from the first score (with 95% probability). For example, consider a score of 40%. If that score were obtained with a 50-item list, there is a 95% probability that a score between 22% and 58% would be obtained on a second 50-item list. In other words, if the initial test score on a 50-item test were 40%, only a score greater than 58% (at least an 18% increase) would represent a significant improvement in performance. For a 25-item test, scores between 16% and 64% would be predicted if the initial test score was 40% and for a 10-item test, scores on a second test may range between 10% and 80%. Table 2 also shows how critical differences change with initial test score. For a 50-item list, if the first score is 80%, only a score greater than 92% (12% improvement) exceeds the critical difference.

To review, two factors that determine variance of speech recognition scores are the score itself and the number of items in the test. The shorter the test list, the larger is the change in performance required to exceed the critical difference. Although decreasing the number of test items presented in a speech recognition test often is suggested as a means of decreasing testing time, one important consequence of shorter test lists is increased test variability. Most important, evaluation of treatment benefit or success with speech recognition scores must be accomplished by estimating the variability associated with repeated test measurement, as described by the critical differences shown in Table 2.

Another important issue concerning interpretation of a speech recognition score is whether a patient's maximum speech recognition score is significantly poorer than expected on the basis of that patient's pure tone thresholds. To make such a determination, it is necessary to consider the normal range (or confidence limit) of PB_{max} associated with a particular set of speech materials and degree of hearing loss. A 95% confidence limit has been defined for PB_{max} from NU-6 speech recognition scores obtained with a large group of persons with confirmed cochlear hearing loss (26). PB_{max} values corresponding to the lower boundary of the confidence limit are provided in tables for a range of PTAs. If PB_{max} determined from a psychometric function is poorer than the table value, PB_{max} may be considered disproportionately poor in rela-

TABLE 2. *Lower and upper limits of the 95% critical differences for percentage scores for 50-item, 25-item, and 10-item test lists*

Score (%)	$n = 50$	$n = 25$	$n = 10$
0	0–4	0–8	0–20
2	0–10		
4	0–14	0–20	
6	2–18		
8	2–22	0–28	
10	2–24		0–50
12	4–26	4–32	
14	4–30		
16	6–32	4–40	
18	6–34		
20	8–36	4–44	0–60
22	8–40		
24	10–42	8–48	
26	12–44		
28	14–46	8–52	
30	14–48		10–70
32	16–50	12–56	
34	18–52		
36	20–54	16–60	
38	22–56		
40	22–58	16–64	10–80
42	24–60		
44	26–62	20–68	
46	28–64		
48	30–66	24–72	
50	32–68		10–90
52	34–70	28–76	
54	36–72		
56	38–74	32–80	
58	40–76		
60	42–78	36–84	20–90
62	44–78		
64	46–80	40–84	
66	48–82		
68	50–84	44–88	
70	52–86		30–90
72	54–86	48–92	
74	56–88		
76	78–90	52–92	
78	60–92		
80	64–92	56–96	40–100
82	66–94		
84	68–94	60–96	
86	70–96		
88	74–96	68–96	
90	76–98		50–100
92	78–98	72–100	
94	82–98		
96	86–100	80–100	
98	90–100		
100	96–100	92–100	80–100

Values within the range shown are not significantly different from the value shown in the percentage score column ($p > .05$).

From Thornton A, Raffin M. Speech discrimination scores modeled as a binomial variable. *J Speech Hear Res* 1978;21:507–518, with permission.

tion to the degree of hearing loss. If a single score obtained at an arbitrary suprathreshold level is poorer than the 95% confidence limit, that score may lead to underestimation of PB_{max}. In that case, speech recognition should be measured at additional speech levels to obtain a more reasonable estimate of the patient's maximum speech recognition.

Auditory Thresholds and the Speech Spectrum

There is a strong relation between magnitude of hearing loss assessed with pure tone thresholds and those assessed with SRTs, such that the SRT may be accurately predicted on the basis of the three-frequency PTA. However, the relation between auditory sensitivity and speech recognition is more complex. As a result, it is difficult to use pure tone thresholds to predict the speech recognition score of a person with a hearing loss. For persons with sensorineural hearing loss of cochlear origin, the speech recognition score is primarily determined by the sensation level of the speech across a wide frequency range and the level and spectrum of any background noise. Predicting speech recognition scores for a particular patient and listening condition is difficult because (a) speech level varies as a function of frequency (see Fig. 1), (b) thresholds of most listeners with hearing losses are not elevated equally across frequency, and (c) each frequency region of the speech spectrum does not provide an equal contribution to recognition. Illustrations of the interactions among speech spectrum, speech level, and auditory thresholds are provided in Figs. 4–6.

Figure 4 displays pure tone thresholds (in dB HL) of a normal-hearing listener and the long-term average spectrum of speech at a level typical for conversational speech. Even the lower limit of speech energy is substantially above the listener's thresholds. For the speech spec-

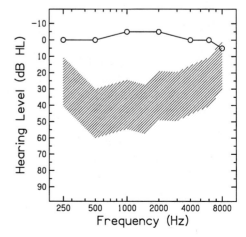

FIG. 4. Auditory thresholds of a normal-hearing listener (○-○) and the long-term average spectrum of speech (*shaded areas*).

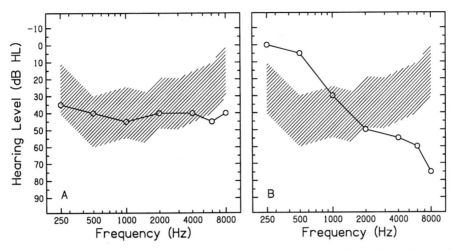

FIG. 5. Auditory thresholds (○-○) of a listener with a hearing loss with a flat audiometric configuration **(A)** and a steeply sloping audiometric configuration **(B)** plotted with the long-term average spectrum of speech.

trum depicted in Fig. 4, this person should achieve an excellent speech recognition score. Figure 5A displays pure tone thresholds (in dB HL) for a person with sensorineural hearing loss of cochlear origin with a relatively flat audiometric configuration. The identical speech spectrum is plotted in Fig. 5B along with thresholds of a person with a steeply sloping audiometric configuration, that is, higher thresholds for higher frequency signals. Several important points are illustrated in this figure. For the person with a flat audiometric configuration (see Fig. 5A), only the more intense speech sounds, such as vowels, are above threshold, although not as much above threshold as for the normal-hearing listener in Fig. 4. Most higher-frequency speech sounds, such as stop and fricative consonants, are below threshold. For the person with a steeply sloping configuration (see Fig. 5B), the lower-frequency speech sounds are substantially above threshold, but

essentially no speech information above 2,000 Hz is audible. For these persons and the speech spectrum depicted, speech recognition scores are likely to be reduced as a result of decreased speech audibility. The same two audiograms are shown in Fig. 6, but there the overall speech level has been increased 20 dB, as might be provided by increasing the output of an audiometer or with a hearing aid with uniform amplification. With speech level increased, all but the highest-frequency speech sounds are audible for the person with a flat audiometric configuration (see Fig. 6A), and the speech recognition score is likely to improve. However, for the person with steeply sloping hearing loss (see Fig. 6B), low-frequency sounds are even louder, but only the highest-intensity high frequency sounds are audible. The speech recognition score may improve only slightly. For this person, selective amplification of the higher-frequency portion of

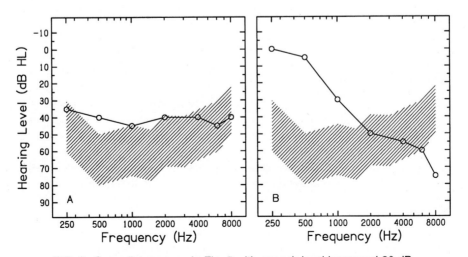

FIG. 6. Same listeners as in Fig. 5 with speech level increased 20 dB.

the speech spectrum would be required to make certain consonant sounds audible.

Summary

Since the speech recognition score was added to the standard audiometric test battery, emphasis has been placed on its diagnostic value. Although the most common clinical practice is to measure speech recognition at a single suprathreshold level, these results have been shown to have limited diagnostic value for differentiating conductive, cochlear, and retrocochlear disorders. Although designed for diagnostic purposes, speech recognition test methods often are criticized when results are poorly correlated with patients' reports of communication difficulties outside the clinic environment. The use of speech recognition scores for other applications may require substantial changes in stimuli and procedures to improve the efficiency and effectiveness of the test for that particular application. For example, the use of sentences or conversational speech as test materials, rather than monosyllabic words, may improve assessment of communicative function. Sentences or running speech may be presented in the soundfield, rather than through an earphone, with a diffuse background of speech-like noise or babble presented from multiple loudspeakers. The value of speech recognition scores in the selection of appropriate amplification devices continues to be controversial because of the poor reliability and sensitivity associated with the tests. The introduction of real-ear probe microphone methods and other objective measures of the electroacoustic characteristics of hearing aids for selecting and verifying amplification parameters has reduced the need for speech tests for this purpose. Other uses of speech stimuli, such as differentiating hearing aids on the basis of paired comparison judgments of the quality of speech, may replace (or more likely be used in addition to) speech recognition scores as part of the hearing aid evaluation test battery. This topic is discussed in more detail in Chapter 37.

MASKING FOR MEASUREMENTS OF SPEECH RECOGNITION THRESHOLD AND SPEECH RECOGNITION SCORE

In Chapter 10 pure tone air conduction results are described in which large differences in thresholds between the right and left ears are obtained (see Chapter 10, Fig. 4). In cases in which the air conduction presentation level in the test ear exceeds the bone conduction threshold in the nontest ear by more than the conservative estimate of intraaural attenuation (40 dB), a masker must be introduced to the nontest ear at a level that will not influence the measurement in the test ear. This same rule applies in the measurement of both the SRT and, more commonly, the speech recognition score. Because of the broad spectral composition of speech stimuli, special considerations apply in judging when masking is needed, selecting a masker, and determining effective masking levels.

The rule for determining the need for masking in the measurement of pure tone air conduction thresholds compares air conduction and bone conduction thresholds at the same pure tone frequency. However, speech contains energy at a broad range of frequencies, and the frequency regions of the speech spectrum are not equally intense (see Fig. 1). To determine the need for masking for measurements with speech stimuli, the difference between the speech presentation level in the test ear and the best (most sensitive) bone conduction threshold in the nontest ear is computed. If that difference exceeds the conservative estimate of intraaural attenuation (40 dB), a masker must be introduced to the nontest ear at a level that will not influence the measurement in the test ear. Because the speech presentation level in the test ear (not the SRT) is one factor that determines the need for masking the nontest ear, masking is needed more often during the measurement of the speech recognition score because the speech presentation level used for that suprathreshold test is necessarily high. Given the characteristics of the speech spectrum, a broadband masker with spectral characteristics similar to speech is used rather than the narrowband masker used in pure tone threshold measurements. Determining effective masking levels is somewhat more difficult for speech stimuli because a masked threshold for speech stimuli (the level to which the SRT is shifted in the presence of a masker) is somewhat more difficult to predict than masked pure tone thresholds. Details of determining effective masking for speech stimuli are beyond the scope of this chapter but are provided elsewhere (16, 27).

OTHER MEASURES OF AUDITORY FUNCTION WITH SPEECH STIMULI

Speech Detection Threshold

Several additional measurements with speech stimuli may be used in the evaluation of the auditory system. The speech detection threshold is obtained instead of the SRT in examinations of patients who cannot provide a response that indicates recognition of the stimulus. Patients are conditioned to respond when they detect the stimulus and do not have to provide correct recognition. This measurement may be used with young children, patients who do not speak English, patients whose exceptionally poor speech recognition ability makes them unable to recognize spondaic words, or patients with profound hearing loss whose SRTs (if measurable) exceed the output limitations of the audiometer. The speech detection threshold is 8 to 9 dB lower (better) than the

SRT (28,29), partly because of differences in the nature of the task (detection versus recognition).

Loudness Discomfort Level

The LDL is the level at which a listener describes an auditory stimulus as uncomfortably loud. This measurement may be made with pure tone, noise, or speech stimuli. Many studies have reported complex effects of instruction set, measurement procedure, stimuli, and magnitude of hearing loss on the LDL. Results obtained by Kamm et al. (30) revealed a nonlinear relation between sensorineural hearing loss and the LDL; LDL increased with hearing loss but only when thresholds exceeded approximately 50 dB HL. Because the LDL does not increase at the same rate as threshold, persons with sensorineural hearing loss must function with a substantially reduced range of hearing (the difference in decibels between threshold and LDL). Most important, large individual differences in LDL often are found among listeners with hearing losses, suggesting that it is difficult to predict LDL from pure tone thresholds or the SRT. Nevertheless, carefully controlled measurement of the LDL with well-established psychophysical procedures provides important information about the ability of a person with a hearing loss to tolerate high-level speech, especially amplified speech.

Most Comfortable Listening Level

The MCL is a range of levels (approximately 20 dB) a listener considers to be comfortable rather than a specific intensity (31). Even when considering that the MCL encompasses a range of levels, large intersubject variability has been observed, making it necessary to measure the MCL directly rather than attempting to predict the MCL from pure tone thresholds or SRTs. Although measurement of the MCL is widely recommended, especially in conjunction with hearing aid evaluations, questions related to its reliability, validity, and rationale have not been thoroughly resolved. For example, selection of gain settings of a hearing aid based on MCL does not take into account the fact that the MCL is a range of levels and that input intensities (conversational speech levels) vary widely (32).

SUMMARY POINTS

- Because speech is the primary means by which persons communicate, it is important that functional evaluation of the auditory system include measurements of the ability to hear and understand speech.
- The speech recognition threshold is an estimate of hearing loss for speech and is strongly associated with the pure tone average among most persons. It is the level, in decibels, at which a person correctly repeats 50% of a list of highly redundant, two-syllable words.
- For some patients, such as young children or those with developmental disabilities, the SRT may be the only method available to obtain a reliable estimate of auditory sensitivity.
- The speech recognition score is used to measure a person's ability to differentiate the sounds of speech at conversational levels. It is the percentage of items correctly repeated by a listener at a particular level and is strongly associated with the audibility of speech sounds across a wide frequency range.

- The speech recognition score may be used for diagnostic purposes, to evaluate receptive communication abilities, or to assess and monitor benefit derived from rehabilitation or other treatment.
- Regardless of the purpose of the test, the speech recognition score is intended to indicate a person's maximum performance. As such, the preferred method is to obtain scores at several speech levels and determine the maximum score (PB_{max}).
- A speech recognition score obtained at a single level selected to estimate PB_{max} is of little diagnostic value because of the wide range of scores obtained within diagnostic or etiologic categories.
- Evaluation of treatment benefit or success with speech recognition scores must take into account the normal variation in scores expected with a particular test and determine the change in score considered statistically significant.

ACKNOWLEDGMENTS

This work was supported in part by grants from the National Institute on Deafness and Other Communication Disorders, National Institutes of Health. The authors thank Jayne B. Ahlstrom and Amy R. Horwitz for editorial contributions.

REFERENCES

1. American National Standards Institute. American national standard specifications for audiometers; ANSI S3.6-1996. New York: ANSI, 1996.
2. American Speech-Language-Hearing Association. Calibration of speech signals delivered via earphones. *ASHA* 1987;29:44–48.
3. Tillman T, Olsen W. Speech audiometry. In: Jerger J, ed. *Modern developments in audiology*. New York: Academic Press, 1973:37–74.
4. Wilson R, Margolis R. Measurement of auditory thresholds for speech stimuli. In: Konkle D, Rintelmann W, eds. *Principles of speech audiometry*. Baltimore: Academic Press, 1983:79–126.
5. Hughson W, Thompson E. Correlation of hearing acuity for speech with discrete frequency audiograms. *Arch Otolaryngol* 1942;36:526–540.
6. Carhart R. Speech reception in relation to patterns of pure tone loss. *J Speech Disord* 1946;11:97–108.

7. Hudgins C, Hawkins J, Karlin J, Stevens S. The development of recorded auditory tests for measuring hearing loss for speech. *Laryngoscope* 1947;57:57–89.

8. Hirsh I, Davis H, Silverman S, Reynolds E, Eldert E, Benson R. Development of materials for speech audiometry. *J Speech Hear Disord* 1952;17:321–337.

9. American Speech-Language-Hearing Association. Guidelines for determining threshold levels for speech. *ASHA* 1988;30:85–89.

10. Fletcher H. A method of calculating hearing loss for speech from an audiogram. *J Acoust Soc Am* 1950;22:1–5.

11. Egan J. Articulation testing methods. *Laryngoscope* 1948;58:955–991.

12. Lehiste I, Peterson G. Linguistic considerations in the study of speech intelligibility. *J Acoust Soc Am* 1959;31:280–286.

13. Tillman T, Carhart R, Wilber L. A test for speech discrimination composed of CNC monosyllabic words (Northwestern University auditory test no. 4); technical report SAM-TDR-62-135. Brooks Air Force Base, TX: USAF School of Aerospace Medicine, Aerospace Medical Division, 1963.

14. Tillman T, Carhart R. An expanded test for speech discrimination utilizing CNC monosyllabic words (Northwestern University auditory test no. 6); technical report SAM-TR-66-55. Brooks Air Force Base, Texas; USAF School of Aerospace Medicine, Aerospace Medical Division, 1966.

15. Olsen W, Matkin N. Speech audiometry. In: Rintelmann W, ed. *Hearing assessment*. Baltimore: University Park Press, 1979:133–206.

16. Bess F. Clinical assessment of speech recognition. In: Konkle D, Rintelmann W, eds. *Principles of speech audiometry*. Baltimore: Academic Press, 1983:127–201.

17. Dirks D, Dubno J. Speech audiometry. In: Jerger J, ed. *Hearing disorders in adults*. San Diego: College Hill Press, 1984:85–113.

18. Kalikow D, Stevens K, Elliott L. Development of a test of speech intelligibility in noise using test materials with controlled word predictability. *J Acoust Soc Am* 1977;61:1337–1351.

19. Carhart R. Problems in the measurement of speech discrimination. *Arch Otolaryngol* 1965;82:253–260.

20. Sanders J, Josey A, Glasscock M. Audiologic evaluation in cochlear and eighth-nerve disorders. *Arch Otolaryngol* 1974;100:283–289.

21. Johnson E. Auditory test results in 500 cases of acoustic neuroma. *Arch Otolaryngol* 1977;103:152–158.

22. Olsen W, Noffsinger D, Kurdziel S. Speech discrimination in quiet and in white noise by patients with peripheral and central lesions. *Acta Otolaryngol* 1975;80:375–382.

23. Jerger J, Jerger S. Diagnostic significance of PB word functions. *Arch Otolaryngol* 1971;93:573–580.

24. Dirks D, Kamm C, Bower D, Betsworth A. Use of performance-intensity functions for diagnosis. *J Speech Hear Disord* 1977;42:408–415.

25. Thornton A, Raffin M. Speech discrimination scores modeled as a binomial variable. *J Speech Hear Res* 1978;21:507–518.

26. Dubno J, Lee F, Klein A, Matthews L, Lam C. Confidence limits for maximum word-recognition scores. *J Speech Hear Res* 1995;38: 490–502.

27. Studebaker G. Clinical masking. In: Rintelmann W, ed. *Hearing assessment*. Baltimore: University Park Press, 1979:51–100.

28. Thurlow W, Silverman S, Davis H, Walsh T. A statistical study of auditory tests in relation to the fenestration operation. *Laryngoscope* 1948; 58:43–66.

29. Chaiklin J. The relation among three selected auditory speech thresholds. *J Speech Hear Res* 1959;2:237–243.

30. Kamm C, Dirks D, Mickey M. Effect of sensorineural hearing loss on loudness discomfort level. *J Speech Hear Res* 1978;21:668–681.

31. Dirks D, Kamm C. Psychometric functions for loudness discomfort and most comfortable loudness levels. *J Speech Hear Res* 1976;19: 613–627.

32. Dirks D, Morgan D. Measures of discomfort and most comfortable loudness. In: Konkle D, Rintelmann W, eds. *Principles of speech audiometry*. Baltimore: Academic Press, 1983:203–229.

The Ear: Comprehensive Otology,
edited by R. F. Canalis and P. R. Lambert.
Lippincott Williams & Wilkins, Philadelphia © 2000.

CHAPTER 12

Tympanometry and Acoustic Reflex Testing

Donald D. Dirks and Donald E. Morgan

Acoustic Immittance
  Physiologic Considerations
  Stiffness, Mass, and
    Friction

Measuring Acoustic Immittance
Tympanometry
Tympanogram Types
Summary

Relative impedance measurements for auditory diagnosis were pioneered by the classic work of Metz (1) in 1946. From these investigations, the objective tests of tympanometry and acoustic reflex measures were developed and have become part of the routine diagnostic strategy for distinguishing between conductive and sensorineural hearing loss, as well as among the various sources for sensorineural hearing loss. Stapedius muscle contraction (acoustic reflex) to a loud sound is indirectly identifiable using acoustic immittance measures and may be differentially affected by conductive, cochlear, eighth cranial nerve, and brainstem disorders.

ACOUSTIC IMMITTANCE

Physiologic Considerations

Acoustic immittance is a generic term that refers to the efficiency of the transmission of energy in an acoustic medium. The transmission of energy in any system can be expressed in terms of the opposition to the flow of energy (impedance) or by the reciprocal of impedance, termed admittance. As applied to the human peripheral auditory system, the transmission of acoustic energy occurs when sound waves in the external ear canal are applied to the tympanic membrane. When sufficient sound pressure is applied, energy is transmitted from the tympanic membrane, via the middle ear system, to the cochlear fluids.

The middle ear plays an especially important role in transmitting the sound waves in the air to the fluid in the cochlea. Sound waves in one medium (air) do not readily pass to another medium (fluid) of different acoustic properties. In such a highly inefficient system, less than 1% of the energy contained in the aerial waves would be transmitted to the fluid. The loss in transmission would amount to nearly 30 dB because of the inherent mismatch in acoustic impedance between the two media. The middle ear system acts as an acoustic transformer to minimize this impedance mismatch. Specifically, the middle ear achieves its transformer action by two processes, the lever action of the ossicular chain and a hydraulic action that arises from the difference in surface area between the tympanic membrane and stapedial footplate. The complex structure of the middle ear makes it difficult to determine the physical basis for the lever action. The lever action of the ossicular chain, as reviewed by Wever and Lawrence (2), is related to the manner of suspension of the malleus, the nature of the joint between the malleus and incus, and the manner in which the incus is anchored. The ossicular lever ratio in man is about 1.31. The anatomic ratio between the drum membrane and the stapes footplate is approximately 21.0 and the effective ratio (as the entire tympanic membrane does not vibrate) is about 14.0. Thus, the transmission provided by the middle ear is a combination of these two ratios or $14.0 \times 1.31 = 18.3$.

Any change in the physical properties of the middle ear system (due to various disease processes) is likely to affect the efficiency with which energy is transmitted through the middle ear. Such changes can be measured at the plane of the tympanic membrane in admittance (or impedance). The practical measurement of acoustic immittance became a reality with the development of an electromechanical

D. D. Dirks: Division of Head and Neck Surgery, University of California, Los Angeles, School of Medicine, Los Angeles, California 90095

D. E. Morgan: Decibel Instruments, Inc., Fremont, California 94555

acoustic impedance bridge by Schuster (3) in 1934. Later, Metz (1) applied impedance measurements to the differential diagnosis of auditory disorders.

In 1946, Metz observed that a change in impedance at the tympanic membrane occurred when a loud sound was applied to the ear contralateral to the test ear fitted with an impedance bridge. This phenomenon was later identified to be a secondary consequence of the reflexive contraction of the middle ear muscles. The tensor tympani (anterior wall of the middle ear to the malleus) and the stapedius (posterior wall of the middle ear to the neck of the stapes) muscles attach directly to the ossicular chain; thus, their contractions lead to a change in energy transfer at the tympanic membrane. In humans, the tensor tympani typically does not contract to acoustic stimulation; thus, the stapedius muscle is primarily responsible for the immittance change at the tympanic membrane when a loud sound is presented to the ear.

Nearly all currently available immittance instruments used in auditory diagnosis measure acoustic admittance. Therefore, the discussion and examples in this chapter focus on admittance rather than impedance measurements. The admittance /Y/ of a system can be measured by applying a known force and measuring the resultant velocity. So, for example, if the same force is applied to two objects, the one with the higher admittance will move at a faster velocity than the object with the lower admittance.

Stiffness, Mass, and Friction

The elements of stiffness (compliance), mass, and friction contribute interactively to the admittance of any mechanoacoustic system. The admittance of a compliant element is called compliant susceptance (Bc). The tympanic membrane, ligaments, and tendons of the middle ear contribute to stiffness. Compliance in admittance terminology is associated with the stiffness of the mechanical system. Examples of mass are the pars flaccida of the tympanic membrane, the middle ear ossicles, and the perilymph in the cochlea. The admittance offered by the mass elements is known as mass susceptance (-Bm). Friction arises primarily from the joints between the bones of the ossicular chain and from the associated membranes, tendons, and ligaments of the middle ear. This element, called conductance (G) in admittance terminology, dissipates or absorbs acoustic energy. In the human ear, friction is a minor contributor to the overall admittance measured at low-frequency probe tones.

Stiffness and mass vary as a function of probe frequency, with stiffness affecting the transmission of low-frequency energy and mass affecting high-frequency transmission. When the admittance of the middle ear is measured with a low-frequency probe tone, the stiffness elements are the major contributors to the admittance measured at the plane of the tympanic membrane. For low frequencies, the middle ear transmission system is

stiffness controlled. Thus, middle ear disorders that increase stiffness, such as otosclerosis and middle ear effusion, have the greatest effect on the transmission of low-frequency signals. When admittance is measured using a high-frequency probe tone, the mass elements are the primary contributors to the admittance measurement. As the mass of the middle ear increases, hearing will decrease in the high frequencies. It may already be intuitive that the measured admittance value provides (a) objective evidence regarding the integrity of the middle ear transmission system (presence or absence of a conductive impairment) and (b) depending on whether the system is stiffness or mass controlled, information regarding the effects of the disorder on the transmission of frequency-specific energy.

Measuring Acoustic Immittance

A simplified block diagram of an acoustic immittance system is shown in Fig. 1. All commercially available clinical instruments use acoustic energy to measure the combined admittance of the ear canal and middle ear. The instrument is coupled to the ear by a probe tip that is hermetically sealed in the ear canal by a soft rubber or foam cuff. The probe tip contains openings connected to three basic subsystems of an immittance measuring instrument. One opening leads to a manometer by which air pressure in the external auditory canal can be controlled. In most commercially available systems, the air pressure in the canal is varied automatically (by electrical pump), and the resulting changes in admittance are synchronized in the analysis system to provide a graphic representation of changes in admittance as a function of changes in ear canal air pressure (in daPa). A second probe tip opening connects to a sound generator and associated transducer to introduce both the probe tone (used to measure admittance) and/or

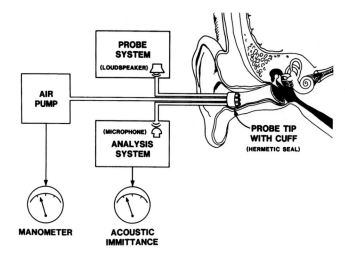

FIG.1. Simplified block diagram of an acoustic immittance system. (From Katz J, ed. *Handbook of clinical audiology.* Baltimore: Williams & Wilkins, 1985:425, with permission.)

the reflex-activating signals. The third opening in the probe tip is connected to the microphone leading to the analysis system, which monitors the sound pressure level changes that occur as the admittance at the tympanic membrane varies due to either changes in the air pressure in the external ear canal or contraction of the stapedius muscle.

In the instrument design shown in Fig. 1, the probe and analysis systems indirectly estimate the acoustic admittance in the ear by monitoring sound pressure levels in the ear canal at the probe tip. The acoustic admittance at the probe tip represents the combined effects of the ear canal, the middle ear structures, and, to a very limited extent, the cochlea. The admittance measured is the complex interaction of stiffness, mass, and friction provided by the physical properties of the middle ear structures and the frequency of the probe tone.

Tympanometry

Tympanometry is the measurement of acoustic immittance at the plane of the tympanic membrane as a function of air pressure change in the external ear canal. The specifications for the terminology and instrumentation used for this measure have been standardized by the American National Standards Institute (ANSI S3.39-1987) (4). The graphic display of the tympanometric data is called a tympanogram. It is used principally to evaluate the integrity of the middle ear transmission system and to estimate middle ear pressure and the equivalent volume of the ear canal and middle ear.

Terkildsen and Thomsen (5) in 1959 were the first investigators to describe tympanograms used originally to estimate middle ear pressure. Fig. 2 shows a representative admittance tympanogram recorded with a low-frequency probe tone of 220 Hz in a normal ear. Changes in acoustic admittance are measured as the air pressure in the sealed ear is varied over a range from +200 to -200 daPa (1 daPa = 1.02 mm H_2O). At high pressures (positive

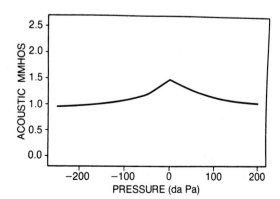

FIG. 2. Mean admittance tympanogram measured with a low-frequency probe tone (220 Hz) for 106 normal ears. (From Katz J, ed. *Handbook of clinical audiology.* Baltimore: Williams & Wilkins, 1985:435, with permission.)

or negative), the tympanic membrane becomes stiff and little acoustic energy flows into the middle ear. Thus, the admittance decreases to a theoretical minimum. As the air pressure approaches atmospheric pressure (0 daPa), the flow of energy into the middle ear is maximized and the admittance reaches a peak value. The maximum flow of energy into the middle ear occurs when the air pressure on each side of the tympanic membrane is equal. The peak (P) of the tympanogram normally will occur at or near 0 daPa. If there is negative pressure in the middle ear, such as in patients with otitis media or eustachian tube dysfunction, the peak of the tympanogram will be observed at a negative pressure. In many patients with otitis media, the tympanograms will have a "flat" appearance, indicating the pressure in the middle ear is extremely negative, and that there is negligible change in relative admittance with ear canal air pressure change.

It is often naively assumed that the tympanogram reflects "tympanic membrane mobility." The "flat" tympanogram can be observed in ears that, on physical examination, may demonstrate some tympanic membrane mobility. This apparent discrepancy can be explained on the basis that a controlled air pressure change is used for tympanometry, but, on physical examination, the air pressure change may exceed that applied for tympanometry. Thus, "movement" of the tympanic membrane seen on physical examination may be seen when "flat" tympanometry is reported.

The physical volume of the sealed ear canal and middle ear also can be estimated from the tympanogram. At high or low negative pressure induced by the air pump, the tympanic membrane becomes extremely stiff and the admittance is minimized. As such, +200 daPa provides an estimate of the ear canal volume only. In normal adult ears, the volume estimate of the ear canal averages 1.1 cm^3. If the tympanic membrane is perforated, the volume estimate will be greater than 2.5 cm^3 because the volume measured includes that of both the ear canal and the middle ear space.

When the tympanic membrane is intact, the admittance of the middle ear without the effect of the ear canal can be estimated from the tympanogram. This value is determined by subtracting the acoustic admittance at high air pressures (e.g., +200 daPa) from the peak admittance value. The equivalent volume of a normal middle ear at 226 Hz averages 0.8 cm^3, with 90% of the normal ears falling within 0.2 to 1.4 cm^3 (ASHA Guidelines 1990) (6). Such static admittance measures are not especially diagnostic, because the normal variability overlaps in some patients with middle ear disorders (for example, stiffness dominated ears due to otosclerosis).

Tympanogram Types

For clinical diagnostic purposes, five basic types of tympanograms measured with a low-frequency tone have

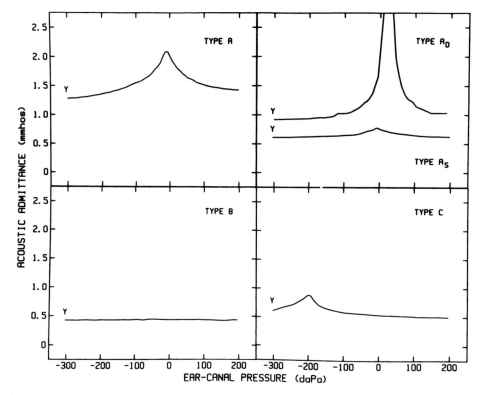

FIG. 3. Five basic types of admittance tympanograms, measured with a 226-Hz probe tone, described by the Liden-Jerger classification system. (From Osguthorpe JD, Melnick W. *The otolaryngologic clinics of North America.* Philadelphia: W.B. Saunders Co., 1991;24(2):308, with permission.)

been described by Liden (7) and Jerger (8). Figure 3 shows representative tympanograms using the Liden-Jerger classification system. Type A is a normal tympanogram. There are two subdivisions of the type A tympanogram. Type A_s is a normal tympanogram except that the peak amplitude is decreased (usually caused by ossicular chain fixation). Type A_d is also a normal tympanogram, but the peak admittance is abnormally high (due to either ossicular chain discontinuity or tympanic membrane pathology such as found in neomembrane or tympanosclerotic plaques).

Also illustrated in Fig. 3 is a type B tympanogram that has a "flat" characteristic shape, suggesting negative pressure in the middle ear and little change in admittance with ear canal air pressure change. It is observed in patients with middle ear effusion, a patent pressure equalization tube, or tympanic membrane perforation. Differentiation among these conditions can be made on the basis of the difference in equivalent ear canal volume. The type B tympanogram shown in Fig. 3 is suggestive of middle ear effusion due to the equivalent ear canal volume of 0.4 cc. A type C tympanogram (also shown in Fig. 3) is characterized by a peak at an extreme negative pressure and may be found in conditions of beginning or resolving middle ear effusion, middle ear cholesteatoma, or eustachian tube dysfunction. Because different pathologies can produce similar tympanometric patterns,

the results must be interpreted in conjunction with the physical examination, the case history, and pure tone test results. Tympanometry is one measurement in a battery of tests used for differential diagnosis of middle ear disorders and provides objective information to complement the physical examination of the ear or bone conduction threshold measurements.

Acoustic Reflex Measurement

Whereas the measurements of static admittance and tympanometry are determined by the status of the external and middle ear, the reflex arc controlling the stapedius muscle contraction is anatomically more complex. Figure 4 shows a schematic representation of the acoustic reflex arc presented by Borg (9) in 1973. The afferent portion includes the cochlea, eighth cranial nerve, and brainstem auditory pathways. The efferent portion includes the brainstem pathways, the seventh cranial nerve, and the stapedius muscle. The contralateral reflex pathway crosses the brainstem, whereas the ipsilateral reflex pathway does not.

The contralateral acoustic reflex arc (Fig. 4B) includes four neurons. From the cochlear sensory cell, impulses are transmitted to the peripheral eighth and the ventral cochlear nucleus and then to the medial superior olive, across the brainstem to the contralateral facial motor

A   IPSILATERAL STAPEDIUS REFLEX PATHWAYS

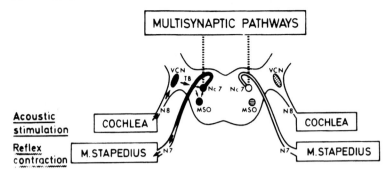

B   CONTRALATERAL STAPEDIUS REFLEX PATHWAYS

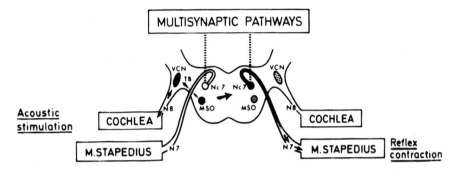

FIG. 4. Schematic diagram of the ipsilateral **(A)** and contralateral **(B)** multisynaptic stapedius reflex pathways. MSO, medial superior olivary complex; N7, facial nerve; N8, acoustic nerve; TB, trapezoid body; VCN, ventral cochlear nucleus. (From Borg E. On the neuronal organization of the acoustic middle ear reflex: a physiological and anatomical study. *Brain Res* 1973;49:101, with permission.)

nucleus. The facial motor nucleus then transmits impulses to the stapedius muscle via the seventh cranial nerve. For the ipsilateral acoustic reflex (Fig. 4A), the cochlear sensory cells transmit impulses to the acoustic nerve and the ventral cochlear nucleus. The majority of axons from the ventral cochlear nucleus pass through the trapezoid body to the ipsilateral facial motor nucleus and then efferently (seventh cranial nerve) to the stapedius muscle.

In the normal auditory system, the stapedius muscle typically contracts to pure tone signals (500 to 4,000 Hz) in the range from 90 to 95 dB sound pressure level (SPL) (10). For broadband noise, the threshold for the reflex is somewhat lower (65 to 75 dB SPL) than for pure tone signals. Whereas the stimulating signal is delivered unilaterally, the reflex contraction is bilateral. Current admittance instruments used in the clinic usually are capable of measuring the ipsilateral and the contralateral acoustic reflex. For the contralaterally activated reflex measurement, the stimulating sound is introduced in the ear contralateral to the ear fitted with a probe tip system used for measuring changes in admittance (as described in Fig. 1). The reflexive contraction of the stapedius muscle is observed indirectly, as a change in admittance, measured at the plane of the tympanic membrane. For the ipsilateral acoustic reflex measurement, both the stimulating tone or noise and the probe tone are presented to the same ear. To avoid the potential interaction between the stimulating and probe signals, commercially available systems use time-sharing circuits (pulsed auditory stimuli) or filtering networks for the ipsilateral measurement of the acoustic reflex.

Considering the order of transmission along the reflex arc, a disorder at any portion of the reflex arc can affect the activation of the stapedius muscle. Therein lies the diagnostic utility of the acoustic reflex measurement. A severe cochlear disorder will result in a reduction of transmission to the brainstem centers and, thus, an absent or elevated ipsilateral and contralateral acoustic reflex. For less severe cochlear losses, the reflex is characteristically present at near-normal sound pressure levels for pure tones. Elevated or absent acoustic reflex measures, in the presence of only mild-to-moderate sensorineural hearing loss, suggests a retrocochlear site of lesion. A seventh nerve disorder (central to the innervation of the stapedius muscle), such as Bell's palsy, will result in the absence of the acoustic reflex in the affected ear no matter which ear is stimulated acoustically. Disorders of the brainstem may result in the loss of both contralateral acoustic reflexes while both ipsilateral acoustic reflexes are preserved (11).

In addition to differentiating among disorders in the afferent, efferent, and brainstem pathways, the acoustic reflex also is sensitive to middle ear disorders. When the probe tip is coupled to an ear with a middle ear disorder, the acoustic reflex usually is absent regardless of the intensity level of the reflex-eliciting signal presented either ipsilaterally or contralaterally. However, when the recording tip is inserted in the normal ear, contralateral to the middle ear disorder, and the reflex-eliciting signal is delivered to the ear with the middle ear disorder, the acoustic reflex threshold will be elevated by the magnitude of the air–bone gap identifiable in the hearing loss secondary to the middle ear disorder. If reflex thresholds are observed at normal presentation levels in both ears, it is safe to conclude that there is no middle ear disorder in either ear.

Middle Ear Disorders

In general, the pattern of admittance results in the ear with a middle ear disorder includes (a) abnormal static admittance, (b) abnormal tympanogram, and (c) absent or elevated acoustic reflexes. In some patients with early otosclerosis, it is possible that both static admittance values and the tympanogram can be normal or near normal. In those patients, the acoustic reflex is usually absent. Terkildsen et al. (12) reported cases in which a reflex was present but was characterized by an abnormal time course, showing a change in admittance at both the onset and offset of the eliciting signal but with no maintenance of the admittance change throughout the duration of the activating signal. This "decoupling" phenomenon has been reported only among patients with early stapes fixation due to otosclerosis. In most patients with other types of middle ear disorders, the reflex will be absent in the ear with the middle ear pathology.

Sensorineural Disorders

A common application of the acoustic reflex is in the differentiation between cochlear and eighth nerve disorder. In these patients, static admittance and the tympanograms usually are normal, because the middle ear is not affected. The acoustic reflex typically is present in ears with a cochlear disorder (depending, as discussed later, on the degree of hearing loss) and characteristically absent or significantly elevated in ears with an eighth nerve disorder. In some patients with an eighth nerve lesion, a reflex may be identifiable but exhibit an abnormal time course with sustained stimulation. The reflex, in such patients, "decays" more rapidly than in those with normal or cochlear-impaired ears (13).

Although the reflex is present in many patients with cochlear disorders, the sensation level (level above audibility threshold) at which the reflex is observed declines in proportion to the degree of hearing loss (14). The prac-

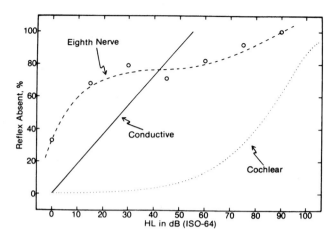

FIG. 5. Relationship between the degree of hearing loss and the likelihood of acoustic reflex absence in patients with conductive, cochlear, and eighth nerve disorders. (From *Arch Otolaryngol* 1974;99:409–413, with permission.)

tical implication of this principle is that, if a patient has a sensorineural hearing loss that does not exceed 55 to 65 dB hearing level (HL), and if the loss is cochlear, a reflex should be present when a sufficiently intense sound is introduced into that ear. If the loss of hearing is greater than 70 dB HL, the absence of a reflex becomes an equivocal finding diagnostically.

An absent acoustic reflex in an ear with mild-to-moderate hearing loss should always raise suspicion of an eighth nerve disorder. Figure 5 shows the relation between the degree of hearing loss and the likelihood of the absence of the reflex in cochlear and eighth nerve disorders (15). When the hearing level is within normal limits, the likelihood of the absence of the reflex in the presence of an eighth nerve disorder is 30%. There is a disproportionate increase in the likelihood of the absence of a reflex with increasing hearing loss. For example, a hearing loss of 20 to 50 dB HL produced by an eighth nerve disorder results in a 70% likelihood of an absent acoustic reflex. Reports by several investigators (16–18) suggest that the accurate identification rate of an eighth nerve disorder by the absence of an acoustic reflex or significant reflex decay to a sustained signal ranges from 77% to 86%.

Brainstem Disorders

For patients with brainstem lesions, several reflex patterns may be observed, depending on the site of the disorder. If, for example, both the ipsilateral and contralateral reflexes are normal in the presence of a brainstem auditory disorder, the results suggest that the lesion is above the level of the central arc in the pons. The presence of normal ipsilateral reflexes but absent contralateral reflexes indicates an interruption in the central reflex arc between the ipsilateral cochlear nucleus and the contralateral facial nucleus. If both contralateral and ipsilateral reflexes are absent, the results suggest an intraaxial brainstem lesion. Variations of these results may be observed in patients with no hearing loss who have multiple sclerosis or other demyelinating diseases of the lower brainstem regions.

SUMMARY

Tympanometry and acoustic reflex measures have become an important tool in the differential diagnosis of auditory disorders. In addition, because the test procedures require no active participation by the patient, they can be used successfully in infants, young children, and difficult-to-test patients. However, immittance measures are not a "stand-alone" differential diagnostic tool but should be included in the battery of auditory diagnostic tests and interpreted in relation to basic audiometric results because they provide no direct information regarding presence or absence of hearing loss.

SUMMARY POINTS

- The efficiency of energy (sound wave) transmission through the middle ear can be assessed indirectly by measuring impedance at the level of the tympanic membrane.
- Impedance is affected primarily by stiffness and mass of the middle ear system and, to a lesser degree, by friction (e.g., resistance of the ossicular joints).
- Stiffness is increased by ossicular fixation (e.g., otosclerosis) or middle ear fluid. Increased stiffness causes greater loss of low-frequency versus high-frequency energy transfer (i.e., predominantly a low-frequency conductive hearing loss). Increased mass (e.g., ossicular abnormality) affects high-frequency conductance.
- Tympanometry and the acoustic reflex are examples of impedance measurements ("acoustic immittance") at the tympanic membrane.
- Tympanometry measurements provide an estimate of middle ear pressure and volume of the external canal and middle ear space.
- Tympanograms can be broadly classified as type A (normal with peak atmospheric pressure), type B (no peak or flat, suggesting middle ear fluid), and type C (peak at negative atmospheric pressure, implying eustachian tube dysfunction).
- The acoustic reflex includes an afferent limb (sound processed by the cochlea, auditory nerve, and brainstem) and an efferent limb (activation of the stapedius muscle by the seventh cranial nerve).
- Contraction of the stapedius muscle can be elicited by a pure tone signal of 90 to 95 dB SPL. Broadband noise or more complex signals, however, can activate the reflex at lower intensity levels (65 to 75 dB SPL). Although the stimulus is delivered unilaterally, the reflex is bilateral.
- The acoustic reflex usually is absent in patients with a conductive hearing loss. An elevated or absent acoustic reflex, or one that "decays" rapidly, in patients with mild-to-moderate sensorineural hearing loss suggests a retrocochlear versus cochlear site of pathology.
- Although tympanometry and acoustic reflex testing are important diagnostic tools, they are best utilized as part of an auditory test battery including pure tone and speech audiometry, auditory brainstem response test, electrocochleography, and otoacoustic emission.

REFERENCES

1. Metz O. The acoustic impedance measured on normal and pathological ears. *Acta Otolaryngol* 1946;63[Suppl]:397–405.
2. Wever EG, Lawrence M. *Physiological acoustics.* Princeton, NJ: Princeton University Press, 1954.
3. Schuster K. Eine methode zum vergleich akusticher impedanzen. *Pyssikalische Z* 1934;35:408–409.
4. American Speech-Language-Hearing Association. Specifications for instruments to measure aural acoustic impedance and admittance (aural acoustic immittance) (ANSI S3.39-1987). New York: ANSI, 1987.
5. Terkildsen K, Thomsen K. The influence of pressure variations on the impedance of the human ear drum. A method for objective determination of middle ear pressure. *J Laryngol Otol* 1959;73:409.
6. American Speech-Language-Hearing Association. Guidelines for screening for hearing impairments and middle ear disorders. *ASHA* 1990;32:17.
7. Liden G. The scope and application of current audiometric tests. *J Laryngol Otol* 1969;83:507–520.
8. Jerger J. Clinical experience with impedance audiometry. *Arch Otolaryngol* 1970;92:311–324.
9. Borg E. On the neuronal organization of the acoustic middle ear reflex: a physiological and anatomical study. *Brain Res* 1973;49:101–123.
10. Wilson R, Margolis R. Hearing assessment. In: Rintleman W, ed. *Acoustic reflex measurement,* 2nd ed. Austin, TX: Pro-Ed, 1990: 247–319.
11. Jerger S, Neely G, Jerger J. Recovery of crossed acoustic reflexes in brain stem and auditory disorder. *Arch Otolaryngol* 1975;101: 329–332.
12. Terkildsen K, Osterhammel P, Bretlau P. Acoustic middle ear muscle reflexes in patients with otosclerosis. *Arch Otolaryngol* 1973;98: 152–155.
13. Anderson H, Barr B, Wedenburg E. Intra-aural reflexes in retrocochlear lesions. In: Hambarger C, Wasall J, eds. *Disorders of the skull base region.* Stockholm: Almquist and Wikesell, 1969:49–55.
14. Jerger J, Hayes D, Anthony L, Mauldin L. Factors influencing prediction of hearing levels from the acoustic reflex. *Monogr Contemp Audiol* 1978;1:1–20.
15. Jerger J, Harford E, Clemis J, Alford B. The acoustic reflex in eighth nerve disorders. *Arch Otolaryngol* 1974;99:409–413.
16. Olsen WO, Noffisinger D, Kurdziel S. Acoustic reflex and reflex decay: occurrence in patients with cochlear and eighth nerve lesions. *Arch Otolaryngol* 1975;101:622–625.
17. Sheehy JL, Inzer BE. Acoustic reflex test in neuro-otologic diagnosis: a review of 24 cases of acoustic tumors. *Arch Otolaryngol* 1976;102: 647–653.
18. Johnson E. An analysis of auditory test results in 500 cases of acoustic neuroma. *Arch Otolaryngol* 1977;103:152–157.

The Ear: Comprehensive Otology,
edited by R. F. Canalis and P. R. Lambert.
Lippincott Williams & Wilkins, Philadelphia © 2000.

CHAPTER 13

Auditory Brainstem Response and Electrocochleographic Testing

Donald D. Dirks, Donald E. Morgan, and Roger A. Ruth

The purpose of clinical auditory testing is to assess the magnitude of the hearing loss and to identify the anatomic location of the auditory disorder. The magnitude of the hearing loss is estimated from pure tone, air conduction audiometry. With few exceptions, little differential diagnostic information can be obtained merely from an air conduction audiogram, because hearing disorders at various anatomic sites may produce similar patterns of sensitivity loss. As a consequence, other test procedures, especially physiologic measures of cochlear and retrocochlear function, are required to determine the anatomic site of lesion and to quantify the functional problems associated with various types of auditory disorders. To provide perspective, this chapter includes a short history of the development of differential diagnostic auditory tests, followed by a more detailed discussion of auditory brainstem response (ABR) testing and electrocochleography (ECochG). Finally, representative cases will be presented to illustrate diagnostic strategies that lead to the differential diagnosis of the anatomic site of an auditory disorder.

D. D. Dirks: Division of Head and Neck Surgery, University of California, Los Angeles, School of Medicine, Los Angeles, California 90095

D. E. Morgan: Decibel Instruments, Inc., Fremont, California 94555

R. A. Ruth: Department of Otolaryngology–Head and Neck Surgery, University of Virginia School of Medicine, Charlottesville, Virginia 22906-0008

HISTORICAL PERSPECTIVE

The potential complexity of auditory diagnosis was apparent as early as 1834, when Ernst Weber (1) observed that bone-conducted signals lateralized to the ear with the greatest air conduction hearing loss in persons with middle ear disorders. In 1855, Heinrich Rinne (2) developed a procedure, still used today, for identifying the presence of a conductive hearing loss by comparing the perceptual duration of a signal by air conduction to the duration of the same signal by bone conduction. The test procedures described by Rinne (2) and Weber (1) were administered by tuning forks and, for nearly a century, remained the primary method for differentiating between a conductive and sensorineural hearing loss.

The development of the electric audiometer set the stage for quantitative tests of auditory sensitivity in which precise control of the amplitude of an acoustic signal could be guaranteed. In 1948, Dix et al. (3) observed that loudness rose more rapidly above threshold in patients with Meniere's disease than in cases with eighth nerve tumors. These investigators measured loudness growth by comparing the loudness in the poorer hearing ear to that in the normal hearing ear of the same subject. This procedure, studied first by E.P. Fowler (4) 10 years earlier in 1937, was called the alternate binaural loudness balance (ABLB) test, and the rapid growth of loudness observed in ears with Meniere's disease was known as "loudness recruitment."

For the next decade, the results of the ABLB test became the validation procedure against which new test methods for auditory differential diagnosis were evaluated. A multitude of test procedures were developed during this period, such as intensity and frequency discrimination, loudness adaptation and fatigue, and masking of tones by noise. The signals used in those procedures were delivered monaurally and, thus, were not dependent on interaural asymmetry, which often limited the use of the ABLB test. In most instances, the diagnostic tests developed during this period for differentiating between cochlear and eighth nerve disorders were characterized as indirect tests of loudness recruitment. As new test procedures were developed, their effectiveness for differential diagnosis was generally based on comparisons between results from the ABLB and the proposed test. As patient data accumulated, the results indicated that numerous patients with eighth nerve tumors also had concomitant cochlear loss and, thus, loudness recruitment often was present. Eventually, it became apparent that the validating criterion for determining the effectiveness of a new test procedure for differential diagnosis should not be the degree to which it compared with results from the ABLB, but rather how well the test predicted site of lesion.

Diagnostic tests introduced between 1955 and 1975 utilized behavioral responses to complex auditory signals, as well as electrophysiologic techniques in which no overt response was required from the patient. In 1947 von Bekesy (5) had developed a self-recording audiometer for measuring changes in auditory sensitivity to temporally interrupted and/or continuous pure tones. The development of this self-recording audiometer provided the tool for investigators (6,7) to measure precisely the phenomenon of adaptation to sustained stimulation. This diagnostic procedure was based on the observation that patients with retrocochlear lesions often evidenced abnormal adaptation at threshold. Because none of the behavioral tests correctly predicted the site of lesion in all patients, the concept of a test battery approach to assessment was advocated. Clinical investigators found that a combination of two or more tests, each sensitive to a different site of disorder, often led to more accurate predictions of the site of the auditory lesion than dependence on results from any single test procedure.

Prior to the 1960s, most auditory tests used for differential diagnosis involved pure tones as the stimulus and required a behavioral response from the patient. The measurement of "discrimination loss" for speech was, however, recognized as a significant measure for a complete auditory evaluation of the receptive capabilities of the patient. It was generally recognized that the maximum word recognition score often was disproportionately poor in relation to the sensitivity loss in patients with eighth nerve disorders. Substantial overlap in maximum word recognition scores of patients with cochlear and eighth nerve disorders, however, effectively limited the diagnostic value of speech recognition testing. In 1971 Jerger and Jerger (8) observed that in patients with retrocochlear lesions, the word recognition score reached a maximum as speech presentation level increased, and then became poorer as speech level was further raised ("rollover" phenomenon). The rollover phenomenon is generally minimal in patients with cochlear disorders, but it may be significant among patients with eighth nerve disorders. Although this procedure improved the differential diagnostic capabilities of word recognition tests, the procedure is time consuming and, as described later, not as predictive of site of lesion as more recently developed objective procedures such as the auditory brainstem evoked response.

Whereas the subjective behavioral tests were among the earliest measures used for differential diagnosis, the modern battery of differential diagnostic tests are objective and usually consist of immittance measures, the ABR, ECochG, and otoacoustic emissions. These tests, although not inclusive of all available auditory diagnostic tests, are widely used and included in most test strategies for differential diagnosis. The remainder of the chapter is devoted to a thorough description of two physiologic measures of cochlear and retrocochlear function—ABR and ECochG.

AUDITORY EVOKED BRAINSTEM RESPONSE

The development of ABR audiometry in the 1970s (9) provided the most powerful electrophysiologic technique for differentiating between a cochlear and eighth nerve disorder. The ABR is one of several clinically useful evoked response potentials that can be recorded in humans. Because the ABR can be obtained without an overt response from the patient, it is widely applied in the identification and quantification of auditory and neurologic disorders in neonates, children, and adults.

Classification of Neural Events

Auditory evoked potentials (AEPs) include a series of neuroelectric responses that are generated at all levels of the auditory nervous system. Using scalp electrodes, as many as 15 different AEP responses have been identified within the first 500 ms following the onset of the acoustic stimulus (10). Although no formal terminology has been standardized in classification of the identifiable AEPs, most methods utilized in clinical practice use as a reference the site of neural generation and the response latency. The latency is the time interval between a reference point of the stimulus and some morphologic characteristic (usually a peak) of the AEP. Amplitude of the peak is often measured from the voltage baseline to the peak or as the difference between the peak of a wave and its subsequent trough.

Recording electrodes used for clinical testing are remote from active neural generators. These electrodes measure the overall electrical fields of many neural units. Therefore, "pinpointing" the anatomic site of the generating neurons for a particular identifiable point on the waveform is complex. Even though it is difficult to make completely accurate inferences about the anatomic origin of a particular AEP response, the usefulness of the AEPs, as empirical correlates of normal or impaired processes, has been satisfactorily demonstrated.

In 1976, Davis (11) grouped the AEPs in order of their latency epoch, which is a range of latencies in which several AEPs may occur. The responses were classified as follows:

First: 0 to 2 ms, which includes the response of the cochlear microphonic (CM), summating potential (SP), and the acoustic nerve

Fast: 2 to 10 ms from the acoustic nerve and lower brainstem

Middle: 8 to 50 ms from the thalamus and auditory cortex

Slow: 50 to 300 ms from the primary and secondary areas of the cerebral cortex

Late: 300 ms and later from the primary and association areas of the cerebral cortex.

Procedural Considerations

For reasons to be developed later, the early evoked responses from the brainstem (0 to 10 ms) are most commonly measured for use in the differential diagnosis of auditory disorders. The waves (created by the peaks and valleys resulting from the amplitude changes over time) of the ABR are recorded by a far-field technique with the recording electrodes placed at approximately the same distance from the brainstem generators, generally the vertex (or another midline head position) and the earlobe of the ear under test. Invariably, the electrodes pick up not only the ABR response, but other, unwanted electrical activity, the latter referred to as "noise." This noise arises from various electrical sources, such as muscle potentials, cardiac and corneoretinal sources, as well as other event-unrelated potentials. All of these sources of electrical noise combine to obscure the ABR responses, which often are small in amplitude. A major issue in most evoked response applications is to use techniques that optimize the detectability of the response within the noise.

Signal averaging is used to extract the potential of interest, freed of the contaminating physiologic noise. As a consequence, the stimulus is presented repetitively, and a series of action potentials (APs) thus produced are added one to the other in an averaging computer. Because the responses to the stimuli have time-locked temporal characteristics, they can be summed to provide an "aver-

age" response. The background or other physiologic activity, however, being in random phase with respect to the activating signal, over time is canceled. The evoked response emerges as a clearly identifiable response.

The stimulus used for ABR and other evoked potential measurements is usually a broadband click or a short tone burst. These stimuli are ideal because of their rapid-onset characteristics. It is the sharpness of the rise time that ensures the greatest synchrony of neural activity. Well-synchronized volleys of evoked potentials generated by clicks and rapid-onset tone bursts are readily recorded by an averager. As the frequency of the signal is decreased, the degree of synchrony at the onset of the stimulus is reduced due to the slow rise time of each cycle (longer wavelength) of the tonal stimulus. This problem is especially prevalent for frequencies below 1,000 Hz. In addition, the rate at which low frequencies are propagated toward the apex of the cochlea becomes somewhat variable and leads to a loss of synchrony between the small evoked potentials generated by each cycle of the low-frequency components of the stimulus. Such asynchronous potentials cannot be extracted satisfactorily by averaging; thus, it is difficult to identify low-frequency contributions to the overall ABR. Thus, for a broadband click stimulus, the resulting ABR is predominantly a measurement of the high-frequency (2,000 to 4,000 Hz) region. Likewise, high-frequency tone pips (1,500 to 4,000 Hz) result in sufficient synchrony of neural activity to produce a replicable averaged response.

The unwanted noise in the overall response also is attenuated by filtering techniques. For ABR measurements, a passband filter extending from 250 to 3,000 Hz often is incorporated within the output amplifier of the measuring system. This removes low-frequency artifacts and any mainline hum (60 Hz). The analysis time selected for the ABR is usually less than 20 ms, which provides ample opportunity to observe all major waves of the ABR. It often is necessary to increase the analysis time for testing of infants, because the ABR waves have prolonged latencies in the normally developed newborn and throughout the first few months of life (12).

For purposes of differential diagnosis of an auditory disorder, most clinics use a repetition rate of less than 30 stimuli/s, with a click stimulus duration of 100 μs. One thousand or more repetitions often are required to obtain a stable averaged waveform even at high-amplitude presentation levels. As the ABR threshold is approached, a larger number of signals must be averaged to extract the response from the noise floor. At a repetition rate of 33.3/s, a series of 1,000 stimuli can be delivered in approximately 30 seconds. Much of the test period is taken up with placing the electrodes properly and, in some instances, waiting for the patient to lie quietly so that muscle artifacts are not so great as to obscure the low-amplitude brainstem potentials. The ABR is not affected by the conscious state of the patient; thus, sedation can be used if replicable recordings cannot be obtained because of hyperactivity or excessive movement.

Clinical Applications

The major clinical applications of the ABR include measures of the functional integrity of the peripheral auditory system in children and adults who cannot be tested by conventional means and for differential diagnosis of the anatomic site of an auditory disorder. Interpolation of the neurologic implications of the ABR is based primarily on the temporal differences in latency measures when compared with average results from a panel of normal hearing subjects.

The ABR latency epoch consists of up to seven identifiable peaks measured within the initial 10 to 14 ms following the onset of the acoustic stimulus. Figure 1 shows the ABR-averaged waveforms from an individual with a normal peripheral auditory system. The signal was a click delivered at presentation levels from 80 to 20 dB above the normal behavioral threshold. Each peak is identified using the standard nomenclature suggested by Jewett and Williston (13).

As shown in Fig. 1, changes in stimulus intensity have a marked effect on the ABR. As stimulus intensity decreases, the individual waves decrease in amplitude and their latencies increase. For example, the latency for wave V decreases from 5.8 ms following stimulus onset at a presentation level of 80 dB to 7.3 ms at a presentation level of 20 dB. Similar latency increases are observed for all waves in an individual with a normal auditory system. At the two higher presentation levels (80 and 60 dB nHL [normal hearing level]), six peaks are clearly identifiable; however, as intensity is reduced below 60 dB nHL, the earlier waves tend to disappear. Wave V remains definable even at the lowest presentation level and is generally the most easily recognizable at

threshold. Clinically, ABR responses may be obtained at several click presentation levels and compared with the results observed on a group of individuals with normal hearing and no neurologic disorders.

Because wave V is usually observable to within 10 or 20 dB of behavioral threshold, the relationship between intensity and wave V latency is stable and reproducible over a wide range of stimulus presentation levels. This latency-intensity relationship can be useful in estimating the magnitude of the hearing loss and in distinguishing between conductive and cochlear hearing loss. Figure 2 shows a schematic representation of the click-elicited wave V latency-intensity function for two hearing-impaired patients (who will be described in detail later) relative to the hatched area, which defines the average normal latency-intensity function (±2 SD). As observed in Fig. 1, wave V latency decreases as the intensity of the stimulus increases for the normal hearing group.

In addition to measures of wave V absolute latency, it is diagnostically insightful to calculate the absolute latency of earlier waves (especially I and III) and to calculate interpeak latencies. Determination of the I–III and I–V interpeak latencies often provides additional differential diagnostic information, especially for patients in whom all waves are present but one or more are delayed, depending on the site of the auditory lesion.

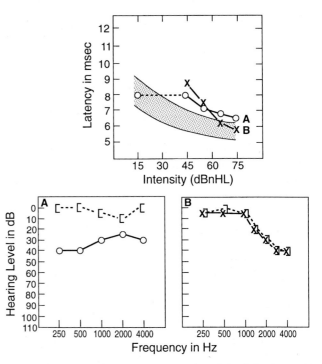

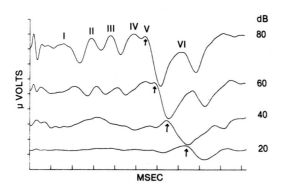

FIG. 1. Effects of decreasing stimulus presentation level on auditory brainstem response wave latency, amplitude, and morphology. The time window is 10 ms. The *arrows* indicate changes in wave V latency. (From Jacobson JT. *The auditory brain stem response.* San Diego: College Hill Press, 1985, with permission.)

FIG. 2. Schematic representation of the click-elicited wave V latency-intensity function **(upper panel)** for two patients. **(A)** A conductive hearing loss. **(B)** A sloping high-frequency sensorineural hearing loss. The *hatched area* represents the average normal function (±1 SD). The audiograms for the patients are shown in the **lower panels**.

Middle Ear Disorders

Although immittance measures are the most sensitive and diagnostically differentiating tests for establishing the presence of a conductive disorder, impairments involving the external and/or middle ear will affect the ABR parameters. The most apparent effect is an increase in the absolute latency of all waves, including wave V relative to the normal ear. Such a result from a patient with conductive hearing loss is shown in Fig. 2 as the latency-intensity function labeled "A." This function was obtained from an adult with a 30-dB HL hearing loss, in the 2,000- to 4,000-Hz range, due to otosclerosis (shown by the audiogram in the lower left panel of Fig. 2). Theoretically, the displacement of the latency-intensity function in patients with middle ear disorders will be proportional to the magnitude of the conductive loss. Consequently, the degree of separation between the normal function and that of the patient is an estimate of the magnitude of the conductive hearing loss. A horizontal dashed line has been drawn from the latency corresponding to a normal ABR threshold (15 dB nHL) until it intersects with the patient's ABR threshold (45 dB nHL). The difference in the stimulus levels producing the two comparable points (threshold) approximates the conductive hearing loss in the 2,000 to 4,000-Hz region. In the example, the conductive loss estimate of 30 dB approximates the air conduction thresholds in this frequency region of the audiogram. Notice, in addition, that the displacement of the patient's latency-intensity curve relative to the normal curve remains equal at all stimulus presentation levels; that is, the slope of the function is normal.

Sensorineural Disorders

Cochlear Site of Lesion

The latency-intensity function for a patient with a sloping, high-frequency hearing loss of cochlear origin is shown in Fig. 2 as curve "B." The audiogram for the patient is illustrated in the lower right panel of the figure. The latency-intensity function in patients with cochlear hearing loss can assume a variety of slopes, depending on the audiometric configuration. However, the majority of individuals with sensorineural loss of cochlear origin evidence either a uniform loss across frequencies or a sloping loss with greater loss in sensitivity for high frequencies relative to low frequencies. The most common characteristic of the slope of the wave V latency-intensity function among persons with high-frequency cochlear loss typically is some variation of curve B in Fig. 2. Near threshold, the latency is greater than for a normal hearing listener at the same stimulus input level. At high (70 to 90 dB nHL) signal levels, the latency more closely approximates that of the normal auditory system. This increased slope in the wave V latency-intensity function can be explained on the basis that at suprathreshold levels, the

area of the cochlea stimulated and the number of hair cell and neural fibers stimulatable are sufficient to provide a normal latency for each of the waves of the averaged response. However, as the elevated threshold is approached (presentation level of clicks is reduced), the number of available neural units decreases rapidly, resulting in a latency response that more closely approximates the latency observed in the normal auditory system at normal threshold levels. The reduced dynamic range of the person with cochlear hearing loss results in a latency-intensity function that is increased in slope by virtue of the reduced signal level range within which the entire slope occurs. For individuals evidencing cochlear hearing loss, the expectation is that at high (75 to 95 dB nHL) signal levels, wave I and all subsequent peaks of the ABR will be observed at latencies comparable to that of the normal auditory system at equal sound pressure levels. Therefore, at high signal levels, absolute latency of wave I and the I–III and I–V interpeak latency will be within normal limits for such patients.

Depending on the magnitude and audiometric configuration of the cochlear hearing loss, there may be variations in the wave V latency-intensity function. For example, Meniere's disease often results in a low-frequency, sensorineural hearing loss with normal or near-normal hearing sensitivity in the 2,000- to 4,000-Hz region. Such a configuration could result in a completely normal ABR throughout the signal level range. Conversely, if an individual evidences profound hearing loss in the 2,000- to 4,000-Hz range and a sharply sloping configuration for frequencies below 2,000 Hz, the click stimulus may be encoded by cochlear structures more apical than those at the basal end of the cochlea. This "shift" in the anatomic site of stimulation will result in an increased latency for wave I (and all subsequent waves). For these patients, the *absolute* latency at which the ABR wave occurs is prolonged, but the interwave latencies will retain normal relationships. For these reasons, interpretation of the ABR requires analysis of both absolute and interwave latencies in the context of the magnitude and configuration of the sensorineural hearing loss.

Retrocochlear Site of Lesion

In 1975, Starr and Achor (14) described the ABR responses from a diverse group of patients with various neurologic disorders. Patients with cortical disorders showed normal ABR responses, whereas one patient with an acoustic tumor, five patients with other retrocochlear tumors, and four patients with demyelinating diseases demonstrated abnormal ABR responses.

The most diagnostic finding in patients with eighth nerve impairment, such as acoustic tumors, is a disruption in the overall pattern of the evoked response. When the first-order neurons of the eighth nerve are affected (e.g., intracanicular tumor), wave I and all subsequent waves within the first 10 ms may be altered. When the lesion affects eighth nerve function (e.g., cerebellopontine angle tumor), wave I may be normal, but the later waves (wave III and subsequent waves) may be affected. The changes in the ABR in patients with eighth nerve disorders may include all or any one of the following characteristics: absence of any identifiable wave, increase in the latency of specific waves, and an increase in interwave latency times.

The most commonly used criteria for an abnormal response are an interaural wave C difference of ≥0.40 ms or an I–V interwave latency difference (same ear) of ≥4.40 ms. Although past experience had shown the ABR to have a detection rate approached 90% to 95% for acoustic tumors (15,16), recent studies have documented a false-negative rate of 10% to 20% for small (intracanalicular) tumors (17–19). These more recent data have become available with the advent of magnetic resonance imaging and the enhanced ability of this imaging modality to detect small tumors. With high-frequency sensorineural hearing loss, wave V latency is prolonged because of the time required for the traveling wave to reach more apical regions of the cochlea that can respond to the stimulus. To compensate for this confounding influence on wave V latency, several investigators have advocated the use of a correction factor based on the degree of hearing loss at 4,000 Hz (20–22). An alternative to this approach is to base the interpretation solely on interpeak (e.g., wave I–V) latencies.

The basis for this wave V latency shift concerns traveling wave time and the fact that synchronization of neural discharges is more easily accomplished from the higher-frequency basal region of the cochlea than from the lower-frequency apical portion. Although a click stimulates the entire basilar membrane, the peak of the basilar membrane displacement is in the 1,000- to 4,000-Hz range. With a higher intensity stimulus, there is sufficient energy in the traveling wave to stimulate effectively the very basal portion of the cochlea. With a lower-intensity stimulus, however, there is no synchronized response from the basal area and the wave must travel apically to the area of maximal basilar membrane displacement before a synchronous discharge occurs. This traveling wave time equates with the increased latency observed in the ABR response.

Figure 3 illustrates the ABR results for a patient with an acoustic neuroma at the cerebellopontine angle, affecting the left ear. The ABR for the right ear (top panel) is within normal limits, with excellent replicability between the test and retest results. The audiogram in the right ear is within normal limits and, interestingly, the audiogram in the left ear reveals only a mild sen-

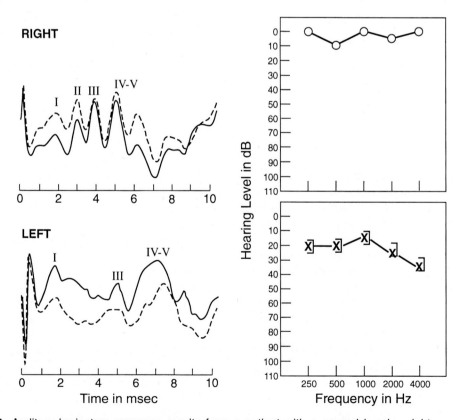

FIG. 3. Auditory brainstem response results from a patient with a normal hearing right ear and an acoustic tumor in the left ear. The *dashed lines* and *solid lines* represent results of two trials with a click presented at 80 dB nHL. The audiogram for each ear is shown in the panels on the **right**.

sorineural hearing loss. Observe that wave I in both ears is normal, but the subsequent waves in the left ear, although present, are delayed and characterized by poor replicability as compared to the right ear results. The left ear waveforms reveal increased absolute latency for waves III and V and, therefore, increased I–III and I–V interpeak latencies.

ELECTROCOCHLEOGRAPHY

Another member of the family of AEPs is ECochG, which is the technique of measuring stimulus-related electrophysiologic potentials of the inner ear and auditory nerve. The electrical potentials associated with this part of the auditory system occur soon after stimulus onset and include the CM, the SP, and the compound AP of the auditory nerve. Although these potentials can, at times, be observed using surface electrode recordings, more precise studies of these events requires placement of electrodes in close proximity to the inner ear.

Even though the CM was first recorded experimentally in animals as early as 1930 (23), the first human AP recordings were not obtained until 1960 (24). These earliest attempts to record from the human peripheral auditory system involved the use of relatively invasive needle electrodes placed through the tympanic membrane onto the promontory wall of the middle ear. Due primarily to this factor, ECochG was soon overshadowed by a rapidly growing interest in the clinical application of the less invasive ABR beginning in the early 1970s. The development over the past several years of various types of noninvasive electrodes has fostered a resurgence of interest in the clinical application of ECochG.

Peripheral Electrophysiology

The CM is an alternating-current response that tends to mirror the waveform of the sound input to the ear (see Chapter 4). It is thought to reflect the displacement-time pattern of the cochlear partition and appears to arise primarily from activity associated with the outer hair cells (25). The magnitude of the CM is dependent on hair cell output and is fairly linear over a sizable range of stimulus intensities.

Unlike the CM, the SP is a direct-current potential. The SP is a complex multicomponent response representing the sum of various nonlinearities associated with cochlear processing (4,26). The SP tends to follow the envelope or on-and-off pattern of the stimulus rather than its waveform. The polarity of the direct-current shift seen with SP measurements may be positive or negative, depending on stimulus frequency, intensity, and electrode recording site. When recorded with noninvasive electrodes in the ear canal or on the eardrum, the SP is generally characterized by a negative shift in baseline that persists for the duration of the evoking stimulus.

The AP reflects the summed response of synchronous discharges from several thousand individual nerve fibers primarily located in the basal region of the cochlea. The AP is represented as an alternating-current voltage. The waveform of the AP is characterized by a relatively large negative deflection referred to as N_1. This component is identical to wave I of the surface-recorded ABR and is thought to arise from the distal most portion of the auditory nerve (27). The AP response often has a subsequent and smaller negative deflection referred to a N_2 that likely arises from the proximal portion of the auditory nerve and corresponds to wave II of the surface-recorded ABR. Both amplitude and latency of the AP are related to the frequency and intensity of the evoking stimulus. For example, smaller AP amplitudes and longer latencies are seen in the presence of lower-intensity and/or lower-frequency signals.

Recording Techniques

ECochG electrodes can be classified as being either invasive or noninvasive, depending on whether the electrode penetrates the skin of the ear canal or eardrum (Table 1). The major advantage of using an invasive electrode is the acquisition of clear and robust waveforms with minimal averaging time due to the superior signal-to-noise ratio, because the recording electrode is very near the generators of the response (hair cells or auditory nerve). Noninvasive or nontraumatic electrodes are, by definition, painless, thus obviating the need for sedation or local anesthetics. One of the more novel approaches to noninvasive ECochG involves the use of a small flexible electrode that rests directly on the tympanic membrane. Such an electrode was first proposed for nontraumatic ECochG recordings more than 20 years ago by Cullen et al. (28). However, it was not until recently that the technique has seen more widespread use in ECochG measurement (29–31). The tympanic membrane electrode is now commercially available from at least one manufacturer of evoked potential instrumentation. However, it can be easily constructed in a clinic or lab with little effort (32).

TABLE 1. *Electrocochleographic electrode types*

Invasive
Transtympanic
Insulated needle electrode
Round window ball electrode
Noninvasive
Extratympanic
Gold foil over foam plug
Plastic leaf with silver ball
Tympanic membrane
Foam or cotton wisp attached to silver wire through flexible tubing

The stimulus and response recording parameters used for ECochG testing are similar in many respects to those used for ABR recordings. The actual parameters used depend to some extent on the particular component of the ECochG waveform of primary interest to the examiner. For example, the AP and SP recordings used for evaluation of patients with endolymphatic hydrops require different stimulus and response parameters than those used to monitor auditory function during surgery or to assess cochlear integrity in the presence of a masking dilemma. The typical stimulus and response parameters used for ECochG measurement are listed in Table 2. As with ABR testing, broadband click stimuli are most often used for ECochG measurements. The primary electrode is located in the ear canal, on the eardrum, or on the promontory wall of the middle ear. The secondary or reference electrode is attached to the contralateral earlobe, mastoid, ear canal, or forehead. When the primary electrode is plugged into the noninverting (+) channel of the differen-

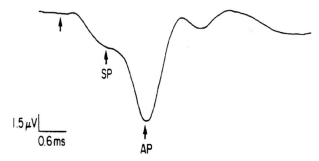

FIG. 4. Normal electrocochleogram recorded from the tympanic membrane in response to alternating polarity clicks at 85 dB HL. The summating potential (SP) and action potential (AP) amplitudes.

TABLE 2. *Electrocochleographic recording parameters*

Stimuli
  Type
    Broadband clicks
    Tone bursts
  Duration (broadband clicks)
    100 μs electrical pulse
  Envelope (tone bursts)
    2–4 ms linear rise per fall
    5–10 ms plateau
  Polarity
    Rarefaction and condensation
    Alternating
  Repetition rate
    11.3/s
  Level
    85–90 dB hearing level (~115–120 dB sound pressure level)
Electrode array
  Primary (+)
    Ear canal/tympanic membrane/promontory/round window
  Second (–)
    Contralateral earlobe/mastoid/ear canal
  Common
    Forehead
Acquisition parameters
  Time base
    5–12 ms
    2–3 ms of prestimulus baseline
  Amplification
    50,000–100,000X (ET-ECochG)
    10,000–25,000X (TT-ECochG)
  Filter bandpass
    1–3,000 Hz
  No. of acquisitions
    1,000–2,000 (ET-ECochG)
    100–200 (TT-ECochG)

ET-ECochG, extratympanic electrocochleography; TT-ECochG, transtympanic electrocochleography.

tial amplifier, the resulting AP response will be pointing down (Fig. 4).

Clinical Applications

ECochG has several clinical applications, including evaluation of Meniere's disease or endolymphatic hydrops, enhancement of wave I in neurodiagnostic assessment, determination of cochlear reserve in patients with maximal conductive components to their hearing loss, and intraoperative monitoring of the peripheral auditory structures at risk for damage secondary to surgically induced trauma.

Meniere's disease

The classic triad of symptoms associated with Meniere's disease includes unilateral sensorineural hearing loss, tinnitus, and episodic vertigo. Patients with these classic findings generally do not present a diagnostic dilemma. However, the hallmark of Meniere's disease is its variable expression from one patient to the next or within the same patient over time. As such, there are many situations in which the certainty of a diagnosis of Meniere's disease is less clear. It is in these patients that ECochG measures may offer additional insight.

The key feature of an ECochG recording in a patient with active Meniere's disease is an enlarged SP amplitude relative to AP amplitude (Fig. 5). The increased endolymphatic fluid volume seen in Meniere's disease alters the mechanical characteristics of basilar membrane motion, which, in turn, causes the natural asymmetry of this action to be enhanced. Because the vibratory asymmetry of the basilar membrane is thought to be related to the production of the SP, enhancement of the asymmetry by hydrops could explain the enlarged SP in Meniere's patients (33). The absolute amplitude of the SP and AP both show considerable variability across subjects. A more stable feature of the response is the SP-to-AP amplitude ratio (34). On the average, an SP-

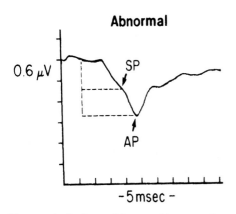

FIG. 5. Abnormal electrocochleographic recording obtained from a patient with active Meniere's disease. Note the enlarged summating potential (SP) amplitude relative to the action potential (AP) amplitude.

patients do not demonstrate this abnormality is unclear. The most likely reason relates to the fluctuant nature of the disorder. If, as we believe, enlarged SP amplitudes reflect increased endolymphatic pressure, then these measures could be expected to normalize as the pressure subsides secondary to rupture of the tectorial membrane. Ferraro et al. (36) found a close relationship between enlarged SP-to-AP amplitude ratio and the presence of aural fullness or pressure in the ear and some degree of hearing loss at the time of the ECochG study. Another reason some patients with Meniere's disease may not have an abnormal SP amplitude relates to the deterioration of outer hair cell function known to occur in more advanced stages of Meniere's disease. Once the outer hair cells are damaged, the apparent source of the SP potential is removed and no longer available for study.

Neurodiagnostic Assessment

Measurement of the elapsed time from ABR component waves I to V is generally considered the most sensitive parameter for assessment of retrocochlear disorder. This is because wave I serves as an indicator or peripheral auditory output, whereas wave V represents activity within the brainstem auditory pathway. The wave I–V interwave interval is not influenced by peripheral hearing loss; thus, its abnormal prolongation is thought to be due to retrocochlear impairment. Of course, wave I must be observed to calculate the I–V interval. In the presence of significant hearing loss, wave I may be absent with routine surface electrode recording procedures. In such cases, the combined use of ECochG and ABR often will allow adequate resolution of wave I and V components (Fig. 7).

to-AP ratio of 0.45 or greater is generally considered abnormal (i.e., SP amplitude ≥45% of SP amplitude). However, Coats (35) has noted that this ratio is not a simple linear relationship. For example, in normal subjects, as the AP amplitude increases from 1 to 4 µV, the normal SP-to-AP ratio decreases from 0.4 to 0.25. Thus, a single ratio differentiating normal from abnormal may not be appropriate. Coats has proposed the use of an "AP-normalized SP" amplitude plot to compensate for this nonlinear behavior and improve test sensitivity (Fig. 6).

Most studies report abnormal SP-to-AP measures in approximately two thirds of patients diagnosed with Meniere's disease. The reason why all Meniere's disease

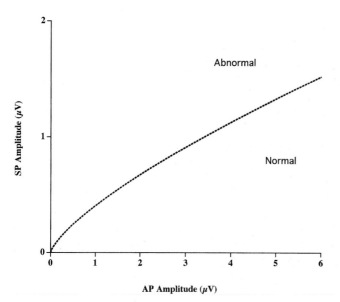

FIG. 6. Method of plotting summating potential (SP) and action potential (AP) amplitudes to determine a normal or abnormal relationship.

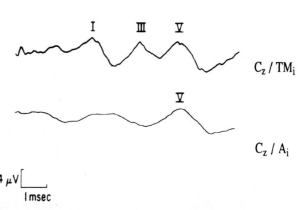

FIG. 7. Auditory brainstem response (ABR) recorded with a vertex (+) to ipsilateral tympanic membrane (-) electrode array (C_z/TM_i) and vertex (+) to ipsilateral earlobe (-) electrode array from a patient with a significant high-frequency hearing loss. Note that wave I is absent from the traditional ABR recording scheme (C_z/A_i) but is present in the combined electrocochleographic/ABR arrangement.

Cochlear Reserve

Otologists may consider knowledge of cochlear reserve essential before deciding whether to operate on a particular ear. Patients with bilateral maximum conductive or mixed-type hearing loss often present a special challenge in this regard due to masking dilemmas. This limitation is related to cross over from the nontest to the test ear of the masking signal at typical levels required to achieve effective masking. In some cases, ECochG can be used effectively to help resolve the integrity of each cochlea because it is considered to be almost exclusively an ipsilateral response. As such, no masking is required to eliminate the participation of the nontest ear.

Intraoperative Monitoring

Virtually any surgical procedure within the posterior fossa places the cochlea and auditory nerve at risk for permanent damage or impairment. In such cases, the surgeon will benefit from ongoing knowledge regarding the status of the inner ear and auditory nerve. When this information is obtained in a timely manner, it can affect the surgical manipulation in such a way as to avoid significant damage. ECochG recording procedures are an important part of such measures when combined with ABR, because they allow for accurate identification of cochlear and distal auditory nerve function in a rapid manner. Further details regarding the use of AEPs for intraoperative monitoring can be found in Chapter 17.

SUMMARY POINTS

- In response to sound, neuroelectric events are generated at various levels within the auditory pathway from cochlea to cerebral cortex. Distinct waveforms occurring within the first 500 ms are termed *auditory evoked potentials.*
- AEPs are recorded by surface electrodes, which are located some distance ("far-field") from their generator sites. Computer averaging of the time-locked responses by a computer is necessary to extract the waveforms of interest from more random background noise of the central nervous system.
- The ABR is a series of five (sometimes up to seven) distinct peaks occurring within the initial 10 to 14 ms following the acoustic stimulus. Waves I and II arise from the distal and proximal parts of the auditory nerve, respectively, and waves III to V from sites within the brainstem.
- The ABR is not affected by state of consciousness; therefore, responses can be recorded from the unconscious patient or from the patient requiring sedation.
- Although the ABR waves can be classified according to latency, amplitude, or morphologic characteristics, latency is the most clinically used parameter.
- Wave V is the most stable and reproducible ABR response, and the one most frequently used in clinical diagnosis.
- There must be a high degree of synchronous firing of cochlear neurons to elicit the ABR. The synchrony is achieved by using a click or high-frequency tone pip as the stimulus. The clinical significance is that the ABR reflects primarily the status of the high-frequency (2,000 to 4,000 Hz) portion of the cochlea.
- There is an inverse relationship between the intensity of the stimulus and the latency of the wave V response. Latency-intensity functions can be useful in estimating magnitude of hearing loss and distinguishing between a conductive and sensorineural hearing loss.
- The ABR is an excellent diagnostic test for eighth nerve lesions (e.g., acoustic neuroma). The anticipated finding is a normal wave I but a delayed wave V.
- For very small (intracanalicular) acoustic neuromas, the false-negative rate for ABR may be as high as 10% to 20%. For larger lesions, sensitivity approaches 90% to 95%.
- The ECochG response consists of an SP, representing cochlear processing, and an AP, reflecting neural discharge from auditory fibers in the more basal portion of the cochlea. The AP is the same response as wave I of the ABR.
- ECochG can be helpful in evaluating Meniere's disease. The key finding is an altered waveform morphology, with an SP amplitude enlarged relative to the AP amplitude. ECochG also is useful in assessing cochlear reserve in patients with bilateral maximal conductive hearing loss (i.e., masking dilemma).

REFERENCES

1. Weber EH. De pulsa, resorpitone, auditu et tactu. De utilitate cochleae in organo auditus. Lipsiae, 1834. In: Feldman H, ed. *A history of audiology: translations of the Beltone Institute for Hearing Research. No. 22.* Chicago: Beltone Institute for Hearing Research, 1970:24.
2. Rinne HA. Beitrage zur Physiologie des menschlichen Ohres. Prager Vierteljahrschr prakt Med 1855:157. In: Feldman H, ed. *A history of audiology: translations of the Beltone Institute for Hearing Research. No. 22.* Chicago: Beltone Institute for Hearing Research, 1970:26.
3. Dix MR, Hallpike CS, Hood JD. Observations upon the loudness recruitment phenomenon, with special reference to the differential diagnosis of disorders of the internal ear and VIII nerve. *J Laryngol Otol* 1948;62:671–686.
4. Fowler EP. The diagnosis of diseases of the neural mechanism of hearing by the aid of sounds well above threshold. *Trans Am Otol Soc* 1937; 27:207–219.
5. von Bekesy GA. New audiometer. *Acta Otolaryngol* 1947;35:411.
6. Reger SN, Cos CM. Clinical measurements and implications of recruitment. *Ann Otol Rhinol Laryngol* 1952;61:810–820.
7. Jerger J. Bekesy audiometry in analysis of auditory disorders. *J Speech Hear Res* 1960;3:275–287.
8. Jerger J, Jerger S. Diagnostic significance of PB word functions. *Arch Otolaryngol* 1971;93:573–580.
9. Hecox K, Galambos R. Brainstem auditory evoked responses in human infants and adults. *Arch Otolaryngol* 1974;99:30–33.
10. Picton TW, Hillyard SA, Krausz HI, Galambos R. Human auditory evoked potentials. I. Evaluation of components. *Electroencephalogr Clin Neurophysiol* 1974;36:179–190.
11. Davis H. Principles of electric response audiometry. *Ann Otol Rhinol Laryngol* 1976;85[Suppl 28]:1-96.
12. Morgan DE, Zimmerman MC, Dubno JR. Auditory brainstem evoked response characteristics in the full-term newborn infant. *Ann Otol Rhinol Laryngol* 1987;96:142–151.
13. Jewett DL, Williston JS. Auditory-evoked far fields averaged from the scalp of humans. *Brain* 1971;94:681–696.
14. Starr A, Achor J. Auditory brainstem responses in neurological disease. *Arch Neurol* 1975;32:761–768.
15. Eggermont J, Don M, Brackmann D. Electrocochleography and auditory brainstem response in humans. *Ann Otol Rhinol Laryngol* 1980; 89[Suppl 75]:1–19.
16. Selters W, Brackmann D. Electrocochleography and auditory brainstem response in humans. *Arch Otolaryngol* 1977;103:15–24.
17. Gordon ML, Cohen NL. Efficacy of auditory brainstem response as a screening test for small acoustic neurons. *Am J Otol* 1995;16:136–139.
18. Chandrasekhar SS, Brackmann DE, Devgan KK. Utility of auditory brain stem response audiometry in diagnosis of acoustic neuromas. *Am J Otol* 1995;16:63–67.
19. Wilson DF, Talbot M, Mills L. A critical appraisal of the role of auditory brain stem response and magnetic resonance imaging in acoustic neuroma diagnosis. *Am J Otol* 1997;18:673–681.
20. Selters WA, Brackmann DE. Acoustic tumor detection with brainstem electric response audiometry. *Arch Otolaryngol* 1977;103: 181–187.
21. Hyde ML, Blair RL. The auditory brainstem response in neuro-otology: perspectives and problems. *J Otolaryngol* 1981;10:117–125.
22. Jerger J, Johnson K. Interactions of age, gender and sensorineural hearing loss on ABR latency. *Ear Hearing* 1988;9:169–175.
23. Wever E, Bray C. Action currents in the auditory nerve in response to acoustic stimulation. *Proc Natl Acad Sci U S A* 1930;16:344–350.
24. Ruben R, Sakula J, Boardly J. Human cochlear response to sound stimuli. *Ann Otol Rhinol Laryngol* 1960;69:459–476.
25. Dallos P. *The auditory periphery.* New York: Academic Press, 1973.
26. Dallos P, Schoeny Z, Cheatham M. Cochlear summating potentials: descriptive aspects. *Acta Otolaryngol* 1972;302[Suppl]:1–46.
27. Moller A, Jannetta P. Interpretation of brain stem auditory evoked potentials: results from intracranial recordings in humans. *Scand Audiol* 1983;12:125–133.
28. Cullen J, Ellis M, Berlin C, Loustear R. Human acoustic nerve action potential recordings from the tympanic membrane without anesthesia. *Acta Otolaryngol* 1972;74:15–22.
29. Stypulkowski P, Staller S. Clinical evaluation of a new EcoG recording electrode. *Ear Hearing* 1987;8:304–310.
30. Ruth A, Lambert P, Ferraro J. Electrocochleography: methods and clinical applications. *Am J Otol* 1988;9:1–11.
31. Ruth R, Lambert P. Comparison of tympanic membrane to promontory electrode recordings of electrocochleographic responses in Meniere's patients. *Otolaryngol Head Neck Surg* 1989;100:546–552.
32. Ruth R. Electrocochleography. In: Katz J, ed. *Handbook of clinical audiology,* 4th ed. Baltimore: Williams & Wilkins, 1994:339–350.
33. Gibson W, Moffat D, Ransden R. Clinical electrocochleography in the diagnosis and management in Meniere's disease. *Audiology* 1977;16: 389–401.
34. Eggermont J. Summating potentials in electrocochleography: relation to hearing disorders. In: Ruben R, Eberling C, Salomon G, eds. *Electrocochleography.* Baltimore: University Park Press, 1976:67–87.
35. Coats A. The normal summating potential recorded from the external ear canal. *Arch Otolaryngol* 1986;112:759–768.
36. Ferraro J, Arenberg I, Hassanein R. Electrocochleography and symptoms of inner ear dysfunction. *Arch Otolaryngol* 1985;111:71–74.

The Ear: Comprehensive Otology,
edited by R. F. Canalis and P. R. Lambert.
Lippincott Williams & Wilkins, Philadelphia © 2000.

CHAPTER 14

Otoacoustic Emissions

Donald D. Dirks and Donald E. Morgan

Classification of Otoacoustic Emissions
Clinical Measurement of Otoacoustic Emissions
Clinical Applications

Cochlear Disorder
Eighth Nerve Disorder
Summary

Although there are many puzzling issues regarding the mechanism of hearing, none has been more baffling than the explanation for the high sensitivity, sharp frequency tuning, and wide perceptual dynamic range observed in psychoacoustic studies in humans and from eighth nerve recordings from some animals. Initially, the cochlea had been viewed as broadly tuned, based principally on early data collected on cadavers (1). The damping characteristics of the cochlea have been explained by a variety of hypotheses, including positive feedback loops or other neural mechanisms that might act to sharpen the response of the cochlea. In 1948, Gold (2) hypothesized that the hair cells might be considered active elements that were capable of modifying the basilar membrane motion via a feedback system, thus providing a sharpened frequency response. This hypothesis was intriguing but remained undocumented until 1978, when Kemp (3) reported the measurement of evoked otoacoustic emissions (OAEs) that could be recorded at very low intensity levels in the external ear canal. Kemp's work suggested that these emissions might be a by-product of cochlear processes, specifically, nonlinear, vibration characteristics at near-threshold intensity levels in the normal ear. Since Kemp's original observations, numerous investigations have confirmed his results and revealed that these emissions result from normal active cochlear processing within the organ of Corti that contributes to the high-sensitivity, sharp frequency response and wide dynamic range of the normal auditory system.

D. D. Dirks: Division of Head and Neck Surgery, University of California, Los Angeles, School of Medicine, Los Angeles, California 90095.

D. E. Morgan: Decibel Instruments, Inc., Fremont, California 94555

Kemp interpreted the emissions to be acoustic energy "leakage" secondary to hair cell activity initiated by the cochlear traveling wave. The energy emanating from the motility of the outer hair cells is released from the cochlea and transmitted via the ossicular chain into the external ear canal. There is now ample evidence that the evoked OAEs are a response to low- and moderate-level stimuli that depend on normal cochlear function and appear to be specific to normal outer hair cell activity. OAEs are not, in and of themselves, essential to hearing; rather, they are a by-product of cochlear processes that are essential to hearing. The evidence supporting such a hypothesis is based primarily on experiments (4–7) that demonstrate that OAEs are preneural and are physiologically vulnerable, depending on the integrity of the outer hair cells. Because the measurement of OAEs is objective and noninvasive, OAEs are particularly useful as a clinical tool to demonstrate a dysfunction associated with the outer hair cells.

CLASSIFICATION OF OAES

OAEs can be broadly classified as spontaneous otoacoustic emissions (SOAEs) or evoked otoacoustic emissions (EOAEs). SOAEs are narrowband signals recorded in the external ear in the absence of external acoustic stimulation. To date, estimates of the prevalence of SOAEs appear to depend on instrumentation and procedural limitations. However, all reports, even from the earliest, are consistent in suggesting that (a) SOAEs are observed only among persons with normal hearing; (b) the spontaneous emission is typically narrow band (often 1 Hz); and, (c) typically the spontaneous emission is stable in amplitude and frequency (8). Reports, however, also are consistent in revealing that the SOAE is subject to influence of contralateral stimulation (9).

In the early 1980s, prevalences of 35% to 40% were common (8); however, as microphone sensitivity, filtering techniques, noise floor control, and other measurement procedures have improved, the reports of SOAE incidence have increased to as high as 72% of persons with normal hearing (10,11). Additionally, recent data have suggested that both gender and racial differences in the incidence of SOAEs may exist, leading to speculation that genetic factors may play a role in the prevalence of SOAEs. Specifically, several studies have identified a higher incidence of SOAEs among normal hearing women than among men (12–14). Whitehead et al. (15) reported differences in prevalence of SOAEs among selected racial groups, supporting the possibility that genetic factors may be a determinant in the incidence of SOAE. The most recent reports (16,17) have identified no differences in the incidence of SOAEs as a function of age, with preterm and full-term neonates showing the same prevalence as normal hearing children and adults. Because SOAEs do not occur in all normal ears, their utility as tools for detection of hearing impairment or in differential diagnosis currently has been limited.

EOAEs are elicited by delivering an acoustic stimulus to the ear. Three types of EOAEs can be usefully categorized based on the stimuli used to evoke them. They include transiently evoked OAEs (TEOAEs) elicited by an acoustic transient such as a click or tone burst; the stimulus-frequency OAEs (SFOAEs) elicited by a single, continuous pure tone; and the distortion product OAEs (DPOAEs) produced in response to two continuous pure tones, separated in frequency.

The TEOAE is a frequency-dispersive response that is evident 4 to 15 ms after presentation of a brief acoustic stimulus such as a click. Nearly all young, normal hearing human ears exhibit TEOAEs. The growth of the TEOAE is nonlinear, increasing less than 1 dB per decibel increase in stimulus level. The TEOAE is absent in ears with sensorineural hearing loss of cochlear origin of 30 to 35 dB hearing level (HL). The TEOAEs tend to be larger in amplitude in infants than adults (18). Because the TEOAE is present in most normal hearing ears and because of the high amplitude of the TEOAE in the infant, there has been great interest in the application of TEOAEs as a hearing screening procedure in infants (19).

The SFOAE is a continuous emission of low-level sound from the cochlea at the frequency of the pure tone stimulus delivered to the ear. SFOAEs apparently are generated by the same mechanism that produces the TEOAEs (20) and appear to be present in nearly all normal hearing ears. Because the stimulus is larger than the emission and simultaneously present at the same frequency in the ear canal, the existence of SFOAEs is observed by sweeping the frequency of the continuous tone. The phase lag of the emission relative to the stimulus increases with increasing frequency, which results in physical interference between the stimulus and the emission. Thus, ripples occur in the otherwise smooth response as the stimulus and the SFOAE moves alternately in and out of phase. There have been only isolated systematic investigations of the practical application of the SFOAE, and there are no current, commercially available systems enabling measurement of the SFOAE.

The DPOAE is an emission from the cochlea at intermodulation distortion frequencies evoked by stimulation of the ear with two pure tones of appropriate frequencies. They are measured by spectral analysis of the energy in the external ear canal. The driving stimuli commonly used to evoke the DPOAE are two pure tones at 65 db sound pressure level (SPL) with an f_2/f_1 ratio of 1.2 to 1.25 (21). The most robust distortion product emission has been observed at the frequency $2f_1 - f_2$ (cubic distortion product). DPOAEs can be detected in most normal hearing humans. Similar to other OAEs, the DPOAE levels typically are low (20), but they can be detected by using either selective amplifiers or averaging techniques with subsequent Fourier analysis.

Since identification of the phenomenon in 1978, research interests have focused on the various OAEs to answer basic physiologic questions regarding cochlear function and to develop clinical tools that may contribute to current audiologic diagnostic tests. Clinical evidence suggests that patients evidencing more than 30 to 40 dB HL thresholds, secondary to a cochlear site of lesion, have no identifiable OAE to transient auditory stimuli. In addition, middle ear lesions typically preclude the measurement of the OAE. Of interest are some patients with retrocochlear disorders with significant sensorineural hearing loss who evidence normal OAEs. As such, the OAE represents the first available auditory function test from which it may be possible to differentiate sensory from neural sites of lesion when the potential exists for only one or the other site to be implicated. A comprehensive review of the use of OAEs for clinical applications can be found in a publication by Robinette and Glattke (22).

CLINICAL MEASUREMENT OF OAES

Because the OAE phenomenon has only recently been discovered and verified, commercially available clinical instruments for its measurement are limited. The instrument with which the predominance of clinical investigations have been conducted is the Otodynamic Analyzer, with software and interfacing hardware developed by Kemp et al. (23). This instrument measures TEOAEs. The "click" stimulus is an 80-μs rectangular pulse stimulus with a frequency response from 600 to 5,000 Hz, and a pulse rate of 50/s. Click stimulus level is under the control of the operator.

The most commonly used strategy for measuring TEOAEs is to present clicks or tone pips via a transducer in a probe fitted to the patient's external ear canal. The probe is coupled to the canal with soft, flexible tips similar to those used in immittance measurements. The emission is measured via a second channel in the probe tip containing a measuring microphone. Responses to two averaged stimulus sets of more than 100 stimuli are averaged and displayed in a 20-ms time-domain window with the initial 2.5 ms blocked to reduce activating signal "artifacts." It is also possible to search for the emission "threshold" with the aforementioned instrumentation or to use moderate-level stimuli where nonlinear growth of the TEOAE is near saturation. Searching for an emission threshold can be especially time consuming and becomes complicated for interpretation, because the threshold

apparently increases with increasing age over 30 years (24).

The results shown in Fig. 1 were obtained by presentations of broadband click stimuli at 80 dB SPL. The resulting acoustic stimulus (as measured by the recording microphone in the probe tip) is presented in the upper left quadrant for Fig. 1A and B and is titled "stimulus." The evoked cochlear emission is characterized in two ways in Fig. 1. The middle panel, titled "cochlear response," reflects the averaged waveform identifiable in the external ear canal as a function of poststimulus time (2.5 to 20 ms).

Following each click presentation, acoustic energy in the ear canal is recorded and delivered to one of two memories

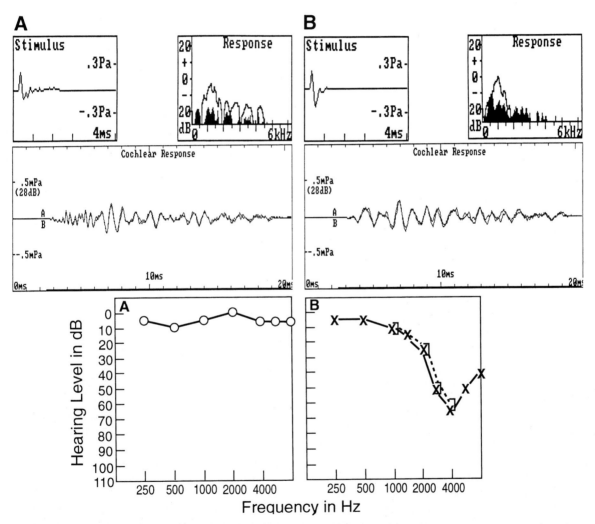

FIG. 1. Transiently evoked otoacoustic emissions **(upper and middle panels)** and audiograms **(lower panel)** for two patients, one with normal hearing **(A)** and the other with a high-frequency sensorineural hearing loss **(B)**. The **upper left panels** (Stimulus) for each patient show the acoustic waveform of the click stimuli as measured in the canal during the test. The **upper right panels** (Response) show the spectrum of the emission (*white area* under the curve) in dB SPL, as a function of frequency, along with the associated noise spectrum (*shaded area*) in the ear canal. The **middle panel** (Cochlear Response) shows emission waveforms as a function of time from 2.5 to 20 ms (poststimulus period). The two cochlear response waveforms (A and B) provide a measure of the replicability of the cochlear emission with repeated click presentations.

(A or B). Time-locked (with respect to the click stimulus) energy will increase in amplitude (to a maximum) as averaging occurs over time. The correlation between the average responses in memories A and B provides a measure of the replicability of TEOAE over time. The waveforms of memories A and B are combined and a Fourier analysis is performed to provide a measure of the frequency specificity of the TEOAE throughout the 20-ms poststimulus period. The upper right quadrants in Fig. 1A and B show the Fourier analysis of the spectrum of the evoked cochlear emission (white area) and of the noise (shaded area) in the ear canal for subjects who evidence audiograms as presented in the bottom panels of Fig. 1A and B.

The left panels (A) in Fig. 1 show the results of the TEOAE and the audiogram from a normal hearing patient with normal middle ear function (demonstrated from tympanometric measurements). Results from a patient with a sharply sloping, high-frequency hearing loss of cochlear origin (noise induced) are shown in Fig. 1B. As shown in Fig. 1B, a TEOAE response is observed throughout the frequency range of 700 to 4,500 Hz for the normal hearing patient. For the patient with a high-frequency sensorineural hearing loss of cochlear origin, an equally replicable TEOAE is present, but it is restricted to the frequency region where the hearing loss is less than 30 dB HL. When interpreting TEOAE data, the presence of emissions suggests normal or near-normal hearing (less than 30 dB HL) throughout the frequency region of the response. The absence of a response in a particular frequency region, however, does not always rule out near-normal hearing sensitivity, because the amplitude and frequency spectrum of the TEOAE response decrease significantly with age and apparently can be affected by other factors not yet identified.

TEOAEs have been observed in some ears with retrocochlear lesions due to acoustic tumors and are absent in others. Because the TEOAE requires viable outer hair cell function but is not dependent on neural integrity, the measurement provides differential diagnostic information regarding the preoperative integrity of the cochlea as reflected in the TEOAE. The TEOAE represents the only current test of auditory test function from which the clinician can differentiate the sensory from the neural component of the loss. This differentiation can be made only in those patients in whom the sensorineural loss exceeds 30 to 35 dB HL and a TEOAE is present. The presence of a TEOAE suggests that outer hair cell function remains intact, despite the sensorineural loss, leading to the conclusion that the loss is predominantly neural in origin, throughout the frequency region of the TEOAE.

In those cases in which a retrocochlear lesion is evident and sensorineural hearing loss is observed but the TEOAE is absent, one cannot rule out a cochlear component contributing to the sensorineural hearing loss. Figure 2 provides an example of a retrocochlear lesion affecting a significant sensorineural hearing loss in

which the TEOAE is present. A practical application of such findings is to provide information that might influence the surgical approach and the potential to maintain postoperative hearing function. To explain, in those instances in which the TEOAE is absent, the portion of the preoperative loss attributable to cochlear function will be unaffected by the surgical outcome; only that portion secondary to the retrocochlear lesion could be affected by the surgery. However, if the preoperative OAE is normal, then the surgical procedure has the potential to affect postoperative hearing both in terms of the positive effect of the procedure on neural integrity and the negative effect on sensory function. During surgical procedures to remove space-occupying lesions affecting the eighth cranial nerve, the most vulnerable anatomy for maintenance of cochlea integrity is the blood supply to the cochlea. When the OAE is present preoperatively (regardless of the presence or absence of hearing loss) but absent postoperatively, it is probable that blood supply to the cochlea has been compromised during (or following) the surgical procedure. Although information regarding the application of the OAE among patients with retrocochlear lesions is rapidly accumulating it is currently incomplete. It is, however, possible that the OAE will provide preoperative and postoperative information regarding cochlear integrity and may provide information leading to more accurate predictions of those patients whose hearing potentially can be maintained or improved during surgical removal of space-occupying lesions affecting the eighth cranial nerve.

CLINICAL APPLICATIONS

This section contains representative results of the differential diagnostic tests discussed in Chapters 12, 13, and 14.

Cochlear Disorder

Figure 3 shows results from a patient with Meniere's disease in the right ear. The patient was a 40-year-old woman with a complaint of unilateral hearing loss, tinnitus, and "fullness" in the right ear associated with a severe attack of vertigo. Radiologic findings were normal. Pure tone thresholds indicated a moderate (50 to 55 dB HL) hearing loss in the right ear with the greatest loss in the low- and mid-frequency region. The bone conduction thresholds in the right ear were elevated and the tympanogram was normal, suggesting the hearing loss was sensorineural in origin.

The acoustic reflex was present in both ears, although slightly elevated when the right ear was stimulated (either ipsilaterally or contralaterally). The presence of the acoustic reflex at near-normal hearing levels, in an ear with sensorineural hearing loss, is consistent with a cochlear disorder.

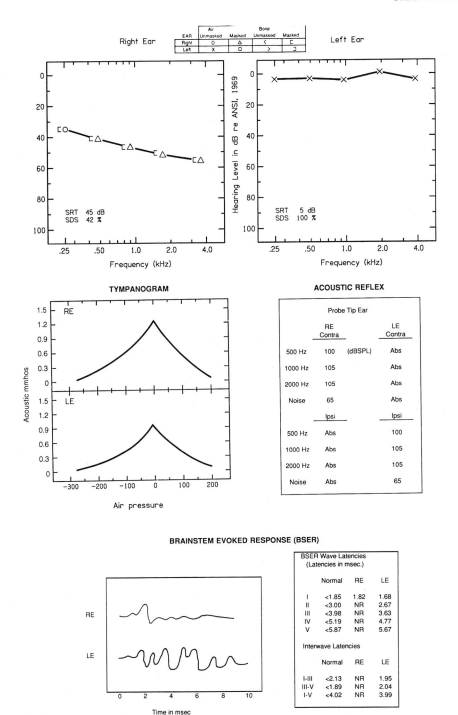

FIG. 2. Auditory diagnostic test results for a patient with a cerebellopontine angle tumor in the right ear. The left ear has normal hearing.

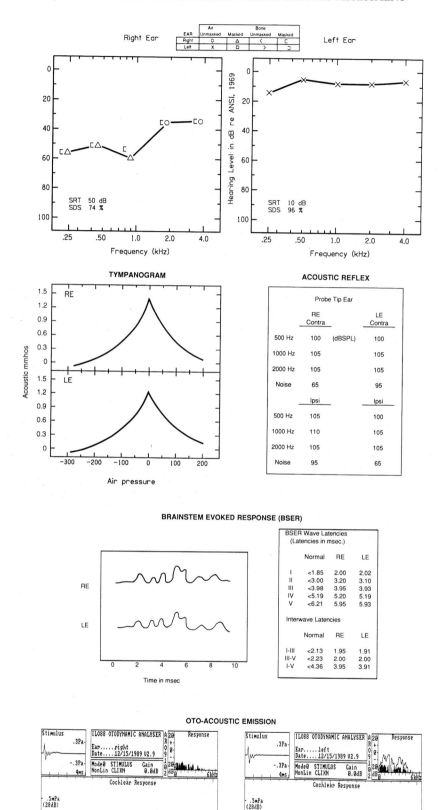

FIG. 3. Auditory diagnostic test results for a patient with Meniere's disease in the right ear. The left ear has normal hearing.

The auditory brainstem response absolute wave latencies, as well as the interwave latencies, for waves I through V were within normal limits for both ears. Finally, the OAE was present for the left ear, with a replicable response throughout the initial 16 ms of the response period with energy throughout the frequency range from 700 to 4,000 Hz. The OAE was absent in the right ear. Recall that OAEs are characteristically absent once the cochlear hearing loss is greater than approximately 30 dB HL.

Eighth Nerve Disorder

Figure 2 illustrates the results from a 48-year-old man with a surgically confirmed eighth nerve tumor. Radiologic evidence indicated that a space-occupying lesion was present in the right cerebellopontine angle. The patient complained of occasional imbalance, tinnitus, and hearing loss in the right ear. The standard auditory tests demonstrated a moderate sensorineural hearing loss in the right ear and normal thresholds in the left ear. The speech recognition score was low (42%). The tympanograms were normal bilaterally, and the acoustic reflex was absent to acoustic stimuli presented to the right ear while normal results were observed for presentations to the left ear.

For the auditory brainstem response test, waves II through V were absent in the right ear, a finding consistent with a retrocochlear lesion. The OAE was present in each ear. The presence of the OAE response is of special interest, because the loss exceeded 30 dB HL in the right ear. The presence of an OAE response in the right ear suggests that the hair cells in the impaired ear were functioning normally despite the presence of the cerebellopontine angle tumor affecting right ear function.

SUMMARY

The fundamental purpose of administering differential diagnostic tests is to identify the site of lesion associated with a particular auditory impairment. The choice of individual test procedures to be conducted should be based on the patient's history, findings on physical examination, and the results of standard auditory tests such as air and bone conduction audiometry, speech recognition measures, and tympanometry. Clinical research and experience has shown that the identification of the site of an auditory lesion is accomplished most effectively by examining the results of several, rather than any single, audiologic measure. The test battery approach to the differential diagnosis of auditory disorders offers several advantages, which include (a) avoiding overgeneralization from a single procedure, (b) a larger database for making predictions, and (c) greater predictive confidence as the number of test results consistently suggests a specific site for the lesion.

As history has shown, differential auditory diagnosis is an evolutionary process. As new procedures are available, their usefulness depends on the accuracy and efficiency with which they contribute to the determination of the anatomic site of auditory lesion. In Chapters 12, 13, and 14 we reviewed the historical, widely used, and evolving measures that are commonly applied in diagnostic audiologic testing.

SUMMARY POINTS

- OAEs result from normal active cochlear processing within the organ of Corti. Specifically, energy from outer hair cell movement is released and transmitted via the ossicular chin into the external auditory canal.
- OAEs can be broadly classified as spontaneous (occurring in the absence of external sound) or evoked (elicited by an acoustic stimulus).
- EOAEs can be elicited by a continuous pure tone or by an acoustic transient such as a click or tone pip. The latter emissions are referred to as "transiently evoked otoacoustic emissions" and occur 4 to 15 ms after the stimulus.
- OAEs are measured via a sensitive microphone placed in the external auditory canal. An evoked emission is the computer-averaged response to several hundred stimuli (e.g., clicks).
- When two pure tones are presented to an ear simultaneously, an evoked emission is observed at an intermediate frequency defined by $2f_1 - f_2$ (where f_1 is the lower of the two frequencies). This evoked response is termed a "distortion product otoacoustic emission."
- TEOAEs and DPOAEs are present in most normal hearing ears, but they are not generated in ears with a cochlear sensorineural hearing loss of more than 30 to 35 dB HL. They are usually absent in ears with a significant conductive hearing loss, as this condition precludes their measurement in the external auditory canal.
- OAEs, especially transiently evoked responses, are being used increasingly as a hearing screening procedure in infants.
- OAEs represent the first auditory function test with the potential for differentiating between a sensory and neural cause for sensorineural hearing loss. For example, a patient with severe sensorineural hearing loss secondary to a neural lesion (e.g., acoustic tumor) may have intact OAEs, because the organ of Corti is unaffected.

REFERENCES

1. von Bekesy G. *Experiments in hearing.* New York: McGraw-Hill Book Company, Inc., 1960.
2. Gold T. Hearing II. The physical basis of the action of the cochlea. *Proc R Acad B* 1948;135:492–498.
3. Kemp DT. Stimulated acoustic emissions from the auditory system. *J Acoust Soc Am* 1978;64:1386–1391.
4. Kemp T, Chum R. Observations on the generator mechanism of stimulus frequency acoustic emissions—two tone suppression. In: van den Brink G, Bilsen F, eds. *Psychophysical, physiological, and behavioral studies in hearing.* Delft: Delft University, 1983:34–42.
5. Lonsbury-Martin BL, Martin GK, Probst R, Coats AC. Acoustic distortion products in rabbit ear canal. I. Basic features and physiological vulnerability. *Hear Res* 1987;28:173–189.
6. Arts H, Norton S, Rubel E. Influence of perilymphatic tetrodoxin and calcium concentration on hair cell function. *Abstracts of 13th Annual Mid-winter Meeting of Association for Research in Otolaryngology* 1990.
7. Siegel J, Kim D. Cochlear biomechanics: vulnerability to acoustic trauma and other alterations as seen in neural responses and ear-canal sound pressure. In: Hamernik D, Henderson D, Salvi R, eds. *New perspectives on noise-induced hearing loss.* New York: Raven Press, 1982:137.
8. Bright KE. Spontaneous emissions. In: Robinette M, Glattke T, eds. *Otoacoustic emissions: clinical applications.* New York: Thieme Medical Publishers, 1997:46–62.
9. Harrison WA, Burns EM. Effects of contralateral acoustic stimulation on spontaneous otoacoustic emissions. *J Acoust Soc Am* 1993;94:2649–2658.
10. Penner MJ, Glotzbach L, Huang T. Spontaneous otoacoustic emissions: measurement and data. *Hear Res* 1993;68:229–237.
11. Talmadge CL, Long GR, Murphy WJ, Tubis A. New off-line method for detecting spontaneous otoacoustic emissions in human subjects. *Hear Res* 1993;71:170–182.
12. Bilger RC, Matthies ML, Hammel DR, Demorest ME. Genetic implications of gender differences in the prevalence of spontaneous otoacoustic emissions. *J Speech Hear Res* 1990;33:418–432.
13. Martin G, Probst R, Lonsbury-Martin BL. Otoacoustic emissions in human ears: normative findings. *Ear Hear* 1990;11:106–120.
14. Strickland AE, Burns EM, Tubis A. Incidence of spontaneous otoacoustic emissions in children and infants. *J Acoust Soc Am* 1985;78:931–935.
15. Whitehead ML, Kamal N, Lonsbury-Martin BL, Martin GK. Spontaneous acoustic emissions in different racial groups. *Scand Audiol* 1993;22:3–10.
16. Burns EM, Arehart KH, Campbell SL. Prevalence of spontaneous otoacoustic emissions in neonates. *J Acoust Soc Am* 1992;91:1571–1575.
17. Bonfils P, Francois M, Avan P, Londero A, Trotuoux J, Narcy P. Spontaneous and evoked otoacoustic emissions in preterm neonates. *Laryngoscope* 1992;102:182–186.
18. Robinette M. Clinical observations with transient evoked otoacoustic emissions with adults. *Semin Hear* 1992;13:1–23.
19. Martin G, Whitehead M, Lonsbury-Martin B. Potential of evoked otoacoustic emissions for infant hearing screening. *Semin Hear* 1990;11:186.
20. Whitehead M, Lonsbury-Martin, Martin G. Relevance of animal models to the clinical applications of otoacoustic emissions. *Semin Hear* 1992;13:81.
21. Durrant J. Distortion-product OAE analysis: is it ready for broad clinical use? *Hear J* 1992;45:42.
22. Robinette M, Glattke T. In: Robinette M, Glattke T, eds. *Otoacoustic emissions: clinical applications.* New York: Thieme Medical Publishers, 1997.
23. Kemp D, Bray P, Alexander L, Brown A. Acoustic emission cochleography—practical aspects. *Scand Audiol* 1986;25[Suppl]:71.
24. Bonfils P, Bertrand Y, Uziel A. Evoked otoacoustic emissions: normative data and presbycusis. *Audiology* 1988;27:27.

The Ear: Comprehensive Otology,
edited by R. F. Canalis and P. R. Lambert.
Lippincott Williams & Wilkins, Philadelphia © 2000.

CHAPTER 15

Differential Diagnosis of Central Auditory System Disorders

Douglas Noffsinger and Charles D. Martinez

The central auditory nervous system (CANS) is an entity whose major parts include the auditory brainstem and the auditory brain. It is not a system that has an agreed-on starting point or end, but it is a system that is functionally very different from its peripheral auditory extensions. For purposes of definition in this chapter, the CANS will be considered to start beyond (central to) the eighth cranial nerve synapses at the cochlear nuclei and to end in auditory processing areas of the posterior temporal lobes.

Tests of CANS integrity and function have many properties and goals that are different from tests designed to investigate peripheral auditory behavior. People with CANS disease uncomplicated by concomitant peripheral auditory damage usually do not have hearing loss for tones or problems hearing or understanding speech, at least as such functions are typically measured. Furthermore, many of the tests that are useful in differentiating one kind of peripheral auditory system damage from another are of little benefit in examining auditory brainstem or brain function. This state of affairs makes detection of CANS damage or disease both interesting and challenging.

This chapter is designed to provide some historical perspective on the differential diagnosis of problems in the CANS, to review test procedures useful in detecting CANS dysfunction, and to illustrate, through case studies, the results that are obtained in typical syndromes of CANS damage. It concentrates by design on test procedures that investigate functions unique to the CANS. As Carhart (1) pointed out, differential diagnosis in the auditory system is successful in direct proportion to the extent to which it incorporates tools that probe functions unique to a particular point in that system. As shall be seen, for the CANS this usually means tests that evaluate either transmission through, or binaural behaviors of, the auditory brainstem, and either transmission through, or speech processing by, the auditory brain.

HISTORICAL PERSPECTIVE

Bocca and his colleagues and students (2–5), the "Italian School" in clinical investigations of hearing function, deserve great credit for work that made known both the manifestations of brain damage in auditory behavior and avenues that would be fruitful in seeking such evidence. Beginning more than 40 years ago, they pointed out that lesions to auditory areas of the brain could be detected by measuring patients' recognition of speech that was made difficult to understand in some way. The ways in which difficulty was added to speech took many forms, and several of them were useful. Noteworthy was the finding that it is the ear on the side opposite brain damage that shows breakdown in performance, e.g., poor word recognition. This was true, however, only when the speech was more

D. Noffsinger and C. D. Martinez: Department of Audiology and Speech Pathology, West Los Angeles VA Healthcare Center, Los Angeles, California 90073

difficult than usual to understand. For most brain-damaged patients, undistorted speech was still comprehended without difficulty.

Although psychoacousticians had been interested in binaural (two-ear) phenomena for many years (6–9), it was clinical investigators associated with the Outpatient Research Center for Sensorineural Deafness at Northwestern University with support from the National Institutes of Health who made apparent that looking at binaural interaction could be profitable in finding and understanding lesions of the auditory system including the auditory brainstem. Carhart and his colleagues and students showed that auditory abilities such as lateralization, binaural sequencing and correlation, and signal detection in noise were clues to the integrity of brainstem structures—and that these functions could be measured clinically (10–14).

Later investigators found different and sometimes better ways to look at the CANS. Procedures such as acoustic reflex threshold and adaptation tests (for review, see Chapter 12) and auditory brainstem response (ABR) measures (15,16) provided information about the intactness of pathways in the brainstem. Auditory evoked potentials of a longer and later time course than the ABR (17,18) and dichotic speech tests (19) gave new insight into the effects of cortical damage and disease. In addition, despite long-standing conventional wisdom that pure tone studies were of little help in evaluating CANS performance, scientists found ways in which perception of tones and tone patterns was affected by brain damage and thus useful to clinicians (20,21). Projecting into time, electrophysiologists allude to a future in which not only auditory events but auditory processes will be measured by simple electrode arrays on the human scalp. However, current technology, particularly when looking at auditory brain function, still usually requires that clinicians present speech or tonal stimuli to patients and that patients voluntarily respond as best they can.

DIFFERENTIAL DIAGNOSTIC TEST PROCEDURES

Auditory Brainstem

Procedures used to examine auditory brainstem function include those that investigate the integrity of transmission lines through the brainstem, those that examine the effects on threshold of binaural interaction, and those that measure the end result of transmission or interaction, usually speech procedures. In the transmission-line category, the most commonly used tests are transbrainstem (also called contralateral or crossed) acoustic reflex measurements and the ABR. Tests of the influence of binaural interaction on threshold that are currently popular include masking level differences for tones and speech. Measures that examine the results of transmission through, or interactions within, the brainstem use speech

discrimination as the key. These include tests requiring fusion of simultaneous or sequential speech segments and tasks that examine understanding of speech made difficult to comprehend by various techniques. Although the speech tasks ultimately depend on speech processing areas of the auditory brain, they first require efficient, undistorted transmission through the brainstem and/or binaural integration of speech parts into a whole by brainstem centers.

Transmission-line Tests

Acoustic Reflexes

The acoustic reflex arc required for a loud sound presented to one ear to trigger an acoustic reflex in both ears includes pathways that cross the low brainstem. Lesions or malfunctions affecting these pathways can prevent the occurrence of the acoustic reflex. In a typical clinical audiologic evaluation, ipsilateral acoustic reflexes, those requiring no cross-brainstem transmission, are also sought. The classic picture resulting from damage within the low intraaxial brainstem is loss of acoustic reflexes that require the transbrainstem passage but retention of the ipsilateral reflex events. This is discussed in Chapter 12 and clearly reviewed by Northern et al. (22). Cortical lesions usually do not affect acoustic reflex behavior (23). A summary of selected lesion sites and their manifestations on acoustic reflex measures is listed in Table 1.

Auditory Brainstem Response

The series of electrical events that occur in the first 10 ms following the presentation of brief, abrupt acoustic signals to the ear is the ABR. In essence, the ABR is a neuroelectric signature of acoustic events as they traverse the eighth cranial nerve and the brainstem. To the extent that each event represents electrical activity at some particular place, abnormalities in expected behavior could point to a location of concern. Although it is becoming increasingly clear from studies of many sorts (24) that the relationship between some potentials and their generator sites is not straightforward, each event in the train of events called the ABR is still thought to represent activity attributable to an area of the eighth cranial nerve or brainstem. Those areas are summarized in Fig. 1, and a good review of the voluminous literature is given by Hall (18). As shown in Fig. 1, the first three waves of the ABR sequence are thought to arise from the eighth cranial nerve and the low brainstem. Later waves IV, V, and VI are associated with ascending tracts (lateral lemniscus) and higher nuclear centers in the brainstem.

It is important to emphasize that characteristic ABR patterns result from various kinds of brainstem disease. Two examples will suffice. (a) Demyelinating diseases such as multiple sclerosis often affect periventricular areas such as those around the fourth ventricle in the

TABLE 1. *Expected acoustic reflex results for both transbrainstem (crossed) and ipsilateral (uncrossed) procedures*

Lesion site	Stimulus ear			
	Ipsilateral to lesion		Contralateral to lesion	
	Crossed	Uncrossed	Crossed	Uncrossed
VII N periph	Present	Present	Present	Present
VII N central	Present	Absent	Absent	Present
VIII N/EABS	Elevated or absent	Elevated or absent	Absent if VII involved	Present
IABS (low)	Elevated or absent	Present	Elevated or absent	Present
IABS (high)	Present	Present	Present	Present
Temporal lobe	Present	Present	Present	Present

The various lesion sites are presumed to be the sole influence on reflex behavior.

VII N periph, seventh nerve peripheral to stapedial branch; VII N central, seventh nerve central to stapedial branch; VIII N/EABS, eighth nerve/extraaxial brainstem; IABS (low), low intraaxial brainstem; IABS (high), high intraaxial brainstem.

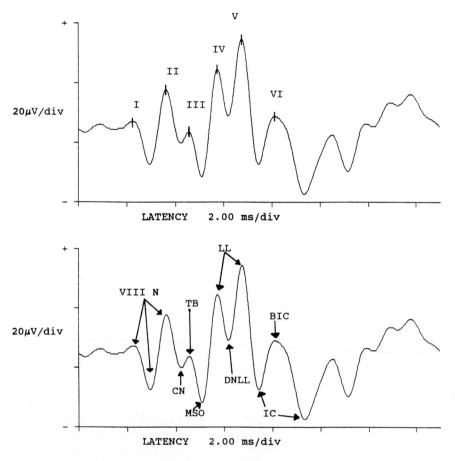

FIG. 1. Top: The auditory brainstem response (ABR) elicited by 2-ms, 4000-Hz tone pips from a young, normal hearing listener. The vertex-positive potentials are labeled in a conventional fashion using Roman numerals I–VI to identify each waveform in sequence of temporal occurrence (16). **Bottom:** The same ABR events with indications of structures from which they may arise [after the discussion and model by Hall (18)]. BIC, brachium, inferior colliculus; CN, cochlear nucleus; DNLL, dorsal nucleus, lateral lemniscus; IC, inferior colliculus; LL, lateral lemniscus; MSO, medial superior olivary nucleus; TB, trapezoid body; VIII N, acoustic branch of eighth cranial nerve.

brainstem. When this occurs, the typical ABR pattern includes the two potentials that arise from the auditory branch of cranial nerve VIII (Jewett waves I and II) (16), but often includes no other normal potentials. Importantly, this may occur in combination with absent transbrainstem (crossed) acoustic reflexes and normal pure tone thresholds, an alliance that is strongly suggestive of low brainstem disorder. (b) Lesions higher in the brainstem, such as damage in the area of the optic chiasm, often leave unaffected the pattern of expected eighth cranial nerve and brainstem potentials except for the late ones, e.g., waves IV and/or V. This finding usually occurs in combination with normal acoustic reflex behavior, an indication that transmission of stimuli through the low brainstem is occurring normally. In a similar vein, lesions in the brain including damage to the temporal lobe usually do not affect the ABR (23).

Binaural Interaction Tasks

Pure Tone Masking Level Difference

When identical low-frequency tones are delivered to the ears in the presence of noise that is also identical at the two ears, reversing the phase of the tone to one ear relative to the phase of the tone in the other ear makes the threshold for the tones better for normal listeners. This release from the effect of the masking noise is called a masking level difference (MLD). As Noffsinger et al. (25) pointed out in their review of this phenomenon, "It is apparent that the binaural masking level difference depends on retrocochlear interaction of signal/masker configurations coming from the two ears, and it seems sensible that such binaural interaction would occur as early as is physiologically possible in the auditory system." Much evidence now exists that the interaction is centered in the caudal pons of the low brainstem (26–28), is unaffected by brain lesions (23), and may not even require brain centers (29).

Pure tone MLDs usually are measured using 500-Hz sinusoids and narrowband noise centered around 500 Hz. These conditions allow large MLDs (8 to 16 dB) when measured clinically (14). Two phase conditions typically are used: a homophasic condition (SoNo) featuring tones at the two earphones that are in phase (So) and noise to the same phones that is also in phase (No); and an antiphasic condition (SπNo) in which the tone to one earphone is 180 degrees out-of-phase with an otherwise identical tone to the other earphone (Sπ), but the noise to the two earphones is in phase (No). The MLD is the threshold difference (in dB) for the tones between the homophasic and antiphasic conditions. Clinically, MLDs are measured using either manual or automatic threshold-seeking methods.

MLD size for tones is influenced by most kinds of auditory dysfunction that produce hearing loss. This is less of a problem than it seems, because MLD procedures are hardly needed to sort one kind of hearing loss from another. More important, MLDs often are greatly reduced or absent in cases of brainstem damage or dysfunction. In the largest series reported to date, Noffsinger (30) reported that half of 140 persons with medically diagnosed brainstem disorders and relatively normal hearing had small or no MLDs. Equally important, virtually all patients with focal lesions of the medullopontine area have abnormal MLDs (27). Most important, many studies (26,28,31) have concluded that "...the coincidence of normal hearing, abnormal MLDs, abnormal transbrainstem acoustic reflexes and an abnormal ABR commencing at potential III is a virtual guarantee that abnormalities of the caudal medullopons area exist" (25).

Speech Masking Level Difference

MLDs can be measured for speech thresholds. Usually, thresholds are measured for spondees in the same manner used for determining speech reception thresholds, except that the phase of the spondees at one earphone is controlled in relation to the phase of the spondees at the other earphone, and noise is present in both phones. Again, the speech MLD is defined by the difference in speech thresholds between SoNo and SπNo signal/masker conditions (see pure tone MLD earlier). MLDs for speech are smaller than for low-frequency tones (12), but still average 8 to 9 dB for normal listeners (32). Abnormal MLDs for speech are slightly more prevalent than abnormal pure tone MLDs in patients with brainstem disorders (14,30) and, thus, the speech MLD's clinical utility is potentially great because patients tend to find it easier to perform than the pure tone procedure. Also valuable to the clinician is the recent production of a compact disk recording that contains materials necessary for quick measurement of a speech MLD as well as several other central auditory tests (33).

Speech Procedures

Monotic Tasks

Speech tests that involve presentation of one or more signals to one ear are called monotic speech tasks. Many such procedures have been developed and used to study CANS function, including several of those used in the pioneering work of Bocca et al. (3). In general, these tasks attempt to make speech difficult to understand in one of two ways: by adding same-ear competition (such as noise), or by altering the character of the primary speech message itself (e.g., through filtering). The goal is to make the materials sufficiently difficult so as to counteract the inherent redundancy of the CANS, thereby producing a clear performance breakdown when the CANS is not working normally.

When brainstem disease or damage is the target, interpreting results of difficult monotic speech tests is complicated not only by the inherent redundancy of the CANS, but also by the fact that the predominant pathway carrying an ear's message toward the brain moves from one side of the brainstem to the other. Thus, a lesion in one place may affect the ear on the side of the damage, a higher level lesion may affect the contralateral ear, and midline low brainstem lesions may disrupt the behavior of both ears. This kind of ambiguity with monotic speech procedures led Olsen et al. (34) to suggest that tests such as the speech-in-noise test are good screening devices for lesions of the CANS, but are not useful "...in suggesting a particular site of involvement as being responsible for the dysfunction." Reviews of the many procedures used are available in any comprehensive audiology textbook. What follows are examples of tests that are used currently.

Synthetic Sentence Index with Ipsilateral Competing Message In 1968, Jerger et al. (35) introduced new materials with which to measure speech discrimination. They called these materials synthetic sentences or a synthetic sentence index (SSI). They are meaningless strings of meaningful words, e.g., "Down by the time is real enough," and much thought went into their composition, length, deviation from standard usage rules, etc. Later, Jerger and Jerger (36,37) modified the test to allow addition of either ipsilateral-ear or contralateral-ear competition that was meaningful running speech. A person's task, whether listening to the sentences without the competing message (SSI), with an ipsilateral-ear competing message (ICM), or with a contralateral-ear competing message (CCM), was to identify the synthetic sentence heard from a closed set of ten such sentences.

The SSI-ICM usually is administered at a level that allows maximum correct understanding of the SSI without competition. The ratio of the level of the competing message to that of the sentences is varied over a range from −20 to +10 dB. Normal listeners do well over that range except at the most unfavorable ratio, −20 dB, where correct identification of the sentences falls to about 50% accuracy. When patients with intraaxial brainstem lesions were tested with the SSI-ICM, all showed breakdown that often was bilateral (36,37). The findings were particularly important, because patients with auditory brain (temporal lobe) lesions fared much better. However, as will be discussed later, the reverse was true for the SSI-CCM. With the contralateral message test, temporal lobe lesion patients fared worse than brainstem lesion cases.

In the authors' experiences, the SSI-ICM may show breakdown via the ear on the side of eighth nerve damage, in one or both ears when the brainstem is damaged, and sometimes in the ear contralateral to a damaged temporal lobe. In combination with the SSI-CCM procedure, however, it is a valuable diagnostic instrument.

Speech-in-noise Test Because it is easy with commercial audiometers to mix speech and noise in the same earphone, speech-in-noise tests have been used frequently to examine everything from lesion effects to aural rehabilitation potential. Of interest to many were reports that speech-in-noise tasks were particularly difficult for persons with CANS damage that was presumed to be primarily located in the brainstem (13,38,39). Patients in these studies were predominantly individuals with multiple sclerosis, although some people with brainstem tumors were included.

Olsen et al. (34) did the most careful study of the value of the speech-in-noise test. Presenting meaningful monosyllabic words at 40 dB above the speech reception threshold and using a signal-to-noise ratio of 0 dB, a common combination of parameters, they studied normal listeners, cochlear-loss groups, eighth nerve tumor victims, patients with multiple sclerosis, and patients with brain lesions due to stroke or surgical intervention. Portions of each of the lesion groups showed breakdown exceeding 40% from their performance levels in quiet. This decrement was greater than that experienced by virtually any of the normal listeners. About 15% of the subjects with multiple sclerosis showed such breakdown, probably because of brainstem demyelination, but as is so often the case with difficult monotic speech tests, no characteristic pattern implicating either a side or site of damage was found.

Other Difficult Monotic Speech Tests Filtered speech materials and time-altered speech materials have received attention as tests of CANS function. Although some data have been reported involving patients with brainstem disease or damage, these approaches have not been particularly fruitful. This may be due to (a) the difficulty in defining and subsequent lack of systematic investigation of appropriate populations, and (b) failure to use appropriate or sufficiently difficult stimulus parameters. Remedy for both situations may be available by study of appropriate populations using normative and psychometric data recently reported for low- and high-pass filtered speech materials (40) and time-compressed speech materials (41).

Binaural Tasks

Other than transmitting signals upward toward the brain, the auditory brainstem also provides the first opportunity for correlation and integration of signals from the two ears. This interaural processing is accomplished in the low brainstem through nuclear areas that receive input directly or via the trapezoid body from the two ears. Knowing that such integration takes place in the brainstem has spurred the development of tests that can demonstrate whether or not the processes are working normally. For speech signals, that usually means putting part of a message in one ear, a different part of the same message in the other, and measuring how well they are combined when both ears are stimulated.

Filtered Speech Several reports (42–45) describe tasks that divide a speech signal, such as monosyllables, into two parts by filtering. For example, one can direct speech through filters to allow only a range of frequencies to pass.

In this way, primarily low-frequency energy can be delivered to one ear and higher-frequency energy to the other ear. Reducing the clues available to the listener in this way can make understanding of either message difficult. Presented separately but simultaneously to the two ears, however, word recognition is much better than it was for either message by itself. Because each message arrives from a separate ear of input, it is the brainstem that is first called on to meld the two into a whole greater than either of the parts. Thus, as shown recently in normal listeners (40), binaural listening may produce performance that outstrips even the sum of the low- and high-pass filtered conditions. Although data (46) suggest that brainstem disease can disrupt the fusion of two filtered speech segments, extensive information relevant to this point does not exist.

Alternating Speech Various investigators (5,10,47) have shown that patients with CANS abnormalities have difficulty understanding speech that is alternated between ears. Typical is the demonstration by Lynn and Gilroy (47) that correct discrimination for sentences that were presented so that the signal alternated between ears every 300 ms was markedly reduced for patients with caudal pontine involvement in the low brainstem. This finding was particularly important in light of the performance of patients with lesions of the higher brainstem or one temporal lobe. Patients in these latter categories had little difficulty with the alternating speech discrimination task. Variations on this theme have appeared in the literature over the past 30 years, but, for many reasons, adequate populations of patients with known brainstem lesion have not been tested. Evaluation of an alternating speech test called VIOECITO (48), which alternates CVC words so that consonants go to one ear and vowels go to the other, is currently under way and may clarify the value of such tests in a wide variety of populations (49).

Auditory Brain

After leaving the medial geniculate body, which is the last major nuclear center in the brainstem where auditory fibers have a synaptic stop, signals from the two ears course along the auditory radiations (geniculotemporal tract) to the temporal lobes. These lobes are thought to be responsible for receiving and analyzing auditory signals and initiating conscious responses to them. Most important to modern man, it is the auditory brain that initiates the response "I hear and I understand," as opposed to the response in the brainstem, which is more likely to be "I sense and I get out of the way."

Lesions to auditory structures of the brain seldom influence threshold sensitivity for tones or speech, although there are rare exceptions reported that are worth study (50,51). Procedures that are of use in seeking damage to the auditory brain fall into three groups: monotic speech tasks, dichotic speech tasks, and tonal pattern tests. Monotic speech tasks are, in most cases, the same

procedures used for evaluation of the auditory brainstem. Dichotic speech tests utilize techniques that pit one ear against the other in a manner that proves difficult for the auditory brain to process completely. Tests using tonal patterns are primarily based on recognition of frequency (pitch) and temporal (duration) information.

Both dichotic speech procedures and tonal pattern tests often call into play not only the temporal lobes but also interhemispheric connections between the two brain hemispheres, predominantly occurring through the corpus callosum. For dichotic speech tests, interhemispheric issues become important because in humans, the two halves of the brain seem to be specialized for (although not exclusively devoted to) different acoustic phenomena (52). Thus, it is often necessary for a signal that arrives first in one hemisphere to get to the other hemisphere to be processed and brought to consciousness. For tonal patterns, events whose perception apparently is not clearly localized to one hemisphere, interhemispheric connections are essential to allow the whole-brain response necessary for the correct verbal report of the patterns.

Speech Procedures

Monotic Tasks

Monotic speech tests were discussed under the same headings in the section on auditory brainstem techniques. Iterating, these tests feature one or more signals to one ear. The usual approach is to make an ordinary speech signal difficult to understand by adding a competing message (noise, speech) to the same ear or by altering the speech signal itself through techniques such as filtering and acceleration.

For patients with damaged or dysfunctional auditory brainstem structures or pathways, monotic speech tests can produce breakdown in the performance of one or both ears, and definitive patterns implicating a particular site or side of lesion are lacking. For patients with damage to the auditory brain (the populations studied have largely been those with temporal lobe damage), the most common result of monotic speech tests is the demonstration of poor performance by the ear on the side opposite the temporal lobe damage. In the abstract, this finding is somewhat surprising, because it is clear that signals to one ear have both contralateral and ipsilateral routes to the brain and, thus, are represented in both halves of the brain. Nevertheless, damage to one temporal lobe produces poor performance by the ear on the other side of the head, a rather convincing testament to the prepotency of the contralateral auditory pathway in human hearing. This is called the contralateral-ear effect. The amount of deviation from normal is variable, probably having to do with both the exact location of the damage and its severity, but the breakdown in performance can be quite marked.

Synthetic Sentence Index–Ipsilateral-ear Competing Message/Speech-in-noise Both tests were discussed in earlier sections of this chapter. When breakdown is seen on these tests, it is in the ear opposite temporal lobe damage or opposite widespread damage to one brain hemisphere that includes the temporal lobe, e.g., major cerebrovascular accident and hemispherectomy. Interpretation of performance breakdown in one ear is complicated by the fact that a similar finding can result from auditory brainstem or from eighth nerve damage (34,53). For the SSI-ICM, it is important to remember that results should be compared with the SSI-CCM. Abnormality will be greater on the CCM task if the lesion is in the brain and greater on the ICM if the lesion is to the brainstem (37).

Time-compressed Speech In the best study of its type, Kurdziel et al. (54) used meaningful monosyllables that were compressed in time by 40% and 60% [see method reported by Beasley et al. (55)] to demonstrate contralateral-ear deficits in 15 patients with damaged or absent temporal lobes on one side. The deficit in the 40% condition was relatively mild, but it was dramatic in the 60% trials: correct understanding was nearly 40% poorer in the contralateral ear than in the ipsilateral ear of the same subjects. A useful control in the study was a population of 16 other patients who had undergone anterior temporal lobe surgery to resect tissue thought responsible for intractable seizures or to remove tumor tissue. For the most part, these people did not have difficulty in either ear with the time-compressed materials. Calearo and Lazzaroni (56) and DeQuiros (57) suggested such findings earlier with less clearly defined test techniques and populations. Mueller et al. (58) found results similar to the discrete anterior temporal lobe group of Kurdziel in a large complement of patients with head injury.

People who studied behavior on time-compressed speech have used methods varying from playing phonograph records at the wrong speed to computer-based software routines. Available now for clinical use are compact disk recordings along with normative data and psychometric function data (41) that should be useful to clinicians who wish to use the technique.

Filtered Speech Dating back to Bocca et al. (3), speech that is filtered to allow only low-frequency information to be heard has been used to study damage to the brain. Usually, filtering was accomplished with cutoff frequencies below 1,000 Hz. Rejection rates for the filters have varied, but they were usually less than 20 dB per octave. The most extensive use of the technique with adults with CANS lesions was by Lynn and Gilroy (47). They demonstrated the expected contralateral-ear breakdown in patients whose brain dysfunction or damage involved the temporal lobe, but no breakdown when the temporal lobe was not involved. The major problem with filtered speech tests is the large variety of test and stimulus conditions that have been used. Such variety has made formulation of guidelines about expected results difficult. Materials and normative data described recently should provide a standard for future work (40).

Dichotic Tasks

When speech segments, words, or sentences are presented to the two ears in a roughly simultaneous fashion and these signals are different in some way, the capacity of the auditory brain to decode them and identify them correctly may be exceeded. For example, if syllables like /pa/ to one ear and /ta/ to the other ear are presented simultaneously, normal listeners will identify over many trials about 70% of the syllables to each ear. This somewhat surprising finding about the limited ability of the auditory system to process short, simultaneous, and different signals has to do with many factors, among them acoustic perception, memory, selective attention, and functional asymmetry of the hemispheres (19,59).

Use of dichotic signals is the most successful auditory approach to seeking lesions of the auditory brain. Tests utilizing dichotic materials can be divided into two classes: casually controlled dichotic tasks and carefully controlled dichotic tasks. The casually controlled tasks may be as unstructured as having a patient listen to pairs of sentences of approximately the same length. The carefully controlled tasks often use signals that have exactly the same onsets, durations, and offsets, and that share many or most features, e.g., the syllable pairs mentioned earlier.

In general, studies of patients with known auditory brain lesions, predominantly temporal lobe insult, have shown that damage to either temporal lobe produces performance reduction in the contralateral ear. In addition, damage to the posterior left temporal lobe can produce breakdown for some speech signals in both ears. Interestingly, lesions to connections between the two hemispheres, particularly to the corpus callosum, can affect perception of left-ear signals. This evidently reflects the necessity of an intact corpus callosum to allow speech signals originating at the left ear and represented first in the right hemisphere to cross to the left temporal lobe for final processing (19,60–63).

Synthetic Sentence Index with Contralateral Competing Message The rationale and composition of the test were described earlier among the brainstem test procedures. In brief, a "synthetic sentence" delivered to one ear must be identified from a closed set of such sentences while a running speech message is delivered to the other ear. Presentation level of the primary message is usually at a level allowing best performance in a noncompeting situation, and the intensity ratio of the signal to the competing message is varied over the range from 0 dB to -40 dB. Normal listeners do well over this range. Patients with temporal lobe damage on one side show breakdown in performance when the sentences are delivered to the contralateral ear (36,37,64). The SSI-CCM is a casually controlled dichotic procedure and is of most use diagnostically when given in combination with the SSI-ICM discussed earlier.

Staggered Spondaic Words Another casually controlled dichotic test is the staggered spondaic word

(SSW) test (65,66), which features presentation of spondees (two-syllables words with equal stress per syllable) to the two ears. The onset-alignment scheme causes the second syllable of the spondee to one ear to overlap in time with the first syllable of the spondee delivered to the other ear. The subject's job is to repeat everything possible. The easiest of the many scoring schemes notes correct responsiveness for both the syllables that are heard without competition in each ear (monotic performance) and for the syllables heard in the ears at the same time (dichotic performance). Mueller (67) provided an excellent review of SSW studies done with various populations and of the many scoring methods that have been proposed. His conclusion that the most useful information from the SSW is the performance of each ear during the dichotic syllable presentation concurs with the authors' experiences. The SSW is quite popular because it is fairly easy for patients to perform and can be administered quickly. Again, the most telling finding is clear breakdown in one ear's performance during the dichotic syllable presentation, an outcome that should arouse suspicion about dysfunction of the contralateral temporal lobe. In addition, surgical interruption of the corpus callosum has been shown to reduce performance via the left ear in a few subjects (68).

Digits Historically, much of the work with digits presented in a dichotic format was undertaken to explain normal processing of speech and hemispheric asymmetries for auditory signals (69,70). Clinical use of digit tests to probe the integrity of the CANS has concentrated on how their perception is affected by temporal lobe lesions (71), but understanding of such altered perception has given rise to models of how the CANS responds when confronted with dichotic signals.

Details of the model vary (60,61,72), but it has come to consist of several parts. (a) Carefully controlled dichotic speech signals cause a suppression of ipsilateral pathways from the ear to the brain. Thus, signals to each ear ascend a contralateral brainstem pathway to the opposite brain hemisphere where they receive preliminary (acoustic/phonetic) processing. (b) Signals that are input through the left ear, after arriving at the right hemisphere, must cross via the corpus callosum to the left hemisphere for final processing. (c) Any lesion along the pathways serving each ear will reduce the involved ear's performance. For the left ear, this includes corpus callosum and left parietal lobe lesions that affect callosal fibers before they reach the left temporal lobe. (d) The final processor for speech is located in the left posterior temporal lobe and perhaps adjacent parietal lobe tissue. Although certain fundamental analysis, recognition, and transmission functions are performed by each anterior temporal lobe, it is the left posterior temporal lobe that is responsible for activity that results in conscious hearing and understanding. Because, under certain dichotic listening conditions, the posterior left temporal lobe is the final destination of

signals from each ear, damage to that brain area can reduce performance accuracy for both ears.

Although the primary reason to perform dichotic digit tasks is to search for temporal lobe lesions, reports by Musiek (53,73) make clear that both brainstem and brain lesions can affect digit perception, and that sometimes only postdiagnostic hindsight makes clear a pattern of results. When digits are used as a test of CANS function, the most common format is to present a series of digits to the ears, e.g., /two/ and /four/ to one ear, /one/ and /nine/ to the other ear. The patient's job is to repeat as many as possible. In this way, a percentage of correct responses for each ear can be tabulated (44). Normative data also are available for single digit pairs (74). If the digits are carefully aligned, lesions of the auditory brain will manifest themselves in the ways summarized in the previous paragraph.

Sentences Although less research and clinical study has been done with dichotic sentences than with syllables and digits, some data have been reported using the synthetic sentences discussed earlier in sections on the SSI-ICM and SSI-CCM. In 1983, Fifer et al. (75) reported results obtained from a new test that took sentences from the SSI (35) and presented them dichotically, a different sentence to each ear, in a roughly simultaneous fashion. The listener tried to identify these from a closed set of such sentences. A version of this test with more carefully controlled sentence onsets, durations, and offsets also has been reported (74). Other investigators have used ordinary, not synthetic, sentences in the same format (76). In general, the little data that exist suggest that damage to one temporal lobe produces reduced ability to recognize the sentences via the contralateral ear, i.e., results usually associated with casually controlled dichotic speech tasks.

Nonsense Syllables (CVs) Over the last 2 decades, perhaps the most popular research and clinical dichotic speech technique has been dichotic nonsense syllables, or CVs, particularly the syllables formed by the stop consonants and the vowel /a/: /pa/, /ta/, /ka/, /ba/, /da/, /ga/ (77,78). As is the case with dichotic digits, the syllable task has been used to explore both normal processing of speech and lesion effects of the CANS, especially of the auditory brain and its interhemispheric connections. Good reviews of such dichotic effects are available (19,74).

Dichotic CVs can be very carefully controlled in time; thus, the amount of competition for processing at the left temporal lobe is keen. Clinically, the test is administered by having a person listen to pairs of the syllables, different ones to each ear, and try to identify both. In general, the effects found due to lesions of the temporal lobes or the corpus callosum, including its course through the left parietal lobe, are those predicted in the model of speech processing discussed earlier in this chapter. The problematic area in interpreting results obtained in a clinic from the nonsense syllable task (and other carefully controlled dichotic speech tasks) is the demonstration of left ear performance breakdown (73,79). This can result from damage to the right temporal lobe, corpus callosum, left parietal lobe (affecting callosal fibers), and left posterior temporal lobe. Usually, an evaluation of difficult monotic, casually controlled dichotic, and carefully controlled dichotic speech tasks, in combination with a good brainstem indicator such as the MLD, will allow this quandary to be cleared up.

Tone Procedures

Frequency Tasks

In 1971, Pinheiro and Ptacek (80) described a test that required a listener to attend to a sequence of three tones (presented monotically). The sequence contained two tones of one frequency and one tone of another frequency. The listener's task was to identify the sequence according to the pitch pattern involved, e.g., low-low-high, high-low-high, etc. In this and other work of Pinheiro (21) and others (53,65,81), it was reported that patients with unilateral temporal lobe lesion on either side of the brain and persons with damage affecting the corpus callosum had great difficulty identifying these simple patterns in either ear.

Complicating matters, Musiek et al. (68) reported pitch pattern results from four patients who were tested before and after complete commissurotomies. None had a problem with the task via either ear before surgery. All of them had severe problems with the task via both ears after surgery. However, neither of a subgroup of two patients had a problem with the task after surgery if allowed to hum rather than verbally report the responses.

By 1985, Musiek (53) concluded that "...it appears that the right hemisphere must recognize the 'acoustic contour' of the pattern and the left hemisphere must convert the pattern to a verbal response.... Both hemispheres must interact appropriately for a correct verbal response to the auditory pattern." Whatever the explanation, frequency pattern recognition is affected for both ears when one or the other temporal lobes or the corpus callosum is damaged. Because the task uses nonverbal stimuli and can use a nonlanguage-based response, it can be valuable in a central auditory test battery.

Duration Tasks

Patterns featuring tones of different durations, although relatively new, may be of value in CANS evaluation (82). Duration tasks are done monotically, and they require that a patient listen to a sequence of three tones, two of which have the same duration and one of which has a different duration. The task is to identify the pattern, e.g., long-long-short, short-long-short, etc. For both the duration and pitch pattern tests, good materials and normative data now are available (81).

Data on duration pattern tasks are sparse, but there is evidence that the procedures are sensitive to lesions in either temporal lobe or in the corpus callosum, and relatively immune to disruption from lesions of the auditory sense organ (cochlea) (82). Musiek (81) points out that "Both the frequency and duration pattern perception tests appear to have a high test efficiency; however, they do not provide laterality information.... Lesions in either hemisphere or the corpus callosum often result in bilateral ear deficits.... The duration pattern test can also detect cerebral lesions which the frequency pattern test can not, but the opposite is also true."

CASE STUDIES

The following case studies were chosen carefully to illustrate the findings that result from classic insults to the CANS, i.e., lesions of the extraaxial brainstem, intraaxial brainstem, ascending auditory brainstem pathways, and right and left temporal lobes. It would be misleading to suggest that lesions in these areas always manifest themselves as clearly as shown in these examples, especially when there is serious involvement of peripheral auditory structures. However, these examples do illustrate expected findings for CANS lesions.

Case 1

Case 1 is a 39-year-old, right-handed man who was seen for an audiologic evaluation due to complaints of gradually decreasing hearing and tinnitus in his left ear over a period of 3 years. The primary complaint was that the hearing loss interfered with his ability to conduct business over the telephone (he used his left ear while writing with his right hand) and made it difficult for him to follow discussions in group meetings. He denied any history of otalgia, otorrhea, vertigo, or noise exposure. Magnetic resonance imaging studies revealed a 10-mm rounded mass lesion in the left cerebellopontine angle apparently adhering to the brainstem.

Audiometric and electrophysiologic test results are given in Fig. 2. Noteworthy are the findings of a unilateral, high-frequency sensorineural hearing loss in the left ear, marked performance breakdown for the left ear on tests of distorted monotic speech recognition (speech-in-noise, SSI-ICM), and reduced MLD size.

Physiologic measures showed abnormal crossed acoustic reflexes for both ears and abnormal uncrossed reflexes for the left ear. ABR measures revealed absent waveforms beginning with wave II in the left ear and normal results for the right ear.

All auditory findings, with the exception of the crossed acoustic reflexes for the right ear, indicate a lesion involving the extraaxial brainstem (and/or cranial nerve VIII) on the left side. That is, the abnormal results are all ipsilateral to the suspected site of lesion. Given the lesion

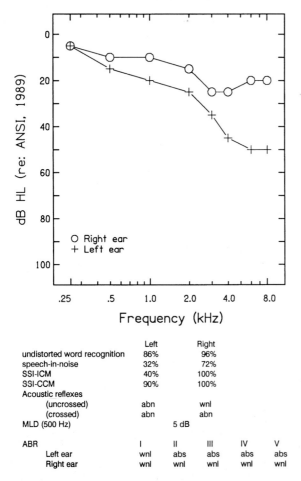

	Left	Right		
undistorted word recognition	86%	96%		
speech-in-noise	32%	72%		
SSI-ICM	40%	100%		
SSI-CCM	90%	100%		
Acoustic reflexes				
(uncrossed)	abn	wnl		
(crossed)	abn	abn		
MLD (500 Hz)		5 dB		
ABR	I	II	III	IV	V
Left ear	wnl	abs	abs	abs	abs
Right ear	wnl	wnl	wnl	wnl	wnl

FIG. 2. Basic hearing test and diagnostic audiology results from a patient with left extraaxial brainstem lesion. Case description and discussion of test results are in the associated text on Case 1. Speech recognition scores are given in percent correct. abn, abnormal; ABR, auditory brainstem response; abs, absent; MLD, masking level difference; SSI-CCM, synthetic sentence index–contralateral-ear competing message; SSI-ICM, synthetic sentence index–ipsilateral-ear competing message; wnl, within normal limits.

size, the abnormal right ear crossed reflexes are probably due to involvement of cranial nerve VII on the left side, preventing the contraction of the left stapedius muscle.

Case 2

Case 2 is a 36-year-old, left-handed man who was diagnosed with multiple sclerosis 5 years prior to audiologic testing. The patient reported that his initial symptoms were weakness of his right leg and "drop" of his right foot. As these symptoms abated, he began to notice blind spots in his visual fields. The patient was confined to a wheelchair at the time of testing due to weakness and lack of coordination of his lower extremities. On careful questioning, he reported difficulty understanding speech in crowded rooms, but he had no complaints of hearing loss.

He denied otalgia, otorrhea, vertigo, or tinnitus. Past history was negative for noise exposure.

Audiometric findings, shown in Fig. 3, revealed hearing for pure tones and undistorted word recognition to be within normal limits. Some breakdown was present in both ears for distorted monotic speech tests. Dichotic listening skills were unaffected. The 500-Hz MLD was abnormally small.

Nonbehavioral measures revealed normal uncrossed acoustic reflexes and abnormal crossed reflexes. ABR results were remarkable for abnormality in waveforms beginning with wave III in both ears.

The audiologic findings in this patient suggest intraaxial brainstem lesion affecting pathways that cross from one side of the brainstem to the other (acoustic reflexes and ABR) or binaural correlation of signals from each ear (MLD). The bilateral breakdown on difficult monotic speech tasks undoubtedly stems from the same source.

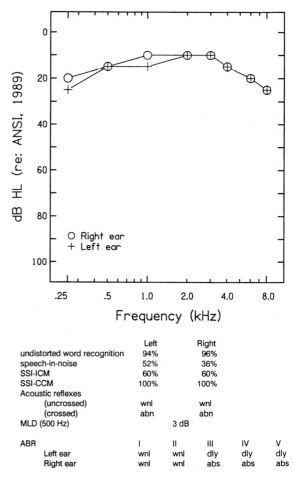

	Left	Right		
undistorted word recognition	94%	96%		
speech-in-noise	52%	36%		
SSI-ICM	60%	60%		
SSI-CCM	100%	100%		
Acoustic reflexes				
(uncrossed)	wnl	wnl		
(crossed)	abn	abn		
MLD (500 Hz)		3 dB		
ABR	I	II	III	IV	V
Left ear	wnl	wnl	dly	dly	dly
Right ear	wnl	wnl	abs	abs	abs

FIG. 3. Basic hearing test and diagnostic audiology results from a patient with intraaxial brainstem lesion. Case description and discussion of test results are in the associated text on Case 2. Speech recognition scores are given in percent correct. abn, abnormal; ABR, auditory brainstem response; abs, absent; dly, delayed; MLD, masking level difference; SSI-CCM, synthetic sentence index–contralateral-ear competing message; SSI-ICM, synthetic sentence index–ipsilateral-ear competing message; wnl, within normal limits.

Case 3

The third case is that of a 52-year-old, left-handed woman with complaints of drooping eyelid, diplopia, hypersensitivity to light, pulsing nonlocalized headache, and some balance disturbance without true vertigo. There were no audiologic complaints, and otologic history was negative. Angiography was consistent with an intracranial aneurysm located on the right posterior communicating artery within the circle of Willis.

Audiometric findings for behavioral tests and for acoustic reflex measures were all within normal limits, as shown in Fig. 4. The only abnormalities found were absent or delayed wave IV or V for each ear on ABR measures.

Although the primary lesion was not located within auditory brainstem pathways, abnormality was found along these pathways. The abnormal ABR findings are likely attributable to compression, displacement, or injury of high brainstem tissue by the aneurysm. Similar cases have been reported (31,83).

Case 4

Case 4 is a 64-year-old, right-handed man whose family reported a 6-month history of seizures and gradual personality changes with increasing forgetfulness and belligerent behavior at home. The patient had surgery of the left lung (lower lobe resection) for primary pulmonary carcinoma 3 years earlier. He reported having ear infections as a child, but otherwise had a negative otologic history. The patient denied any auditory symptoms or history of noise exposure. Five months prior to audiologic testing, the patient underwent craniotomy for exci-

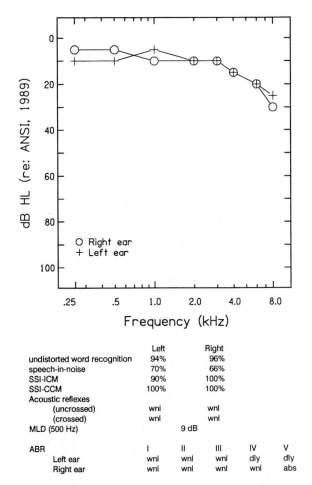

	Left	Right			
undistorted word recognition	94%	96%			
speech-in-noise	70%	66%			
SSI-ICM	90%	100%			
SSI-CCM	100%	100%			
Acoustic reflexes					
(uncrossed)	wnl	wnl			
(crossed)	wnl	wnl			
MLD (500 Hz)		9 dB			
ABR	I	II	III	IV	V
Left ear	wnl	wnl	wnl	dly	dly
Right ear	wnl	wnl	wnl	wnl	abs

FIG. 4. Basic hearing test and diagnostic audiology results from a patient with high brainstem insult. Case description and discussion of test results are in the associated text on Case 3. Speech recognition scores are given in percent correct. ABR, auditory brainstem response; abs, absent; dly, delayed; MLD, masking level difference; SSI-CCM, synthetic sentence index–contralateral-ear competing message; SSI-ICM, synthetic sentence index–ipsilateral-ear competing message; wnl, within normal limits.

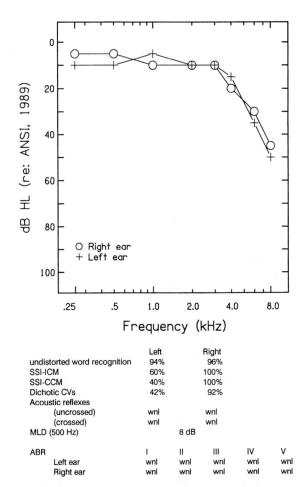

	Left	Right			
undistorted word recognition	94%	96%			
SSI-ICM	60%	100%			
SSI-CCM	40%	100%			
Dichotic CVs	42%	92%			
Acoustic reflexes					
(uncrossed)	wnl	wnl			
(crossed)	wnl	wnl			
MLD (500 Hz)		8 dB			
ABR	I	II	III	IV	V
Left ear	wnl	wnl	wnl	wnl	wnl
Right ear	wnl	wnl	wnl	wnl	wnl

FIG. 5. Basic hearing test and diagnostic audiology results from a patient with right temporal lobe lesion. Case description and discussion of test results are in the associated text on Case 4. Speech recognition scores are given in percent correct. ABR, auditory brainstem response; CVs, nonsense syllables; MLD, masking level difference; SSI-CCM, synthetic sentence index–contralateral-ear competing message; SSI-ICM, synthetic sentence index–ipsilateral-ear competing message; wnl, within normal limits.

sion of metastases located in the right frontal and temporal lobe regions. He had completed a course of radiation therapy prior to audiologic testing.

Audiometric results, shown in Fig. 5, revealed a bilateral, mild-to-moderate, high-frequency sensorineural hearing loss. All auditory tests of cranial nerve VIII and brainstem function (MLD, acoustic reflexes, and ABR) were within normal limits. A degraded monotic speech test (SSI-ICM) and both measures of dichotic listening performance (SSI-CCM, dichotic CVs) revealed breakdown in left ear performance, i.e., a contralateral-ear effect. Here, unlike cranial nerve VIII or extraaxial brainstem lesions, the poor auditory performance is reflected in the ear opposite the site of temporal lobe lesion. (See the earlier text on dichotic speech tests for discussion of other brain lesions that can give a picture featuring performance breakdown in the left ear.)

Case 5

Case 5 is a 57-year-old, right-handed man who was hospitalized with sudden onset of seizures following a long period of unremitting headache. The patient had no previous history of neurologic disease. He reported difficulties understanding speech in crowds and in noisy environments. He described bilateral tonal tinnitus of long standing. The patient had a 30-year history of noise exposure from his work as a carpenter. Computed tomographic scan revealed a circumscribed mass located on the left anterior temporal lobe. Surgical intervention subsequent to the audiometric tests revealed a meningioma.

Audiometric findings (Fig. 6) revealed a bilateral, mild-to-moderate, notch-shaped sensorineural hearing loss, consistent with the history of noise exposure. Word recognition ability, 500-Hz MLD, crossed and uncrossed acoustic reflexes, and ABR measures were all within normal limits for both ears.

The SSI-ICM, SSI-CCM, and dichotic CV results exhibited performance breakdown in the right ear, consistent with the expected findings of contralateral-ear effects in cases of temporal lobe damage. These results differ from those found when the posterior left temporal lobe is damaged, as illustrated in Case 6.

Case 6

Case 6 is a 68-year-old, right-handed man who was hospitalized following sudden onset of right-sided paralysis and aphasia. The patient had a long history of poorly controlled hypertension and coronary artery disease. Cerebral angiography revealed occlusion of the middle cerebral artery on the left affecting the posterior parietal, angular, and posterior temporal branches of the middle cerebral artery. Computed tomographic scan revealed an area of infarction extending from the left posterior temporal lobe into the parietal lobe. Although

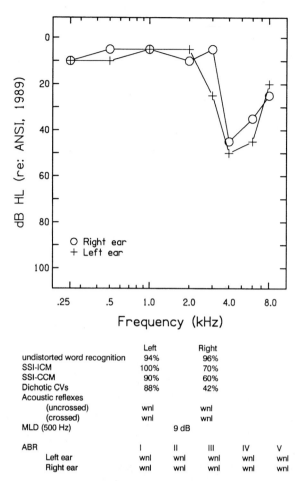

	Left	Right		
undistorted word recognition	94%	96%		
SSI-ICM	100%	70%		
SSI-CCM	90%	60%		
Dichotic CVs	88%	42%		
Acoustic reflexes				
(uncrossed)	wnl	wnl		
(crossed)	wnl	wnl		
MLD (500 Hz)		9 dB		

ABR	I	II	III	IV	V
Left ear	wnl	wnl	wnl	wnl	wnl
Right ear	wnl	wnl	wnl	wnl	wnl

FIG. 6. Basic hearing test and diagnostic audiology results from a patient with left anterior temporal lobe lesion. Case description and discussion of test results are in the associated text on Case 5. Speech recognition scores are given in percent correct. ABR, auditory brainstem response; CVs, nonsense syllables; MLD, masking level difference; SSI-CCM, synthetic sentence index–contralateral-ear competing message; SSI-ICM, synthetic sentence index–ipsilateral-ear competing message; wnl, within normal limits.

the patient's symptoms had improved by the time of the audiologic evaluation, he continued to exhibit moderate aphasia characterized by word-finding difficulties. According to the patient's family, there had been no recent otologic problems, and there was no history of noise exposure.

Audiometric findings (Fig. 7) revealed a bilateral, mild, high-frequency sensorineural hearing loss. Acoustic reflexes, 500-Hz MLD, and ABR measures were within normal limits for both ears.

The SSI-ICM and the SSI-CCM results exhibited performance breakdown in the right ear, consistent with the expected findings of contralateral-ear effect in cases of temporal lobe damage. However, dichotic nonsense syllables (dichotic CVs) revealed performance breakdown in both ears, suggesting that the final processing areas for verbal stimuli (for both ears) were affected by the lesion.

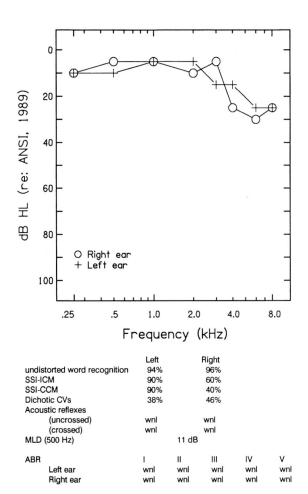

	Left	Right
undistorted word recognition	94%	96%
SSI-ICM	90%	60%
SSI-CCM	90%	40%
Dichotic CVs	38%	46%
Acoustic reflexes		
(uncrossed)	wnl	wnl
(crossed)	wnl	wnl
MLD (500 Hz)	11 dB	

ABR	I	II	III	IV	V
Left ear	wnl	wnl	wnl	wnl	wnl
Right ear	wnl	wnl	wnl	wnl	wnl

FIG. 7. Basic hearing test and diagnostic audiology results from a patient with left posterior temporal lobe lesion. Case description and discussion of test results are in the associated text on Case 6. Speech recognition scores are given in percent correct. ABR, auditory brainstem response; CVs, nonsense syllables; MLD, masking level difference; SSI-CCM, synthetic sentence index–contralateral-ear competing message; SSI-ICM, synthetic sentence index–ipsilateral-ear competing message; wnl, within normal limits.

SUMMARY POINTS

- Disorders of the CANS are those that affect auditory centers or pathways in the brainstem and brain.
- Some of these disorders disrupt transmission of acoustic signals and some affect processing of the signals.
- The diagnostic chore is to be able to identify either of these types of disruption and to label correctly the level and side of the insult.
- Transmission-line tests and tests of tone pattern recognition have considerable value in this regard. Also useful are tests that probe functions unique to the auditory brainstem and brain, namely, binaural (two-ear) interaction procedures (brainstem) and difficult speech processing tasks (brain).

REFERENCES

1. Carhart R. Special hearing tests for otoneurologic diagnosis. *Arch Otolaryngol* 1969;89:38–41.
2. Bocca E, Calearo C, Cassinari V. A new method for testing hearing in temporal lobe tumors. *Acta Otolaryngol* 1954;44:219–221.
3. Bocca E, Calearo C, Cassinari V, Migliavacca F. Testing "cortical" hearing in temporal lobe tumors. *Acta Otolaryngol* 1955;45:289–304.
4. Bocca E. Clinical aspects of cortical deafness. *Laryngoscope* 1958;68:301–309.
5. Bocca E, Calearo C. Central hearing processes. In: Jerger J, ed. *Modern developments in audiology.* New York: Academic Press, 1963:337–370.
6. Hirsh I. The influence of interaural phase on interaural summation and inhibition. *J Acoust Soc Am* 1948;20:536–544.
7. Licklider J. The influence of interaural phase relation upon the masking of speech by white noise. *J Acoust Soc Am* 1948;20:150–159.
8. Colburn H, Durlach N. Models of binaural interaction. In: Carterette E, ed. *Handbook of perception, volume 4.* Orlando, FL: Academic Press, 1978:467–518.
9. Durlach N, Colburn H. Binaural phenomena. In: Carterette E, ed. *Handbook of perception, volume 4.* Orlando, FL: Academic Press, 1978:365–466.
10. Jerger J. Observations on auditory behavior in lesions of the central auditory pathways. *Arch Otolaryngol* 1960;71:797–806.
11. Jerger J. Auditory tests for disorders of the central auditory mechanism. In: Fields W, Alford B, eds. *Neurological aspects of auditory and vestibular disorders.* Springfield, IL: Charles C Thomas, 1964:77–93.
12. Carhart R, Tillman TW, Dallos PJ. Unmasking for pure tones and spondees: interaural phase and time disparities. *J Speech Hear Res* 1968;11:722–734.
13. Noffsinger D, Olsen WO, Carhart R, Hart CW, Sahgal V. Auditory and vestibular aberrations in multiple sclerosis. *Acta Otolaryngol* 1972;[Suppl] 303:1–63.
14. Olsen WO, Noffsinger D, Carhart R. Masking level differences encountered in clinical populations. *Audiology* 1976;15:287–301.
15. Sohmer H, Feinmesser M. Cochlear action potentials recorded from the external ear in man. *Ann Otol Rhinol Laryngol* 1967;76:427–435.
16. Jewett DL, Williston JS. Auditory-evoked far fields averaged from the scalp of humans. *Brain* 1971;94:681–696.
17. Davis H, Yoshie N. Human evoked cortical responses to auditory stimuli. *Physiologist* 1963;6:164.
18. Hall J. *Handbook of auditory evoked responses.* Needham Heights, MA: Allyn and Bacon, 1992:3–40.
19. Berlin C, McNeil M. Dichotic listening. In: Lass N, ed. *Contemporary issues in experimental phonetics.* New York: Academic Press, 1976:327–387.
20. Bosatra A, Russolo M. The diagnostic value of tonal tests in peripheral and central auditory lesions. In: Stephens ES, ed. *Disorders of auditory function.* London: Academic Press, 1976:243–252.
21. Pinheiro M. Auditory pattern perception in patients with left and right hemisphere lesions. *Ohio J Speech Hear* 1977;12:9–20.
22. Northern J, Gabbard S, Kinder D. The acoustic reflex. In: Katz J, ed. *Handbook of clinical audiology.* Baltimore: Williams & Wilkins, 1985:476–495.
23. Mueller H, Beck W. Brainstem level test results following head injury. *Semin Hear* 1987;8:253–260.
24. Moller AR. Origin of latency shift of cochlear nerve potentials with sound intensity. *Hear Res* 1985;17:177–189.
25. Noffsinger D, Martinez C, Schaefer A. Puretone techniques in evaluation of central auditory function. In: Katz J, ed. *Handbook of clinical audiology.* Baltimore: Williams & Wilkins, 1985:337–354.
26. Michaud D. *Masking level differences in patients with brainstem lesions.* Unpublished dissertation. Detroit, MI: Wayne State University, 1980:1.
27. Lynn GE, Gilroy J, Taylor PC, Leiser RP. Binaural masking-level differences in neurological disorders. *Arch Otolaryngol* 1981;107:357–362.
28. Hannley M, Jerger JF, Rivera VM. Relationships among auditory brainstem responses, masking level differences and the acoustic reflex in multiple sclerosis. *Audiology* 1983;22:20–33.
29. Konishi M. Listening with two ears. *Sci Am* 1993;268:66–73.
30. Noffsinger D. Clinical applications of selected binaural effects. *Scand Audiol* [Suppl] 1982;15:157–165.
31. Noffsinger D, Martinez CD, Schaefer AB. Auditory brainstem responses and masking level differences from persons with brainstem lesion. *Scand Audiol* [Suppl] 1982;15:81–93.

32. Wilson RH, Zizz CA, Sperry JL. Masking-level difference for spondaic words in 2000-msec bursts of broadband noise. *J Am Acad Audiol* 1994;5:236–242.

33. Noffsinger D, Wilson RH, Musiek FE. Department of Veterans Affairs compact disc (VA-CD) recording for auditory perceptual assessment: background and introduction. *J Am Acad Audiol* 1994;5:231–235.

34. Olsen WO, Noffsinger D, Kurdziel S. Speech discrimination in quiet and in white noise by patients with peripheral and central lesions. *Acta Otolaryngol* 1975;80:375–382.

35. Jerger J, Speaks C, Trammell JL. A new approach to speech audiometry. *J Speech Hear Disord* 1968;33:318–328.

36. Jerger J, Jerger S. Auditory findings in brainstem disorders. *Arch Otolaryngol* 1974;99:342–350.

37. Jerger J, Jerger S. Clinical validity of central auditory tests. *Scand Audiol* 1975;4:147–163.

38. Dayal VS, Tarantino L, Swisher LP. Neuro-otologic studies in multiple sclerosis. *Laryngoscope* 1966;76:1798–1809.

39. Morales-Garcia C, Poole JP. Masked speech audiometry in central deafness. *Acta Otolaryngol* 1972;74:307–316.

40. Bornstein SP, Wilson RH, Cambron NK. Low- and high-pass filtered Northwestern University Auditory Test No. 6 for monaural and binaural evaluation. *J Am Acad Audiol* 1994;5:259–264.

41. Wilson RH, Preece JP, Salamon DL, Sperry JL, Bornstein SP. Effects of time compression and time compression plus reverberation on the intelligibility of Northwestern University Auditory Test No. 6. *J Am Acad Audiol* 1994;5:269–277.

42. Matzker J. Two new methods for the assessment of central auditory functioning in cases of brain disease. *Ann Otol* 1959;68:1185–1196

43. Ivey R. *Tests of CNS auditory function.* Unpublished thesis. Fort Collins, CO: Colorado State University, 1969:1.

44. Mueller H. Monosyllabic procedures. In: Katz J, ed. *Handbook of clinical audiology.* Baltimore: Williams & Wilkins, 1985:355–382.

45. Lukas R, Genchur-Lukas M. Spondaic word tests. In: Katz J, ed. *Handbook of clinical audiology.* Baltimore: Williams & Wilkins, 1985:383–403.

46. Smith BB, Resnick D. An auditory test for assessing brainstem integrity: preliminary report. *Laryngoscope* 1972;82:414–424.

47. Lynn G, Gilroy J. Evaluation of central auditory dysfunction in patients with neurological disorders. In: Keith R, ed. *Central auditory dysfunction.* New York: Grune and Stratton, 1977:177–221.

48. Wilson RH, Arcos JT, Jones HC. Word recognition with segmented-alternated CVC words: a preliminary report on listeners with normal hearing. *J Speech Hear Res* 1984;27:378–386.

49. Wilson RH. Word recognition with segmented-alternated CVC words: compact disc trials. *J Am Acad Audiol* 1994;5:255–258.

50. Jerger J, Lovering L, Wertz M. Auditory disorder following bilateral temporal lobe insult: report of a case. *J Speech Hear Disord* 1972;37:523–535.

51. Martinez C, Morgan D, Dobkin B, Kenworthy D. Subcortical lesions resulting in loss of auditory perception. *ASHA* 1993;35:244.

52. Benson F, Zaidel E, eds. *The dual brain. Hemispheric specialization in humans.* New York: Guilford Press, 1985.

53. Musiek F. Application of central auditory tests: an overview. In: Katz J, ed. *Handbook of clinical audiology.* Baltimore: Williams & Wilkins, 1985:321–336.

54. Kurdziel S, Noffsinger D, Olsen W. Performance by cortical lesion patients on 40 and 60% time-compressed materials. *J Am Audiol Soc* 1976;2:3–7.

55. Beasley D, Forman B, Rintelmann W. Intelligibility of time-compressed CNC monosyllables by normal listeners. *J Aud Res* 1972;12:71–75.

56. Calearo D, Lazzaroni A. Speech intelligibility in relation to the speed of the message. *Laryngoscope* 1957;67:410–419.

57. DeQuiros J. Accelerated speech audiometry; an examination of test results. *Transl Beltone Inst Hear Res* 1964;17:1.

58. Mueller H, Beck W, Sedge R. Comparison of the efficiency of cortical level speech tests. *Semin Hear* 1987;8:279–298.

59. Beasley D, Rintelmann A. Central auditory processing. In: Rintelmann W, ed. *Hearing assessment.* Baltimore: University Park Press, 1979:321–349.

60. Cullen J, Berlin C, Hughes L, Thompson C, Samson D. Speech information flow: a model. In: Sullivan M, ed. *Central auditory processing disorders.* Lincoln, NE: University of Nebraska Press, 1975:108–127.

61. Sparks R, Geschwind N. Dichotic listening in man after section of neocortical commissures. *Cortex* 1968;4:3–16.

62. Milner B, Taylor L, Sperry RW. Lateralized suppression of dichotically presented digits after commissural section in man. *Science* 1968;161:184–186.

63. Noffsinger D, Kurdziel S. Assessment of central auditory lesions. In: Rintelmann W, ed. *Hearing assessment.* Baltimore: University Park Press, 1979:351–377.

64. Speaks C. Dichotic listening: a clinical or research tool? In: Sullivan M, ed. *Central auditory processing disorders.* Lincoln, NE: University of Nebraska Press, 1975:2–25.

65. Katz J. The use of staggered spondaic words for assessing the integrity of the central auditory nervous system. *J Aud Res* 1962;2:327–337.

66. Katz J. *SSW workshop manual.* Buffalo, New York: Allentown Industries, 1978.

67. Mueller H. The staggered spondaic word test: practical use. *Semin Hear* 1987;8:267–277.

68. Musiek F, Kibbe K, Baran J. Neuroaudiological results from split-brain patients. *Semin Hear* 1984;5:219–229.

69. Broadbent D. The role of auditory localization of attention and memory span. *J Exp Psychol* 1954;47:191–196.

70. Kimura D. Cerebral dominance and the perception of verbal stimuli. *Can J Psychol* 1961;15:166–171.

71. Kimura D. Some effects of temporal-lobe damage on auditory perception. *Can J Psychol* 1961;15:156–165.

72. Sparks R, Goodglass H, Nickel B. Ipsilateral versus contralateral extinction in dichotic listening resulting from hemisphere lesions. *Cortex* 1970;6:249–260.

73. Musiek FE. Results of three dichotic speech tests on subjects with intracranial lesions. *Ear Hear* 1983;4:318–323.

74. Noffsinger D, Martinez CD, Wilson RH. Dichotic listening to speech: background and preliminary data for digits, sentences, and nonsense syllables. *J Am Acad Audiol* 1994;5:248–254.

75. Fifer RC, Jerger JF, Berlin CI, Tobey EA, Campbell JC. Development of a dichotic sentence identification test for hearing-impaired adults. *Ear Hear* 1983;4:300–305.

76. Willeford J. Sentence tests of central auditory dysfunction. In: Katz J, ed. *Handbook of clinical audiology.* Baltimore: Williams & Wilkins, 1985:404–420.

77. Berlin C, Lowe S. Temporal and dichotic factors in central auditory testing. In: Katz J, ed. *Handbook of clinical audiology.* Baltimore: Williams & Wilkins, 1972:280–312.

78. Berlin CI, Lowe-Bell SS, Janetta PJ, Kline, DG. Central auditory deficits after temporal lobectomy. *Arch Otolaryngol* 1972;96:4–10.

79. Olsen WO. Dichotic test results for normal subjects and for temporal lobectomy patients. *Ear Hear* 1983;4:324–330.

80. Pinheiro ML, Ptacek PH. Reversals in the perception of noise and tone patterns. *J Acoust Soc Am* 1971;49:1778–1782.

81. Musiek FE. Frequency (pitch) and duration pattern tests. *J Am Acad Audiol* 1994;5:265–268.

82. Musiek FE, Baran JA, Pinheiro ML. Duration pattern recognition in normal subjects and patients with cerebral and cochlear lesions. *Audiology* 1990;29:304–313.

83. Noffsinger D, Schaefer A, Martinez C. Behavioral and objective estimates of auditory brainstem integrity. *Semin Hear* 1984;5:337–349.

The Ear: Comprehensive Otology,
edited by R. F. Canalis and P. R. Lambert.
Lippincott Williams & Wilkins, Philadelphia © 2000.

CHAPTER 16

Auditory Assessment of Pediatric Patients

Annelle V. Hodges, Shelly Dolan-Ash, and Stacy L. Butts

Behavioral Testing
  Behavioral Observation Audiometry
  Conditioned Response Audiometry
Objective Measures
  Immittance Measures
  Tympanometry
  Physical Volume
  Acoustic Reflex

  Auditory Brainstem Response
  Otoacoustic Emissions
Speech Perception Testing
  Threshold Speech Tests
  Suprathreshold Speech Tests
  Tests of the Central Auditory
    Nervous System
Summary

The identification and treatment of childhood hearing loss, whether mild, profound, or in between, is vital to the social and intellectual development of the affected child. Although only one in 1,000 children is born with a severe-to-profound hearing loss, another two will acquire deafness in early childhood. In addition, nearly 100% of children will experience some period of transient hearing loss associated with middle ear infections before the age of 11 years (1). Sixteen of 1,000 students have hearing losses ranging from mild to severe (2). There is little argument that undetected and untreated sensorineural hearing loss can have serious lifelong consequences. The long-term effects of mild fluctuating hearing loss due to middle ear infections are less clear cut, but studies have suggested that recurrent otitis media can have a significant impact on educational achievement (3–6). Although treatment of the infection is primary, accompanying hearing loss should not be ignored.

The purpose of pediatric hearing assessment is to identify the presence of a hearing loss, quantify the degree of hearing loss, establish the type of loss, and monitor progress of intervention strategies when a hearing loss is present. A test battery approach consisting of both behavioral and objective measures will provide the most comprehensive and reliable assessment of auditory status. The "cross-check" principle provided by use of several

supporting measures has been described as an important factor in pediatric auditory evaluation (7).

Only in recent years have the behavioral testing techniques and technology been available that can allow accurate auditory evaluation of very young and difficult to test children. Prior to the introduction of conditioned response audiometry techniques, behavioral testing of infant hearing was based on observation of the child's behavior in response to noisemakers. Such testing could provide only a gross estimate of the child's actual hearing and often was compromised by factors other than hearing. Many professionals believed that young children simply could not be tested until they reached school age. However, conditioned response techniques have been used successfully with children as young as 5 months of age (8). Different types of conditioned response and response-reward paradigms have been developed for children of differing age and interest levels. Such techniques can be used successfully with the vast majority of young children. Behavioral audiometry is the only means by which a hearing loss can be fully quantified and, as such, remains the primary tool in pediatric hearing assessment.

Technologic advances, including immittance measures, evoked response audiometry, and, more recently, otoacoustic emissions (OAEs), have enabled testers to obtain objective data with which to corroborate behaviorally obtained results and to test those from whom no responses could be obtained otherwise. Although not specifically a test of hearing, evoked potential testing,

A. V. Hodges, S. Dolan-Ash, and S. L. Butts: Department of Otolaryngology, University of Miami, Miami, Florida 33129

most often the auditory brainstem response (ABR), can provide an excellent starting point from which to obtain more specific behavioral results. However, successful ABR testing requires a very quiet (sleeping) child, and as such its use is generally limited to very young infants or settings in which the child may be sedated for testing. OAEs have the distinct advantage of being very quick to complete, so the child need only remain quiet for a brief period of time. OAEs can be measured easily in any clinical setting. However, as with the ABR, OAEs are not a test of hearing per se, and they should be used in conjunction with behavioral testing. The primary advantage to these measures is that when a normal response is obtained on these two measures, the hearing health professional and the family can feel relatively comfortable that hearing is normal. Conversely, if an abnormal response is obtained on either measure, the family and professionals know that they must proceed until complete audiologic information is obtained.

Although testing techniques and technology are important instruments in pediatric hearing assessment, the most valuable tool is a good pediatric audiologist. Unless the audiologist can establish a rapport with both the child and parents, the behavioral test session may be over before it begins. In addition, the pediatric audiologist must have the ability to read and understand the way in which each particular child responds. The good pediatric audiologist must understand the technology so that equipment problems do not result in inaccurate or misinterpreted results. Finally, the audiologist must be able to critically observe the behaviors of the child and reconcile test results with other pertinent information to provide a true picture of auditory functioning.

The means to identify and quantify hearing loss in children have made great leaps forward in recent decades. Advances in treatment of profound deafness, most specifically through the multichannel cochlear implant, have made it as important to reach beyond quantification of the degree of hearing loss. The benefits of digital hearing aid technology for children cannot be determined without sensitive measures of speech recognition. Assessment of the quality of residual hearing in very young children is currently one of the major challenges in pediatric audiology. A number of test measures for assessment of suprathreshold hearing abilities in children have been introduced in recent years.

A final area of pediatric auditory assessment involves those children who have no quantifiable hearing loss, but who nevertheless are unable to effectively use auditory information. Evaluation of auditory processing has not become a well-accepted part of the standard audiologic evaluation. However, there is clearly a need for professionals who are interested in the assessment and treatment of central auditory processing disorders.

This chapter will discuss the current state of pediatric audiometric evaluation, including the commonly used behavioral techniques as well as the application of objective measures in the identification and quantification of hearing loss in children.

BEHAVIORAL TESTING

Despite the physiologic tests available that provide objective information on various portions of the auditory system, measures of frequency-specific sensitivity and suprathreshold auditory functioning are dependent on behavioral test procedures. Reliable voluntary audiometric responses can be obtained beginning at around the age of 6 months if cognitive and motoric development are normal (9). Several procedures have been developed specifically to take advantage of the interests and abilities of children of different ages. According to Wilson and Thompson (10), behavioral test measures are based on either overt nonreinforced responses or on shaped, reinforced responses. Those that do not use reinforcement to shape a response behavior are called behavioral observation audiometry (BOA), whereas techniques that use a reward to shape a response are commonly referred to as conditioned response audiometry.

Behavioral Observation Audiometry

The earliest attempts to test children were based on the normal tendency of infants to react in some manner to a novel auditory stimulus. No attempt was made to train or condition the child to react; rather, any overt action that occurred following presentation of a sound was observed and recorded. It was up to the "observer" to determine if the action was tied to presentation of the stimulus.

Research has helped to make BOA a more standardized and reliable measure through careful studying and recording of the responses exhibited by children of different developmental levels to varying types and intensities of sound (11). The important factor in BOA is to establish an activity baseline and then determine if the activity changes in response to the sound presentation. For example, the baby may be observed to be quietly sucking on a pacifier in the test setting. When a sound is presented, the baby may momentarily cease sucking or may briefly suck harder. The observer then must judge if the change in activity is related to the auditory stimulus. Infants may respond in many ways, most of them very subtle. Actions such as eye widening, eye blinking, eye shift, raising of the eyebrows, arousal from inactivity, or quieting from activity may constitute response to sound by an infant.

Northern and Downs (1) review several studies which conclude that the chance for false-positive responses is too great in an awake baby and suggest that the most valid method of testing an infant is with the child in a light sleep (12,13). This may present a problem in the clinical setting, because a strange setting and unknown people may keep the baby from sleeping easily.

BOA techniques are most useful with children in the 0- to 6-month age range or children who are not developmentally capable of the head control necessary for conditioned response techniques. BOA may be the only means of obtaining behavioral responses to auditory stimulation in children with severe mental retardation (10).

BOA techniques have severe limitations in testing infant hearing. In general, frequency-specific information and accurate sensitivity levels cannot be obtained using BOA alone. Children tend to habituate to the stimuli rather quickly, and they are more sensitive to broadband signals such as speech and music. Stimuli that are sufficient to cause a change in the child's behavior are likely to be considerably above the actual threshold of hearing. Rather than threshold, it has been suggested that responses obtained during BOA testing be labeled as minimum response levels (14).

Despite its limitations, Northern and Downs (1) report that at least 95% of children can be identified successfully as having normal hearing using noisemakers in a behavioral observation procedure when the testing is performed in an appropriate setting by experienced testers. BOA provides a gross measure of auditory sensitivity, and a lack of response should serve to alert the tester of the need for aggressive follow-up with more accurate tests.

Conditioned Response Audiometry

Based on techniques of operant conditioning, several variations of stimulus-response-reward audiometry procedures have been developed to appeal to children at different developmental levels. Conditioned response techniques can first be used with infants who have reached a developmental level of 5 to 6 months, and they are useful until the child is developmentally ready to do standard audiometry. In conditioned response audiometry, a child's response to an auditory stimulus is shaped, and some type of reward is used to maintain the response behavior. In all such procedures, the audiologist must observe the child and question the parent prior to testing to determine at what level testing should begin. All behavioral procedures should begin with stimulus levels at 40 to 50 dB above threshold for conditioning or training procedures. Conditioned response audiometry can be used to obtain frequency-specific responses that are generally 10 to 15 dB worse than those exhibited by adults (10). By the age of 18 months, responses should approximate adult levels. Studies have shown that responses obtained using conditioned response audiometry are reliable and stable (15,16).

Conditioned Orientation Response Audiometry

Conditioned orientation response audiometry (COR) was described by Suzuki and Ogiba (17) as a method for testing children below the age suitable for play audiometry techniques in use at the time. Suzuki and Ogiba based their method on the natural tendency for an infant to turn toward a novel stimulus, a response called the "orientation reflex." The original report indicated that the method

worked especially well with children between the ages of 1 and 3 years. In children below the age of 1 year, slightly less than one half of children could be tested successfully, whereas results were obtained in close to 90% of those between 1 and 3 years. Beyond the age of 3, the child's interest could no longer be held by the toy long enough to obtain complete data. The method was reported to have test-retest reliability within 5 dB in 88% of the test trials.

The COR task requires that the child detect the sound and make a head turn toward the sound source. Auditory stimuli are presented through one of two loudspeakers. The child is seated, usually on a parent's lap, between the two loudspeakers. A visual reinforcer, usually some type of toy placed in a darkened plexiglass box, is located on or near each speaker. The tester controls a switch that illuminates the box, making the toy visible.

Initially, illumination of the toy serves as the unconditioned stimulus, which is paired with the auditory or conditioned stimulus. Presentation of the toy is immediately preceded by presentation of an auditory stimulus judged to be significantly above the hearing level of the child. The two stimuli then remain on simultaneously for several seconds. The procedure is repeated using the other speaker and reinforcer. Three to four presentations are viewed as sufficient to condition the child to turn toward the illuminated toy as soon as the sound is heard. At this point, the visual stimulus has become the reward. Sound intensity and frequency then are varied to determine hearing sensitivity.

One of the major drawbacks of the COR method is that no ear-specific information is obtained, because all testing is done in the sound field through loudspeakers. In addition, the method works well with normally hearing children, but it has been reported as less successful with hearing impaired children (18). Nevertheless, COR remains a useful tool for obtaining initial behavioral indications of auditory status in cases where the child refuses to tolerate inserts, earphones, or a bone oscillator.

Visual Reinforcement Audiometry

In an attempt to overcome limitations of the COR procedure, Liden and Kankkunen (19) reported on a modification of the procedure, which they called visual reinforcement audiometry (VRA) (19). The test setup was similar to that used in COR. However, speakers were set at 90 degrees azimuth while the visual reinforcer was placed in front of the child. The reinforcer was used primarily to add interest to the task and keep the child participating for longer periods. The ear not being tested was plugged in an attempt to test one ear at a time. Rather than a head turn toward the reinforcer, several types of responses, somewhat reminiscent of BOA procedures, were considered acceptable. The report indicated that acceptance of various types of responses made it possible to obtain results from more children, but at the same time it increased the chances for subjective bias.

These original procedures form the basis for currently used visual response audiometry techniques. The procedures described by Gravel (20) are both a combination and modification of COR and VRA. Figure 1 shows a common two-tester VRA setup. According to Gravel, the signal need not have any intrinsic interest, thus making it possible to obtain responses to auditory signals that may include speech, music, narrowband noise, or warbled pure tones, or even standard pure tone stimuli.

One modification that increases the child's period of cooperation and reduces the chances of false responses is the use of a second tester. The role of the assistant is to attract the child's attention toward the midline between stimulus presentations. The assistant and whatever is used as a distracter must not be interesting enough to completely divert the child's interest from the listening task. The assistant also may provide social reward to the child and may help judge the validity of responses.

Another important modification is the use of either earphones or insert receivers instead of, or in addition to, sound field stimulus presentation. Obtaining ear-specific information is necessary for both medical treatment and habilitative measures. Many children today are familiar with earphones and are willing to tolerate their use. Insert receivers offer an alternative. Some children who will not allow the use of one will inexplicably accept the other. Use of ear-specific transducers does not change the basic procedure. Presentation to a given ear is associated with the same-side reinforcer. Unlike the original VRA procedure, the only acceptable response is a turn of the head or eyes toward the reinforcer on the stimulated side.

If a child does not respond to the sound stimulus, it is often difficult to determine if it is because the child has not heard the sound, or because he or she does not understand the task. A helpful procedure in such a case is to condition the child using the bone oscillator. Presentation of a bone-conducted, 250- or 500-Hz tone at 50 dB is easily felt, if not heard. The oscillator may be placed on the mastoid or even in the child's hand, and a conditioning procedure conducted. If the child conditions to the tactile stimulation but not the auditory, it is likely that hearing is decreased. On the other hand, if the child cannot be conditioned to respond to the tactile stimulation, repeated test sessions may be necessary. Objective measures such as acoustic reflexes, OAEs, or ABR should be used immediately.

A recent modification has been development of a computerized VRA system (21,22). One such system, intelligent visual reinforcement audiometry (23), uses a Bayesian mathematical theory to classify response patterns of children for both screening and assessment purposes (23). Such systems are particularly useful when the option of having a second tester is not available. However, there is inherent inflexibility in the system, which makes it less useful for more problematic children.

Tangible Reinforced Operant Conditioning Audiometry

Tangible reinforced operant conditioning audiometry (TROCA), described by Lloyd et al. (24), reinforces the child using food or some other small tangible reward rather than the visual stimulus. The procedure is more challenging and interesting for the child, because he or she is required to push a button when the sound is heard. A typical TROCA device is shown in Fig. 2. The unit includes a light source that can be paired with the auditory stimulus in initial conditioning trials as well as a response bar or button. Inside is a revolving tray composed of small compartments into which the reinforcers are placed. Distribution of the reward is controlled by a test assistant when there is agreement between presentation of the signal and the response. Initially, a suprathreshold sound cou-

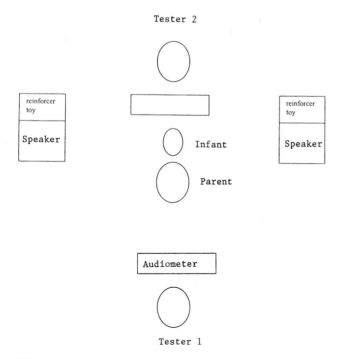

FIG. 1. Standard two-tester visual reinforcement audiometry setup.

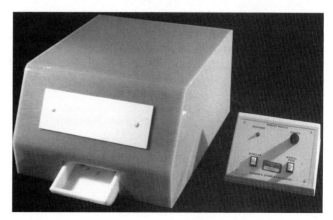

FIG. 2. Tangible reinforced operant conditioning audiometry device.

pled with a light source is used to train the child to press the response bar to receive the reward. The light is gradually removed so that response is made only to the sound stimulus. It is important to determine something that is appealing to the child to be used as the reward. Cereal, candy, pennies, stickers, or a combination often are effective in keeping the child's attention focused. TROCA is particularly helpful with children who are too young for play audiometry, but for whom VRA toys no longer hold interest. Children between the ages of 2 and 4 years often fall into this category. Another group for whom TROCA frequently proves useful is older children whose developmental level is not adequate for play audiometry. The authors have found TROCA to be a valuable tool in cochlear implant programming, during which the child's attention must be maintained for long periods of time.

Conditioned Play Audiometry

Play audiometry techniques were described as early as 1947 (25), and for children approaching the age of 3, has become the test technique of choice. In a study reported by Thompson and Weber (26), only 2% of children less than 24 months of age could be tested using play audiometry. That number had increased to 70% between the ages of 24 and 29 months. By the age of 3 years, 96% of the children evaluated could be tested successfully using play audiometry.

Play audiometry can be used to obtain a complete ear-specific air and bone conduction audiogram in many children. The procedure requires that the child perform a simple task, such as dropping a block in a bucket or putting a peg into a pegboard, in response to the sound. Verbal praise generally is sufficient reward to motivate the developmentally appropriate child to complete the task. In other cases, intermittent use of the toys normally used in VRA procedures can be used to reinforce the response.

Some children may need to be trained to do the task by having the tester or an assistant physically prompt the child in performing the task several times or modeling the correct response. Others may simply be instructed on the procedure. A single tester can often do play audiometry by sitting in the sound suite with the child and using a portable audiometer. More difficult to test children may require the use of two testers, one inside the sound booth with the child while the other sits at the audiometer.

Standard Audiometry

By the time a child has reached a developmental age of 4 years, he or she generally is capable of performing standard techniques such as hand raising. However, in cases requiring long testing sessions to obtain both air and bone conduction thresholds, children up to 5 years may benefit from having a task to perform. Beyond 5 years, social reward presented less frequently as age increases may remain helpful in maintaining the child's attention and focus.

The ultimate goal of all behavioral audiometric assessment is to determine threshold levels at frequencies of 250 to 8,000 Hz in each ear. In reality, pediatric assessment involves obtaining as much information as possible, as quickly as possible, based on the child's developmental age and behavioral state. For difficult to test children, numerous visits may be necessary, with little pieces of information obtained at each visit. Normal hearing children are most likely to be easily tested because they are already attuned to sound. Hearing impaired, multihandicapped, or mentally challenged children may require variations and combinations of behavioral test methods, together with patience, flexibility, and ingenuity on the part of the audiologist. Table 1 shows test procedures categorized by age appropriateness.

TABLE 1. *Age-appropriate test procedures for auditory assessment of pediatric patients*

Age (mo)	Objective test measure	Behavioral test measure	Difficult to test
0–6	ABR OAE Tympanometry[a]	BOA	NA
7–36	Tympanometry Acoustic reflexes OAE	VRA COR	ABR (sedated)
36–60	Tympanometry Acoustic reflexes OAE	Conditioned play TROCA	ABR (sedated) VRA TROCA
60+	Tympanometry Acoustic reflexes OAE	Standard audiometry	Conditioned play TROCA ABR (sedated)

Column 4 shows the measures that might be the child's developmental age used if the age is significantly below the chronological age.

[a]Tympanometry should be interpreted with caution in infants <7 months of age.

ABR, auditory brainstem response; BOA, behavioral observation audiometry; COR, conditioned orientation response audiometry; NA, not applicable; OAE, otoacoustic emission; TROCA, tangible reinforced operant conditioning audiometry; VRA, visual reinforcement audiometry.

OBJECTIVE MEASURES

Each of the objective measures currently used in pediatric hearing assessment is discussed in detail elsewhere in this chapter. However, because these tests are an integral part of the pediatric test battery, the application of such measures will be discussed briefly. Objective evaluation of the auditory system commonly includes immittance measures, evoked potentials, most specifically the ABR, and OAEs. Each of these measures may be used for large-scale pediatric screening purposes or may be used on an individual basis to obtain more specific information on a given child.

I\mmittance Measures

Pure tone air and bone conduction testing using one of the techniques described earlier is necessary to identify and quantify conductive hearing losses due to middle ear disorders. However, the tests that comprise the immittance battery appear to be more useful in the identification of middle ear disease than is the pure tone hearing test (27). Middle ear disease is the most common reason for visits to the doctor among children, and otitis media is the most common form of middle ear disease (28). Consensus on the long-term consequences of chronic middle ear disease has yet to be achieved, but indications of the fluctuating hearing loss often associated with chronic otitis media are too strong to ignore. Although many experienced otologists and otolaryngologists feel that immittance testing is not necessary in the diagnosis of middle ear pathology, not all pediatricians and general practitioners are as accomplished with the otoscope or the pneumatic otoscope. Tests including tympanometry, physical volume, and acoustic reflexes can provide a quick and noninvasive means of assessing the middle ear status of young children when applied with appropriate understanding of the limitations associated with the procedures.

Tympanometry

Tympanometry is a procedure that measures changes in the compliance of the middle ear system in response to air pressure changes in the ear canal, providing information on middle ear pressure and mobility. Middle ear pressure is known to fluctuate frequently among children, and pressures ranging from 50 to -150 decapascals are generally considered within the normal range. Among children, static immittance or measures of mobility are considered normal between 0.2 and 0.9 ml (29).

The use of tympanometry in infants below the age of 6 to 7 months should be approached with caution because of a high false-negative rate (30). It has been assumed that the lack of rigidity of the infant ear canal translates as movement of the middle ear system, although this assumption has not been proven (31). Several age-related changes in tympanometric results were described by Holte et al. (32). These studies demonstrated that the middle ear system of the infant differs in several ways from that of the adult, confirming that tympanometry in infants should be interpreted in conjunction with competent otoscopy (32). However, with growing support for the use of OAEs in infant hearing screening programs, the use of tympanometry may deserve another look. Because the absence of emissions can be associated with either middle ear disorders or cochlear hearing loss, an accurate tool for identifying middle ear abnormalities in neonates has obvious value.

Tympanometry is limited in its usefulness with children by the transient nature of middle ear status in children. Studies have shown that tympanometric results can change on a daily basis (33). These researchers reported that both normal tympanograms and those showing negative middle ear pressure had a greater than 25% chance of being different on 2 subsequent days. Tympanograms consistent with stiff middle ear systems were found to be least likely to vary over time. Tos and his colleagues (34) reported that although the incidence of middle ear effusion is high among children between the ages of 6 months and 2 years, many of these episodes resolve spontaneously. Consequently, medical referrals based on tympanometry alone, most particularly a single test, should be avoided. However, Orchik and MacKimmie reported that the presence of hearing loss, together with abnormal tympanometry. confirms a middle ear disorder in 90% of cases, and they suggest that tympanometry should be used in conjunction with behavioral audiometry whenever possible (35). For those children who have been established as otitis prone, tympanometry can be used on a regular basis to monitor the middle ear status and to document the effects of treatment.

Physical Volume

When the probe tip of the impedance system is hermetically sealed into the ear canal, a space is created between the end of the probe and the tympanic membrane. The size of the cavity can be estimated based on the relationship between the measured sound pressure level of the probe tone and the size of the cavity. In a normal pediatric ear canal, the equivalent volume reading is between 0.4 and 1.0 cc (29).

If the tympanic membrane is disrupted by a perforation or a pressure equalization (PE tube), the cavity being measured will include the middle ear space, resulting in a volume reading three to four times greater than normal. The physical volume test can confirm the presence of a difficult to visualize perforation. The functional status of PE tubes also can be evaluated, because blockage of the tube will result in a normal volume reading as opposed to the larger reading produced by an open tube. A volume reading smaller than normal should alert the tester to the presence of significant cerumen or foreign body in the canal.

Acoustic Reflex

The acoustic reflex is a measurement of change in middle ear compliance resulting from contraction of the stapedius muscles. Elicitation of the response in either ear results in a bilateral reflex. As the muscles contract, the middle ear systems stiffen, resulting in a change in stiffness properties. Acoustic reflexes occur at predictable sensation levels in both normal ears and frequently in ears with cochlear hearing loss. Absence of acoustic reflexes may be indicative of middle ear disorder, retrocochlear hearing loss, or severe-to-profound sensorineural hearing loss. Used with both tympanometry and behavioral audiometry, acoustic reflexes are a useful component of the cross-check principle.

In pediatric evaluation, the presence of acoustic reflexes in the absence of other indicators prepares the tester to expect normal hearing. Presence of reflexes, together with concerns about speech and language development, should alert the tester to the possibility of cochlear hearing loss of mild-to-moderate degree. Absence of the reflex, together with normal tympanometry and parental concerns, suggests the possibility of sensorineural hearing loss of severe to profound degree. Finally, absence of acoustic reflexes associated with abnormal tympanometry generally is indicative of conductive involvement. Freyss et al. (36) reported that the presence or absence of the acoustic reflex was more sensitive to the presence of middle ear effusion than is tympanometry.

As with tympanometry, measurement of acoustic reflexes in infants must be approached with caution. Keith (37) reported the measurement of a clear acoustic reflex in only 33% of trials among 40 infants in a well-baby nursery. Four of these infants had no reflexes, but they were later found to have normal hearing. Several studies have reported a higher incidence of present reflexes among infants when a higher-frequency probe tone is substituted for the typically used 226-Hz tone (38–40). Measurement of reflexes using high-frequency probe tones has not become a commonly used clinical tool. The ease with which more specific information can be obtained from ABR and OAE testing has perhaps lessened the potential value of acoustic reflexes in infant testing.

Auditory Brainstem Response

The ABR has become the most widely used of the auditory evoked potentials in assessment of both hearing and neurologic status of the auditory system. The ABR consists of a series of seven positive peak waveforms that normally occur within 10 ms of an auditory stimulus presentation. ABR waveforms represent the synchronous neural discharges of multiple generator sites from the eighth cranial nerve and the brainstem auditory nuclei and are not a direct test of hearing (41). However, ABR waveforms are highly correlated with pure tone thresholds of 2 to 4,000 Hz. Identifiable waveforms generally are present at 10 to 20 dB above behavioral threshold. In the hearing assessment of infants, presence of wave V, generally the most robust of the peaks, is the primary response criterion. The ABR response can be obtained using low-level stimuli, thus providing a closer approximation of actual hearing levels than infant behavioral screening techniques. ABR also has the advantage of providing ear-specific information, because stimuli are presented to each ear individually via earphones or insert receivers. ABR requires no cooperation from the infant, and it is most effectively obtained in a sleeping subject. Evoked responses occurring later in time, including the middle latency response, the 40-Hz steady-state potential, and the cortical responses, have been studied, but they have not been found to be as accurate and reliable as the ABR in estimation of hearing status (42,43).

An important consideration in the use of ABR testing with infants is maturation of the response. Although present as early as 30-weeks gestational age (44), prior to the age of 18 months, the response may differ significantly from the mature waveform. In preterm infants, latencies are prolonged and thresholds elevated as compared to the full-term infant (45). Therefore, it is necessary that testers use age-specific norms in interpretation of infant responses. In addition, when an abnormal or absent response is obtained from a preterm infant, no conclusions beyond the need for further testing should be drawn. Finitzo-Hieber (45) suggests that a premature infant can exhibit an abnormal response that may show partial-to-complete recovery as the infant's neurologic system matures, making ABR follow-up as well as behavioral testing imperative before a definitive diagnosis is made.

Another consideration that must be kept in mind when using the ABR as a hearing assessment tool is that the typical stimulus is a broadband click. The response obtained is most closely correlated with behavioral thresholds of 2 to 4,000 Hz. Lack of an ABR response cannot be equated with a lack of residual hearing. Numerous attempts have been made to develop methods for obtaining more frequency-specific information through ABR testing. Several such procedures have been described, but they are beyond the capabilities of most clinics (46–49). Therefore, when interpreting ABR results for anxious parents, caution should be exercised, and the need for further quantification of the loss is emphasized.

Figure 3 shows a threshold search ABR performed on a 3-week-old infant during natural sleep in the audiology clinic. A pediatric nurse made note of a small patch of white hair at a 2-week follow-up visit. This led the family to seek hearing evaluation. Questionable behavioral responses were obtained to speech and music presented at 80 dB in the sound field. As shown, repeatable ABR responses were obtained at 10 dB normalized hearing level

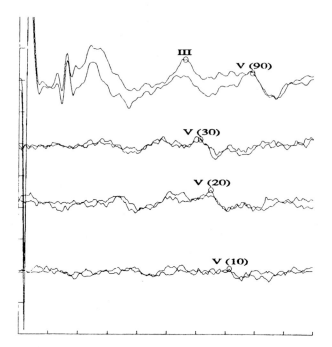

FIG. 3. Auditory brainstem response (ABR) tracings in a 3-week-old infant during natural sleep. The tracings represent the stimulus responses at 90, 30, 20, and 10 dB nHL. Repeatable ABR responses at 10 dB nHL indicated normal threshold.

(nHL) in this infant. Her transient OAEs, shown in Fig. 4, corroborate the ABR results.

Protocols for use of ABR as a screening tool differ from those used in follow-up testing. The Joint Committee on Infant Hearing (50), which included representatives from otolaryngology, speech and hearing, and pediatrics, published a recommended protocol for infant screening using ABR. This committee recommended that ABR be used to screen the hearing of all children who exhibit any of a group of factors that place an infant at risk of hearing loss. Information on the high-risk factors can be found in several sources (1). The committee recommended that a response to a click stimulus at 40 dB nHL or less in each ear be considered the criterion for passing. If no response is obtained at 40 dB nHL, the tester may or may not, based on time and protocol, perform an additional test at a higher level. Either way, the infant who does not pass at the criterion level of 40 dB nHL will be referred for follow-up testing. The failure rate among neonatal intensive care unit screenings ranges from 3% to 10% based on the pass-fail criterion used (44).

If a child fails an infant screening, or if other reasons exist that create suspicion of the hearing status in an infant, ABR testing can be used to obtain a more specific estimation of auditory status. As illustrated in Fig. 3, the stimuli are presented at decreasing intensity levels until a response is no longer judged to be present. If desired, a bracketing technique can be used to obtain even more specific levels. As mentioned earlier, such a procedure provides information related primarily to high-frequency hearing and must be supplemented by behavioral testing or other physiologic techniques, such as OAE testing.

Otoacoustic Emissions

OAEs, first recorded by Kemp (51) in 1978, are measurements of a low-level sound most likely produced by outer hair cells of the cochlea. The responses travel back-

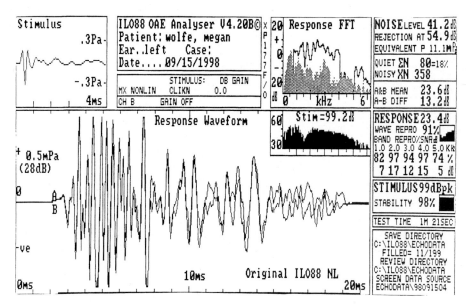

FIG. 4. Transient otoacoustic emission response consistent with probable normal hearing from the same patient shown in Fig. 3.

ward from the cochlea through the middle ear system. OAEs may be either spontaneous or evoked by auditory stimulation. Spontaneous emissions occur in approximately one half of normal hearing persons. It is possible to record spontaneous emissions, but to date they have not proven to be of significant diagnostic use. Evoked OAEs can be recorded through placement of a probe containing both a stimulus source and a pickup microphone into the ear canal. Evoked emissions have been shown to be present in 80% to 90% of normal hearing ears (52–54).

Evoked emissions are of two types, transiently evoked (TEOAE) and distortion product. TEOAEs are absent in ears in which hearing loss exceeds 30 dB. Distortion product OAEs are absent in ears in which hearing loss exceeds 50 dB. Lonsbury-Martin et al. (55) and Lonsbury-Martin and Martin (56) report that evoked emissions are systematically reduced or absent in the presence of sensorineural hearing loss. Consequently, the presence of evoked OAEs strongly correlates with normal hearing. One drawback to the use of OAEs in children is that the presence of middle ear disorders renders the response unrecordable (57). Therefore, the middle ear status of the child must be assessed to interpret correctly the absence of OAEs.

Early studies such as those by Bonfils et al. (58) and Stevens et al. (59) demonstrated excellent agreement between the absence of transient OAEs and absence of an ABR at levels greater than 30 dB HL. All infants with ABR responses present at 30 dB HL and lower also exhibited present TEOAEs. Bonfils et al. reported that recording of TEOAE responses required approximately 5 minutes, whereas determination of ABR thresholds required closer to 40 minutes to complete.

The TEOAEs obtained from the 3-week-old infant suspected of having Waardenburg's syndrome are shown in Fig. 4. In this case, ABR (shown in Fig. 3) and TEOAE responses are in agreement, and they are consistent with probable normal hearing even though no clear behavioral responses could be obtained.

As with ABR, OAEs can be used as either a screening tool in a large-scale program or, as illustrated in this chapter, they can be used effectively in the pediatric audiometric evaluation. Studies such as the Rhode Island Hearing Assessment Project showed that OAEs could be a cost-effective and effective tool in a hearing screening program (60). Such findings led the National Institutes of Health Consensus Committee to recommend implementation of a universal screening program that uses TEOAEs as the first-level screening (61).

SPEECH PERCEPTION TESTING

Every auditory assessment of pediatric patients should include at least some measure of speech perception. Threshold tests of speech can be used to verify pure tone results. In children with normal hearing, suprathreshold tests of speech perception can be helpful in assessing the need for speech and language referrals. The child's hearing, chronologic age, and both speech reception and speech production should all be in agreement. If not, it is the responsibility of the hearing health care professional to refer the child for appropriate follow-up evaluations. For children identified with hearing loss, speech perception measures can be used to determine the suitability of amplification and to monitor progress over time. As is the case with many severely to profoundly hearing impaired adults, the quality of hearing in children can vary significantly. Acceptable responses on the aided audiogram do not necessarily equate with good sound quality. Improvements in hearing aids and cochlear implants make it more necessary than ever to consider quality as well as quantity of residual hearing in children. Traditional speech measures have included the speech reception threshold (SRT), speech awareness threshold (SAT), and measures of monosyllabic word recognition. Newer tests applicable to younger children include measures of pattern perception abilities and understanding of sentence materials. These types of speech perception testing are considered tools to assess peripheral auditory function. Interest in assessment of the function of higher auditory centers have led to the development of a battery of tests aimed at evaluation of central auditory processing.

Threshold Speech Tests

The SRT is the lowest level at which words with two equally stressed syllables, such as baseball or hotdog, can be correctly identified with 50% accuracy. Identification may be either by repeating the word or by pointing to a picture. For children who are unable to either point to or repeat words due to delayed language or other disorders, an SAT can be obtained using behavioral audiometry techniques. In obtaining an SAT, the child need only respond if the word is heard in the same manner used to obtain responses to other stimuli. The SAT is used often with severely to profoundly hearing impaired children who have insufficient speech and language abilities to perform an SRT task.

As with adults, the threshold of speech recognition or awareness can provide validation for pure tone responses. If the SRT or SAT is inconsistent with the pure tone audiogram, there is good reason to suspect the results. The SRT can be expected to be approximately 5 to 6 dB above the pure tone average of thresholds obtained at 500, 1,000, and 2,000 Hz (62). The SAT should approximate the level of the best frequency response.

Suprathreshold Speech Tests

Suprathreshold tests are measures that are presented at a listening level that is comfortably above the SRT. In standard clinical evaluation, measures of speech discrimination are presented at 40 dB above the SRT. In certain situations, such as assessment of benefits provided by an amplification system, the materials may be presented at a standard listening level, such as 70 dB sound pressure level. Standardized words lists used with adults, such as the NU6 (63) or CID W-22 (64), are appropriate for most children above the age of 10 years (65). Speech discrimination measures designed specifically for young children have been available since Haskins (66) introduced the phonetically balanced kindergarten (PBK) word lists in 1949. Speech tests for children may be classified as either closed set or open set. Closed set measures provide the listener with a small group of words or pictures from which to choose. Closed set measures will always have a chance score that may be obtained through guessing. Open set measures provide no choices for the listener, and guessing is not a factor.

The most commonly used open set test of single word recognition for young children has been the PBK lists. The words were selected on the basis of familiarity for children of kindergarten age in the late 1940s. However, a recent study suggested that the word lists may be outdated, as only 31% of the PBK words are actually familiar to very young or language-limited children (67).

More recently developed open set tests of word recognition are the Lexical Neighborhood Monosyllabic Word Test and the Multisyllabic Lexical Neighborhood Test. These two tests were developed at the University of Indiana to evaluate the speech recognition abilities of children with cochlear implants (68). The authors were concerned that monosyllabic tests, such as PBK, which is based primarily on the ability to discriminate consonant sounds, would most likely underestimate the abilities of implanted children. A lexical "neighborhood" consists of words that differ by only one phoneme. Words also can be categorized into neighborhoods based on the frequency of occurrence of the words in language usage and by the number of words within the lexical neighborhood. Two sets of words—easy word with high frequency of occurrence from a "sparse" lexical neighborhood, and hard word with low frequency of occurrence from a "dense" neighborhood—comprise the test items. Although perhaps not sufficient to test the hearing abilities of children with lesser degrees of hearing loss, these words do seem to give a better picture of the day-to-day word recognition abilities of young severely to profoundly hearing impaired children.

Closed set monosyllabic word recognition tests include the Word Intelligibility by Picture Identification (WIPI) (69) and the Northwestern University Children's Perception of Speech (NU-CHIPS) Test (70). Both WIPI and NU-CHIPS use a picture pointing task. The WIPI is appropriate for children between the ages of 4 and 6 years. The test consists of 25 monosyllabic words. The words are presented on a picture plate, which contains six alternatives from which to select. Chance score on the WIPI is 16%. NU-CHIPS consists of 50 test items pre-

sented in a four-picture format. This test has been standardized on hearing impaired children as young as 2.8 years of age. Chance score on the NU-CHIPS is 25%.

The often extremely low language level and, in particular, the limited vocabulary development of young deaf children are significant problems in the administration of these tests. Geers and Moog (71) introduced a speech perception evaluation tool called the Early Speech Perception Test Battery (71). Their test is based on earlier tests developed to assess simpler aspects of speech, including the Glendonald Auditory Screening Procedure (72), the Auditory Numbers Test (73), and the Monosyllable, Trochee, Spondee Test (74). The test is designed to go below the word recognition level and assess emerging speech discrimination ability. Test items were selected based on their familiarity to deaf children below the age of 6 years. There are three subtests, including pattern perception, spondee word recognition, and monosyllabic word recognition. A picture pointing task is used for each. However, the pattern perception subtest also has a low verbal version that uses familiar objects for those children whose vocabulary is insufficient for the standard version. The test is available in a recorded version.

Several tests of sentence materials for children have been developed. The first, Bamford-Kowal-Bench Sentence Lists for Partially Hearing Children (75), was developed in an attempt to assess speech recognition in a normal language usage format. The sentences of these lists are based on language samples obtained from hearing impaired children between the ages of 8 and 15 years. Two groups of sentences were developed. The standard version consists of 21 lists of 16 sentences and 50 key words that are presented with no visual information. The second group consists of 11 lists of 16 sentences that have corresponding pictures designed to be used with children whose auditory abilities are below that required to complete the auditory only task. The sentences were developed for, and standardized on, English children. They have not been widely used in the United States.

The need for sentence materials appropriate for children in the United States has been recognized. The Common Phrases Test (76) was developed at Indiana University School of Medicine primarily for use with children with cochlear implants. There are six lists of ten sentences. The vocabulary and grammatical structures are drawn from materials familiar to young, profoundly hearing impaired children. The test is presented in a live voice format and may be subject to influence by the tester.

A recently developed sentence test for children is the Hearing-in-Noise Test (HINT) (77), which is considered appropriate for children age 6 to 12 years. Children above the age of 12 perform as adults on the HINT. Younger children were found to require increased signals as compared to competing noise to achieve results comparable to adults. The test consists of 13 lists of ten sentences, which are available on compact disk. The sentences may be used without the competing noise simply as a measure of sen-

TABLE 2. *Materials commonly used in evaluating speech threshold and speech recognition in pediatric patients*

Speech measure	Test material
Speech awareness threshold (SAT)	Nonsense syllables
	Words
Speech reception threshold (SRT), closed set	Spondee picture cards
	Body parts
Speech reception threshold (SRT), open set	Live voice or recorded spondees
Word recognition, closed set	NU-CHIPS
	WIPI
	MLNT
	GASP words
Speech recognition sentence level, open-set	BKB
	Common phrases
	GASP sentences
	HINT sentences

BKB, Bamford-Kowal-Bench Sentence Lists for Partially Hearing Children; GASP, Glendonald Auditory Screening Procedure; HINT, Hearing in Noise Test; MLNT, Multisyllabic Lexical Neighborhood; NU-CHIPS, Northwestern University Children's Perception of Speech; WIPI, Word Intelligibility by Picture Identification.

tence understanding for children whose abilities surpass the Common Phrases Test. Table 2 shows tests that are commonly used to obtain measures of speech threshold and speech recognition abilities in children.

Tests of the Central Auditory Nervous System

The speech tests discussed thus far test primarily the peripheral auditory system. Tests such as the Illinois Test of Psycholinguistic Abilities (78) and the Wepman Test of Auditory Discrimination (79) were early attempts to assess auditory processing abilities. These tests were primarily used by either psychologists or speech language pathologists. Test results were heavily influenced by factors such as language abilities. Attempts to isolate and test the higher auditory pathways were reported by Bocca et al. (80). Developed for adults, these tests were aimed at identifying the site of a space-occupying lesion. With today's advanced imaging techniques, such measures are receiving less attention. However, other researchers have applied the concepts behind these tests to the identification and evaluation of auditory processing dysfunction in children (81–83). These researchers recognized that there are children who demonstrate normal responses on tests of hearing and simple speech recognition, but who are unable to decode speech in a normal manner.

The earliest tests used with children were adaptations of tests that had been developed for adults. Measures included filtered speech, speech in noise, time-compressed speech, and dichotic presentation of CVs or digits. These tests have not achieved widespread clinical use with children for several reasons, including time required for administration, complexity of the tasks, effects of language level and attention span of the child, and difficulty in interpreting the results (65).

One measure that was developed specifically for children is the SCAN (84). Designed as a screening measure,

the SCAN requires a short period of time to administer. The battery consists of three subtests including filtered speech, auditory figure ground, and competing words. Normative data have been obtained on children from 3 to 11 years of age. The test author reported that the SCAN is useful in identifying children with attention deficit disorders (85). More research is needed both in the identification of disorders of the central auditory nervous system and in the intervention appropriate with children who exhibit such dysfunctions.

SUMMARY

Auditory assessment of pediatric patients may be undertaken for several reasons. Identification of hearing loss that may interrupt normal language development in infants and the quantification of such losses for the purposes of implementing appropriate intervention strategies are primary. Hearing evaluation may be used by otologists or otolaryngologists in selecting and monitoring the course of treatment in medically related auditory disorders. Audiologic evaluation is necessary to select the appropriate amplification for children with sensorineural hearing loss or for those with conductive losses in whom surgical intervention is deferred. Children who undergo treatment with ototoxic antibiotics or chemotherapeutic agents need to have their hearing evaluated and monitored. Simple monitoring of middle ear status and management of related fluctuating hearing loss can have a positive impact on classroom performance.

Regardless of the reason for auditory evaluation, it is important to keep in mind that every child can be tested. Younger or more difficult to test children may require several sessions to obtain a complete evaluation, but difficulty in testing is not a reason to wait. A combination of ABR, OAE, and BOA testing can identify those children who need further evaluation. Children who exhibit abnormal responses on these measures should be enrolled immediately in an intervention program. If the audiologist does not provide the therapy, he or she should be in close contact with the therapist so that decisions regarding amplification can be made quickly. Ongoing therapeutic evaluation should be used to monitor the appropriateness of amplification and to modify it as necessary.

By the age of 5 to 6 months, attempts to obtain unaided and aided responses to pure tone and speech stimuli can be initiated using conditioned response audiometry techniques. Children who have been participating in auditory therapy are especially prepared to respond in the test situation.

Speech tests as simple as the Ling six sounds can provide helpful information in the selection and evaluation of appropriateness of amplification. Even before a child is able to repeat words, his or her emerging ability to decode the speech signal can be assessed using measures such as the low-verbal version of the Early Speech Perception Battery. Progress in auditory development should be monitored with age- and ability-appropriate speech perception measures.

It is important to keep in mind that no one test measure alone is adequate. A combination of pure tone testing, appropriately selected physiologic measures, and speech perception measures is necessary to provide a complete picture in the auditory assessment of pediatric patients.

SUMMARY POINTS

- Every child, regardless of chronologic or developmental age, can undergo audiometric evaluation.
- With difficult cases or very young children, several test sessions may be necessary to obtain adequate results.
- ABR and OAE tests are not tests of hearing, but they are excellent indicators that further hearing evaluation is necessary, especially in very young or difficult to test children.
- Evaluation and therapy should proceed hand in hand in the hearing impaired child with active interaction between therapists and hearing health care providers.
- No one test measure is adequate to provide a complete picture of a child's auditory status and capabilities.
- The "cross-check" principle—use of a test battery approach is most effective for testing children.
- Adequate evaluation of hearing impaired children should include both unaided and aided results, including a measure of the child's ability to receive the speech signal.

REFERENCES

1. Northern JL, Downs MP. *Hearing in children*. Baltimore: Williams & Wilkins, 1991:139–187.
2. Paul PV, Quigley SP. *Education and deafness*. New York: Longman, 1990:56.
3. Friel-Patti S, Finitzo T, Conti G. Language delay in infants associated with middle ear disease and mild fluctuating hearing impairment. *Pediatr Infect Dis J* 1982;1:104–109.
4. Friel-Patti S, Finitzo T, Meyerhoff W, Hieber J. Speech-language learning and early middle ear disease: a procedural report. In: Kavanagh J, ed. *Otitis media and child development*. Parkton: York Press, 1986:129–138.
5. Friel-Patti S, Finitzo T. Language learning in a prospective study of otitis media with effusion in the first two years of life. *J Speech Hear Res* 1990;33:188–194.
6. Roberts JE, Burchinal MR, Zeisel SA, et al. Otitis media, the caregiving environment and language and cognitive outcomes at two years. *Pediatrics* 1998;102:346–354.
7. Jerger J, Hayes D. The cross check principle in pediatric audiology. *Arch Otolaryngol* 1976;102:614–620.
8. Moore JM, Wilson WR, Thompson G. Visual reinforcement of head turn responses in infants under twelve months of age. *J Speech Hear Disord* 1977;42:328–334.
9. Widen JE. Behavioral screening of high-risk infants using visual reinforcement audiometry. *Seminars in Hearing* 1990;11:342–356.
10. Wilson WR, Thompson G. Behavioral audiometry. In: Jerger J, ed. *Pediatric audiology*. San Diego: College Hill Press, 1984:1–44.
11. Eisenberg RB, Griffin EJ, Coursin DB, Hunter MA. Auditory behavior in the human neonate. *J Speech Hear Res* 1964;7:245–269.
12. Ling D, Ling AH, Doering DG. Stimulus response and observer variables in the auditory screening of newborn infants. *J Speech Hear Res* 1970;13:9–18.
13. Menchef GT. Screening infants for auditory deficits: University of Nebraska Neonatal Hearing Project. *Audiology* 1972;11[Suppl]:69.
14. Matkin N. Assessment of hearing sensitivity during the preschool years. In: Bess FH, ed. *Childhood deafness*. New York: Grune and Stratton, 1977:117–131.
15. Nozza RJ, Wilson WR. Masked and unmasked puretone thresholds of infants and adults: development of auditory frequency selectivity and sensitivity. *J Speech Hear Res* 1984;27:613–622.
16. Diefendorf AO. Behavioral evaluation of hearing impaired children. In: Bess FH, ed. *Hearing impairment in children*. Parkton: York Press, 1988:133–151.
17. Suzuki T, Ogiba Y. Conditioned orientation audiometry. *Arch Otolaryngol* 1961;74:192–198.
18. Reddell RC, Calvert DR. Conditioned audio-visual response audiometry. *Proceedings of the Conference on Oral Education of the Deaf* 1967;1:502–506.
19. Liden G, Kankkunen A. Visual reinforcement audiometry. *Acta Otolaryngol* 1969;67:281–292.
20. Gravel JS. Behavioral audiologic assessment. In: Lalwani AK, Grundfast KM, eds. *Pediatric otology and neurotology*. Philadelphia: Lippincott-Raven, 1998:103–111.
21. Eilers RE, Widen JE, Urbano R, Hudson T, Gonzales L. Optimization of automated hearing test algorithms: a comparison of data from simulations and young children. *Ear Hear* 1991;12:199–204.
22. Eilers RE, Ozdamar O, Steffins ML. Classification of audiograms by sequential testing: reliability and validity of an automated behavioral hearing screening algorithm. *J Am Acad Audiol* 1993;4:172–181.
23. Ozdamar O, Eilers RE, Miskiel E, Widen J. Classification of audiograms by sequential testing using a dynamic Bayesian procedure. *J Am Acoust Soc Am* 1990;88:2171–2179.
24. Lloyd L, Spradlin J, Reid M. An operant audiometric procedure for difficult-to-test patients. *J Speech Hear Disord* 1968;33:236–245.
25. Dix M, Hallpike C. The peep show: a new technique for pure tone audiometry in young children. *Br Med J* 1947;1:719–723.
26. Thompson G, Weber B. Responses of infants and young children to behavioral observation audiometry (BOA). *J Speech Hear Disord* 1974;39:140–147.
27. Bluestone C, Beery Q, Paradise J. Audiometry and tympanometry in relation to middle ear effusion in children. *Laryngoscope* 1973;83:594–604.
28. Goin D. Acute inflammatory disease of the middle ear and mastoid. In: English G, ed. *Otolaryngology*. New York: Harper and Row, 1975:157–166.

29. Margolis RH, Heller JW. Screening tympanometry criteria for medical referral. *Audiology* 1987;26:197–201.
30. Paradise JL, Smith CG, Bluestone CD. Tympanometric detection of middle ear effusion in infants and young children. *Pediatrics* 1976;59: 198–210.
31. Hall JW, Chandler D. Tympanometry in clinical practice. In: Katz J, ed. *Handbook of clinical audiology.* Baltimore: Williams & Wilkins, 1994: 283–299.
32. Holte L, Margolis RH, Cavanaugh RM. Developmental changes in multifrequency tympanograms. *Audiology* 1991;30:1–24.
33. Lewis N, Dugdale A, Canty A, Jerger J. Open-ended tympanometric screening: a new concept. *Arch Otolaryngol* 1975;101:722–725.
34. Tos M, Poulson G, Hancke A. Screening tympanometry during the first year of life. *Arch Otolaryngol* 1979;88:388–394.
35. Orchik DJ, MacKimmie KS. Immittance audiometry. In: Jerger J, ed. *Pediatric audiology.* San Diego: College Hill Press, 1984:45–69.
36. Freyss G, Narcy P, Manac'h Y. Acoustic reflex as a predictor of middle ear effusion. *Ann Otol Rhinol Laryngol* 1980;89:196–199.
37. Keith RW. Middle ear functions in neonates. *Arch Otolaryngol* 1975; 101:376–379.
38. McCandless GA, Allred PL. Tympanometry and emergence of the acoustic reflex in infants. In: Harford ER, Bess FH, Bluestone CD, eds. *Middle ear disease in children.* New York: Grune and Stratton, 1978: 56–57.
39. McMillan P, Bennett M, Marchant C, Shurin P. Ipsilateral and contralateral acoustic reflexes in neonates. *Ear Hear* 1985:320–324.
40. Sprague B, Wiley T, Goldstein R. Tympanometric and acoustic-reflex studies in neonates. *J Speech Hear Res* 1985;28:265–272.
41. Picton RW, Hillyard SA, Frauz HJ, Galambos R. Human auditory evoked potentials. *Electroencephalogr Clin Neurophysiol* 1974;36: 179–190.
42. Brown DD, Shallop JK. A clinically useful 500 Hz evoked response. *Nicolet Potentials* 1982;1:9–12.
43. Kileny P, Shea SL. Middle latency and 40 Hz auditory evoked responses in normal-hearing subjects. *J Speech Hear Res* 1986;29: 20–28.
44. Weber BA. Comparison of auditory brainstem response latency norms for premature infants. *Ear Hear* 1992;3:257–262.
45. Finitzo-Hieber T. Auditory brainstem response: its place in infant audiological evaluations. *Semin Speech Lang Hear* 1982;3:76–87.
46. Don M, Eggermont JJ, Brackman DE. Reconstruction of the audiogram using brainstem responses and high-pass noise masking. *Ann Otol Rhinol Laryngol Suppl* 1979;88:1–20.
47. Gorga MP, Kaminski JR, Beauchaine KA. Auditory brainstem responses to high-frequency tone bursts in normal hearing subjects. *Ear Hear* 1987;8:221–226.
48. Stapells DR. Thresholds for short-latency auditory evoked potentials to tones in notched noise in normal hearing and hearing impaired subjects. *Audiology* 1990;29:262–274.
49. Stapells DR, Gravel JS, Martin BA. Thresholds for auditory brainstem responses to tones in notched noise from infants and young children with normal hearing or sensorineural hearing loss. *Ear Hear* 1995;16: 361–371.
50. Joint Committee on Infant Hearing. Position statement. *ASHA* 1991;33 [Suppl 5]:3–6.
51. Kemp DT. Stimulated acoustic emissions from within the human auditory system. *J Acoust Soc Am* 1978;64:1386–1391.
52. Cope Y, Lutman ME. Otoacoustic emissions. In: McCormick B, ed. *Paediatric audiology 0–5 years.* London: Taylor and Francis, 1988: 221–245.
53. Norton SJ, Neely ST. Tone burst otoacoustic emissions from normal hearing subjects. *J Acoust Soc Am* 1987;81:1860–1872.
54. Bonfils P, Uziel A. Clinical applications of evoked acoustic emissions: results in normally hearing and hearing impaired subjects. *Ann Otol Rhinol Laryngol* 1989;98:326–331.
55. Lonsbury-Martin BL, Harris P, Stagner BB, Hawkins MD, Martin GK. Distortion product emissions in humans. *Ann Otol Rhinol Laryngol* 1990;99:3–14.
56. Lonsbury-Martin BL, Martin GK. The clinical utility of distortion product otoacoustic emissions. *Ear Hear* 1990;11:144–154.
57. Anderson SD, Kemp DT. The evoked cochlear mechanical response in laboratory primates. *Arch Otorhinolaryngol* 1979;224:47–54.
58. Bonfils P, Uziel A, Pujol R. Screening for auditory dysfunction in infants by otoacoustic emissions. *Arch Otolaryngol Head Neck Surg* 1988;114:887–890.
59. Stevens JC, Webb HD, Hutchins J, Connell J, Smith MF, Buffin JT. Click evoked otoacoustic emissions in neonatal screening. *Ear Hear* 1990;11:128–133.
60. White KR, Vohr BR, Behrens TR. Universal newborn hearing screening using transient evoked otoacoustic emissions: results of the Rhode Island Hearing Assessment Project. *Semin Hear* 1993;14:18–29.
61. National Institutes of Health. *Early identification of hearing impairment in infants and young children. NIH consensus statement.* Bethesda, MD: National Institutes of Health, 1993;11:1–24.
62. Hodgson WR. *Basic audiologic evaluation.* Baltimore: Williams & Wilkins, 1980.
63. Tillman TW, Carhart R. *An expanded test for speech discrimination utilizing CNC monosyllabic words: Northwestern University auditory test number 6. Technical report number SAM-TR-66-55.* Brooks Airforce Base, TX: USAF School of Aerospace Medicine, 1966.
64. Hirsch IJ, Davis H, Silverman SR, Reynolds EG, Eldeft E, Benson RW. Development of materials for speech audiometry. *J Speech Hear Disord* 1952;17:321–337.
65. Stelmachowicz PG, Gorga MP. Audiology: early identification and management of hearing loss. In: Cummings CW, Frederickson JM, Harker LA, Krause CJ, Schuller DE, Richardson MA, eds. *Pediatric otolaryngology head and neck surgery* St. Louis: Mosby, 1998: 401–417.
66. Haskins HA. *A phonetically balanced test of speech discrimination for children.* Master's thesis. Evanston, IL: Northwestern University, 1949.
67. Logan JS. *A computational analysis of young children's lexicons. Research on spoken language processing technical report number 8.* Bloomington IN: Indiana University, 1992.
68. Kirk KI, Pisoni DB, Osberger MJ. Lexical effects on spoken word recognition by pediatric cochlear implant users. *Ear Hear* 1992;15: 470–481.
69. Ross M, Lerman J. A picture identification test for hearing impaired children. *J Speech Hear Res* 1970;13:44–53.
70. Katz DR, Elliott LL. Development of a new children's speech discrimination test. Paper presented at the American Speech Language Hearing Association Convention, Chicago, Illinois, 1978.
71. Geers AE, Moog JS. *Early speech perception battery.* St. Louis: Central Institute for the Deaf, 1990.
72. Erber N-P. *Auditory training.* Washington DC: Alexander Graham Bell Association for the Deaf, 1982.
73. Erber NP. Use of the auditory numbers test to evaluate the speech perception ability of hearing-impaired children. *J Speech Hear Res* 1980; 17:194–202.
74. Erber NP, Alencewica C. Audiologic evaluation of deaf children. *J Speech Hear Disord* 1976;41:256–267.
75. Bench J, Kowal A, Bamford J. The BKB sentence lists for partially hearing children. *Br J Audiol* 1979;13:108–112.
76. Robbins AM, Renshaw JJ, Osberger MJ. *Common phrases test.* Indianapolis, IN: Indiana University School of Medicine, 1988.
77. Nilsson MJ, Soli SD, Gelnett DJ. *Development and norming for a hearing in noise test for children.* House Ear Institute Internal Report, 1996.
78. Kirk S, McCarthy J, Kirk W. *Illinois test of psycholinguistic abilities.* Urbana IL: University of Illinois Press, 1968.
79. *Wepman test of auditory discrimination.* Chicago: Language Research Associates, 1958.
80. Bocca E, Calearo C, Cassinari V. A new method for testing hearing in temporal lobe tumors. *Acta Otolaryngol* 1954;44:219–221.
81. Willeford JA. Central auditory function in children with learning disabilities. *Audiol Hear Educ* 1976;2:12–20.
82. Jerger SW, Johnson K, Loiselle L. Pediatric central auditory dysfunction: comparison of children with confirmed lesions versus suspected processing disorders. *Am J Otol* 1988;9:63–71.
83. Musiek FE, Geurkink NA, Keitel S. Test battery assessment of auditory perceptual dysfunction in children. *Laryngoscope* 1982;92:251–257.
84. Keith RW. *SCAN, a screening test for auditory processing disorders.* San Antonio, TX: The Psychology Corporation, 1986.
85. Keith RW, Rudy J, Dona PA, Katbamna B. Comparison of SCAN results with other auditory and language measures in a clinical population. *Ear Hear* 1989;10:382–386.

The Ear: Comprehensive Otology,
edited by R. F. Canalis and P. R. Lambert.
Lippincott Williams & Wilkins, Philadelphia © 2000.

CHAPTER 17

Intraoperative Monitoring of Cranial Nerves

Bruce M. Edwards and Paul R. Kileny

Intraoperative cranial nerve monitoring (IOM) is composed of procedures that evaluate sensory function via the optic and auditory nerves and motor nerve function by observing free-running and electrically triggered electromyographic (EMG) activity from cranial nerves III through VII and IX through XII. Facial and auditory nerve monitoring comprise the most common IOM modalities in ear-related surgical cases. Monitoring EMG from the mandibular division of the trigeminal nerve via the masseter muscle helps to differentiate cranial nerve V from VII activity in cases of large skull base or internal auditory canal lesions (see Chapter 53). Table 1 lists cranial nerves, optimal sites for recording electrodes, and recommendations for monitoring.

IOM usually requires a team approach, with the audiologist and surgeon contributing their respective skills to this dynamic field (1–3). The team must possess a thorough understanding of electrophysiologic science, recognize the impact of pharmacologic techniques and physiologic variables on monitored activity (Table 2), and be prepared to differentiate between changes in IOM related to anesthetic intervention and those related to surgical events.

INSTRUMENTATION

Present-day instrumentation manufactured for IOM ranges from simple dual-channel systems to personal

computer-based, multichannel, multimodality equipment with sophisticated software packages that permit recording and stimulating parametric changes, maintain a permanent log of IOM events, and complete a printed report before the patient is wheeled to recovery. Regardless of the system's sophistication, certain minimal requirements are necessary. At least two channels need to be available for monitoring free-running EMG activity. An electrical stimulator circuit, isolated and discretely controlled through a range of intensity levels, is mandatory, as is a good-quality visual display of monitored activity.

Complex skull base cases often call for multimodality monitoring of numerous cranial nerves. Equipment must allow recording in four or more channels with multiple and independent time bases, variable display and acquisition sensitivities, and utilizing different stimulus modalities with adjustable parametric features (Figs. 1 and 2). System maneuverability is key in IOM practices that require equipment to be transported to numerous operating rooms (ORs) located throughout a large medical complex. Compared to bulky multicomponent apparatus of the past (Fig. 3), a self-contained unit housed in a sturdy yet reasonably sized cart best fulfills this need.

Before IOM is instituted, planners should consider the neuroanatomic pathways through which surgery is to be monitored (e.g., auditory, visual, or motor pathways) and the form of electrophysiologic stimulus and stimulator type used to generate responses (e.g., click and insert earphone, flash and LED goggles, or rectangular electrical pulse and hand-held stimulator). Likewise, the data acquisition mode should be predetermined (e.g., averaged, free-running, or triggered). Other

B. M. Edwards and P. R. Kileny: Department of Otolaryngology–Head and Neck Surgery, University of Michigan Health System, Ann Arbor, Michigan 48109-0312

TABLE 1. *Cranial nerve monitoring*

Cranial nerve	Recording site(s)	Monitoring comments
III (oculomotor)	Medial, superior, inferior rectus[a]	Monitored during cavernous sinus cases
IV (trochlear)	Superior oblique[a]	Difficult to access
V (trigeminal)	Masseter (mandibular [V3] division)	Adjunct to monitoring cranial nerve VII in cases of large CPA lesions
VI (abducens)	Lateral rectus[a]	See comments for cranial nerve III
VII (facial)	A. Upper (frontalis/orbicularis oculi), lower divisions (nasolabial/mentalis) for CPA surgery, or B. Four branches (temporal, zygomatic, buccal, marginal mandibular) for parotidectomy	Most often monitored branchial motor nerve

VIII (auditory)	Active electrode: vertex, high forehead
	Ground electrode: shoulder, contralateral ear
	Reference electrode:
	  ABR: ipsilateral ear, anterior to tragus
	  ECochG: medial ear canal, promontory
	  Direct nerve potential: nerve VIII
		Used in planned hearing preservation cases, vestibular neurectomy, microvascular decompression, endolymphatic sac procedures, selected skull base surgery

IX/X (glossopharyngeal/vagus)	Soft palate, pharyngeal wall (IX), posterior cricoarytenoid (X), or thyroarytenoid	Surface electrode to monitor recurrent laryngeal nerve
XI (accessory)	Trapezius, sternocleidomastoid	Monitored in radical neck dissections
XII (hypoglossal)	Lateral tongue	Used in combination with IX/X in posterolateral cranial base surgery

[a]Care warranted during insertion in patients with elevated intraocular pressures.
ABR, auditory brainstem response; ECochG, electrocochleography; CPA, cerebellopontine angle; CN, cranial nerve.

important preoperative decisions include the type of recording electrodes to be used (Fig. 4), the specific locations for those electrodes, and how stimulating or recording electrodes will be attached so as to remain fixed without interfering with patient access by either anesthesiology or surgery. The stimulator device and stimulation parameters need to be considered (e.g., monopolar vs. bipolar stimulation, constant current vs. constant voltage modes). Importantly, patient grounding issues must be addressed.

TABLE 2. *Influences on intraoperative cranial nerve monitoring (4–7)*

Pharmacologic agent	Effect
Modality: auditory brainstem response	
Enflurane	Up to 1-ms latency shift in wave V
Halothane	Delay of up to 0.5 ms in wave V latency
Isoflurane	After 1.5% end-tidal concentration, >0.5-ms prolongation of wave I–V interpeak latency (inhibitory effects on evoked potentials vary among volatile anesthetics)
Lidocaine	Amplitude reduction and absolute latency delay of wave V
Thiopental	At 20 mg/kg or greater dose, increase in absolute latency wave V; larger doses result in amplitude reductions
Pentobarbital	After 9 mg/kg, latencies increase and amplitudes are reduced
Modality: facial electromyogram	
Local anesthetics (lidocaine, bupivacaine, cocaine, tetracaine)	Delayed latencies and reduced amplitudes due to impaired propagation of potentials
Neuromuscular blockers (pancuronium, atracurium, mivacurium, vecuronium)	Spontaneous, free-running, and evoked responses may be abolished for lengthy periods

Physiologic event	Effect
Local or systemic hypothermia	Prolongation of absolute and interpeak latencies of auditory brainstem response components; neurotonic stimulation of electromyographic activity
Tissue compression, retraction	Response delay, amplitude diminution, and degradation of waveform morphology
Inadequate ventilation, hemodilution, systemic hypotension, regional ischemia	Altered oxygen supply causing reduction in endocochlear potential, decreased cochlear output

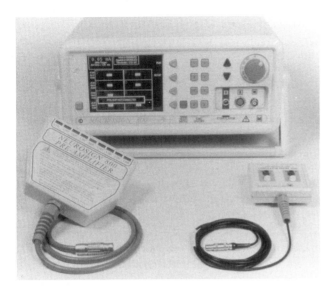

FIG. 1. Compact eight-channel electromyographic device used for intraoperative cranial nerve monitoring. (Courtesy of Magstim Company Ltd.)

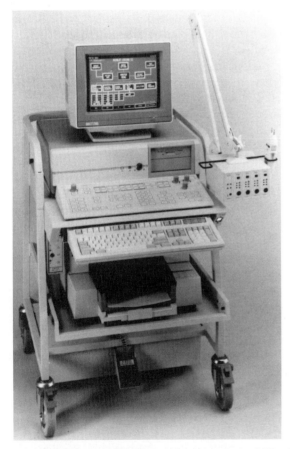

FIG. 2. Portable multimodality intraoperative monitoring device utilized for intraoperative cranial nerve monitoring. (Courtesy of Nicolet Biomedical Inc.)

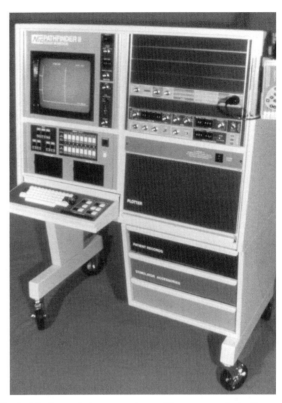

FIG. 3. Early mainframe-style multicomponent device used for intraoperative cranial nerve monitoring. (Courtesy of Nicolet Biomedical Inc.)

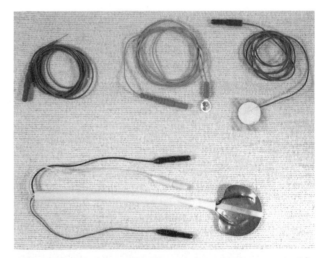

FIG. 4. Electrodes used to record cranial nerve activity intraoperatively. Clockwise, from **top left**: subdermal needle electrode, silver cup-style surface recording electrode, self-adhering surface recording electrode, paddle-style electrode for the posterior cricoarytenoid space placed by direct laryngoscopy.

FACIAL NERVE MONITORING

Technologic advances have resulted in significant improvements in both mortality and morbidity rates associated with resection of acoustic tumors. For example, mortality rates that ranged from 20% to 43.5% early in this century are presently less than 1% because of technologic advances that aid in earlier diagnoses, improvements in microsurgical management, and postoperative care (8,9). Facial nerve monitoring (FNM) has similarly benefited from improved basic and clinical research, technologic development, and production. One of the earliest reports of FNM utilized standard EMG and surface electrodes attached with collodion to observe frontalis muscle activity in 14 patients who had suboccipital resections of acoustic neuromas (10). A specially designed Teflon-coated silver wire shaped to resemble a bayonet forceps was utilized to deliver an electrical stimulus of up to 30 V, resulting in an evoked response from the frontalis muscle (Fig. 5). Twelve patients had normal facial mobility 1 week postoperatively. The significance of this early report was that in departing from the method of direct observation of the patient's face using a mirror or an assistant under the surgical drapes, the technique of observing facial muscle evoked responses appreciably reduced the margin of error for misunderstanding visually observed facial muscle contractions. Since this early report, others have investigated the feasibility and reliability of FNM (11–31). In 1991, IOM of the facial nerve received the official recognition of the National Institutes of Health in a Development Conference Consensus Statement that read, in part, "... routine intraoperative monitoring of the facial nerve should be included in surgical therapy for vestibular schwannoma"(32).

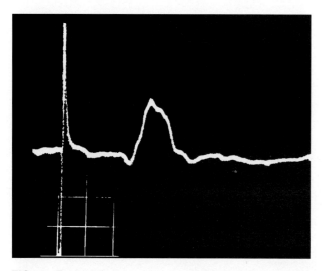

FIG. 5. Evoked facial nerve response recorded over the frontalis muscle after intracranial stimulation. Ordinate, 70 µv/division; abscissa, 5 ms/division. (From Delgado TE, Buchheit WA, Rosenholtz HR, Chrissian S. Intraoperative monitoring of facial muscle evoked responses obtained by intracranial stimulation of the facial nerve: a more accurate technique for facial nerve dissection. *Neurosurgery* 1979;4: 418–421, with permission.)

Wiegand and colleagues (33) reviewed surgical data of 1,579 patients with unilateral acoustic nerve lesions submitted to the Acoustic Neuroma Registry in a 5-year period ending in February 1994. They reported that FNM was used 94% of the time in 1,579 translabyrinthine, posterior, and middle cranial fossa cases. At the time of hospital discharge, 56% of patients had unchanged or improved facial function. In 805 patients available for 1-year follow-up examination, 79% (634) had facial grades of I to II using the House-Brackmann scale. A variety of uncontrolled factors including multiple surgeons and monitoring personnel of disparate experience and skill undoubtedly influence such aggregate studies.

Individual centers have analyzed intraoperative results in attempts to predict long-term facial function (26, 28–31,34–36). For example, two large studies reported postoperative facial mobility as a function of electrical stimulus threshold. Lalwani et al. (35) reported that 90% of 129 patients who received FNM during translabyrinthine and retrosigmoid approaches to acoustic neuromas had House-Brackmann grades of I to II 1 year after surgery. Further, 98% of patients with proximal electrical thresholds of 0.2 V or less had grade I or II function as compared to 50% of patients who had stimulus thresholds greater than 0.2 V. Nissen and colleagues (36) described how intraoperative median electrical stimulus thresholds of 0.1 V at the root entry zone predicted postoperative House-Brackmann grades of I to II in 81 patients. They reported statistically significant differences between tumor size groups, and they believed that FNM was a good predictor of postoperative facial nerve function.

The observation of intraoperative facial EMG involves two simultaneously conducted measures: (a) continuous monitoring of ongoing or free-running EMG (motor potential activity) sampled from muscle groups served by peripheral facial nerve branches, and (b) regular use of electrical stimulation to obtain a compound facial muscle action potential. These methods can be used to monitor EMG of any of the cranial motor nerves (Table 1). After placement of paired intramuscular needle electrodes in the upper and lower divisions of the face, one observes the free-running EMG after determining that the patient is not paralyzed. The underlying principle of free-running EMG monitoring is that normal muscle tissue at rest is electrically quiet. Motor unit potentials that occur as a change in this baseline activity elicited by facial nerve manipulation need to be reported to the surgical team. Often, alterations in ongoing facial EMG will be observed with manipulation of neighboring tissue prior to direct observation of the facial nerve (Fig. 6). Such an event alerts the surgical team of their proximity to this structure.

We previously reported our FNM protocol and preferences for electrical stimulation (1,6,13). We prefer to use a flush-tipped probe for monopolar stimulation using constant-current rectangular pulses delivered at a rate of 2 to 3 Hz over an intensity range from 0.1 to 2.0 mA. Compound muscle action potential amplitudes are com-

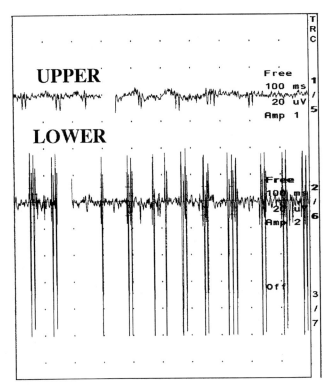

FIG. 6. Strong spasm in the lower division of the face recorded during dissection of vestibular schwannoma in the internal auditory canal.

pared following proximal and distal stimulation at suprathreshold levels. Differences between stimulation sites in excess of 20% are considered significant, suggesting reduced facial mobility, at least in the short term.

AUDITORY NERVE MONITORING

Intraoperative monitoring of the eighth cranial nerve is used in otologic, neurotologic, and neurosurgical cases as a means of observing and protecting the functional status of the operated ear. A preoperative audiologic workup should include pure tone and speech audiometry, immittance measures, auditory electrophysiology, and otoacoustic emission evaluation. These measures help in two ways: first, they determine the patient's preoperative hearing function, and second, they assist in planning the most effective mode of auditory monitoring. For example, in planned hearing preservation cases, when the preoperative auditory brainstem response (ABR) suggests poor waveform repeatability, intraoperative electrocochleography (ECochG) obtained concurrently with the ABR will at least allow assessment of the distal portion of the auditory nerve.

Standard clinical evoked potential systems may be used with caution, but a system that permits multimodality recording and stimulation is preferable if IOM is requested by a variety of surgical services. System components, such as the headboard and amplifiers, must be able to withstand

the rigors of use in an electrically hostile environment such as the OR. Those who monitor electrophysiologic activity in the OR would be well served by a consultation with their respective system manufacturer to determine the suitability of equipment to be used in IOM.

To perform intraoperative auditory monitoring, subdermal needle electrodes are placed where appropriate to the form of monitoring (Table 1) and secured with surgical tape. The acoustic transducer is positioned on the patient's chest below the monitored ear, and a soft insert phone is placed deeply in the external ear canal (Fig. 7). The transducer, connector tube, and insert earphone are fastened securely for the duration of the case. Importantly, the ear canal should be sealed using bone wax and surgical tape to prevent the entry of surgical scrub solutions into the ear canal. Nonsterile electrode leads and the earphone cable should be directed away from the surgical field, a process that obviously must be completed before the ear is prepped and draped for surgery. A preincision ABR should be obtained to verify the integrity of the auditory setup and provide baseline measures of stimulus threshold and suprathreshold latency. Attending to the technical details of the IOM setup will ensure its stability and allow the monitoring clinician to confidently report on the electrophysiologic status of the patient.

Planned hearing preservation procedures benefit from various forms of auditory nerve monitoring (Table 3). Each has unique strengths and shortcomings.

The ABR is an exogenous, averaged far-field response that represents afferent activity of the eighth cranial nerve

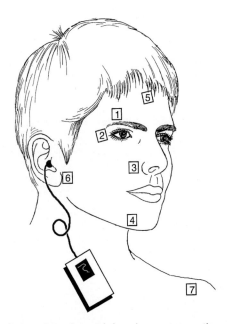

FIG. 7. Setup for planned hearing preservation surgery. Insert-style earphone, connector tubing, and transducer for delivery of monaural acoustic stimuli to right ear. Numbered sites for intramuscular electrodes: *1–2,* upper division and *3–4,* lower division for facial nerve monitoring; *5,* active electrode and *6,* reference electrode for auditory brainstem responses; *7,* ground electrode.

TABLE 3. *Surgical procedures that benefit from intraoperative monitoring of auditory evoked potentials*

1. Planned hearing preservation surgery
2. Large tumor debulking wherein contralateral auditory brainstem response is requested (to monitor brainstem function via auditory pathway)
3. Vestibular nerve section
4. Microvascular decompression of trigeminal or facial nerve
5. Cochlear implantation, electric auditory brainstem response

from the distal auditory nerve (wave I) to the lateral lemniscus in the brainstem (wave V). It is the technique most often used to monitor cochlear function during planned hearing preservation procedures, in part because of the ease with which the response can be obtained. Typically, a single-channel, click-evoked ABR from the affected ear is recorded, although one may choose to monitor the ABR from the nonaffected ear to serve as a control measure during surgery. In cases of large intracranial lesions that compress the brainstem, one may record an ABR from the nonaffected ear to assess brainstem function. Indices of interest include absolute and interpeak latencies as well as amplitude measures of ABR wave V (Fig. 8).

Early reports found the ABR simple to record in patients undergoing posterior fossa exploration of vascular or neoplastic lesions, microvascular decompression, vestibular nerve section, and acoustic neuroma resection. Changes in intraoperative ABRs were associated with postoperative morbidity in these studies (37,38). In a large series, Radtke and colleagues (39) attributed improvements in postoperative hearing ability to the use of intraoperative cochlear monitoring after retrospectively examining 222 patients who had microvascular decompressions of either the fifth or seventh cranial nerve. Significant differences were reported between monitored and unmonitored patient groups operated on by the same surgeon. Kemink and colleagues (40) reported similar differences in hearing 3 months postoperatively between monitored and unmonitored patients undergoing suboccipital acoustic neuroma resection. No patient with a tumor larger than 1.5 cm had

serviceable hearing postoperatively after total tumor extirpation when speech reception thresholds and word recognition scores were poorer than 30 dB or 70%, respectively. Further, they found that maintenance of ABR wave V correlated well with postoperative hearing when prolongation of the absolute latency of wave V (relative to baseline measures) was less than 3 ms (Fig. 9). Hecht and associates (41) reported that in patients undergoing middle fossa or retrosigmoid approaches for resection of acoustic tumors, those with tumors smaller than 1.5 cm had an approximate 50% hearing preservation rate. Conversely, hearing preservation occurred in only 16% of cases when maximum tumor dimension exceeded 1.5 cm.

Moller (42) and Harner et al. (43) reported that, in skull base surgery, monitoring of auditory function may help reduce postoperative deficits, particularly in cases of larger mass lesions. Harner et al. reported that in 144 consecutive cases of complete tumor resection, 26% (38 of 144) had pure tone averages equal to or better than 60 dB 3 months postoperatively. Moller (44) suggested that surgeons variably benefit from auditory monitoring based on their individual level of experience and skill in planned hearing preservation procedures.

One notable weakness of the ABR is that it requires approximately 1 minute of averaging; during tumor dissection close to the eighth cranial nerve, this could prevent the quick relay of information to the surgeon regarding significant iatrogenic events that might alter the outcome of a planned hearing preservation case. Because of the need for speedier indicators of auditory function during tumor dissection, near-field methods of recording auditory potentials have been examined (45–48). Moller and Jannetta (49) recorded compound action potentials from cranial nerve VIII during microvascular decompressions. An example of the effects of retraction on distally recorded cranial nerve VIII compound action potentials is shown in Fig. 10.

Moller (50) demonstrated a method in which the recording electrode was positioned on the floor of the fourth ventricle and cranial nerve VIII compound action potentials were recorded in close proximity to the cochlear nucleus. This technique was reportedly a good predictor of postop-

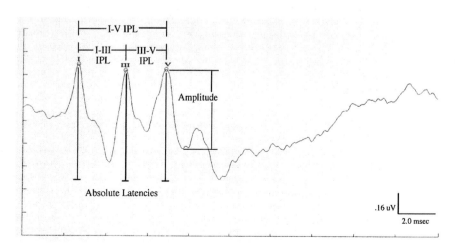

FIG. 8. Auditory brainstem response interpeak latencies (IPL), absolute latencies, and wave V amplitude measurements observed during intraoperative auditory nerve monitoring.

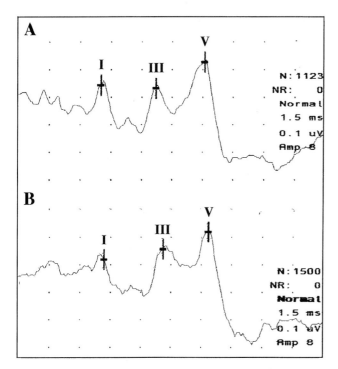

FIG. 9. Preincision **(A)** and closing **(B)** auditory brainstem responses following total extirpation of a small auditory nerve lesion.

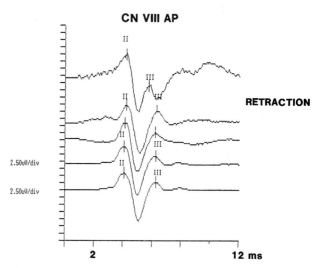

FIG. 10. Intraoperative electrocochleography demonstrating effect of retraction on distally recorded cranial nerve VIII compound action potential. Note shift of III.

erative hearing. Matthies and Samii (51) described their experience using a modified retractor placed at the cerebellomedullary junction, attached to which was a recording electrode placed close to the anterior cochlear nucleus. They successfully used such nuclear auditory evoked potentials to identify large-amplitude response components with increased speed, as only a small number of stimuli are required to generate a response given the proximity of generator and recording sites. The technique's value as a tool for reporting changes related to surgical manipulations was suggested, largely due to the small number of stimuli required to generate a response. Such a tool could be advantageous because the recording location would be well removed from surgical locations in many cases. The authors used their technique in cases of microvascular

decompression and acoustic tumor resection, reporting no false results in 34 cases.

ECochG is a recording of stimulus-related components of early auditory evoked potentials. It may be used in hearing preservation cases requiring quick samplings of distal auditory function or in cases where ABR components are poorly formed (52). The strength of the ECochG lies in the proximity of recording sites (medial ear canal or promontory) and the response generator (distal auditory nerve). Schwaber and Hall (53) suggested that speedier ECochG averaging was related to improved surgical results in planned hearing preservation cases. Simultaneous recording of the ECochG and the ABR is possible (Fig. 11). When this technique is used, distal cranial nerve VIII action potentials and more proximal wave V activity can be monitored simultaneously (54). The placement of the recording electrode, whether in the external ear canal close to the tympanic membrane or on the promontory through the tympanic membrane, will influence action potential amplitudes, with the latter position resulting in larger amplitudes (55).

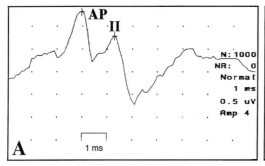
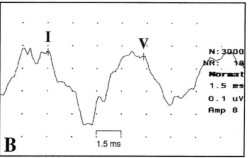

FIG. 11. Simultaneously recorded electrocochleography **(A)** and auditory brainstem responses (ABR) **(B)** during planned hearing preservation surgery. Note the amplitude differences between the electrocochleographic response and the ABR and the number of stimuli used to obtain each response. See text for explanation.

ECochG and direct cranial nerve VIII compound action potentials have been examined to determine their sensitivity and reliability for predicting postoperative hearing function. Zappia et al. (56) analyzed intraoperative events and postoperative hearing outcomes utilizing ECochG and direct recording from the cochlear nerve in 26 patients who were candidates for planned hearing preservation procedures. Patients were divided into two groups based on the technique used. For ECochG the promontory was approached transtympanically, while direct recordings were obtained by placing a cotton wick attached to a multistrand electrode on the exposed eighth cranial nerve. All other technical parameters remained constant. Zappia et al. documented the benefits and disadvantages of each technique. For example, ECochG allowed for auditory monitoring from the outset of the case, although technical problems such as displaced promontory electrodes affected reliability measures. Direct nerve recordings could not be obtained until the eighth cranial nerve was exposed well into the case, but they proved to be very sensitive to surgical changes. These authors found a trend toward better postoperative hearing function, although they reported no statistically significant differences between the near-field techniques.

The electric ABR (EABR) is a useful diagnostic tool for cochlear implant ear selection and for establishing the stimulability of selected implant electrodes. It is quickly becoming important in the perioperative assessment of adults and pediatric patients undergoing cochlear implantation (57). In young children, transtympanic EABRs are obtained in the OR on the day of surgery after the patient has been placed under general anesthesia. Neuromuscular blockade is administered to negate myogenic artifacts associated with possible electrical stimulation of the facial nerve. Subdermal needle electrodes are placed at the anterior tragus to serve as the indifferent electrode for promontory stimulation, and at the vertex, contralateral earlobe or nape of the neck to record the EABR. The forehead serves as the site for a ground electrode. Stimuli are balanced biphasic current pulses (200 μs/phase) generated by a customized stimulator, battery powered and triggered by the clinical evoked potential system. EABRs are amplified, filtered, and stored. Alternating the onset polarity of the biphasic pulses can minimize artifacts. Stimulus current levels may reach 1 mA, and threshold measures are obtained for at least the preferred ear (based on temporal bone anatomy and the results of preoperative hearing testing). Special techniques are required to avoid overloading the digital-to-analog converters; for example, stimulus artifacts are blocked digitally during response averaging. Postaveraging digital filtering (30 to 100 Hz, zero phase) may improve response detection.

In a recent report, EABRs were successfully obtained in 41 of 43 patients aged 2 to 14 years (58). Mean EABR thresholds of 406.5 and 472 μA were obtained for 31 patients with patent cochleas and for 10 patients with cochlear ossification, respectively. Twenty-five patients

had each ear evaluated successfully; in nine cases responses were present from only one ear, which then was implanted. Notably, two of these patients had bilateral labyrinthitis ossificans, and a third had bilateral Mondini malformation. In the remaining 16 patients, the ear with the lowest threshold response was implanted. Threshold differences between ears ranged from 25 to 200 μA.

Following insertion of the implant electrode array and after the implant receiver is seated, a supplemental EABR is obtained by stimulating selected electrodes to verify implant function and establish effective stimulus delivery. Transmission to the implant is achieved via a coil placed in a sterile arthroscopy sleeve. Triggered pulses are delivered in a common ground mode (for a Cochlear Corporation device) so as to approximate behavioral threshold measures at the time of initial programming in the bipolar +1 mode.

DEVELOPING AN INTRAOPERATIVE MONITORING PROGRAM

An effective IOM program requires that certain considerations be made well in advance of the actual provision of services. Although no recognized standards exist, virtually each technical and professional organization involved in IOM has promulgated guidelines to assist in the development of intraoperative protocols. Several manufacturers supply well-constructed educational opportunities for pro-

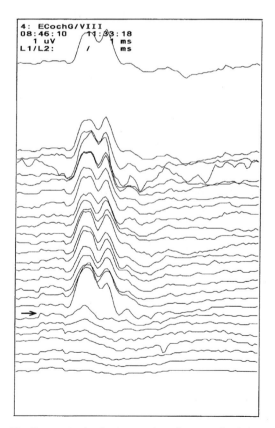

FIG. 12. Curve stack of averaged auditory evoked potentials recorded during a planned hearing preservation case. Note evoked potential diminution following tumor dissection (*arrow*).

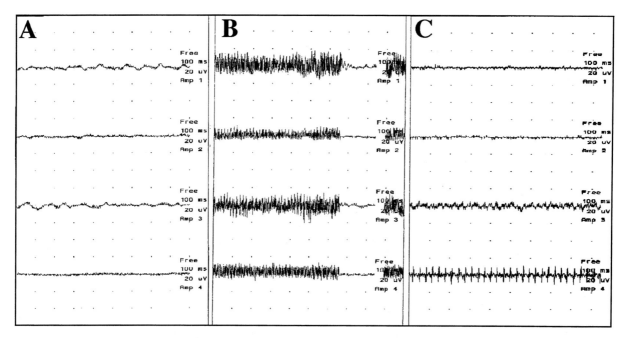

FIG. 13. Examples of intraoperatively recorded facial electromyographic activity. **A:** Quiescent baseline activity. **B:** Typical display of electrocautery-induced noise overlying baseline activity. **C:** Spasm in marginal mandibular branch of facial nerve seen in lowermost channel.

fessional consumers, whereas others limit their support to after-sale assistance. As we have stated, the value of an IOM service lies in the preparation of the individuals involved in its deliverance. Likewise, a considered approach to the needs of the patient, as well as those of the other professionals involved, will help to establish a collegial environment that allows for quality planning, cooperation, and improved postoperative outcomes.

Institution-recognized protocols for specific types of surgical procedures requiring IOM are necessary. Within each protocol, certain standards and criteria assist the clinician involved in IOM to provide a level of service that will maximize surgical outcomes. For instance, one may find assistance in planning for monitoring by using a guide that reviews key elements (Appendix 1). Several comments may exemplify both the need to plan and to make effective use of available technology. It is suggested that, when surgical cases require extensive time commitments, monitoring clinicians should rotate periodically to remain focused and able to contribute maximally. However, this requires that the relief person become acquainted with individual events and overall trends up to that point. A written or computer-generated log of comments is helpful for updating the case, as is a graphics package that generates curve stacks and trend plots used to display, for example, the history of averaged auditory responses from the beginning of the case (Fig. 12). Such planning ensures that intraoperative neurophysiologic patterns not easily verbalized are clear to each team member throughout the case. It also serves as a precise instructional tool for residents and fellows, and it may be important in litigation cases.

Technology is not a substitute for vigilance by the monitoring professional. Rather, observation of ongoing activity is required to determine its significance to operative events. For example, alterations from baseline activity related to the use of electrocautery devices are common and must be distinguished from actual and potentially significant changes in monitored activity related to surgical manipulation (Fig. 13). Two aspects of electrically triggered facial nerve stimulation need consideration. One may wish to know how well the facial nerve stimulates at closing by comparing the triggered compound muscle action potential with those obtained before tumor dissection is well under way (Fig. 14). Further, one should evaluate the

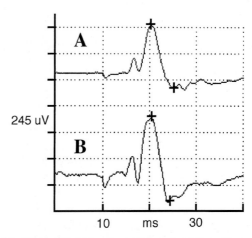

FIG. 14. Compound muscle action potentials with constant current stimulation of proximal facial nerve before **(B)** and after **(A)** resection of acoustic neuroma.

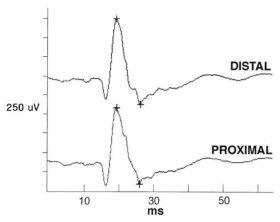

FIG. 15. Compound muscle action potentials from facial nerve distal and proximal to site of resected tumor.

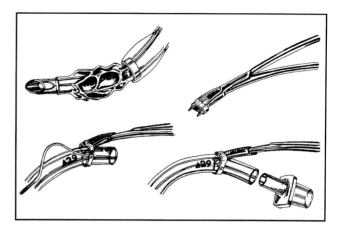

FIG. 16. Preparation of a sized endotracheal tube for laryngeal EMG recording. (From Mermelstein M, Nonweiler R, Rubenstein EH. Intraoperative identification of laryngeal nerves with laryngeal electromyography. *Laryngoscope* 1996;106:752–756, with permission.)

effects of resection by comparing the compound muscle action potential following nerve stimulation at sites proximal and distal to the point of tumor resection (Fig. 15).

During auditory monitoring, response quality needs to be examined from the outset. Although an experienced clinician may be able to make a quick, visual determination of the relative presence of noise in a recording, another somewhat more objective manner in which to estimate the magnitude of noise in averaged responses is to utilize the plus/minus method of averaging (59,60). While an averaged evoked potential response is obtained, successive samples of the potentials are placed into separate positive and negative buffers. After subtraction of the two stored responses, that which remains (i.e., that which cannot be canceled by subtraction) represents the noise present in that averaging portion (61). A signal-to-noise ratio can be calculated by dividing reference variances into response variances. Further, digital filtering can be fabricated through which the remainder of the averaging may be routed (62). Alternately, one may opt to reanalyze the patient setup, manipulating hardware or software parameters to reduce the amplitude of spurious noise elements. To reiterate, improved signal-to-noise ratios result in smaller degrees of averaged variability, which is paramount when attempting to identify significant IOM events.

MONITORING OF LOWER CRANIAL NERVES

Although not routine, monitoring of lower cranial nerves is becoming more common in certain posterior cranial fossa procedures and in the resection of lateral skull base tumors. Monitoring of the tenth cranial nerve usually is accomplished by observing free-running EMG activity from muscles innervated by the laryngeal nerves.

Several methods have been developed to record recurrent laryngeal nerve activity. Some are based on pressure changes as recorded through an endotracheal tube cuff placed between the vocal cords (63) and others rely on EMG recordings of the laryngeal muscles (64–66). Pressure-based methods can be traumatic to the endolaryn-

geal structures and are not advisable in lengthy skull base cases. EMG techniques may be performed with external or internal electrodes. Transcutaneous electrodes require experience for accurate placement. When used in infratemporal approaches, they may be located within the surgical field where they could be displaced. Placement of internal needle electrodes is predicated on a perfect view of the endolarynx. They are less subject to displacement, but correct positioning requires considerable experience and skill. To obviate these problems, two laryngeal surface devices are available. In the first case, an indwelling paddle-style electrode (Fig. 4) produced by RLN Systems (Jefferson City, MO) is placed by direct laryngoscopy in the postcricoid hypopharynx. The second device consists of an endotracheal tube with surface electrodes and is produced by Xomed-Treace (Jacksonville, FL). Attempting to

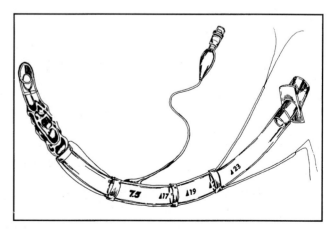

FIG. 17. Endotracheal tube with Silastic rings, Teflon tubing, and recording stainless steel wire used to monitor free-running and electrically triggered laryngeal electromyogram. (From Mermelstein M, Nonweiler R, Rubenstein EH. Intraoperative identification of laryngeal nerves with laryngeal electromyography. *Laryngoscope* 1996;106:752–756, with permission.)

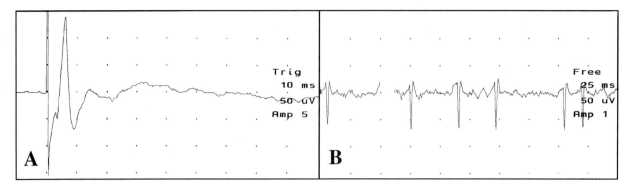

FIG. 18. A: Evoked laryngeal electromyographic response from recurrent laryngeal nerve triggered with constant-current stimulation at 1.5 mA using monopolar hand-held probe. **B:** Motor potential activity from recurrent laryngeal nerve with surgical manipulation of thyroid tissue containing neural structures.

improve the reliability of electrode positioning, Mermelstein et al. (67) introduced a modification of the Xomed-Treace device, which is prepared before surgery based on the anatomic requirements of the patient (Figs. 16 and 17). However, if the endotracheal tube is inadvertently twisted, electrode contact may be lost. Therefore, the authors prefer the paddle-shaped electrode that would seem to offer longer-term stability.

After electrodes are connected to the recording apparatus and once an electrical circuit is established, the location of the nerve may be explored with either monopolar or bipolar electrical stimulation (Fig. 18A). Recurrent laryngeal nerve activity may be detected with high sensitivity and reliability when surgical manipulation occurs in proximity to the vagal trunk (Fig. 18B).

Monitoring of the twelfth cranial nerve is done infrequently, but it has a role when approaching craniocervical junction lesions, especially tumors involving the anterior portion of the occipital foramen and hypoglossal canal. Electrodes are placed into the ipsilateral half of the tongue. EMG recordings can be obtained readily, but it often is dif-

ficult to maintain the electrodes in place, as repeated tongue contractions tend to extrude them. Sutures through the tongue surface and around the electrodes are sometimes helpful in preventing electrode extrusion.

Monitoring of the eleventh accessory nerve follows the same techniques as for the seventh and twelfth cranial nerves. However, the intracranial portion of this nerve stimulates readily and function can be detected by observation of the shoulder movements when an EMG channel is not available in multichannel devices.

CRANIAL NERVE MONITORING CASE STUDIES

Case 1

A 59-year-old man who underwent left suboccipital resection of an acoustic neuroma presented with left ear fullness and tinnitus. Magnetic resonance imaging showed a 5- to 6-mm enhancing lesion in the left internal auditory canal between the facial and vestibular nerves. Audiometry demonstrated sensorineural hearing loss in the left ear (Fig. 19A). Left ear ABR showed mildly prolonged wave

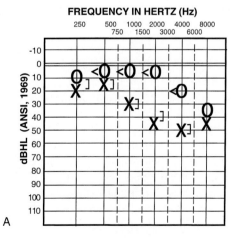

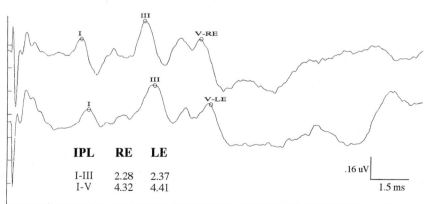

FIG. 19. A: Preoperative audiogram of patient from Case 1 shows a moderate mid- to high-frequency sensorineural hearing loss in the left ear. Contrast-enhanced imaging demonstrated a 5- to 6-mm tumor in the left internal auditory canal. **B:** Preoperative auditory brainstem response interpeak latencies from the left (affected) ear are outside laboratory's norms. Right ear results are normal.

I–III and I–V interpeak latencies and good waveform morphology (Fig. 19B). Facial evoked EMG was normal. Physical examination was otherwise unremarkable.

Subdermal needle electrodes were placed in frontalis and orbicularis oculi muscles, and in the nasolabial fold and mentalis muscle. Subdermal electrodes were inserted preauricularly and at the vertex representing reference and active recording sites for ABR recording. A flexible gel-tipped tympanic membrane electrode (Fig. 20) was placed against the eardrum under direct microscopy to

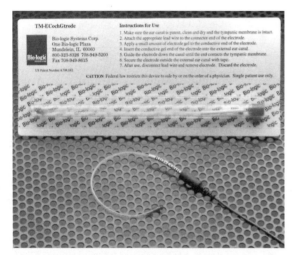

FIG. 20. A flexible gel-tipped tympanic membrane electrode used to obtain intraoperative electrocochleographic responses. (Courtesy of Biologic Systems Corp.)

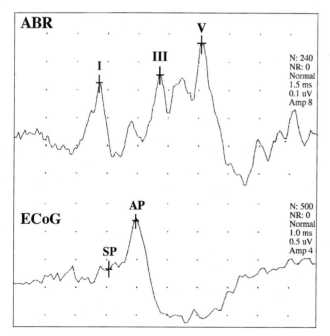

FIG. 21. Electrocochleography (ECoG) and auditory brainstem responses (ABR) obtained during suboccipital resection of 7-mm right acoustic neuroma. The patient's postoperative hearing function was unchanged relative to preoperative results.

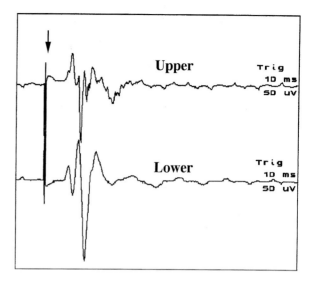

FIG. 22. Proximal electrical stimulation of the facial nerve reveals upper and lower division responses at 0.1 mA after tumor dissection was complete. *Arrow* indicates stimulus onset.

serve as reference for ECochG recordings after being wedged into place with a foam insert plug connected to an acoustic transducer. The ear canal was sealed with bone wax and taped over to prevent fluids from entering the stimulating/recording site.

Baseline measures of the ABR, ECochG, and freerunning facial EMG were obtained. A left suboccipital craniotomy was performed, the posterior wall of the internal auditory canal was removed, and the tumor was exposed. New baseline ABR and ECochGs were obtained. Regular electrical stimulation was used to distinguish tumor from nerve fibers. Resection was performed from medial to lateral, with no significant alterations in auditory responses (Fig. 21). After tumor removal, proximal stimulation of the facial nerve at 0.1 mA confirmed its functional integrity (Fig. 22). Postoperatively, the patient's hearing was unchanged relative to preoperative threshold levels.

Case 2

A 49-year-old woman presented with a large right petroclival meningioma with extension into the cavernous sinus and jugular foramen. Significant brainstem compression and encasement of the basilar artery and the fourth cranial nerve were noted. She had severe sensorineural hearing loss in the right ear, with a 72% word recognition score. Midfrequency hearing in the right ear and left ear hearing sensitivity were within normal limits (Fig. 23A). ABRs were abnormal bilaterally, representing both the effects of the lesion on the right auditory tract and brainstem compression on the nonaffected left ear (Fig. 23B).

The patient underwent a right petrosal approach for planned partial tumor resection. Multimodality IOM was carried out during the case. Intramuscular needle elec-

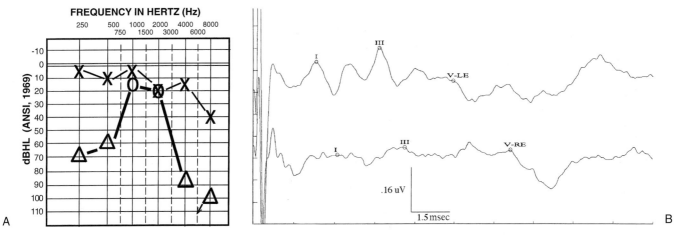

FIG. 23. A: Preoperative audiometric results for patient in Case 2. Severe-to-profound sensorineural hearing loss in the low and high frequencies was present in the right ear. Interestingly, mid-frequency hearing in the affected ear was normal, as were left ear thresholds through 4,000 Hz. **B:** Preoperative auditory brainstem responses from patient in Case 2 showed prolonged wave I–V interpeak latencies for each ear (right ear 6.51 ms, left ear 5.13 ms) compatible with intracranial effects of his large right petroclival meningioma.

trodes were placed in the left lateral rectus and contralateral forehead to monitor the sixth cranial nerve activity, and a left ear click-evoked ABR and two-channel FNM was provided to monitor activity originating from cranial nerves VIII and VII, respectively.

With the exception of a slight increase in the absolute latency of wave V during drilling, the contralateral ABR remained stable. Monitored facial EMG remained quiet throughout the mastoid drillout. The facial nerve stimulated at 0.3 mA through bone. At the onset of tumor dissection, a mild spasm of the lower face occurred (Fig. 24). The facial nerve continued to stimulate at 0.1 to 0.3 mA throughout the case. Postoperatively, the patient had mildly decreased sensation in the maxillary division of

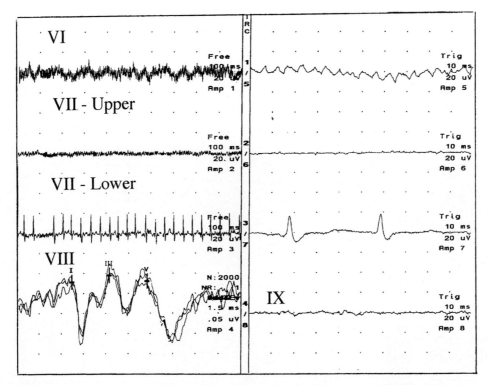

FIG. 24. Multimodality intraoperative monitoring of cranial nerves VI, VII, VIII, and IX. Note the lower facial spasm during tumor dissection (VII-Lower). Auditory responses are superimposed on earlier baseline average (VIII). See text for description of recording sites and methods of stimulation.

the trigeminal nerve, nystagmus, imbalance, and a mild increase in right ear hearing loss. She had a temporary right facial weakness and some swallowing difficulty that quickly improved. Corneal reflexes and sensation remained intact.

PERSPECTIVE

Much progress has been made in the area of IOM, thereby increasing safety and cranial nerve preservation in neurotologic and skull base procedures, although further advances are needed and expected. These include the real-time recording of auditory function. The time interval from stimulus onset to acquiring an ABR is often critical during dissections around the auditory nerve. Presently, information regarding signs of functional damage may reach the surgeon too late to prevent morbid complications. Refinements in monitoring cranial nerve motor responses would further increase the utility of these highly valuable techniques. Motor nerves are often found markedly flattened by tumor growth, and intraoperative stimulation of areas carrying few fibers may not produce the expected EMG response. Improvements in bipolar stimulating electrodes, such as finer tips, and uniformly accepted prognostic indicators could facilitate monitoring under difficult conditions.

SUMMARY POINTS

- Audiologists who are properly qualified and experienced can perform intraoperative monitoring of cranial nerves.
- Pathologic and pharmacologic variables can significantly affect intraoperative monitoring of cranial nerves.
- Attended and nonattended intraoperative monitoring of cranial nerves is differentiated.
- Intraoperative monitoring continues to benefit from technologic improvements.
- Facial nerve monitoring is formally recognized by the National Institutes of Health.

- Auditory monitoring is valuable in planned hearing preservation procedures. Several techniques for monitoring the auditory system are available, including ABR, ECochG, and direct cranial nerve VIII recordings.
- Recognized protocols and preoperative planning help to maximize the potential of intraoperative monitoring of cranial nerves.
- Intraoperative monitoring of cranial nerves may result in significantly improved postoperative outcomes and is applicable in a variety of ear-related surgical procedures.
- Lower cranial nerve monitoring is gaining importance in skull base cases.

APPENDIX 1

Elements in a Planned, Standardized Intraoperative Cranial Nerve Monitoring Program

I. Recording Issues
  A. Estimated procedure duration
  B. Electrodes
    1. Surface, subdermal, paddle
    2. Matched impedances
    3. Patient monitoring ground
  C. System parameters
    1. Amplifiers
    2. Filters
    3. Averaging mode(s)
  D. Dealing with artifacts
    1. Isolating source(s)
    2. Recognizing magnitude in ongoing activity

II. Stimulation Issues
  A. Trigger source
    1. Internal
    2. External
      a. Synchronization
  B. Electrodes
    1. Exposed tip
    2. Flush tip
    3. Lead extensions
  C. Electrical stimulus
    1. Monopolar, bipolar
    2. Constant current, constant voltage
    3. Increment, intensity, duration rate, mode
  D. Auditory
    1. Signal: click, tone, filtered noise
    2. Envelope: linear, Blackman, Gaussian, Hanning

APPENDIX 1 *(CONT.)*

3. Intensity, increment, polarity, duration, ramp, plateau

III. Anesthesia Issues
A. Use of specific agents before/within procedure
B. Team communication to prevent unintended patient condition
C. Reversing anesthetic state

IV. Monitoring Hardware
A. Averager
  1. Multiple, independent time bases
  2. Variable display sensitivities
  3. Flexible mode designations (noise estimation)
B. Monitor
  1. Multiple waveform display
  2. Assorted information environment
    a. Waveforms, cursors, text, graphics supported
C. Grounding/safety procedures
  1. System ground connection in line power cord
  2. Measurement of leakage current to ground
  3. Gauging leakage current of patient isolation section (amplifier)

4. Electrosurgical unit to return electrode positioned properly
D. Physical location in the operating room
  1. Sharing loudspeaker output with team
  2. Able to view video images from operating microscope
  3. Opportunity to communicate regularly with team members

V. Defining Responses
A. Accepted degree/characteristics of variability (quantify reproducibility)
B. Significant change regarding baseline activity
C. Recognizing false-negative/false-positive events
D. Marking waveforms

VI. Data Management
A. Storage medium: hard drive, disk, tape
B. Printed copies of events, reports
  1. Report deadline
  2. Canned versus individualized by case
    a. Supplemental material
  1. Dictated surgical report
  2. Preoperative studies
    a. Physical examination
    b. Tests of function: audiologic, vestibular
    c. Test of structure: imaging studies

ACKNOWLEDGMENT

This work is dedicated to the memory of the brother and mentor of the first author.

REFERENCES

1. Edwards BM, Kileny PR. Intraoperative monitoring. *Curr Opin Otolaryngol Head Neck Surg* 1996;4:360–366.
2. Edwards BM, Kileny PR. Audiologists in intraoperative neurophysiologic monitoring. *Semin Hear* 1998;19:87–95.
3. Jackler RK, Selesnick SH. Indications for cranial nerve monitoring during otologic and neurotologic surgery. *Am J Otol* 1994;15:611–615.
4. Hogan K. Neuroanesthesia techniques for intraoperative monitoring. In: Kartush JM, Bouchard KR, eds. *Neuromonitoring in otology—head and neck surgery.* New York: Raven Press, 1992:61–79.
5. Kinsella SB. Anesthesia and intraoperative monitoring. In: Beck D, ed. *Handbook of intraoperative monitoring.* San Diego: Singular Publishing Group, 1994:227–238.
6. Kileny PR, Niparko JK. Intraoperative monitoring of auditory and facial functions in neurotologic surgery. *Adv Otolaryngol Head Neck Surg* 1988;2:55–88.
7. Kileny PR, Niparko JK. Neurophysiologic intraoperative monitoring. In: Jacobson J, ed. *Principles & applications in auditory evoked potentials.* Boston: Allyn and Bacon, 1994:447–476.
8. Chang CYJ, Cheung SW. Complications after acoustic neuroma surgery. In: House WF, Luetje CM, Doyle KJ, eds. *Acoustic tumors: diagnosis and management,* 2nd ed. San Diego: Singular Publishing Group, 1997:283–300.
9. Ojemann RG. Management of acoustic neuromas (vestibular schwannomas). *Clin Neurosurg* 1992;40:498–535.
10. Delgado TE, Buchheit WA, Rosenholtz HR, Chrissian S. Intraoperative monitoring of facial muscle evoked responses obtained by intracranial stimulation of the facial nerve: a more accurate technique for facial nerve dissection. *Neurosurgery* 1979;4:418–421.
11. Benecke JE, Calder HB, Chadwick G. Facial nerve monitoring during acoustic neuroma removal. *Laryngoscope* 1987;97:697–700.
12. Silverstein H, Smouha E, Jones R. Routine identification of facial nerve using electrical stimulation during otological and neurotological surgery. *Laryngoscope* 1988;98:726–730.
13. Niparko JK, Kileny PR, Kemink JL, Lee HM, Graham MD. Neurophysiologic intraoperative monitoring: II. Facial nerve function. *Am J Otol* 1989;10:55–61.
14. Wolf SR, Schneider W, Hofman M, Haid CT, Wigand ME. Intraoperative monitoring of the facial nerve in transtemporal surgery of acoustic neuroma. *HNO* 1993;4:179–184.
15. Fisher RS, Raudzens P, Nunemacher M. Efficacy of neurophysiological monitoring. *J Clin Neurophysiol* 1995;12:97–109.
16. Calder HB, White DE. Facial nerve EMG monitoring. *Am J END Technol* 1996;36:28–46.
17. Kartush JM, Niparko JK, Bledsoe SC, Graham MD, Kemink JL. Intraoperative facial nerve monitoring: a comparison of stimulating electrodes. *Laryngoscope* 1985;95:1536–1540.
18. Gantz BJ. Intraoperative facial nerve monitoring. *Am J Otol* 1985;S58–S61.
19. Leonetti JP, Matz GJ, Smith PG, Beck DL. Facial nerve monitoring in otologic surgery: clinical indications and intraoperative technique. *Ann Otol Rhino Laryngol* 1990;99:911–918.
20. Kwartler JA, Luxford WM, Atkins J, Shelton C. Facial nerve monitoring in acoustic tumor surgery. *Otolaryngol Head Neck Surg* 1991;104:814–817.
21. Silverstein H, Rosenberg S. Intraoperative facial nerve monitoring. *Otolaryngol Clin N Am* 1991;24:709–725.

22. Uziel A, Benezech J, Frerebeau P. Intraoperative facial nerve monitoring in posterior fossa acoustic neuroma surgery. *Otolaryngol Head Neck Surg* 1993;108:126–134.

23. Silverstein H, Rosenberg SI, Flanzer J, Seidman MD. Intraoperative facial nerve monitoring in acoustic neuroma surgery. *Am J Otol* 1993; 14:524–532.

24. Sterkers JM, Morrison GA, Sterkers O, El-Dine MM. Preservation of facial, cochlear, and other nerve functions in acoustic neuroma treatment. *Otolaryngol Head Neck Surg* 1994;110:146–155.

25. Magliulo F, Petti R, Vingolo GM, Cristofari P, Ronzoni R. Facial nerve monitoring in skull base surgery. *J Laryngol Otol* 1994;108:557–559.

26. Esses BA, LaRouere MJ, Graham MD. Facial nerve outcome in acoustic tumor surgery. *Am J Otol* 1994;15:810–812.

27. Prass RL. Iatrogenic facial nerve injury: the role of facial nerve monitoring. *Otolaryngol Clin N Am* 1996;29:265–275.

28. Grey PL, Moffat DA, Palmer CR, Hardy DG, Baguley DM. Factors which influence the facial nerve outcome in vestibular schwannoma surgery. *Clin Otolaryngol* 1996;21:409–413.

29. Magliulo G, Zardo F. Intra-operative facial nerve monitoring. Its predictive value after skull base surgery. *J Laryngol Otol* 1997;111:715–718.

30. Zeitouni AG, Hammerschlag PE, Cohen NL. Prognostic significance of intraoperative facial nerve stimulus thresholds. *Am J Otol* 1997;18: 494–497.

31. Nissen AJ, Sikand A, Welsh JE, Curto FS, Gardi J. A multifactorial analysis of facial nerve results in surgery for cerebellopontine angle tumors. *Ear Nose Throat J* 1997;76:37–40.

32. National Institutes of Health. *Consensus statement.* National Institutes of Health Consensus Development Conference, December 11–13, 1991, Bethesda, MD, 1991;9:1–24.

33. Wiegand DA, Ojemann RG, Fickel V. Surgical treatment of acoustic neuroma (vestibular schwannoma) in the United States: report from the acoustic neuroma registry. *Laryngoscope* 1996;106:58–66.

34. Beck DL, Atkins JS, Benecke JE, Brackmann DE. Intraoperative facial nerve monitoring: prognostic aspects during acoustic tumor removal. *Otolaryngol Head Neck Surg* 1991;104:780–782.

35. Lalwani AK, Butt FY, Jackler RK, Pitts LH, Yingling CD. Facial nerve outcome after acoustic neuroma surgery: a study from the era of cranial nerve monitoring. *Otolaryngol Head Neck Surg* 1994;111:561–570.

36. Nissen AJ, Sikand A, Curto FS, Welsh JE, Gardi J. Value of intraoperative threshold stimulus in predicting postoperative facial nerve function after acoustic tumor resection. *Am J Otol* 1997;8:249–251.

37. Raudzens PA. Intraoperative monitoring of evoked potentials. *Ann N Y Acad Sci* 1982;388:308–326.

38. Grundy BL. Intraoperative monitoring of sensory evoked potentials. In: Nodar RH, Barber C, eds. *Evoked potentials II*. Boston: Butterworth Publishers, 1983:624–631.

39. Radtke RA, Erwin CW, Wilkins RH. Intraoperative brainstem auditory evoked potentials: significant decrease in postoperative morbidity. *Neurology* 1989;39:187–191.

40. Kemink JL, LaRouere ML, Kileny PR, Telian SA, Hoff JT. Hearing preservation following suboccipital removal of acoustic neuromas. *Laryngoscope* 1990;100:597–602.

41. Hecht CS, Honrubia VF, Wiet RJ, Sims HS. Hearing preservation after acoustic neuroma resection with tumor size used as a clinical prognosticator. *Laryngoscope* 1997;107:1122–1126.

42. Moller AR. Neuromonitoring in operations in the skull base. *Keio J Med* 1991;40:151–159.

43. Harner SG, Harper CM, Beatty CW, Litchy WJ, Ebersold MJ. Far-field brainstem response in neurotologic surgery. *Am J Otol* 1996;17: 150–153.

44. Moller AR. Intra-operative neurophysiologic monitoring in neurosurgery: benefits, efficacy, and cost-effectiveness. *Clin Neurosurg* 1995;42:171–179.

45. Moller AR, Jannetta P, Bennett M, Moller MB. Intracranially recorded responses from the human auditory nerve: new insights into the origin of brain stem evoked potentials (BSEPs). *Electroencephalogr Clin Neurophysiol* 1981;52:18–27.

46. Moller AR, Jannetta P, Moller MB. Intracranially recorded auditory nerve responses in man. New interpretations of BSER. *Arch Otolaryngol* 1982;108:77–82.

47. Moller AR, Jannetta PJ. Monitoring auditory nerve potentials during operations in the cerebellopontine angle. *Otolaryngol Head Neck Surg* 1984;92:434–439.

48. Jannetta PJ, Moller AR, Moller MB. Technique of hearing preservation in small acoustic neuromas. *Ann Surg* 1984;200:513–523.

49. Moller AR, Jannetta PJ. Monitoring auditory function during cranial nerve microvascular decompression operations by direct recording from the eighth nerve. *J Neurosurg* 1983;59:493–499.

50. Moller AR. Monitoring auditory functions during operations to remove acoustic tumors. *Am J Otol* 1996;17:452–460.

51. Matthies C, Samii M. Direct brainstem recording of auditory evoked potentials during vestibular schwannoma resection: nuclear BAEP recording. Technical note and preliminary results. *J Neurosurg* 1997; 86:1057–1062.

52. Ferraro J, Ruth RA. Electrocochleography. In: Jacobson J, ed. *Principles and applications in auditory evoked potentials*. Boston: Allyn and Bacon, 1993:101–122.

53. Schwaber MK, Hall JW. Intraoperative monitoring. In: Kartush J, Bouchard K, eds. *Neuromonitoring in otology—head and neck surgery*. New York: Raven Press, 1992:215–228.

54. Kileny PR, Kemink JL, Tucci DL, Hoff JT. Neurophysiologic intraoperative facial and auditory function monitoring in acoustic neuroma surgery. In: Tos M, Thomsen J, eds. *Proceedings of the First International Conference on Acoustic Neuroma*. Amsterdam, NY: Kugler Publications, 1992:569–574.

55. Winzenburg SM, Margolis RH, Levine SC, Haines SJ, Fournier EM. Tympanic and transtympanic electrocochleography in acoustic neuroma and vestibular nerve section surgery. *Am J Otol* 1993;14:63–69.

56. Zappia JJ, Wiet RJ, O'Connor CA. Intraoperative auditory monitoring in acoustic neuroma surgery. *Otol Head Neck Surg* 1996;115:98–106.

57. Kileny PR, Zwolan TA, Boerst A, Telian SA. Electrically evoked auditory potentials: current clinical applications in children with cochlear implants. *Am J Otol* 1997;18:S90–S92.

58. Kileny PR, Zwolan TA, Zimmerman-Phillips S, Telian SA. Electrically evoked auditory brain-stem response in pediatric patients with cochlear implants. *Arch Otolaryngol Head Neck Surg* 1994;120:1083–1090.

59. Schimmel, H. The +/- reference: accuracy of estimated mean components in average response studies. *Science* 1967;157:92–93.

60. Wong P, Bickford K. Brain stem auditory evoked potentials: the use of noise estimates. *Electroencephalogr Clin Neurophysiol* 1980;50:25–34.

61. Hall JW, Rupp KA. Auditory brainstem response: recent developments in recording and analysis. In: Alford BR, Jerger J, Jenkins HA, eds. *Electrophysiologic evaluation in otolaryngology*. Basel: Karger, 1997:21–45.

62. Jacobson GP, Balzer GK. Basic considerations in intraoperative monitoring: working in the operating room. In: Kartush JM, Bouchard KR, eds. *Neuromonitoring in otology—head and neck surgery*. New York: Raven Press, 1992:21–60.

63. Donati F, Plaud B, Meistelman C. A method to measure elicited contraction of laryngeal adductor muscles during anesthesia. *Anesthesiology* 1991;74:827–832.

64. Basmajian JV, Stecko G. A new bipolar electrode for electromyography. *J Appl Physiol* 1962;17:849.

65. Lipton RJ, McCaffrey TV, Litchy WJ. Intraoperative electrophysiologic monitoring of laryngeal muscle during thyroid surgery. *Laryngoscope* 1988;98:1292–1296.

66. Rice DH, Cone-Wesson B. Intraoperative recurrent laryngeal nerve monitoring. *Oto Head Neck Surg* 1991;105:372–375.

67. Mermelstein M, Nonweiler R, Rubenstein EH. Intraoperative identification of laryngeal nerves with laryngeal electromyography. *Laryngoscope* 1996;106:752–756.

The Ear: Comprehensive Otology,
edited by R. F. Canalis and P. R. Lambert.
Lippincott Williams & Wilkins, Philadelphia © 2000.

CHAPTER 18

Temporal Bone Imaging

J. Pablo Villablanca, Alexandra R. Borges, and Robert B. Lufkin

The temporal bone is affected by a broad range of pathologic conditions, many of which are clinically difficult to evaluate and necessitate imaging studies to aid in diagnosis and treatment planning. In imaging of the temporal bone, any modality must provide precise localization and high-resolution depiction of bone, air, and soft-tissue structures and serve as an effective tool to survey the general region. These requirements may necessitate use of several imaging modalities to fully characterize a single entity.

J. P. Villablanca and A. R. Borges: Department of Radiological Sciences/Neuroradiology, UCLA Medical Center, Los Angeles, California 90095

R. B. Lufkin: Department of Radiology, University of California, Los Angeles, School of Medicine, Los Angeles, California 90095-1721

When deciding between computed tomography (CT) or magnetic resonance (MR) as the imaging modality for a particular clinical question, it is helpful to keep several general considerations in mind. CT is the study of choice when the pathologic process primarily involves the bones or air spaces of the temporal bone. CT also is useful in the evaluation of soft-tissue masses when these are separated from normal structures by fatty tissue planes and for the detection but usually not the characterization of solid soft-tissue masses when they alter the contours or tissue density of normal anatomic features. In contrast, MR imaging cannot be used to differentiate cortical bone from air when these lie immediately adjacent to each other because both provide signal voids. This limits the sensitivity and specificity of MR imaging when a pathologic processes primarily involves air spaces, cortical bone adjacent to air, or small bones devoid of a marrow cavity. Because of the inherent signal characteristics of normal tissues, MR imaging is superior to CT in the evaluation of soft-tissue structures. Blood vessels, bone with fatty marrow, and spaces filled with cerebrospinal fluid (CSF) are better evaluated with MR imaging.

Because CT and MR imaging are generally complementary, both modalities frequently are used in the evaluation of temporal bone disorders. Factors other than imaging considerations may determine which modality to use. Some of these include cost, continuity with historical studies, patient weight limits, claustrophobia, the presence of implanted metal medical devices, and allergies to intravenously administered contrast agents. This chapter includes a discussion of the relative merits of both imaging modalities for most pathologic entities presented.

NORMAL ANATOMY

A thorough knowledge of normal anatomy is prerequisite to a deep understanding of temporal bone abnormalities. The normal high-resolution CT anatomy of the temporal bone is illustrated in detail in both axial and coronal planes in Figs. 1 through 22, which are annotated in Keys 1 and 2. Temporal bone anatomy as depicted with high-resolution MR imaging is shown in Figs. 23 through 25, which are annotated in Key 3. The images demonstrate that the main advantage of MR over CT in temporal bone imaging is the ability of MR imaging to depict inner ear structures, including the membranous labyrinth and semicircular canals, and directly the nerves within the internal auditory canals. The images were obtained at 1.5 T with dual phased-array coils applied to the temporal regions, large matrix, small field of view, and 3-mm contiguous sections.

IMAGING STRATEGIES: A GENERAL APPROACH

Imaging strategy generally is determined by the type of hearing loss or other clinical deficit and by the patient's age. Temporal bone MR imaging with contrast enhancement is the imaging study of choice to evaluate patients for sensorineural hearing loss (SNHL). The routine protocol calls for a standard head coil and includes T1-weighted and T2-weighted whole-brain imaging in the axial plane. This is followed by axial T1-weighted sequences before administration of contrast material and axial and coronal thin sections through the temporal bones after administration of contrast material. Temporal bone sequences are generally 3-mm contiguous sections. Optional high-resolution dual phased-array coils can be used to generate T2-weighted axial sequences with larger matrix size, 2 to 4 signal aver-

ages, and 3-mm intersection gap. This protocol provides fine resolution of the nerves in the internal auditory canal and of the membranous labyrinth. Some facilities are performing T2-weighted scanning with 0.8-mm section thickness in scan planes parallel and perpendicular to the internal auditory canal (IAC).

The CT protocol for patients with SNHL includes 1-mm contiguous sections in the axial and coronal planes through the temporal bones, filmed with both soft-tissue and bone-window techniques. Intravenous administration of contrast material should be used in all examinations of adults to optimize detection of acoustic schwannoma and other enhancing tumors of the cerebellopontine angle (CPA). For children with SNHL, thin-bone–algorithm CT technique is sufficient, and intravenous administration of contrast material is not routine.

Patients with conductive hearing loss benefit from high-resolution CT in the axial and coronal planes with a bone-window algorithm. Most conductive hearing loss is a consequence of a degenerative or inflammatory disorder or a neoplastic process, hence the epicenter and extent of processes in the middle ear cavity are generally more important clues in CT diagnosis than is the enhancement pattern. Contrast material is administered intravenously only when extratemporal extension of temporal bone neoplasms is suspected. MR imaging is not routinely used as the first imaging study in evaluations of patients with conductive hearing loss.

Evaluation of patients with mixed hearing loss usually begins with CT. This includes imaging with a high-resolution bone algorithm for the conductive component and contrast-enhanced imaging of the temporal bone, internal auditory canal, and brain with a soft-tissue algorithm for the SNHL component. If the SNHL is the more prominent feature of the disorder that caused the mixed hearing loss, MR imaging may be the more appropriate first study.

CONGENITAL PATHOLOGIC CONDITIONS

Anomalies of the Outer Ear

Stenosis of the external auditory canal may be focal or segmental and is often associated with severe microtia (1,2). Atresia of the auditory canal is caused by aplasia of the tympanic ring and may be unilateral or bilateral, partial or complete. It ranges from complete bony atresia (Fig. 26) to a membrane or soft-tissue plug of variable thickness. Atresia may be associated with posterior migration of the temporomandibular joint (Fig. 27), fusion of the neck of the malleus to the atresia plate (3), or cholesteatoma. In patients with atresia of the external auditory canal (EAC) complicated by congenital or acquired cholesteatoma, CT may show a dysplastic, non-aerated middle ear cavity or opacification with bony wall erosion and ossicular destruction (4). CT can be used to evaluate surgical outcome.

(text continues on page 302)

FIGS. 1–22. High-resolution CT anatomy of the temporal bone in axial and coronal planes. See Keys 1 and 2 for annotation.

Key 1. Numerals: *1,* facial nerve, mastoidal segment; *2,* caroticojugular spine; *3,* petrotympanic fissure (glaserian fissure); *4,* sigmoid sinus plate; *5,* mastoid air cells; *6,* tympanosquamous suture; *7,* vidian canal; *8,* petrooccipital synchondrosis; *9,* squamosphenoid suture; *10,* tympanic annulus; *11,* cochlear aqueduct; *12,* tensor tympani muscle; *13,* basal turn of cochlea; *14,* round window niche; *15,* sinus tympani; *16,* stapedius tendon; *17,* vestibular aqueduct; *18,* squamosal temporal bone; *19,* cochleariform process; *20,* malleus, head; *21,* uncudomalleal joint; *22,* incus, body; *23,* incus, short process; *24,* sinus tympani; *25,* pyramidal eminence; *26,* facial nerve recess; *27,* facial nerve, posterior genu; *28,* incudal fossa; *29,* mesotympanum; *30,* facial nerve, tympanic (horizontal) segment; *31,* cochlea, apical turn; *32,* cochlea, basal turn; *33,* modiolus; *34,* groove for greater superficial petrosal nerve (nervus intermedius); *35,* horizontal semicircular canal; *36,* horizontal semicircular canal, anterior limb; *37,* superior semicircular canal; *38,* posterior semicircular canal; *39,* facial nerve, labyrinthine (meatal) segment; *40,* facial nerve, geniculate ganglion; *41,* aditus ad antrum; *42,* epitympanum; *43,* mastoid antrum; *44,* incus, long process; *45,* incudostapedial joint; *46,* Koerner's septum; *47,* stapes superstructure; *48,* oval window; *49,* eustachian tube, bony segment; *50,* facial nerve, anterior genu; *51,* malleus, long process; *52,* Bill's bar; *53,* crista falciformis; *54,* tegmen tympani; *55,* arcuate eminence.

Key 2. Lower-case letters: *cc,* cervical carotid canal; *fl,* foramen lacerum; *fo,* foramen ovale; *fr,* foramen rotundum; *fs,* foramen spinosum; *fv,* foramen of Vesalius; *jb,* jugular bulb; *jf,* jugular fossa; *mc,* mandibular condyle; *oc,* occipital condyle; *pa,* petrous apex; *pcc,* petrous carotid canal; *ss,* sigmoid sinus.

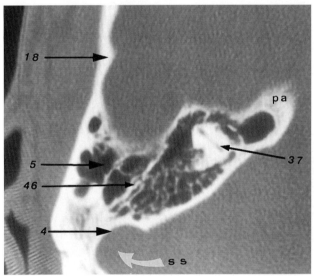

FIG. 1.

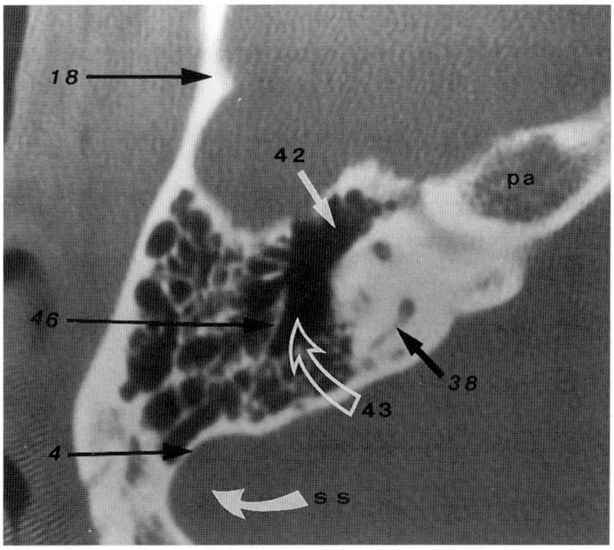

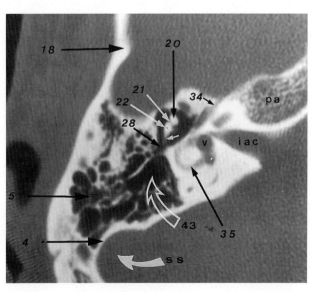

FIG. 2.

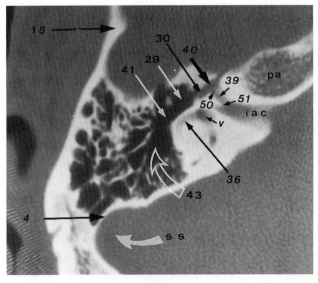

FIG. 3.

FIG. 4.

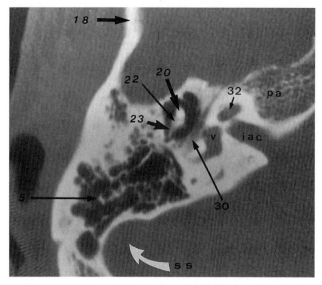

FIG. 5.

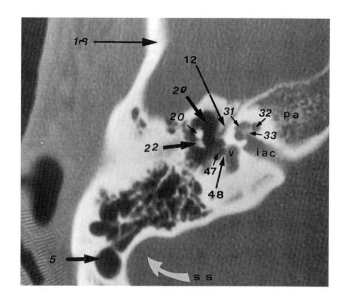

FIG. 6.

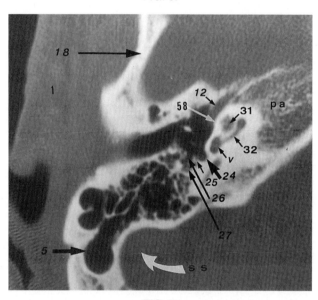

FIG. 7.

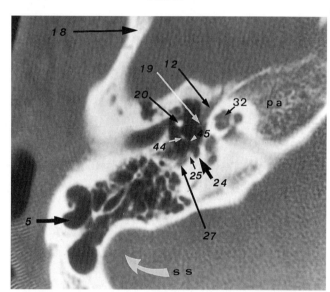

FIG. 8.

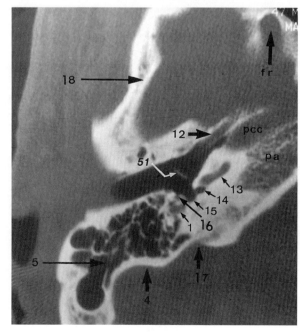

FIG. 9.

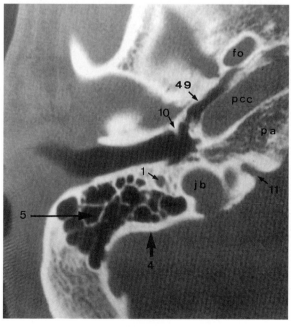

FIG. 10.

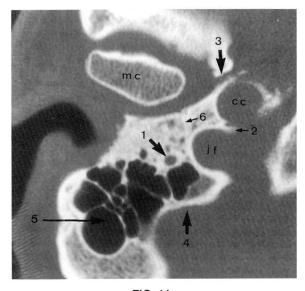

FIG. 11.

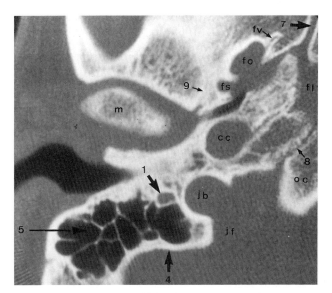

FIG. 12.

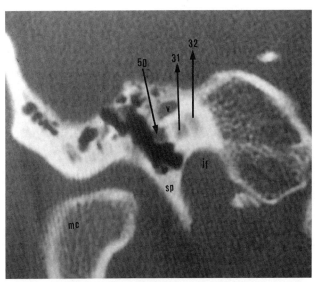

FIG. 13.

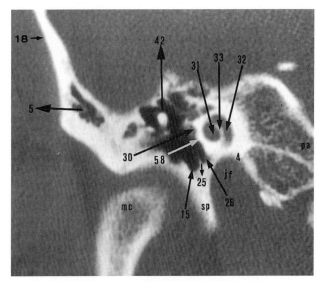

FIG. 14.

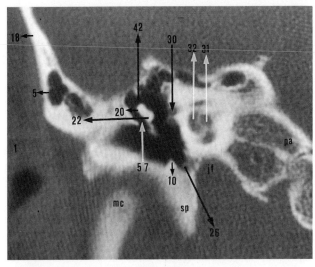

FIG. 15.

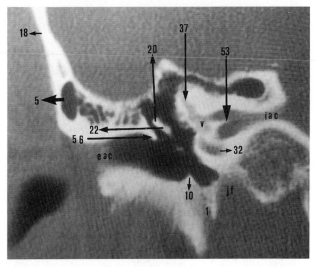

FIG. 16.

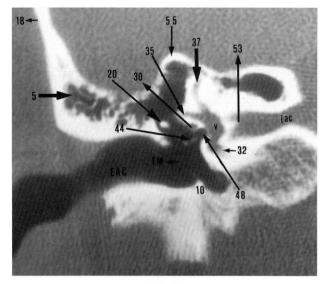

FIG. 17.

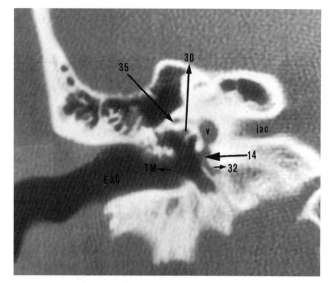

FIG. 18.

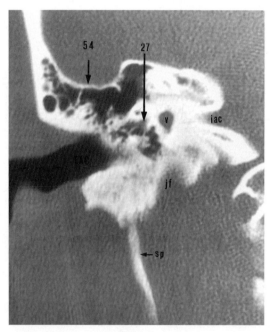

FIG. 19.

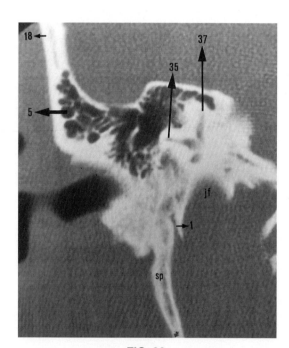

FIG. 20.

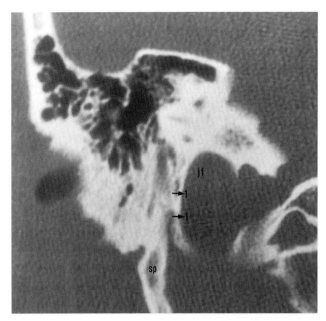

FIG. 21.

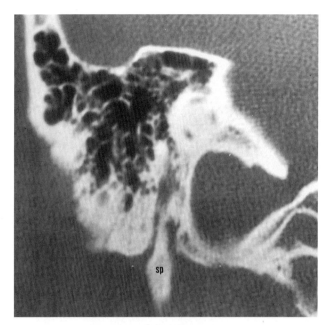

FIG. 22.

FIGS. 23–25. High-resolution MR anatomy of the temporal bone.
Key 3. Upper-case letters: *A,* cochlea, apical turn, axial plane; *B,* cochlea, basal turn, axial plane; *C,* cochlea, coronal plane; *CN,* cochlear nerve, internal auditory canal; *IVN,* inferior vestibular nerve; *LC,* lateral semicircular canal; *PC,* posterior semicircular canal; *SC,* superior semicircular canal; *V,* vestibule.

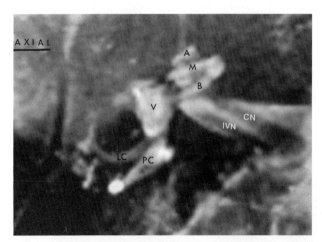

FIG. 23.

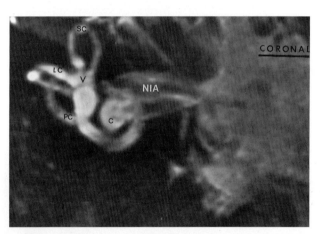

FIG. 24.

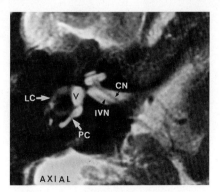

FIG. 25.

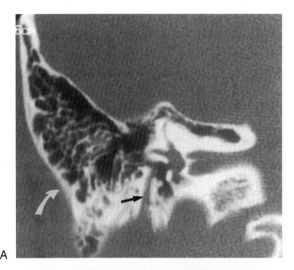

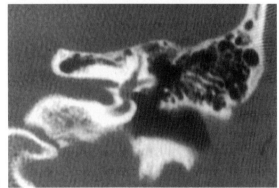

FIG. 26. Atresia of the external auditory canal. Coronal CT image. **A:** Right side. Image at plane of vestibule. *White arrow* indicates where ear should be. Middle ear cavity is absent. The mastoidal segment of the facial nerve (*black arrow*) is anteriorly displaced. **B:** Left side is normal. Facial nerve is not visible at this corresponding plane.

Anomalies of the Middle Ear

Minor middle ear anomalies generally are associated with dysplasia of the tympanic ring, which often is seen among patients with canal stenosis. The middle ear cavity may be of normal size. Partial fusion of the ossicles to each other or the walls of the mesotympanum is common (Fig. 28).

In atresia of the EAC, the mastoid segment of the facial nerve exits more anteriorly, near the temporomandibular joint, rather than posteromedially to the styloid process of the mastoid as is normal. The joint space is posteriorly displaced, and the glenoid fossa may contact the anterior wall of the mastoid process. When the tympanic ring fails to form, the neck of the malleus is fused to the atretic plate (see Fig. 28). The mesotympanum is usually small but may be normal or on rare occasion larger than normal. Absence of the ossicles is rare. The mastoids generally are well pneumatized (5).

Anomalies of the Inner Ear

Anomalies of the inner ear are a heterogeneous group of malformations that defy easy classification. The spectrum of anomalies ranges from complete aplasia to subtle dysplasia of one anatomic component (6,7). The cochlea may be hypoplastic (Fig. 29), and the cochlea, vestibule, and semicircular canals may be dysplastic (Fig. 30), fused (Fig. 31), or absent. The cochlea, vestibule, and semicircular canals may be a single sac, likely a persistent primitive otic vesicle (see Fig. 31) (8). Types of cochlear dysplasia include a small or large common sac, fusion of the middle and apical turns, and hypoplasia. Cochlear hypoplasia may be associated with a facial

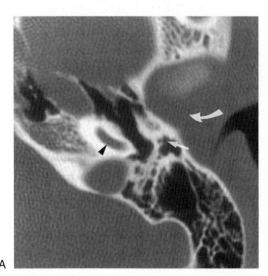

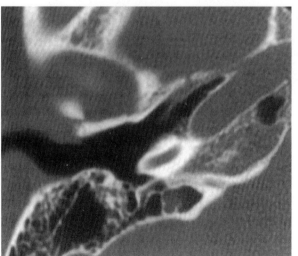

FIG. 27. Atresia of the external auditory canal. Axial CT image at level of basal turn of cochlea (*arrowhead*). **A:** Left side. Image shows absent posterior wall of glenoid fossa (*curved arrow*) and anterior displacement of mastoidal segment of the facial nerve canal (*arrow*). **B:** Right side is normal.

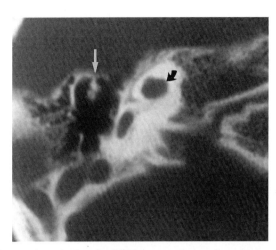

FIG. 28. Dysplasia of middle ear cavity and ossicular dysplasia, inner ear anomaly. Axial CT image of the left side shows an enlarged middle ear cavity and ossicular dysplasia with the head of malleus fused to the anterior wall of the mesotympanum (*white arrow*). The cochlea is dysplastic, visible here as a single cavity (*black arrow*). The semicircular canals are absent.

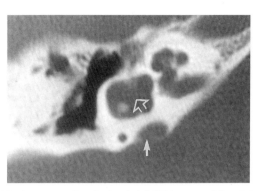

FIG. 30. Inner ear dysplasia. Axial CT image of the right side shows fused semicircular canals and enlarged vestibule (*open arrow*). The cochlea appears well formed. The vestibular aqueduct is enlarged (*white arrow*).

nerve running in an anterior and medial position (9). Of the three semicircular canals, the horizontal semicircular canal completes development last and is the most frequently abnormal (9). It may be dysplastic or fused to a hypoplastic vestibule.

Dilatation of the vestibular aqueduct is associated with progressive hearing loss in childhood and adulthood (10). Measurements of the diameter of the normal vestibular aqueduct vary widely depending on the technique used and the site selected for measurement. The diameter of a normal aqueduct should generally not exceed the diameter of one crus of the adjacent normal semicircular canal

(10). Dilatation of the vestibular aqueduct may be isolated or accompany cochlear and vestibular anomalies. Congenital perilymphatic fistula is abnormal communication between the inner and middle ear cavities that allows passage of perilymph into the middle ear. CT scans frequently show associated abnormalities. The vestibular aqueduct may be dilated, and the cochlea or vestibule may be anomalous (9,10). The stapes may be monopod or show anomalous asymmetric crura (10).

Vascular Anomalies

Complete Absence of the Carotid Artery

Complete absence of the carotid artery is very rare and is believed to arise during embryogenesis; some experts

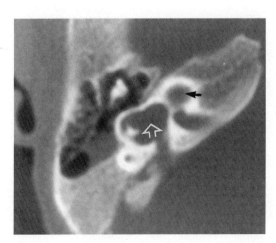

FIG. 29. Inner ear dysplasia. Axial CT image of the right side shows dilated vestibule and fused semicircular canals (*open arrow*). The cochlea is dysplastic with a single chamber. The modiolus is absent (*black arrow*).

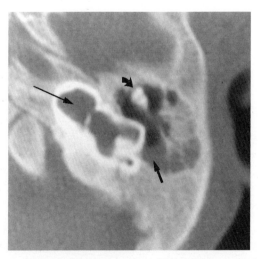

FIG. 31. Inner ear dysplasia. Axial CT image of the left side shows partially fused cochlea and vestibule. The cochlea is a single chamber (*long arrow*). The ossicles are fused to the anterior wall of the middle ear cavity (*curved arrow*). There is soft tissue in the mastoid air cells (*short arrow*), but no bony destruction is visible.

suspect a mechanical cause, such as amniotic adhesions (11). The anomaly may be unilateral or bilateral. CT of the temporal bones shows absence of the bony petrous and cervical internal carotid artery canals. Cerebral angiography shows absence of the internal carotid arteries, usually with persistent inferior tympanic or hyoid-caroticotympanic arteries. The finding often is incidental.

Lateral (Aberrant) Course of the Internal Carotid Artery

A lateral course of the internal carotid artery is seen on less than 1% of temporal bone studies performed for all indications (12). It has a marked female predominance and is generally seen on the right side (12). Congenital failure of ossification of the lateral carotid canal is the suspected cause. The cervical internal carotid artery becomes tortuous with age, allowing the vessel to protrude through the bony defect. CT shows a soft-tissue mass in the hypotympanum with extension into the oval window region (Fig. 32). The carotid artery may displace the tympanic membrane laterally or cause remodeling of the cochlear promontory. Axial and coronal views show absence of the lateral bony canal wall of the vessel. Angiography shows deviation of the internal carotid artery lateral to a line drawn tangential to the lateral margin of the vestibule. The artery is usually larger than the normal opposite vessel. An associated persistent stapedial artery is frequently seen.

Partial Absence of the Carotid Artery

The vertical portion of the intrapetrous carotid artery may be atretic. Consequently blood alternately courses

through the inferior tympanic and hyoidal arteries to enter the hypotympanic cavity through Jacobson's canal as a large inferior tympanic artery. The artery then courses inferior and anterior to the stapes, below the cochlear promontory, and anteriorly within the petrous segment of the carotid canal (13). CT studies show a soft-tissue density in the middle ear that looks like an aberrant internal carotid artery. Cerebral angiography reveals the true vascular anomaly. MR angiography (MRA) may help detect it depending on the size of the inferior tympanic artery.

High-riding Jugular Bulb

High-riding jugular bulb is the most common vascular anomaly of the temporal bone. It is found in approximately 5% of histologic specimens (14) and is defined as a jugular bulb that has an apex on axial CT images at or above the plane of the basal turn of the cochlea (Fig. 33) (15). It is more common among patients with poorly pneumatized mastoids, in whom the jugular fossa tends to be deep, the sigmoid sinus more anterior, and the jugular dome higher than usual. The bony covering of the jugular bulb may be thinner than normal, potentially exposing the jugular bulb to traumatic or iatrogenic injury.

Protruding Jugular Bulb

The jugular bulb may protrude into the hypotympanum through a dehiscence in the floor of the middle ear. This is the second most common vascular anomaly of the temporal bone. Patients may report pulsatile tinnitus and sometimes hearing loss caused by mechanical impinge-

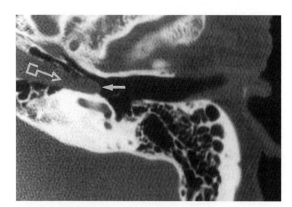

FIG. 32. Dehiscent carotid artery. Axial CT image of left temporal bone above plane of cervical carotid canal shows lack of bony covering (*white arrow*) over lateral aspect of petrous segment of the internal carotid artery (*open arrow*). Carotid artery margin protrudes a small distance into hypotympanum. Middle ear cavity and otic capsule are intact.

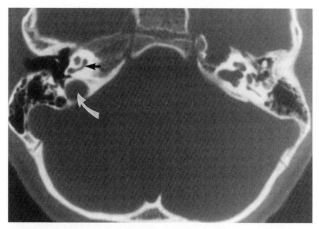

FIG. 33. High-riding jugular bulb. Axial CT image obtained with bone-window technique shows right side. Rounded area of hypodensity represents apex of jugular bulb (*white arrow*). Apex of jugular bulb is at the same plane as the basal turn of the cochlea (*black arrow*).

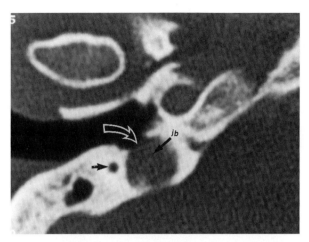

FIG. 34. Dehiscent jugular bulb. Axial noncontrast CT scan of the temporal bone on the right side shows a defect (*curved arrow*) in the anterolateral wall of the jugular bulb (*long arrow*). The fallopian canal lateral to jugular bulb is normal (*short arrow*).

ment of the ossicles or tympanic membrane by the jugular bulb (15). The appearance is usually a retrotympanic bluish mass. CT scans show a bony defect in the floor of the hypotympanum above the jugular bulb (Fig. 34). Contrast images show an enhancing mass in the middle ear cavity. Similar findings may be seen with jugular venography in nonsubtracted views. A jugular diverticulum is differentiated from a protruding jugular bulb by its more posterior and medial location in the petrous bone. This anomaly does not protrude into the middle ear and is not visible at routine examinations.

TEMPORAL BONE FRACTURES

High-resolution CT is the study of choice in the evaluation of patients with temporal bone trauma and related complications (16,17). Acquisition of axial and coronal contiguous sections 1.0- or 1.5-mm thick usually is advised. MR imaging generally is reserved for problem cases, in which facial nerve paralysis and vestibular syndromes are present but the CT study does not reveal the cause. For example, MR imaging may show a hematoma or edema of the facial nerve or labyrinthine hemorrhage (18).

Longitudinal Fractures

Longitudinal fractures occur along the long axis of the temporal bone (19,20). They constitute about 80% of all temporal bone fractures. The fracture line usually spares the labyrinth and passes anterior or posterior to it. The fracture typically begins in the temporal squamosa, passes through the superior and posterior walls of the EAC, crosses the roof of the middle ear, passes through

the petrous apex, and usually terminates near the foramen lacerum (Fig. 35). Lacerations of the EAC and tympanic membrane are not infrequent but are difficult to demonstrate with CT. Ossicular chain dislocations or fractures also are frequent and are readily demonstrated with CT. Delayed or transient facial nerve paralysis is present in as many as 20% of cases. It is usually caused by facial nerve injury just distal to the geniculate ganglion and anterior genu (21) and is detectable with CT. CSF leaks are usually caused by disruption of the tegmen tympani or dura above the posterior mastoid or petrous air cells (see later).

Transverse Fracture

Transverse fractures have a principal axis that is perpendicular to the petrous bone. They constitute approximately 20% of temporal bone fractures (21). The fracture line may be medial or lateral to the arcuate eminence (18). It typically begins at the foramen magnum, passes across the occipital bone, jugular fossa, petrous pyramid, and body of the sphenoid, usually sparing the middle ear cavity. As the transverse fracture passes into the floor of the middle cranial fossa, the petrous segment of the internal carotid canal may be fractured, leading to laceration or occlusion of this vessel. The facial canal is involved in 30% to 50% of these fractures, leading to damage of the nerve (22). The most common site of facial nerve injury as demonstrated with high-resolution CT is the labyrinthine segment proximal to the geniculate ganglion. Transverse temporal bone fractures may involve the otic capsule and labyrinth and cause complete SNHL. Extension of the fracture through the round or oval window or into the footplate of the stapes is a cause of perilymphatic fistula. Pneumolabyrinth may result from transverse fractures that create a communication between the middle ear cavity or mastoid air cells and the vestibule, cochlea, or semicircular canals or from dislocation of the footplate of the stapes. These abnormalities are demonstrable with CT.

Dehiscence of the Tegmen Tympani and Cerebrospinal Fluid Fistula

Axial and coronal CT scans of the temporal bone obtained after intrathecal injection of nonionic contrast material are now routine in the evaluation of patients with suspected CSF fistulas. The CT images may show the defect in the roof of the temporal bone. The defect may be caused by traumatic, congenital, surgical, inflammatory, or neoplastic conditions (23) and may be associated with a meningocele. The dura over a tegmen tympani fracture can be directly visualized. Posttraumatic encephalocele can be visualized with MR imaging (24).

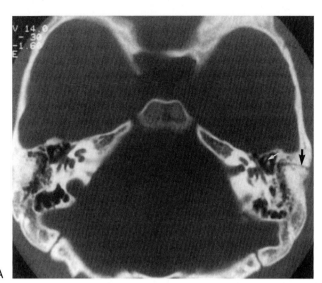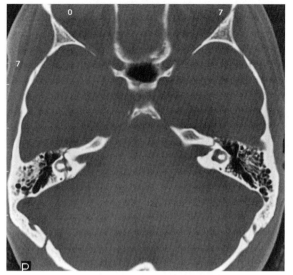

FIG. 35. Fractures of the temporal bone. **A:** Axial bone-window CT image shows longitudinal fracture. Linear lucency extends through long axis of left temporal bone (*black arrow*) into the middle ear cavity. The distance between the head of the malleus and the body of the incus is wider than normal, compatible with incudomalleal dislocation (*white arrow*). **B:** Axial bone window CT image shows transverse fracture. Linear lucency extends transversely through the labyrinth.

INFLAMMATORY DISEASES

Acute Mastoiditis

Imaging usually is not needed to establish the diagnosis of acute mastoiditis. In uncomplicated disease, images show fluid or soft-tissue densities and in some cases air-fluid levels in the mastoid air cells and middle ear cavity without bone destruction. Complications of acute mastoiditis that can be detected with MR imaging or CT include subperiosteal abscess, meningitis, parenchymal abscess, petrous apicitis, and venous sinus thrombosis. High-resolution CT is the study of choice in the evaluation of bony change (25). Attention must be given to excluding cortical disruption in the postauricular area, where the trabecular bone is thin, and excluding the presence of a subperiosteal abscess. If the posterior root of the zygomatic bone is pneumatized, anterior extension of the inflammatory process may lead to formation of an anterior preauricular abscess. A Bezold's abscess may result when the infection spreads caudally into the mastoid tip and along the sternocleidomastoid muscle (25).

Sigmoid sinus thrombophlebitis, sigmoid and petrosal vein thrombosis, and epidural or intracerebral abscesses are evaluated by means of contrast CT and MR imaging with coronal sections (26). In sinus thrombosis, contrast CT may show failure of uniform enhancement within the sinus, whereas MR imaging may show absence of flow signal intensity on T2-weighted or gradient echo images. MRA shows marked reduction or interruption of flow and helps confirm the diagnosis. Pneumatization of the petrous portion of the temporal bone is seen among as many as 30% of patients. Infection causes petrous apicitis or acute inflammation of the air cells. Osteomyelitis of the petrous apex occurs when nonpneumatized bone is involved (27). CT reveals opacified petrous apex air cells, destruction of bony septa, and possibly lysis of bony cortex. MR findings include opacification, abnormal marginal or internal enhancement of the petrous bone, and possibly dural enhancement or empyema.

Secretory Otitis Media

Although rarely needed, CT is the best modality for evaluating chronic serous otitis media (28). In a completely opacified system, where fluid levels are not present, the diagnosis of middle ear effusion is not possible. However, when an air-fluid level is seen in two planes, the diagnosis can be made with confidence (29). Pressure equalization tubes, unless they are of equal density to adjacent debris, are well visualized on CT scans (30,31).

Chronic Otitis Media

CT is the modality of choice in the evaluation of otitis media. Images show variable opacification of the middle ear and mastoid air cells without bone resorption or ossicular destruction. Air-fluid levels are occasionally seen when air-space opacification is incomplete. Another finding is ossicular erosion, usually involving the long and lenticular process of the incus and the stapes. These changes can be seen on both axial and coronal CT images. Axial images are optimal for visualization of the ossicular chain, except for the long process of the incus and malleus, which are best seen on coronal images (32). Images also may show widening of the incudostapedial joint caused by erosion and replacement with fibrous tissue. Ossicular abnormalities may be difficult to appreciate when the middle ear is opacified.

Cholesteatoma

CT scans can reliably demonstrate tympanic membrane thickening and retraction (33). Retraction of the pars tensa is more readily visible on CT scans than that of the pars flaccida because it occupies a larger area (34). Acquired cholesteatoma arises in Prussak's space and generally grows upward into the attic and aditus ad antrum, because this path offers little resistance (35) (Fig. 36). These lesions generally displace the head of the malleus and body of the incus medially and tend to erode the bony process at the junction of the lateral attic wall and EAC, called the *scutum*. Because the scutum and head of the malleus are well depicted on coronal images, cholesteatoma of Prussak's space is most easily demonstrated on coronal CT sections (36).

In contradistinction, cholesteatoma of the pars tensa is best seen on axial CT images, because for the most part they arise from posterosuperior tympanic membrane retractions that initially involve the sinus tympani medially and facial nerve recess laterally. These two tympanic cavity recesses are best seen on axial images (37). When superior extension into the mesotympanum, epitympanum or aditus ad antrum has occurred, choles-

teatoma of the pars tensa generally displaces the ossicles laterally.

The CT density of cholesteatoma is nonspecific and is usually equal to that of the surrounding soft tissue (38). Therefore secondary defining features such as ossicular or other bony erosion, the epicenter of the process, and displacement of normal structures are sought to establish the diagnosis of cholesteatoma (Fig. 37). As many as 90% of cholesteatomas of the pars tensa and approximately 75% of cholesteatomas of the pars flaccida show ossicular destruction (39). Cholesteatoma of the pars flaccida destroys the head of the malleus and body of the incus (Fig. 38). Other findings associated with cholesteatoma include remodeling of the lateral wall of the epitympanum and erosion of the inferior border of the glaserian fissure (anterior tympanic spine). The MR signal characteristics of cholesteatoma are nonspecific. Generally, both T1 and T2 relaxation times are prolonged, and the lesion is depicted as hypointense on T1-weighted and hyperintense on T2-weighted images (40). Intravenous administration of contrast material may help to differentiate cholesteatoma, which as a rule does not become enhanced, from other enhancing lesions, such as granulation material and neoplasms (41).

A serious complication of cholesteatoma is labyrinthine fistula with resultant pneumolabyrinth (Fig. 39). This generally is caused by erosion of the cochlear promontory and lateral semicircular canal (42). At CT the defect can be identified on axial or coronal images. Erosion of the tegmen tympani superiorly or the sigmoid sinus plate posteriorly is a potentially serious complication of cholesteatoma. Involvement tegmen tympani is seen best on coronal CT images, whereas erosion through the sigmoid sinus plate is most evident on axial CT images (43). When bony breach at these sites occurs and superinfection is suspected, contrast-enhanced MR imaging is recommended to exclude or confirm meningitis, epidural or cerebral abscess, subdural empyema, and venous thrombophlebitis.

The condition of the facial canal is best evaluated with CT. However, because the tympanic segment of the facial nerve beneath the horizontal semicircular canal may be variably covered by a thin film of bone, CT in some cases may not depict subtle invasion by cholesteatoma. Gross invasion generally is well demonstrated on coronal CT sections that include the most commonly involved segments of the seventh nerve: the anterior genu and the posterior genu (44). After surgical intervention CT scans may be needed to evaluate causes of persistent drainage.

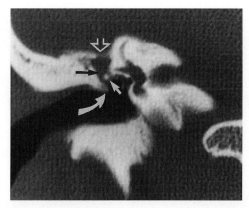

FIG. 36. Pars flaccida cholesteatoma. Coronal noncontrast CT image of right temporal bone obtained with bone-window technique shows soft-tissue density in epitympanic recess (*black arrow*), ossicular erosion (*straight white arrow*), and blunted scutum (*curved white arrow*). The tegmen tympani is thinned but intact (*open white arrow*).

Tympanosclerosis

CT findings that suggest tympanosclerosis include variable amounts of material with nonspecific soft-tissue

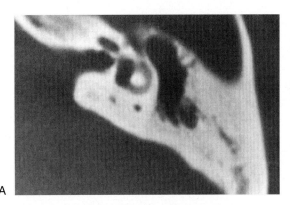

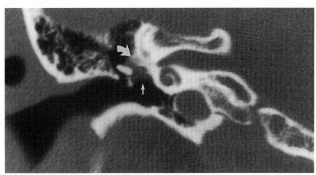

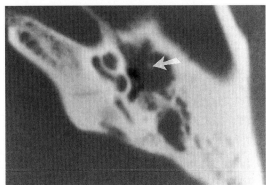

FIG. 37. Congenital cholesteatoma. **A:** Axial CT image of the left side obtained with bone-window technique shows complete opacification of the epitympanum and mastoid antrum. The aditus ad antrum is enlarged. **B:** Axial CT image in a slightly higher plane than in **A** shows opacified middle ear cavity and small ossicular remnants (*arrowhead*). **C:** Coronal CT image of a different patient obtained with bone-window technique shows soft-tissue density interposed between the ossicles and the cochlear promontory (*straight arrow*). Mild erosion of otic capsulae bone is present (*curved arrow*). There is no evidence of ossicular destruction.

density mainly in the oval window niche and epitympanum and a thickened tympanic membrane. These fibrous tissue deposits and bands may encase the ossicles and suspensory ligaments and gradually calcify. The advanced CT appearance is large, calcified plaques that appear as punctate or linear densities within the tympanic membrane and suspensory ligaments and tendons of the ossicles (Fig. 40). Conduction deficits caused by tympanosclerosis may sometimes be corrected with an ossicular prosthesis.

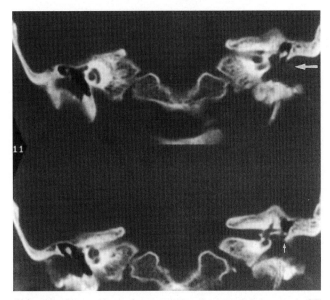

FIG. 38. Bilateral cholesteatoma. Sequential coronal CT cuts obtained with bone-window technique show soft-tissue masses in left external auditory canal and middle ear with bony debris (*large arrow*) and mild ossicular erosions. The tip of the scutum is blunted (*small arrow*). Right side exhibits soft tissue in external auditory canal with clear middle ear cavity and intact ossicles.

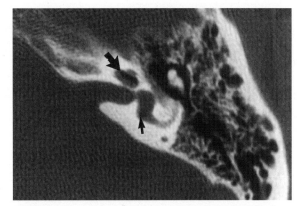

FIG. 39. Air in cochlea, pneumolabyrinth. Axial CT image at plane of cochlea shows band of very low hypodensity within the basal turn of the cochlea (*large arrow*) and in the common crus of the horizontal and posterior semicircular canals (*small arrow*), indicating the presence of air within the inner ear.

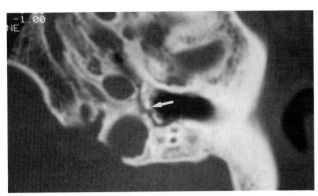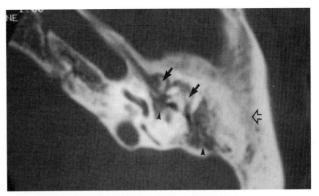

A   B

FIG. 40. Tympanosclerosis. **A:** Axial CT image of left temporal bone obtained with bone-window technique shows thickened, grossly calcified, retracted tympanic membrane (*white arrow*). **B:** Axial CT image of the plane of the middle ear cavity of the patient in **A** shows calcific masses (*black arrows*) and soft-tissue density within the middle ear cavity. Soft tissue is present in the sinus tympani and mastoid air cells (*arrowheads*). Early bone resorption is visible along the lateral aspect of the mastoid bone; this sign is compatible with the presence of a chronic inflammatory process (*open arrow*).

Otosclerosis

The value of CT in the management of otosclerosis is limited to assessment of cochlear involvement (Fig. 41) and problems related to prosthesis placement (Fig. 42). MR imaging has no practical role in the evaluation of this disorder.

Labyrinthitis

Abnormal enhancement of the membranous labyrinth on MR images has been reported among patients with acute or subacute labyrinthitis (45). Correlation between patient symptoms and imaging findings appears to be high (46). Findings consist of intense enhancement of the cochlea and vestibule and variable enhancement of the semicircular canals (Fig. 43). Chronic labyrinthitis leads to fibrosis and eventual calcification of the mem-

branous labyrinth, which is best visualized with noncontrast CT.

Cholesterol Granuloma

Cholesterol granuloma can occur anywhere in the middle ear or petrous apex (47). The lesion is a foreign-body response to cholesterol crystals. The dominant feature is a hemorrhagic component, which causes the typical MR signal characteristics of the lesion (48). The lesion is filled primarily with extracellular methemoglobin, which causes a characteristic heterogenous hyperintense signal on both T1-weighted and T2-weighted MR sequences

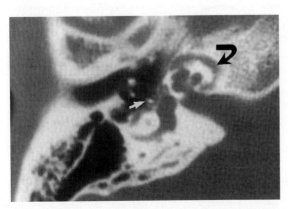

FIG. 41. Cochlear otosclerosis. Axial bone-window CT image shows well-defined halo of lucency surrounding right cochlea (*black arrow*). An incidental finding is a piston-type prosthesis through the right oval window (*white arrow*).

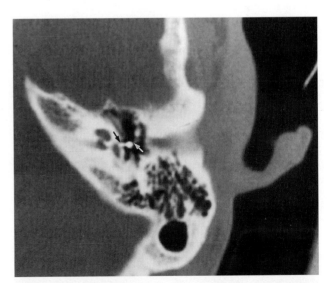

FIG. 42. Stapedial prosthesis. Axial CT image of the left side shows small piston with thin shaft entering oval window (*black arrow*). The head of the prosthesis articulates with the long process of the incus (*white arrow*).

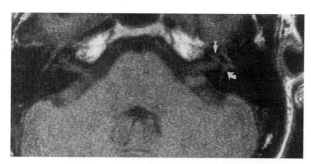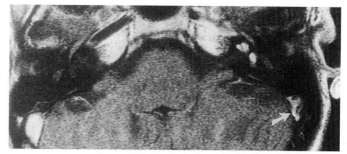

A

B

FIG. 43. Labyrinthitis. Axial MR images. **A:** Axial precontrast T1-weighted image shows normal isointense signal in the cochlea (*straight arrow*) and vestibule (*curved arrow*). **B:** Axial postcontrast T1-weighted axial image shows intense contrast enhancement of cochlea and vestibule. Enhancement of the sigmoid sinuses is normal (*arrow*).

(Fig. 44). The presence of hemosiderin may produce areas of central hypointensity on T1-weighted and T2-weighted images (49). Enhancement is not seen on CT or MR studies unless vascular granulation tissue is present (49). The lesions generally cause little mass effect and have a smooth expansile quality (50). CT shows a lobulated mass of variable density in the petrous apex or middle ear and smooth bony remodeling. Imaging studies may be helpful in differentiating cholesterol granuloma from cholesteatoma, paraganglioma, aberrant internal carotid artery, or dehiscent internal jugular vein.

Malignant Otitis Externa

Malignant otitis externa is usually a *Pseudomonas* infection typically occurring among susceptible elderly patients, persons with diabetes, and patients' compromised immune function. It begins at the osteocartilaginous junction and may extend rapidly along the skull base as a process of progressive osteitis. Facial nerve paralysis occurs when the infection involves the infratemporal fossa at the stylomastoid foramen. Intracranial invasion with abscess formation, cerebral infarction, and dural sinus thrombosis is infrequently seen and is best evaluated with MR imaging. MR imaging also provides excellent delineation of abnormalities of the infratemporal fossa and stylomastoid region. CT frequently shows enhancing abnormal soft tissue in the EAC, infratemporal fossa, and frequently the mastoid region (Fig. 45). CT with technetium 99m or gallium may help to establish the diagnosis and is valuable in assessment of resolution of the process after therapy.

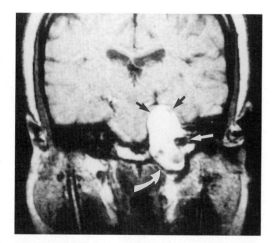

FIG. 44. Cholesterol granuloma. T1-weighted MR image shows a large hyperintense mass in the left cerebellopontine angle cistern that has remodeled the skull base (*curved white arrow*). The lesion was hyperintense on T2-weighted images (not shown). This signal intensity pattern is characteristic of cholesterol granuloma. The mass does not enter the internal auditory canal (*straight white arrow*). A mass effect is visible on the brainstem and mesial temporal lobe (*black arrows*).

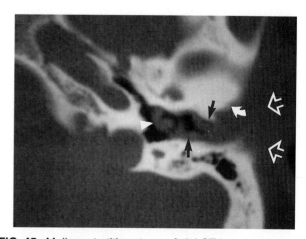

FIG. 45. Malignant otitis externa. Axial CT image of left temporal bone obtained with bone-window technique shows thickening of the periauricular soft tissues (*open arrows*) and soft tissue filling the external auditory canal (*black arrows*). The tympanic membrane is thickened (*arrowhead*). Early erosion of the inferior lip of the external auditory canal is visible (*curved arrow*). The appearance is nonspecific, and requires clinical correlation.

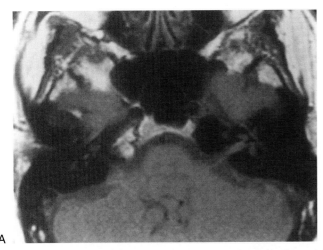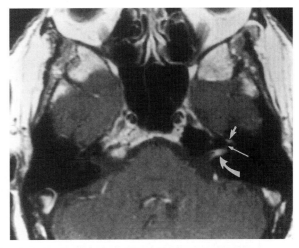

A

B

FIG. 46. Ramsay Hunt syndrome. **A:** Axial T1-weighted precontrast image shows normal appearance of internal auditory canal, cochlea, vestibule, and tympanic segment of the facial nerve. **B:** Axial post-contrast T1-weighted image shows definite enhancement in fundic aspect of the internal auditory canal (*curved arrow*), labyrinthine segment of the facial nerve (*long white arrow*), and geniculate ganglion (*short white arrow*).

FACIAL PARALYSIS

Radiologic studies in the management of facial paralysis are helpful in the evaluation of Bell's palsy (MR imaging), trauma (CT), herpes zoster (MR imaging), central nervous system disease (MR imaging) congenital causes (CT), and neoplasia (CT and MR imaging). Facial nerve paralysis may be caused by malignant tumors arising from or involving the temporal bone, parotid gland, CPA cistern, and skull base (51). If the cause of facial palsy is localized clinically to the parotid gland, IAC, CPA, or pons, enhanced MR imaging is the preferred imaging modality. If a seventh-nerve lesion is clinically nonlocalized, enhanced MR imaging also is the imaging modality of choice. If the abnormality is clinically localized to the tympanic cavity or mastoid facial canal, high-resolution CT with bone-window and level settings and enhanced MR imaging both may be used. Gadolinium-enhanced MR imaging is the modality of choice in the evaluation of acute facial nerve palsy (52).

Inflammatory Diseases

On MR images intralabyrinthine facial nerve enhancement or thickening in conjunction with facial palsy is seen with herpes zoster oticus, or Ramsay Hunt syndrome (Fig. 46). The geniculate, tympanic, and fundic segments of the facial nerve may show enhancement, and there may occasionally be associated enhancement of the eighth cranial nerve at the fundus of the IAC. These findings are intense compared with the mild enhancement of the facial nerve usually seen on contrast MR images, which is probably caused by brightening of the perineural vascular plexus that surrounds the intratemporal nerve segments. Bell's palsy may exhibit similar findings (Fig. 47).

Neoplasia

Tumor growth can occur anywhere along the course of the seventh cranial nerve. The geniculate ganglion is the most frequent intratemporal site (Fig. 48) (53). Facial schwannomas generally are rounded in the IAC and cigar shaped in the tympanic segment and fallopian canal (Fig. 49). Facial schwannoma occurs in the IAC and may be radiographically identical to acoustic schwannoma (54). Occasionally an eccentric location within the IAC may help to differentiate facial from acoustic schwannoma (55).

For accurate localization relative to local bony anatomy, high-resolution CT is the study of choice for facial schwannoma, and contrast MR imaging helps in general location (56). The tumors generally are well circumscribed and isodense to brain on unenhanced images. Contrast-enhanced images show homogeneous enhancement. The differential diagnosis of facial schwannoma

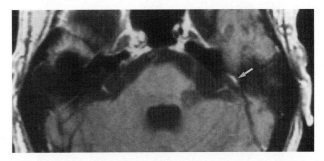

FIG. 47. Bell's palsy. Axial contrast enhanced T1-weighted MR image of temporal bones shows intense enhancement of the tympanic segment of the left facial nerve (*arrow*). This enhancement extended to the posterior genu and down the fallopian canal (not shown).

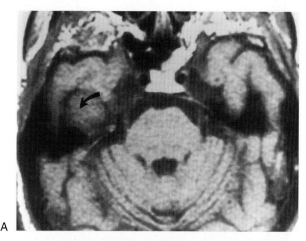

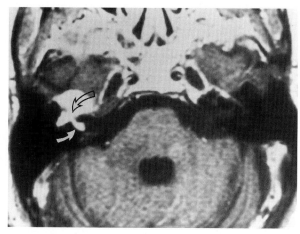

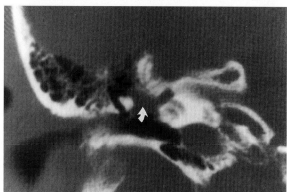

FIG. 48. Schwannoma of the geniculate ganglion. **A:** Axial precontrast MR image shows rounded soft-tissue mass near right petrous apex (*arrow*). Lesion is isointense to brain on T1-weighted images. **B:** Axial contrast-enhanced T1-weighted MR image shows mass centered at the geniculate ganglion (*open arrow*) and intense, homogeneous enhancement. Medially projecting tail (*white arrow*) represents tumor extension through labyrinthine segment into internal auditory canal. **C:** Coronal bone-window CT image of right side shows soft tissue in the middle ear cavity that displaces the ossicles laterally (*arrow*) and erosion of the medial wall of the epitympanum. The tympanic segment of the facial nerve was not visualized.

includes hemangioma, epidermoids, and primary brain tumors. Hemangiomas usually have indistinct borders and may contain calcium (Fig. 50) (57). Epidermoids usually have very well-circumscribed margins, are isodense or hypodense on precontrast images, and do not enhance after intravenous administration of contrast material (58).

When large, schwannoma of the geniculate ganglion may invaginate into the brain and mimic primary tumors of the temporal lobe of the brain or parenchymal metastatic lesions (59). A soft-tissue mass in the region of the proximal tympanic segment of the seventh cranial nerve caused by persistence of a stapedial artery may be misinterpreted as schwannoma of the facial nerve (58). This misdiagno-

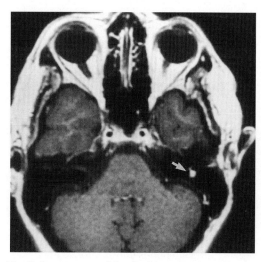

FIG. 49. Schwannoma of the facial nerve. Axial T1-weighted contrast image at level of mastoid facial nerve segment shows intense enhancement of enlarged nerve (*arrow*).

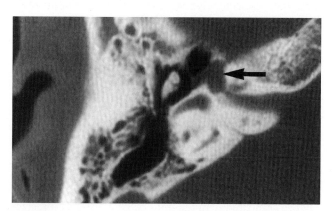

FIG. 50. Facial nerve hemangioma. Axial bone-window axial CT scan shows smooth enlargement of the fossa of the geniculate ganglion (*arrow*). CT appearance is nonspecific. The internal auditory canal is normal. The middle ear cavity shows no mass, and the ossicles are normal.

sis can be avoided with documentation of the absence of an ipsilateral foramen spinosum.

BENIGN LESIONS OF THE CEREBELLOPONTINE ANGLE

Masses found in the CPA cistern include neural, vascular, osseous, or meningeal lesions (Fig. 51). When a retrocochlear lesion is the suspected cause of vestibulocochlear symptoms, gadolinium-enhanced MR imaging is the modality of choice. MR imaging depicts the intrinsic signal characteristics and enhancement pattern of a lesion, gives evidence of local disruption of the blood-brain barrier, and allows multiplanar, fat-suppression, thin-section, high-resolution, and angiographic sequences. Cerebral and cervical angiography generally is reserved for evaluation of tumor vascularity, preoperative embolization, and detection of vascular anomalies.

Acoustic Schwannoma

Most acoustic schwannomas measure 1 to 4 cm in greatest dimension when first detected with CT or MR imaging. A small percentage are purely intracanalicular and measure less than 1 cm. Very large tumors are uncommon. Eighty-five percent of schwannomas show acute angles at the bone-tumor interface, and about 75% of meningiomas show obtuse bone-tumor angles (60). Arachnoid cysts may occur in association with larger acoustic schwannomas (61), but gross hemorrhage and calcification are rare (62). Larger tumors, accounting for approximately 20% of lesions, may contain central xan-

thomatous degeneration, cystic change, or hypocellularity and produce irregular peripheral enhancement (63).

At CT, more than half of all acoustic schwannomas are isodense to brain on noncontrast images (60). The others are of variable or mixed density. As many as two thirds of lesions enhance homogeneously and strongly after intravenous administration of contrast material (62). Enlargement of the ipsilateral IAC is common.

At MR evaluation, small and medium tumors generally are homogeneous in signal intensity, and larger tumors tend to show an irregular core. On T1-weighted images, acoustic schwannoma is mildly hypointense in two thirds of cases and isointense to brain tissue in the rest. On T2-weighted images acoustic schwannoma generally is mildly to markedly hyperintense relative to brain parenchyma. A distinct tumor-brain interface usually is found (see Fig. 38). The lesion is reliably centered on the IAC (Figs. 52, 53).

Bilateral acoustic tumors are seen with neurofibromatosis type 2 along with other cranial nerve schwannomas (37), meningiomas, and nonneoplastic intracranial calcifications, particularly of the choroid plexus. The trigeminal is the cranial nerve second most frequently involved in neurofibromatosis type 2 (64) (Fig. 54). The signal characteristics and enhancement pattern of nerve sheath tumors in neurofibromatosis type 2 are similar to those of isolated lesions.

Angiographic findings in schwannoma are variable. Most tumors appear as hypovascular or avascular lesions the presence of which is inferred on the basis of vascular displacement with draping or stretching of adjacent arter-

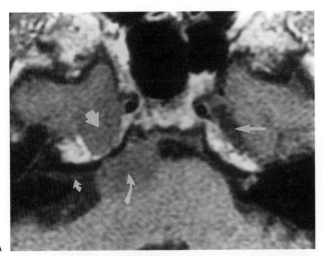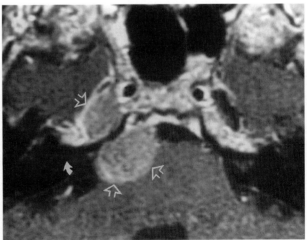

A B

FIG. 51. Trigeminal schwannoma. **A:** Axial T1-weighted precontrast MR image shows mass isointense to brain within the anterior aspect of the right cerebellopontine angle (CPA) cistern (*long curved arrow*) and effaces cerebrospinal fluid within the cistern. Mass is centered at level of Meckel's cave, and the normally low signal intensity of cerebrospinal fluid within that structure is not visible (*short arrow*). Contralateral Meckel's cave is normal (*long arrow*). The right internal auditory canal (IAC) is normal (*short curved arrow*). **B:** The borders of the mass in the right CPA cistern and right Meckel's cave are easier to appreciate after intravenous infusion of contrast agent (*open arrows*). There is no abnormal enhancement at the right IAC (*curved arrow*).

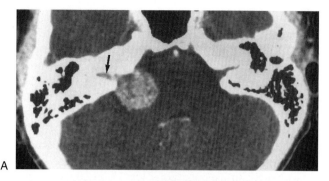

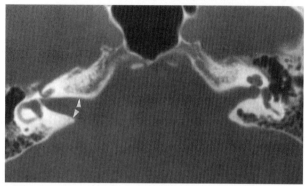

FIG. 52. Acoustic schwannoma. **A:** Axial contrast-enhanced CT image of temporal bones obtained with soft-tissue–window technique shows a rounded mass within the right cerebellopontine angle cistern and centered at the right internal auditory canal (IAC). The tumor exhibits heterogeneous enhancement. The enhancement extends into the fundic aspect of the IAC (*arrow*), a finding characteristic of schwannoma. **B:** Bone-window image of patient in **A** shows mild widening of the right IAC (*arrows*). There is no calcification of the tumor mass and no hyperostosis of the bone. Both are features of meningioma, not schwannoma.

ies and veins. Benign and malignant nerve sheath tumors cannot be reliably differentiated on the basis of angiographic patterns.

Meningioma

Meningioma is the most common nonglial primary extraaxial tumor. It accounts for 15% of all intracranial tumors and approximately 7% of all tumors of the CPA. The posterior surface of the petrous bone and clivus are the most common posterior fossa locations. Different from acoustic schwannoma, which generally is spherical or ovoid, most meningiomas are hemispherical and have a broad base against a dural surface. The tumors generally are sharply circumscribed and show a cleft of CSF and invaginated arachnoid where they indent into the surrounding brain parenchyma (65). Approximately 75% of meningiomas show an obtuse tumor-bone interface (66). The IAC is rarely enlarged.

On CT images, meningiomas are mildly hyperdense (75%) or isodense (25%) to brain on noncontrast images. As many as 25% of meningiomas are variably calcified, sometimes densely (66), and enhance homogeneously after intravenous administration of contrast medium (66). Peritumoral edema is seen in 60% of cases (67). Hyperostosis of the underlying bone is not frequent, but when present is highly characteristic (67).

At MR imaging, meningioma of the CPA is variable in signal intensity on T2-weighted images, but isointensity or mild hypointensity usually is seen. On T1-weighted images meningioma of the CPA is isointense. The signal variability of these lesions is a reflection of their variable histologic subtypes and the possible presence of calcification. Meningioma with primarily angioblastic or syncytial elements tends to be hyperintense to brain on T2-weighted images. Primarily fibro-

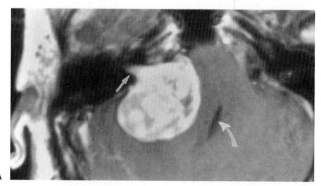

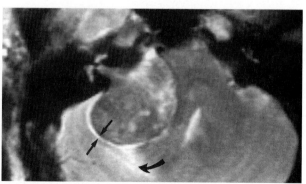

FIG. 53. Large right acoustic schwannoma. **A:** Axial contrast enhanced T1-weighted image shows tumor entering the right internal auditory canal (*straight arrow*). Image shows mass effect on brainstem and partial effacement of fourth ventricle (*curved arrow*), which is shifted to the left of midline. **B:** Axial T2-weighted image shows the subarachnoid space as a thin rim of hyperintensity surrounding the tumor (*straight arrows*), confirming the extraaxial location of the tumor. Mild peritumoral edema is visible as an area of T2-weighted high signal intensity posterior to the tumor (*curved arrow*).

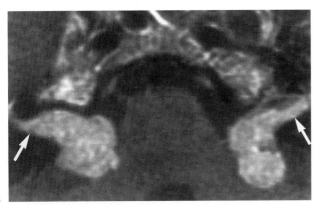
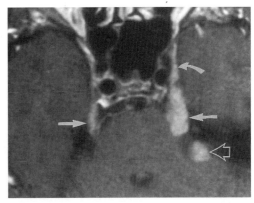

FIG. 54. Neurofibromatosis. **A:** Axial T1-weighted contrast-enhanced image through the posterior fossa shows bilateral nerve sheath tumors with dominant masses centered in the cerebellopontine angle (CPA) cisterns and tumor extension deep into the internal auditory canals (*arrows*). **B:** Same patient as in **A**. Image at level of porus trigeminus shows bilateral enhancing tumors of the fifth cranial nerve that extend from the trigeminal nerve root exit zone in the pons to Meckel's caves (*straight arrows*) and inferior cavernous sinuses (*curved arrow*). Dome of left acoustic tumor is visible in the left CPA cistern (*open arrow*).

blastic, calcific, or transitional tumors tend to be hypointense to normal brain on all sequences. Thickening and enhancement of the dura adjacent to a meningioma are seen in as many as 70% of cases and are believed to be a reaction to the presence of the tumor rather than tumor infiltration (67). This "dural tail" sign is not specific to meningioma and may be seen with a number of other tumors, including metastatic lesions (67). Cerebral angiograms of moderate-sized meningiomas show a primarily dural arterial supply. On images of large tumors, the pial supply also may been seen (68). A principal dural feeder usually supplies the tumor in a typically radial pattern. Late arterial and capillary phase images show a characteristic prolonged vascular blush. Intratumoral hemorrhage is rarely seen.

Meningioma has to be differentiated from schwannoma, lymphoma, leptomeningeal metastatic lesions, sarcoma, and localized inflammatory processes such as tuberculosis, sarcoidosis, Lyme disease, and idiopathic pachymeningitis (69).

Epidermoid Tumors

Epidermoid tumors represent 1% of all intracranial tumors and are the third most common mass of the CPA. As many as 50% of all epidermoid tumors occur in the CPA region. Ninety percent of these tumors are intradural; 10% are extradural, usually intradiploic (70). Intradural epidermoid tumors are uncommon in the temporal bone.

On CT scans, most epidermoid tumors appear as well-circumscribed, hypodense, lobulated lesions. The density of these tumors generally is similar to that of CSF. Intratumoral hemorrhage, fatty saponification, or densely proteinaceous debris may cause a hyperdense appearance on noncontrast images (71). Epidermoid tumors do not usually become enhanced, although marginal enhancement

occasionally is seen. Calcification is seen in less than one fourth of tumors (72).

Epidermoid tumors generally have long T1-weighted and T2-weighted values and tend to follow CSF signal on T1-weighted and T2-weighted sequences (Fig. 55). Epidermoids with a high lipid content occasionally may be hyperintense on T1-weighted images. These tumors are sometimes called "white epidermoids." Epidermoids

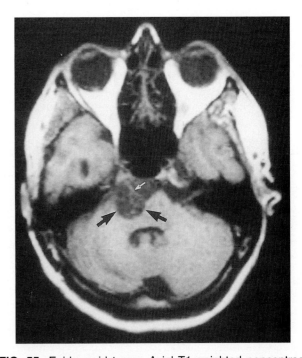

FIG. 55. Epidermoid tumor. Axial T1-weighted noncontrast MR image of temporal bones shows hypointense mass within right cerebellopontine angle cistern. The lesion causes smooth invagination into the pons and cerebellar peduncle (*black arrows*) and characteristically nondisplaced cranial nerves that traverse the lesion (*white arrow*).

with a low lipid content have very long T1-weighted values and are called "black epidermoids." Enhancement usually is not seen.

Arachnoid Cysts

Arachnoid cysts may resemble epidermoids. However, whereas epidermoids engulf structures so that vessels and cranial nerves are frequently seen traversing them, arachnoid cysts displace these structures (73). Arachnoid cysts may be associated with scalloping of the adjacent inner bony table, whereas epidermoid tumors are not. Diffusion-weighted scanning may be useful in differentiating these two lesions. Diffusion sequences show that arachnoid cysts have a low signal intensity, similar to that of water, whereas epidermoid tumors have apparent diffusion coefficients similar to those of brain parenchyma (74). Proton-density–weighted sequences may show slight hyperintensity of the epidermoid contents compared with the CSF in the basal cisterns and ventricles. Arachnoid cysts exhibit signal characteristics equal to those of CSF in all sequences. Arachnoid cysts may sometimes develop from arachnoid invagination associated with a CPA tumor, characteristically meningioma (Fig. 56).

Lipoma

Intracranial lipoma rarely is identified in the CPA on CT or MR images. They are congenital malformations resulting from maldifferentiation of the meninx primitiva, an embryologic structure that normally forms the leptomeninges. These lesions are nearly always incidental findings. The signal intensity follows that of fat on all MR pulse sequences and shows no enhancement after intravenous administration of contrast material. Lipoma rarely

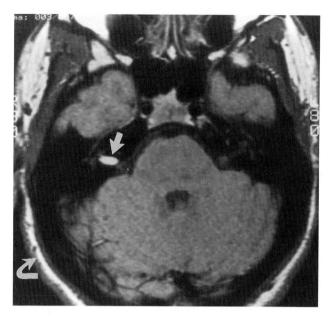

FIG. 57. Intracanalicular lipoma. Axial T1-weighted noncontrast MR of the temporal bone shows sausage-shaped, well-circumscribed area of hyperintensity (*straight arrow*) within normal-sized and fundic aspects of right internal auditory canal (IAC). Contralateral findings are normal. Signal intensity of lesion within IAC matches that of fat (*curved arrow*) on all sequences.

may occur within the IAC, where it can be confused with a small intracanalicular schwannoma (Fig. 57).

Vascular Lesions

Ectasia of the basilar and vertebral arteries may be the most common posterior fossa vascular lesion to cause compressive cranial deficits. Vertebrobasilar ectasia is defined as a cross-sectional diameter of the basilar artery larger than 4.5 mm. The basilar artery is considered tortuous and elongated if the basilar tip is above the plane of the suprasellar cistern and extends lateral to the body of the clivus, or the dorsum sella. If symptoms are present, patients with elongated but nondilated vertebrobasilar systems tend to have mononeuropathy, whereas those with dolichoectasia of these vessels may have polyneuropathy and other central nervous system symptoms.

MR imaging is the study of choice for evaluation of the vertebrobasilar system, because the vascular flow voids are well depicted on axial T2-weighted images. MRA with three-dimensional time-of-flight or phase-contrast techniques can provide an angiographic view of these vessels and has largely replaced cerebral digital subtraction angiography (75). Helical contrast-enhanced CT with or without three-dimensional reconstruction is proving useful in evaluating partially thrombosed ectatic basilar arteries; this study depicts both the patent and thrombosed portions of the vessel (Fig. 58), and the possibility of MR-related flow phenomena is eliminated.

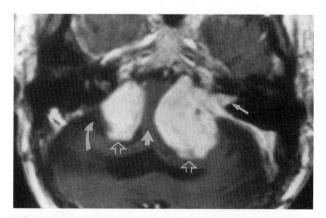

FIG. 56. Neurofibromatosis. Axial T1-weighted postcontrast MR image of posterior fossa shows large, heterogeneous enhancing masses centered at IACs (*open arrows*). The left-sided mass is entering the IAC (*long arrow*). Both masses markedly compress interposed brainstem (*short arrow*). The right-sided tumor has an associated arachnoid cyst posterior to the lesion (*curved arrow*).

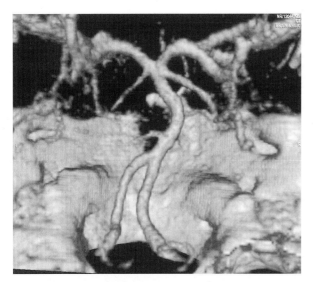

FIG. 58. Vertebrobasilar ectasia. Coronal, curved, multiplanar, reformatted CT image shows dilated, ectatic vertebral artery containing calcifications and a very mild mass effect on the adjacent brain.

Giant aneurysms are those larger than 2.5 cm in maximal diameter. These lesions, which are frequently partly thrombosed, may cause compressive or ischemic symptoms. Enhanced CT images typically show a nonenhancing, isodense, crescentic mural thrombus and an eccentric, patent lumen. A calcified rim may be present (Fig. 59). MR imaging shows a flow void in a patent lumen, peripheral thrombus with variable signal intensities, and occasionally a hemosiderin-laden T2-weighted hypointense rim.

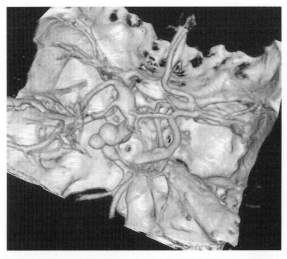

FIG. 59. Basilar artery aneurysm. Axial single-section multiplanar reformatted CT image shows 4-cm aneurysm of the vertebrobasilar junction with marked mass effect on the adjacent pons and medulla.

Loops associated with the anterior inferior cerebellar artery (AICA) may occasionally be associated with acoustic nerve dysfunction. The vascular loop may be found adjacent to the facial and acoustic nerves within the CPA cistern, porus acusticus, or IAC. CT cisternography with intrathecal administration of contrast material demonstrates well the cisternal course of the anterior superior cerebellar artery. MRA does not consistently demonstrate the AICA. Thin-section T2-weighted images may show the cisternal AICA.

BENIGN TUMORS AND TUMOR-LIKE LESIONS

Exostosis and Osteoma of the External Auditory Canal

Exostosis of the EAC is most frequently associated with long-term exposure to cold water (76). Exostosis differs from osteoma both radiographically and histologically. Exostosis is a sessile proliferation of dense lamellar bone; osteoma is a pedunculated growth of mature bone that contains fibrovascular spaces and often an attachment to suture lines (Fig. 60). As shown at CT, the bony growth in exostosis is frequently bilateral, is located in the osseous portion of the EAC, usually is broad based, and arises along the tympanomastoid or tympanosquamous suture lines. Osteoma usually is congenital and unilateral and can arise from any portion of the temporal bone (77).

The radiographic differential diagnosis of bony lesions of the EAC includes atresia of the EAC, chondroid tumors, fibrous dysplasia, and Paget's disease. Congenital atresia of the EAC is discussed earlier. Dysplasia can lead to stenosis of the EAC, but the bony changes are typically more extensive and may involve other portions of the temporal bone and skull.

Fibrous Dysplasia

Fibrous dysplasia is a benign focal skeletal disorder of fibroblasts that replaces the normal intramedullary contents of lamellar bone with proliferative, vascular, fibrocellular tissue and abnormal immature woven bone (78). The temporal bone is infrequently affected. CT findings may vary, but the typical appearance is expanded, sclerotic bone with intact cortices and a homogeneous ground glass appearance of the medullary space. In the early active stage of the disease, the medullary space may have a fairly lucent appearance. Some lesions may exhibit a mixture of lucent and sclerotic changes. Variable enhancement is seen after intravenous administration of contrast material (79).

At MR examinations the abnormal bone appears homogeneously isointense on T1-weighted images and heterogeneously hypointense on T2-weighted images. Gadolinium-enhanced sequences show heterogeneous enhancement that is variable between lesions and proportional to the presence of vascular components in the lesion (Fig. 61).

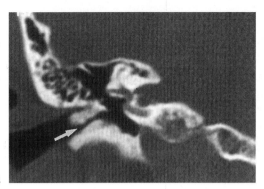 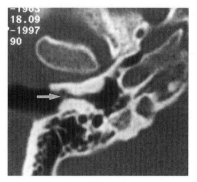

FIG. 60. Exostosis. Coronal **(A)** and axial **(B)** bone-window CT sections of right temporal bone show segmental thickening of bony walls of right external auditory canal with marked narrowing of canal lumen (*arrows*). The process is bilaterally symmetric (not shown). Other otic structures are normal.

Glomus Tumors

Paraganglioma is the second most common tumor of the temporal bone (80). CT and MR imaging are complementary in the evaluation of these tumors; CT shows the bony changes, and MR imaging shows the soft-tissue extent. Mass effect may cause demineralization of the jugular plate or lateral caroticojugular spine with a characteristic "moth-eaten" pattern on CT scans (81). Larger tumors have a characteristic heterogeneous pattern of T1-weighted hypointensity and T2-weighted hyperintensity (82). Branching flow voids reflective of the highly vascular nature of these tumors also are seen. Care should be taken not to confuse flow-related high signal intensity in the jugular bulb with abnormal signal intensity arising from a glomus jugulare tumor. Radionuclide scintigraphy with indium 111 octreotide and iodine 123 metaiodobenzylguanidine have proved useful in evaluations for recurrent disease (83).

Tumors of the glomus tympanicum appear as well-defined, intratympanic soft-tissue masses without bone or ossicular destruction (Fig. 62) (84). High-resolution CT is the imaging study of choice for describing tumor extent and for surgical planning. These tumors are hypervascular and therefore enhance well after intravenous infusion of contrast material. MRA does not reliably demonstrate the characteristic vascularity of the tumor.

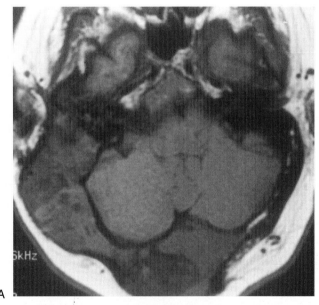 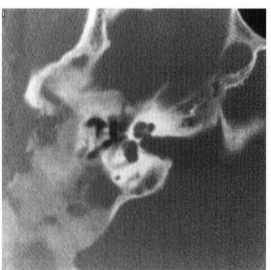

FIG. 61. Fibrous dysplasia. **A:** Axial T1-weighted image at level of mastoid temporal bone shows marked focal expansion of medullary space of right mastoid, sphenoid, and occipital bones by soft tissue of heterogeneous signal intensity. **B:** Axial CT image obtained with bone-window technique shows the lesion has expanded the bone without destroying cortex and shows a characteristic ground glass appearance.

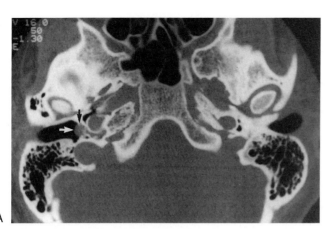
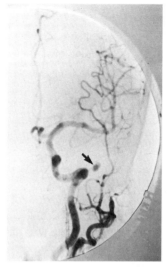

A　　　　　　　　　　　　　　　　　　　　　　　　　B

FIG. 62. Glomus tympanicum. **A:** Axial noncontrast CT image obtained with bone-window technique shows small, well-circumscribed soft-tissue mass (*white arrow*) at level of inferior tympanic annulus (*black arrow*). The small bluish mass was visible at otoscopic examination. **B:** Right internal common carotid artery injection, mid–arterial phase, digital subtraction angiogram in anteroposterior projection shows small, rounded intense contrast blush at level of tympanic membrane characteristic of glomus tympanicum tumor (*arrow*).

Hemangioma

Hemangioma may occasionally arise (in order of frequency) in the geniculate ganglion, posterior genu of the facial nerve, middle ear, and IAC (Fig. 63). Hemangioma of the tympanic membrane is rare (Fig. 64). Hemangiomas are usually small at time of diagnosis. Small tumors are frequently missed on CT scans, particularly when they are in the IAC (85). Hemangiomas of the IAC are well characterized at MR imaging, but those of the anterior genu may be more easily detected with CT,

which shows mild expansion and bone erosion (55). These lesions are markedly hyperintense on T2-weighted images and generally are isointense on T1-weighted images. Larger tumors are well seen on CT scans obtained with bone-window techniques and MR images obtained with T2-weighted sequences. CT scans may show a honeycomb appearance of the bone adjacent to the tumor, whereas MR images demonstrate only heterogeneous osseous signal intensities.

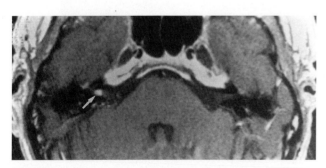

FIG. 63. Hemangioma of internal auditory canal (IAC) in a 58-year-old woman without auditory symptoms. Axial T1-weighted postcontrast MR image of right temporal bone shows small, rounded, intensely enhancing mass in fundic aspect of the IAC (*white arrow*). The lesion was isointense to brain on the precontrast T1-weighted images and mildly hyperintense on the T2-weighted images. There is no enlargement of the IAC or enhancement of the dura of the canal wall. The geniculate and tympanic segments of the right seventh cranial nerve are normal.

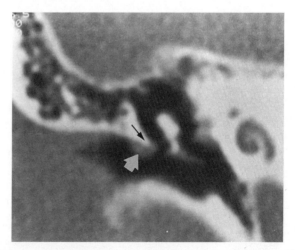

FIG. 64. Hemangioma of tympanic membrane. Coronal CT image obtained with bone-window technique shows small soft-tissue density within medial aspect of right external auditory canal (*white arrow*) adjacent to scutum (*black arrow*). The mass was bluish at otoscopy. The CT appearance is nonspecific. The tympanic membrane is not visible.

MALIGNANT TUMORS

General Findings

The cardinal CT and MR findings of an aggressive malignant tumor are an infiltrating, poorly marginated mass that obliterates fascial planes and replaces rather than displaces structures in its path (Fig. 65). Contrast-enhanced MR imaging is the modality of choice for evaluation of the skull base. The most common sites of intrusion are the petroclinoid fissure and foramen lacerum; temporal bone involvement is seen less often.

T1-weighted MR images generally reveal a mass that is isointense to muscle. T2-weighted images show a mass hyperintense to both muscle and bone and fairly homogeneous enhancement. Cortical bone destruction can be detected at MR imaging by means of identifying disruption of the thin curvilinear contour and the normally low T1-weighted and T2-weighted signal intensity of intact cortex. Bone marrow invasion should also be sought and is best seen on noncontrast T1-weighted images, which show replacement of the normal hyperintense fatty marrow signal with bland tissue that is T1-weighted isointense to muscle and enhances after intravenous adminis-

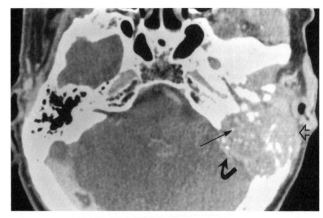

FIG. 65. Squamous cell carcinoma metastatic to temporal bone. Axial contrast-enhanced CT image through the temporal bones shows enhancing mass centered in the left temporal bone. The mass has an aggressive appearance with destruction of the otic capsule (*straight arrow*), epidural tumor extension (*curved arrow*), and cortical breach with invasion of the subcutaneous soft tissues (*open arrow*).

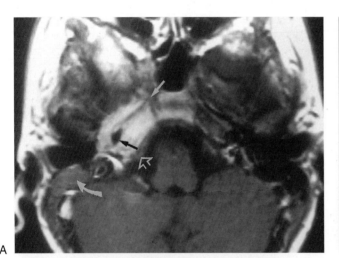

A

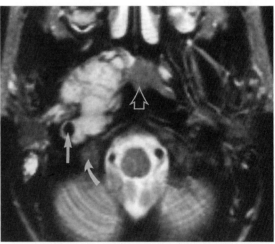

B

C

FIG. 66. Alveolar rhabdomyosarcoma. **A:** Axial contrast-enhanced T1-weighted image of temporal bones shows enhancing mass in the right petrous apex, Rosenmüller's fossa (*straight white arrow*), and petroclival fissure region. The petrous segment of the carotid artery is encased by tumor (*black arrow*). There is nonenhancing abnormal signal in right mastoid air cells (*curved white arrow*). Tumor is visible in the epidural space of the right cerebellopontine angle cistern (*open white arrow*). **B:** Axial T2-weighted image at level of clivus shows mass is hyperintense to brain and appears lobulated. True extent of tumor is better depicted than on T1-weighted images. Image shows encased cervical internal carotid artery (*straight arrow)* and normal marrow signal within the clivus (*open arrow*) and right occipital condyle (*curved arrow*). **C:** Same patient as in **A** and **B**. Axial bone-window CT image shows petrous apex and petroclival fissures have been destroyed by the infiltrative mass. Small bone fragments are visible within the tumor bed (*solid arrows*), indicating a very aggressive lesion. Presence of sphenooccipital synchondrosis (*open arrow*) indicates skeletal immaturity.

tration of contrast material. Central necrosis may be seen in the primary tumor or, more commonly, in nodal metastatic lesions. CT is superior to MR imaging in identifying small areas of bone destruction. MR imaging is superior in detection of perineural tumor spread. It provides excellent definition of soft-tissue planes and allows more sensitive detection of enhancement related to malignant invasion of nerves (86).

Rhabdomyosarcoma

Rhabdomyosarcoma is a rare malignant tumor of mesenchymal origin (87). One third of these tumors involve the head and neck. Skull base invasion is common. On CT images, rhabdomyosarcoma appears as an infiltrating soft-tissue mass that may cause skull base destruction. The MR features of rhabdomyosarcoma are similar to those of squamous cell carcinoma. On T2-weighted images the signal intensity of rhabdomyosarcoma is frequently more heterogeneous than that of squamous cell carcinoma (Fig. 66) (88). Enhancement generally is moderate and somewhat heterogeneous.

Regional Extensions

Nasopharyngeal carcinoma may gain access to the temporal bone through the sinus of Morgagni, which is a defect in the superolateral aspect of the pharyngobasilar fascia through which the cartilaginous eustachian tube and tensor veli palatini muscle pass. Tumor extension by this route is well delineated on MR images as abnormal signal intensity and enhancement.

Chloroma

Patients with acute myelogenous leukemia may have focal infiltrates of leukemic cells called *granulocytic sarcoma*. The term *chloroma* also is frequently applied to such deposits because of the elaboration of myeloperoxidase by the tumor cells, which on visual examination imparts a greenish hue to the tissue. Densely cellular tumors such as chloroma and tumors with high nucleus to cytoplasmic ratios are electron rich and therefore have high attenuation values on noncontrast CT studies. Chloroma appear as a hyperdense dura-based lesion on unenhanced CT scans (Fig. 67). Postcontrast images typically show homogeneous enhancement of the tumor. Permeative changes of the underlying bone are possible but not common. MR image scans show a lesion that is isointense to brain on T1-weighted sequences. The hypercellularity typical of these tumors is reflected as hypointensity relative to brain tissue on T2-weighted images, an indication of the lower water content of highly cellular tumors. Homogeneous and prominent enhancement is typical after intravenous administration of contrast material (81).

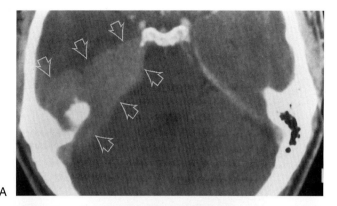

A

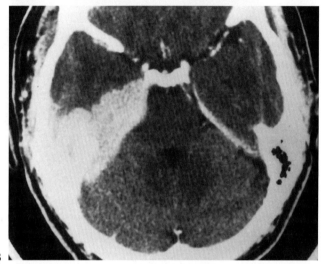

B

FIG. 67. Chloroma. **A:** Axial noncontrast soft-tissue–window CT image shows mass hyperdense to normal brain and centered within the right temporal bone and petrous ridge. There is a mass effect on the adjacent temporal lobe and cerebellum (*arrows*). **B:** Same patient as in **A**. Postcontrast axial CT image obtained with soft-tissue window shows intense homogeneous enhancement of soft-tissue mass.

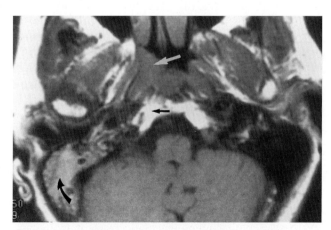

FIG. 68. Lymphoma. Axial noncontrast T1-weighted image of posterior fossa shows asymmetric mass in right nasopharynx effacing right Rosenmüller's fossa (*white arrow*). The mastoid air cells are opacified (*curved black arrow*) by more hyperintense material because of mechanical effacement of the eustachian tube. The signal intensity of the marrow within the occipital condyles is normal, indicating no invasion (*straight black arrow*).

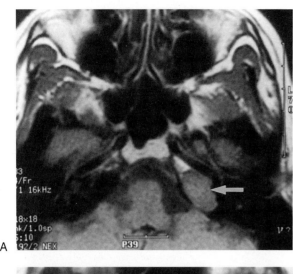

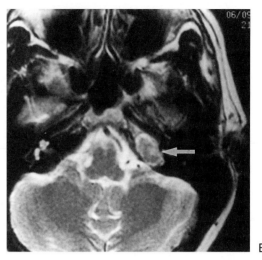

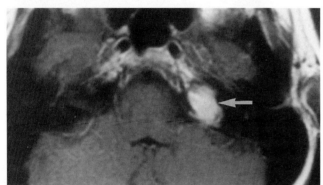

FIG. 69. Meningioma of the petrous apex. **A:** Axial T1-weighted images show an oval, smoothly marginated soft-tissue mass in the left cerebellopontine angle cistern (*arrow*). The mass depresses the left seventh and eight cranial nerve complexes and has caused smooth remodeling of the left petrous apex. **B:** Axial T2-weighted images show lesion is heterogeneous in signal intensity (*arrow*). **C:** After intravenous infusion of contrast medium the mass enhances homogeneously and strongly (*arrow*).

Lymphoma

Lymphoma may be neural, leptomeningeal, or primary (89). Nasopharyngeal lymphoma may involve the temporal bone through mechanical obstruction of the eustachian tube with secondary opacification (Fig. 68) or may extend through the foramen of Morgagni into the middle ear cavity and mastoid region. Direct invasion is less common. Primary temporal bone lymphoma is rare. The CT appearance of extranodal lymphoma is nonspecific. MR imaging of highly cellular tumors such as lymphoma may reveal low T2-weighted signal intensity relative to adjacent brain. Enhancement generally is moderate to intense and usually is homogeneous (Fig. 69).

Carcinomatous Meningitis

Seeding of CSF by malignant cells from a metastatic tumor may lead to neoplastic coating of the cranial nerves and basal leptomeninges. Focal deposits of malignant cells accumulating in the IAC may mimic a small acoustic schwannoma (Fig. 70). Contrast-enhanced MR imaging is the study of choice. CT with or without administration of contrast material generally lacks the resolution necessary to detect subtle temporal deposits.

The correct diagnosis usually can be established with documentation of abnormal leptomeningeal enhancement elsewhere in the posterior fossa and basal cisterns. The differential diagnosis includes bacterial, mycobacterial, and fungal meningitis.

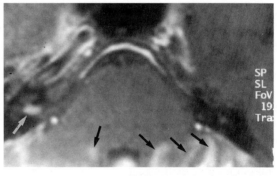

FIG. 70. Carcinomatous meningitis. Axial postcontrast T1-weighted image through skull base shows abnormal leptomeningeal enhancement within the cerebellar sulci and right lateral recess of the fourth ventricle (*black arrows*). Abnormal enhancement also is visible within the right internal auditory canal (*white arrow*). The appearance is nonspecific. Cytologic examination of the cerebrospinal fluid revealed metastatic carcinoma of the breast.

SUMMARY POINTS

- A thorough knowledge of the normal cross-sectional anatomy of the temporal bone is a prerequisite to understanding the imaging appearance of pathologic conditions that affect the temporal bone.
- CT is the imaging tool of choice when the pathologic process involves primary bones or air spaces.
- MR imaging is superior to CT in imaging soft tissues such as blood vessels, bone with fatty marrow, and CSF spaces.
- Temporal bone MR imaging with intravenous infusion of contrast medium generally is the imaging study of choice for adult patients with SNHL.
- Patients with conductive hearing loss benefit from noncontrast high-resolution CT of the temporal bones.
- Mixed hearing loss usually is evaluated first with high-resolution bone-algorithm CT. If the sensorineural component of the mixed defect predominates, MR imaging may be the more appropriate first study.
- Congenital ear anomalies and vascular anomalies are best evaluated with CT. Intravenous infusion of contrast medium is routinely used for vascular anomalies.
- Temporal bone trauma associated with hearing loss, vertigo, facial nerve paralysis, CSF leakage, or delayed complications such as cholesteatoma is best evaluated with high-resolution CT. MR imaging generally is reserved for problem cases in which facial paralysis and vestibular syndromes are present but unexplained with CT findings.
- Both CT and MR imaging are effective tools in the evaluation of complications resulting from inflammatory disease of the temporal bone; CT generally is sufficient.
- Because of superior soft-tissue characterization, MR imaging generally is preferred in the evaluation of malignant and nonmalignant masses involving the temporal bone.

REFERENCES

1. Dastidar P, Pertti R, Karhuketo T. Axial high-resolution CT, 2D and MIP reconstruction in temporal bone lesions. *Acta Otolaryngol Suppl (Stockh)* 1997;529:43–46.
2. Mayer TE, Bruecekmann H, Siegert R, Witt A, Weerda H. High resolution CT of the temporal bone in dysplasia of the auricle and external auditory canal. *AJNR Am J Neuroradiol* 1997;18:53–65.
3. Swartz JD, Faerber EN. Congenital malformations of the external canal and middle ear. *AJNR Am J Neuroradiol* 1985;6:501–506.
4. Weissman JL. Hearing loss. *Radiology* 1996;199:593–611.
5. Brookhouser, PE. Sensorineural hearing loss in children. In: Cummings CW, Fredrickson JM, Harker AL, Krause CJ, Schuller DE, eds. *Otolaryngology–head and neck surgery,* 2nd ed. St. Louis: Mosby–Year Book, 1993:3080–3102.
6. Jackler RK, Luxford M, House WF. Congenital malformations of the inner ear: a classification system based on embryogenesis. *Laryngoscope* 1987;97:2–14.
7. Hasso AN, Broadwell RE. The temporal bone: congenital anomalies. In: Som PM, Bergerton RT, eds. *Head and neck imaging,* 2nd ed. St. Louis: Mosby–Year Book, 1991:960–992.
8. Lowe LH, Vezina LG. Sensorineural hearing loss in children. *Radiographics* 1997;17:1091–1093.
9. Curtin HD. Congenital malformations of the ear. *Otolaryngol Clin North Am* 1988;221:317–336.
10. Okumura T, Takahashi H, Honjo I, Takagi A, Mitamura K. Sensorineural hearing loss in patients with large vestibular aqueduct. *Laryngoscope* 1995;105;289–293.
11. Quint D, Silbergleit R. Congenital absence of the left internal carotid artery. *Radiology* 1992;182:477–481.
12. Anderson JM, Stevens JL, Sundt TM Jr, et al. Ectopic internal carotid artery seen initially as middle ear tumor. *JAMA* 1983;249:2228–2230.
13. Sinnreich AI, Parisier SC, Cohen NL, et al. Arterial malformations of the middle ear. *Otolaryngol Head Neck Surg* 1984;92:194–206.
14. Vignaud J, Jardin C, Rosen L. *The ear: diagnostic imaging.* Paris: Masson Publishing, 1986;104–145.
15. Ford KL 3rd. Aunt Minnie's corner: high-riding jugular bulb. *J Comput Assist Tomogr* 1998;22:508.
16. Schubiger O, Valavanis A, Stuckman G, et al. Temporal bone fractures and their complications: examination with high resolution CT. *Neuroradiology* 1986;28:93–99.
17. Lee D, Honrado C, Har-El G, Goldsmith A. Pediatric temporal bone fractures. *Laryngoscope* 1998;108:816–821.
18. Zimmerman RA, Bilianuk LT, Hackney DB, et al. Magnetic resonance imaging in temporal bone fracture. *Neuroradiology* 1987:29:246.
19. Guerrissi JD. Facial nerve paralysis after intratemporal and extratemporal blunt trauma. *J Craniofacial Surgery* 1997;8:431–437.
20. Ghorayeb BR, Yeakley JW. Temporal bone fractures: longitudinal or oblique? The case for oblique temporal bone fractures. *Laryngoscope* 1992;102:129–134.
21. Fisch U. Facial paralysis and fractures of the petrous bone. *Laryngoscope* 1974;84:2141–2154.
22. Aguilar EA III, Yeakley JW, Ghorayeb BY, et al. High resolution CT scan of temporal bone fractures: association of facial nerve paralysis with temporal bone fractures. *Head Neck Surg* 1987;9:161–166.
23. Neely JG, Neblett CR, Rose JE. Diagnosis and treatment of spontaneous cerebrospinal fluid otorrhea. *Laryngoscope* 1982;92:608–612.
24. Gentry LR. Temporal bone trauma: current perspective for diagnostic evaluation. *Neuroimaging Clin N Am* 1991;1:319–340.
25. Mafee MF, Singleton EL, Valvassori GE, et al. Acute otomastoiditis and its complications: role of CT. *Radiology* 1985;155:391–423.
26. Holliday RA. MRI of mastoid and middle ear disease. *Radiol Clin North Am* 1989;27:283–299.
27. Murakami T, Tsubaki J, Tahara Y, Nagashima T. Gradenigo's syndrome: CT and MRI findings. *Pediatr Radiol* 1996;26:684–685.
28. Bluestone CD, Cantekin EI. Eustachian tube dysfunction. In: English GM, ed. *Otolaryngology.* New York: Harper & Row, 1979.
29. Buckingham RA. Cholesteatoma in chronic otitis media following middle ear intubation. *Laryngoscope* 1981;91:1415–1456.
30. Pratt LL, Murray J. The placement of middle ear ventilation tubes: some indications and complications. *Laryngoscope* 1973;83:1022–1026.
31. Swartz JD, Goodman RS, Russell KB, et al. High resolution computed tomography of the middle ear and mastoid, III: surgically altered anatomy and pathology. *Radiology* 1983;148:461–464.
32. Swartz JD, Berger AS, Zwillenberg S, et al. Ossicular erosions of the dry ear: CT diagnosis. *Radiology* 1987;163:765–765.
33. Swartz JD, Goodman RS, Russell KB, et al. High resolution computed tomography of the middle ear and mastoid, II: tubotympanic disease. *Radiology* 1983;148:455–459.
34. Cummings CW, Fredrickson JM, Harker LA, Krause CJ, Schuller DE, eds. *Otolaryngology–head and neck surgery.* St. Louis: Mosby, 1986.

35. Garber LZ, Dort JC. Cholesteatoma: diagnosis and staging by CT scan. *J Otolaryngol* 1994;23:121–124.

36. Mafee MF, Kumar A, Heffner DK. Epidermoid cyst (cholesteatoma) and cholesterol granuloma of the temporal bone and epidermoid cysts affecting the brain. *Neuroimaging Clin N Am* 1994;4:561–578.

37. Phelps PD, Lloyd GAS. The radiology of cholesteatoma. *Clin Radiol* 1980;31:501–512.

38. Phelps PD, Lloyd GA. Vascular masses in the middle ear. *Clin Radiol* 1986;37:359–364.

39. Sade J, Berco E, Buyanover D. Ossicular damage in chronic middle ear inflammation. In: Sade J, ed. *Cholesteatoma and mastoid surgery.* Amsterdam: Kugler, 1982:347–358.

40. Ishi K, Takahashi S, Matsumoto K. Middle ear cholesteatoma extending into the petrous apex. *AJNR Am J Neuroradiol* 1991;12:719–724.

41. Larson TL, Wong ML. Primary mucocele of the petrous apex. *AJNR Am J Neuroradiol* 1992;13:203–204.

42. Silver AJ, Janecka I, Wazen J, et al. Complicated cholesteatomas: CT findings in inner ear complications of middle ear cholesteatomas. *Radiology* 1987;164:47.

43. Sade J. Pathogenesis of attic cholesteatoma. *J R Soc Med* 1978;71:716–732.

44. Swartz JD. Cholesteatomas of the middle ear: diagnosis, etiology and complications. *Radiol Clin North Am* 1984;22:15–35.

45. Mark AS, Seltzer S, Nelson-Drake J, et al. Labyrinthine enhancement on GD MRI in patients with sudden hearing loss and vertigo. *Ann Otol Rhinol Laryngol* 1992;101:459–464.

46. Belai A Jr, Ylikoski J. Poststapedectomy dizziness: a histopathologic agent. *Am J Otol* 1982;3:187–191.

47. Muckle RP, Delacruz A, Lo WM. Petrous apex lesions. *Am J Otol* 1998;19:219–225.

48. Gomori JM, Grossman RI. Mechanisms responsible for the MR appearance and evolution of intracranial hemorrhage. *Radiographics* 1988;8:427.

49. Martin N, Sterkers O, Nahum H. Chronic inflammatory disease of the middle ear cavities: Dg-DTPA enhanced MR imaging. *Radiology* 1990;176:399–405.

50. Khang P, Fagan PA, Atlas MD, Roche J. Imaging destructive lesions of the petrous apex. *Laryngoscope* 1998;108:599–604.

51. Latack JT, Gabrielsen TO, Knake JE, et al. Facial nerve neuromas: radiologic evaluation. *Radiology* 1983;149:731–739.

52. Chen JM, Moll C, Wichmann W, Kurrer MO, Fisch U. Magnetic resonance imaging and intraoperative frozen sections in intraoperative facial schwannomas. *Am J Otol* 1995;16:68–74.

53. Fagan PA, Misra SN, Doust B. Facial neuroma of the cerebellopontine angle and the internal auditory canal. *Laryngoscope* 1993;103:442–446.

54. Kuzma BB, Goodman JM. Pitfalls in facial nerve enhancement on MRI. *Surg Neurol* 1997;48:636–637.

55. Lo WWM, Shelton C, Waluch VM, et al. Intratemporal vascular tumors: detection with CT and MR imaging. *Radiology* 1989;171:443–449.

56. Kallmes DF, Provenzale JM, Cloft HJ, McClendon RE. Typical and atypical MR imaging features of intracranial epidermoid tumors. *AJR Am J Roentgenol* 1997;169:883–887.

57. Kienzle GD, Goldenberg MH, Just NW, et al. Facial nerve neurinoma presenting as middle cranial fossa mass: CT appearance. *J Comput Assist Tomogr* 1986;10:391–394.

58. Pahor AL, Hussain SSM. Persistent stapedial artery. *J Laryngol Otol* 1992;106:254–257.

59. Saeed SR Sr, Birzgalis AR, Ramsden RT. Intralabyrinthine schwannoma shows by magnetic resonance imaging. *Neuroradiology* 1994;36:63–64.

60. Bilianuk LT. Adult infratentorial tumors. *Semin Roentgenol* 1990;25:155–173.

61. Nezmek WR. The trigeminal nerve. *Top Magn Reson Imaging* 1996;8:132–154.

62. Kim SH, Youn JY, Song SH, Kim Y, Song KS. Vestibular schwannoma with repeated intratumoral hemorrhage. *Clin Neurol Neurosurg* 1998;100:68–74.

63. Cohen LM, Schwartz AM, Rockoff SD. Benign schwannomas: pathologic basis for CT inhomogeneities. *AJR Am J Roentgenol* 1986;147:141–143.

64. Thomas NW, King TT. Meningiomas of the cerebellopontine angle: a report of 41 cases. *Br J Neurosurg* 1996;10:59–68.

65. Sheporaitis L, Osborn AG, Smirniotopoulos JG, Clunie DA, Howieson J, D'Agostino AN. Intracranial meningioma. *AJNR Am J Neuroradiol* 1992;13:29–37.

66. Valavanis A, Schubiger O, Hayek J, et al. CT of meningiomas on the posterior surface of the petrous bone. *Neuroradiology* 1981;22:111–121.

67. Rubenstein LJ. Tumors of the central nervous system. In: Friminger HI, ed. *Atlas of tumor pathology,* 2nd series, fascicle 6. Washington, DC: Armed Forces Institute of Pathology, 1972:169–292.

68. Osborn AG. The external carotid artery. In: *Introduction to cerebral angiography,* Hagerstown, MD: Harper & Row, 1980:49–86.

69. Phillips ME, Ryals TJ, Kambhu SA, et al. Neoplastic vs inflammatory meningeal enhancement with Gd-DTPA. *J Comput Assist Tomogr* 1990;14:536–542.

70. Ruge JR, Tomashitas T, Naidich TP, et al. Scalp and calvarial masses of infants and children. *Neurosurgery* 1988;22:1037–1042.

71. Tekok IH, Cataltepe O, Saglam S. Dense epidermoid cyst of the cerebellopontine angle. *Neuroradiology* 1991;33:255–257.

72. Gao PY, Osborn AG, Smirniotopoulus JG, Harris CP. Epidermoid tumor of the cerebellopontine angle. *AJNR Am J Neuroradiol* 1992;13:863–872.

73. Quint DJ. Retroclival arachnoid cysts. *AJNR Am J Neuroradiol* 1992;13:1503–1504.

74. Maeda M, Kawamura Y, Tamagawa Y, et al. Intravoxel incoherent motion (IVIM) MRI in intracranial, extracranial tumors and cysts. *J Comp Assist Tomogr* 1992;16:514–518.

75. Ballantine ES, Page RD, Meaney JFM, et al. Coexistent trigeminal neuralgia, hemifacial spasm, and hypertension. *J Neurosurg* 1994;80:559–563.

76. Deleyiannis FW, Cockcroft BD, Adlam EF. Exostoses of the external auditory canal in Oregon surfers. *Am J Otolaryngol* 1996;17:303–307.

77. Denia A, Perez F, Canalis RR, et al. Extracanalicular osteomas of the temporal bone. *Arch Otolaryngol* 1979;105:706.

78. Leeds NE, Seaman WB. Fibrous dysplasia of the skull and its differential diagnosis. *Radiology* 1962;78:570–578.

79. Casselman JW, DeJonge I, Neyt L, et al. MRI in craniofacial fibrous dysplasia. *Neuroradiology* 1993;35:234–237.

80. Batsakis JG. *Tumors of the head and neck: clinical and pathological considerations,* 2nd ed. Baltimore: Williams & Wilkins, 1979:369–380.

81. Caldemyer KS, Mathews VP, Azzarelli B, Smith RR. The jugular foramen: a review of anatomy, masses and imaging characteristics. *Radiographics* 1997;17:1123–1139.

82. Olsen WL, Dillon WP, Kelly WM, et al. MR imaging of paragangliomas. *AJR Am J Roentgenol* 1987;148:201–204.

83. Kwekkeboom DJ, Van Urk H, Paun BKH, et al. Octreotide scintigraphy for the detection of paragangliomas. *J Nucl Med* 1993;34:873–878.

84. Larson TC III, Reese DF, Baker HL Jr, et al. Glomus tympanicum chemodectomas: radiologic and clinical characteristics. *Radiology* 1987;163:801–806.

85. Lo WWM, Horn KL, Carberry JN, et al. Intratemporal vascular tumors: evaluation with CT. *Radiology* 1986;159:181–185.

86. Mendenhall WM, Million RR, Mancuso AA, et al. Nasopharynx. In: Million RR, Cassisi NJ, eds. *Management of head and neck cancer: a multidisciplinary approach.* Philadelphia: JB Lippincott, 1994:603–626.

87. Canalis RF, Jenkens HA, Hemenway WG, et al. Nasopharyngeal rhabdomyosarcoma: a clinical perspective. *Arch Otolaryngol Head Neck Surg* 1978;104:122–126.

88. Scotti G, Harwood-Nash DC. Computed tomography of rhabdomyosarcomas of the skull base in children. *J Comput Assist Tomogr* 1982;6:33–39.

89. Berciano J, Jimenez C, Figols J, et al. Primary leptomeningeal lymphoma presenting as cerebellopontine angle lesion. *Neuroradiology* 1994;36:369–371.

The Ear: Comprehensive Otology,
edited by R. F. Canalis and P. R. Lambert.
Lippincott Williams & Wilkins, Philadelphia © 2000.

CHAPTER 19

Diseases of the Auricle and Periauricular Region

Ian S. Storper, Rinaldo F. Canalis, and Paul R. Lambert

Lesions of the external ear are common and may be grouped into any of the basic categories of disease. They may be congenital, infectious, traumatic, inflammatory, autoimmune, neoplastic, or idiopathic. Although auricular lesions may be localized to the area of appearance, there may be warning signs of contiguous pathologic processes in the external auditory canal, middle ear, mastoid, scalp, skull, neck, parotid gland or temporomandibular joint. Disease of the pinna may be a sign of systemic illness, as in systemic lupus erythematosus, relapsing perichondritis, or gout.

ANATOMY

The auricle develops from the six hillocks of His, which are derived from the first and second branchial arches (1).

I. S. Storper: Department of Otolaryngology–Head and Neck Surgery, College of Physicians and Surgeons, Columbia University, New York, New York 10032

R. F. Canalis: Department of Surgery, University of California, Los Angeles, School of Medicine, Los Angeles, California 90095-1624.

P. R. Lambert: Department of Otolaryngology–Head and Neck Surgery, University of Virginia Health Sciences Center, Charlottesville, Virginia 22908-0430

The first arch contributes three hillocks, which give rise to the tragus, and the root and superior part of the helix. The three hillocks derived from the second arch give rise to the antihelix, the antitragus, and the lobule. The first branchial groove forms the external auditory meatus and the concha.

The external ear lies laterally, between the superior orbital rim and the nasal spine, and protrudes 30 degrees from the skull. The normal distance between the upper portion of the helix and the temporal skin is 2 cm or less (2). There usually are three extrinsic and six intrinsic muscles of the external ear. The *extrinsic muscles* are the *anterior auricular muscle,* which originates from the epicranial aponeurosis and inserts on the helical spine; the *superior auricular muscle,* which originates from the epicranial aponeurosis and inserts on the cranial side of the cartilage opposite the triangular fossa; and the *posterior auricular muscle,* which is thicker and arises from the base of the mastoid process and inserts on the ponticulus, which is on the cranial side of the concha (1). The anterior and superior auricular muscles are innervated by the *temporal branch* of the facial nerve; the posterior auricular muscle is innervated by the *posterior auricular (*or *occipital) branch* of the facial nerve.

The *sensory innervation* of the auricle is mainly by the *greater auricular nerve,* which arises from C2-3 near the posterosuperior portion of the sternocleidomastoid muscle and courses anterosuperiorly toward the auricle. This nerve divides into an anterior branch, which supplies the lower lateral part of the auricle, and a posterior branch, which supplies the inferior portion of the cranial surface of the auricle. The *auriculotemporal nerve* supplies the superolateral portion of the auricle and the skin on the anterior and superior surfaces of the external auditory canal. The superior cranial surface of the ear is usually supplied by branches of the *lesser occipital nerve.* Arnold's branch of the vagus nerve supplies the skin of the concha and the posterior portion of the external auditory canal.

The *arterial supply* of the auricle is relatively constant. The *posterior auricular branch of the external carotid artery* travels with the occipital branch of the facial nerve on the posterior belly of the digastric muscle. The main supply to the posterior auricle is from the *occipital artery* more than 90% of the time (3,4). The posterior auricular artery supplies the parotid gland, the mastoid cells, the tympanic cavity, the posterior auricle, and the postauricular skin. The retroauricular branch sends a branch to the lobule and another to the concha. In half of cases, the branch continues into the temporoparietal region; in the other half, it terminates on the postauricular surface. The lateral portion of the auricle is supplied by the *superficial temporal artery* in addition to those mentioned earlier.

The *venous drainage* of the auricle courses just deep to the greater auricular nerve, to meet the *external jugular vein.* There also may be a communication with the sigmoid sinus through the *mastoid emissary vein.* The superior part of the auricle may drain into the *superficial temporal* and *retromandibular veins.*

The *lymphatic system* differs from the vascular supply of the auricle (5). The concha and external auditory meatus drain into the preauricular and infraauricular nodes. The cranial portion of the auricle and the external auditory canal drain into the mastoid and infraauricular nodes. For additional information and illustrations pertinent to the anatomy of this region see Chapter 2.

EXAMINATION OF THE AURICLE

Proper examination of the auricle requires good lighting, ear specula, and suction tips. The patient's head should be supported by a head rest while the auricle is inspected and palpated. Both sides are examined; bimanual palpation is recommended if the ear is not too tender. The evaluation is extended to the postauricular, preauricular, and supra- and infraauricular extents of the lesions.

CONGENITAL MALFORMATIONS

Congenital Auricular Malformations

Total auricular aplasia (anotia) is uncommon. When it occurs, anotia is most frequently associated with defects of the external auditory meatus and canal. Associated malformations of the tympanic membrane and middle ear often accompany auricular malformations. A number of congenital syndromes with combined malformations of the ear and other structures are discussed in Chapter 20. The problems of auricular aplasia, lop ear, prominent auricle, and other malformations and the advantages and disadvantages of reconstructive auriculoplasty are discussed in Chapters 21 and 22.

The problems of combined auricular, external meatal, canal, and middle ear malformations necessitate collaborative otosurgical and reconstructive surgical approaches. Surgical reconstruction of combined ear malformations should be staged with primary attention directed at canaloplastic procedures for external meatal and canal atresia and tympanoplastic procedures for middle ear reconstruction. If the auricular malformation is severe, staged auricular reconstruction is begun first, and canaloplasty and tympanoplasty are performed once an auricle has been constructed.

Conchal Blockade (Physiologic Effect of Malformation of the Concha)

A "collapsed," anteriorly displaced conchal fold and cartilage abutting the posteromedial surface of the tragus may be responsible for blockade of the external auditory meatus (6) and intermittent conductive hearing loss (Reger effect). The condition is usually bilateral, and some patients learn that they hear better if the auricle is pulled backward and upward, pulling the conchal fold away from the tragal contact area. Among some patients, hearing loss is present only when there is additional obstruction by cerumen, moisture, or the swelling of external otitis. This deformity may be similar to the displacement of the anterior edge of the concha that sometimes occurs after otoplasty, canal-wall-down mastoidectomy with inadequate meatoplasty, or rhytidectomy. Surgical correction of these acquired deformities is the same as that described later for congenital blockage.

Some patients with conchal blockage need frequent cerumen removal but no further treatment. In severe cases meatoplasty involving subtotal removal of the anterior conchal lip usually resolves the problem (Fig. 1). The operation may be performed under local anesthesia. After a low endaural incision, the anterior edge of the conchal cartilage is exposed. Skin and perichondrium are elevated as needed, and semilunar resection of the obstructive portion of the cartilage is carried out along with removal of excess skin. In some cases, removal of additional superior conchal skin in the meatal portion of the endaural incision is necessary. It is often advisable to suture an indwelling arterial polyester (Dacron) tube (1 cm by 2 cm) to the upper wound margins during the 2-week healing period.

Preauricular Pits and Sinus Tracts

Preauricular pits with or without sinus tracts occur commonly among children, although the exact incidence is not well documented (Fig. 2). These anomalies are

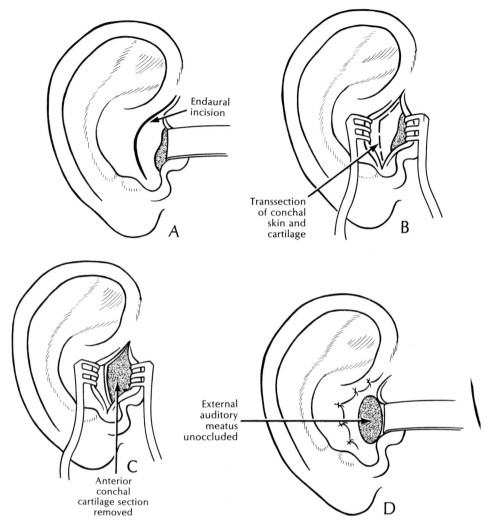

FIG. 1. Surgical correction of conchal obstruction (congenital or acquired). **A, B:** Skin and cartilage incisions. **C, D:** Cartilage resection and closure.

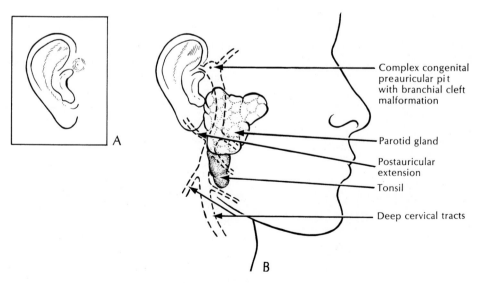

FIG. 2. A: Preauricular pit. **B:** Possible paths for preauricular fistula formation.

thought to develop from fusion abnormalities of the hillocks of His. They can be unilateral or bilateral and appear as pit-like depressions in front of the helix or above the tragus. If the pit is followed medially, there often is an epithelium-lined track that may communicate with a cyst. Some patients have an intermittent, scant, malodorous discharge.

Also associated with faulty fusion of the hillocks of His are preauricular and sometimes postauricular skin tags, which may contain cartilage (7) (Fig. 3). All of these lesions may be removed for cosmetic or therapeutic reasons. If a preauricular pit is symptomatic, once the infection has been controlled with antibiotics, surgical resection of the cyst and its sinus track is recommended. Initial incision and drainage of an acutely inflamed lesion is best avoided, because the resultant scarring will make surgical resection difficult (Fig. 4). Otic pits are removed through an elliptic incision. Sinus tracts are excised in continuity down to the cartilage. Injection of methylene blue into the sinus tract may facilitate identification and decrease the probability of incomplete resection (8).

First Branchial Cleft Cysts

Anomalies of the first branchial cleft are caused by incomplete fusion of the first and second branchial arches. They represent a spectrum of congenital defects. First branchial cleft deformities have been grouped into four categories: aplasia, atresia, stenosis, and duplication (9). Of these, only the duplication deformities are discussed in this chapter. Anomalies of the first branchial

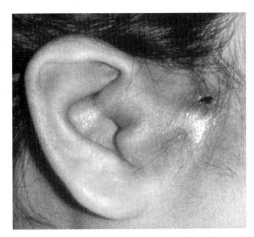

FIG. 4. Infected preauricular fistula.

cleft are considerably less common than those of the second branchial cleft. The paired branchial arches appear between the third and fourth weeks of embryonic development. These mesodermal structures are separated by ectodermal clefts and endodermal pouches. The first cleft persists as the external auditory canal; the other clefts are obliterated by the growth of mesoderm. The dorsal portion of the first ectodermal cleft forms the external ear canal proper; the middle portion gives rise to the cavum conchae; and the ventral portion is normally obliterated. Failure of this ventral portion to become completely obliterated is thought to result in anomalies of the first branchial cleft (10). Work (10,11) has provided the most frequently used classification of first branchial cleft anomalies, dividing them into two types (Fig. 5). In both types, the external auditory canal is present and well formed, but an epithelial track extends from the skin to the external auditory canal or middle ear cleft. Type I anomalies are of ectodermal origin and represent duplication of the membranous external canal. Type II anomalies arise from ectodermal elements of the first branchial cleft and mesodermal elements of the first and second branchial arches. They are regarded as duplication anomalies of both the membranous and cartilaginous external canal.

The anatomic location and histologic appearance of branchial cleft anomalies can be predicted on the basis of their embryogenesis (12). Ectodermal type I anomalies stay close to the external canal, because they are not influenced by the growth of mesodermal elements of the first and second branchial arches. No adnexal structures are expected within a type I anomaly. Type II anomalies, however, contain mesodermal elements necessary for adnexal development, and they are pulled medially and inferiorly away from the external canal as other structures of the first and second branchial arches (mandible and hyoid) develop. Both type I and type II anomalies are linked histologically with keratinizing squamous epithe-

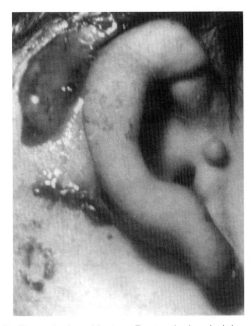

FIG. 3. Preauricular skin tag. Postauricular draining granuloma from recurrent mastoid fistula also is present.

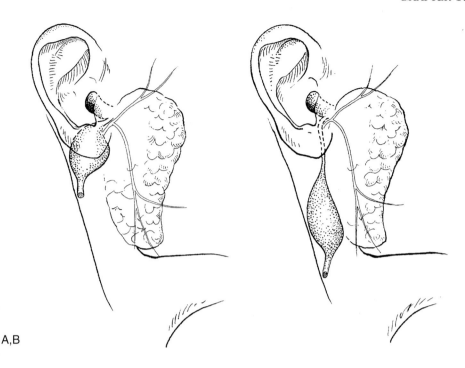

FIG. 5. First branchial cleft cyst. **A:** Type I anomaly represents a duplicated membranous external canal. **B:** Type II anomaly is a duplication of the cartilaginous and membranous external canal. (From Lambert PR, Dodson EE. Congenital malformation of the external auditory canal. *Otolaryngol Clin North Am* 1996;29:741–760, with permission.)

A,B

lium and exhibit a variable amount of acute and chronic inflammation. Type II anomalies contain hyaline cartilage, adnexal structures, or both.

The usual location of a type I branchial cleft anomaly is posterior, inferior, and medial to the conchal cartilage and pinna with a sinus tract paralleling the external canal. The tract may also lie within normal parotid tissue and is usually but not always lateral to the facial nerve. Although rare, extension of the tract into the middle ear has been reported (5,9). Type I anomalies typically present as a cyst or fistula near the concha or pretragal region. A frequently encountered history is recurrent periauricular swelling or abscess formation, often managed with incision and drainage. In many instances, the correct diagnosis is delayed many years.

Type II branchial cleft cysts are less common than type I and usually present in the first years of life as a superficial cyst or sinus below the angle of the mandible in the anterior triangle of the neck. Drainage, either periauricular or from the ear canal, is common. These anomalies may contain cartilage, hair follicles, and glandular (sweat and sebaceous) elements. The cyst tract courses through the parotid gland in close association with the facial nerve, usually terminating at the bony cartilaginous junction of the external canal.

Rare cases of malignant degeneration of branchial cleft cyst epithelium into branchial cleft carcinoma have been reported (13). Martin et al. (14) described four criteria for diagnosis of branchial cleft carcinoma, as follows: (a) the tumor should occur where branchial clefts are found, that is, along a line extending from the tragus, over the sternocleidomastoid muscle, and down to the clavicle; (b)

the histologic appearance of the lesion should be consistent with tissue known to be present in branchial vestiges; (c) the patient must survive for 5 years with consistent examinations and no evidence of a primary focus; and (d) there should be histologic proof that the tumor arises directly from the normal cyst epithelium. The last criterion is the sine qua non for the diagnosis of branchial cleft carcinoma. Therapy for this tumor is oncologic resection followed by radiotherapy.

Complete surgical excision is the treatment of patients with first branchial cleft cysts, sinuses, and fistulas (Fig. 6). High-resolution computed tomography (CT) may be helpful in preoperative planning. CT is preferred over magnetic resonance imaging because of its ability to delineate bony detail and to help determine the cystic nature of the lesion (15). Surgical intervention should be performed when the patient is free of infection. The presence of considerable inflammation may obscure important planes of dissection and increase the risk for both incomplete excision and injury to adjacent structures, such as the facial nerve. Because of the variable course of the sinus or fistulous tract as it relates to the facial nerve, most patients need superficial parotidectomy with identification of the facial nerve. Facial nerve monitoring may be useful, particularly when a patient has undergone previous surgical treatment or has had chronic or recurrent infection. Any communication with the external ear canal or middle ear space must be completely excised, and excision must be followed by reconstruction of the canal, tympanic membrane, or middle ear structures by means of standard tympanoplasty techniques.

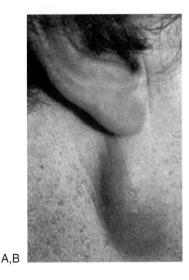
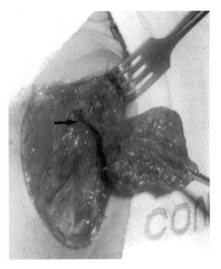

FIG. 6. A: First branchial cleft cyst, type II. **B:** Intraoperative photograph of cyst shows tract (*arrow*), which was found to end in the external auditory canal.

A,B

INFECTIONS

Cellulitis and Erysipelas

Erysipelas is an infectious disease of the skin caused by β-hemolytic streptococci (Fig. 7). The auricle becomes erythematous, tender, and indurated. The border of the infection is well demarcated. *Cellulitis* is an infection of the skin and subcutaneous tissue most often caused by a streptococci or staphylococci. The usual mode of infection is superficial abrasion or laceration. Constitutional symptoms can accompany either infection. In general, patients with erysipelas may be treated with penicillin G or erythromycin. Patients with cellulitis are best treated with a penicillinase-resistant penicillin.

Furunculosis

Furunculosis is a circumscribed infection of the hair follicles in the cartilaginous portion of the external audi-

tory meatus. The medial portion of the canal usually is normal. If the anterior canal is involved, there may be severe pain with mastication. *Staphylococcus aureus* is the most common pathogen in the early phases of infection, and oral administration of an antistaphylococcal antibiotic is recommended. If an abscess is present, incision and drainage are performed.

Herpes Zoster Oticus (Ramsay Hunt Syndrome)

Herpes zoster oticus is a recurrent outbreak of the varicella zoster virus along the portion of the auricle supplied by the sensory fibers of the auriculotemporal nerve in addition to the seventh and eighth cranial nerves (Fig. 8).

FIG. 7. Erysipelas of the auricle.

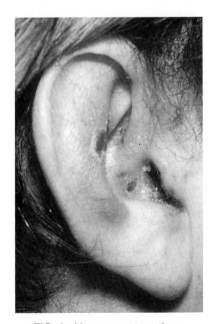

FIG. 8. Herpes zoster oticus.

It is manifested by extreme pain and cutaneous vesicular eruptions along the auricle or external auditory canal. Pain usually precedes the eruption by several hours and occasionally by a day or more. Facial paralysis, hearing loss, and vertigo can occur alone or in various combinations. Intravenous acyclovir is generally recommended for Ramsay Hunt syndrome; corticosteroids are added if cranial neuropathy exists in a host with normal immune function.

Auricular Perichondritis

Infection of the auricular perichondrium and cartilage most frequently occurs after surgical procedures, traumatic lacerations, burns, and frost bite (see Chapter 49). Infection also can be introduced during aspiration of a pseudocyst of hematoma, after ear piercing or acupuncture of the overlying cartilage, or as a complication of otitis externa. Diabetes may be a predisposing factor (16). The auricle initially becomes erythematous and painful. Progression causes edema, a subperichondrial abscess, and necrosis of the underlying cartilage. The most common organism is *Pseudomonas aeruginosa*.

In the very early stages, perichondritis may be managed with oral antibiotics, local cleansing, and daily evaluation. Unless a specific gram-positive organism is suspected, ciprofloxacin is the drug of choice. If a clear therapeutic response is not reported in the first 24 to 36 hours or if the case is initially severe, intravenous antipseudomonal coverage is necessary. Once an abscess

has formed, prompt incision and drainage should be performed and repeat cultures obtained. If chondritis exists, débridement of necrotic cartilage and soft tissue should be undertaken with careful preservation of the overlying skin.

Tropical Disease

Numerous diseases prevalent in tropical regions can have effects on the auricle. Examples of those occasionally seen in the United States are leprosy and leishmaniasis (Fig. 9).

AUTOIMMUNE DISEASE

Relapsing Polychondritis

Relapsing polychondritis is characterized by inflammation and progressive destruction of the auricular cartilages, the nose, and the laryngotracheal structures. The pathogenesis of this disease is thought to be mediated by antibodies reactive with type II collagen. The most common symptoms are chondralgia (especially of the auricles), arthralgia, nasal septal inflammation with bleeding and deformity, scleritis, and asymmetric, migratory nondestructive arthritis (17,18). Dyspnea may be caused by bronchiolar involvement (19). The differential diagnosis of auricular chondritis includes trauma, infectious perichondritis, cellulitis, Wegener's granulomatosis, and syphilis (20).

In 1966 it was found that serum of patients with relapsing polychondritis reacts with cartilage (21). Before 1980, the diagnosis of relapsing polychondritis was purely clinical; three of the following criteria had to be met: recurrent bilateral ear chondritis, inflammation of the nasal cartilage, laryngeal and tracheal chondritis, nonerosive inflammatory polyarthritis, ocular inflammation, and vestibulocochlear involvement (22). In 1980 it was shown that there are changes in granular immunoreactant deposition of the chondrofibrous junction, suggesting a pathogenic role of type II antibodies in the disease (23). Circulating type II antibodies have been implicated in the development of chondritis, but some authors have questioned whether they are specific. Helm et al. (18) proposed that direct immunofluorescence may be used to diagnose this ailment in its early stages. They proposed that a positive test result shows diffuse granular immunoglobulin G (IgG) and C3 at the chondrofibrous junction in perichondrial fibrous tissue. Biopsy is preferably avoided, because it may exacerbate the disease. If performed, a biopsy shows chondrolysis, chondritis, and perichondritis.

Relapsing polychondritis may appear in association with other collagen vascular disorders, such as rheumatoid arthritis, systemic lupus erythematosus, ulcerative colitis, Wegener's granulomatosis, Behçet's disease,

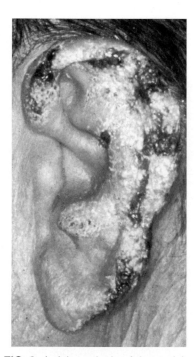

FIG. 9. Leishmaniasis of the auricle.

Churg-Strauss syndrome, and primary biliary cirrhosis (17,24). Therapy for relapsing polychondritis is administration of a glucocorticoid for both acute exacerbations and chronic maintenance to prevent exacerbations. Dapsone, indomethacin, and aspirin may be useful.

Chronic Discoid Lupus Erythematosus

Chronic discoid lupus erythematosus is a disease of the skin characterized by raised, erythematous lesions of the cheeks and nose (butterfly pattern), neck, scalp, upper chest, and ears (25). The incidence is highest among women in their third decade and is more common than systemic lupus erythematosus. Sunlight, cold exposure, burns, trauma, and genetic factors have been implicated in the development of this disease. The lack of antibodies to double-stranded DNA and normal complement levels make an autoimmune cause questionable (26).

The lesions are dull red in color and sharply limited. They are slightly raised. The papules grow slowly and are pruritic. The disease progresses from erythema to hyperkeratosis and atrophy. Direct immunofluorescence shows a deposition of immunoglobulin and complement at the dermoepidermal junction. Topical steroids improve the lesions; systemic antimalarial agents are effective in scar prevention. Five percent of patients also have systemic lupus erythematosus.

Wegener's Granulomatosis

Wegener's granulomatosis is a necrotizing, granulomatous disease affecting the upper and lower respiratory tracts and the kidney, where it is associated with focal glomerulonephritis (27,28). Although the cause of the disease is unknown, it is generally believed to be an autoimmune disease or vasculitis brought on by altered immune function; the anti-neutrophil cytoplasmic antibody test is positive among a large proportion of patients. There are four forms of otologic involvement: serous otitis media causing conductive hearing loss; suppurative otitis media; sensorineural hearing loss; and red, tender, brawny, diffuse swelling of the pinna that resembles relapsing polychondritis and occurs during active phases of the disease (29). Approximately one of every seven patients with Wegener's granulomatosis has ear symptoms (30). The typical histopathologic findings are inflammation of the mucosa and submucosa, necrosis, ulceration, vasculitis, and granuloma formation. Tissue diagnosis is difficult and usually is obtained from upper airway biopsy, even for patients with ear symptoms. A positive anti-neutrophil cytoplasmic antibody test result is highly suggestive of the diagnosis. Treatment in limited disease is trimethoprim-sulfamethoxazole or cyclophosphamide. In more extensive disease, prednisone and cyclophosphamide are used together.

AURICULAR MANIFESTATIONS OF SYSTEMIC DISEASE

Acquired Immunodeficiency Syndrome

More than 100,000 cases of acquired immunodeficiency syndrome have been reported in the United States, and there have been more than 59,000 deaths (31,32). It is the leading cause of death among men 25 to 44 years of age (33). Human immunodeficiency virus infection may be a predisposing factor for otitis externa, acute otitis media, otitis media with effusion, chronic otitis media, Ramsay Hunt syndrome, sensorineural hearing loss, otosyphilis (34), and auricular Kaposi's sarcoma. Aside from Kaposi's sarcoma, it is still being investigated whether these infections are causally related or coincidental to human immunodeficiency virus infection.

Gout

Gout is a severe type of monoarticular arthritis associated with hyperuricemia, which is caused by deposition of urates in tissue (35). Gout accounts for 5% of all cases of arthritis in the United States. It is most commonly found among men and is aggravated by alcohol use. The incidence is highest among Filipino-Americans. The disease is metabolic, inherited, and related to deficiencies in purine metabolism. One of these enzymes, hypoxanthine-guanine phosphoribosyltransferase, is deficient in a severe form of the disease, and the deficiency is found in Lesch-Nyhan syndrome. Some forms of gout have been associated with overactivity in synthesis of purines rather than inability to degrade them. In the auricle, gouty tophi may be found on the helix. If compressed, they exude a chalky material, which is a urate salt. Negatively birefringent crystals are seen when biopsy specimens or aspirates are examined in polarized light. Surgical therapy is contraindicated for the tophaceous deposits on the auricles, because the decreased vascular supply may compromise healing. Acute attacks are managed with colchicine; allopurinol is commonly prescribed for maintenance between attacks.

Chondrodermatitis Nodularis Helicis Chronica

Also known as Winkler's disease, chondrodermatitis nodularis helicis chronica is characterized by small, extremely painful nodules on the free border of the helix. It is primarily seen among men older than 50 years. The male-to-female ratio is 10:1 (36). Chondrodermatitis nodularis helicis chronica tends to occur where blood supply is poor and where skin is stretched tightly over cartilage. In rare instances the antihelix, antitragus, concha, or tragus may be involved. The nodules usually are unilateral, but bilateral disease has been reported. This disease most commonly occurs in the right ear, perhaps because most people sleep on this side with pressure being a causative agent. This finding is corroborated by a higher incidence of the disease among telephone operators and nuns, both of whom wear constrictive headpieces on their auricles.

The lesions of chondrodermatitis nodularis helicis chronica are solitary, firm, and 3 mm to 3 cm in size, with an average diameter of 4 to 7 mm. Pathologic changes involve the epidermis, dermis, perichondrium, and cartilage. In the epidermis, there is a horny parakeratotic plug or ulceration with a scaly crust. In the dermis, there is homogenization, edema, and fibrinoid necrosis of collagenous connective tissue. The perichondrium usually has a thick proliferation of fibrocartilage. Granulation tissue in this region can encase small nerve bundles and cause pain. There may be focal cell loss and hyalinization of the auricular cartilage, representing the end stage of this chronic inflammatory process. Diagnosis is largely clinical, but biopsy of the lesions may be performed if the diagnosis is not obvious. The differential diagnosis includes actinic keratosis, keratoacanthoma, cutaneous horn, and verruca vulgaris (37). There are two treatment modalities: steroid injection as initial therapy and surgical excision for treatment failures.

Ochronosis

Ochronosis is a congenital defect in the metabolism of aromatic compounds. It occurs most commonly among eastern Europeans and is inherited autosomally. The metabolic defect is the absence of homogentisic acid oxidase, which results in accumulation of homogentisic acid. This acid is oxidized to a black substance that concentrates on the auricle. A blue color is present on the skin of the pinnae, the tip of the nose, the sclerae, costochondral junctions, and extensor tendons of the hands. Patients have alkaptonuria, characterized by the urine's turning black on exposure to sunlight. Treatment is a low-protein diet to prevent metabolite accumulation (38).

CYSTS AND TUMORS OF THE AURICLE

Benign Lesions

Sebaceous Cysts

Sebaceous cysts develop from sebaceous gland entrapment and occur frequently in the lobule and postauricular region (Figs. 10, 11). Cysts that arise from hair follicles are called *pilar cysts*. They are generally soft and mobile and often have a visible punctum. Most of these lesions remain asymptomatic, but they may occasionally become infected. When asymptomatic, the cysts may be excised for cosmetic reasons. If a cyst is infected (with subsequent resolution) or if the diagnosis is unclear, excision is recommended. Regardless of the indication, complete

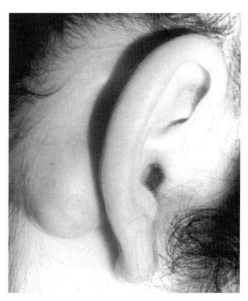

FIG. 10. Large postauricular sebaceous cyst.

excision with an intact capsule is the only sure way to prevent recurrence.

Dermoid Cysts

Dermoid cysts are congenital and appear as round, spongy eruptions behind the pinna over the upper part of the mastoid process. They are a type of teratoma composed of a fibrous wall lined with stratified squamous epithelium and containing sebaceous glands, sweat glands, and hair follicles. Although the precise cause is unknown, dermoid cysts are thought to derive from displacement or entrapment of ectodermal tissue during

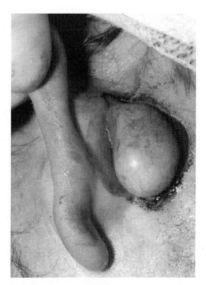

FIG. 11. Intraoperative photograph shows excision of sebaceous cyst.

fetal development. These lesions are surgically excised for diagnostic and cosmetic reasons.

Epidermal Implantation Cyst

Epidermal implantation cysts are also called *incisional cysts.* They are frequently thought to occur from traumatic implantation of squamous epithelium into subcutaneous tissue during a surgical procedure. They are generally asymptomatic unless they become infected or large enough to compress surrounding structures. Therapy is surgical removal when the cysts produce cosmetic deformity, pain, or compressive symptoms or when there is a question of malignancy.

Pseudocyst

Pseudocysts present as asymptomatic unilateral swellings in the upper antihelix of middle-aged men (39,40) and are characterized by intracartilaginous accumulation of fluid. There are two etiologic theories. The first is abnormal formation of auricular cartilages during development, and the second is release of lysosomal enzymes that cause tissue resorption. The second theory is more widely accepted, because these lesions appear later in life. Because the cysts lack an epithelial lining, treatment involves removing the fluid and preventing recurrence. Effective methods include excision of the anterior cartilaginous leaflet and suturing the skin, incision and drainage followed by a compression dressing, and possibly aspiration followed by instillation of one drop of 1% iodine. Simple aspiration is associated with a very high incidence of recurrence.

Keloid

A keloid is a benign, often pigmented, hypertrophic connective-tissue lesion that appears smooth, spherical, and scar like (Fig. 12). It generally follows trauma or a skin incision and frequently appears in the ear lobule after ear piercing. Keloids are thought to result from a defect in collagenase that leads to hypertrophic deposition of immature collagen. Koonin (41) suggested that an aberration in metabolism of melanocyte-stimulating hormone may be the cause. He found deeply pigmented people of all races more prone to keloid formation than those with fair skin. Keloids are more prevalent in areas away from the midline of the body, such as the ears. Therapy for small lesions occasionally may be accomplished with steroid injections, but large or resistant lesions are difficult to manage. Complete surgical excision followed by steroid injection along the incision line is performed and frequently is followed by multiple postoperative injections of triamcinolone acetonide (Kenalog). A Dermajet device is useful for applying steroids in the area. In recurrent and resistant cases, postoperative low-dose irradia-

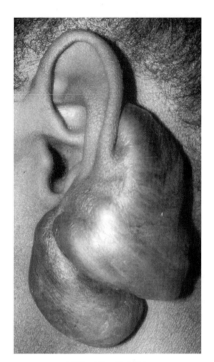

FIG. 12. Keloid.

tion should be considered; the patient's age and the possible oncogenic risks of this treatment must be taken into account. Carbon dioxide laser excision has been used with some success. Frequent, short treatments tend to give the best results.

Seborrheic Keratosis

Seborrheic keratosis is proliferation of basal cells and formation of epithelial cysts and hyperkeratosis. Melanin pigment or melanocytes may be present, imparting a color to the lesions that varies from yellow to black. The lesions usually are elevated and oily, and parts can flake off, which causes bleeding. Seborrheic keratosis has no malignant potential. If the lesions are cosmetically disturbing or if there is a question about the diagnosis, the lesions should be excised.

Senile Keratosis

Lesions of senile keratosis are common results of sun exposure and are precancerous. They have the same color as lesions of seborrheic keratoses but lack furrows on the surface. Lesions of senile keratosis usually are less than 10 mm in diameter and are treated with topical application of 5-fluorouracil.

Papilloma

Papilloma is the same type of verrucous wart found in other areas of the body. This lesion is caused by a DNA

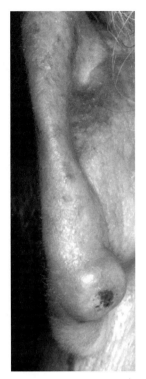

FIG. 13. Keratoacanthoma.

virus. Pathologic examination reveals papillary hypertrophy of the skin. Papilloma usually appears as an exophytic outgrowth of the pinna. Treatment is with carbon dioxide laser therapy or local excision.

Keratoacanthoma

Keratoacanthoma is a benign lesion that clinically resembles squamous cell carcinoma. it often grows rapidly to 1 cm or more in diameter and appears as a mound-like soft-tissue swelling in sun exposed areas (Fig. 13). Surgical removal is always recommended, so that squamous cell carcinoma is clearly excluded. There may be some use for retinoids in the management of these lesions (6).

Adenoma

Adenoma is a benign tumor of glandular origin, usually thought to arise from sebaceous glands in the fibrocartilaginous part of the external auditory canal. Adenoma is small, compressible, and asymptomatic unless it blocks the entire meatus. Treatment is surgical excision followed by cauterization of the tumor bed. A rare type of adenoma that may be present on the auricle is pleomorphic adenoma (42). The tissue of origin of this lesion is unclear. Sebaceous glands, ceruminous glands, and aberrant salivary gland tissue are the likely sources.

Vascular Tumors

A variety of benign vascular tumors can occur on the auricle. Congenital lesions may be grouped into dermoid tumors and angiomas, which consist of hemangiomas and lymphangiomas. A strawberry mark is an immature angioma present at birth but often more visible at the age of 3 months. This lesion may grow throughout childhood but usually involutes after puberty (Fig. 14). In general treatment of this lesion is watchful waiting. Laser treatments are used if there is repeated hemorrhage, obstruction of the ear canal, or massive cosmetic deformity.

Cavernous hemangioma is a red-to-purple, raised, compressible lesion that appears cavernous on histopathologic section. It enlarges with a Valsalva maneuver. These lesions may be watched, but they have less of a tendency to involute than do angiomas, although they may remain

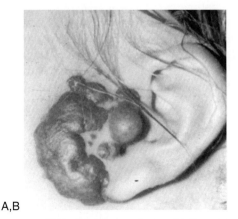
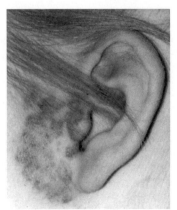
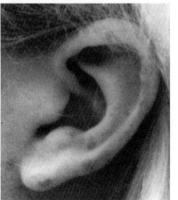

A,B   C

FIG. 14. Hemangioma of left auricle. **A:** Age 8 months. **B:** Age 2 years. **C:** Age 8 years. Near complete resolution.

stable for a long time. Surgical treatment with possible use of a laser may be performed if a lesion is disfiguring or debilitating (43).

Lymphangiomas are rare on the pinna. When present they usually represent extensions from a primary neck site. Because these lesions do not involute with time, surgical excision is recommended, depending on the site of origin and structures involved.

Calcinosis

Calcinosis, also known as petrified auricle, occurs when the auricle loses its elasticity and becomes a rigid unit. It is caused by ectopic calcification of the auricular cartilage and may occur after trauma, external irradiation, or in association with certain endocrine disorders such as Addison's disease, hypopituitarism, hypothyroidism, or parathyroid dysfunction. Auricular ossification occurs when the elastic cartilage of the ear is replaced by bone. This entity is known to develop after frostbite; its possible occurrence after continued cold water swimming among patients with exostosis has been discussed (44,45).

Other Benign Lesions

Many benign lesions occasionally may be found on the pinna. These include nevi, lipoma, xanthoma, myxoma, fibroma, chondroma, neurofibroma (46), angiolymphoid hyperplasia (47), and eosinophilic granuloma (48).

Malignant Lesions

Malignant lesions of the auricle can be derived from the skin or its appendages. Treatment varies with lesion.

Malignant Lesions of the Skin

Approximately 6% of all malignant lesions of the skin are found on the pinna. Although squamous cell carcinoma is the most common of these lesions, basal cell carcinoma, melanoma, and other lesions may occur.

Squamous Cell Carcinoma

Squamous cell carcinoma of the pinna is most common among elderly white men, which is consistent with the observation that it is related to exposure to ultraviolet radiation (49) (Fig. 15). It represent 45% of all ear carcinomas, with an incidence of 40% for the auricle and 60%

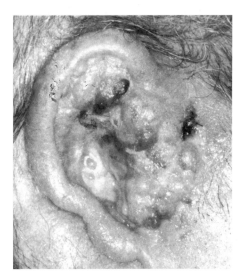

FIG. 15. Advanced squamous cell carcinoma of the auricle.

for the external auditory canal. Chen and Dehner (50) reported a mean age at diagnosis of 75 years with an age range of 37 to 88 years. The most common initial manifestation is a sessile mass or ulcer on the helix. Tumors are solitary with an average size of about 2 cm. The mean delay from occurrence to presentation is 2.3 years. The surface epithelium is characteristically ulcerated with indurated margins and peripheral erythema. Regional lymph node metastases occur among 12% to 18% of patients (51). The most common sites are the parotid nodes, followed in order of frequency by the upper jugulodigastric and upper posterior cervical nodes and the mid-jugulodigastric and midposterior cervical nodes. Distant metastasis is unusual; 12% is the highest incidence in reported series (52). Ninety percent of these tumors are well to moderately well differentiated (50). In addition to biopsy, evaluation includes CT of the temporal bone to assess medial extension of disease and cervical adenopathy.

Treatment options are surgical resection or radiation therapy. Although results may be similar with either modality for small neoplasms, surgery followed by radiation therapy usually is indicated for large tumors. For lesions confined to the pinna, wide local excision with a 1-cm cuff of normal surrounding tissue is mandatory. The simplest option for lesions of the helical rim, helix, and antihelix is through-and-through wedge excision. The advantage of this approach is one-stage removal. Cosmetic results are good, although the ear is made smaller. Other options include stellate excision to minimize cup deformity and excision of the posterior auricle with a postauricular advancement flap of skin and subcutaneous tissue. These techniques offer excellent cosmetic results.

For large lesions, auriculectomy with a split-thickness skin graft for closure is indicated. A prosthetic auricle may be used later. For lesions that extend into the external auditory canal and medially, modified temporal bone resection is needed (see Chapter 52). Neck dissection and postoperative irradiation are indicated when regional adenopathy is present. For lesions confined to the pinna, there is a 94% 5-year survival rate; for lesions involving the external auditory canal, the prognosis is considerably worse.

Basal Cell Carcinoma

Basal cell carcinoma is the most common malignant tumor of the skin with an 80% incidence in the head and neck region. Most patients are in the fifth or sixth decade of life. In the ear the most common sites of involvement are the preauricular, postauricular, and retroauricular areas, although lesions also occur on the anterior pinna (Fig. 16). Early lesions appear as nodules or plaques with surrounding inflammation; as the lesion grows, the center ulcerates. The prognosis is excellent for small lesions, but it worsens if the external auditory meatus is involved. Metastasis is rare with approximately 250 reported cases to date; 75% of these involve regional lymph nodes (53).

For small lesions, there are several treatment options. These include surgical resection (as described earlier), irradiation, Mohs' chemosurgery, cryosurgery, electrodesiccation, and curettage. Surgical excision is indicated when cartilage is involved. When the lesion invades bone, modified temporal bone resection usually is needed for complete resection. Niparko et al. (54) described a method to use Mohs' margin analysis in temporal bone resection to help assure eradication of disease.

Melanoma

Malignant melanoma of the auricle represents 7% of melanomas of the head and neck (55). Survival from melanoma has been found to correlate most accurately with thickness of the lesion. Melanoma, a tumor of melanocytes in the skin, should always be regarded as a systemic illness; it is therefore important to obtain oncologic consultation. For small lesions, wedge resection may adequately remove the tumor. For larger lesions, temporal bone resection and parotidectomy may be needed. Chemotherapy, biologic response modifiers, and immunotherapy have proved useful. It has been shown that for end-stage disease, external beam irradiation provides benefit (56).

Malignant Tumors of the Sebaceous Glands

Malignant tumors of the sebaceous glands arise in the conchal skin, which has an abundance of sebaceous glands. Two lesions are recognized: basal cell carcinoma with sebaceous differentiation and sebaceous carcinoma. These neoplasms are treated with wide local excision. Recurrence rates are high, but metastasis is unusual. These tumors are considered radioresistant.

Malignant Tumor of the Soft Tissues: Merkel Cell Carcinoma

Merkel cell carcinoma, also known as neuroendocrine carcinoma of the skin, primary small-cell carcinoma of the skin, and endocrine carcinoma of the skin, usually is seen early on sun-exposed regions of the head and neck (57). It is characterized by very rapid growth (58). At histologic examination this lesion resembles metastatic oat cell carcinoma, anaplastic carcinoma, Ewing's sarcoma, and neuroblastoma. Local recurrences and metastasis are common: 40% of patients have recurrent disease within 6 months; 55% present with regional metastases; and 49% have distant metastases within 2 years. The overall 3-year survival rate is 55%. Current recommendations for therapy include aggressive excision with 3 to 5 cm margins and systemic chemotherapy for extensive local disease, metastasis, or recurrence. The value of conventional irradiation remains unclear.

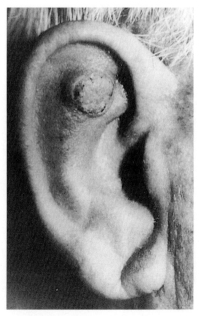

FIG. 16. Basal cell carcinoma of the auricle.

SUMMARY POINTS

- Congenital auricular malformations are commonly associated with middle ear abnormalities.
- Preauricular pits and skin tags are thought to develop from abnormal development of the hillocks of His.
- Type I branchial cleft cysts parallel the external canal and involve the lower portion of the parotid gland. Type II cysts present below the angle of the mandible and course posterosuperiorly in the parotid gland.
- Infections of the auricle include erysipelas caused by β-hemolytic streptococcus, furunculosis usually caused by *S. aureus,* and perichondritis usually caused by *P. aeruginosa.*
- Herpes zoster oticus is caused by the varicella zoster virus and affects the fibers of the auriculotemporal, facial, and eighth cranial nerves.
- Autoimmune diseases involving the auricle include relapsing polychondritis lupus and Wegener's granulomatosis. Relapsing polychondritis is thought to be mediated by antibodies reactive with type II collagen.
- Systemic diseases involving the auricle include gout, which presents as helical tophi containing urate salts and ochronosis, a congenital defect of the metabolism of aromatic compounds.
- Chondrodermatitis nodularis helicis chronica occurs most commonly among men older than 50 years and is characterized by small, painful nodules of the helix.
- Auricular cysts are common. They may be sebaceous, teratomatous (dermoid), or incisional. Pseudocysts are swellings in the antihelix produced by intracartilaginous accumulation of fluid.
- Keloids generally follow trauma and are most frequent in the lobule. They may be caused by an anomaly of melanocyte-stimulating hormone. Other benign lesions include seborrheic keratosis, papilloma caused by a DNA virus, keratoacanthoma, adenoma, dermoid cyst, and angioma.
- Squamous cell carcinoma of the pinna represents 45% of all ear cancers. It most commonly involves the helix.
- Basal cell carcinoma is most frequent in the fifth and sixth decades of life. The prognosis is excellent for small lesions; prognosis worsens if the meatus is involved.
- Seventy-nine percent of melanomas of the head and neck occur in the auricle.

REFERENCES

1. Holmes EM. Congenital malformations of the ear. In: Ferguson CF, Kendig EI, eds. *Pediatric Otology,* 2nd ed. Philadelphia: WB Saunders, 1972.
2. Allison GR. Anatomy of the auricle. *Clin Plast Surg* 1990;17:209–212.
3. Park C, Shin KS, Kang HS, et al. A new arterial flap from the postauricular surface: its anatomic basis and clinical application. *Plast Reconstr Surg* 1988;82:498–505.
4. Wada M, Fujino T, Terashima T. Anatomic description of the free retroauricular flap. *J Microsurg* 1979;1:108–110.
5. Mounsey RA, Forte V, Friedberg J. First branchial cleft sinuses: an analysis of current management strategies and treatment outcomes. *J Otolaryngol* 1993;22:457–461.
6. Smith R, Dickinson JT, Teachey WS. Medial conchal excision in otoplasty. *Laryngoscope* 1975;85:738–750.
7. DiBartolomeo JR, Paparella MM, Meyerhoff WL. Cysts and tumors of the external ear. In: Paparella MM, Shumrick DA, Gluckman JL, Meyerhoff WL, eds. *Otolaryngology,* 3rd ed. Vol 2. Philadelphia: WB Saunders, 1991.
8. Prasad S, Grundfast K, Milmoe G. Management of congenital preauricular pit and sinus tract in children. *Laryngoscope* 1990;100:320–321.
9. Karmody CS. A classification of the anomalies of the first branchial groove. *Otolaryngol Head Neck Surg* 1979;97:334–338.
10. Work WP. Newer concepts of first branchial cleft defects. *Laryngoscope* 1972;82:1581–1593.
11. Work WP. Cysts and congenital lesions of the parotid glands. *Otolaryngol Clin North Am* 1977;10:339–344.
12. Aronsohn RS, Batsakis JG, Rice DH, et al. Anomalies of the first branchial cleft. *Arch Otolaryngol* 1976;102:737–740.
13. Park SS, Karmody CS. The first branchial cleft carcinoma. *Arch Otolaryngol Head Neck Surg* 1992;118:969–971.
14. Martin H, Morfit HM, Erlich H. The case for branchogenic cancer (malignant branchioma). *Ann Surg* 1950;132:867–887.
15. Mukherji SK, Tart RP, Slattery WH, et al. Evaluation of first branchial anomalies by CT and MR. *J Comput Assist Tomogr* 1993;17:576–581.
16. Bassiouny A. Perichondritis of the auricle. *Laryngoscope* 1981;91:422–431.
17. Hager MH, Moore ME. Relapsing polychondritis syndrome associated with pustular psoriasis, spondylitis and arthritis mutilans. *J Rheumatol* 1987;14:162–164.
18. Helm TN, Valenzuela R, Glanz S, Parker L, Dijkstra J, Bergfeld WF. Relapsing polychondritis: a case diagnosed by direct immunofluorescence and coexisting with pseudocyst of the auricle. *J Am Acad Dermatol* 1992;26:315–318.
19. Arnold HL, Odom RB, James WD. Andrew's disease of the skin, 8th ed. Philadelphia: WB Saunders, 1990.
20. Cohen PR, Rapini RP. Relapsing polychondritis. *Int J Dermatol* 1986;25:280–285.
21. Dolan DL, Lemmon GB, Teitelbaum SL. Relapsing polychondritis: analytic literature review and studies on pathogenesis. *Am J Med* 1966;41:285–299.
22. McAdam LP, O'Hanlan MA, Bluestone R, et al. Relapsing polychondritis: prospective study of 23 patients and a review of the literature. *Medicine (Baltimore)* 1976;55:193–215.
23. Valenzuela R, Cooperrider PA, Gogate P, et al. Relapsing polychondritis: immunomicroscopic findings in cartilage of ear biopsy specimens. *Hum Pathol* 1980;11:19–22.
24. Hughes GB, Kinney SE, Barna BP, Calabrese LH. Autoimmunity in otology. *Am J Otolaryngol* 1986;7:197–199.
25. Prystowsky SD, Gilliam JN. Discoid lupus erythematosus as part of a larger disease spectrum: correlation of clinical features with laboratory findings in lupus erythematosus. *Arch Dermatol* 1975;11:1448–1452.
26. Tuffanelli DL. Cutaneous immunopathology: recent observations. *J Invest Dermatol* 1975;65:143–153.
27. McDonald TJ. Manifestations of systemic disease. In: Cummings CW,

Fredrickson JM, Harker LA, Krause CJ, Schuller DE, eds. *Otolaryngology—head and neck surgery.* Vol 4. St. Louis: Mosby, 1986.

28. Illum P, Thorling K. Otological manifestations of Wegener's granulomatosis. *Laryngoscope* 1982;92:801–804.

29. McDonald TJ, DeRemee RA. Wegener's granulomatosis. *Laryngoscope* 1983;93:220–231.

30. McCaffrey TV, McDonald TJ, Facer GW, et al. Otologic manifestations of Wegener's granulomatosis. *Otolaryngol Head Neck Surg* 1980;88:586–593.

31. Morris MS, Prasad S. Otologic disease in the acquired immunodeficiency syndrome. *Ear Nose Throat J* 1990;69:451–453.

32. Centers for Disease Control and Prevention. First 100,000 cases of acquired immunodeficiency syndrome—United States. *MMWR Morb Mortal Wkly Rep* 1989;38:561–563.

33. Centers for Disease Control and Prevention. Mortality attributable to HIV infection among persons aged 25–44 years —United States, 1991 and 1992. *MMWR Morb Mortal Wkly Rep* 1993;42:869–872.

34. Smith ME, Canalis RF. Otologic manifestations of AIDS: the otosyphilis connect. *Laryngoscope* 1989;99:365–372.

35. Wyngaarden JB, Kelley WN. *Gout and hyperuricemia.* New York: Grune & Stratton, 1976.

36. Cannon CR. Bilateral chondrodermatitis helicis: case presentation and literature review. *Am J Otol* 1985;6:164–166.

37. Silva G, Martins O, Picoto A, et al. Bone formation in chondrodermatitis nodularis helicis. *J Dermatol Surg Oncol* 1980;6:582–585.

38. LaDu BN. Alkaptonuria. In: Stanbury JB, Wyngaarden JB, Fredrickson DS, eds. *The metabolic basis of inherited disease,* 2nd ed. New York: McGraw-Hill, 1966.

39. Cohen PR, Grossman ME. Pseudocyst of the auricle. *Arch Otolaryngol Head Neck Surg* 1990;116:1202–1204.

40. Harder MK, Zachary CB. Pseudocyst of the ear: surgical treatment. *J Dermatol Surg Oncol* 1993;19:585–588.

41. Koonin AJ. The aetiology of keloids: a review of the literature and a new hypothesis. *S Afr Med J* 1964;39:913.

42. Ito A, Nakashima T, Kitamura M. Pleomorphic adenoma of the auricle. *J Laryngol Otol* 1982;96:1137–1140.

43. Kemink JL, Graham MD, McClatchey KD. Hemangioma of the external auditory canal. *Am J Otol* 1983;5:125–126.

44. DiBartolomeo JR. The petrified auricle: comments on ossification, calcification and exostoses of the external ear. *Laryngoscope* 1985;95:566–576.

45. Talmi YP, Cohen AM, Bar-Ziv J, Finkelstein Y, Floru S, Zohar Y. Ossified auricle in Addison's disease. *Ann Otol Rhinol Laryngol* 1990;99:499–500.

46. Stevenson TR, Zavell JF, Anderson RD. Neurofibroma of the ear. *Ann Plast Surg* 1986;17:151–1154.

47. Ferlito A, Caruso G. Angiolymphoid hyperplasia with eosinophilia of the external ear (Kimura's disease). *ORL J Otorhinolaryngol Relat Spec* 1985;47:139–144.

48. Green I, Behar AJ, Shanon E, Gorsky M. Multifocal extraosseous eosinophilic granuloma of the head and neck. *Arch Otolaryngol Head Neck Surg* 1988;114:561–563.

49. Conley J, Schuller DE. Malignancies of the ear. *Laryngoscope* 1976;86:1147–1163.

50. Chen KTK, Dehner LP. Primary tumors of the external and middle ear, I: introduction and clinicopathologic study of squamous cell carcinoma. *Arch Otolaryngol* 1978;104:247–252.

51. Blake GB, Wilson JSP. Malignant tumors of the ear and their treatment, I: tumors of the auricle. *Br J Plast Surg* 1974;27:67–76.

52. Freedlander E, Chung FF. Squamous cell carcinoma of the pinna. *Br J Plast Surg* 1983;36:171–175.

53. Bryarly RC, Veach SR, Kornblut AD. Metastasizing auricular basal cell carcinoma. *Otolaryngol Head Neck Surg* 1980;88:40–43.

54. Niparko JK, Swanson NA, Baker SR, Telian SA, Sullivan MJ, Kemink JL. Local control of auricular, periauricular and external canal cutaneous malignancies with Mohs' surgery. *Laryngoscope* 1990;100:1047–1051.

55. Byers RM, Smith JC, Russel N, et al. Malignant melanoma of the external ear: review of 102 cases. *Am J Surg* 1980;140:518–521.

56. Storper IS, Lee SP, Abemayor E, Juillard G. The role of radiation therapy in the treatment of head and neck cutaneous melanoma. *Am J Otolaryngol* 1993;14:426–431.

57. Hanke CW, Conner AC, Temofeew RK, Lingeman RE. Merkel cell carcinoma. *Arch Dermatol* 1989;125:1096–1100.

58. Weymuller ET Jr., Marks M, Ridge D. Merkel cell carcinoma of the ear. *Head Neck* 1991;13:68–71.

The Ear: Comprehensive Otology,
edited by R. F. Canalis and P. R. Lambert.
Lippincott Williams & Wilkins, Philadelphia © 2000.

CHAPTER **20**

Diseases of the External Auditory Canal

Thomas C. Kryzer and Paul R. Lambert

The external auditory canal (EAC) allows sound to reach the tympanic membrane and middle ear and protects those delicate structures. The physical properties of the EAC augment sound in the important frequencies of 2 to 4 kHz. These properties are related to the shape of the canal, which is an elongated, blind tube lined with keratinizing epithelium. Disorders of the EAC are common in clinical otology (Table 1). Successful treatment requires understanding of the anatomy, physiology, and bacteriology of the EAC.

ANATOMY

The EAC is an S-shaped tube approximately 2.5 cm in length from concha to tympanic membrane; the anteroin-

ferior canal wall is about 5 mm longer than the superior wall of the canal. The extreme lateral third of the canal is cartilaginous, and the medial two thirds are osseous. The skin covering the cartilaginous portion is supported by a delicate subcutaneous tissue layer that contains sebaceous and apocrine adnexa. These structures are associated with hair follicles and are collectively called *apopilosebaceous units* (Fig. 1). The cartilaginous portion of the canal has an anterior concavity, which can be lessened by pulling the pinna in a posterior, superior, and lateral direction to allow easier inspection of the canal and tympanic membrane. The cartilaginous segment of the canal contains dehiscences called *fissures of Santorini,* which may allow infection to spread from the canal to the soft tissue of the periparotid area and the temporomandibular joint and vice versa. The junction of the cartilage and bony segments of the EAC is its most narrow portion and is called the *isthmus.*

The osseous portion of the EAC is slightly concave posteriorly. It has no supporting subcutaneous tissue, and

T. C. Kryzer: Department of Surgery, University of Kansas School of Medicine, Wichita, Kansas 67214-4917

P. R. Lambert: Department of Otolaryngology–Head and Neck Surgery, University of Virginia Health Sciences Center, Charlottesville, Virginia 22908-0430

TABLE 1. *Disorders of the external auditory canal*

Dermatologic disorders
    Essential pruritus
    Dermatitis: contact, allergic, infectious eczematoid
Infectious diseases
    Bacterial otitis externa
    Skull base osteomyelitis (malignant otitis externa)
    Otomycosis
Trauma
    Laceration, burns
Benign tumors
    Seborrheic keratosis
    Osteoma
    Exostosis
    Hemangioma
    Angiolymphoid hyperplasia with eosinophilia
    Ceruminal gland adenoma
Malignant tumors
    Basal cell carcinoma
    Squamous cell carcinoma
    Adenoidcystic carcinoma
    Ceruminal gland adenocarcinoma
Other
    Hyperceruminosis
    Foreign body
    Acquired stenosis
    Herniation of temporomandibular joint
    Keratosis obturans
    External auditory canal cholesteatoma

the epidermis, which rests on the periosteum, is continuous with the squamous epithelium of the tympanic membrane. There are no melanocytes in the deep EAC. The osseous portion of the EAC is formed by growth of the tympanic bone that fuses with both the squamous part of the temporal bone superiorly (tympanosquamous suture) and the mastoid part of the petrous bone inferiorly (tympanomastoid suture) (1). In children from 1 to 4 years of age there is an anterior dehiscence in the tympanic bone called *Huschke's foramen,* which occasionally persists in adults (Fig. 2). This dehiscence may allow spread of infection from the deep canal to the preauricular space.

The EAC is innervated by cranial nerves V, VII, IX, and X. The exact distribution of the nerves is variable, but some generalizations can be made. The *auriculotemporal branch* of the mandibular division of the trigeminal nerve supplies the anterior and superior walls of the EAC and a corresponding portion of the tympanic membrane. The *vagus, glossopharyngeal,* and *facial nerves* supply the posterior and inferior walls of the canal and the posterior half of the tympanic membrane. These nerves enter the EAC through the tympanomastoid suture with the auricular branch (Arnold's nerve) of the vagus nerve from the superior (jugular) ganglion. The medial aspect of the

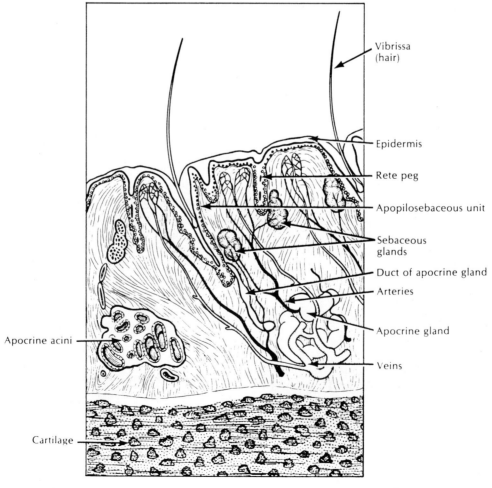

FIG. 1. Normal epidermis in cartilaginous portion of the external auditory canal.

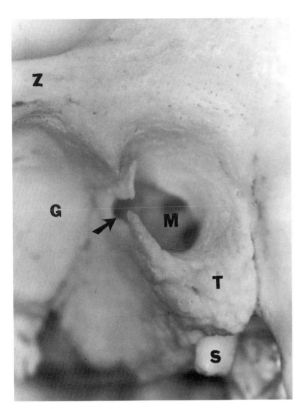

FIG. 2. Photograph shows lateral surface of the left temporal bone of an adult skull. A persistent Huschke's foramen is present (*arrow*). *T*, Tympanic bone; *M,* middle ear; *Z,* zygomatic arch; *G,* glenoid fossa; *S,* styloid process.

tympanic membrane is supplied with fibers from the tympanic branch (Jacobson's nerve) of the glossopharyngeal nerve (2,3).

The lymphatic drainage of the inferior EAC passes to the infraauricular nodes just posterior to the angle of the mandible. The lymphatic vessels from the posterior aspect of the canal drain to the deep cervical nodes. Those from the anterior canal pass to the parotid nodes then to the superficial and deep cervical nodes.

PHYSIOLOGY

The sebaceous and apocrine glands and hair follicles are contained in the cartilaginous portion of the EAC. Sebaceous glands lie in clusters, several alveolar ducts emptying into a single hair follicle space. The central portion of the alveolus is filled with fat-laden cells that eventually break down into fatty debris. The resulting oily substance is secreted into the hair follicles and extruded onto the surrounding skin. Modified apocrine sweat glands form an outgrowth of the hair follicle and are composed of three portions: coiled secretory portion, secretory duct, and terminal duct. Myoepithelial cells form a single layer that covers the coiled portion of the gland. In the apocrine glands, cells contain lipid and pigment granules, which are excreted into the hair follicle space. The secretions of the sebaceous and apocrine

glands mix with the exfoliated stratum corneum of the more medial canal and tympanic membrane to produce a waxy, water-resistant substance with an acidic pH. Infection in the EAC often can be traced to a breakdown of this protective covering (4).

The physiologic processes involving the skin of the EAC differ from those of skin elsewhere. Dead epithelial elements and keratin are removed from other parts of the body by means of friction. Because this is not possible in the EAC, migration of squamous epithelium is the primary way dead skin and debris are removed from the depth (5,6). Stratum corneum cells of the tympanic membrane move radially toward the annular area of the tympanic membrane and laterally along the surface of the deep EAC. The cells continue moving laterally until they reach the junction with the cartilaginous canal and are shed. The absence of rete pegs and subepithelial glands and the presence of a smooth basement membrane allow movement of the epidermis of the deep canal to the lateral canal, where rete pegs and adnexa appear (7). This movement of desquamated epithelium from the deep to lateral canal contributes to the natural cleaning mechanism of the EAC, and dysfunction may lead to disease.

HYPERCERUMINOSIS

Hyperceruminosis is defined as abnormal accumulation of cerumen. It can be caused by defective production or defective clearance. Excess production of cerumen may be related to infection, although in most cases the cause is not known. Plugs from patients with cerumen impaction show excessively long sheets of unseparated keratin that resemble the stratum corneum of the deep canal skin (8). Abnormal keratinocyte separation, perhaps from low steroid sulfatase activity in the stratum corneum of the deep canal, has been suggested as a possible cause of cerumen accumulation (7). Steroid sulfatase is thought to promote keratinocyte separation by means of deactivating cholesterol sulfate, which binds together the cells of the stratum corneum. The level of steroid sulfatase in the stratum corneum of the osseous canal has been shown to be higher than the level in the cartilaginous canal (7). A deficiency of steroid sulfatase may prevent normal keratinocyte separation in the stratum corneum of the osseous canal and cause accumulation of unseparated sheets of keratinocytes.

Cerumen accumulation can be caused by anatomic obstruction of the canal. An overly tortuous canal and narrow isthmus can block natural migration of the stratum corneum from the medial portion of the canal. In elderly persons, downward migration of the auricle occasionally causes partial occlusion of the external meatus and prevents normal elimination of cerumen. Acquired stenosis of the EAC after trauma, chronic infection, or surgical intervention may hinder cerumen elimination. Foreign bodies and tumors are other potential causes of obstruction.

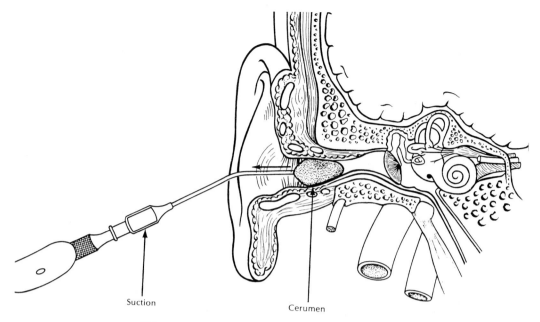

FIG. 3. Removal of cerumen by means of suction.

Before impacted cerumen is removed, patients should be asked about a history of perforation of the tympanic membrane, previous operations on the ear, or a history of acute or chronic otitis media. Depending on the consistency of the cerumen, a wire loop, blunt right-angle hook, or suction may be used to clean the external canal (Figs. 3, 4). Irrigation must be used with caution, especially when the condition of the tympanic membrane is not known. This structure may be damaged when attenuated; the middle and even the inner ear may be damaged when the drum is absent. Adequate illumination and binocular magnification facilitate removal of cerumen and minimize trauma to the underlying epithelium. After all debris is removed, it is important to inspect the canal for any pathologic condition that might predispose to hyperceruminosis and to examine the tympanic membrane to ascertain its integrity.

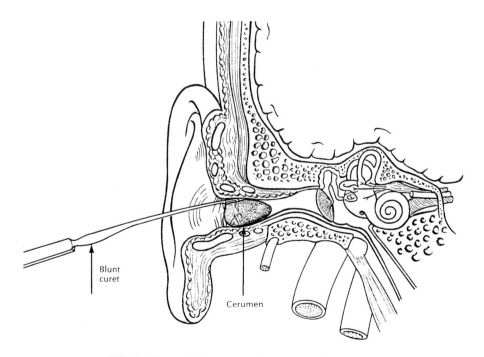

FIG. 4. Removal of cerumen by means of curettage.

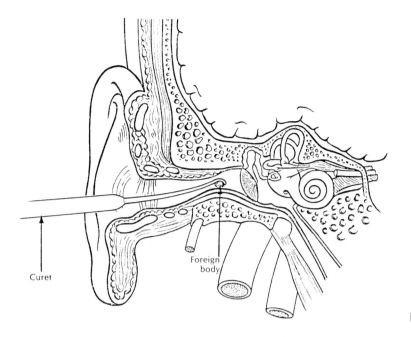

FIG. 5. Removal of unimpacted foreign body.

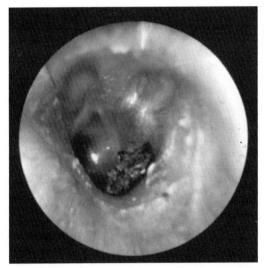

FIG. 6. A small rock as an unimpacted foreign body.

FOREIGN BODIES

Unimpacted foreign bodies such as crayons, beads, and small rocks are the most common type of objects encountered in the EAC and generally can be removed easily (Figs. 5, 6). Impacted foreign bodies are more difficult to manage because an instrument cannot be easily inserted behind them for extraction (Fig. 7). Organic foreign bodies are prone to impaction because they absorb moisture from the external canal and swell. The use of general anesthesia may be necessary depending on the foreign body and the level of patient cooperation. It is more prudent to remove a difficult foreign body under general anesthesia than to risk injury to the tympanic membrane and ossicles from sudden, unanticipated movement of an uncooperative patient. On rare occasions it may be necessary to make a canal incision to remove the foreign

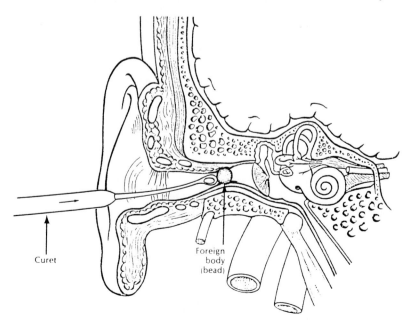

FIG. 7. Impacted foreign body; anesthesia needed for safe removal.

body. An antibiotic containing otic drops may be used if there is a large amount of canal skin erythema or excoriation after the foreign body has been removed.

Unusual foreign bodies such as button batteries, concrete, iron slag, and insects call for different treatments because of their potential for causing severe trauma. Insects may be rendered motionless with instillation of alcohol, chloroform, or mineral oil and removed. Hot iron slag causes burns of the EAC that may have to be débrided of devitalized tissue and packed with gauze or gelatin foam containing an antibiotic medication. Small watch batteries are a particular problem and should be removed as soon as possible. They cause damage by leaking alkali into the canal and producing an electric current in the canal, which causes tissue electrolysis (9). The extent of damage is not apparent initially, and frequent reassessment and débridement of devitalized tissue are necessary. Depending on the extent of tissue loss, the canal may have to be stented with packing to avoid stenosis.

DERMATOLOGIC DISEASES

Essential Pruritus

Primary or essential pruritus is a sense of itching experienced by the patient for which there is no discernible cause. Local factors that may lead to this symptom include lack of cerumen, lichen planus and other dermatoses, and contact with irritants such as hair spray and soap. Once all causes of pruritus have been excluded, the patient should be reassured. A steroid cream or ointment may provide some relief. Essential pruritus may be associated with inhalant or food allergies. Systemic diseases such as diabetes mellitus, hepatic or renal disease, and lymphoma or leukemia may have to be excluded.

Dermatitis

Contact dermatitis is an inflammatory response of the skin caused by contact with an irritating agent. Depending on the strength of the irritant, a single exposure may be sufficient to cause a skin reaction, although repeated exposure usually is necessary before a noticeable response occurs. A common cause of contact dermatitis is the material used to make hearing aid molds. For sensitive patients, hypoallergenic materials are available and frequently are helpful.

Allergic dermatitis is a delayed type of hypersensitivity reaction of the skin of sensitized persons caused most frequently by simple compounds of low molecular weight such as hair spray, shampoo, solvents used for cleaning hearing aid molds, and topical medicines. Approximately 1.0% of the population has a hypersensitivity reaction to neomycin (skin erythema, rash or scaling), which is a common component of many antibiotic ear drops. Frequently there is no apparent skin response on the first

contact with the offending chemical. On subsequent exposures, however, the skin response may be brisk. Treatment consists of removing the offending agent, cleaning the EAC with saline or a mild acetic acid solution, and applying a corticosteroid ointment. In especially severe cases, systemic steroids and antipruritic agents may be necessary.

Infectious eczematoid dermatitis is a condition caused by contact of the skin of the EAC with purulent middle ear exudate draining through a tympanic membrane perforation. The canal skin becomes erythematous in the area of drainage, often with yellowish plaques that extend to the concha. Treatment is directed at the otitis media with supportive care (suction cleaning, topical antibiotics and steroids) to the canal. A steroid-containing cream applied to the conchal bowl helps when considerable crusting and excoriation is caused by the drainage.

INFECTIOUS DISEASES

Bacterial Otitis Externa (Acute Diffuse Otitis Externa)

Bacterial otitis externa is characterized by inflammation of the skin and subepithelial tissue of the cartilaginous portion of the external canal. The bacterial infection may spread to involve the osseous canal in more severe cases.

High humidity and high temperature act as cofactors that may predispose a patient to bacterial otitis externa. As the humidity in the EAC increases, the cartilaginous portion of the stratum corneum absorbs water, and intracellular edema occurs. Edema leads to blockage of the apopilosebaceous units, and the excretion of cerumen decreases. A low cerumen content increases the pH of the EAC and reduces the water-repellent covering of the canal skin (4). The exposed skin becomes vulnerable to maceration, and the higher pH gives bacteria, particularly *Pseudomonas* organisms, a more favorable environment for growth (10). Multiplying bacteria can penetrate the dermis through the apopilosebaceous units after superficial breakdown or after minor trauma such as that produced by scratching with cotton swabs.

Bacteriologic studies indicate that skin colonization by exogenous bacteria is important in bacterial otitis externa. The most common isolates from a normal EAC are *Staphylococcus epidermidis* and *Corynebacterium* species. *Staphylococcus aureus* organisms are occasionally isolated and *Pseudomonas* organisms are rarely recovered from a normal canal. The latter two bacteria are the most commonly cultured organisms in bacterial otitis externa, suggesting that exogenous bacterial colonization and host and environmental factors play a critical role in the development of this infection (10,11). Gram-negative bacteria are most commonly cultured from diseased canals; *Pseudomonas* organisms are isolated in 33% to 66% of cases. *Enterobacter* and *Proteus mirabilis* organisms also are frequently cultured. *S. aureus* is the most common gram-positive organism isolated and the second most common pathogen cultured overall. Fungi and yeast usually are not clinically significant in acute bacterial external otitis, although they are cultured in about 10% of cases (4,11) (Fig. 8: see color plate 1 following page 484).

Initial symptoms of otitis externa usually are pruritus and aural fullness. Progression to ear pain occurs rapidly and may become extreme and seem out of proportion to the degree of apparent inflammation. Depending on the extent of infection, purulent otorrhea and hearing loss caused by canal edema and occluding debris may be presenting symptoms. Examination generally reveals an inflamed and erythematous cartilaginous canal and a variable degree of involvement of the osseous canal (Fig. 9). As the infection worsens, pain may preclude adequate examination of the deeper canal and tympanic membrane. Inflammation of the pre- and postauricular soft tissues and regional lymphadenopathy may occur in severe infections. The tympanic membrane initially is not affected, but with continued infection this structure and the medial portion of the canal become involved and often appear granular. In such instances, pneumatic otoscopy is needed to rule out concomitant otitis media.

Initial treatment step is to thoroughly clean the EAC of all purulent material and squamous debris. This is best performed with the aid of a surgical microscope and may have to be repeated frequently during the usual 7 to 10 day course of infection. Ototopical drops or powders containing antibiotics or acidifying agents, often combined with a corticosteroid, are needed for most bacterial infections of the canal. Drops containing a combination of polymyxin B, neomycin, and hydrocortisone are a frequent first choice. Polymyxin B is effective against

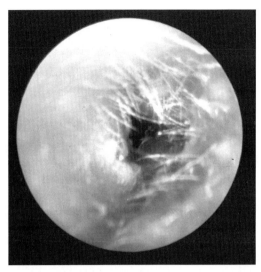

FIG. 9. Otitis externa causing edema of the cartilaginous portion of the ear canal.

Pseudomonas aeruginosa and neomycin against *S. aureus*. The steroid component reduces inflammation and edema. Severe edema may preclude instillation of otic drops or prevent penetration to the deeper portions of the canal. In such cases a wick should be placed in the membranous canal and removed or replaced every 48 to 72 hours until the edema resolves. Drying agents such as boric acid in 95% ethyl alcohol and 2% acetic acid solutions are effective in controlling the infection because *Pseudomonas* organisms grow best in a moist, alkaline environment. Application of powders such as boric acid or the combination of chloramphenicol, Fungizone or amphotericin B, and sulfanilamide also is useful. Liquid or powdered quinolones are very effective against *Pseudomonas* infection.

Oral antibiotics may be necessary to manage infections with periauricular involvement. Adequate coverage usually requires ciprofloxacin (used only to treat adults because of the potential for damage to cartilage in the weight-bearing joints of children). A second-generation cephalosporin, or erythromycin for patients allergic to cephalosorins, may be of benefit for any cellulitic process. Adequate pain management is always part of the management of diffuse external otitis and usually consists of nonsteroidal antiinflammatory agents or codeine-hydrocodone–containing compounds. Strict water precautions for the involved ear are critical to successful management of the infection. The patient should be carefully instructed in the use of ear plugs.

Care must be exercised when ototopical drops are used to treat patients with perforation of the tympanic membrane. Cochlear toxicity has been documented in chinchillas after instillation of ototopical drops in the middle ear, apparently from round window transport of the med-

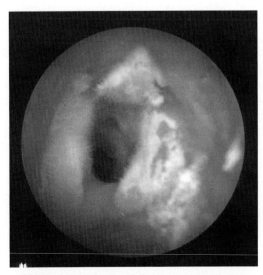

FIG. 8. Fungal otitis externa. (Courtesy of Dr. Armando Lenis.)

ication (12). Similar data on humans are lacking (see Chapter 25).

Chronic Stenosing External Otitis (Medial Canal Fibrosis)

A rare complication of chronic otitis externa is stenosis of the medial portion of the external canal. Initially there is thickened, erythematous skin often associated with a thin mucoid discharge and intense pruritus. Thereafter the canal skin becomes extremely thickened, showing hyperkeratosis and acanthosis (Fig. 10) and eventually mature fibrosis. Conductive hearing loss is the main symptom (13,14). Recognition of the process is important in the early stages when antibiotic and topical steroids may be helpful. Once stenosis is present, excision of the involved skin and relining with split-thickness skin grafts are required. Depending on the bony contours of the EAC, enlargement of the canal with a drill may be necessary (15).

Otomycosis

Otomycosis is an infection of the EAC caused by fungi or yeast. The disease has the same predisposing factors as bacterial otitis externa. Senturia et al. (4) showed that prolonged use of ototopical drops can foster development of otomycosis. Most episodes of otomycosis are caused by opportunistic (saprophytic) organisms. The most common are *Aspergillus niger,* Mucoraceae, dermatophytes, and *Actinomyces* organisms (16).

Symptoms of otomycosis include pruritus, pain, otorrhea, and hearing loss. The debris filling the EAC may be gray, black, or white; hyphae and mycelia often are evident (Fig. 11). Topical antifungal agents are effective in

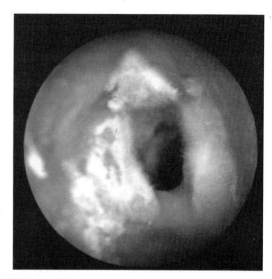

FIG. 11. Otomycosis showing fine white mycelia.

the management of these infections, but adequate and frequent aural cleaning is an essential part of successful therapy. A commonly used preparation is 2% acetic acid solution, either alone or combined with aluminum sulfate and calcium carbonate (modified Burow's solution). Other ototopical drops effective against fungal infections include m-cresyl-acetate (Cresylate), aluminum acetate (Burow's solution), tolnaftate, clotrimazole, nystatin and vital dyes such as gentian violet and sudan red. Chronic or recurrent otomycosis should prompt the physician to search for underlying causes, such as compromised immune function, other local infections, dermatitis (eczema), and chronic use of antibiotic drops.

Malignant External Otitis (Skull Base Osteomyelitis)

Meltzer and Keleman (17) in 1959 were the first to describe a potentially lethal, progressive, necrotizing infection of the skull base caused by *P. aeruginosa.* Chandler (18,19) later coined the term *malignant external otitis* and showed that surgical treatment alone was not adequate and long-term antibiotic therapy was necessary. Although the term *malignant otitis externa* is customarily used, *skull base osteomyelitis* is preferred because there is no neoplastic element to the disease. Osteomyelitis of the skull base almost always occurs among elderly patients with diabetes; however, it may occur in any age group of patients with compromised immune function. Osteomyelitis of the skull base should be considered when any patient with diabetes or compromised immune function has otitis externa or any patient with otitis externa does not respond to adequate therapy. Often a history of chronic diffuse external otitis can be elicited. The infection spreads to the soft tissues adjacent to the deep external canal, osteitis of the surrounding tympanic bone

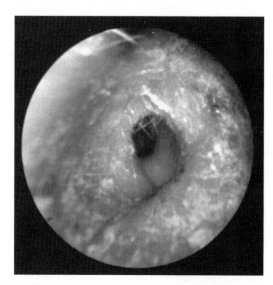

FIG. 10. Chronic otitis externa showing thickening and scaling of the skin of the cartilaginous portion of the ear canal.

occurs, and involvement of the marrow spaces of the skull base produces osteomyelitis. As the process progresses to involve the soft tissues of the skull base, cranial neuropathy develops (20). The facial nerve is the most common cranial nerve affected, and paralysis results from extension of the inflammation to the stylomastoid foramen and periparotid area. Involvement of the lower cranial nerves (IX, X, XI) is caused by progression of the infective process to the jugular foramen (21). In the past, multiple cranial neuropathies were associated with a mortality rate as high as 60%, but aggressive therapy with parenteral antipseudomonal antibiotics has improved outcome (20).

Patients with osteomyelitis of the base of the skull report deep-seated, intense otalgia with discharge. Examination reveals severe inflammation of the EAC with granulation tissue in the deep inferior canal and possibly exposed bone. The presence of granulation tissue at the osteocartilaginous junction of the canal is a cardinal sign. After a thorough history and physical examination, culture and biopsy are advised. To assess the presence and extent of involvement of the temporal bone and skull base, imaging studies are performed. Computed tomography (CT) and magnetic resonance (MR) imaging can help define the extent of soft-tissue involvement of the skull base (22,23). CT tends to yield more information about both bone and soft-tissue involvement and is the first study performed. Technetium 99m and gallium 67 bone scans offer information on the presence or absence of osteomyelitis (24). In the presence of osteomyelitis a ^{99m}Tc scan, which images bone reaction to inflammation, shows abnormal findings; the scan remains abnormal for an extended time. A ^{67}Ga bone scan, which images white blood cells and proteins associated with acute infection, is abnormal only during active osteomyelitis and reverts to normal after adequate therapy.

The mainstay of therapy for osteomyelitis of the base of the skull is long-term administration of antibiotics, frequent aural examination and cleaning, and strict control of the diabetes and immunocompromising disorders. Antibiotic therapy usually is continued for at least 6 weeks with intravenous, late-generation cephalosporins or aminoglycosides. Newer oral cephalosporins active against *Pseudomonas* species or fluoroquinolones such as ciprofloxacin may be substituted after an initial 2 to 3 weeks of intravenous therapy. Success with starting with oral ciprofloxacin has been reported (25). In general, a conservative role for surgery is advised. Obviously devitalized tissue or bone sequestra should be débrided and any abscesses drained. Hyperbaric oxygen therapy has been used with success as adjunctive therapy on a limited basis (26). A multidisciplinary approach with contributions from an otolaryngologist, endocrinologist, radiologist, and infectious disease consultant is important in treating patients with this aggressive, potentially lethal infection. After the active disease has been resolved, it is prudent to periodically examine patients with diabetes because they are prone to recurrent otitis externa because of the high pH of their cerumen (27).

S. aureus, S. epidermidis, Proteus, and *Salmonella* organisms have been reported to cause isolated cases of skull base osteomyelitis. Culture results should direct appropriate antibiotic therapy. Special attention should be paid to culture results that show *Aspergillus* species (*flavus* and *fumigatus*) when there is poor response to what should be adequate therapy. Although unusual, invasion of the skull base by *Aspergillus* organisms has been reported and necessitates long-term treatment with amphotericin B (28).

Furunculosis (Acute Localized Otitis Externa)

Furunculosis is an abscess of the hair follicle that occurs after obstruction of the apopilosebaceous units. This infection usually responds to application of warm compresses and administration of antibiotics effective against *S. aureus*. Occasionally the abscess necessitates incision and drainage.

TRAUMA

Injuries to the EAC are relatively uncommon because of the protected position of the canal. Lacerations can occur with penetrating or blunt trauma, often in association with a temporal bone fracture (see Chapter 49). In rare instances the EAC can be injured when a condyle fracture disrupts the anterior wall. These lacerations usually require no specific therapy, but cholesteatoma from skin entrapped in the fracture line has been described (29). Canal abrasions can predispose a patient to diffuse external otitis or cause a significant loss of canal skin and secondary stenosis.

Chemical, thermal, and electrical burns of the EAC can occur and present special problems. Caustic chemicals must be diluted and washed from the canal as soon as possible. Thermal burns and electrical burns may be very destructive and cause large amounts of tissue injury. Devitalized tissue must be removed and the canal inspected frequently under adequate magnification, because the true extent of the burn may not be apparent initially. Packing the ear with gelatin foam soaked with antibiotic solution can help prevent secondary infection. If there has been circumferential trauma, canal stenting for 10 to 14 days with 0.25-inch gauze packing impregnated with antibiotic ointment may help prevent stenosis.

ACQUIRED STENOSIS

The causes of acquired stenosis are varied. They include chronic diffuse external otitis (see earlier), trauma, otologic operations, and dermatologic diseases. Early treatment with stenting and antibiotic-steroid solutions may prevent stricture formation in selected

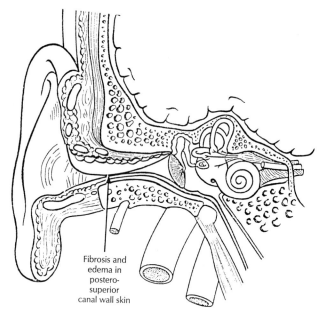

FIG. 12. Acquired stenosis of the external ear canal.

instances. Once stenosis has developed, canaloplasty and, if needed, meatoplasty are necessary (Fig. 12). The diseased canal skin is removed, and a split-thickness skin graft is placed freely in the canal or sutured to the enlarged meatus (15). Enlargement of the bony canal with a drill often is required (Fig. 13). The newly lined EAC is stented for 10 to 14 days with hydrated Merocel wicks or 0.25-inch gauze coated with antibiotic ointment (Fig. 14)

TUMOR-LIKE LESIONS OF THE EXTERNAL AUDITORY CANAL

Herniated Temporomandibular Joint Soft Tissue

Soft-tissue masses of the EAC may be infectious, neoplastic, or, rarely, may represent herniation of temporomandibular joint contents. The retrodiscal tissue of the temporomandibular joint inserts on the bony anterior canal wall, and if bony dehiscence exists this tissue can directly contact the subepithelial tissue of the EAC. Defects in the bony anterior wall may be traumatic (e.g., mandibular condyle fracture dislocation), iatrogenic (e.g., temporomandibular joint surgery or diagnostic arthroscopy of the joint) or congenital in origin.

Congenital dehiscences of the anterior canal wall have been ascribed to persistence of Huschke's foramen, which forms during development of the tympanic bone. As the leading edges of the tympanic ring grow toward each other, they fuse laterally before fusing medially, creating a foramen in the medial aspect of the anterior canal wall. This foramen normally closes by the fourth year; however, it may persist into adulthood (see Fig. 2). Persistence of this foramen may allow herniation of temporomandibular joint soft tissue into the external canal (30).

The diagnosis of herniated soft tissue of the temporomandibular joint can be made on the basis of physical examination. With the mouth closed, the retrodiscal tissue herniates into the canal through the anterior canal wall defect to produce a smooth, rounded mass covered with normal canal epithelium (Fig. 15: see color plate 2 following page 484). With the mouth opened, this soft tissue is pulled forward in the glenoid fossa and retracted out of the EAC (Fig. 16: see color plate 3 following page 484).

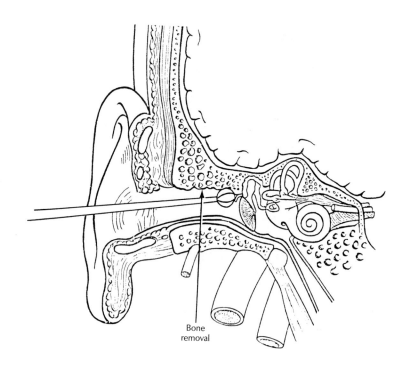

FIG. 13. Repair of acquired stenosis of the ear canal. Removal of canal skin and bone enlarges the canal, which is relined with a split-thickness skin graft.

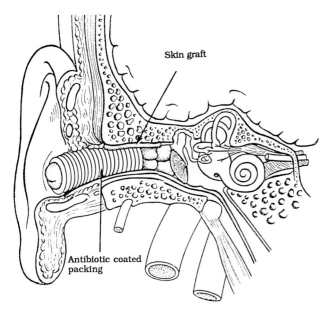

FIG. 14. Repair of acquired stenosis of the ear canal. Gauze packing with antibiotic ointment or wicks moistened with an antibiotic suspension are placed in the canal for 10 days.

Hearing loss or infection are not expected unless the mass is large enough to obstruct the canal. The diagnosis should be confirmed with imaging. CT shows the defect in the anterior canal wall. MR imaging delineates the soft tissue of the temporomandibular joint. If there is any suggestion of bony erosion or soft tissue infiltration, a biopsy to rule out neoplasia is warranted.

Inflammatory Polyp

Inflammatory polyps that occlude the EAC almost always originate from the middle ear through a perforation in the tympanic membrane. Only rarely do they originate from the wall of the canal or from the lateral surface of the tympanic membrane (see Chapter 25). Examples of polyps of the EAC or tympanic membrane are those that occur after surgical intervention or trauma, especially if there has been loss of squamous epithelium and exposure of underlying cartilage. Polyps usually are smooth, pale, well circumscribed, and pedunculated. They are most commonly seen in response to chronic otitis media or cholesteatoma; however, polyps may be the first sign of squamous cell carcinoma or glomus tumor of the middle ear. Often there is purulent discharge around the polyp.

Management of an inflammatory polyp involves identification of the underlying cause. Polyps prevent examination of the tympanic membrane and deeper canal; their attachment to ossicles, facial nerve, or a cholesteatoma over a labyrinthine fistula cannot be ascertained. Therefore, polyps should not be avulsed from the canal. Topical antibiotic-steroid preparations in conjunction with aural cleaning reduce the size of the polyp and may allow adequate examination. Cauterization of the polyp with silver nitrate also can be used for this purpose. Polyps that do not respond to conservative medical approaches require surgical removal. In most cases, the operation should be performed in conjunction with middle ear exploration so that the underlying pathologic condition can be managed. Pathologic examination is advised for removed polyps of uncertain origin to rule out the possibility of a neoplasm.

Keratosis Obturans

Keratosis obturans and EAC cholesteatoma are separate entities. Keratosis obturans usually appears in younger patients, and although the cause is unknown, faulty migration of canal epithelium and chronic hyperemia have been implicated (31). Keratosis obturans is associated with bronchiectasis and chronic sinusitis and usually occurs bilaterally (32,33). Patients usually have

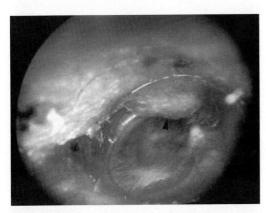

FIG. 15. Herniation of temporomandibular joint contents into the ear canal. With the patient's mouth closed this lesion is seen as an anterior soft-tissue mass (*arrow*).

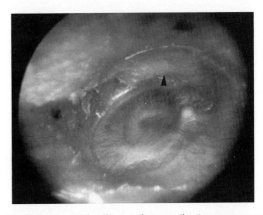

FIG. 16. With the patient's mouth open the temporomandibular joint contents are retracted back into the joint, leaving a slight depression in the wall of the ear canal (*arrow*).

otalgia, hearing loss, or both caused by a mass of keratin debris that fills the EAC. After the keratin mass is removed, generalized widening of the osseous portion of the external canal such that the tympanic membrane and annulus stand out in relief often is apparent (Fig. 17). Marked inflammation, vascular dilatation, and bone erosion may be seen in more severe cases. Treatment consists of removing the plug of desquamated squamous epithelium, frequent cleaning to minimize accumulation of debris, and ototopical drops containing steroids to control the inflammation (34). In unusual cases, excision of the skin of the external canal is needed with skin grafting and enlargement of the bony canal to facilitate cleaning.

Cholesteatoma of the External Auditory Canal

Cholesteatoma of the EAC is the accumulation of exfoliated keratin that originates from a circumscribed area of the external canal. The cause of these uncommon lesions is unknown; however, trauma has been implicated (29). This condition usually occurs among older patients and is unilateral. Inflammation and subepithelial vascular changes are confined to the area of the cholesteatoma sac. Dull pain and otorrhea are the usual presenting symptoms. Examination shows an area of accumulated squamous debris in the posterior or inferior aspect of the osseous canal with purulent drainage deeper in the canal. Unlike the situation with keratosis obturans, the desquamated epithelium does not form a plug that occludes the canal but is seen as loose squamous debris that protrudes from the involved canal wall (Fig. 18). After removal of the loosely packed keratin debris, there is usually a localized area of erosion of the bony canal, which may extend into the mastoid (32,33).

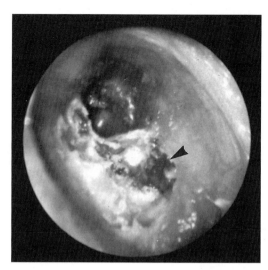

FIG. 18. Cholesteatoma of the external canal. Posteroinferior canal wall erosion is filled with squamous debris (*arrow*).

Treatment depends on the extent of the disease. Only removal of keratin debris may be needed followed by topical administration of antibiotics and periodic inspection. In many cases, however, the involved bone has to be removed with a drill and the defect covered with a split-thickness skin graft. If the bone loss is extensive, reconstruction with autologous cartilage or bone graft is necessary.

BENIGN TUMORS OF THE EXTERNAL AUDITORY CANAL

Skin Lesions

Skin lesions of the EAC may be pigmented (Fig. 19) or nonpigmented and have the same differential diagnosis as skin lesions in other regions of the body. Although

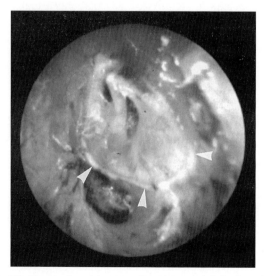

FIG. 17. Keratosis obturans. Squamous debris has been removed, and the annulus is visible in relief (*arrows*).

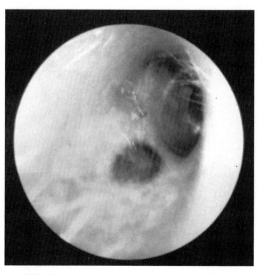

FIG. 19. Nevus of the external ear canal.

melanocytes are absent from the osseous portion of the EAC (2), melanomas do occur in the cartilaginous external canal. Biopsies should be performed on most skin lesions in the EAC to rule out a malignant lesion.

Seborrheic Keratosis

Although a common benign epithelial lesion of the head and neck, seborrheic keratosis is unusual in the EAC. These lesions occur most commonly in the fifth to sixth decades, and are located most frequently on the face, neck, and upper torso. Symptoms of seborrheic keratosis within the canal are related to its propensity for bulky growth and obstruction of the canal, which can become secondarily infected (Fig. 20). Histologic features of seborrheic keratosis include a thickened epidermis caused by accumulation of immature keratinocytes and keratin tunnels or cysts in the epithelium (34,35). These lesions can be confused with verrucous carcinoma and squamous cell carcinoma, especially when inflammation alters the histologic appearance by causing maturation of the keratinocytes and increasing mitosis (35). Seborrheic keratosis requires local excision with skin grafting as necessary (15).

Osteoma

Osteoma of the EAC is a pedunculated, bony tumor that occurs among middle-aged adults. The tumor usually is unilateral and tends to be laterally placed (Fig. 21: see color plate 4 following page 484). It commonly arises on the tympanosquamous suture and less frequently on a tympanomastoid suture (Fig. 22). The cause of canal osteomas is unknown. Histologic examination reveals normal bone formation with mature cortex and marrow spaces (34). Occasional osteomas grow to a size that impedes the egress of cerumen (Fig. 23). If this occurs the osteoma can be removed through a transcanal approach with a chisel or drill, and the underlying bone

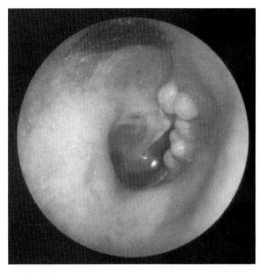

FIG. 21. Multiple osteomas involving the ear canal. (Courtesy of Dr. Armando Lenis.)

smoothed with either a drill or curette. Skin loss is usually small, and skin grafting rarely is needed.

Exostosis

Exostosis is the presence of multiple, broad-based bony lesions deep in the EAC. The condition is thought to be caused by chronic inflammation of the periosteal layer of the bony canal. The most common offending agent is cold water. Histologic examination of the lesions of exostosis show layers of bone laid down by the periosteum and forming a compact mass. Marrow spaces and cortical bone are not present (34). Treatment is indicated if the lesions become sufficiently large to block the self-

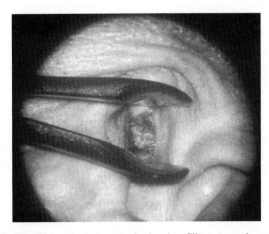

FIG. 20. Seborrheic keratosis. Lesion fills external canal.

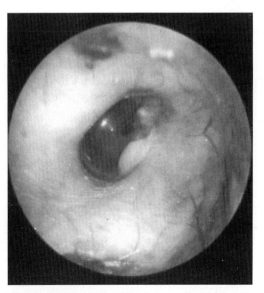

FIG. 22. Osteoma of the external ear canal arising from the tympanomastoid suture.

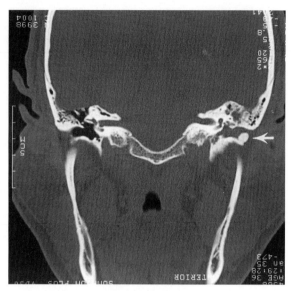

FIG. 23. CT scan shows obstructing osteoma of the right external canal. The patient had severe otitis externa and eventually needed surgical excision of the osteoma.

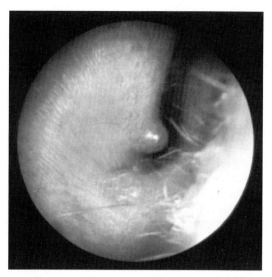

FIG. 24. Angiolymphoid hyperplasia with eosinophilia in the cartilaginous portion of the ear canal.

cleaning action of the canal or to cause hearing loss. With a postauricular incision, the overlying skin is elevated and reflected and the exostoses are removed with a drill. Distortion of the canal anatomy due to new bone growth places the mastoid portion of the facial nerve at risk, especially as the abnormal bone is removed in the posterior inferior aspect of the canal. The use of ear plugs can help prevent external canal exostosis among persons who frequently swim in cold water.

Hemangioma

Hemangioma originating in the EAC is unusual. It usually is seen soon after birth and may grow in the first 2 years of life. Hemangioma of the external canal appears as a smooth or slightly lobulated bright red or bluish lesion, depending on how deeply it originates in the subepithelial tissue. Obstruction, ulceration, and bleeding occur as the lesion grows. Hemangioma in the EAC has the same histologic patterns as that located elsewhere in the head and neck. Hemangioma usually shows some involution after the age of 2 or 3 years, and most require no intervention. When a lesion does not involute or when bleeding or infection becomes a problem, treatment may be needed. Systemic steroid therapy may help reduce the size of a lesion or arrest growth. Surgical excision, cryotherapy, and injection with sclerosing agents have been used successfully (4).

Angiolymphoid Hyperplasia with Eosinophilia

Angiolymphoid hyperplasia with eosinophilia is an uncommon benign inflammatory lesion that often is man-

ifested in the head and neck. Although originally thought to be synonymous with Kimura's disease, it is now considered to be a separate entity (36). The hallmarks of this disease are small to medium-sized (5 mm to 5 cm) vascular lesions in the dermis and subcutaneous tissues (Fig. 24). Histologic examination shows well-circumscribed aggregates of vascular channels and lymph vessels. As the nodules age, the predominate vascular nature is lost and replaced by perivascular lymphocytic and plasma cell infiltrates. Peripheral eosinophilia and lymphadenopathy frequently occur. The clinical course of this disease is self limited but prolonged. It is important to be aware of this disease so that a malignant tumor, especially angiosarcoma, is not mistakenly diagnosed. Angiolymphoid hyperplasia with eosinophilia requires only local removal; laser excision, electrodesiccation, steroid injection, cryotherapy, and routine surgical excision have been described (37).

Ceruminal Gland Adenoma (Ceruminoma, Hidradenoma)

Ceruminal gland adenoma is a benign growth of the apopilosebaceous units within the cartilaginous canal. The term *ceruminoma* may be confused with other more aggressive lesions (ceruminal gland adenocarcinoma) and therefore the name *ceruminal gland adenoma* is preferred (34). These tumors are more common among persons 40 to 60 years of age and show a 3:1 male predominance. The lesions usually are asymptomatic unless obstruction of the EAC and secondary infection occur. Ceruminal gland adenoma appears as a nonulcerated, epithelial covered nodule in the lateral canal. Histologic section shows the tumor nodule to be grayish red, often cystic, and lacking a well-defined capsule. The glandular component may be varied, even within the same tumor but usually contains an outer layer of cuboidal or spindle-shaped cells that may represent the myoepithelial cells of normal glands. Individual cells have a benign appearance without evidence of invasion (34). Treatment involves local excision of the lesion with skin grafting as needed. Recurrences are common in cases of incomplete excision.

MALIGNANT TUMORS OF THE EXTERNAL AUDITORY CANAL

Basal Cell Carcinoma

Basal cell carcinoma is uncommon in the EAC and generally more difficult to manage than that involving the skin of the face because of their late detection and difficulty in achieving complete resection. Presenting symptoms tend to be more insidious than those of squamous cell carcinoma, but otalgia and otorrhea are common. The histologic features are similar to those of basal cell carcinoma elsewhere in the head and neck. Treatment requires wide excision of the tumor. For large lesions, auriculectomy and en bloc resection of the EAC may be necessary. Metastasis is rare with this lesion.

Squamous Cell Carcinoma

Squamous cell carcinoma is the most common neoplasm of the EAC (34). Patients have otalgia and a discharge that often is bloody. The presence of facial nerve paralysis indicates advanced disease and is a poor prognostic sign. Examination shows an area of ulceration, a polyp, or a mass. Often there is a history of chronic otitis externa for which persistent therapy has failed and biopsy is performed. Cholesteatoma occasionally is present when carcinoma involves the middle ear space (38). The histologic features of the tumor are the same as those of squamous cell carcinoma elsewhere in the head and neck (34).

Early squamous cell carcinoma arises in the cartilaginous portion of the external canal (38). Access through the fissures of Santorini in the cartilaginous canal may allow these tumors to spread to the tissues of the preauricular space. High-resolution CT has been used to assess extension of the tumor to surrounding structures for staging purposes (39). MR imaging can provide information about adjacent soft-tissue involvement (40). Although CT helps with preoperative planning, actual tumor extent and surgical margins have to be confirmed at operation.

Squamous cell carcinoma limited to the external canal and adjacent soft tissues and not involving the middle ear or facial nerve may be managed with en bloc resection of the cartilaginous and bony external canal, tympanic membrane, and, as necessary, parotid gland (40). For car-

cinoma that involves the middle ear, mastoid, facial nerve, or more medial structures, more complete resection of the temporal bone is indicated. In this case the mandibular condyle, squamous and petrous portions of the temporal bone, and any involved middle fossa dura are included in the resection (38,40–42). Control rates for tumors confined to the EAC and managed with en bloc resection are generally in the range of 80% to 85% and for tumors with limited extension beyond the external canal 60% to 70% (40,43). When a tumor has widely extended beyond the external canal and involves the skull base, control rates fall sharply, and the survival value of extended temporal bone resection is uncertain (40,43). Postoperative radiation therapy usually is added for lesions that have progressed to involve the middle ear, mastoid, and more medial structures of the temporal bone (44).

Adenoidcystic Carcinoma

Adenoidcystic carcinoma is the most common glandular malignant tumor of the EAC (45). It occurs most frequently among middle-aged patients and shows no sex predilection. The presenting symptom usually is sharp pain located deep in the canal that radiates to the preauricular area. Examination reveals a lesion in the medial portion of the canal that may variously appear as granulation tissue, a polyp, or a subepithelial mass. CT and MR imaging are used to determine tumor extent and may aid in the diagnosis (39). Adenoidcystic carcinoma of the external canal may exhibit cribriform, tubular, and solid growth patterns as seen elsewhere in the head and neck. These tumors are slow growing but have a propensity for perineural invasion. Treatment involves wide excision of the tumor by means of en bloc excision of the external canal or formal temporal bone resection with postoperative radiation therapy. If involved, the facial nerve should be resected and grafted when clear margins are obtained. It is not unusual for patients to live many years with recurrent or residual disease.

Ceruminal Gland Adenocarcinoma

Ceruminal gland adenocarcinoma occurs among middle-aged or older persons and has a male predominance (34,45). It is the malignant counterpart of benign ceruminal gland adenoma. Symptoms include otalgia, aural discharge that often is bloody, and hearing loss. Examination reveals erythema and ulceration of the involved canal. Histologic examination shows the same general architecture as that of the benign lesion but with mitotic activity and invasion (34). Treatment is similar to that of adenoidcystic carcinoma; postoperative radiation therapy plays an important role. Recurrence rates of 10% to 50% are not uncommon, but metastasis is unusual.

SUMMARY POINTS

- Sebaceous and apocrine glands and hair follicles (collectively called *apopilosebaceous units*) are located in the cartilaginous portion of the EAC. These units secrete a protective, lipid-rich, water-resistant substance with an acid pH.
- The normal EAC flora includes *S. epidermidis* and *Corynebacterium* species. The most commonly cultured bacteria in otitis externa are *P. aeruginosa* and *S. aureus*.
- Management of otitis externa involves thorough cleaning of the EAC, instillation of antibiotic or acidifying otic drops (often containing a corticosteroid), possible administration of oral antibiotics for severe cases (especially those with associated cellulitis), possible stenting of the canal with a wick, pain management, and dry-ear precautions.
- Malignant otitis externa (skull base osteomyelitis) should be considered when any patient with diabetes or compromised immune function has otitis externa that does not respond to usual therapies. CT, MR imaging, and technetium and gallium scans can be helpful in diagnosing and following the course of this potentially lethal condition.
- Acquired stenosis of the EAC can result from chronic otitis externa, dermatologic disease, penetrating or blunt trauma (including temporal bone fracture), and otologic operations.
- A polyp within the EAC usually originates from the middle ear and often heralds underlying cholesteatoma. Less commonly, a neoplasm, such as glomus tumor or squamous cell cancer can present as a canal polyp.
- Keratosis obturans and EAC cholesteatoma are two distinct causes of keratin debris accumulation within the external canal and erosion of the bony canal.
- Benign epithelial tumors in the EAC include seborrheic keratosis, ceruminal gland adenoma, and hemangioma.
- Benign bony tumors of the EAC include osteoma and exostosis. Osteoma usually is unilateral, pedunculated, and located superiorly, along the tympanosquamous suture line. Exostoses tend to be bilateral and broad based and occur on the posterior and anterior canal wall; advanced lesions can occlude the canal.
- The most common malignant tumor of the EAC is squamous cell carcinoma. Early lesions limited to the canal itself can be managed with en bloc resection; the expected cure rate is approximately 80%.

REFERENCES

1. Proctor B. Connections of the four temporal bone constituents. In: *Surgical Anatomy of the Ear and Temporal Bone.* New York: Thieme Medical Publishers, 1989.
2. Hollinshead WH. The ear. In: *Anatomy for surgeons: the head and neck,* 3rd ed. Vol. 1. Philadelphia: Harper & Row, 1982.
3. Lambert PR. Referred otalgia. In: Britton BH, ed. *Common problems in otology.* St. Louis: Mosby–Year Book, 1991.
4. Senturia BH, Marcus MD, Lucente FE. Diseases due to infection. In: *Diseases of the external ear: an otologic-dermatologic manual,* 2nd ed. New York: Grune & Stratton, 1980.
5. Smelt G, Hawke M. A paradigm for tympanic epithelial dispersion. *J Otolaryngol* 1986;15:336–343.
6. Johnson A, Hawke M, Berger G. Surface wrinkles, cell ridges, and desquamation in the external auditory canal. *J Otolaryngol* 1984;13: 345–354.
7. Weinberger J, Hawke M, Clark JTR, Warren IB. Steroid sulfatase activity in the skin of the external ear canal. *J Otolaryngol* 1990;19:83–85.
8. Robinson AC, Hawke M, Naiberg J. Impacted cerumen: a disorder of keratinocyte separation in the superficial external ear canal. *J Otolaryngol* 1990;19:86–90.
9. Capo JM, Lucente FE. Alkaline battery foreign bodies of the ear and nose. *Arch Otolaryngol Head Neck Surg* 1986;112:562–563.
10. Cassisi N, Cohn A, Davidson T, Witten BR. Diffuse otitis externa: clinical and microbiological findings in the course of a multicenter study on a new otic solution. *Ann Otol Rhinol Laryngol* 1977;86[Suppl 39]:1–16.
11. Hawke M, Wong J, Krajden S. Clinical and microbiological features of otitis externa. *J Otolaryngol* 1984;13:289–295.
12. Wright CG, Meyerhoff WL. Ototoxicity of otic drops applied to the middle ear in the chinchilla. *Am J Otolaryngol* 1984;5:166–176.
13. Slattery WH, Saadat P. Postinflammatory medial canal fibrosis. *Am J Otol* 1997;18:294–297.
14. Birman CS, Fagan PA. Medial canal stenosis–chronic stenosing external otitis. *Am J Otol* 1996;17:2–6.
15. McCary WS, Kryzer TC, Lambert PR. Application of split-thickness skin grafts for acquired diseases of the external auditory canal. *Am J Otol* 1995;16:801–805.
16. Mugliston T, O'Donoghue G. Otomycosis: a continuing problem. *J Laryngol Otol* 1985;99:327–333.
17. Meltzer P, Kelemen G. Pyocyaneous osteomyelitis of the temporal bone, mandible, and zygoma. *Laryngoscope* 1959;69:1300–1316.
18. Chandler JR. Malignant external otitis. *Laryngoscope* 1968;78: 1257–1294.
19. Chandler JR. Malignant external otitis: further considerations. *Ann Otol Rhinol Laryngol* 1977;86:417–428.
20. Damiani JM, Damiani KK, Kinney SE. Malignant external otitis with multiple cranial nerve involvement. *Am J Otol* 1979;1:115–120.
21. Bernheim J, Sadé J. Histopathology of the soft parts in 50 patients with malignant external otitis. *J Laryngol Otol* 1989;103:366–368.
22. Ruben J, Curtin HD, Yu VL, Kamerer DB. Malignant external otitis: utility of CT in diagnosis and follow-up. *Radiology* 1990;174:391–394.
23. Gherini SG, Brackman DE, Bradley WG. Magnetic resonance imaging and computerized tomography in malignant external otitis. *Laryngoscope* 1986;96:542–548.
24. Noyek AM, Kirsch JC, Greyson HD, et al. The clinical significance of radionucleotide bone and gallium scanning in osteomyelitis of the head and neck. *Laryngoscope* 1984;94[Suppl 34]:1–21.
25. Hickey SA, Ford GR, Eykyn SJ, Sonksen PH, Fitzgerald-O'Connor AF. Treating malignant otitis externa with oral ciprofloxacin. *BMJ* 1989; 299:550–551.
26. Davis JC, Gates GA, Lerner C, et al. Adjuvant hyperbaric oxygen in

malignant external otitis. *Arch Otolaryngol Head Neck Surg* 1992;118: 89–93.

27. Driscoll PV, Ramachandrandrula A, Drezner DA, et al. Characteristics of cerumen in diabetic patients: a key to understanding malignant otitis externa? *Otolaryngol Head Neck Surg* 1993;109:676–679.

28. Kountakis SE, Kemper JV, Chang CY, et al. Osteomyelitis of the base of the skull secondary to Aspergillus. *Am J Otolaryngol* 1997;18: 19–22.

29. Brooks GB, Graham MD. Post traumatic cholesteatoma of the external auditory canal. *Laryngoscope* 1984;94:667–670–679.

30. Heffez L, Anderson D, Mafee M. Developmental defects of the tympanic plate: case reports and review of the literature. *J Oral Maxillofac Surg* 1989;47:1336–1340.

31. Corbridge RJ, Michaels L, Wright T. Epithelial migration in keratosis obturans. *Am J Otolaryngol* 1996;17:411–414.

32. Piepergerdes JC, Kramer BM, Behnke EE. Keratosis obturans and external canal cholesteatoma. *Laryngoscope* 1980;90:383–390.

33. Farrior J. Cholesteatoma of the external ear canal. *Am J Otol* 1990;11: 113–116.

34. Hyams VJ, Batsakis JG, Michaels L. Neoplasms of the external ear. In: *Tumors of the upper respiratory tract.* Washington, DC: Armed Forces Institute of Pathology, 1988.

35. Lambert PR, Fechner RE, Hatcher CP. Seborrheic keratosis of the ear canal. *Otolaryngol Head Neck Surg* 1987;96:198–201.

36. Sharp JF, Rodgers MJC, MacGregor FB, Mehan CJ, McLaren K. Angiolymphoid hyperplasia with eosinophilia. *J Laryngol Otol* 1990; 104:977–979.

37. Thompson JW, Colman M, Williamson C, Ward PH. Angiolymphoid hyperplasia with eosinophilia of the external ear canal: treatment with laser excision. *Arch Otolaryngol* 1981;107:316–319.

38. Lewis JS. Squamous carcinoma of the ear. *Arch Otolaryngol* 1973;97: 41–42.

39. Arriaga M, Curtin HD, Takahashi H, Kirsch BE, Kamerer DB. Staging proposal for external auditory meatus carcinoma based on preoperative clinical examination and computed tomography findings. *Ann Otol Rhinol Laryngol* 1990;99:714–721.

40. Kinney SE. Squamous cell carcinoma of the external ear canal. *Am J Otol* 1989;10:111–116.

41. Crabtree JA, Britton BH, Pierce MK. Carcinoma of the external auditory canal. *Laryngoscope* 1976;86:405–415.

42. Arena S. Tumor surgery of the temporal bone. *Laryngoscope* 1974;84: 645–670.

43. Arriaga M, Hirsch BE, Kamerer DB, Myers EN. Squamous cell carcinoma of the external auditory meatus. *Otolaryngol Head Neck Surg* 1989;101:330–337.

44. Austin JR, Stewart KL, Fawzi N. Squamous cell carcinoma of the external auditory canal. *Arch Otolaryngol Head Neck Surg* 1994;120: 1228–1232.

45. Hicks GW. Tumors arising from the glandular structures of the external auditory canal. *Laryngoscope* 1983;93:326–340.

The Ear: Comprehensive Otology,
edited by R. F. Canalis and P. R. Lambert.
Lippincott Williams & Wilkins, Philadelphia © 2000.

CHAPTER 21

Management of Congenital Aural Atresia

Dennis R. Maceri and Paul R. Lambert

The first accurate description of atresia of the ear was made by Paulus of Aegina in the seventh century (1). Simple incision when possible was the recommended treatment. Today's advances in audiologic and radiographic testing and in microsurgical technique provide precision in the diagnosis and the potential for hearing restoration. Still, the otologist's clinical acumen and surgical abilities are challenged by congenital aural atresia. The initial decision process centers on the need for amplification. Surgical candidacy must next be assessed. If surgery is recommended, a thorough understanding of the abnormal development of the temporal bone is essential so that complications such as facial nerve or labyrinthine injury can be avoided. This chapter reviews the concepts

and protocols of preoperative evaluation, surgical therapy, and postoperative care of patients with congenital aural atresia.

EPIDEMIOLOGY

Atresia of the ear canal with middle ear anomalies can occur in isolation or in association with microtia or craniofacial dysplasia. The reported incidence is 1 in 10,000 to 20,000 births. Genetic transmission occurs in many of the syndromes that include aural atresia, such as Treacher Collins syndrome, but it is rare in cases of isolated atresia. In approximately one third of cases aural atresia is bilateral, and each side can vary in complexity (2).

EMBRYOLOGY

A brief review of embryology is necessary to understand the developmental defects in aural atresia and the

D. R. Maceri: Department of Otolaryngology–Head and Neck Surgery, University of Southern California School of Medicine, Northridge, California 91325

P. R. Lambert: Department of Otolaryngology–Head and Neck Surgery, University of Virginia Health Sciences Center, Charlottesville, Virginia 22908-0430

altered surgical anatomy. All three germ layers take part in the formation of the pinna, external ear canal, tympanic membrane, and inner ear structures. The embryologic development of the first pharyngeal pouch, the first and second branchial arches, and the first branchial cleft is particularly germane to the discussion of aural atresia. The auricle, external ear canal, tympanic membrane, and otocyst are ectodermal derivatives. The mesenchyme of the first (Meckel's cartilage) and second (Reichert's cartilage) branchial arches gives rise to the ossicles and middle ear muscles. The eustachian tube and middle ear cavity arise from the first branchial pouch endoderm. The external ear auricle develops from six knob-like hillocks situated around the primitive meatus at about the sixth week of intrauterine life.

The external ear canal is derived from the first branchial cleft. During the second intrauterine month, a solid core of epithelium migrates inward from the rudimentary pinna toward the lateral end of the first branchial pouch (Fig. 1). This tissue is the precursor of the external auditory canal. The plate of tissue (presumptive meatal plate) formed by the inward and outward migration of tissue ultimately becomes the tympanic membrane. At the same time, the malleus and incus are taking shape from the upper end of the first branchial arch cartilage, while the stapes superstructure forms from the second arch cartilage. The ossicles attain their final shape by the end of the fourth intrauterine month. By the end of the seventh or eighth month, the expanding middle ear cleft (endoderm) surrounds the ossicles and lines them with mucous membrane.

The external auditory canal starts to hollow out (recanalize) during the sixth intrauterine month. At this point, absorption of the epithelial cells begins and progresses in a medial to lateral direction. If this canalization process is arrested prematurely, it is possible to have a normal tympanic membrane and bony external ear canal associated with an atretic or stenotic membranous canal. This situation predisposes to the development of a canal cholesteatoma as trapped squamous epithelium within the medial canal continues to desquamate.

Because the recanalization sequence is a second trimester event, inner ear development is complete and cochlear and vestibular function are expected to be normal. Middle ear structures have been formed but full maturation has not occurred. Arrested growth of the ossicular chain can leave the ossicles at various stages of formation. For example, the stapes often is misshapen but usually is mobile. The incus and malleus are fused. Variations in the anatomic course of the facial nerve, most notably an acute bend at the external genu with the mastoid segment coursing in a more anterior and lateral direction, is common.

As recanalization of the external ear canal takes place, the developing mastoid process becomes separated from the mandible by the bony tympanic ring, which causes the mastoid to grow in a posterior-inferior direction. This is a key step in development, because the mastoid carries with it the middle ear structures and facial nerve to their ultimate anatomic locations. This posterior migration may be arrested at any point form the beginning of development of the tympanic bone deep over the middle ear

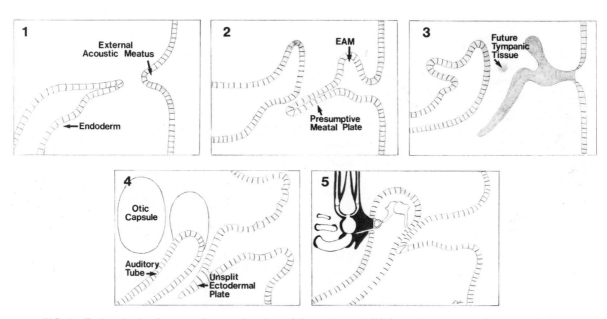

FIG. 1. Embryologic diagram shows migration of tissue inward **(1)** from the presumptive meatal plate **(2)**. Future tympanic tissue gives rise to the ossicles **(3)**. Ectoderm of the external canal begins to recanalize **(4)**. By the eighth month, endoderm surrounds the ossicles in the tympanic cavity **(5)**.

from the tympanic bone, continues its lateral growth during the first and second postnatal years.

CLASSIFICATION OF DEFORMITIES

Colman (3) divided congenital ear malformations into three anatomic types: minor, moderate, and severe aplasia. Severe aplasia is an osseous deformity that consists of complete absence of the external canal. The mass of compact tympanic bone fails to recanalize. This mass of bone forms the lateral wall of the middle ear cavity, which itself is very small and situated anteriorly beneath the temporomandibular joint. The ossicles, if discernible, usually appear as an amorphous mass. The stapes is not well defined at computed tomography (CT). The pinna is usually severely deformed or absent, or there is no evidence of an ear canal. These cases often are a part of a complex syndrome of craniofacial dystocia and must be thoroughly evaluated. Surgical therapy for hearing restoration rarely is indicated.

In moderate aplasia, there is a significant defect in canalization of the tympanic bone. The pinna is usually abnormal or severely deformed, and the membranous external canal is absent or ends in a pinpoint fistula-like opening. The bony canal is narrowed severely or completely atretic (see Fig. 2). The ossicles are deformed, and the malleus and incus are fused. The neck of the malleus typically is fused to the atretic bone. The lateral ossicular mass may or may not articulate with the stapes, which is usually small and misshapen. Concomitant craniofacial abnormalities may be present. This is the most commonly encountered type of atresia, and it may be amenable to surgical correction.

In minor aplasia the tympanic bone and eardrum are developed, but the recanalized external canal is smaller than normal because of the thickness of the bone (see Fig. 3). The ear canal ends at a tympanic membrane that frequently is small. Complex middle ear abnormalities may be present, including absence or deformity of one or more ossicles or ossicular chain fixation (4). The pinna is normal or only slightly deformed. This type of minor aplasia may go unnoticed until the conductive hearing loss is identified and evaluated.

PREOPERATIVE PATIENT ASSESSMENT

Approximately 40% of patients with aural atresia are not candidates for surgical correction. The proper selection of patients maximizes the opportunity for hearing recovery and minimizes the potential for surgical complications. The patient evaluation includes a physical examination, audiometric assessment, and CT of the temporal bone. In most cases, the findings at radiographic evaluation of the middle ear determine candidacy for surgical treatment.

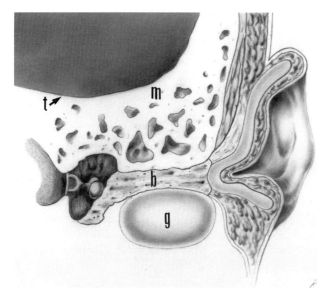

FIG. 2. Tympanic bone (*b*) of left ear has failed to recanalize, leaving a solid core of bone. Glenoid fossa (*g*) remains lateral to tympanic cavity because posterior migration of mastoid process (*m*) has been arrested. Tegmen (*t*) is visible.

(Fig. 2) to a stage at which canalization extends completely to the outer meatus (Fig. 3). At any time cessation of development can cause a spectrum of types of atresia ranging from a complete lack of tympanic bone to an almost completely normal relation between the tympanic bone and the mastoid process and condyle of the mandible. A normal osseous ear canal, which is derived

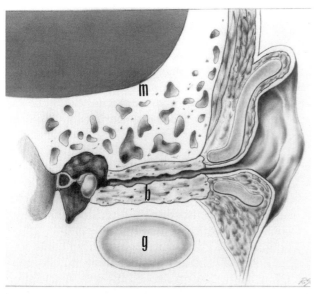

FIG. 3. Partial recanalization of tympanic bone (*b*) of left ear with more posterior displacement of the mastoid (*m*). This results in a more anteriorly placed glenoid (*g*). Canal remains stenotic.

History

An initial history and physical examination by an otologist are usually part of a craniofacial team evaluation of an infant. Because this is a most anxious and difficult time for parents, sufficient time must be allowed for a thorough examination, counseling, question answering, and reassurance. A complete and accurate pregnancy history through delivery is obtained, including questions about infections, drugs taken, trauma, and family history. Genetic counseling is recommended for those with a family history of craniofacial or otologic disorders.

Physical Examination

The physical examination should uncover any other craniofacial anomalies, such as Treacher Collins syndrome, hemifacial microsomia, or facial paralysis. The size, shape, and type of pinna are recorded, and special attention paid to the relation between the pinna and the temporomandibular joint. The caliber of the external canal should be graded as normal, stenotic, blindly ending, or atretic. A small pinpoint meatus or fistula may mean a partially developed tympanic bone and trapped epithelium, which may give rise to drainage or development of a cholesteatoma (Fig. 4). A rounded or blunt canal implies absence of a tympanic bone (Fig. 4). A well-developed mastoid tip often is associated with a well-pneumatized mastoid.

In the care of a young child, achievement of neurologic milestones, such as speech and ambulation, are assessed through history and direct observation. All divisions of the facial nerve are carefully assessed and any weakness recorded. It is rare to encounter paresis or paralysis involving the entire hemiface, although occasional involvement of the lower face or lip area may be seen. The most common anomaly of facial function is congenital absence of the depressor anguli oris muscle.

Audiologic Evaluation

Atresia of the external canal causes a 50 to 60 dB conductive hearing loss. Sensorineural function is normal in most instances. If the atresia is unilateral, audiologic assessment is straightforward. Most children can undergo behavioral audiometry, although auditory brainstem response testing may be necessary for infants or children who are difficult to test.

Patients with bilateral atresia present a masking dilemma. It is essential in examinations of these patients to determine the level of cochlear function in each ear to prevent operating on a patient's only hearing ear or an ear with little or no potential for hearing improvement. Bone conduction auditory brainstem response testing can be used to help resolve this masking problem (5). Wave I of the auditory brainstem response is generated by the distal portion of the auditory nerve and is most robust when measured with a recording electrode placed on the ear being stimulated. In simultaneous recording in both ears with surface electrodes, any wave I response recorded reflects primarily the activity from the underlying ipsilateral cochlea. Although a bone conduction signal cannot stimulate each ear independently, differential assessment of cochlear function is possible because of the relative specific wave I response.

Computed Tomography

The standard for preoperative assessment is the high-resolution CT in the coronal and axial planes. Axial projections (parallel to the line from the infraorbital rim to the external meatus) delineate the malleus and incus, the incudostapedial joint, and the round window. Coronal projections (parallel to the ramus and the mandible) show the stapes, the oval window, and vestibule. Both projections are necessary to follow the course of the facial nerve. Three-dimensional CT is of little help in resolving the complex temporal bone anatomy. Magnetic resonance imaging also does not provide any useful additional information.

The timing of CT is dictated by the timing of the surgical procedure. Because most infants need sedation, routine CT is not performed for patients with unilateral or bilateral atresia until they are about 5 years of age. The one exception is a child who is believed to have sensorineural hearing loss in either ear as result of a cochlear anomaly.

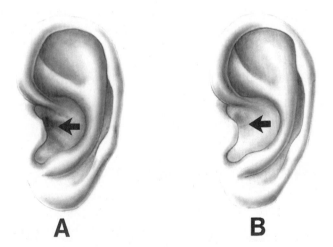

FIG. 4. A: Left ear with slit-like conical opening into the external canal (*arrow*). This type of meatus heralds a stenotic canal that frequently ends in a blind pouch. **B:** Left ear with flat thumb-print–like depression where the canal should be (*arrow*). The presence of this type of meatus suggests complete absence of the tympanic bone.

Once CT images have been obtained, several points of anatomy must be evaluated. First the presence and extent of the tympanic bone and the degree of canalization are assessed. The extent of middle ear and mastoid development are determined. In general, risk for surgical complications is minimized and the chances for successful hearing are increased if the size of the middle ear and mastoid size is at least two thirds of normal.

The ossicular anatomy is defined, and the presence of an intact stapes and patent oval window is documented. The course and degree of bony covering of the facial nerve are examined. The relation between the condyle and the middle ear space and mastoid is determined. A grading system that quantifies the developmental status of the ear on the basis of radiographic criteria has been developed. Postoperative hearing results have been shown to correlate with this grading system (6). Patients with a score of 8 or above are excellent surgical candidates, and those with a score of 4 or 5 or below are poor surgical candidates (Figs. 5, 6).

Although normal development of the cochlea and vestibular labyrinth is anticipated in patients with aural atresia, their appearance on CT scans should be recorded. In rare instances an abnormality of the horizontal semicircular canal or vestibule is identified. In such cases, surgical repair of the atresia can proceed; however, manipulation of the stapes should be minimized because of the possibility of abnormal communication between the perilymph and cerebrospinal fluid.

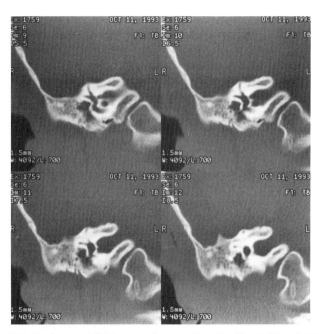

FIG. 6. Coronal CT images from patient in Fig. 5. The right ear shows poor middle ear and mastoid development, no definable ossicular mass, and a closed oval window. This ear is not a candidate for surgical therapy (score of 3).

MEDICAL MANAGEMENT

Unilateral Atresia

Unilateral atresia is about six times more common than its bilateral counterpart. If the uninvolved ear has normal hearing, little functional disability should arise in the development of speech and language. However, it is extremely important to make sure that the normal ear is normal. It is not unusual to find a middle ear conductive hearing loss or even a sensorineural hearing loss in what was thought to be a normal ear. This is especially true once the patient is old enough to undergo thorough audiometric evaluation.

A hearing aid for the atretic ear is not recommended because of poor acceptance by most children and the small benefit it affords to overall audition. As a child enters school, preferential seating is advised. In classrooms with unavoidable noise, an auditory trainer can be useful. The consequences of unilateral atresia often are found by teenagers and adults to be a problem in social settings and at work, and these persons may more readily accept a hearing aid. In cases of atresia of the ear canal, a bone conduction hearing aid must be used. If the canal is only stenotic, an air conduction aid is preferred because of cosmesis, better sound localization, broader frequency response, and less sound distortion.

Bilateral Atresia

For infants with bilateral atresia, early amplification is paramount. Audiologic and medical evaluations can be

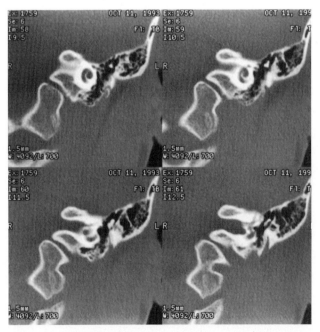

FIG. 5. Coronal CT images of a patient with bilateral microtia and canal atresia. The left ear shows good middle ear and mastoid air cell development, a prominent ossicular mass with the malleus and incus heads fused but distinct, and an open oval window. This ear is an excellent candidate for surgical therapy (score of 8).

completed within the first few months of life and a bone conduction hearing aid fitted soon thereafter.

SURGICAL MANAGEMENT

General Considerations

Although most otologic surgeons would consider repair in bilateral cases of atresia, many are reluctant to operate when only one ear is involved. The issue is not simply the unilateral hearing loss, because there is little controversy involving middle ear exploration for a child with a large conductive hearing loss from other causes. The reluctance is based on expectations of hearing recovery, potential lifetime care of a mastoid cavity, and surgical risks, especially to the facial nerve and labyrinth. These concerns have prompted many surgeons to recommend delaying surgery for unilateral atresia or the second ear in bilateral atresia until adulthood, when the person is old enough to participate in decision making.

In addressing the foregoing concerns, the following factors should be considered. To eliminate the disability of unilateral hearing loss, a speech-hearing threshold of 25 dB or better is required. Although this degree of hearing improvement cannot be achieved by all patients selected for surgery, approximately 55% to 65% have this hearing level in the long term. A mastoid cavity can be avoided if the anterior surgical approach is used, and this approach reduces the need for frequent cavity cleaning after the operation. Risk of facial nerve injury is minimized if the surgeon understands the abnormal development of this structure and performs intraoperative facial nerve monitoring. We and others believe that the benefits of binaural hearing and the possibility of achieving that goal are sufficiently great to offer corrective surgery to carefully selected children with unilateral atresia. The selection process is critical. Approximately 40% of patients with unilateral atresia are not surgical candidates. Included in this category are patients with severe aplasia, such as most patients with Treacher Collins syndrome.

Patients with bilateral atresia present less of a surgical dilemma. Their goal is to restore sufficient hearing so that amplification is no longer necessary. In contradistinction to ear selection for most other otologic disorders, the better ear (as determined with CT evaluation) is selected for the initial surgical procedure. In most cases, the initial ear is operated on as the child approaches school age. Depending on the hearing result, the second ear is treated within the next several years. Although the selection criteria are slightly less stringent in bilateral cases, careful patient screening is essential for satisfactory results.

Timing of Surgery

Surgical correction of atresia is usually performed after 6 or 7 years of age. By that time, accurate audiometric tests have been performed, pneumatization of the temporal bone is well advanced, and most children are able to cooperate with postoperative care. This timing also allows time for repair of microtia. For patients with microtia who need extensive reconstruction of the external ear, it is recommended that reconstructive surgery proceed first (see Chapter 22). This assures a surgical field free of scars or comprised blood supply and optimizes survival of the implanted rib cartilage framework. The overall appearance will be better without the restriction of having to reconstruct an auricle around the bony canal that has been drilled in the temporal bone. Later, during atresia repair, the reconstructed auricle can be repositioned with appropriate undermining to align the meatus and external canal.

Canal Cholesteatoma

Canal cholesteatoma can develop in ears with minor aplasia as desquamated squamous epithelium accumulates in the stenotic ear canal. Cole and Jahrsdoerfer (7) reviewed the cases of 50 patients with a canal diameter of 4 mm or less and found a 50% incidence of cholesteatoma. Patient age and canal size were important variables in predicting disease. Cholesteatoma was not found among patients younger than 3 years but were increasingly encountered as children reached adolescence. Bone erosion or middle ear involvement from canal cholesteatoma did not occur among patients younger than 12 years. The preponderance of cholesteatoma developed in canals 2 mm or less in diameter. The usual presenting symptom was drainage from the ear canal or from a postauricular fistula tract. Given these data, it is judicious to obtain CT scans of patients with severe stenosis of the external ear canal by the age of 5 or 6 years. Surgical treatment is indicated if cholesteatoma is found. If cholesteatoma is not detected, several options are available. For patients with CT findings that are favorable with regard to hearing improvement, canal and middle ear operations can be considered. Canaloplasty is offered alone to patients with unfavorable middle ear findings. Periodic CT is not needed by patients with complete atresia of the ear canal because of the rarity of cholesteatoma in that setting.

SURGICAL TECHNIQUE

For patients with minor aplasia and a developed external auditory canal, the canal is surgically widened and any ossicular abnormalities or eardrum problems are corrected. These patients usually experience good hearing results and few complications.

For patients with moderate aplasia (and the rare patient with severe aplasia), there are two basic surgical approaches: the mastoid (or posterior) approach and the anterior approach. In the mastoid approach, the sinodural angle is identified and then the antrum (8,9). The facial recess is opened and the incudostapedial joint separated. Atretic bone is removed. Often the lateral ossicular mass (malleus and incus complex) also is removed, and ossicular reconstruction is accomplished with cartilage, bone, or alloplastic material.

In the anterior approach, the middle ear is exposed directly through the atretic bone itself with limited opening into the mastoid air cells. Among properly selected patients, there is sufficient access through this area to construct an ear canal (Fig. 7). This approach obviates a mastoid cavity with its attendant problems of debris accumulation and infection. There also is less surgical manipulation in the area of the vertical segment of the facial nerve. The more cylindrical contours of the new canal achieved in the anterior approach facilitate placement of a split-thickness skin graft. The following are the salient features of the anterior approach.

Incision

A postauricular incision is used to expose the mastoid bone. The soft tissues are elevated anteriorly until a depression in the surface of the mastoid bone is encountered. In most cases of severe aplasia, this depression is the temporomandibular joint, although occasionally a stenotic bony ear canal is found. Dissection within this area may rarely be necessary to differentiate between the two, but any manipulation should be limited because the facial nerve frequently exits the skull into the glenoid fossa.

Canal Drilling

Landmarks for drilling the external canal are the middle cranial fossa superiorly, the glenoid fossa anteriorly, and the mastoid air cells posteriorly. These structures delimit the atretic bone, which lies lateral to the middle ear space. The tympanic bone remnant occasionally is apparent and clearly demarcated from the surrounding cortex. The bone removed is usually solid but may be cellular in areas. The posterior wall of the glenoid fossa (anterior wall of the new ear canal) is kept as thin as possible to allow access to the anterior half of the middle ear space. As the dural plate of the middle cranial fossa is followed medially, the epitympanum is the first portion of the middle ear space encountered. The fused heads of the malleus and the incus are identified (Fig. 8). Concentrat-

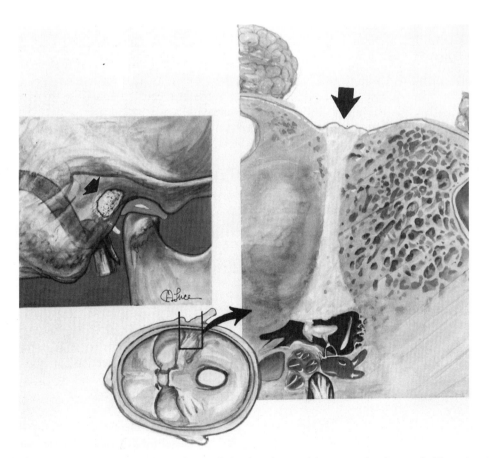

FIG. 7. Schematics show atretic bone from a lateral and an axial perspective (*arrows*). (From Lambert PR. Major congenital ear malformations: surgical management and results. *Ann Otol Rhinol Laryngol* 1998;97:641–649, with permission.)

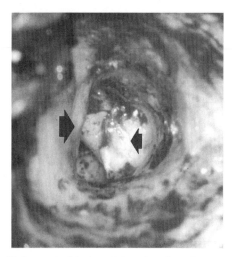

FIG. 8. Right ear with fused heads of malleus and incus (*large arrow*) exposed in the epitympanum. The rest of the middle ear is covered by atretic bone (*small arrow*). (From Lambert PR. Major congenital ear malformations: surgical management and results. *Ann Otol Rhinol Laryngol* 1998:97: 641–649, with permission.)

ing on drilling superiorly along the middle cranial fossa has the advantage of protecting the facial nerve because that structure always lies medial to the ossicular mass in the epitympanum. Drilling in a posterior-inferior direction brings the dissection closer to the facial nerve. Because of the more anterior and lateral course of the vertical segment of the facial nerve, it is vulnerable to injury in this area.

Middle Ear Operation

Atretic bone lateral to the fused malleus incus complex is removed circumferentially around the ossicular mass (Fig. 9). Fixation of the ossicular chain to the atretic bone

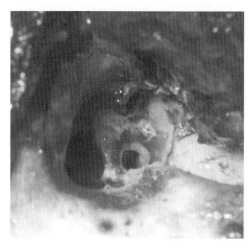

FIG. 9. Right ear with ossicular chain fully exposed.

is usually at the neck of the malleus. The stapes may be partially obscured because of the small middle ear cavity, malformed lateral ossicular mass, or overlying facial nerve. Enough of the stapes usually can be seen to assess its mobility and the integrity of the incudostapedial joint. A normal oval window and stapes footplate are anticipated, but the stapes may be fixed in as many as 5% of cases. An inadequate incudostapedial connection is encountered in 5% to 7% of cases. In such instances, ossicular reconstruction with or without stapedectomy is necessary. In most cases, however, the ossicular chain is intact and maintained in position. Long-term hearing results may be better among patients who do not need a prosthesis (10).

Tympanic Membrane Grafting

A thin temporalis fascia graft is placed over the mobilized ossicular chain. Because the manubrium of the malleus is either absent or very deformed, it is difficult to anchor the graft beneath this ossicle. Lateralization of the tympanic membrane graft is a potential complication. Several techniques can be used to help avoid this problem. First, the graft can be tucked beneath anterior and superior bony ledges of the canal wall, or a sulcus can be drilled in the anterior canal wall medial to the level of the ossicles. A second technique to avoid lateralization involves covering the fascial graft with the split-thickness skin graft of the canal and placing over the covered ossicles a polymeric silicone (Silastic) button that has been contoured to the circumference of the canal (11).

Meatoplasty

A circular meatal opening about twice the normal size is made in the reconstructed auricle. The alignment of the meatus in the bony external canal is assessed. The meatus frequently is offset anteriorly or inferiorly. In such cases, the auricle is undermined so that it can be repositioned in a more favorable location.

Skin Grafting

A thin split-thickness skin graft (0.008 to 0.010 inches) is harvested from the upper thigh or medial upper arm. A graft size of approximately 4 cm by 6 cm is required. To facilitate graft placement at the level of the tympanic membrane, multiple small wedges are excised from that portion of the graft.

With the ear retracted forward, the split-thickness skin graft is positioned in the bony canal and allowed to overlay the fascial graft (Fig. 10). The skin graft is stabilized with Merocel ear wicks placed in the canal and hydrated with Cortisporin suspension (Fig. 11). After the bony

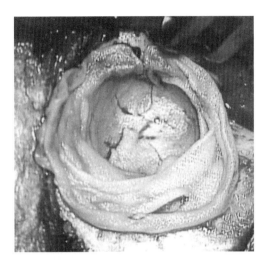

FIG. 10. Split-thickness skin graft positioned within the bony canal.

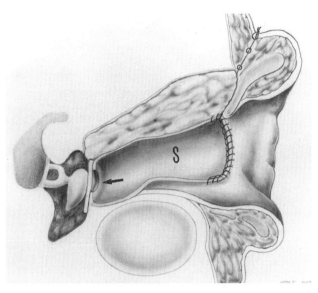

FIG. 12. Left ear with completed atresia repair. Skin graft (*s*) is sutured to the margin of the new meatus. The graft overlaps the fascial graft (*arrow*).

canal is packed, the auricle is returned to its normal anatomic position. The surgeon, working through the meatus, unfolds the lateral edge of the skin graft and sutures it to the meatal skin edge (Fig. 12). Additional Merocel packing is used to fill the lateral soft tissue portion of the canal.

Postoperative Care

Approximately 10 days postoperatively, the ear canal packing is removed with the silicone button, if used. Complete take of the split-thickness skin graft is anticipated at this time. If any granulation tissue is present, Cortisporin-soaked pieces of gelatin foam are placed within the canal, and the patient instructed to keep these moist for the next 1 to 2 weeks.

SURGICAL FINDINGS

Ossicles

In the moderate and severe types aplasia, the malleus and incus are deformed and fused. The malleus is typically more deformed than the incus, and the manubrium is short or absent (Fig. 13). Ossicular fixation occurs most often between the malleus neck and the atretic bone. Stapedial abnormalities also are common. The superstructure is usually small with delicate, misshapen crura. Stapedial fixation and incudostapedial joint incompetence or discontinuity may be encountered.

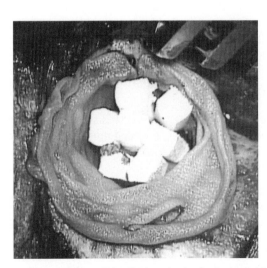

FIG. 11. Merocel ear wicks (before hydration) placed in the bony canal to stabilize the skin graft.

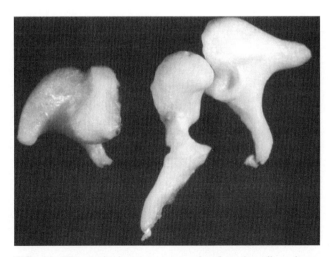

FIG. 13. The typical appearance of a fused malleus-incus complex (*left*). These fused ossicles are small compared with normal ossicles (*right*), and the malleus is more deformed than the incus.

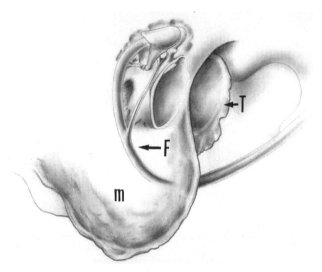

FIG. 14. Normal tympanic ring (*T*) and normal course of the facial nerve (*F*). Mastoid process (*m*) is in normal anatomic position.

Facial Nerve

In the normal course of development, posterior migration of the mastoid process carries the facial nerve with it. The facial nerve ultimately exits the skull beneath the temporal bone. At this point, the nerve has descended in its vertical segment and crosses the mandibular ramus at an angle of about 120 degrees relative to the descending portion (Fig. 14). The angle between the horizontal and vertical segments (external genu) is obtuse. In the atretic ear, the facial nerve makes a more abrupt anterior and lateral turn (less than 90 degrees) at the second genu. The result is that the nerve covers a portion of the posterior mesotympanum and crosses the condyle rather than the ramus (12) (Fig. 15). As a consequence, the round window usually is obscured, and access to the oval window may be partially

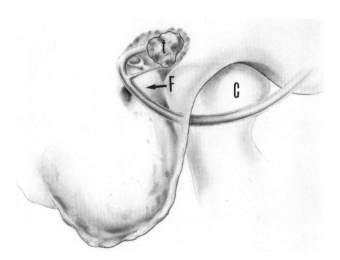

FIG. 15. Complete developmental arrest. Course of the facial nerve (*F*) is altered; the nerve turns more abruptly across the condyle of the mandible. Remnant of tympanic bone (*t*) is present. Condyle (*C*) is adjacent to mastoid.

obstructed. The more distal portion of the vertical segment of the facial nerve actually is lateral to the middle ear space. In addition to this abnormal course of the mastoid segment, bony dehiscence of the tympanic segment and inferior displacement of the tympanic segment often are encountered. A higher incidence of facial nerve abnormalities has been found among patients with more severe microtia; thus the extent of external ear deformity may provide some indication of facial nerve status (10,13).

HEARING RESULTS

It is difficult to compare hearing results from various series because of differences in classification of congenital ear malformations, selection criteria in reporting of hearing results, and length of follow-up periods. In general, a postoperative hearing level of 30 dB or better can be achieved by 50% to 75% of patients with moderate or severe aplasia. A hearing level of 20 dB or better is possible among 15% to 50% of patients. Bellucci (14) reported a hearing level of at least 30 dB among 55% of 71 patients observed a minimum of 2 years. Schuknecht (15) reported similar results for 30 patients with a mean follow-up period of 1.3 years; 30% of patients in this series had a hearing level of 20 dB or better. Nager and Levin (16) reported a hearing level of at least 30 dB among 70% of 23 patients. De la Cruz et al. (17) described 56 patients with a 6-month follow-up period and found that 53% had a conductive deficit of 20 dB or less and 73% had a deficit of 30 dB or less; similar results were found for a follow-up series of 24 patients (18). Jahrsdoerfer et al. (6) reported a postoperative hearing level 1 month after treatment of 25 dB or better among 71% of 86 patients. Lambert (19) reported both early (less than 1 year) and late (more than 1 year; mean 34 months) follow-up results for 50 patients with atresia. In the early postoperative period, 60% of the patients achieved a speech reception threshold (SRT) of 25 dB or better; almost half of achieved an SRT of 10 to 15 dB. These results diminished to 46% as the follow-up period extended beyond the first year. Long-term results after revision surgery were 53% with an SRT of 25 dB or better and 64% with an SRT of 30 dB or better (19).

COMPLICATIONS

In most series, the rate of revision surgery is approximately 30%. Revision is needed most commonly because of restenosis, graft migration or failure, and inadequate hearing results.

Conductive Hearing Loss

The causes of a persistent or recurrent conductive hearing loss are varied. They include inadequate mobilization of the ossicular mass from the atretic bone, unrecognized incudostapedial joint discontinuity, a fixed stapes footplate, or regrowth of bone with refixation of the ossicular chain. Wide exposure of the ossicular mass during the operation is necessary to ensure chain mobility and to prevent refixation. Lateralization or perforation of the tympanic membrane can cause a recurrence of conductive hearing loss. The incidence of graft failure or middle ear adhesions approximates that encountered in routine tympanoplasty procedures.

Canal Stenosis

Postoperative narrowing of the new external canal develops in as many as 25% of patients, particularly in the membranous segment or at the meatus. The development of marked stenosis results in chronic infection from trapped squamous epithelium. Attempts to dilate the canal with hard or soft stents rarely are effective, and canaloplasty-meatoplasty with skin grafting is needed. In some patients, the lateral ear canal may be narrowed by displacement of the pinna rather than by fibrous tissue formation. It is common at the time of the operation for the meatus to be offset anteriorly and inferiorly relative to the bony canal. This misalignment is corrected during the operation by means of undermining the auricle and removing a strip of postauricular skin.

Facial Nerve Injury

Perhaps the most feared complication in congenital ear surgery is facial nerve injury. The abnormal development of temporal bone described earlier, which obscures normal otologic landmarks, places the frequently anomalous facial nerve at risk. In these patients, however, facial nerve anomalies encountered are predictable; this fact and the use of facial nerve monitoring enable the surgeon to proceed with confidence. In a study of more than 1,000 operations for congenital anomalies of the ear, facial nerve paresis or paralysis occurred among less than 1% (20). For an experienced surgeon, the incidence of a facial nerve injury approximates that in operations for chronic ear disorders.

Labyrinthine Injury

High-frequency sensorineural hearing loss has been found postoperatively among some patients, although marked loss in the speech frequencies is rare (10,18,21). Because the ossicular mass is connected to atretic bone, energy from drilling is transmitted to the inner ear whether or not the anterior or posterior approach is used. Care in removing the final portion of atretic bone from the ossicular chain is particularly important with the anterior approach, because the incudostapedial joint is not disarticulated. In general, the incidence of substantial sensorineural hearing loss is similar to that during operations on the stapes.

SUMMARY

The objective in surgical therapy for congenital aural atresia is to construct a functional pathway by which sound can reach the cochlear fluid. This type of surgery presents a challenge to otologic surgeons. Thorough knowledge of the anatomic variations that can occur with abnormal development of temporal bone is essential to minimize intraoperative and postoperative complications. Consistently excellent hearing results cannot yet be achieved in operations for atresia; however, restoration of serviceable hearing can be anticipated among almost two thirds of properly selected patients.

SUMMARY POINTS

- The cochlea and vestibular labyrinth are derived from the ectodermal otocyst, and the critical aspects of development precede those of the external and middle ear. Inner ear function therefore is expected to be normal among patients with aural atresia.
- Disruption of the recanalization process of the external auditory canal during the late second trimester can result in a spectrum of canal anomalies from stenosis to atresia.
- Congenital malformations of the ear can be divided into minor, moderate, and severe aplasia. Minor or moderate aplasia is potentially amenable to surgical correction.
- The CT appearance of the temporal bone, especially size of the middle ear and development of the ossicles, is the most critical factor in patient selection for surgical treatment.
- Patients with unilateral atresia, if properly selected, may be considered for surgical treatment. Overall, approximately two thirds of patients with aural atresia are candidates for operative intervention.
- The facial nerve often is aberrant in aural atresia. Dehiscence of the tympanic segment, with or without inferior displacement, is commonly encountered. The mastoid segment of the facial nerve usually makes a more acute angle at the second genu, resulting in anterior and lateral displacement; it may obscure the round window.
- In congenital atresia, the malleus and incus are deformed and fused. Ossicular fixation usually involves the neck of the malleus and the atretic bone. The stapes usually is mobile but is small with delicate, misshapen crura.
- With proper patient selection, a long-term hearing level of 25 dB or better can be achieved by 50% to 60% of patients, and a level of at least 30 dB by two thirds to three fourths of patients.
- Revision operations are needed most often for canal stenosis. Refixation of the ossicular chain, an unrecognized stapes or incudostapedial joint problem, or graft lateralization can result in persistence or recurrence of conductive hearing loss. The incidence of facial nerve injury (less than 1%) approximates that for operations for chronic ear problems.

REFERENCES

1. Politzer A. *History of otology.* Milstein S, Portnoff C, Coleman A, translators. Phoenix: Columella Press, 1981.
2. Jafek BW, Nager GT, Strife J, et al. Congenital aural atresia: an analysis of 311 cases. *Trans Am Acad Ophthalmol Otolaryngol* 1975;80: 588–592 (abst).
3. Colman BH. Congenital atresia: aspects of surgical care. *Acta Otorhinolaryngol Belg* 1971;25:929–933.
4. Lambert PR. Congenital absence of the oval window. *Laryngoscope* 1990;100:37–40.
5. Tucci DL, Ruth RA, Lambert PR. Use of the bone conduction ABR wave I response in determination of cochlear reserve. *Am J Otolaryngol* 1990;11:119–124.
6. Jahrsdoerfer RA, Yeakley JW, Aguilar EA, et al. Grading system for the selection of patients with congenital aural atresia. *Am J Otolaryngol* 1992;13:6–12.
7. Cole RR, Jahrsdoerfer RA. The risk of cholesteatoma in congenital aural stenosis. *Laryngoscope* 1990;100:576–578.
8. Crabtree JA. Congenital atresia: case selection, complications, and prevention. *Otolaryngol Clin North Am* 1982;15:755–761.
9. Glasscock ME III, Schwaber MK, Nissen AJ, et al. Management of congenital ear malformations. *Ann Otol Rhinol Laryngol* 1983;92:504–509.
10. Lambert PR. Major congenital ear malformations: surgical management and results. *Ann Otol Rhinol Laryngol* 1988;97:641–649.
11. Jahrsdoerfer RA, Cole RR, Gray LC. Advances in congenital aural atresia. *Adv Otolaryngol Head Neck Surg* 1991;5:1–15.
12. Crabtree JA. The facial nerve in congenital ear surgery. In: Graham MD, House WF, eds. *Disorders of the facial nerve.* New York: Raven Press, 1982:389–395.
13. Jahrsdoerfer RA. Congenital atresia of the ear. *Laryngoscope* 1978;88[Suppl 13]:1–46.
14. Bellucci RJ. Congenital aural malformations: diagnosis and treatment. *Otolaryngol Clin North Am* 1981;14:95–124.
15. Schuknecht HG. Congenital aural atresia. *Laryngoscope* 1989;99: 908–917.
16. Nager GT, Levin LS. Congenital aural atresia: embryology, pathology, classification, genetics, and surgical management. In: Paparella MM, Shumrick D, eds. *Otolaryngology.* Philadelphia: WB Saunders, 1980: 1303–1344.
17. De la Cruz A, Linthicum FH Jr, Luxford WM. Congenital atresia of the external auditory canal. *Laryngoscope* 1985;95:421–427.
18. Malony TB, De la Cruz A. Surgical approaches to congenital atresia of the external auditory canal. *Otolaryngol Head Neck Surg* 1990;103: 991–1001.
19. Lambert PR. Congenital aural atresia: stability of surgical results. *Laryngoscope* 1998;108:1801–1805.
20. Jahrsdoerfer RA, Lambert PR. Facial nerve injury in congenital aural atresia surgery. *Am J Otol* 1998;19:283–287.
21. Jahrsdoerfer RA. Congenital malformation of the ear. *Ann Otol Rhinol Laryngol* 1980;89:348–352.

The Ear: Comprehensive Otology,
edited by R. F. Canalis and P. R. Lambert.
Lippincott Williams & Wilkins, Philadelphia © 2000.

CHAPTER 22

Reconstruction of the Congenitally Deformed Auricle

Robert O. Ruder

Reconstruction of severe congenital deformities of the external ear requires extensive experience and a sound understanding of the normal anatomy and supporting elements of the pinna. Most persons have differences in size, configuration, and position of the ears that are not conspicuous. The literature abounds with descriptions of numerous malformations and procedures to correct them (1,2). Much of this information has caused considerable confusion because of a lack of standardization of the components of each specific deformity. The terms *prominent, cupped, hooded, lidded, cryptic,* and *peanut ear* often are used interchangeably and incorrectly. It is essential to become familiar with the anatomic subunits of the auricle and be able to differentiate dysmorphic and dysplastic malformations. Many severe-appearing anomalies can be easily repaired if most elements are present but misshapen. Microtia is the result of the most catastrophic form of arrested auricular development. Repair demands well-planned and individually tailored operations.

EMBRYOLOGIC CONSIDERATIONS

The anlage of the external ear is first seen by the fourth week of gestation as a slit beneath the developing mandible. The auricle arises from the first and second branchial arches and the fundus (slit) lying between them (3). Three separate accumulations of mesoderm and epiderm, called *hillocks,* develop from each of these two arches (see Chapter 2). Classic microtia represents arrested differentiation of these six accumulations during the second intrauterine month. Hillocks 1 to 3 on the first branchial arch become the lobule, tragus, and root of the helix. Hillocks 4 through 6 on the second (hyoid) arch develop into the superior and anterior aspects of the ear as the antihelix, scapha, and antitragus. The more com-

R. O. Ruder: Department of Head and Neck Surgery, UCLA Medical Center Beverly Hills, California 90024; and Head and Neck Surgery, Cedars Sinai Medical Center, Los Angeles, California 90211-1715

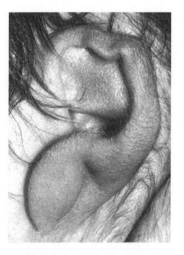

FIG. 1. Dysmorphic ear anomalies result from abnormal intrauterine positioning that causes pressure on the developing auricle.

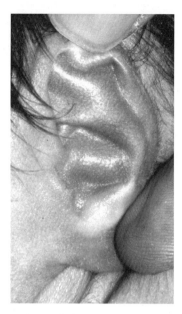

FIG. 2. A finger "opens" the ear to reveal that all anatomic subunits are present.

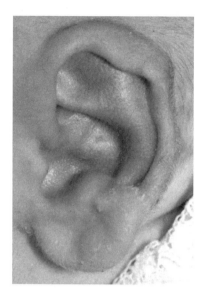

FIG. 4. Appearance 10 days after sculpturing by means of a nonsurgical technique.

mon developmental problems occur with arrested development of this second arch, which produces small, constricted ears that seem to fall over on themselves because of inadequate tissue and support. By the second intrauterine month the developing auricle begins its migration toward the mastoid process. By the twentieth week of gestation, the ear has attainted its adult configuration, although the size and location are still infantile.

Several other organ systems are rapidly forming during the first trimester. Even the most subtle adverse genetic or environmental factors can severely influence this dramatic sequence of change and cause catastrophic malformations. Almost 50% of patients with microtia have additional anomalies. Maldevelopment of the first and second branchial arch and groove derivatives can produce auricular appendages, weakness or paralysis of the facial nerve, microsomia, canal stenosis or atresia, and middle and inner ear dysplasia. Distant anomalies of the urinary tract, ribs, cervical spine, and heart also can occur. It is critical for the otologist and facial plastic surgeon to develop a closely coordinated team with consultants in pediatrics, genetics, dentistry, orthodontics, prosthodontics, nursing, audiology, speech pathology, psychiatry, and social work to handle other concomitant problems.

Adverse factors after the twentieth week can be troublesome even after the auricle has reached its adult-like configuration. Although all components are present, the ear may be deformed by either abnormal intrauterine positioning or cervical masses that compress the ear. These dysmorphic deformities can be corrected easily by means of remolding the ear with cotton and tape within the first week after birth (Figs. 1–4). The high concentration of maternal estrogen circulating within a neonate makes the auricular fibroelastic cartilage especially pliable in this period. At birth the ear is almost two thirds of adult size but is still slightly rounder (rather than oval) and is more inferior in location than the mature pinna.

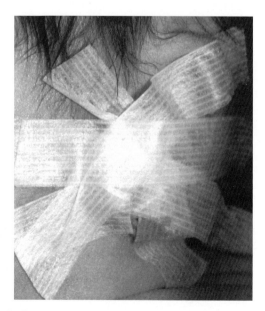

FIG. 3. Dysmorphic ears can be remolded with cotton and tape.

PHILOSOPHY OF RECONSTRUCTION

Microtia is one aspect of a multifaceted otologic and craniofacial problem. Unlike a dysmorphic ear, a microtic ear must have all parts reconstructed. Both the inadequate cartilage framework and skin envelope must be addressed. Proper placement of the reconstructed ear

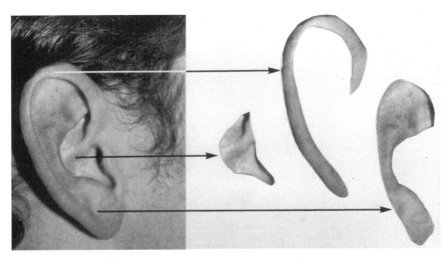

FIG. 5. The auricle can be conceptualized as three layers: concha, scapha, and helix. The scapha is the main buttress and structural support.

is the essential criterion. Even the most delicately constructed ear will look abnormal if it is not properly positioned in relation to other facial structures. This multi-countoured flap-like structure must lie between the eyebrow and base of the columella. It should not be vertical, but inclined 20 degrees and parallel to the axis of the nose. Ideal lateral placement is the distance of the vertical height of the normal ear (5.5 to 6 cm) from the lateral aspect of the orbit. Farkas (4) meticulously assessed the morphologic features of the ear and detailed uniform standard measurements for planning reconstruction. It is perhaps best to integrate his standards with one's own aesthetic guidelines. In unilateral microtia, the normal side is an ideal model for proper size, position, and configuration. However, with bilateral microtia, the surgeon must have an even sounder knowledge of facial proportions, shape, and orientation.

The auricle can be conceptualized as a three-layered oval structure that protrudes from the skull (Fig. 5). The concha is the most interior layer and surrounds the opening of the external canal (5). The scapha is the middle tier and is the main structural support. When weak or deficient, the ear folds over on itself causing lack of vertical height. The helix is the most lateral layer and delineates the delicate peripheral silhouette.

Auricular deformity can be better understood in a context of one of three grades of deformity (6). Grade I deformity represents ears with all anatomic subunits present but misshapen (see Fig. 1). A prominent or cup ear with its unfurled antihelical fold and excessively deepened, overly angulated concha are dysmorphic anomalies. Ears with grade II deformities are constricted in size. Anatomic subunits are either deficient or absent (Fig. 6). Arrested development of the scapha with absence of the fossa triangularis causes lidding in the

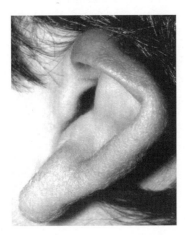

FIG. 6. Class II deformities are constricted and small. These ears lack anatomic subunits.

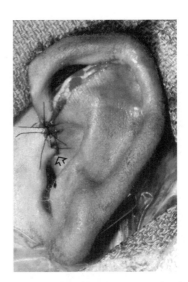

FIG. 7. Low-lying foreshortened crus on the helix must be repositioned to a higher level.

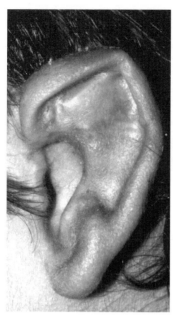

FIG. 8. Completed repositioning of the helix and composite chondrocutaneous grafts.

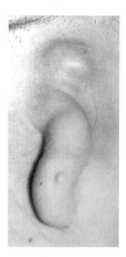

FIG. 9. Class III (microtia) deformities have an inferior fibroadipose lobule and a nubbin of cartilage in the superior remnant.

superior aspect with foreshortening and flattening of the helical rim. Reconstruction often requires chondrocutaneous and full-thickness skin grafts (Figs. 7, 8). Ears with grade III deformities are dysplastic and microtic. Almost no normal remnants are present except the lobule (Fig. 9). These ears are usually positioned higher than the normal side, and have a deficient cartilage framework and skin envelope.

CLASSIC MICROTIA

The typical appearance of microtia is a vertically oriented appendage with a superior nubbin of cartilage and an inferior fibroadipose lobule. Although small, the rem-

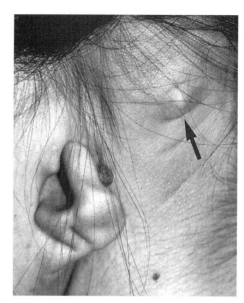

FIG. 10. The developing auricle has failed to migrate to the mastoid process. It lies on the mandible. *Arrow* indicates mastoid where adult auricle should lie.

nant of cartilage can be developed well enough to resemble an auricle. The fibroadipose lobule is the most consistent and best developed subunit. These ears usually lie at different levels from the normal side. If microtia occurs within the first weeks of development, migration toward the mastoid process may be interrupted, and the ear may lie almost anywhere along this path, even under the mandible (Fig. 10).

Sequence and Timing of Operation

Auricular repair ideally should precede temporal bone surgery. Reconstruction usually involves four stages at 3-month intervals. The first step is sculpturing and implantation of ribs grafts into the shape of an ear. The second is posterior positioning of the remaining fibroadipose remnant into an earlobe. Third, a tragus is formed with skin and composite grafts. The last step is construction of a postauricular sulcus. The age at which to begin the surgical procedures depends on the physical and emotional maturity of the patient. Studies have suggested that these patients often suffer severe psychologic distress (7,8). Most children become extremely sensitive to their body image by 5 years of age, a period when any deformity or difference becomes an object of curiosity to playmates. The negative emotional effect of undue attention and jokes may cause shame, anguish, and withdrawal.

By 6 years of age, most patients begin asking their parents for help either orally or in behavioral changes. They are more motivated to cooperate with their postoperative care. The size and configuration of the chest wall must be large enough to allow harvesting the cartilage portions of three to four ribs without causing additional deformity at the donor site. Small, shallow, underdeveloped ribs are difficult to sculpture. Although the age of 8 or 9 years may be ideal, most children have an adequately developed chest wall to begin reconstruction by 6 years of age. Patients with severe hemifacial microsomia and bilateral microtia present additional problems (9). If craniofacial reconstruction is necessary and cannot be delayed until auricular reconstruction is completed, the teams must be well coordinated. The craniofacial team should attempt to make their scars peripheral to the ear site by using coronal and intraoral incisions.

Framework

Several different implant materials have been used. Gilles (10) described use of allografts of cartilage sutured together. These frameworks often resorbed and definition was soon lost. Cronin and Ascough (11,12) used premolded polymeric silicone (Silastic) implants. The ease of using these grafts reduced the morbidity of harvesting costal cartilage. However, the frequency of graft extrusion dampened initial enthusiasm. Ohmori and Sekiguchi (13) modified the polymeric silicone framework with a Dacron polyester mesh backing. They reported a high incidence of extrusion and an infection rate of 25% among 175 patients. Tanzer (14) popularized the use of autogenous rib cartilage sculptured into a three-layered framework. Gorney (15) used conchal cartilage from the opposite ear to repair partial and complete deformities. This technique is demanding for surgeons who only occasionally treat patients with microtia. It requires considerable experience and artistic skill. Brent (16) also used autogenous costal cartilage. He initially constructed an open framework, but it lacked stability to maintain a permanent contour. He now constructs a three-layered framework (17), as I have been doing for 10 years.

The question of growth of donor cartilage is controversial. At birth the ear is 66% of adult size. By 8 years of age it is almost 85%; by 10 years of age it approaches full size. Growth of the reconstructed ear seems to keep up with that of the opposite ear (17). It is unclear whether this is growth of the donor cartilage or of the soft tissue. Brent (17) believes that 48% of his patients' ears grew at an even pace with the opposite normal ear. Forty-one percent of the ears grew several millimeters larger, and 10% lagged several millimeters behind the normal side. I therefore make the ear slightly smaller than the normal side for the youngest patients and the same size for patients older than 10 years.

Preoperative Plan

The prospect of four operations with rib and cartilage grafts can be overwhelming to a young family. Both the parents and the child should be present at consultations to establish a warm and comforting connection, foster confidence, and alleviate fears.

Auricular repair should begin before correction of the atretic canal (Fig. 11). Previous operations in this area

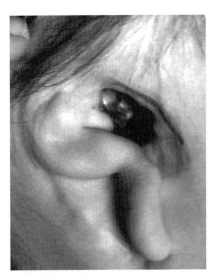

FIG. 11. Construction of the external canal has left a large, malpositioned cavity with excessive scarring. This prevents successful auricular construction.

violate skin vascularity and produce undesired scarring. A nonscarred elastic skin pocket is essential to accommodate the subtle convolutions of the three-dimensional cartilage graft. If the atresia and auricular reconstructive teams are not well coordinated, the auricle and canal may be on different levels.

Two templates of exposed radiographic film are made to ensure proper placement and symmetry of the reconstructed ear (18). The first template is made for configuration and size. The film is placed over the opposite ear, and its silhouette is traced (Fig. 12). This mold is cut a

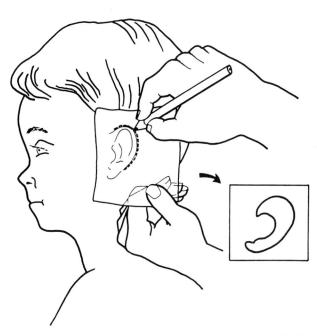

FIG. 12. Template of normal pinna made of radiographic film to determine size and configuration of the microtic ear. The template is drawn slightly smaller to allow for skin thickness.

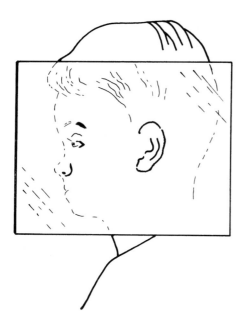

FIG. 13. A second template of radiographic film is made from the normal side with the eyebrow, lateral canthus, nostril, and lip as landmarks to ensure proper positioning.

few millimeters smaller in all dimensions to allow for the thickness of the skin and soft tissue. A second template is constructed to assure proper alignment in axial, vertical, and anterior-posterior positions (Fig. 13). Normal facial landmarks of the ear to eyebrow, ear to nostril, and ear to corner of the mouth are drawn. The template is reversed and tattooed onto the microtic side with methylene blue. Proper placement often is more difficult with severe hemifacial microsomia. The differences in height and anterior-posterior dimensions of each side may be dramatic. The reconstructed ear should be aligned with the superior pole of the normal pinna. The anterior-posterior placement must be a compromise but not arbitrary. The vestige should not be too close to the eye or too far back on the head.

A low hairline can cause problems (19). One should never compromise proper location because of hairline considerations. The reconstructed ear occasionally is made smaller to compensate for a low hairline. The opposite normal ear is reduced by excising the scaphal cartilage at the time of tragal construction. With bilateral microtia, both ears are made slightly smaller to minimize hair growth on the upper helical rim.

Operative Technique

Sculpturing and Placement of Rib Graft

Rib cartilage is taken from the side opposite the ear being constructed to take advantage of the natural curvature that conforms to the sculptured ear. An incision is made 2 cm above and parallel to the inferior costal margin. The rectus muscle and sheath are divided and dissected until the ribs are visualized. The interior aspect of

the ribs is elevated in a supraperichondral plane by means of meticulous dissection to prevent perforation of the closely adherent pleura. The templates are used to determine the amount of cartilage needed (Fig. 14). Although every chest wall is different, the synchondrotic region of the sixth and seventh ribs is usually ample for the framework. The first free-floating rib is harvested to form a helix (20). While the assistant is closing the chest wall, the surgeon sculptures the cartilage block on a separate dissecting table. It is imperative to leave as much perichondrium intact as possible for nourishment of the graft and to prevent postoperative infection and absorption. A three-layered auricle is sculptured into a concha, scapha, and helical rim (Fig. 15). Several elements must be exaggerated in depth and height when the overlying skin is thick or if the hairline is low. A common error is to make the framework too wide rather than too long.

The eighth or floating ninth rib is ideal for the helical rim. This rib must be thinned to a gentle curvature while enough height is maintained to exaggerate the rim. To preserve perichondrium, this rib is sculptured only on its concave (outer) side to cause deliberate bending. The helical rim should be sutured to the base with 4-0 clear nylon horizontal mattress sutures with the knots buried on the undersurface of the framework. The helix extends a few millimeters beyond the base anteriorly as a crural helix and reaches the level of the antitragus to resemble a caudal helix inferiorly. The fossa triangularis and scapha are excavated with gouges and scalpels (21). Drills can cause chondrocytic damage and cartilage absorption and must be avoided. This three-layered monoblock framework is far superior to an "expansile" open-faced framework, which tends to flatten and dissolve with time.

The second template is tattooed onto the microtic side to assure proper placement of the neoauricle. An incision

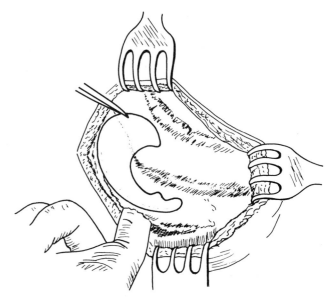

FIG. 14. Template placed over dissected seventh and eighth cartilaginous ribs.

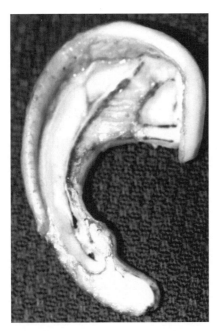

FIG. 15. Three-layered auricular framework is sculptured into a concha, scapha, and helix.

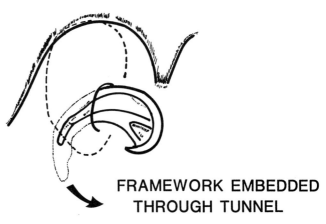

FRAMEWORK EMBEDDED THROUGH TUNNEL

FIG. 17. The framework is inserted into the skin pocket through an anterior incision.

is made anterior to the microtia nubbin, and a thin, elastic, well-vascularized subdermal pocket is made. Vasoconstrictors are avoided so that any blanching of the skin will be an early warning that the pocket is under excessive tension and that necrosis may occur. Dissection is extended 2 cm superior and lateral to the tattooed outline, and 5 mm inferior to it to gain enough skin laxity to lie within the sculptured sulci (Fig. 16). Vestigial cartilage in the superior aspect of the microtic nubbin is discarded. After meticulous hemostasis, the graft is inserted into the pocket and rotated into place (Fig. 17). If blanching occurs, the pocket must be enlarged to avoid necrosis of

the skin. Two 10F drains are inserted and attached to wall suction at 80 mm Hg for 3 days to control the inevitable accumulation of serum. Continuous suction also helps skin-to-cartilage coaptation and avoids the use of bolsters, mattress sutures, and tight dressings, which can cause skin necrosis. The sulci are loosely packed with petrolatum gauze dressings and covered with sterile eye pads. Antibiotics are continued for 1 week until the packing and sutures are removed.

Construction of the Lobule

Construction of the earlobe is performed 3 months after placement of the framework. Although some surgeons include this stage with framework insertion, it is safer and more accurate to develop the lobule in a separate procedure (Fig. 18). The remaining fibroadipose

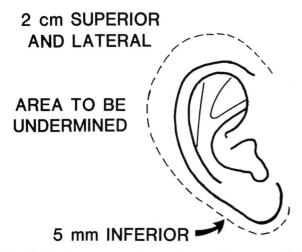

2 cm SUPERIOR AND LATERAL

AREA TO BE UNDERMINED

5 mm INFERIOR

FIG. 16. A subdermal pocket is dissected 2 cm superiorly and 5 mm inferiorly beyond the tattooed outline framework to gain skin laxity to lie in the newly made convolutions without tension.

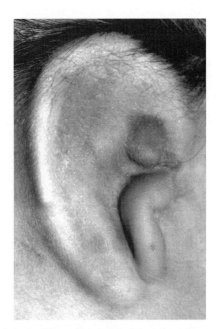

FIG. 18. Inferior fibroadipose lobular remnant remains in an abnormal vertical axis.

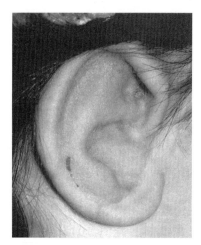

FIG. 19. The lobule has been transposed to its proper location.

remnant is dissected as an inferiorly based flap and rotated posteriorly onto the framework. Brent (17) has cleverly suggested filleting and "splicing" the lobule. He elevates the tail of the framework without exposing the underlying cartilage. The lobular remnant is transposed over and under the tip of the cartilage. No additional internal support is necessary; however, any excessive tension on the flap causes shrinkage and disappearance of the earlobe. Redundant skin in the superior aspect of the neoauricle is excised and discarded (Fig. 19).

Tragus Reconstruction and Conchal Excavation

At this stage there is now relative asymmetry of the ears. The microtic ear is closely adherent to the skull, and the normal side appears to be protruding. Construction of a tragus, deepening of the conchal bowl, and formation of a neointroitus of an external canal are performed in one procedure. A 15 mm by 40 mm composite chondrocutaneous graft is taken from the vertical portion of the contralateral concha. The normal ear is retracted anteriorly, and a full-thickness postauricular skin graft 2 cm in diameter is harvested. Closure of these donor defects

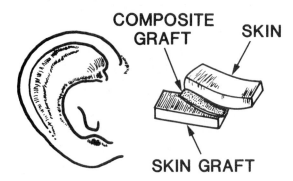

FIG. 20. A J-shaped incision is made at the proposed site of the tragus. The chondrocutaneous graft is sutured to the facial skin anteriorly and the free skin graft posteriorly.

COMPOSITE GRAFT   SKIN

SKIN GRAFT

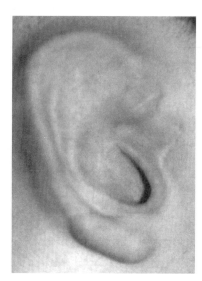

FIG. 21. The tragus is constructed, and the conchal bowl is deepened.

brings the normal ear closer to the scalp and improves the relative protrusion of this side (22).

On the microtic side a J-shaped incision is made in the concha at the proposed area of the posterior aspect of the tragus (Fig. 20). Thick soft tissue under the posterior flap is excavated to deepen the concha. The composite graft is sutured to the anterior skin, and the full-thickness postauricular skin graft is sutured to the composite graft. These three tissues (facial skin, composite graft, and skin graft) are then folded in an accordion like manner. With the supporting composite graft on the undersurface of the anterior skin, a tragus and neomeatus are formed. The deepened conchal bowl and shadow formed by the tragus resemble a meatus (Fig. 21). There is no shrinkage of this firm, cartilage-supported tragus as there is with other techniques in which soft-tissue advancement flaps are used (23,24). The bowl and meatus are packed with bismuth tribromophenate (Xeroform) gauze for 1 week to prevent blunting. In repair of bilateral microtia no tissue is available for a composite chondrocutaneous graft. One must compromise with less predictable soft-tissue advancement flaps for tragus repair.

Elevation of the Auricle and Construction of a Postauricular Sulcus

The ear may lack adequate projection because of its cryptotic appearance. Patients often are frustrated fitting sunglasses and hearing aids because they have no shelf on which to rest them. Construction of a sulcus can be performed while the otologist begins canalplasty or implantation of a bone conduction hearing aid (25–31). A peripheral incision is made 5 mm behind the posterior margin of the helix. A 6- to 7-cm scalp flap is elevated in a subgaleal plane. Inferiorly the fibers of the sternomastoid muscle are sectioned with electrocoagulating current. The framework is carefully elevated above the mas-

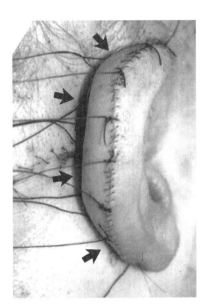

FIG. 22. Additional protrusion is obtained through a scalp advancement flap and a skin graft. The *arrows* indicate the direction of the scalp flap advancement to create a postauricular sulcus.

toid periosteum without exposure of bare cartilage, because denuded cartilage does not accept skin grafts. If the framework is exposed, it must be covered with soft tissue, or the procedure must be postponed until a later time. The ear is elevated to, but not beyond, the concha. Excessive dissection weakens stabilization and causes the superior pole to shift forward. The scalp flap is advanced anteriorly beneath the framework and secured under tension to the periosteum with 2-0 polyglactin 910 (Vicryl) sutures. This advancement of the scalp and hairline increases protrusion of the neoauricle and decreases visibility of the skin graft on lateral profile.

The denuded posterior surface of the auricle is covered with a full-thickness skin graft from the inguinal area. Bolsters of bismuth tribromophenate packing are sutured into place to avoid tenting of the sulcus and to prevent potential dead space with hematoma formation, graft loss, and cartilage exposure. This technique gains additional protrusion and better harmony with the normal ear (Fig. 22).

ATYPICAL MICROTIA

Thickened nonpliable scarring from operations or trauma often produces inferior results. This unusable tissue must be excised and replaced with skin grafts. Because bare cartilage does not nourish a graft, a well-vascularized bed of tissue must be interposed between the cartilage and skin. A temporoparietal fascial flap (TPFF) can adequately cover the avascular cartilage framework and simultaneously nourish the skin graft (32–34). The TPFF is abundant, accessible, thin, well vascularized, and hairless. It is continuous with the superficial musculoaponeurotic fascia that inserts on the zygomatic arch. The TPFF must not be confused with the underlying, less

vascular temporalis fascia, which lies deep to the arch and inserts on the mandibular condyle. A TPFF is supplied by the superficial temporal and postauricular arteries and veins. These vessels lie in the fascia beneath the subcutaneous fat and hair follicles. The vessels extend almost 12 cm above the ear, where they become superficial and fuse with the subdermal vascular plexus. Twelve centimeters is therefore the maximum superior boundary of TPFF dissection. The anterior border is limited by the temporal branch of the facial nerve as it crosses the zygomatic arch. The posterior edge is the area of the posterior branches of the superficial temporal artery and vein.

The subdermal pocket made for implantation of the sculptured rib cartilage is similar to that made in operations on nonscarred microtic ears (Fig. 23). The framework is inserted in the pocket, and unusable scarred skin is excised. The amount of flap coverage is measured, and a vertical incision up to 12 cm long is made above the cartilage graft. The parietal scalp is elevated just to the depth of the base of the subcutaneous hair follicles. Dissecting too superficially damages the bulbs and causes alopecia. Too deep a dissection injures the axial arrangement of vessels in the TPFF. This tedious dissection must be accomplished without vasoconstrictors to allow adequate blood flow at the distal margins of the flap.

The TPFF is measured to adequately cover the exposed cartilage and to lie within the convolutions and sulci without tension. At the superior margin, a 6-cm transverse incision is made and connected to two vertical incisions to free the TPFF from the temporalis fascia. The

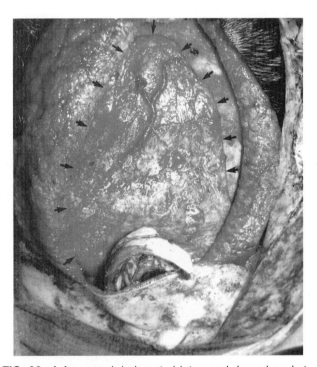

FIG. 23. A framework is inserted into a subdermal pocket. Nonusable, scarred skin is discarded. The temporoparietal fascial flap (TPFF) is measured for adequate coverage and elevated. *Arrows* indicate the TPFF border.

flap is easily dissected from the underlying temporalis fascia and is rotated downward to cover cartilage. It is sutured to the undersurface of the superior margins of the skin pocket in a pants-over-vest manner (Fig. 24). A 10F drain is inserted under the framework and attached to wall suction. A 0.016-inch (0.4 mm) skin graft is placed over the TPFF and secured with bismuth tribromophenate bolsters (Fig. 25). A second closed-suction drain is placed under the scalp. After 3 days the drains are removed, and stages of elevation of the framework and creation of a tragus are followed in proper sequence.

SUMMARY

Correction of microtic and constricted ears requires thorough analysis of the missing components and an understanding of the techniques available to correct them. The plastic, otologic, and craniofacial surgical teams must act in concert to prevent excessive scarring and to avoid poorly coordinated procedures. Problems with skin coverage, pliability of the ear, and graft material will continue to stimulate our creativity until the ideal implant is found. However, auricular reconstruction should no longer be an intraoperative exercise in frustration. Excellent results can be consistently reproducible, natural appearing, and long lasting (Figs. 26, 27).

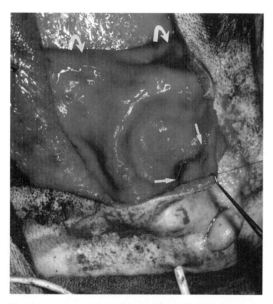

FIG. 24. A temporoparietal fascial flap (TPFF) is folded over *(curved arrow)* to cover the exposed cartilage framework. *Straight arrows* indicate where the TPFF is sutured to the undersurface of the inferior skin.

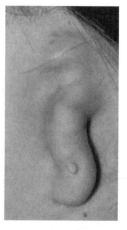

FIG. 26. Preoperative view of patient with microtia.

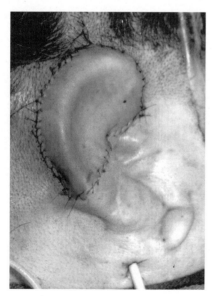

FIG. 25. A 0.016-inch (0.4 mm) skin graft covers the temporoparietal fascial flap, and suction drainage is inserted for 3 days.

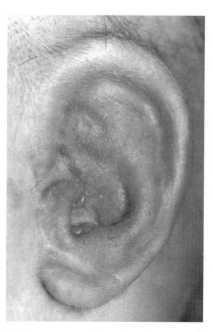

FIG. 27. Appearance after microtia reconstruction.

SUMMARY POINTS

- Microtia reconstruction requires a well-coordinated team to help child and parents with the physical, psychologic, and developmental problems associated with craniofacial deformities.
- Dysmorphic auricles with all anatomic subunits present can be corrected with nonsurgical means within 1 week of birth. Tape is applied for 2 weeks.
- Infants with microtia must be evaluated with brainstem audiometry and for other possible anomalies of the heart, neck, and kidneys.
- Repair of unilateral microtia usually is started at 6 years of age, when the chest wall is large enough to harvest ribs without leaving a donor site deformity.
- Reconstruction of the auricle is best begun *before* temporal bone surgery to prevent unnecessary scarring of the mastoid skin.
- Thickened, scarred, nonpliable mastoid skin will not adequately conform to the sculptured cartilage framework. It must be removed and replaced with a temporal fascial flap and skin graft.
- The three or four reconstructive procedures are staged at 3-month intervals.
- Tragal reconstruction encompasses a chondrocutaneous skeletal framework and postauricular skin graft from the opposite auricle.

REFERENCES

1. Berghaus A, Toplak F. Surgical concepts for reconstruction of the auricle: history and current state of the art. *Arch Otolaryngol Head Neck Surg* 1986;112:338–397.
2. Brent B. The correction of microtia with autogenous cartilage grafts, I: the classical deformity? *Plast Reconstr Surg* 1980;66:1–12.
3. Anson B, Blast T. Developmental anatomy of the ear. In: Shambaugh G Jr, Glasscock M, eds. *Surgery of the ear,* 3rd ed. Philadelphia: WB Saunders, 1980.
4. Farkas LG. Anthropomometry of normal and anomalous ears. *Clin Plast Surg* 1978;5:401–412.
5. Tolleth H. A hierarchy of values in the design and construction of the ear. *Clin Plast Surg* 1990;17:193–197.
6. Cosman B. The constricted ear. *Clin Plast Surg* 1988;5:389–394.
7. Ruder RO, Maceri D, Crockett D. Congenital aural atresia and microtia. In: Meyerhoff W, Rice D, eds. Otolaryngology–head and neck surgery. Philadelphia: W.B. Saunders Co., 1992.
8. MacGregor FC. Ear deformities: social and psychological implications. *Clin Plast Surg* 1978;5:347–350.
9. Lauritzen C, Munro IR, Ross RB. Classification and treatment of hemifacial microsomia. *Scand J Plast Surg* 1985;19:33–39.
10. Gilles H. *Plastic surgery of the face.* London: Frowde, Hodder & Stoughton, 1920.
11. Cronin T. Use of a silastic frame for total reconstruction of the external ear: preliminary report. *Plast Reconstr Surg* 1966;37:399–405.
12. Cronin TD, Ascough BM. Silastic ear construction. *Clin Plast Surg* 1978;5:367–378.
13. Ohmori S, Sekiguchi H. Follow-up study of the reconstruction of microtia using Silastic frame. *Aesthet Plast Surg* 1984;8:1–6.
14. Tanzer RC. Reconstruction of microtia: a long term follow-up. In: Goldwyn RM, Murray JE, eds. *Long term results in plastic and reconstructive surgery.* Boston: Little, Brown: 1980.
15. Gorney M. Ear cartilage. In: Davis J. *Aesthetic and reconstructive otoplasty.* New York: Springer-Verlag: 1987.
16. Brent B. Ear reconstruction with an expansible framework of autogenous rib cartilage. *Plast Reconstr Surg* 1978;5:351.
17. Brent B. Auricular repair with autogenous rib cartilage grafts: two decades of experience with 600 cases. *Plast Reconstr Surg* 1993;90:355–374.
18. Ruder RO. New concepts in microtia repair. *Arch Otolaryngol Head Neck Surg* 1988;114:1016–1019.
19. Richards RN, McKenzie MA, Meharg G. Electroepilation (electrolysis) in hirsutism: 35,000 hours experience on the face and neck. *J Am Acad Dermatol* 1986;15:693–697.
20. Aguilar EA. The surgical repair of congenital microtia and atresia. *Otolaryngol Head Neck Surg* 1988;98:600–606.
21. Ruder RO, Maceri D, Crockett D. Management of congenital aural atresia and microtia. In: Johnson J, Mandell-Brown M, Newman R, eds. *Instructional courses,* vol 4. St. Louis: Mosby, 1991.
22. Brent B. Cartilage and perichondrial grafting. In: McCarthy JC, ed. *Plastic surgery.* Philadelphia: WB Saunders, 1990.
23. Kirkham HLD. The use of preserved cartilage in ear reconstruction, *Ann Surg* 1940;111:896.
24. Distant F, Morgon A. Correction des microties en deux temps. *Pediatrie* 1993;48:407.
25. Cole RR, Jahrsdoerfer RA. Congenital aural atresia. *Clin Plast Surg* 1990;17:376–371.
26. Crabtree JA. Congenital atresia: case selection complications, and prevention. *Otolaryngol Clin North Am* 1982;15:755–762.
27. Crabtree JA. The facial nerve in congenital ear surgery. In: Graham MD, House WF, eds. *Disorders of the facial nerve.* New York: Raven Press, 1982.
28. Derlacki EL. The role of the otologist in the management of microtia and related malformations of the hearing apparatus. *Arch Otolaryngol* 1969;72:980.
29. Gill NW. Congenital atresia of the ear: a review of the surgical findings in 83 cases. *J Laryngol Otol* 1969;83:551–587.
30. Jahrsdoerfer RA. Congenital ear atresia. In: Tanzer RC, Edgerton MT, eds. Symposium on reconstruction of the auricle. St. Louis: Mosby, 1974.
31. Rousch J, Rauch SD. Clinical application of implantable bone conduction hearing device. *Laryngoscope* 1990;100:281–285.
32. Brent B, Byrd HS. Secondary ear reconstruction with cartilage grafts covered by axial, random, and free flaps of temporoparietal fascia. *Plast Reconstr Surg* 1983;72:141–152.
33. Ruder RO. Injuries of the pinna. In: Gates G. *Current therapy in otolaryngology–head and neck surgery.* St. Louis: Mosby, 1993.
34. Ruder RO. Microtia reconstruction. In: Papel I, Nachlas N, eds. *Facial plastic surgery.* St. Louis: Mosby, 1992.

The Ear: Comprehensive Otology,
edited by R. F. Canalis and P. R. Lambert.
Lippincott Williams & Wilkins, Philadelphia © 2000.

CHAPTER 23

Otitis Media with Effusion

Steven D. Handler and Thomas M. Magardino

Otitis media with effusion (OME) is an inflammatory condition of the middle ear and mastoid air cell system characterized by accumulation of fluid in the middle ear without signs or symptoms of acute infection. OME occurs as a result of decreased ventilation of the middle ear or mastoid air cell system through the eustachian tube. Also known by numerous other names such as *serous otitis media, glue ear,* and *nonpurulent otitis media,* OME is one of the most commonly occurring disorders among children. It is the most common diagnosis made by physicians treating children younger than 15 years and accounts for a large number of referrals to otolaryngologists (1–4). OME may occur as an innocuous short-term manifestation of an upper respiratory infection (URI), or it may appear as a chronic process with marked hearing loss, delayed development of speech and language, balance disorders, or structural changes of the tympanic membrane and ossicles. Because OME is primarily a childhood disease, this chapter concentrates on the diagnosis and management of OME among children. The special case of OME among adults is discussed at the end of the chapter.

PATHOGENESIS

Any process that interferes with normal opening of the proximal (nasopharyngeal) end of the eustachian tube or mucociliary clearance mechanism causes a situation that can lead to OME. Pharyngeal edema and inflammation from a URI, allergy (5–7), or smoking (8) affects both mucociliary transport and normal eustachian tube opening. Barotrauma, pressure on the torus tubarius by nasopharyngeal masses (such as neoplasms or large or infected adenoids), or abnormal eustachian tube anatomy, as with cleft palate deformities, can impair eustachian tube function. Foreign bodies such as nasogastric or nasotracheal tubes often are associated with OME.

OME often follows an episode of acute otitis media (AOM). AOM is defined as fluid in the middle ear accompanied by signs and symptoms of acute illness, including fever, irritability, lethargy, anorexia, vomiting, diarrhea, ear pain, bulging tympanic membrane, and perforation with purulent drainage. It most commonly results from bacterial infection of the middle ear cleft with *Streptococcus pneumoniae, Haemophilus influenzae,* or *Moraxella catarrhalis.* The associated inflammation causes anatomic and functional obstruction of the eustachian tube, which delays clearance of the middle ear effusion.

Effusion typically persists in the middle ear for weeks to months after an episode of AOM. Studies have shown that 41% to 85% of children have OME when examined

    S. D. Handler and T. M. Magardino: Department of Pediatric Otolaryngology, The Children's Hospital of Philadelphia, Philadelphia, Pennsylvania 19104

2 weeks after resolution of AOM, 23% to 67% continue to have middle ear fluid 1 month later, and 5% to 25% have chronic OME, defined as an effusion present for at least 3 months (9). Factors associated with persistence of OME 1 month after a bout of AOM include age younger than 2 years, bilateral infection, tendency to otitis (more than than three episodes of AOM in 6 months), and presence of *S. pneumoniae* organisms in the effusion (10).

The organisms commonly cultured from AOM often are found in effusions associated with OME. *S. pneumoniae, H. influenzae,* or *M. catarrhalis* can be detected in a large proportion of effusions from children with OME. In one study, 30% of middle ear effusions were culture positive, and with polymerase chain reaction techniques, bacterial DNA was identified in 48% of effusions that were culture negative (11). This finding suggests that the presence of these bacteria in effusions may be important in the development or persistence of OME despite our inability to culture them with routine techniques.

The data suggest that acute otitis media is one etiologic factor in the development of OME. Although antibiotics are effective in treating many children with OME, not all children respond to this therapy. It is uniformly accepted that the pathogenesis of OME is multifactorial. Risk factors that increase a child's risk for chronic OME are related in part to the anatomy and physiology of the eustachian tubes.

THE EUSTACHIAN TUBE

The eustachian tube is essential in maintaining a healthy, well-aerated middle ear. It ventilates the middle ear, protects it from pathogenic organisms in the nasopharynx, equilibrates pressure across the tympanic membrane, and allows drainage of secretions from the middle ear into the nasopharynx. At rest, the eustachian tube is closed because of passive recoil of the cartilaginous torus tubarius (nasopharyngeal orifice) and the pressure applied on it by surrounding soft tissue. During swallowing, yawning, or sneezing, the torus transiently opens primarily through contraction of the tensor veli palatini muscle. Although the levator veli palatini and salpingopharyngeus muscles insert onto the torus tubarius, their contribution to tubal opening is minimal.

The anatomy of the eustachian tubes of infants is different from that of the tubes of adults. In an infant, the eustachian tube lies in a plane parallel to the skull base approximately 10 degrees off horizontal; it is 13 to 18 mm long and cylindrical. The torus tubarius descends with the palate during development, attaining a 45-degree angle with respect to the horizontal by the age of 7 years, and lies 2.0 to 2.5 cm below the middle ear orifice. The eustachian tube elongates to 31 to 38 mm and assumes the shape of two cones connected by the narrow ends. This narrow midportion of the eustachian tube is called the *isthmus*. It is thought that infantile eustachian tube

anatomy is inherently dysfunctional because of the horizontal orientation, shorter length, and patulous configuration (12–14).

Evaluation of eustachian tube function is critical to understanding its dysfunction. Three methodologic components must be met to effectively study eustachian tube function. The technique must not interfere with the normal physiologic mechanisms; it should allow manipulation of standardized ambient pressure conditions; and the tympanic membrane must be in free ambient air contact at all times (15).

The Valsalva maneuver is the most commonly used eustachian tube function test. It enables quick and easy evaluation of the ability of the eustachian tube to open passively when pressure in the nasopharynx increases. The physician visualizes the tympanic membrane with an otoscope while the patient performs the maneuver. A positive test result occurs when the tympanic membrane moves or air bubbles are seen through a perforation. Unfortunately, a positive test result allows one to state that the eustachian tube can be forced open. It does not give information about physiologic, active tubal function. It also cannot be used in examinations of children or adults who are unable to perform a proper Valsalva maneuver (16).

The nine-step *inflation-deflation test* described by Bluestone et al. (3) involves tympanometry to evaluate active tubal opening capacity. A tympanogram is obtained to record resting middle ear pressure. The external auditory canal then is exposed to positive or negative pressure. After the patient swallows, a tympanogram is obtained to record the ability of the eustachian tube to equilibrate the applied pressure. A classification system correlates the performance of the eustachian tube on this test with active tubal function (14). Results of the nine-step test are inaccurate, however, if an effusion is present in the middle ear at the time of testing.

Sonotubometry is a noninvasive technique that provides information on the extent and duration of active eustachian tube opening. A tone is presented to the nose, and a recording of that tone is taken from within the external auditory canal. The sound transmission from the nasal cavity into the external canal is louder during eustachian tube opening. The level and duration of sound transmission correlate with the extent and duration of tubal opening. Measurements taken in normal and diseased ears have yielded information on active tubal function, but interpretation of these data is difficult because of the error introduced by accessory sounds produced in the nasopharynx during swallowing (17,18).

The *photoelectric technique* is used to measure luminosity transmitted through the eustachian tube. A fiberoptic scope is placed at the torus tubarius to provide a light source, and a highly-sensitive photodiode records the luminosity within the external auditory canal. This system also records the extent and duration of tubal opening and provides direct visualization of the torus tubarius during eustachian tube opening. Further studies of this technique are needed to assess its utility in evaluation of tubal function (19).

Correlations between results of eustachian tube function tests and "normal" and "abnormal" eustachian tube function have been difficult because these tests measure the ability or inability to open the eustachian tube. Normal eustachian tube function is derived from more than its ability to open; it comprises a dynamic equilibrium of tubal opening and closing with continuous intratubal mucociliary activity. Improper functioning of these mechanisms results in poor ventilation of the middle ear cleft.

Air, composed predominately of oxygen, carbon dioxide, nitrogen, and water vapor, normally fills the middle ear cleft. Of these gases, nitrogen plays an important role in pressure equilibration across the tympanic membrane. Because it does not participate in metabolic processes and has the slowest rate of diffusion from the middle ear into the surrounding circulation, nitrogen maintains the highest partial pressure of the gases (water vapor, oxygen, carbon dioxide) within the middle ear–mastoid system (20). Over time, however, nitrogen does diffuse out of the middle ear cleft. As ventilation of the middle ear decreases, a pressure imbalance develops between the middle ear–mastoid system and the ambient environment (external ear canal, nasopharynx). As the pressure in the middle ear–mastoid system becomes more negative with respect to the ambient environment, the tympanic membrane retracts medially. Increased negative middle ear pressure collapses the pliable cartilaginous torus tubarius, making aeration increasingly more difficult. Fluid, consisting of passive transudate and active exudate, fills the middle ear–mastoid system (21). The fluid ranges from thin and watery to thick, almost gelatinous, mucoid material.

Resolution of OME depends on return of normal eustachian tube function. As middle ear ventilation is restored, the pressure differential between the middle ear and the ambient environment is reduced. Mucociliary transport becomes effective in moving the middle ear fluid through the eustachian tube to the nasopharynx. OME is marked by a high degree of spontaneous resolution (1,22). Middle ear fluid resolves without treatment in as many as two thirds of patients observed for 1 month. However, OME also is characterized by a high rate of recurrence; between 28% and 38% of preschool children experience recurrence of OME (1). Eustachian tube dysfunction among children is common and transient, often recurs throughout early childhood, and typically normalizes by the age of 7 to 10 years. The factors that predispose some children to the development of chronic OME are complicated and controversial.

EPIDEMIOLOGY

Efforts to define the population of patients with OME are hampered by the facts that many children with OME have no symptoms and that often there is no clear-cut beginning or end of an episode of OME (3). Studies of incidence (occurrence over time) have shown that between 35% and 70% of preschool children have at least one episode of OME (1,23). This large variation is related to the frequency and interval between observations, the criteria for diagnosis of OME, and the population studied. For example, OME detected on two occasions may represent one prolonged episode or two distinct bouts of OME. The prevalence (occurrence at one point in time) of SOM has been reported from 5% to 35% of preschool children (1,2,22). This number depends on the season of the year and the presence of concurrent URIs. Higher prevalence is found in the winter months, when more bouts of OME are associated with concurrent URI.

The effect of age on OME is unclear (3). OME is uncommon among children younger than 1 year, unlike AOM, which has its highest incidence among infants. The incidence of OME among preschool children appears fairly constant from the ages of 2 to 6 years (35% to 70%, depending on the study) and decreases dramatically as the children approach 10 years of age. OME is uncommon among adults without predisposing conditions such as nasopharyngeal neoplasm, sinusitis, barotrauma, or cleft palate deformity.

Although sex has been related to the incidence of AOM (more boys than girls), no such association has been determined for OME (3). The high incidence of AOM among American Indians, Alaskan Inuits, and Hispanic people has not been reflected in increased incidence of OME in these populations.

The high incidence of OME among patients with cleft palate, Down syndrome, and other craniofacial abnormalities is well known. It is thought to be related to abnormalities in palatonasopharyngeal anatomy and function that cause chronic eustachian tube dysfunction (3). The incidence of OME appears to decrease among these patients as the defects (e.g., cleft palate) are repaired.

The relation between OME and socioeconomic status is not clear. There is, however, a higher incidence of OME among children in day care settings than among those cared for at home (2). Household smoking has been found to be associated with OME in several studies, but the association is controversial (24,25).

DIAGNOSIS

The diagnosis of OME is difficult because the process is often asymptomatic, so-called silent otitis media (1,3). With the absence of signs of acute infection (pain, fever, discharge), OME may go undetected by the parent, teacher, or even the child. The diagnosis of OME is usually made at *physical examination* of the ear with the detection of fluid behind the normally translucent tympanic membrane. Otoscopic examination of the ear of a child with OME reveals the tympanic membrane to be retracted, dull, and opaque (Fig. 1: see color plate 5 following page 484). The color of the tympanic membrane can range from light pink (clear, thin fluid that allows visualization of the mucosa over the promontory) to amber and even dark blue (if there has been hemorrhage into the fluid). The short process of the malleus appears very prominent as the long process is retracted medially with the tympanic membrane. The presence of air bubbles or air-fluid levels makes the diagnosis more evident (Fig 2: see color plates 6A and 6B following page 484). Often the findings in OME are subtle and may be missed in a cursory examination by an inexperienced observer.

Pneumatic otoscopy is important in the diagnosis of OME. A closed speculum is inserted snugly into the ear canal, and gentle positive and negative pressure is applied to the tympanic membrane. In a normal ear, the tympanic membrane moves visibly with the air pressure. With OME, the tympanic membrane does not move or moves only slightly with negative pressure. Pneumatic otoscopy performed by an experienced otoscopist is the most accurate means of diagnosing OME. This technique has been reported as having a sensitivity as high as 90% with 80% specificity (3). However, because many physicians are unfamiliar with pneumatic otoscopy, their ability to diagnose OME by means of physical examination is decreased.

In an effort to identify asymptomatic OME, which may account for 10% of cases (26), several screening techniques have been developed. The first is *impedance audiometry (tympanometry)*, which is used to measure changes in acoustic impedance of the tympanic membrane–middle ear system with changes in air pressure in the external auditory canal. This test is simple and rapid and is the most commonly used method of screening for middle ear disease.

Tympanometry or audiometry is currently recommended at the beginning of school and 1 year later to screen 5- and 6-year-old children to identify the 10% with asymptomatic OME. Pneumatic otoscopy is not recommended because of the variability of results dependent on the skill level of the observer. Middle ear pressure more negative than −200 decapascals (type C) or a flat tympanometric curve (type B) is classified as a failure. A child who fails tympanometry of both ears and has at least a 20 dB hearing loss at 1, 2, or 4 kHz should be referred to a physician for evaluation. A child who fails screening in one ear or fails tympanometry in both ears without marked hearing loss (less than 20 dB) should be retested 2 months later. If that child fails the second screening, a physician should evaluate him or her. Hearing, speech, and language should be assessed and appropriate referrals made early if delays are found with concurrent OME (26).

Although tympanometry has a very high degree of sensitivity (more than 90%), its low specificity can cause a high number of false-positive findings (3,27). Ten to fourteen percent of children with low-compliance tympanograms have only tympanic membrane retraction or thickening without effusion (14,27). Technical difficulties such as occlusion of the probe by cerumen or the child's crying can cause invalid results.

Acoustic reflectometry has been developed to screen for OME among children (3,28,29). An acoustic otoscope inserted into the ear canal generates a swept tone (1.8 to 7.0 kHz) and records the sound reflected from the tympanic membrane. This technique involves use of the cancellation effect of the sound wave reflected by the tympanic membrane on the incident sound wave produced by the acoustic otoscope. The louder the reflected sound, the greater is the chance that an effusion is present in the middle ear. This test is rapid, easy to perform, does not require an airtight seal in the ear canal, and is not affected by the presence of cerumen or crying. The sensitivity and specificity of this test depend on the breakpoint chosen by the user. The breakpoint is defined as the level of sound reflectivity thought to correlate with the presence of a middle ear effusion. A lower breakpoint is associated with increased false-positive results, whereas a higher breakpoint results in a higher number of false-negative findings. Acoustic reflectometry also gives inaccurate results in ears with an air bubble, air-fluid level, high negative pressure, or tympanosclerosis (30,31). Because of variability in interpretation of the information it provides, acoustic reflectometry has not become widely accepted among otolaryngologists.

Pure tone audiometric screening has been used to detect middle ear fluid in children (3). However, this technique is time consuming and requires expensive equipment and trained personnel to perform correctly. Screening levels commonly used, such as 30 dB, miss a large proportion of children with OME who have only a very mild hearing loss.

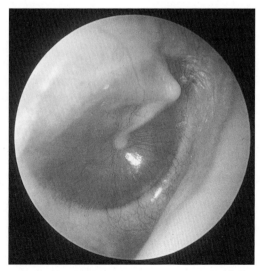

FIG. 1. Dull, retracted tympanic membrane characteristic of otitis media with effusion. Short process of malleus is prominent. (Courtesy of Dr. Armando Lenis.)

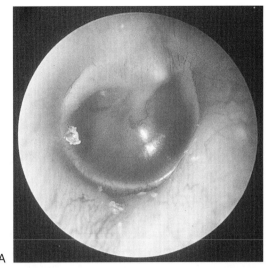 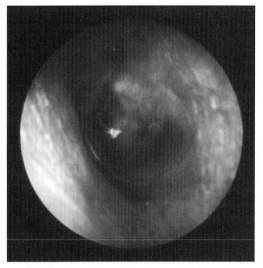

FIG. 2. Air-fluid level **(A)** or the presence of air bubbles **(B)** makes diagnosis of otitis media with effusion obvious. (Courtesy of Dr. Armando Lenis.)

TREATMENT

Treatment of patients with OME is directed at restoring normal middle ear ventilation. For a large percentage of patients, this occurs naturally, usually as the frequently associated URI resolves. Incidence and prevalence studies have shown that many of the episodes of OME are brief (1 month or less) and that many resolve spontaneously (1–3,22,23). These brief, infrequent bouts of OME cause little morbidity to the child and require no treatment. Growth plays a large role in the treatment of patients with chronic OME. As the child ages, eustachian tube function improves and the incidence of OME decreases; the child outgrows OME.

If OME is related to specific predisposing factors, avoidance or elimination of the factors can play a role in resolution of the middle ear fluid. If barotrauma was the cause of the OME, the potential for further barotrauma, such as flying or scuba diving, should be avoided. Eliminating household smoking, removing the child from child care facilities, and avoidance of known environmental and food allergens have been proposed as initial nonmedical, nonsurgical therapy for OME. Because most effusions resolve spontaneously and the hearing loss from OME may be substantial, some physicians advocate the use of hearing amplification while awaiting spontaneous resolution of the effusion (32).

Medical Treatment

Treatment of patients with long-standing or symptomatic OME is indicated to avoid sequelae of chronic OME. Because OME frequently is accompanied by a URI, antihistamines or decongestants often are recommended to clear the middle ear fluid. The rationale behind this treatment rests on the analogy of comparing the middle ear and mastoid system to a paranasal sinus. Because antihistamines or decongestants help clear sinonasal secretions and congestion, it would seem logical that they should be able to do the same for OME. If allergy is an etiologic agent in OME, these same drugs should have a beneficial effect on OME. Unfortunately, this is not the case; good, controlled studies have not demonstrated any efficacy of these compounds in the course of OME (4,21,33).

The mainstay of medical therapy for OME rests with antimicrobial agents. Although it is not a true infection, OME often follows bouts of AOM, and bacterial isolates have been found in many samples of OME fluid (11,21). The most common organisms include *S. pneumoniae,* nontypable *H. influenzae, M. catarrhalis,* and group A streptococci. *Staphylococcus aureus* and many other organisms have been cultured from middle ear fluid (34). Controlled studies have shown that antibiotics such as amoxicillin, amoxicillin-clavulanate, cefaclor, erythromycin, trimethoprim-sulfamethoxazole, or erythromycin-sulfisoxazole can improve clearance of the effusion in 1 month (4,35). Treatment may include prophylactic dosing. The prophylactic dose is one-half the daily dose used to treat an acute infection. This method of dosing may be continued longer than 1 month if the child begins to show signs of resolution and is not having complications of OME, such as recurrent bouts of AOM, symptomatic hearing loss, or severe tympanic membrane retraction. Long-term therapy with prophylactic dosing of antibiotics is currently under scrutiny given the dramatic increase in resistant strains of bacteria. Although it has been shown to be efficacious in OME, prophylactic dosing of antibiotics coupled with attendance in day care is associated with a higher prevalence and increasing incidence of resistant bacterial species.

From 1980 to 1989, the prevalence of β-lactam–resistant strains of *H. influenzae* increased from 17% to 34%

and of β-lactam-resistant strains of *M. catarrhalis* increased from 61% to 90%. This resistance has been overcome by the use of β-lactamase–stable antibiotics such as amoxicillin-clavulanate, cephalosporins, and loracarbef, but development of resistance to these antibiotics may pose a serious problem in the future. Of more concern is the increasing prevalence of *S. pneumoniae* organisms resistant to penicillins by virtue of their penicillin-binding proteins, which also provide resistance to β-lactamase–stable antibiotics. Vancomycin is currently the only antibiotic available to which all species of *S. pneumoniae* are sensitive. Concern over development of bacterial resistance has led to heated debate over proper antibiotic management of OME (36,37).

In 1994, the American Academy of Pediatrics, the American Academy of Family Physicians, and the American Academy of Otolaryngology–Head and Neck Surgery with the review and approval of the Agency for Health Care Policy and Research of the U.S. Department of Health and Human Services reviewed the research literature and scientific knowledge available on OME and the efficacy of current medical and surgical therapy. After the review, these groups published the clinical practice guideline Managing Otitis Media with Effusion in Young Children to provide recommendations on the management of OME among children 1 to 3 years of age with no craniofacial or neurologic abnormalities or sensory deficits (4).

Once the diagnosis of OME is made, the guideline allows 3 months of observation or antibiotic therapy and counseling on environmental risk factors before further evaluation. The guideline states that exposure to passive smoking, bottle feeding, and day care are associated with an increased risk for OME. However, the studies reviewed by the panel did not find a significantly decreased incidence of OME with breastfeeding or removal from day care. There is no recommendation on passive exposure to smoke.

A patient who has had persistent OME for 3 months should be referred for hearing evaluation. A bilateral hearing loss of at least 20 dB should be treated with oral antibiotic therapy or myringotomy with tube placement. If there is bilateral hearing loss less than 20 dB or unilateral hearing loss, the guideline recommends continued observation or antibiotic therapy. If OME is present after 4 to 6 months with a history of bilateral hearing loss (at least 20 dB), the guideline recommends bilateral myringotomy with tube placement (4).

Some investigators have advocated corticosteroids in the medical management of OME (38,39). It is postulated that these compounds reduce the inflammatory response in the nasopharynx–eustachian tube complex and may stimulate a surface-active agent in the eustachian tube to facilitate air and fluid movement through the eustachian tube. The results of many controlled studies of both oral and topical (nasal) corticosteroids, however, are mixed. In the 1994 clinical guideline, steroids with concurrent antibiotic use in the treatment of 1- to 3-year-old children improved clearance of OME at 1 month by 25%. Steroids alone may increase resolution of the effusion by 4.5%. Unfortunately, steroid use has only short-term success with a high rate of recurrence of effusion over time. Because there is no significant long-term efficacy and there is risk for infectious sequelae with corticosteroids, routine use of these compounds is not recommended (4).

Because allergy often has been cited as a cause of OME, allergy treatment in the form of antihistamines and decongestants, avoidance of allergens, and desensitization has been recommended (5–7,40,41). However, there is no evidence that the middle ear is an allergy target organ, and the lack of documented efficacy of allergy treatment makes this type of management controversial.

Some research has been performed with mucolytic agents and their effect on middle ear effusion (42). The theory behind use of these agents is to alter the viscoelastic properties of the middle ear mucus to improve mucous transport from the middle ear, through the eustachian tube, and into the nasopharynx. At present, however, mucolytic agents do not play a role in the management of OME.

Because OME among children is often directly or indirectly related to viral or bacterial infection, vaccination is a promising therapeutic approach. The pneumococcal vaccine currently available is not effective against OME because the polysaccharides in the vaccine do not correlate with the pneumococcal types normally present in OME. Studies are currently underway to identify the antigens of the most common bacterial pathogens found in effusions (*S. pneumoniae,* nontypable *H. influenzae, M. catarrhalis*) that could be used to develop vaccines. Immunization to these bacteria may prevent many cases of OME. Because OME often accompanies a viral URI, development of antiviral vaccines may reduce or eliminate many cases of OME (43).

There is a controversy regarding physical manipulation of the eustachian tube in the management of OME. Some clinicians recommend politzerization (or self-politzerization) of the nose to blow open the eustachian tube and reestablish middle ear ventilation. Others, however, believe this maneuver will blow infected debris from the nasopharynx into the middle ear and either cause AOM or prolong OME (21). Similar lack of agreement exists with respect to bottle feeding. Although there is a theoretic possibility of nasopharyngeal reflux of milk into the eustachian tube during bottle feeding, this does not appear to be an appreciable risk among most infants. Most clinicians agree, however, that allowing a child to feed in the supine position can let formula or milk enter and remain in the nasopharynx for extended periods and lead to inflammation in that area.

Surgical Treatment

Surgical management is indicated for cases of OME that have not resolved spontaneously or responded to medical therapy (21). The length of medical therapy before surgical management of OME is controversial. Some situations, however, justify early surgical intervention. Factors that should alert a physician to consider early surgical management to prevent further speech or language delay and possible permanent structural changes in the ear are hearing loss that affects communication skills, coexisting developmental delay or disabilities such as visual impairment, severe tympanic membrane retraction with or without ossicular erosion, balance disorder, unilateral external canal atresia, and sensorineural hearing loss (44).

The simplest form of surgical therapy for OME is drainage of the fluid. Myringotomy is performed and the fluid aspirated from the middle ear. Proponents of this technique believe this procedure can be performed easily in the office setting without anesthesia. However, the procedure usually results in only temporary clearing of the condition (45). If eustachian tube function continues to be impaired after the myringotomy site heals, the fluid reaccumulates. The pain and extremely loud suction noises (ranging from 74 to 117 dB) (46) associated with this procedure can cause the child to fear further encounters with the otolaryngologist or other medical personnel.

Effective treatment is directed at providing permanent or long-term clearing of OME. Attempts to ventilate the middle ear–mastoid system have been concentrated on providing an alternative route of aeration until eustachian tube function has returned to normal. Because simple myringotomy heals within several days, techniques have been developed to try to keep the site open and prolong the period of ventilation. Searing the edges of the tympanic membrane incision by means of cauterization or laser treatment has been somewhat successful in preventing early closure of the perforation. However, results are irregular and unreliable (47).

Politzer used rubber grommets in the late 1800s to provide long-term middle ear ventilation. However, the tympanic membrane rejected the foreign bodies after a short time. Armstrong (48) reintroduced ventilation tubes in 1954. Their use has increased to the point that myringotomy and tube insertion is second only to circumcision as the most commonly performed operation in the United States (49,50). Numerous styles, designs, and materials have been used to manufacture ventilation tubes in an effort to avoid the complications of early extrusion, recurrent otorrhea, and occlusion of the tube lumen. Although each surgeon has his or her favorite tube, there does not appear to be any one tube that is superior to any of the rest (Fig. 3). The most commonly used tube is the collar-button or grommet style made of silicone or polytetrafluoroethylene (PTFE; Teflon). Tubes made of other materials such as gold, titanium, or carbon coating offer no advantages over the conventional silicone tubes (51–54). The T tube or larger-flanged grommet-style tubes stay in place longer but have a higher rate of perfo-

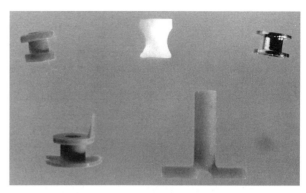

FIG. 3. Examples of commonly used ventilation tubes. *Top row:* Collar button styles (*left to right*) include Paparella (silicone), Shepard (Teflon), Reuter Bobbin (stainless steel). *Bottom row:* Longer lasting tubes include Paparella no. 2 (silicone) (*left*) and T tube (silicone).

ration after spontaneous extrusion, and many of them have to be surgically removed (54).

In an effort to provide long-term ventilation, so-called permanent ventilation tubes have been developed (55). Insertion of these long tubes necessitates elevation of a tympanomeatal flap and drilling of a notch in the bony annulus for proper placement. Removal necessitates a second operation with general anesthesia. Eustachian tube stents have been proposed to provide long-term ventilation (56). These tubes require exploratory tympanotomy for placement and can lead to permanent scarring of the eustachian tube.

Audiometric evaluation should be performed before surgical intervention. This is to determine the conductive hearing loss caused by the middle ear fluid and detect the presence of any preexisting sensorineural hearing loss (53). If a conventional behavioral or visually reinforced (play audiometry) audiogram cannot be obtained, consideration should be given to performing evoked response audiometry before surgical intervention.

For children, ventilation tubes usually are placed in a surgical procedure with general anesthesia. Although many adults tolerate this procedure under local anesthesia, the often-painful injections in the ear canal or the unreliable anesthesia obtained with iontophoresis makes this technique less in the care of children. To avoid the potential complications of general anesthesia, some practitioners advocate performing insertion of ventilation tubes without any anesthesia for young children. This technique is strongly discouraged.

The external ear canal is inspected and cleared of all cerumen and other debris. All quadrants of the tympanic membrane are viewed to make sure that there is no other pathology condition, such as cholesteatoma, high-riding jugular bulb, or a retraction pocket. A 2- to 3-mm myringotomy is made in the anterior-superior or anterior-inferior quadrant. Studies have shown that ventilation tubes in these quadrants tend to remain in place longer than those in other sites (57). The posterior-superior quadrant is to be avoided to prevent potential damage to the underlying ossicles and facial nerve. Tympanosclerotic portions of the tympanic membrane are poor sites for tube placement. Myringotomy is difficult in these areas, and a tube placed in the middle of a tympanosclerotic plaque is resistant to spontaneous extrusion and may have to be removed surgically. Atrophic areas of the tympanic membrane (so-called monomers) are to be avoided because they heal very poorly after extrusion of ventilation tubes and may cause postoperative perforation.

After the myringotomy is performed, middle ear fluid (if present) is suctioned out (Fig. 4). An attempt is made to remove as much fluid as possible to maximize immediate hearing improvement and to minimize the potential for early occlusion of the ventilation tube lumen by the secretions. The ventilation tube is placed in the myringotomy site, and any remaining secretions and blood are gently suctioned out of the ear. Any tympanic membrane retraction at the incision site should be gently elevated with a small suction tube. Otic or ophthalmic drops often are used (at the end of the procedure and for 2 or 3 days postoperatively) to prevent early occlusion of the tube lumen and to reduce the incidence of postoperative infection.

Postoperative water precautions are discussed. Use of ear molds or plugs usually is recommended for children who will undergo a great deal of water exposure, such as swimming under water. Lesser degrees of water exposure such as bathing (unless the head is completely immersed) probably do not require such protection (58). In the event of unintentional water exposure, otic or ophthalmic drops have been effective in reducing risk for a subsequent ear infection with discharge.

If a ventilation tube remains in place for a prolonged period, usually more than 3 years, and it is thought that the child may have outgrown the eustachian tube dysfunction and no longer needs the artificial middle ear

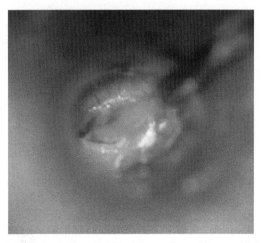

FIG. 4. Thick, viscous fluid being suctioned from middle ear after myringotomy.

ventilation, the tube may have to be surgically removed. Factors to be considered when contemplating removal of a long-standing ventilation tube include age, absence of nasopharyngeal abnormalities, and repair of cleft palate, all of which affect the incidence of OME. If a child has a tube in place in one ear and the contralateral ear is normal and has not had episodes of AOM or OME for 1 year, it can be assumed that both eustachian tubes can ventilate their respective middle ears, and the remaining tube can be removed. The tube may be removed in the office if the child is cooperative or in the operating room. If an ear has had multiple tubes or a large tube has been removed, consideration should be given to freshening the edges of the perforation (with a pick or trichloroacetic acid) and placing a paper patch over the resulting perforation to aid healing.

Complications of Treatment

Postoperative otorrhea is the most common complication of placement of ventilation tubes (45,54). Use of otic or ophthalmic drops in the postoperative period (2 to 3 days) has been advocated to reduce the incidence of early otorrhea. Approximately 20% of children with collar-button style tubes experience episodes of drainage through their tubes. This number rises to 50% among children with T tubes. Some of these episodes are related to concurrent URI and represent acute ear infections. Others are probably a result of water contamination of the tube and middle ear from unprotected swimming or bathing.

Otorrhea through a ventilation tube usually is managed with a 10-day course of topical otic or ophthalmic drops. The parent should clean the outer meatus of as much discharge as possible to allow the drops to reach the infected ventilation tube. Suctioning the ear with the aid of an operating microscope often speeds resolution of the infection. Oral antibiotics are given to children whose otorrhea does not respond to topical treatment or who have a fever or other symptoms of an associated URI.

The incidence of long-standing *perforation* after extrusion of a ventilation tube varies with the type of tube (54). Some clinicians believe that because the goal of therapy is long-term ventilation, persistent perforation is not a complication but actually a benefit. However, any condition resulting from surgical intervention that necessitates a reparative procedure (tympanoplasty) is more properly considered a complication. Conventional collar-button tubes usually have an incidence of perforation that is less than 1%. Longer-lasting tubes such as a T tube or large grommet-style tube have been reported to have perforation rates of 10% to 20%.

Hearing loss caused by ventilation tube placement has been reported as a reason to avoid use of tubes. The theory behind the hearing loss is the development of tympanosclerosis, a calcified hyaline deposit in the middle fibrous layer of the tympanic membrane. In rare, severe cases, tympanosclerosis can occur in the middle ear and involve the middle ear ossicles. Opponents of use of ventilation tubes point out that tympanosclerotic plaques have been reported in as many as 59% of ventilated ears (59,60). However, tympanosclerosis also has been found in as many as 13% of nonventilated ears, presumably related to recurrent bouts of AOM (45,59). The relation between tympanosclerosis and ventilation tubes is unclear because many plaques appear to be separate from the ventilation tube in the tympanic membrane (Fig. 5: see color plate 7 following page 484). The location and size of the tympanosclerotic plaques in the child's ear can vary over time, and many plaques ultimately disappear (60). In long-term studies children have been observed for as long as 7 years after tube placement. Only a 0.5 to 2.5 dB difference in hearing sensitivity compared with control ears has been found (45,59,60). Hearing loss does not appear to be a serious complication of ventilation tube placement.

Granulation tissue may form around a tube as part of a foreign body reaction. This condition often responds to topical administration of otic or ophthalmic drops that contain corticosteroids, especially dexamethasone. In some cases, however, the granulation tissue becomes so exuberant that removal of the ventilation tube is required.

Early occlusion of the tube lumen with wax or secretions prevents middle ear ventilation. For cooperative children, the occluding material can be gently removed from the tube lumen with the aid of a microscope in the office. Otic or ophthalmic drops may be used to clear the tube lumen. Hydrogen peroxide (also present in Debrox or Murine ear drops) is especially helpful in dissolving and loosening wax, blood, or serum (61). Successful opening of a tube is indicated when the child suddenly expresses discomfort as the water formed from the peroxide enters the middle ear and the nasopharynx.

Early extrusion of a ventilation tube is a problem for a child who continues to have eustachian tube dysfunction. The need to replace an extruded or blocked ventilation tube often is cited as a complication of insertion of ventilation tubes. However, this really reflects the chronicity of the eustachian tube dysfunction that causes OME. Conventional collar-button tubes tend to remain in place 6 to 12 months (54). Modified tubes such as T tubes or larger, flanged grommet-style tubes can remain in the tympanic membrane for 1 to 3 years or even longer. However, these tubes have a higher incidence of perforation after extrusion, and many must be removed in a surgical procedure with general anesthesia (54).

Cholesteatoma is an infrequent complication of ventilation tube placement. It occurs among less than 1 percent of patients (54). When cholesteatoma does occur, the tube and the lesion must be removed and tympanoplasty with or without mastoidectomy performed.

ADENOIDS

The adenoids have long been thought to play a role in the development of OME and AOM. Obstruction of the eustachian tube by enlarged adenoids, release of allergic inflammatory mediators from adenoidal mast cells (62), and adenoid tissue acting as a reservoir for pathogenic bacteria are some of the proposed mechanisms for this association. Studies have shown benefit of adenoidectomy in the natural course of OME, especially in shortening the length of time effusion is present and reducing relapse rates of OME and AOM (63–65). Because improvement was not correlated with adenoid size, the proposed association of adenoid removal with improvement in OME is thought to be related to decreasing the number of pathogenic bacteria in the nasopharynx. Adenoidectomy may benefit patients with allergies by removing the source of inflammatory mediators produced by activated mast cells in adenoidal tissue. Because the morbidity of adenoidectomy is higher than that associated with ventilation tube insertion alone, adenoidectomy usually is not suggested as initial surgical therapy for OME unless other symptoms, such as upper airway obstruction or sleep apnea, are present. Adenoidectomy generally is reserved for patients with recurrent OME who need a second or third insertion of ventilation tubes. Myringotomy with or without tube insertion generally is performed at the same time as adenoidectomy. Because of a lack of data on the efficacy of adenoidectomy in the care of 1- to 3-year-old children, the clinical practice guideline discussed earlier does not recommend adenoidectomy for management of OME in children 1 to 3 years of age. Although tonsillectomy usually is performed with adenoidectomy to treat patients with upper airway obstruction or recurrent adenotonsillitis, there is no evidence to indicate any benefit of tonsillectomy in the management of OME (4).

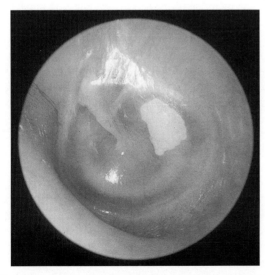

FIG. 5. Tympanosclerotic plaque in tympanic membrane.

CLEFT PALATE

Cleft palate deformity is commonly associated with the development of OME. Eustachian tube dysfunction in this population occurs as a result of the structural abnormalities of the torus tubarius and malinsertion of the tensor veli palatini muscle onto the torus. The torus tubarius of a child with cleft palate has a decreased curvature and an increased elastin density that make it floppy (66). These anatomic abnormalities increase risk for tubal obstruction. Anatomic studies have shown that the tensor veli palatini muscle does not insert onto the torus in 40% of children with cleft palate. Though the tensor veli palatini does have some insertion onto the torus in 60% of these children, it functions poorly because of infiltration of its tendon by adipose and connective tissue. Only 20% of middle ear effusions clear after surgical repair of the cleft palate. Most children with cleft palate, however, continue to suffer from middle ear disease because of the presence of persistent eustachian tube dysfunction. Ninety-six percent of children with cleft palate need placement of bilateral myringotomy tubes for management of middle ear disease (66).

RELATED NASAL CONDITIONS

Nasopharyngeal masses other than adenoids are rare among children but must be considered as a possible cause of OME. Rhabdomyosarcoma, lymphoma, and rarely squamous carcinoma of the nasopharynx in a child cause OME due to blockage or infiltration of the torus tubarius. In these cases, local excision of the malignant lesions (as the first step in treatment that also includes chemotherapy and radiation therapy) often facilitates resolution of OME. Benign lesions such as antral-choanal polyps and nasopharyngeal dermoids may present as OME. Surgical removal of the lesions usually leads to resolution of OME.

Other nasal conditions in the upper airway may affect the nasopharynx and contribute to the development of OME. Sinusitis, nasal septal deformities, turbinate hypertrophy, and choanal atresia or stenosis can affect the passage of air through the nasopharynx. However, the role of surgical therapy for these conditions in the management of OME is unclear.

If OME is related to the presence of a nasogastric or nasotracheal tube, removal of the tube is the first step in the management of middle ear fluid. A short course of antibiotics may be needed to manage the residual inflammatory process in the nasopharynx even after the tube is removed.

COMPLICATIONS OF OTITIS MEDIA WITH EFFUSION

Physicians spend billions of health care dollars each year treating patients with OME even though the 1994 clinical practice guideline recommends observation for up to 3 months after diagnosis of a middle ear effusion (4). The eagerness to provide aggressive medical or surgical management of OME is related to physician concern over the effect of hearing loss commonly associated with middle ear effusion. OME is the most common cause of conductive hearing loss among children. Although hearing level with OME is commonly reported as approximately 25 dB, losses up to 40 dB are not uncommon (67–69). Most clinicians agree that congenital or early-onset hearing loss is associated with delay in speech development and language acquisition. Because OME most commonly affects children in this period of development, even a temporary hearing loss during this time may have a profound effect on development of language, speech, and cognitive ability.

Studies have shown that children with hearing loss from OME are less attentive and less responsive to verbal cues. They also have been found to use nonverbal cues to communicate more frequently than children with normal hearing. Poor receptive vocabulary skills and unintelligibility of speech also are associated with a history of OME. Even children with long-standing unilateral hearing loss and OME have difficulty with speech identification in the presence of background noise (70). These studies have been criticized for their retrospective design, evaluation of relatively small numbers of children, and failure to control for confounding factors.

Teele et al. (71) prospectively observed a large number of children to determine the effect of middle ear effusion on development of speech, language, cognitive ability, and intelligence. They observed 205 children for the first 3 years of life and recorded total time spent with middle ear effusion. These children underwent testing with standard speech and language tests at 3 years of age. Children who spent little time with middle ear effusions significantly outperformed the children who spent more time with middle ear effusions. Time spent with middle ear effusion during a child's first year of life most significantly correlated with poor performance on speech and language tests at 3 years of age.

Teele et al. (72) conducted a separate study in which they prospectively observed 498 children until 7 years of age, again recording time spent with middle ear effusion. The children who spent more time with a middle ear effusion during their first 3 years of life had lower scores on tests of speech, language, cognitive ability, and school performance when tested at 7 years of age. Time with middle ear effusion after the third year of life did not have any effect on test scores.

Unfortunately, the studies by Teele et al. are based only on the presence or absence of OME. The investigators did not perform any hearing tests on the children; therefore, the effect of hearing loss associated with OME cannot be determined from these studies. Not all children have hearing loss in the presence of an effusion, and children with hearing loss from OME most likely clear the effusion spontaneously and again have normal hearing within a few weeks. One cannot conclude from these studies that hearing loss associated with OME adversely affects speech and language development, only that there is an association between time spent with OME and poor performance on the tests administered.

Despite the evidence suggesting a detrimental effect of OME on speech, language, and cognitive development, many studies have been performed that have not shown this association (70). It is extremely difficult to control for confounding factors, which may contribute to poor performance on standardized testing. Language is a reflection of culture; to study language one must address the cultural diversity of the study participants. Age, sex, parental intelligence, socioeconomic status, even day care all may have an effect on the development of language and cognitive ability. On the basis of a thorough review of the literature, the 1994 clinical guideline states that recommendations for managing OME are tempered by failure to find rigorous, methodologically sound research to support the theory that untreated OME results in speech and language delays or deficits (4). Some researchers have looked at more objective psychoanalytic and electrophysiologic measures of language, yet the effect of hearing loss on these measures and the correlation of the data with effect on communication remains unclear. Because of a paucity of data, it is not known whether any of these early effects of OME on speech and language persist into adulthood (70).

Overall, the current literature does support an association between the hearing loss of OME and delay in development of speech, language, and cognitive ability (70, 73). Regardless, until more defined measures are developed with which we can isolate the individual effect of this hearing loss on childhood development, clinical management should favor the well-being of the child. Multiple prolonged courses of antibiotics may be a long-term detriment to the child because of the development of resistant strains of bacteria. Placement of myringotomy tubes effectively clears the effusion, restores normal hearing, and reduces or eliminates the need for antibiotics.

Balance Mechanisms

Parents have reported poor balance and clumsiness as a symptom of the presence of middle ear fluid in their children. Studies have confirmed the observations by finding that the presence of middle ear fluid is associated with increased body sway and impaired gross motor skill. These conditions improve with insertion of ventilation tubes (74,75).

Middle Ear Structure

Long-term OME can lead to structural changes in the tympanic membrane and middle ear. Atelectasis of the tympanic membrane with formation of a retraction pocket

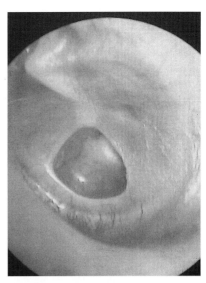

FIG. 6. Retraction pocket associated with serous otitis media.

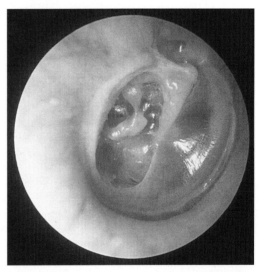

FIG. 7. Severe tympanic membrane retraction with erosion of incudostapedial joint. (Courtesy of Dr. Armando Lenis.)

can result from OME (Fig. 6). Erosion of the incudostapedial joint (Fig. 7: see color plate 8 following page 484), tympanic membrane perforation, and cholesteatoma have been reported as sequelae of long-term OME (76,77).

HIGH NEGATIVE PRESSURE

High negative pressure (HNP) is a form of OME that requires special mention (1,22). This condition is manifested by negative middle ear pressures more than -200 mm water without middle ear effusion. HNP occurs as an early stage in the development of OME and is the last stage before the middle ear returns to normal. HNP rarely causes problems more than a vague feeling of fullness or mild pressure in the ear. Occasionally, however, HNP may be a source of problems for the patient. The tympanic membrane retraction associated with HNP is usually very mild, but in some instances, severe atelectasis and incudostapedial joint erosion may occur (see Fig. 7). In rare instances, this condition may progress to cholesteatoma formation. The hearing loss associated with HNP is generally very mild (less than 10 dB), but some ears manifest hearing losses of up to 30 dB. If the negative pressure and resulting hearing loss do not clear (either spontaneously or after medical treatment), ventilation tube placement is indicated.

OTITIS MEDIA WITH EFFUSION IN ADULTS

OME in adults is less common than in children and may represent a far more serious condition, such as neoplastic infiltration of the nasopharyngeal orifice of the eustachian tube. Although mild negative middle ear pressure often accompanies URI in adults, fluid accumulation in the middle ear is uncommon. OME in an adult, especially unilateral, may represent primary nasopharyngeal carcinoma or lymphoma. Nasopharyngeal carcinoma represents approximately 18% of all carcinomas among the Chinese (even higher in Taiwan) (78); therefore unilateral OME in a patient of Asian descent should raise the suspicion of a nasopharyngeal tumor. Nonneoplastic processes such as Wegner's granulomatosis and malignant otitis externa also can present as OME. An otolaryngologist treating an adult with unilateral OME must examine the nasopharynx carefully using endoscopic techniques and appropriate imaging as clinically indicated.

Benign causal factors associated with OME among adults include paranasal sinus disease, adenoidal hypertrophy, the presence of a nasogastric or nasotracheal tube, and barotrauma. Purulence from acute or chronic sinusitis flows through the nasopharynx over the eustachian tube orifice. Inflammation of the torus tubarius causes eustachian tube dysfunction and OME. Treatment with antibiotics and appropriate nasal sprays (decongestants, steroid sprays) is associated with clearance of the middle ear fluid. Tympanocentesis or myringotomy with tube placement may be performed to alleviate temporarily the symptoms of pain, fullness, and hearing loss associated with the effusion until the underlying process resolves.

Adenoidal hypertrophy is associated with smoking and the human immunodeficiency virus (HIV) infection. An adult with OME and enlarged adenoids at nasal endoscopy should undergo HIV testing. If HIV test results are positive, adenoidectomy should be performed to rule out lymphoma. The adenoidectomy often promotes clearance of the effusion. Smokers should be encouraged to stop smoking (79).

Nasogastric and nasotracheal intubation are commonly used in the care of patients in intensive care units. Otolaryngologists frequently are consulted to evaluate and manage OME, which is commonly diagnosed by means of computed tomography of the head. OME occurs as a result of physical obstruction of the eustachian tube orifice by the tubes and associated nasopharyngeal inflammation. Most of these patients have concurrent sinusitis from obstruction of the osteomeatal complex, which contributes to nasopharyngeal inflammation. The tubes should be removed from the nose and placed orally, though it may be more uncomfortable for the patient. A nasal decongestant spray used short term (e.g., oxymetazoline for 3 days) with a nasal steroid spray, nasal saline spray, and appropriate course of antibiotics typically clears the OME and sinusitis.

BAROTRAUMA

Barotrauma can cause OME. It is more common during transition from low to high pressure (descent). During transition from high to low pressure (ascent), air in the middle ear passively escapes through the eustachian tube into the nasopharynx. However, during transition from low- to high-pressure regions, pressure in the nasopharynx increases, requiring active opening of the torus for equilibration. If pressure equilibration does not occur, nasopharyngeal pressure continues to increase, eventually compressing the cartilaginous torus tubarius, making it increasingly more difficult for the eustachian tube to open. Barotrauma occurs as middle ear pressure becomes acutely negative compared with atmospheric pressure. A middle ear transudate forms and occasionally is mixed with blood from rupture of small vessels (20).

The symptoms of barotrauma include otalgia, fullness, hearing loss, and occasionally tinnitus and vertigo. With extreme pressure changes, the tympanic membrane may perforate, and the perforation causes hearing loss, tinnitus, or vertigo. At otoscopy, the tympanic membrane is typically amber or bluish (if hemorrhage has occurred), but occasionally the examiner sees tympanic membrane perforation and otorrhea.

The Toynbee maneuver, which gently increases nasopharyngeal pressure with swallowing during occlusion of the nasal and oral cavities, or the more aggressive Valsalva maneuver, which increases nasopharyngeal pressure with forceful expiration against a closed nasal and oral cavity, can be performed periodically during a pressure transition to promote tubal opening and equilibration of pressure. Taking pseudoephedrine or using oxymetazoline nasal spray 1 hour before air travel or scuba diving has been shown to prevent or minimize the symptoms of barotrauma. Persons with allergies may benefit from use of antihistamines (80,81). When barotrauma does occur, it is usually self-limited and resolves on its own, provided that no further barotrauma occurs. Antimicrobial agents occasionally are prescribed to prevent acute infection of the middle ear fluid. Drainage rarely is needed. Persons prone to barotrauma whose livelihoods depend on air travel can undergo myringotomy with placement of tubes. Before an adult undergoes myringotomy with tube insertion, the nasopharynx must be inspected to rule out a nasopharyngeal mass.

SUMMARY POINTS

- Otitis media with effusion is an inflammatory condition of the middle ear and mastoid air cell system characterized by accumulation of fluid without signs or symptoms of acute infection.

- Any process that interferes with normal opening of the eustachian tube or the mucociliary clearance mechanism can cause OME.

- The incidence of OME among children 2 to 6 years of age is 35% to 75%. It decreases dramatically after 7 years of age.

- Diagnosis of OME usually is made with pneumatic otoscopy. Tympanometry and audiometry are used to confirm the diagnosis and assess hearing loss.

- OME resolves spontaneously in most cases.

- Antibiotics improve the clearance of the effusion, but their use has been linked to increased bacterial resistance.

- The clinical practice guideline Managing Otitis Media with Effusion in Young Children was developed in 1994 to guide management of OME among children 1 to 3 years of age with no craniofacial or neurologic abnormalities or sensory deficits.

- Surgical therapy is indicated for OME refractory to medical management. Early surgical intervention is indicated in the following situations: substantial hearing loss, coexisting developmental delay or disabilities (e.g., sensorineural hearing loss, vision impairment), balance disorder, severe tympanic membrane retraction, or ossicular erosion.

- High negative pressure, manifested by negative middle ear pressures more than -200 mm water, is associated with tympanic membrane retraction, which can erode the incudostapedial joint or progress to cholesteatoma.

- OME in an adult may be the only manifestation of a malignant tumor of the nasopharynx.

REFERENCES

1. Casselbrant ML, Brostoff LM, Flaherty MR, et al. Otitis media with effusion in preschool children. *Laryngoscope* 1985;95:428–436.
2. Birch L, Elbrond O. Prospective epidemiological study of secretory otitis media in children not attending kindergarten: a prevalence study. *Int J Pediatr Otorhinolaryngol* 1986;11:191–197.
3. Bluestone CD, Fria TJ, Arjona SK, et al. Controversies in screening for middle ear disease and hearing loss in children. *Pediatrics* 1986;77: 57–70.
4. Stool SE, Berg AO, Berman S, et al. Managing otitis media with effusion in young children: quick reference guide for clinicians; AHCPR Publication No. 94–0623. Rockville, MD: Agency for Health Care Policy and Research, Public Health Service, U.S. Department of Health and Human Services, 1994.
5. Gungor A, Corey JP. Relationship between otitis media with effusion and allergy. *Curr Opin Otolaryngol Head Neck Surg* 1997;5:46–48.
6. Mattucci KF, Greenfield BJ. Middle ear effusion–allergy relationships. *Ear Nose Throat J* 1995;74:752–758.
7. Bernstein JM. Role of allergy in eustachian tube blockage and otitis media with effusion: a review. *Otolaryngol Head Neck Surg* 1996;114: 562–568.
8. Agius AM, Wake M, Pahor AL, Smallman LA. Smoking and middle ear ciliary beat frequency in otitis media with effusion. *Acta Otolaryngol* 1995;115:44–49.
9. Teele DW, Klein JO, Rosner B and the Greater Boston Otitis Media Study Group. Epidemiology of otitis media during the first seven years of life in children in greater Boston: a prospective, cohort study. *Infect Dis* 1989;160(1):83–94.
10. Jero J, Virolainen A, Virtanen M, Eskola J, Karma P. Prognosis of acute otitis media: factors associated with poor outcome. *Acta Otolaryngol* 1997;117:278–283.
11. Post JC, Preston RA, Aul JJ, et al. Molecular analysis of bacterial pathogens in otitis media with effusion. *JAMA* 1995;273:1598–1604.
12. Bluestone CD, Rood SR, Swarts JD. Anatomy and physiology of the eustachian tube. In: Cummings CW, Fredrickson JM, Harker LA, Krause CJ, Schuller DE, eds. *Otolaryngology–head and neck surgery.* St Louis: Mosby–Year Book, 1993:2548–2565.
13. Schucknecht HF. *Pathology of the ear.* Philadelphia: Lea & Febiger, 1993.
14. Bluestone CD, Klein JD. *Otitis media in infants and children.* Philadelphia: WB Saunders, 1988.
15. Ingelstedt S, Ivarsson A. The physiology of the eustachian tube: a nontraumatic method. In: Munker G, Arnold W, eds. *Physiology and pathophysiology of eustachian tube and middle ear.* New York: Thieme-Stratton, 1980:8–18.
16. Tos M. Tympanomastoiditis: management and treatment. In: Alberti PW, Ruben RJ, eds. *Otologic medicine and surgery.* New York: Churchill Livingstone, 1988:1203–1239.
17. Kumazawa T, Iwano T, Ushiro K, Kinoshita T, Hamada E, Kaneko A. Eustachian tube function tests and their diagnostic potential in normal and diseased ears. *Acta Otolaryngol* 1993;[Suppl 500]:10–13.
18. McBride TP, Derkay CS, Cunningham MJ, Doyle WJ. Evaluation of noninvasive eustachian tube function tests in normal adults. *Laryngoscope* 1988;98:655–658.
19. Yagi N, Haji T, Honjo I. Eustachian tube patency detected by a photoelectric method. *Laryngoscope* 1987;97:732–736.
20. Sade J, Ar A. Middle ear and auditory tube: middle ear clearance, gas exchange, and pressure regulation. *Otolaryngol Head Neck Surg* 1997; 116:499–524.
21. Healy GB, Smith HG. Current concepts in the management of otitis media with effusion. *Am J Otolaryngol* 1981;2:138–144.
22. Tos M. Epidemiology and natural history of secretory otitis. *Am J Otol* 1984;5:459–462.
23. Birch L, Elbrond O. Prospective epidemiological study of secretory otitis media in children not attending kindergarten: an incidence study. *Int J Pediatr Otorhinolaryngol* 1986;11:183–190.
24. Kraemer MJ, Richardson MA, Weiss NS, et al. Risk factors of persistent middle-ear effusions: otitis media, catarrh, cigarette smoke exposure, and atopy. *JAMA* 1983;249:1022–1025.
25. Blakely BW, Blakely JE. Smoking and middle ear disease: are they related? a review article. *Otolaryngol Head Neck Surg* 1995;112: 441–446.
26. Gates GA, Stewart IA, Northern JL. Diagnosis and screening. *Ann Otol Rhinol Laryngol* 1994;103[Suppl 164]:53–57.
27. Finitzo T, Friel-Patti S, Chinn K, Brown O. Tympanometry and otoscopy prior to myringotomy: issues in diagnosis of otitis media. *Int J Pediatr Otorhinolaryngol* 1992;24:101–110.
28. Teele DW, Teele J. Detection of middle ear effusion by acoustic reflectometry. *Pediatr* 1984;104:832–838.
29. Schwartz DM, Schwartz RH. Validity of acoustic reflectectometry in detecting middle ear effusion. *Pediatrics* 1987;79:739–742.
30. Babonis T, Weir MR, Kelly P, Krober MS. Progression of tympanometry and acoustic reflectometry: findings in children with acute otitis media. *Clin Pediatr (Phila)* 1994;33:593–600.
31. Douniadakis DE, Nikolopoulos TP, Tsakanikos MD, Vassiliadis SV, Apostolopoulos NJ. Evaluation of acoustic reflectometry in detecting otitis media in children. *Br J Audiol* 1993;27:409–414.
32. Flanagan PM, Knight LC, Thomas A, Browning S, Aymat A, Clayton MI. Hearing aids and glue ear. *Clin Otolaryngol* 1996;21:297–300.

33. Cantekin EI, Mandel EM, Bluestone CD, et al. Lack of efficacy of a decongestant-antihistamine combination for otitis media with effusion ("secretory" otitis media) in children. *N Engl J Med* 1983;308: 297–301.

34. Kenna MA. Otitis media with effusion. In: Bailey B, ed. *Head and neck surgery–otolaryngology.* Philadelphia: Lippincott-Raven, 1993: 1592–1606.

35. Corwin MJ, Weiner LB, Daniels D: Efficacy of oral antibiotic for the treatment of persistent otitis media with effusion. *Int J Pediatr Otorhinolaryngol* 1986;11:109–112.

36. Giebink GS, Meyerhoff WL, Canafax DM, et al. Treatment. *Ann Otol Rhinol Laryngol* 1994;103[Suppl 64]:58–66.

37. Paradise JL. Managing otitis media: a time for change. *Pediatrics* 1995; 96:712–715.

38. Rosenfeld RM, Mandel EM, Bluestone CD. Systemic steroids for otitis media with effusion in children. *Arch Otolaryngol Head Neck Surg* 1991;117:984–989.

39. Podoshin L, Fradis M, Ben-David Y, Faraggi D. The efficacy of oral steroids in the treatment of persistent otitis media with effusion. *Arch Otolaryngol Head Neck Surg* 1990;116:1404–1406.

40. Bernstein JM, Lee J, Conboy K, Ellis E, Li P. The role of IgE mediated hypersensitivity in recurrent otitis media with effusion. *Am J Otol* 1983;5:66–69.

41. Doyle WJ, Takahara T, Fireman P. The role of allergy in the pathogenesis of otitis media with effusion *Arch Otolaryngol* 1985;111: 502–506.

42. Brown DT, Potsic WP, Marsh RR, Mitchell-Litt D. Drugs affecting clearance of middle ear secretions: a perspective for the management of otitis media with effusion. *Ann Otol Rhinol Laryngol Suppl* 1985;117:3–15.

43. Ogra PL, Barenkamp SJ, Mogi G, et al. Microbiology, immunology, biochemistry, and vaccination. *Ann Otol Rhinol Laryngol* 1994;103 [Suppl 164]:27–43.

44. Handler S. Current indications for tympanostomy tubes. *Am J Otolaryngol* 1994;15:103–108.

45. Bonding P, Tos M. Grommets versus paracentesis in secretory otitis media: a prospective, controlled study. *Am J Otol* 1985;6:455–460.

46. Wetmore RF, Henry WJ, Konkle DF. Acoustical factors of noise created by suctioning middle ear fluid. *Arch Otolaryngol Head Neck Surg* 1993;119:762–766.

47. Goode RL, Schulz W. Heat myringotomy for the treatment of serous otitis media. *Otolaryngol Head Neck Surg* 1982;90:764–766.

48. Armstrong B. A new treatment of chronic serous otitis media. *Arch Otolaryngol* 1954;59:653–654.

49. Heald MM, Matkin ND, Meredith KE. Pressure-equalization (PE) tubes in treatment of otitis media: national survey of otolaryngologists. *Otolaryngol Head Neck Surg* 1990;102:334–338.

50. Gates GA. Cost effectiveness considerations in otitis media treatment. *Otolaryngol Head Neck Surg* 1996;114:525–530.

51. Handler SD, Potsic WP, Marsh RR. A trial of Biolite ventilation tubes in children: is further use warranted? *Otolaryngol Head Neck Surg* 1983;91:437–440.

52. Handler SD, Miller L, Potsic WP, Wetmore RF, Marsh RR. A prospective study of titanium ventilating tubes. *Int J Pediatr Otorhinolaryngol* 1988;16:55–60.

53. Handler SD, Miller L, Potsic WP, et al. A controlled study of a "new" ventilation tube: the gold standard? *Int J Pediatr Otorhinolaryngol* 1986;12:33–38.

54. Weigel MT, Parker MY, Goldsmith MM, Postma DS, Pillsbury HC. A prospective randomized study of four commonly used tympanostomy tubes. *Laryngoscope* 1989;99:252–256.

55. Silverstein H. Permanent middle ear aeration. *Arch Otolaryngol* 1970; 91:313–318.

56. Wright JW. Preliminary results with use of an eustachian tube prosthesis. *Laryngoscope* 1977;87:207–214.

57. Alberti PW. Epithelial migration on the tympanic membrane. *J Laryngol Otol* 1964;78:808–830.

58. Salata JA, Derkay CS. Water precautions in children with tympanostomy tubes. *Arch Otolaryngol Head Neck Surg* 1996;122:276–280.

59. Tos M, Stangerup SE. Hearing loss in tympanosclerosis caused by grommets. *Arch Otolaryngol Head Neck Surg* 1989;115:931–935.

60. Moller P. Tympanosclerosis of the ear drum in children. *Int J Pediatr Otorhinolaryngol* 1984;7:247–256.

61. Brenman AK, Milner RM, Weller CR. Use of hydrogen peroxide to clear blocked ventilation tubes. *Am J Otol* 1986;7:47–50.

62. Berger G, Ophir D. Possible role of adenoid mast cells in the pathogenesis of secretory otitis media. *Ann Otol Rhinol Laryngol* 1994;103: 632–635.

63. Sade J, Luntz M. Adenoidectomy in otitis media. *Ann Otol Rhinol Laryngol* 1991;100:226–231.

64. Gates GA, Avery CA, Priholda TJ. Effect of adenoidectomy upon children with chronic otitis media with effusion. *Laryngoscope* 1988;98: 58–63.

65. Gates GA. Adenoidectomy for otitis media with effusion. *Ann Otol Rhinol Laryngol Suppl* 1994;163:54–58.

66. Muntz HR. An overview of middle ear disease in cleft palate children. *Facial Plast Surg* 1993;9(3):177–180.

67. Hunter LL, Margolis RH, Giebank GS. Identification of hearing loss in children with otitis media. *Ann Otol Rhinol Laryngol* 1994;163:59–61.

68. Baldwin RL. Effects of otitis media on child development. *Am J Otol* 1993;14(6):601–604.

69. Fria TJ, Cantekin EI, Eichler JA. Hearing acuity of children with otitis media with effusion. *Arch Otolaryngol* 1985;111:10–16.

70. Ruben RJ, Bagger-Sjoback D, Chase C. Complications and sequelae. *Ann Otol Rhinol Laryngol* 1994;103[Suppl 164]:67–80.

71. Teele DW, Klein JO, Rosner BA and The Greater Boston Otitis Media Study Group. Otitis media with effusion during the first three years of life and development of speech and language. *Pediatrics* 1984;74(2): 282–287.

72. Teele DW, Klein JO, Chase C, Menyuk P, Rosner BA and The Greater Boston Otitis Media Study Group. Otitis media in infancy and intellectual ability, school achievement, speech, and language at age seven years. *The Journal of Infectious Diseases* 1990;162:685–694.

73. Teele DW. Long term sequelae of otitis media: fact or fantasy? *Pediatric Infection Disease Journal* 1994;13:1069–1073.

74. Orlin MN, Handler SD. Effect of otitis media with effusion on gross motor skill ability in preschool-aged children: preliminary findings. *Pediatrics* 1997;99:334–337.

75. Jones NS, Radomskij P, Prichard AJ, Snashall SE. Imbalance and chronic secretory otitis media in children: effect of myringotomy and insertion of ventilation tubes on body sway. *Ann Otol Rhinol Laryngol* 1990;99:477–481.

76. Tos M, Stangerup SE, Larsen P. Dynamics of eardrum changes following secretory otitis. *Arch Otolaryngol Head Neck Surg* 1987;113: 380–385.

77. Sade J. Bone resorption. *Otitis media with effusion and its sequelae.* New York: Churchill Livingstone, 1979;171–183.

78. Neel HB. Benign and malignant neoplasms of the nasopharynx. In: Cummings CW, Fredrickson JM, Harker LA, Krause CJ, Schuller DE, eds. *Otolaryngology—head and neck surgery.* St Louis: Mosby–Year Book, 1993:1355–1371.

79. Finkelstein Y, Ophir D, Talmi YP, Shabtai A, Strauss M, Zohar Y. Adult-onset otitis media with effusion. *Arch Otolaryngol Head Neck Surg* 1994;120:517–527.

80. Brown TP. Middle ear symptoms while flying: ways to prevent a severe outcome. *Postgrad Med* 1994;96:135–142.

81. Csortan E, Jones J, Haan M, Brown M. Efficacy of pseudoephedrine for the prevention of barotrauma during air travel. *Ann Emerg Med* 1994;23:1324–1327.

The Ear: Comprehensive Otology,
edited by R. F. Canalis and P. R. Lambert.
Lippincott Williams & Wilkins, Philadelphia © 2000.

CHAPTER 24

Acute Suppurative Otitis Media and Mastoiditis

Rinaldo F. Canalis and Paul R. Lambert

This chapter focuses on the clinical and pathologic features of acute bacterial infections of the middle ear cleft and mastoid process. Acute bullous myringitis (ABM), which involves the lateral middle ear boundary, and acute fungal infections of the middle ear, mastoid, and skull base are discussed briefly.

ACUTE OTITIS MEDIA

Definition

Acute otitis media (AOM), or acute suppurative otitis media, is an infectious process of the middle ear cleft and, to a variable extent, of the mastoid air cell system.

R. F. Canalis: Department of Surgery, University of California, Los Angeles, School of Medicine, Los Angeles, California 90095-1624

P. R. Lambert: Department of Otolaryngology–Head and Neck Surgery, University of Virginia Health Sciences Center, Charlottesville, Virginia 22908-0430

Epidemiology

Acute suppurative otitis media affects patients of all ages, but it is predominantly a disease of infants and young children. Numerous current studies exploring the natural history of the disease and encompassing several thousand patients have reported that 47% to 60% of all children experience their first episode of AOM during the first year of life and that 60% to 70% do so by their fourth birthday (1–3). In a recent, highly representative study, Pukander et al. (4) surveyed all documented cases of AOM occurring in a Finnish population of more than 146,000 people for a period of 1 year. They collected 6,158 episodes occurring in 4,582 patients for a residence-adjusted incidence of 4.08%. The incidence for children under 16 years of age was 16.6% and for children under 10 was 25.3%. The highest annual incidence (73.5%) was found in a subgroup of patients whose age was between 6 and 11 months.

Undoubtedly several factors are operative in increasing the susceptibility of young children to AOM. Among these, the frequency of upper respiratory infections affecting the pediatric population and developmental alterations of the eustachian tube are discussed most often. Other factors, such as poor nutrition, lower socioeconomic status, and systemic allergies, also appear to play a contributory role.

Etiology

The most common etiologic factor in AOM is an upper respiratory infection. The mucosa of the pharyngeal end of the eustachian tube is part of the mucociliary system of the middle ear. Its interference by edema, tumor, or negative intratympanic pressure facilitates direct extension of infection from the pharynx, resulting in otitis media. Mechanical factors that may alter the mucosal surface of the middle ear also are important. Among these, foreign material entering the middle ear cleft either through a tympanic membrane perforation or the eustachian tube, as is the case with regurgitated esophageal contents, must be considered. Barometric pressure changes that alter the normal middle ear pressure may produce surface mucosal alterations that, in turn, can facilitate the development of local infection.

Bacteriology

The high degree of correlation between AOM and upper respiratory infections suggests that viruses are likely to have a role in the development of otitis media. During epidemics and in isolated situations, the respiratory syncytial virus, influenza A and B, and parainfluenza viruses have been cultured from middle ear exudates (5,6). However, it is not known if these agents can cause otitis media by themselves or if they facilitate the development of a bacterial infection.

A review of several large studies of middle ear cultures obtained during the course of AOM identified *Streptococcus pneumoniae* (±48%), *Haemophilus influenzae* (±31%), and group A streptococci (±11%) as the most frequently encountered bacteria, with close to 30% of all cultures failing to produce any growth (7). Recently, *Moraxella catarrhalis* has risen as a significant pathogen in the development of AOM in children (8) and may account for up to 20% of cases. Notable exceptions to this distribution are encountered in children under 6 weeks of age in whom bacteriologic findings favor gram-negative enteric organisms and *Staphylococcus aureus*. In adults and in children 5 years of age or older, the relative incidence of the pneumococcus group increases, with *H. influenzae* being of less significance (9). The incidence of β-hemolytic streptococcus, which was high during the epidemics of childhood eruptive illnesses, has, at least in the industrialized nations, significantly decreased following widespread immunization programs. As a consequence, acute necrotizing processes resulting in large

tympanic membrane perforations and ossicular chain destruction are now seen infrequently. In the authors' experience, *Pseudomonas aeruginosa* is an uncommon cause of AOM, but it must be considered in the immunocompromised patient and in patients who fail to respond to apparently adequate treatment.

Pathology

AOM starts as a mucosal inflammation of the eustachian tube, middle ear, and tympanic membrane. Polymorphonuclear and lymphocytic infiltrates accompany the initial edema, with periostitis involving the promontory of the tympanic cavity and surface mucositis producing diffuse ciliary paralysis. The middle ear cavity fills with serous, hemorrhagic, or purulent exudate. The tympanic membrane is thickened by inflammatory edema and frequently ruptures spontaneously.

Symptoms

Ear symptoms, primarily otalgia, can occur within hours of the onset of upper respiratory infection or may be delayed days or, rarely, weeks. Ear stuffiness and hearing loss may precede or follow otalgia, which can vary from slight discomfort to severe pain, spreading to the temporal area. Pain is rarely completely relieved by analgesics. Fever usually is present, but it may be masked by analgesics or antibiotics.

Physical Findings

Examination of the nose and nasopharynx usually demonstrates vascular congestion and edema. Crusting and purulent discharge may be present. The external ear usually reveals no abnormalities. At the onset of the disease, manipulation of the auricle seldom causes discomfort, in contrast with the findings of acute external otitis. However, as the infection progresses, tympanic membrane swelling may spread to involve the tissues of the external auditory canal, resulting in edema, erythema, and auricular pain. Mastoid tenderness is common in early otitis media and is not a diagnostic sign of mastoiditis.

The diagnosis of AOM usually is made on otoscopic examination. Adequate visualization requires careful removal of cerumen and epithelial debris. Typical findings include increased vascularization of the tympanic membrane, frequently spreading beyond the annulus to the skin of the external auditory canal (*erythematous phase*). In early AOM, the two primary bony landmarks, the malleal short process and the umbo, are visible, although they may be distorted by intense arteriolar and venous engorgement (Fig. 1: see color plate 9 following page 484). As the infection proceeds from mucositis to marked submucosal edema and progressive closure of the eustachian tube, rapid middle ear exudation occurs

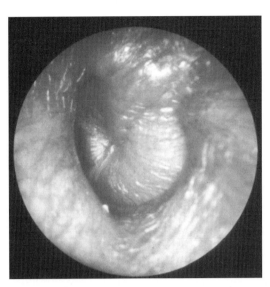

FIG. 1. Acute suppurative otitis media, early stage. Note erythema and bulging of tympanic membrane. The malleal short process and umbo are still visible. (Courtesy of Dr. Armando Lenis.)

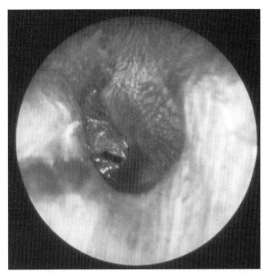

FIG. 3. Acute suppurative otitis media with spontaneous tympanic membrane rupture (anteroinferior quadrant). Note decompression of middle ear exudate with return of malleal landmarks. (Courtesy of Dr. Armando Lenis.)

(*exudative* phase). The exudate rapidly changes from serous to purulent. Blurring of the malleal short process, due to epitympanic mucositis, is followed by edema and bulging of the pars flaccida (*suppurative* phase) (Fig. 2: see color plate 10 following page 484).

The progression to mesotympanic involvement and the development of friable fibrosis results in loculation of the tympanic exudate. Swelling of the tympanic membrane may be generalized or limited to the anterior, posterior, or posterosuperior quadrants. These differences usually are due to tympanic fibrosis resulting from previous episodes of suppurative otitis media. Additional spread of edema to the tympanic annulus can blur the boundaries between

the tympanic membrane and the external auditory canal so that no definitive tympanic membrane landmarks are recognizable. At any time during the suppurative phase the tympanic membrane may rupture, releasing the middle ear contents. Decompression results in retraction of the pars flaccida into a more normal position and visualization of some landmarks, especially the malleus (Fig. 3: see color plate 11 following page 484).

Laboratory Tests

Plane mastoid radiographs generally are not indicated, but when taken they will reveal a haziness in the periantral cells that occasionally may extend to the entire mastoid. A computed tomographic (CT) or magnetic resonance imaging (MRI) scan is necessary for the rare patient with a serious complication (e.g., meningitis or brain abscess). Blood counts usually will show leukocytosis with polymorphonuclear elevation.

Hearing Tests

The degree of conductive hearing loss will depend on the amount and viscosity of the middle ear exudate, middle ear fibrosis, and tympanic membrane edema. Thus, it may vary from 10 to 50 dB, with predominant involvement of the low frequencies (Fig. 4A). Hearing loss may be mixed if there is labyrinthine extension, which is relatively rare (Fig. 4B).

Clinical Course

AOM is a self-limiting disease in approximately 80% of cases, with acute symptoms sometimes abating sponta-

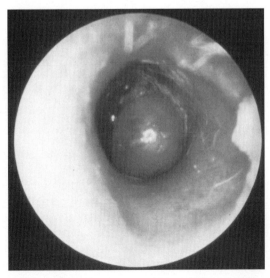

FIG. 2. Acute suppurative otitis media, advanced stage. Note severe bulging of tympanic membrane with loss of landmarks. (Courtesy of Dr. Armando Lenis.)

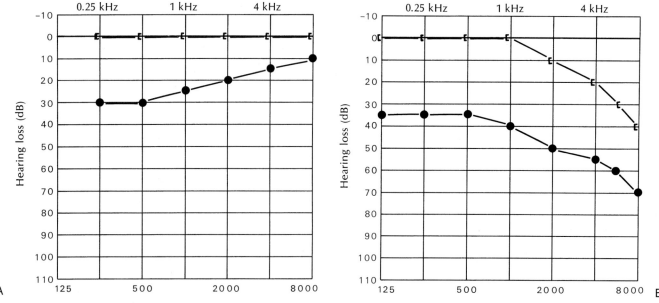

FIG. 4. A: Conductive hearing loss in acute otitis media. **B:** Mixed hearing loss in complicated acute otitis media.

neously as early as 24 to 72 hours after onset. However, the process may progress rapidly to spontaneous tympanic membrane rupture and otorrhea, which may be serous, serosanguineous, or purulent. The duration of aural discharge varies but usually is brief. In a retrospective study of nearly 3,000 cases, most of which were not treated or managed with myringotomy alone, suppuration stopped within 30 days in 88% of cases (10). In nearly two thirds of cases, discharge ceased by the eighth day. If pain, fullness, and hearing loss are not relieved by spontaneous otorrhea, either intratympanic purulent loculation has occurred, or there is marked severity of the infectious process, or both.

Medical Treatment

The general treatment of AOM is that of any potentially serious infection. Bed rest, hydration, a light diet, and avoidance of irritants (smoking) are important. Nasal and/or systemic decongestants may be symptomatically helpful, but there is no evidence that they alter the course of the disease. A cool mist humidifier is helpful in relieving mucosal dryness and crusting. Warm steam vaporizers tend to increase congestion and are best avoided.

The introduction of sulfonamide therapy in the late 1930s and shortly thereafter the discovery of penicillin revolutionized the treatment of AOM by permitting effective management without surgery. Ideally, and certainly when a complication is present, antibiotic therapy should be specifically determined by bacteriologic cultures and antibiotic sensitivity tests. However, in most cases, immediate treatment can be instituted against the most commonly isolated etiologic agents: the pneumococcus group and, especially in children 5 years old or younger, *H. influenzae*. Until relatively recently the drug most commonly used was amoxicillin, but the growing incidence of β-lactamase–producing bacteria has begun to limit its effectiveness. The addition of clavulanic acid to amoxicillin or the use of second-generation cephalosporins (such as cefaclor or cefuroxime) have been used increasingly because of emerging bacterial resistance. The combination drugs trimethoprim-sulfamethoxazole and erythromycin-sulfisoxazole or the newer macrolide antibiotics (e.g., clarithromycin or azithromycin) have been shown to sterilize the middle ear when *H. influenzae* was the causative agent. These antibiotics also are effective in the management of *M. catarrhalis*, a known β-lactamase producer, and they can be used in penicillin-allergic patients.

Once culture results and sensitivities are available, therapy should be modified accordingly and maintained for 10 to 14 days. Close follow-up is mandatory with discontinuation of therapy only when followed by resolution of all symptoms, return to normal otoscopic findings, and restoration of normal hearing.

Surgery: Myringotomy

There is considerable debate as to the benefit of myringotomy in the management of AOM. In a comprehensive review, Gates (11) noted that many retrospective and prospective studies were at least partially flawed because of incomplete statistical analysis and failure to stratify patients by age or to separate them in groups with multiple or isolated attacks, as well as unilateral or bilateral disease. He concluded that there was no evidence to support the routine use of myringotomy, but that in severe cases it provides prompt pain relief and accelerates the resolution of the process. In addition, it is a critical step in the management of complicated disease.

In general agreement with these concepts, we believe that when otitis is rapidly progressive with a red, bulging tympanic membrane, severe otalgia, and fever, treatment should include antibiotics and *immediate myringotomy*. Indications for myringotomy in purulent middle ear locations are the same as for incision and drainage of pus in any closed cavity or viscus. When purulent secretions are retained in the middle ear cleft, pressure will result in spread of the infection following areas of less resistance. Tympanic rupture and loculation of pus within the mastoid air cells occur commonly. Less frequently, the labyrinthine windows, the perineurium of the facial nerve, or the subarachnoid space may be involved.

In infants and very young children, a myringotomy may be done without anesthesia. With good illumination, magnification, and adequate restraint, the procedure can be performed rapidly. In older children general anesthesia is preferred. In adults an endomeatal lidocaine-epinephrine block or topical anesthesia with phenol usually provides adequate analgesia. The patient should be lying comfortably on an examining table. Assistance to keep the patient's head immobilized should be available to prevent unexpected, potentially dangerous movement.

The ear should be examined under the surgical microscope. A bimanual technique is recommended, in which the speculum is held in one hand and the myringotomy knife in the other. A beveled speculum is preferred and it should allow for the cartilaginous canal to be straightened while its tip should reach the bony portion. Following gentle removal of cerumen and epithelial debris with fine suction tips and metal forceps, the tympanic membrane is inspected. The incision site should be based on the location of the major tympanic membrane swelling, taking care to stay within the limits of the pars tensa and avoiding injury to the ossicular chain in the posterosuperior quadrant. The incision should be approximately 2.5 to 4 mm in length (Fig. 5).

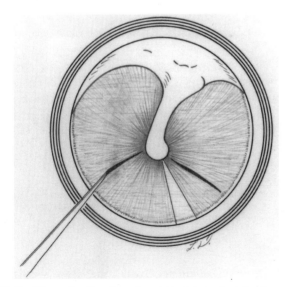

FIG. 5. Alternative locations for myringotomy incision in acute otitis media.

Purulent material is aspirated and sent to the laboratory in a sterile tube for culture and sensitivity tests. The external auditory canal is kept lightly closed with sterile cotton, which should be changed every few hours for as long as otorrhea continues. The external canal should not be irrigated.

Follow-up Care

Regardless of the response to initial therapy, close follow-up is of the highest importance in AOM. Care must be taken to detect an unresolved secretory process, bearing in mind that in many cases of adequately treated AOM effusion may persist for 2 to 6 weeks or even longer.

The most common sequel of AOM is persistent, painless, middle ear fluid that may be serous or mucoid. This finding nearly always is associated with a variable degree of conductive hearing loss. Left untreated it may lead to recurrent suppurative otitis media. Management may require repeated cultures, extended antibiotic treatment, or myringotomy with insertion of pressure equalization tubes for middle ear fluid that persists beyond 3 months (see Chapter 23). The patient with AOM in whom all acute symptoms have subsided should be reexamined by otoscopy and audiometric tests 3 to 4 weeks following apparent resolution of the acute infection. Normal otoscopic and audiometric findings should precede the patient's release from care.

Complications

Despite its usually benign course, otitis media occasionally may result in acute or chronic complications. Among these complications, acute mastoiditis, facial nerve paralysis, labyrinthitis, meningitis, and brain abscess are seen occasionally. In addition to aggressive antibiotic therapy, most acute complications require at least a myringotomy to decompress the middle ear suppuration and to obtain material for culture and sensitivity studies. Other surgical procedures to provide drainage include insertion of a ventilation tube and/or a simple mastoidectomy. Chronic complications include tympanic membrane perforations, cholesteatoma, tympanosclerosis, ossicular necrosis, toxic or suppurative labyrinthitis, and less frequently intracranial suppuration. These and other problems resulting from suppurative ear disease are discussed in Chapter 26.

ACUTE BULLOUS MYRINGITIS

ABM is a self-limiting disease usually characterized by the rapid onset of ear pain and the development of one or more vesicles in the tympanic membrane (Fig. 6: see color plate 12 following page 484). ABM usually is unilateral and occurs most frequently in adolescents and young adults. Spontaneous rupture of the vesicles results in transient clear yellow or bloody tinged otorrhea. Conductive hearing loss, when present, usually is mild.

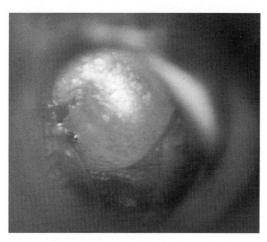

FIG. 6. Acute bullous myringitis. Note one large vesicle obscuring more than one half of the tympanic membrane. (Courtesy of Dr. Armando Lenis.)

Marked conductive loss is indicative of an associated middle ear process. Wetmore and Abramson (12) reviewed 22 cases of ABM and discussed seven patients who experienced a variable degree of sensorineural hearing loss. Hearing returned to predisease level in all patients, except one who was a diabetic with severe labyrinthitis. These authors concluded that sensorineural hearing loss in bullous myringitis probably is more common than previously estimated.

The etiologic agent in ABM has been sought for more than 7 decades. Chanock et al. (13) and Rifkind et al. (14) reported a high incidence of myringitis following the inoculation of 27 sera-negative volunteers with *Mycoplasma pneumoniae*. Tympanic membrane findings, however, were typical of ABM in only 2 of 12 volunteers who developed myringitis. Following these studies there have been multiple reports of negative complement fixation tests in patients with ABM (12,15). In the study by Wetmore and Abramson (12), no change in acute and convalescent titers for *Mycoplasma pneumoniae* and several respiratory viruses were encountered.

The major lesion in ABM usually is limited to the tympanic membrane, where all layers undergo rapid inflammatory edema with bullae forming under the external epithelial layer. The infection may then spread to the middle ear cleft. Secondary bacterial infection is common.

ABM usually resolves rapidly. Treatment is symptomatic. Oral analgesics usually suffice for pain control. In our experience and that of others (15), uncapping vesicles usually produces no significant pain relief. The patient should protect the ear from water contact. Antibiotic therapy should be reserved for secondary bacterial infections.

ACUTE MASTOIDITIS

Definition

Acute mastoiditis is an infection of the mastoid, characterized by diffuse osteitis followed by rarefaction and breakdown of the bony septae that compartmentalize its air cell system. Pus formation and mucoperiosteal edema of the air cells, often found in AOM, do not constitute clinical mastoiditis.

Incidence

Although the incidence of acute mastoiditis has declined markedly by virtue of ever-improving antibiotic therapy, it continues to be a serious clinical problem. At present, there is no statistical information regarding the true incidence of acute mastoiditis. Most recently reported series surveying the current epidemiology of the disease consist of groups of 40 to 70 patients collected over periods of 10 years or more in hospitals serving large metropolitan areas (16–18). These series represent an approximate frequency of 4 to 5 patients per 100 major surgical ear cases, which correlates well with our own experience in two large teaching institutions.

Acute mastoiditis occurs most commonly as a sequela of incompletely treated suppurative otitis media and is prevalent in children. The majority of available studies address the pediatric population (birth to 18 years) and reveal a median age of approximately 3 years and an average age of 3 ± 0.5 years. In a study of 34 patients surveying all ages, the mean was 15 years, with a range of 1 to 77 years (18). Until recently, the disease was believed to be more frequent in patients with a history of recurrent ear infection. More current studies, however, dispute this view. In the series by Rubin and Wei (18), 76% (26/34) of patients had previously normal ears; in the series by Hawkins et al. (16), 74% (40/54) had no previous history of otitis media. Mastoiditis occasionally may be the initial presentation of a congenital cholesteatoma.

Bacteriology

Streptococcus pyogenes is the leading etiologic agent in acute mastoiditis. In the series of 54 cases of acute mastoiditis in children reported by Hawkins et al. (16), cultures were obtained in 21 instances either by myringotomy or at mastoidectomy. *S. pyogenes* was cultured in 9 patients, *S. pneumoniae* in 6, *H. influenzae* in 12, and the rest included enterococci/anaerobes and *Mycobacterium tuberculosis*. In a composite review of this series and two other series (17,18), for a total of 157 cases, the results of positive cultures were available in 47. Of these, 15 were due to *S. pyogenes* (32%), 8 to *S. pneumoniae* (17%), 6 to coagulase-negative staphylococcus (13%), 5 to *H. influenzae* (11%), and the remaining 13 cases (27%) to various other bacteria, including *P. aeruginosa* (8.5%), proteus (8.5%), anaerobic agents (5%), and *M. tuberculosis* (5%).

Pathology

In acute mastoiditis complicating otitis media the process spreads from the aditus ad antrum through the

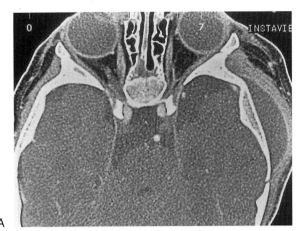
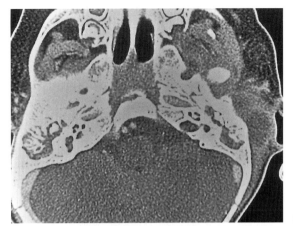

FIG. 7. Axial computed tomographic scans in acute mastoiditis showing subtemporal **(A)** and postauricular **(B)** abscess.

diploic and marrow spaces into the mastoid air cell system. There may be involvement of squamous, petrous, and perilabyrinthine cell groups. In addition, extension occurs to hypotympanic, peritubal, digastric, and retrosinus cell groups. This initial phase of mastoiditis is followed by the changes characteristic of the disease: (a) obstruction by edema, inspissated pus, and early formation of granulation tissue; and (b) osteitis with breakdown of the bony framework of the air cell septae.

Obstruction results in rapid increase of pressure against the air cell septae and widespread cellular necrosis. This osteitic process is associated with an alteration in local pH, which fosters decalcification and softening of the organic matrix of the mastoid bone. Removal of the decaying matrix is facilitated by phagocytes and possibly by certain bacteria. The mastoid rapidly loses its structural form, with coalescence of multiple cell spaces, and it continues to fill with the products of its own breakdown. The eventual course is contingent on several factors, among which the virulence of the offending agent, the immunologic status of the patient, the reestablishment of natural drainage, and medical intervention play significant roles.

In untreated cases, spread to the mastoid cortex and its periosteum follows the described events. Erosion through the cortex results in the formation of a subperiosteal abscess (Fig. 7), which is a relatively late development of the disease. Subperiosteal abscesses also may result from extension of the infection along the vessels passing through the cribriform area.

Symptoms

The symptoms of acute mastoiditis may follow those of AOM, with or without a symptom-free interval of a few days to several weeks or more. The most salient features of acute mastoiditis are otalgia, aural discharge, and conductive hearing loss. Headache and general malaise frequently are present.

Physical Findings

Fever usually is measurable on presentation, and it may fluctuate from a slight elevation to 39°C or higher. Otoscopy will demonstrate obliteration of the malleal short process. A swelling of the superior tympanic membrane and contiguous canal skin will result in "sagging" of the posterosuperior wall of the external auditory canal, with narrowing of its lumen. Otorrhea may be absent. When present, it may be serous, seropurulent, or mucopurulent. It can be pulsatile as a result of transmitted middle ear fluid pressure. A tympanic membrane perforation frequently is present, but it may be obscured by intense edema of this structure and of the external auditory canal. The postauricular area first demonstrates erythema and tenderness, rapidly followed by pitting edema, obliteration of the postauricular crease, and abscess formation with auricular displacement (Fig. 8). A variable degree of subcutaneous fluctuance appears, as liquefaction of inflammatory products takes place and tension increases. Weber's and Rinne's tuning fork tests usually indicate a conductive hearing loss in the affected ear.

Laboratory Tests

Leukocytosis of a variable degree usually is present, with white blood cell counts fluctuating between a slight elevation and 25,000/mL or more.

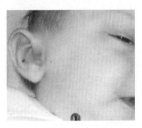

FIG. 8. Marked lateral inferior auricular displacement in acute mastoiditis with subperiosteal abscess.

Auditory Tests

Audiometric evaluation should be performed early in the course of the disease to establish a point of reference. It usually will confirm the clinical impression of conductive hearing loss, but changes in bone conduction may be present indicating a mixed loss. Small changes (15 dB or less) in bone conduction thresholds are usually of a "mechanical" type and not due to cochlear involvement. Patterns are similar to those noted in AOM (Fig. 4). However, in severe, protracted, acute mastoiditis, the patient may have true cochlear hearing loss due to inner ear involvement via the oval and round windows. In such cases, speech discrimination scores will drop, an indication of true labyrinthitis (see Chapter 26).

Radiographic Evaluation

When the clinical history and findings are as described, especially in the presence of posterosuperior canal wall collapse and subperiosteal abscess, radiographs offer little more than confirmatory evidence of coalescent mastoiditis. Diffuse opacification and, in advanced disease, rarefaction and structural breakdown of bone are the expected findings.

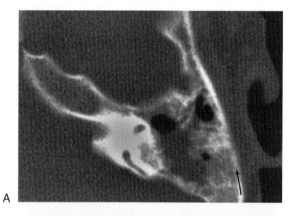

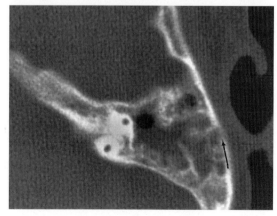

FIG. 9. A,B: Sequential axial computed tomographic scan projection in acute mastoiditis. Note diffuse rarefaction of bone and breakdown of cellular septae. *Arrow* indicates periostitis with area of impending cortical breakdown.

CT scanning has value in the evaluation of those cases of acute mastoiditis where the typical picture has been obscured or modified by antibiotic therapy (Fig. 9). Since the advent of wide spectrum antibiotics, this form of masked mastoiditis is seen with increasing frequency and must be considered in all cases of unresolved otitis media (19).

Medical Management

From a therapeutic standpoint acute mastoiditis has two distinct phases: (a) osteitic and (b) coalescent. During the osteitic phase, the infection has yet to progress to the formation of an abscess and may be treated conservatively with intravenous antibiotics and immediate myringotomy. The latter should be performed in all cases where aural drainage is absent or impaired and may, on occasion, need to be repeated.

Cultures taken at presentation or at myringotomy are of paramount importance in the management of acute mastoiditis. Intravenous antibiotics should be started promptly and aimed at the control of the most commonly found bacteria. Therapy should be modified according to culture and sensitivity results. *S. pyogenes* and *S. pneumoniae* must be covered initially and, despite its relatively low incidence, *H. influenzae* should be considered in the initial therapeutic plan. Therefore, a good single drug initial plan should include a second-generation cephalosporin or (provided no allergy exists) one of the augmented penicillins that also can be useful against *P. aeruginosa*.

Intravenous antibiotic therapy should be maintained for at least 24 to 48 hours after the resolution of symptoms, and then followed with oral antibiotics for 2 weeks on an outpatient basis, with frequent reexaminations including audiometry.

Surgical Management

Approximately two thirds of all cases of acute mastoiditis presenting in the osteitic phase respond to medical therapy and myringotomy, showing signs of improvement within the first 48 to 72 hours of treatment. In patients with persistent purulent drainage, otalgia, and fever, surgery should be considered. CT scan of the temporal bones is of value in cases where the evolution of mastoiditis is unclear.

Patients with subperiosteal abscesses have entered the coalescent phase of mastoiditis and are considered surgical candidates. It often is practical to incise the subperiosteal abscess at presentation to decompress its contents. This step frequently results in abatement of the more acute local and systemic changes and subsequently permits a more controlled surgical procedure (20). The following are signs that, alone or in combination, indicate the advisability of mastoid surgery: (a) CT changes documenting destruction of bony cell walls; (b) persistent fever, leukocytosis, and systemic symptoms; (c) progressive sagging of the posterosuperior wall of the external auditory canal; and (d) subperiosteal abscess.

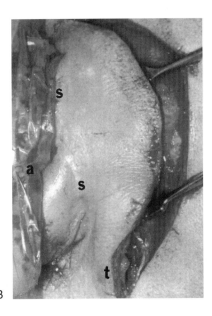 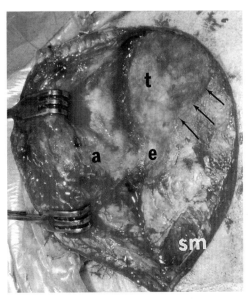

A,B

FIG. 10. A: The postauricular incision is placed away from the sulcus (*S*) in cases where exposure of the sigmoid and retrosigmoid sinus air cells is needed. *a*, auricle folded anteriorly; *t*, mastoid tip. B: Flap elevation and anterior auricular displacement demonstrating wide exposure of the mastoid cortex and surrounding areas. *Arrows* indicate the temporal line. *a*, auricle; *e*, external ear canal; *sm*, insertion of the sternocleidomastoid muscle at the mastoid tip; *t*, temporalis muscle.

Selected subperiosteal abscesses presenting in children without previous history of ear disease and responding rapidly to incision, drainage, and antibiotic therapy may be treated without mastoidectomy. This conservative attitude is safe in the hands of experienced ear surgeons and predicated on complete clinical resolution with CT scanning demonstrating re-aeration of the middle ear and mastoid. Because cholesteatoma may present as acute mastoiditis, prolonged follow-up and optimal patient compliance are essential.

TECHNIQUE OF SIMPLE MASTOIDECTOMY

The objectives of mastoidectomy in acute mastoiditis are removal of infected soft tissue and bone, restoration of tubotympanic-mastoid continuity, and prevention of serious complications. These goals often can be achieved with a simple cortical mastoidectomy and antrostomy, without undertaking all the steps herein described.

The operation is preferably done through a postauricular incision placed approximately 2 cm away from the postauricular sulcus to allow easy exposure of the mastoid cortex and surrounding areas (Fig. 10). The postauricular incision needs to be modified in children 2 years of age or younger, because the lack of mastoid tip development leaves the trunk of the facial nerve unprotected. Therefore, the incision is done so that it slants obliquely in a posterior, rather than inferior, direction (Fig. 11).

The mastoid cortex is exposed, taking care to identify the zygomatic root, insertion of the sternocleidomastoid muscle, spine of Henle, cribriform area, and posterosuperior margins of the bony external canal. The posterior canal skin and tympanic membrane are left undisturbed. The periosteum overlying the mastoid, when identifiable, is divided as a T, with the upper bar paralleling the temporal line inferior to the insertion of the temporalis muscle and extending into the root of the zygoma. The periosteum is

elevated and folded anteriorly and posteriorly. The cortex is opened with cutting burrs of variable sizes, and Koerner's septum is removed to open the antrum (Fig. 12). Special care must be taken to open the aditus ad antrum, as this area often is blocked by edematous mucosa and granulation tissue. Usually the procedure for drainage in acute mastoiditis is terminated at this point. The following technical steps pertain to a complete "canal-wall-up" mastoidectomy. The lateral semicircular canal is identified. The tegmen mastoideum and the sigmoid sinus plate are skeletonized and the sinodural angle developed. The attic

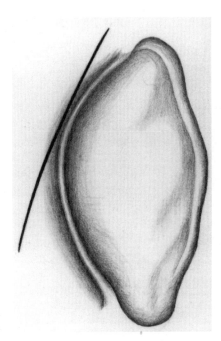

FIG. 11. Modification of the postauricular incision in infants and young children (left ear). Posterior slanting prevents dissection in the region of the unprotected trunk of the facial nerve.

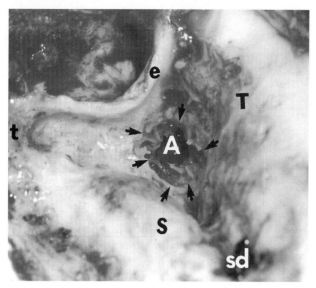

FIG. 12. Intraoperative photograph (right ear) in canal-wall-up mastoidectomy. *e,* posterior wall of the external ear canal; *s,* sigmoid sinus; *sd,* sinodural angle; *t,* mastoid tip; *T,* mastoid tegmen. The antrum (*A*) has been opened. *Arrowheads* indicate limits of Koerner's septum. In most cases of acute mastoiditis, this dissection level suffices for drainage and control of the acute process.

is entered, exposing the incus. Care is taken to remove all infected tissue and to exenterate, or open, all involved air cells. This may require inclusion of those of the mastoid tip, and perifacial and retrofacial systems (Fig. 13).

It bears reemphasizing at this point that meticulous exenteration of air cells, as described, *is not always possible or indicated* in acute mastoiditis. When the infection is severe and the tissues profusely hemorrhagic, it is best to establish drainage of the antrum and cortical air system

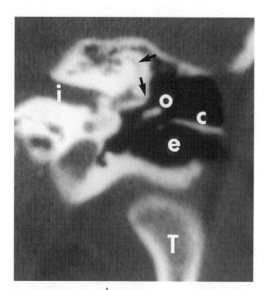

FIG. 13. Computed tomographic scan (coronal projection) following complete canal-wall-up mastoidectomy. *c,* canal wall; *e,* external canal; *i,* internal auditory canal; *o,* ossicles; *T,* mandibular condyle. *Arrows* point to superior and lateral semicircular canals. Note excellent aeration of the mastoid cavity and middle ear.

and consider a secondary procedure if the process does not resolve completely.

Following exenteration of involved cell groups, the incision is closed loosely. The mastoid cavity is not packed. A Penrose drain or soft silicone rubber tube is placed in the antrum for drainage. If the tympanic membrane is intact, myringotomy and placement of a pressure equalization tube usually are indicated.

Postoperative care includes maintenance of antibiotic therapy and repeated cultures. Antibiotic therapy should be continued until there is no drainage from the middle ear and the patient is asymptomatic.

Follow-up audiologic studies are important. Failure to normalize a conductive hearing loss is an indication of continued mucositis or ossicular disease. The ear then must be examined at monthly intervals for a period of 6 months. The patient should be discharged from care only when there is a healed tympanic membrane, return of normal hearing, and resolution of all symptoms.

TEMPORAL BONE FUNGAL INFECTION

Although *P. aeruginosa* is responsible for more than 98% of cases of necrotizing otitis externa, fungal infections occasionally can spread beyond the confines of the external auditory canal and involve the middle ear, mastoid, and skull base. Aspergillus species have been the most commonly identified invasive fungi (ten case reports) (21–29). Mucor, cryptococcus, and candida also have been reported to involve the temporal bone, and specifically the middle ear and inner ears (30–33). These fungi are more likely to have spread from the nasopharynx and eustachian tube (usually secondary to sinonasal involvement), from a primary infection in the middle ear, or from the meninges, rather than from an external auditory canal infection, which is typical for the aspergillus cases. A menogenic route of spread has been postulated in one case of a candida labyrinthitis (30).

Fungi, *Staphylococcus epidermidis,* and diphtheroids often can be cultured as normal external ear canal flora. Aspergillus species are ubiquitous in nature, occurring in the soil and especially in decaying organic material. Candida species and *Aspergillus niger* are common fungi producing routine otitis externa. There are no reports of these pathogens becoming invasive and causing otitis media, mastoiditis, or skull base osteomyelitis. Two aspergillus species, *A. fumigatus* and *A. flavus,* however, are capable of aggressive infection. Several factors predispose to aspergillus becoming invasive (24,25). Most important is a breakdown of the host's immunologic defenses by an underlying systemic disease and/or by the administration of cytotoxic drugs. Prior administration of broad spectrum antibiotics also may promote fungal growth. A local point of entry, such as a traumatized external auditory canal or a perforated tympanic membrane, then initiates the deeper tissue infection.

Necrotizing otitis externa secondary to aspergillus may be difficult to diagnose initially for several reasons.

First, the clinical picture resembles a bacterial infection: persistent ear pain, otorrhea, and canal edema despite local care and application of otic drops; possible cranial nerve involvement (especially cranial nerve VII); and an immunocompromised state. Second, the external auditory canal culture may fail to reveal aspergillus; a deep tissue biopsy often is necessary. Alternatively, the culture may reveal several pathogens, including bacteria and aspergillus. In this setting, the fungus may be misinterpreted as simply an opportunistic colonization. Last, the radiographic findings, including CT, MRI, gallium, and technetium 99m scans are nondiagnostic. Most of the reported cases of aspergillus skull base osteomyelitis were initially misdiagnosed as a pseudomonas infection.

Several findings may be helpful in suggesting the correct diagnosis. First, in the patients with invasive aspergillus of the temporal bone, the immunocompromised state most commonly was caused by neutropenia secondary to a myeloproliferative disease (or secondary to the chemotherapy for the disease). Consistent with this observation is a report on invasive aspergillosis from the National Cancer Institute, which found that almost 90% of affected patients had a hematologic or lymphoreticular disease (25). Diabetes was the risk factor for several patients with skull base osteomyelitis secondary to aspergillus, but it does not appear to play as dominant a role as it does in patients with pseudomonas osteomyelitis. Second, a facial paralysis was present in more than 80% of the reported cases, a percentage that is higher than that reported for bacterial skull base osteomyelitis. Last, a culture of *A. flavus* or *A. fungatus* should be considered a true pathogen and not a superimposed infection.

To summarize, it would appear appropriate to initiate antipseudomonal therapy in suspected invasive otitis externa/skull base osteomyelitis while awaiting culture results. The patient's clinical response and the radiographic findings (especially sequential MRI and gallium scans) are followed. Failure to culture *P. aeruginosa* or a poor response to medical therapy should prompt surgical intervention to remove tissue from the external auditory canal and/or mastoid for diagnostic purposes. Surgical specimens are submitted for culture and histology. Identification of septate hyphae with dichotomous branching suggests aspergillus. Histologic examination is important to rule out an underlying malignant process. The early culture of *A. flavus* or *A. fungatus* from an external canal exudate should prompt immediate surgical biopsy, before assessing the response to antipseudomonal therapy. Treatment for fungal osteomyelitis consists of intravenous amphotericin B. A review of the cases reported suggests that a total dose of 2 to 3 g administered over many weeks to months was successful in resolving the osteomyelitis in most cases, although recovery of any cranial nerve deficit was unusual. Nephrotoxicity is the major concern with amphotericin B, and serum creatinine and blood urea nitrogen levels must be monitored closely. As with pseudomonas skull base osteomyelitis, surgical debridement of devitalized tissue may be necessary.

SUMMARY POINTS

- AOM is principally a disease of childhood, with two thirds of children by age 4 experiencing at least one episode.
- Although viral, upper respiratory infections are a frequent precursor to AOM, the middle infection is bacterial. The most common pathogens are *S. pneumoniae*, *H. influenzae*, *M. catarrhalis*, and group A streptococci.
- The bacterial pathogens causing AOM differ for neonates versus older children. In children under several months of age, gram-negative enteric organisms and *S. aureus* predominate.
- Once a diagnosis of AOM is confirmed otoscopically, treatment is begun with antibiotics directed against the anticipated bacterial pathogens. Obtaining material for cultures is only necessary in patients exhibiting a complication, the neonate, or the patient not responding to initial antibiotic therapy.
- Myringotomy should be considered in patients with severe otalgia or when cultures are desired. Evacuation of middle ear pathogens is essential in patients exhibiting a complication such as labyrinthitis, facial paralysis, or central nervous system involvement.
- ABM is characterized by the appearance of one or more vesicles on the tympanic membrane. The etiology is undetermined and rapid resolution is anticipated. Treatment is symptomatic, directed primarily at pain control.
- Acute mastoiditis is characterized by osteitis with breakdown of the air cell septae and filling of the mastoid space with products of the infection. A subperiosteal abscess occurs as the infection erodes through the mastoid cortex.
- The most common pathogen cultured from acute mastoiditis is *S. pyogenes*. Bacteria common to AOM, gram-negative enteric bacilli, and various anaerobic species also can be etiologic agents.
- Early in the evolution of acute mastoiditis, intravenous antibiotics and myringotomy may resolve the process. More frequently, the addition of a simple mastoidectomy is necessary to drain the infection.
- Fungi, including *A. fumigatus* and *A. flavus*, mucor, cryptococcus, and candida, can involve the middle ear, mastoid, and skull base. Usually these infections occur in an immunocompromised patient (e.g., those with diabetes, neutropenia secondary to chemotherapy, or a myeloproliferative disease).

REFERENCES

1. Ingvarsson L, Lundgren K, Olofsson B. Epidemiology of acute otitis media in children—a cohort study in an urban population. In: Lim AL, Bluestone CD, Klein JO, Nelson JD, eds. *Recent advances in otitis media with effusion.* Philadelphia: BC Decker, 1984:19–22.

2. Ingvarsson L, Lundgren K, Stenstrom C. Occurrence of acute otitis media in children: cohort studies in an urban population. *Ann Otol Rhinol Laryngol Suppl* 1990;149:17–18.

3. Pukander J, Karma P, Sipila M. Occurrence and recurrence of acute otitis media among children. *Acta Otolaryngol (Stockh)* 1982;94:479–486.

4. Pukander J, Sipila M, Kataja M, Karma P. Estimating the risk of acute otitis media among urban children. *Ann Otol Rhinol Laryngol Suppl* 1990;149:18–20.

5. Henderson FW, Collier AM, Sanyal JA, et al. A longitudinal study of respiratory viruses and bacteria in the etiology of acute otitis media with effusion. *N Engl J Med* 1982;306:1377–1383.

6. Sarkinen H, Ruuskaneno, Meorman O, et al. Identification of respiratory virus antigens in middle ear fluids of children with acute otitis media. *J Infect Dis* 1985;151:444–448.

7. McCabe W. The correlation of in vitro tests with the outcome of antimicrobial therapy for otitis media. *Pediatr Ann* 1984;13:365–368.

8. Shurin PA, Marchant CA, Kim CH. Emergence of beta-lactamase-producing strains of Branhamella catarrhalis as important agents of acute otitis media. *Pediatr Infect Dis* 1983;2:34–38.

9. Wright PF. Indication and duration of antimicrobial agents for acute otitis media. *Pediatr Ann* 1984;13:377–379.

10. Diamant U, Diamant B. Abuse and timing of use of antibiotics in acute otitis media. *Arch Otolaryngol* 1974;100:226–232.

11. Gates GA. The role of myringotomy in acute otitis media. *Pediatr Ann* 1984;13:391–397.

12. Wetmore SJ, Abramson M. Bullous myringitis with sensorineural hearing loss. *Otolaryngol Head Neck Surg* 1979;87:66–70.

13. Chanock RM, Rifkind D, Kravetz HM, et al. Respiratory disease in volunteers infected with Eton agent: a preliminary report. *Proc Natl Acad Sci U S A* 1961;47:887–890.

14. Rifkind A, Chanock RM, Kravetz HM, et al. Ear involvement (myringitis) and primary atypical pneumonia following inoculation of volunteers with Eton agent. *Am Rev Respir Dis* 1962;85:479–489.

15. Merifield DO, Miller GS. The etiology and clinical course of bullous myringitis. *Arch Otolaryngol* 1966;84:487–489.

16. Hawkins DB, Dru D, House JW, Clark RW. Acute mastoiditis in children: a review of 54 cases. *Laryngoscope* 1983;93:568–572.

17. Rosen A, Ophir A, Marshak G. Acute mastoiditis: a review of 69 cases. *Ann Otol Rhinol Laryngol* 1986;95:222–224.

18. Rubin JS, Wei WL. Acute mastoiditis: review of 34 patients. *Laryngoscope* 1985;95:963–965.

19. Holt RG, Gates GA. Masked mastoiditis. *Laryngoscope* 1983;93:1034–1037.

20. Hawkins DB, Dru A. Mastoid subperiosteal abscess. *Arch Otolaryngol* 1983;109:369–371.

21. Cunningham M, Yu VL, Turner, J, Curtin H. Necrotizing otitis externa due to Aspergillus in an immunocompetent patient. *Arch Otolaryngol Head Neck Surg* 1998;114:554–556.

22. Petrak RM, Pottage J, Levin S. Invasive external otitis caused by Aspergillus fumigatus in an immunocompromised patient. *J Infect Dis* 1985;151:196.

23. Stanley RJ, McCaffrey TV, Weiland LH. Fungal mastoiditis in the immunocompromised host. *Arch Otolaryngol Head Neck Surg* 1988;114:198–199.

24. Menachof MR, Jackler RK. Otogenic skull base osteomyelitis caused by invasive fungal infection. *Otolaryngol Head Neck Surg* 1990;102:285–289.

25. Bickley LS, Betts RF, Parkins CW. Atypical invasive external otitis from aspergillus. *Arch Otolaryngol Head Neck Surg* 1988;114:1024–1028.

26. Phillips P, Bryce G, Shepard J, Mintz D. Invasive external otitis caused by aspergillus. *Rev Infect Dis* 1990;12:277–281.

27. Strauss M, Fine E. Aspergillus otomastoiditis in acquired immunodeficiency syndrome. *Am J Otol* 1991;12:29–53.

28. Hanna E, Hughes G, Eliachar I, et al. Fungal osteomyelitis of the temporal bone: a review of reported cases. *Ear Nose Throat J* 1993;72:532–541.

29. Kountakis SE, Kemper JV, Chang CYJ, DiMaio DJM, Stiernberg CM. Osteomyelitis of the base of the skull secondary to aspergillus. *Am J Otol* 1997;18:19–22.

30. Meyerhoff WL, Paparella MM, Oda M, Shea D. Mycotic infections of the inner ear. *Laryngoscope* 1979;89:1725–1734.

31. Bergstrom L, Hemenway WG, Barnhart RA. Rhinocerebral and otologic mucormycosis. *Ann Otol Rhinol Laryngol* 1970;79:70–81.

32. Gussen R, Canalis RL. Mucormycosis of the temporal bone. *Ann Otol* 1982;91:27–32.

33. Yun MW-D, Lui C-C, Chen W-J. Facial paralysis secondary to tympanic mucormycosis: case report. *Am J Otol* 1994;15:413–414.

The Ear: Comprehensive Otology,
edited by R. F. Canalis and P. R. Lambert.
Lippincott Williams & Wilkins, Philadelphia © 2000.

CHAPTER **25**

Chronic Otitis Media and Cholesteatoma

Rinaldo F. Canalis and Paul R. Lambert

CHRONIC OTITIS MEDIA

Definition

Chronic otitis media (COM) is an unresolved inflammatory process of the middle ear and mastoid. The disease nearly always is associated with a tympanic membrane perforation and may be active when infection and otorrhea are present, or quiescent when they are absent. The length of active and quiescent periods varies from patient to patient. Individuals prone to upper respiratory infections and allergies tend to experience more frequent and lengthier episodes of active disease.

Etiology

Although the source of ongoing debate, COM is believed to usually result from an unresolved middle ear effusion that may be purulent, serous, or mucoid in nature.

R. F. Canalis: Department of Surgery, University of California, Los Angeles, School of Medicine, Los Angeles, California 90095-1624

P. R. Lambert: Department of Otolaryngology–Head and Neck Surgery, University of Virginia Health Sciences Center, Charlottesville, Virginia 22908-0430

The basis for this hypothesis, advanced 2 decades ago by John et al. (1), rests on the careful scrutiny of many temporal bone specimens and a vast multiinstitutional clinical experience. This evidence suggests that an initially uncomplicated inflammatory process of the middle ear may evolve over time to produce persistent effusion and irreversible mucosal changes (2–8). Additional evidence suggests that chronic middle ear fluid contains enzymes capable of altering the mucosal lining of the middle ear (9,10), including the lateral surface of the tympanic membrane and its fibrous layer (11). This structure is altered further by the direct action of invading pathogens that produce a chronic inflammatory response predominantly affecting the pars flaccida and the annular and manubrial regions of the pars tensa (12,13). Repeated insults will then diffusely or segmentally weaken the tympanic membrane, rendering it susceptible to collapse or chronic perforation (see following, Pathogenesis of Cholesteatoma).

In addition to the middle ear cleft, the mastoid air cells experience similar changes that lead to persistent fluid accumulation. Mucosal edema and polypoid degeneration (see following) produce partial or complete obliteration of air cells. These changes are especially important as they involve the antrum. Obstruction of the narrow communication between the antrum and the attic, the aditus, results in a condition termed *aditus block*, which prevents aeration of the mastoid and resolution of the infection (14).

Bacteriology

The bacteriology of active COM is different from that of acute otitis media. Most current studies show *Pseudomonas aeruginosa* as the prevalent etiologic agent in COM, with an incidence of 40% to 65%; *Staphylococcus aureus* follows, with a 10% to 20% prevalence (15–17). Other aerobic bacteria found in pure or associated forms are *Escherichia coli,* proteus, and *S. epidermidis.* Among anaerobic agents, *Bacteroides,* especially *B. melaninogenicus* and *B. fragilis,* predominate in the gram-negative bacilli group. Peptostreptococcus is prevalent among aerobic gram-positive cocci (16,17). The incidence of (aerobic and anaerobic) β-lactamase–producing bacteria has been estimated to be as high as 70% (18). Occasionally, local and systemic mycosis may complicate the bacteriologic picture of the disease. *Mycobacterium tuberculosis* and nontuberculous mycobacteria are rare causes of COM (see following).

Pathology

The temporal bone changes of COM are similar in ears with or without tympanic membrane perforations (19). During the active phase, the middle ear mucosa exhibits an extensive infiltrate of acute and chronic reparative cells. Lymphocytes and plasma cells predominate. Intraepithelial bacteria occasionally are found. Chronic edema often results in pronounced polypoid changes, with marked proliferation of brittle new capillaries and the development of granulation tissue (Fig. 1) (7). Sade (4) has shown that, in chronic inflammation, the middle ear mucosa is lined by secretory epithelium forming glandlike structures (Fig. 2). This change is irreversible and widespread (Figs. 3 and 4), and is responsible for the persistence of mucoid or mucopurulent secretions. In addition, surface breakdown can produce various degrees of ulceration and exposure of the underlying bony capsule, which may result in areas of chronic osteitis and periostitis (Fig. 5) (20). Repeated infections followed by quiescent reparative periods lead to the formation of fibrous bands that extend from the undersurface of the tympanic membrane to the promontory. Similar adhesions and scars of variable thickness also occur in the epitympanum and around the ossicles (21). The tympanic membrane undergoes a variety of changes, resulting in chronic perforation or diffuse loss of the collagenous layer, in turn producing its collapse against the medial wall of the middle ear cleft (Fig. 6) (22). This sequela is termed *adhesive otitis media* and is associated with total impairment of eustachian tube function (23).

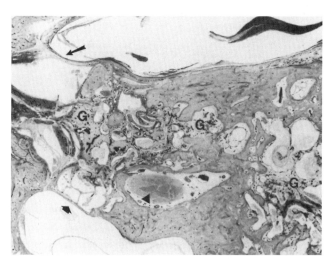

FIG. 1. Granulation tissue. Intact tympanic membrane (*arrow*). Active granulation tissue (*G*) fills the posterior middle ear and mastoid (original magnification × 10). *Arrowhead* indicates stapes footplate; *triangle* indicates facial nerve. (From daCosta SS, Paparella MM, Schachern PA, Yoon TH, Kimberly BP. Temporal bone histopathology in chronic infected ears with intact and perforated tympanic membranes. *Laryngoscope* 1992;102:1229–1236, with permission.)

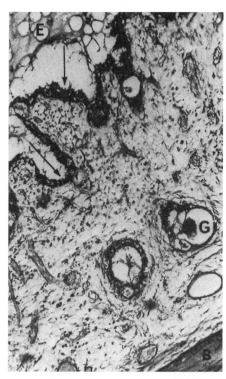

FIG. 2. Temporal bone histologic section from a patient with chronic otitis media showing thick submucosa with glands (*G*) in it. The mucosa is hyperplastic (*arrows*), and there is mucous in the middle ear (*E*). *B*, bone. (From Sade J. The biopathology of secretory otitis media. *Ann Otol Rhinol Laryngol* 1974;83[Suppl 11]:59–70, with permission.)

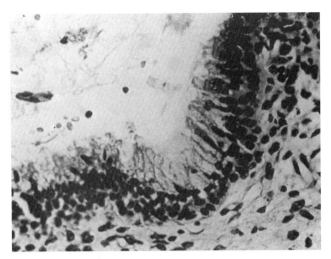

FIG. 3. Glue ear: biopsy from the middle ear. Note pseudo-stratified secretory columnar epithelium.

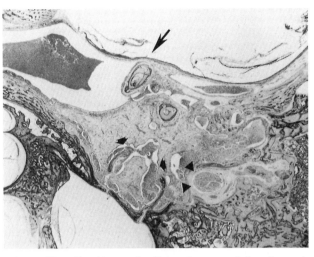

FIG. 5. Chronic otitis media. Extensive granulation tissue is seen behind an intact tympanic membrane (*arrow*) (original magnification × 10). Also note severe osteitic changes to the otic capsule including the facial canal (*triangles*) and oval window. The stapes suprastructure is partially destroyed (*arrowheads*). (From Paparella MM, Kimberly BP, Alleva M. The concept of silent otitis media: its importance and implications. *Otolaryngol Clin North Am* 1991;24:763–774, with permission.)

Hyalinization or *tympanosclerosis* appears to be a healing response occurring during the evolution of otitis media and mastoiditis. Characteristically, it occurs during quiescent periods and results in the formation of tympanic membrane plaques and amorphous middle ear masses that may envelop the entire ossicular chain. These lesions are formed by fused collagenous fibers, which are hardened by the deposition of calcium and phosphate crystals (Fig. 7). Tympanic membrane plaques often are thin and do not produce functional impairment. Conductive hearing loss usually is associated with masses restricting ossicular mobility. On occasion, aggressive hyalinization envelopes an ossicle, most frequently the stapes (Fig. 8) (24–26).

Ossicular erosion is frequent in COM. It may be due to the infectious process per se or to necrosis following vascular thrombosis. It most commonly affects the lenticular

process of the incus and/or the head of the stapes (Fig. 9), which often is replaced by fibrous tissue. In addition, the ossicles may be subject to periostitis and osteitis followed by osteoclastic changes, decalcification, and matrix loss (Fig. 5). Bone changes are prominent in the mastoid and are characterized by both destruction and repair (20). Initially breakdown predominates, but as the disease progresses reparative changes take over. Increased osteoneo-

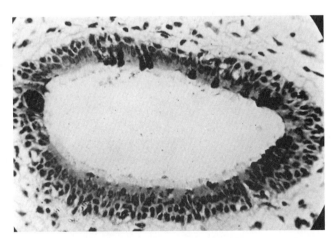

FIG. 4. Mastoid cell lined by ciliated columnar epithelium containing goblet cells in chronic mastoiditis (original magnification × 144). (From Friedmann I. *Pathology of the ear.* Oxford, UK: Blackwell Scientific Publications, 1974:81, with permission.)

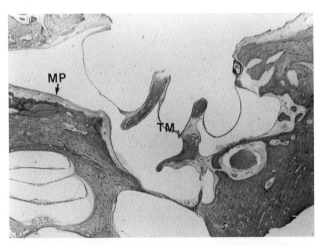

FIG. 6. Silent otitis media and atelectasis. Note a thin collapsed tympanic membrane (*TM*) draping over the ossicles. The mucoperiosteum (*MP*) is thickened (original magnification × 10). (From Paparella MM, Kimberly BP, Alleva M. The concept of silent otitis media: its importance and implications. *Otolaryngol Clin North Am* 1991;24:763–774, with permission.)

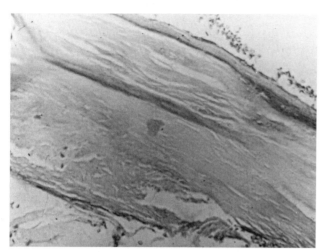

FIG. 7. Middle ear tympanosclerosis (fibrosis and hyalinized collagen) (hematoxylin and eosin, original magnification × 60). (From Goodhill V, ed. *Ear diseases, deafness and dizziness.* Hagerstown, MD: Harper and Row Publishers, 1979: 336, with permission.)

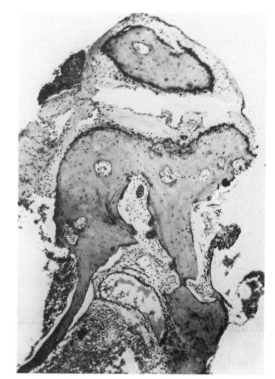

FIG. 9. Head of the stapes completely destroyed by inflammatory granulation tissue. The intercrural space is filled with inflammatory exudate containing many foam cells. The thickened mucosa is lined by columnar cells in places (original magnification × 100). (From Friedmann I. *Pathology of the ear.* Oxford, UK: Blackwell Scientific Publications, 1974:65, with permission.)

genesis following destructive episodes eventually leads to the formation of sclerotic bone. This abnormal bone lacks haversian canals and shows multiple lines of apposition in a glacierlike pattern with markedly irregular cement lines that give the area the appearance of a mosaic (Fig. 10). These changes are responsible for the narrow, dense mastoids often encountered in the course of surgery for chronic ear disease. Ossification may become extreme, occupying every free space of the temporal bone except the labyrinth.

Ossification of the labyrinth or *labyrinthitis ossificans* is an uncommon process characterized by often extensive bone formation within the spaces of the membranous labyrinth, and deafness (Fig. 11). Labyrinthitis ossificans

is usually a sequela of suppurative meningitis. Bacteria reach the inner ear by way of the internal auditory canal and cochlear aqueduct, producing widespread destruction of the membranous labyrinth (27,28). Ossification is preceded by a fibroblastic stage occurring 2 to 3 weeks after

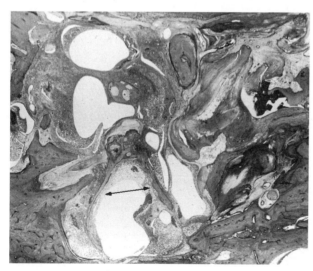

FIG. 8. Severe tympanosclerosis involving the stapes. *Arrow* indicates crura.

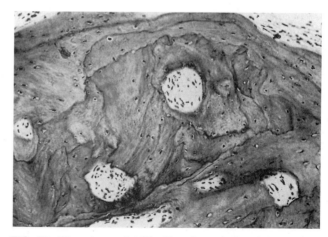

FIG. 10. Chronic mastoiditis. Note irregularity of the cement lines forming a mosaic pattern (sclerotic bone) (original magnification × 184). (From Friedmann I. *Pathology of the ear.* Oxford, UK: Blackwell Scientific Publications, 1974:62, with permission.)

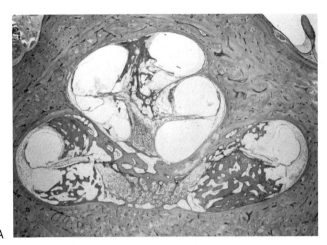 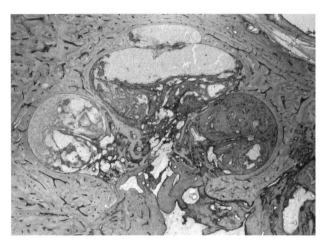

A   B

FIG. 11. Labyrinthitis ossificans. Midmodiolar section left temporal bone (hematoxylin and eosin, original magnification × 10). **A:** Mild ossification (involving primarily the scala tympani and scala vestibuli of basal turn). **B:** Severe ossification.

the acute purulent phase (29). The source of new bone formation is unknown, but it may develop from fibrous tissue (metaplastic type) and/or from the denuded otic capsule (osteoplastic type). The basal turn of the cochlea tends to be involved first, and the extent of bone formation seems to depend on the infecting organism. Pneumococcal infection results in the most extreme degree of ossification. Meningococcus also produces ossification, but *Haemophilus influenzae* usually fails to induce it (30). Brodie et al. (31) recently showed, in Mongolian gerbils, osteogenesis following intralabyrinthine injection of the polysaccharide capsule antigens of *Streptococcus pneumoniae*. These authors also demonstrated labyrinthine osteoneogenesis in a group of animals receiving two intrathecal injections of *S. pneumoniae* organisms. These findings suggest that the propensity of pneumococcus to induce labyrinthine bone formation may be related to the immunologic characteristics of its polysaccharide capsule.

Another frequent surgical finding in COM is the presence of yellowish masses surrounded by granulation tissue, edematous mucosa, and fibrous tissue. These lesions, originally termed *cholesterol granulomas* (CG) by Friedmann (32), tend to occur in clusters scattered throughout the mastoid and less frequently in the middle ear. They usually are surrounded by a brownish exudate suggestive of recent focal hemorrhage. Diffuse, extensive involvement of temporal bone spaces may occur, but it is rare. Cholesterol granulomas do not represent a specific entity, but are part of the general pathology of COM. Microscopically, they consist of granulation tissue containing many cholesterol crystals and foreign body giant cells (Fig. 12). A fibrous background is present. The pathogenesis of cholesterol granulomas is not entirely understood, but it appears that focal hemorrhage plays a significant role in its production. Breakdown of extravasated blood resulting in clustering of cholesterol crystals most likely

triggers a severe inflammatory reaction followed by the proliferation of foreign body giant cells (32–34).

Evidence of focal hemorrhage as the inciting event in cholesterol granuloma formation may be encountered in *idiopathic hemotympanum* or *"blue drum."* The pathogenesis of this entity also is unclear, but some of its pathologic changes resemble those seen in COM, including effusion, proliferation of granulation tissue, mucosal glandular

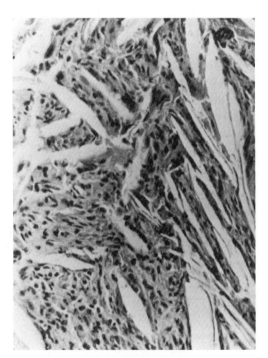

FIG. 12. Cholesterol granuloma exhibiting the characteristic clefts of the lesion (hematoxylin and eosin, original magnification × 90). (From Goodhill V, ed: *Ear diseases, deafness and dizziness.* Hagerstown, MD: Harper and Row Publishers, 1979:332, with permission.)

changes, and frequently cholesterol granulomas (35). Sheehey and Linthicum (36) have proposed that idiopathic hemotympanum results from negative middle ear pressure producing intercellular fluid exudation, capillary rupture, and hemorrhage. Breakdown of extravasated blood with the resulting accumulation of cholesterol crystals then will result in the described changes.

Additional support for this theory is found in the common observation, during mastoid revision operations, of areas of granuloma formation in direct proximity to hemorrhage and necrotic tissue resulting from surgical trauma. These areas often trap decaying blood products, such as cholesterol crystals, and produce a reaction identical to the one described. These *necrobiotic granulomas* (Fig. 13) are not limited to the temporal bone and can be seen in joint spaces and elsewhere in the body following surgery.

Sensorineural Hearing Loss

Despite a number of clinical and histologic studies on the relationship between COM and sensorineural hearing loss (SNHL), questions persist. The majority of studies have concluded that COM is associated with some degree of SNHL and that elements of COM (e.g., bacterial toxins) are the causative agents. Differences exist regarding the severity of the SNHL and whether there is a correlation between the severity of the SNHL and related COM parameters such as middle ear mucosal status, presence of cholesteatoma, duration of disease, etc. Paparella et al. (37–41) have repeatedly discussed the significance of SNHL in COM, reporting absolute bone conduction losses between 18 and 33 dB across the frequency range (500 through 4,000 Hz). Others have found the SNHL with COM to be smaller, ranging from 5.6 to 12.8 dB across speech frequencies (42).

Recently, Noordzij et al. (43) reported a study of 69 patients, aged 4 to 46 years (mean 22), who met the following selection criteria: unilateral COM and no history of head trauma, meningitis, posttraumatic tympanic membrane perforation, labyrinthine fistula, noise exposure, previous ear surgery involving bone drilling, stapes fixation at the time of surgery, or systemic disease that might affect hearing. The contralateral ear served as a control, as it eliminated other etiologies such as hereditary or congenital SNHL, noise, and presbycusis. The threshold differences (diseased ear minus control ear) ranged from 0.5 to +4.4 dB across frequencies, with the differences being statistically significant at 2,000 and 4,000 Hz. In these results, greater SNHL occurred at the higher frequencies. This observation correlates with histopathologic findings by Paparella (38) and Walby et al. (44), who showed that human temporal bones with premortem otitis media had serofibrinous precipitates and inflammatory cells mainly localized in the scala tympani near the round window. More recently, Lundman, et al. (45) showed that *P. aeruginosa* exotoxin A can cross the round window membrane of chinchillas and cause irreversible loss of cochlear hair cells, primarily in the basal turn. It must be noted, though, that little is known about the occurrence and importance of this and other exotoxins in human COM.

History and Physical Findings

Intermittent, often malodorous, otorrhea and hearing loss are the two most common complaints in COM. Otalgia is not common, except during acute exacerbations. Persistent otalgia, especially when associated with headache, suggests central nervous system involvement (e.g., epidural or brain abscess). Vertigo is unusual; when present, it should raise the suspicion of labyrinthitis or labyrinthine fistula.

Most patients relate a history of multiple earaches during childhood, followed by bilateral ear problems with or without asymptomatic periods. Some patients may have had a middle ear and mastoid operation, with reactivation of aural discharge following accidental contamination by water while bathing or swimming.

Otoscopic findings vary greatly. Although the examination often begins with the hand-held otoscope, the surgical microscope is recommended for atraumatic manipulation and accuracy of findings. The external canal should be inspected for inflammatory changes, fistulas, and crusts. Aspiration of mucoid and/or purulent secretions from tympanic membrane perforations may provoke vertigo. Occasionally, spontaneous nystagmus will follow instrumentation, suggesting a possible labyrinthine fistula.

A defect in the pars tensa of the tympanic membrane, or of the pars flaccida, or both, is present in most cases (Fig. 14: see color plate 13 following page 484). Atelectatic lesions are seen in the pars tensa, but they are more common in the pars flaccida. The entire membrane may be absent (Fig. 15: see color plate 14 follow-

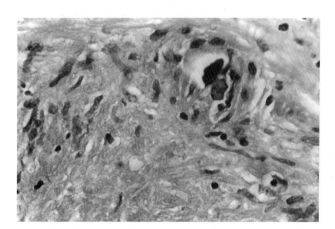

FIG. 13. Necrobiotic granuloma from mastoidectomy specimen (hematoxylin and eosin, original magnification × 60).

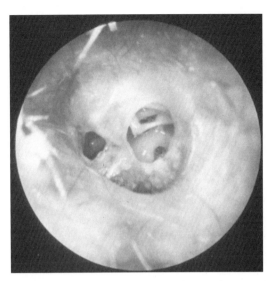

FIG. 14. Anterior and posterior tympanic membrane perforations (left ear). Note the incudostapedial joint, stapes, facial nerve, and round window. (Courtesy of Dr. Armando Lenis.)

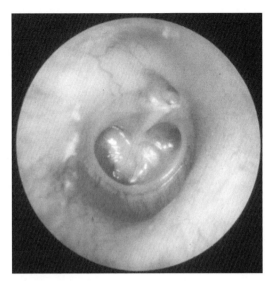

FIG. 16. Severe atelectasis of monomeric tympanic membrane (end-stage adhesive otitis media) of the right ear. (Courtesy of Dr. Armando Lenis.)

ing page 484), or it may appear to be absent because of severe atelectasis and adherence to the medial tympanic wall (Fig. 16: see color plate 15 following page 484). Squamous epithelial invasion may continue from the external auditory canal into the middle ear and fuse with the ossicles or the promontory (Figs. 17 and 18: see color plates 16 and 17 following page 484). In some cases, ossicular lesions (Fig. 19: see color plate 18 following page 484), granulomas, polyps (Figs. 20 and 21: see color plates 19 and 20 following page 484), tympanosclerotic plaques, and middle ear effusion (Fig. 22: see color plate 21 following page 484) are visible.

Occasionally, the tympanic membrane may be intact and vary from edematous to relatively normal in appearance. However, its normal translucency usually is lost, as is its mobility on pneumatic otoscopy. Tuning fork tests will be consistent with a conductive hearing loss, although a sensorineural component may predominate in advanced disease.

Results of head and neck examination frequently are normal in patients with COM. Infected tonsils and adenoids, paranasal sinusitis, nasal polyposis, cervical lymphadenopathy, and other manifestations of recurrent upper respiratory disease may be present.

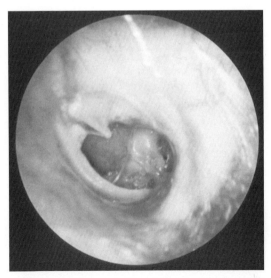

FIG. 15. Near-total perforation of the pars tensa (left ear). Note medial displacement of the malleus. (Courtesy of Dr. Armando Lenis.)

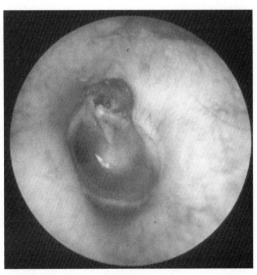

FIG. 17. Chronic otitis media (left ear). Early retraction pocket precursor of cholesteatoma. (Courtesy of Dr. Armando Lenis.)

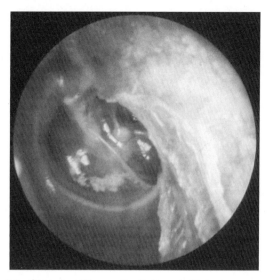

FIG. 18. Chronic otitis media (left ear). Note tympanosclerotic changes of the pars tensa and posterior mesotympanic collapse of the pars tensa over the stapes. A fibrous union at the incudostapedial joint and the stapedial tendon is noticeable. (Courtesy of Dr. Armando Lenis.)

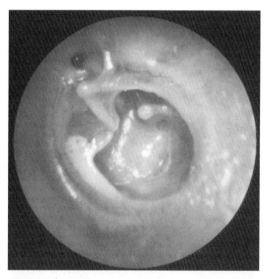

FIG. 19. Chronic otitis media (left ear). Note collapse of monomeric pars tensa, anterior tympanosclerotic plaque, anteromedially displaced malleal handle, absent (eroded) long process of the incus, and prominent head of the stapes. (Courtesy of Dr. Armando Lenis.)

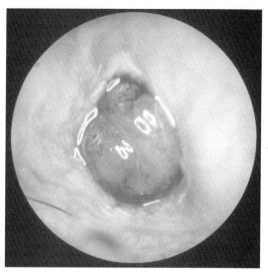

FIG. 20. Chronic otitis media. Note inflammatory polyp filling the external ear canal. (Courtesy of Dr. Armando Lenis.)

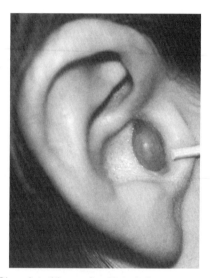

FIG. 21. Chronic otitis media. Note inflammatory polyp protruding through the external meatus.

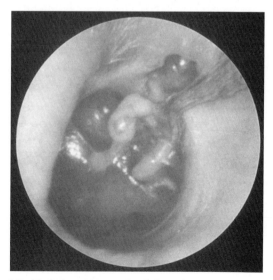

FIG. 22. Chronic otitis media (left ear). Note pars flaccida retraction pocket, partial collapse of the pars tensa with retraction pocket anterior to the malleus handle, exposure of incus long process, deformed malleus handle, and middle ear fluid. (Courtesy of Dr. Armando Lenis.)

Audiologic Examination

Audiometry in COM usually shows a conductive or mixed hearing loss, the degree of which is related to the severity of the middle ear lesion. Tympanic membrane defects, ossicular discontinuity or stiffness, and middle ear fluid are additive. In most cases, there is a consistent relationship between the severity of the lesion and the degree of conductive hearing loss. A significant sensorineural component may be present in advanced disease.

Vestibular Evaluation

Vestibular studies are of limited value in the majority of patients with COM. When vertigo is present, tests for sinusoidal rotation, spontaneous and positional nystagmus, and a fistula test with eyes opened and closed may add to a better understanding of a complex case.

Radiographic Evaluation

With the advent of high-resolution computerized axial tomography, plane mastoid films have lost their practical value in the assessment of COM. The disease stage (active vs. inactive) often can be estimated without radiographic evaluation; generally, radiographic assessment in uncomplicated tympanic membrane perforations is not indicated. Imaging is valuable in the presence of uncontrollable aural discharge, when complications such as facial nerve dysfunction and labyrinthine disturbances are present, and when central nervous system involvement is suspected. In the latter case, magnetic resonance imaging should be considered.

Medical Treatment

Medical management of COM is aimed at infection control and stabilization of the process to prevent further irreversible damage and the development of serious complications. Local therapy that includes cleaning and topical otic preparations is the mainstay of therapy. Oral, and rarely parenteral, antibiotics also play a role. Ear drops used most commonly for COM contain one or more antibiotics (e.g., neomycin, tobramycin, gentamycin, polymyxin B, ciprofloxacin) with or without a corticosteroid. When a perforation is present, an otic drop with a more neutral pH is preferred to diminish burning with application to the mucosa. Ophthalmic drops usually have a pH closer to 7 than otic preparations, and they often are preferred for this reason. Although neomycin is a frequent component of ear drops, the clinician should be aware that a small percentage of patients (approximately 0.1% to 1.0%) will have a hypersensitivity reaction (primarily skin erythema, rash, or scaling) to this antibiotic (46). If the tympanic membrane is intact, nonantibiotic acidifying ear

drops (e.g., boric acid) can be efficacious in local infection control. Powders containing antibiotics or boric acid also can be used. Otic drops will be most effective if they can be applied directly to the mucosal surface and not on to a blanket of mucopus. Therefore, periodic cleaning (e.g., weekly or biweekly) using a microscope and suction may be necessary initially. Although not performed routinely, a sample of the otorrhea can be taken for culture and sensitivity studies. This is especially important in immunocompromised patients or recalcitrant cases.

It should be noted that many otic drop preparations contain an aminoglycoside, raising the possibility of ototoxicity (see Chapter 35). Although several studies have documented ototoxicity following topical administration of antibiotic preparations in animal models, there is only anecdotal evidence of this in humans (47–49). In a recent national survey (50), only 3.4% of more than 2,235 otolaryngologists had witnessed irreversible SNHL attributable to the use of topical agents. The authors state, however, that these responses were "opinions" and were not verified by objective tests.

In the experimental studies of ototoxicity due to topical antibiotics referenced previously, both electrophysiologic alterations and hair cell loss were noted. In general, the findings were more dramatic in rodents than in higher primates. It also should be noted that the experimental conditions did not always mimic the clinical setting. For example, antibiotics were applied through a large tympanic membrane perforation or directly into the round window niche, sometimes at concentrations higher than those used in humans. In a clinical setting, there are a several factors, aside from natural tolerance, which may help protect the human cochlea from ototoxic antibiotics applied to the middle ear. Among these, the inflamed mucosa may limit penetration of the antibiotic to the round window membrane. Second, an overhanging bony niche and thick adhesions over the round window membrane are likely to prevent diffusion of the antibiotic into the inner ear (51–53).

To conclude, there is no doubt that currently used topical medications have produced middle and inner ear damage under experimental conditions and possibly in rare clinical situations. Therefore, they should be used when clearly indicated and the patient should be alerted to the onset of tinnitus and/or dizziness as a possible indication of ototoxicity.

Tuberculous Otomastoiditis

Tuberculosis is an uncommon cause of COM. *M. tuberculosis* is believed to reach the middle ear and mastoid by the hematogenous route. Palva et al. (54) reported a 0.9% incidence of tuberculosis in a retrospective study of 1,638 cases of COM. Most patients were in the 30- to 40-year-old group. In our 20-year experience with an indigent population of more than 4,000 surgical cases of chronic suppurative ear disease, only four cases (approximately 0.1%) of tuberculous OM were diagnosed. Three patients were foreign born and PPD positive; three had active pulmonary disease and one (a 2-year-old child) had no bronchopulmonary involvement. The classically described findings of multiple perforations and fetid, creamy aural discharge were not present, and the offending agent was unsuspected prior to culture and histopathologic study.

The largest current series of tuberculous ear disease was reported in 1986 by Samuel and Fernandes (55). These authors studied 23 cases in South Africa. Of these, 17 (73%) were under 13 years of age and 16 (70%) had active pulmonary tuberculosis. Of the pediatric cases, 9 presented with facial nerve paralysis, 6 with acute mastoiditis, and 2 with meningitis. Other findings were profound hearing loss, postauricular cutaneous fistulas, abundant granulation tissue, and osteomyelitis with multiple bony sequestra. The high incidence of childhood disease in this series probably is due to the use of unpasteurized milk.

The histopathology of tuberculous otomastoiditis is similar to that of the infection affecting other sites (56). The tissue involving the mastoid usually is densely packed and contains granulomas made up of epithelioid cells, lymphocytes, and Langhans' giant cells. Caseation usually is seen late in the course of the disease. Destruction of the bony framework of the mastoid occurs early and usually is extensive (Fig. 23).

Treatment is based on the management of the systemic infection with multiple antituberculosis agents. Surgery may play a diagnostic role in the unsuspected case, because presentation may mimic that of acute or coalescent mastoiditis; otherwise, it should be limited to the management of complications and, possibly, to reconstruction after the disease has been controlled by medical means and the activity of the ear process has ceased for sometime.

Nontuberculous Mycobacteria and COM

Nontuberculous mycobacteria infections are being diagnosed with increased frequency in the United States. Otologic infection caused by *M. fortuitum* and *M. avium* have been reported occasionally over the past 2 decades (57–59), and more recently several cases of COM cholesteatoma resulting from *M. abscessus*, a rapidly growing mycobacterium, have been discussed in the literature (60,61). Otitic nontuberculous mycobacteria infections are rarely considered but should be suspected in chronically draining ears refractory to traditional treatment. Trauma and foreign bodies, such as pressure equalization tubes, and the use of steroid-containing ear drops have been shown to be associated with nontuberculous mycobacteria, especially *M. abscessus* (56). The manifestations of the infection vary from persistent ear drainage to abscess formation and bone destruction. The diagnosis is made by positive culture identification. The species grows well in routine and mycobacterium media, but colonies are likely to develop several days after plating. Biopsies reveal acute and chronic inflammation and microabscesses. Noncaseating granulomas often are present. Therapy is by surgical debridement and long-term antibiotic therapy, often for up to 6 months. Nontuberculous mycobacteria is not susceptible to standard antituberculosis drugs. *M. fortuitum* usually is susceptible to fluorinated quinolones, sulfonamides, tetracycline, and amikacin (56). *M. abscessus* is susceptible to amikacin,

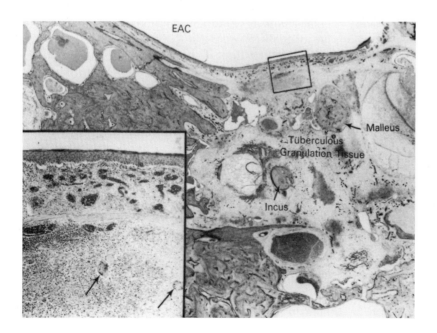

FIG. 23. Acute tuberculous otitis media and mastoiditis. The middle ear is filled with tuberculous granulation tissue. The tympanic membrane **(inset)** is intact but greatly thickened by granulation tissue composed of typical epithelioid cells, round cells, and multinucleated giant cells (*arrows*). The inner ear shows no tubercular involvement (original magnification × 6.4; inset original magnification × 49). (From Schuknecht HF. *Pathology of the ear.* Philadelphia: Lea & Febiger, 1993: 201, with permission.)

and high doses of erythromycin, clarithromycin, and cefoxitin (62).

Wegener's Granulomatosis

Wegener's granulomatosis is characterized by necrotizing granulomas and vasculitis of small arteries. The respiratory tract and kidneys are the principal sites involved, although any organ system can be affected. Otologic manifestations occur in 19% to 61% of patients (63–66).

Based on the study by McCaffrey et al. (67) and subsequent case reports (66–70), otologic involvement can be classified, in order of prevalence, as follows: serous otitis media, SNHL, COM or mastoiditis, and facial nerve paralysis.

More than 90% of patients with otologic symptoms will have unilateral or bilateral serous otitis media. Nasopharyngeal inflammation causing eustachian tube dysfunction is the presumed mechanism. Almost half of the patients will experience SNHL, often asymmetric, which may be severe. Vasculitis of cochlear vessels, granulomatous involvement of the cochlear nerve, and deposition of immune complexes in the cochlea have been postulated as possible mechanisms (63,71,72). Facial nerve involvement occurs in 5% to 10% of patients. Both the facial paralysis and the SNHL may improve significantly with medical therapy of Wegener's granulomatosis.

COM and/or mastoiditis occurs in approximately 25% of patients with otologic symptoms. It can present as otalgia, a thickened and inflamed tympanic membrane, a tympanic membrane perforation with mucopurulent otorrhea, or a tympanic membrane perforation with granulationlike tissue extruding through it. Computed tomographic (CT) and magnetic resonance imaging scans typically show middle ear and mastoid opacification without bony destruction. A delay in diagnosing Wegener's granulomatosis is common, because the clinical picture is nonspecific. Tuberculous otitis media often is diagnosed when the patient fails to respond to routine therapy for presumed bacterial otitis media. Mastoid and/or middle exploration with biopsy frequently yields nonspecific findings.

The key to the correct diagnosis of Wegener's granulomatosis limited to the ear is a high index of suspicion. A serologic marker, antineutrophil cytoplasmic autoantibody, is highly specific for this disease and can be invaluable in establishing a correct diagnosis. The cellular immunofluorescent staining pattern for antineutrophil cytoplasmic autoantibody can be subtyped as cytoplasmic or perinuclear; the cytoplasmic pattern offers 99% specificity for Wegener's granulomatosis.

In approximately one third of cases, Wegener's granulomatosis is locoregional in presentation. Within several months to several years, however, it progresses to the generalized form, which usually runs a forminant course if untreated. The early diagnosis of Wegener's granulomato-

sis, when it is limited in scope (e.g., COM), offers the best chance for clinical remission. It should be noted that although the cytoplasmic pattern for antineutrophil cytoplasmic autoantibody is a highly specific serologic marker, its sensitivity when the disease is locoregional is only 60%; its sensitivity is greater than 90% for generalized disease. Prednisone and cyclophosphamide are the mainstays of therapy. Potential complications to cyclophosphamide include bone marrow suppression, hemorrhagic cystitis, induction of neoplasm, and sterility.

CHOLESTEATOMA

Definition

Cholesteatomas are cystlike, expanding lesions of the temporal bone, lined by stratified squamous epithelium and containing desquamated keratin and purulent material (Fig. 24). They most frequently involve the middle ear and mastoid, but they may develop anywhere within the pneumatized portions of the temporal bone. They may be congenital (infrequently) or acquired. The term cholesteatoma was first used in 1838 by Mueller to define a "pearly tumor" originally described by Cuveilhier (73). Because the lesion does not contain cholesterol, some authorities favor the term keratoma as more accurate (74); however, time and custom have enfranchised the original misnomer and we will use it throughout this chapter.

Pathology and Pathogenesis of Acquired Cholesteatoma

The precise nature of acquired cholesteatoma and the sequence of events leading to its development remain

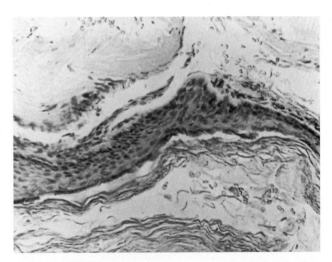

FIG. 24. Cholesteatoma squamous epithelium overlying layers of laminated keratin (hematoxylin and eosin, original magnification × 60). (From Goodhill V, ed: *Ear diseases, deafness and dizziness.* Hagerstown, MD: Harper and Row Publishers, 1979:335, with permission.)

controversial. The prevailing view is that, excluding trauma with direct implantation of squamous epithelium (see Chapter 49), cholesteatomas result from complications of chronic middle ear infections.

Two processes appear central to the development and progression of cholesteatoma: *mucosal invasion by squamous epithelium* and *bone destruction*. Although the first of these changes is believed to initiate the sequence of events leading to the formation of a cholesteatoma, the process is not linear in nature (75). It is modified by a variety of factors, such as the site of initial involvement, reactivation and severity of acute infections, local and systemic immunologic factors, and medical or surgical intervention.

Mucosal Invasion by Squamous Epithelium

The mechanics of mucosal transformation and epithelial ingrowth have been the focal point of cholesteatoma theory for more than a century. The following is an account of the most significant observations that contributed to our current understanding of this process.

Habermann (76) in 1889 stated that cholesteatomas resulted from epithelial migration from the edge of a peripheral perforation, and Bezold (77) first related eustachian tube dysfunction to the formation of a chronically infected epithelial cyst. In more modern times, Ruedi (78) integrated these theories and postulated that inward growth of the surface epithelium follows papillary proliferation of the germinative layer of the pars flaccida. Eventually an open pouch is formed, which later tunnelizes into the attic and mastoid (Fig. 25). The theory of epithelial migration has gained support in recent monoclonal antibody studies by Van Blitterswike and Grote (79). These authors showed that specific cytokeratin subtypes of the external ear canal skin and tympanic membrane also are present in the matrix of cholesteatomas suggesting a common origin. However, Sade (80) has challenged the concept that squamous epithelium in the middle ear mucosa derives exclusively from migration from areas peripheral to it and has shown in temporal bone specimens areas of squamous metaplasia surrounded by normal appearing mucosa (Fig. 26). In subsequent studies of tissue cultures of middle ear mucosa cells, Sade et al. (81) showed that although epithelium migrates freely when unopposed, it stops when it encounters another epithelium *(contact inhibition)*. This finding would explain why cholesteatoma arises rarely from central perforations and led these authors to conclude that metaplasia from pseudostratified ciliated columnar epithelium to stratified squamous epithelium plays a major role in cholesteatoma formation.

Whether by migration, metaplasia, or a combination of the two, epithelial invasion is followed by its invagination or tunnelization into the middle ear cleft and mastoid. Several incompletely understood mucosal changes con-

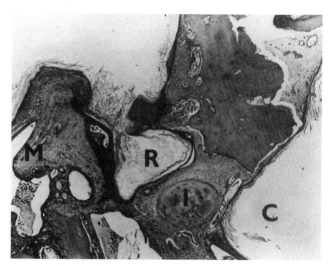

FIG. 25. Retraction pocket (*R*) arising from pars flaccida of tympanic membrane and extending medially as far on the incus (*I*). The pocket shows downgrowths of its epithelium. Deep to the incus there is a cholesteatoma sac (*C*). There are numerous small gland structures in relation to the middle ear mucosa, a manifestation of chronic otitis. The handle of the malleus (*M*) and the long process of the incus are eroded (hematoxylin and eosin, original magnification × 43). (From Michaels L. Biology of cholesteatoma. *Otolaryngol Clin North Am* 1989;22:869–881, with permission.)

tribute to this process. Based on surgical and histologic observations, Juers (82) postulated that the formation of fibrous bands sealed off the attic, isolating this space from the rest of the middle ear. Over time, other fibrous bands would attach to an incipient cholesteatoma and, aided by negative pressure, retract it into the mastoid. A similar concept was advanced by Draper (83) in a study

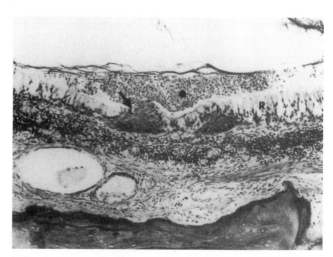

FIG. 26. Intraepithelial budding of stratified squamous epithelium (*arrow*) amidst a middle ear mucosa with an inflammatory exudate alone (•) and an inflammatory infiltrate in the submucosa (*R*). (From Sade J, Babiacki A, Pinkus G. The metaplastic and congenital origin of cholesteatoma. *Acta Otolaryngol* 1983;96:119–129, with permission.)

of 540 children with secretory otitis media followed into adolescence. This author hypothesized that the formation of middle ear adhesions introduces an element of irreversibility in chronic ear disease that sets the stage for the formation of cholesteatoma. Extensive surgical and clinical observations led Smyth (6) to propose that all forms of COM, including cholesteatoma, derive from a single cause, which is an unresolved middle ear effusion, resulting from prolonged eustachian tube dysfunction. This concept is supported experimentally by the work of Aberg et al. (84), who documented the morphologic events of cholesteatoma formation in a group of Mongolian gerbils that had undergone eustachian tube ligation. These authors identified four progressive pathologic stages. In the first stage, middle ear effusion was followed by the formation of an orthokeratotic plug in the external ear canal. In the second and third stages, the tympanic membrane underwent progressive retraction followed by the accumulation of middle ear granulation tissue. In the fourth stage, bone destruction occurred. Clinically this view also is supported by El Saifi (85) in a study of 416 children with otitis media and effusion followed for 15 years. These patients had an incidence of 1.6% retraction pockets, 0.9% ossicular necrosis, 0.8% COM with mastoiditis, 0.6% cholesteatoma, 0.6% perforation, and 0.45% atelectasis. Because these children were under continuous medical supervision, the findings do not represent the natural course of the disease, but they are significant because these sequelae are likely to be more frequent in severe and neglected cases.

In addition to changes affecting the middle ear cleft, loss of elasticity and thinning of the tympanic membrane are major factors in the genesis of epithelial ingrowth. Abramson and Huang (11) and Iwanaga et al. (86) documented that both chronic effusion and granulation tissue contain enzymes capable of inducing lysis of the collagen fibers of the tympanic membrane. The result of this injury is total or segmental atelectasis of this structure and/or perforation. This mechanism may operate both in the pars tensa, rich in elastic fibers, and the pars flaccida, which has only a scant network of disorganized collagen elements and no elastic fibers. This difference may contribute to the higher incidence of cholesteatomas arising in the epitympanum (87). In addition, Smyth (8) proposed that negative pressure may be a factor limited to the attic, presumably when scar tissue and adhesions seal off this compartment from the rest of the middle ear cleft.

The following summarizes the various steps resulting in epithelial ingrowth (Fig. 27). It must be emphasized that they do not take place successively and that, once the initial changes become chronic, progressive alterations tend to occur simultaneously.

A. Eustachian tube dysfunction, increased negative pressure, repeated infection, and chronic middle ear effusion.
B. Loss of collagen fibers and structural support of the tympanic membrane.
C. Segmental collapse of the tympanic membrane and formation of a chronically retracted pocket.
D. Development of granulation tissue and fibrous bands medial to the collapsed segment leading to further retraction of the pocket.
E. Complicating factors are chronic infection, pocket rupture, epithelial migration, and metaplasia.

Bone Destruction

Bone destruction in COM with or without cholesteatoma has been, and continues to be, the focus of much research. Three groups of factors appear to be involved in this process: (a) *mechanical*, related to pressure generated by the expansion of cholesteatoma as it accumulates increasing amounts of keratin and purulent debris, (b) *biochemical*, due to bacterial elements (endotoxins), products of the host's granulation tissue (collagenase, acid hydrolases) and substances related to the cholesteatoma itself (growth factors, cytokines), and (c) *cellular*, predominantly induced by osteoclastic activity. It is likely that bone destruction in cholesteatoma results from a combination of all or some of these factors, but clarification is needed regarding their specific roles.

Because *keratin accumulation* is a primary characteristic of cholesteatoma, several theories related to this sub-

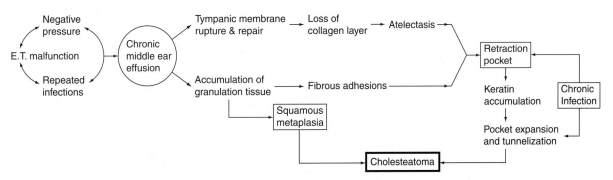

FIG. 27. Pathogenesis of cholesteatoma according to present theory. E.T., eustachian tube.

stance are currently discussed (88–90), including the following: (a) keratin acts as a foreign body producing a granulomatous response, with macrophage activity resulting in bone breakdown; (b) increasing amounts of trapped keratin produce pressure on the surrounding bone, inducing cortical devascularization and resorption; (c) the accumulation of keratin prevents removal of destroyed cells, which results in a high concentration of lysosomal enzymes and the accumulation of bacteria and their decay products; and (d) epithelial cells or their products stimulate the proliferation of subepithelial mesenchymal cells (fibroblastlike elements that release enzymes capable of stimulating the breakdown of bone) and granulation tissue.

Evidence supporting *enzymatic activity* in this process was advanced by Abrahamson and Huang (11), who demonstrated a high collagenase content in samples of patients with cholesteatoma. However, Moriyama et al. (91) noted that collagenase has no effect on bone that has not undergone demineralization. These authors demonstrated that, in rat epithelial cultures, epithelial cells stimulate fibroblastlike elements to release collagenase, but they also noted that infection or inflammation was needed to produce demineralization and bone breakdown.

The effects of *pressure* by cholesteatoma have been studied by Chole et al. (92) and Orisek and Chole (93). The latter authors used implantable pressure gauges in gerbilline cholesteatomas. Pressures between 1.31 and 11.8 mm Hg were recorded, and osteoclastic bone resorption was noted in areas of documented pressure. In an effort to more precisely identify the role of pressure in bone destruction, Macri and Chole (94) implanted barriers between the cholesteatoma and the promontory of Mongolian gerbils. These barriers eliminated direct contact between the cholesteatoma and the otic capsule, theoretically preventing factors other than pressure to act on the underlying bone. Because erosion of the otic capsule resulted, these authors concluded that pressure alone could be responsible for bone resorption, at least under the experimental conditions presented.

The majority of recent research points toward the active participation of a *cellular component* in cholesteatoma-related osteolysis. The work of Chole (95,96) and Chole et al. (92) has provided considerable evidence to support the idea that the osteoclast may be the basic vehicle for this process. However, precise documentation of the osteoclast role remains elusive because this cell is difficult to identify in temporal bone sections, it has a relatively short life span, and its activity probably varies depending on the stage of the disease. Chole (97) found subepithelial osteoclasts in 11 of 24 intraoperative samples of patients with cholesteatoma. Osteoblasts also were noted, raising the possibility that they may participate in osteoclast activation. A proposed mechanism involves the release of cytokine by osteoblasts, which exposes the mineral in the bone surface preparing it for osteoclastic activity and breakdown of its matrix. These findings are at odds with those of Thomsen et al. (89) and Thomsen (98) and Thomsen et al. (99), who failed to show osteoclasts in cholesteatomas with active and widespread bone resorption.

To conclude, the available information tends to support a multifactorial theory in cholesteatoma-induced bone destruction, with several agents acting simultaneously. The following list and Fig. 28 summarize the key events in this process.

1. Keratin accumulation produces increased pressure on the involved bone surfaces. This results in superficial erosion, probably enhanced by interference with capillary blood flow, and sets the stage for demineralization.
2. Epithelial cells and cellular decay products trapped in the cholesteatoma stimulate the proliferation of subepithelial (fibroblastlike) mesenchymal cells and granulation tissue. Collagenase and other enzymes (acid phosphatase, lysosomes) are released.
3. Demineralization is induced by infection and probably by the participation of cytokine-secreting cells, such as osteoblasts. Pressure directly applied to bone

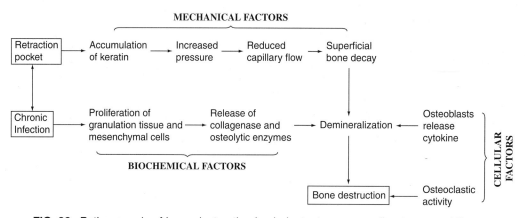

FIG. 28. Pathogenesis of bone destruction in cholesteatoma according to present theory.

by a growing cholesteatoma may have a contributory role.

4. The demineralized bone is broken down by collagenase and other osteolytic enzymes, and by the activity of osteoclasts.

Growth Patterns of Cholesteatoma

Although there are many variables involved, the mechanics of cholesteatoma growth and its limitations are closely related to the anatomy of the middle ear and especially to the structural elements forming and surrounding the attic, pars flaccida, and posterior portion of the mesotympanum (Fig. 29). It is in this region where the majority of acquired cholesteatomas develop. Within this area the attic is a small, self-contained space with limited communication with the rest of the middle ear cleft and the mastoid. Inferiorly it is separated from the mesotympanum by Proctor's fibroosseous diaphragm constituted by the ossicles, their supporting ligaments, and an intricate system of membranous folds that allows for only two restricted pathways or isthmuses (100). Beyond this the attic is completely surrounded by bone, except for the narrow passage into the mastoid constituted by the aditus ad antrum.

Epitympanic Cholesteatomas

These arise from either *Prussak's space* (most commonly) or the anterior *epitympanic recess* (Fig. 29B).

Prussak's space is a very shallow pouch situated in the posterior portion of the pars flaccida. It lies between this structure and the neck of the malleus and is limited superiorly by the lateral malleal fold and inferiorly by the lateral process of this ossicle. The anterior epitympanic recess is limited by the anterior insertion of the lateral malleal fold and the malleal head superiorly, the annular rim anteriorly, and the anterior malleal fold and the facial nerve inferiorly. Cholesteatomas developing in the pars flaccida overlying Prussak's space extend posteriorly along the lateral surface of the body of the incus, eventually reaching the antrum and through it the mastoid (Fig. 30). Anterior epitympanic cholesteatomas are infrequent and tend to grow anteriorly along the cochleariform process and inferiorly into the supratubal recess. They may extend into the mesotympanum through the anterior pouch of von Tröltsch.

The anterior epitympanic space or supratubal recess is limited anteriorly by the middle cranial fossa, the petrous tip, and the root of the zygoma, posteriorly by a bony ridge, termed the *cog*, extending to the cochleariform process, superiorly by the middle cranial fossa, and laterally by the tympanic bone and chorda tympani nerve. The anterior epitympanic space may be divided into two spaces by the supratubal ridge (85% of temporal bones) or present as a single cavity (15% of temporal bones) (Fig. 31) (101). The space between the cochleariform process and the cog is the entrance to the recess. Removal of the cog exposes the recess, which contains the distal portion of the horizontal segment of the facial nerve

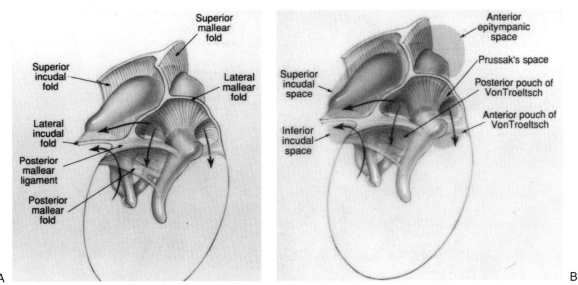

FIG. 29. A: The ligaments and folds of the mesotympanum and epitympanum. These structures constitute barriers that tend to channel cholesteatoma growth along characteristic anatomic pathways. The *larger arrows* indicate these typical pathways. **B:** Ligaments and folds compartmentalize the middle ear into spaces and pouches (*stippled areas*). The *larger arrows* indicate the typical pathways for cholesteatoma growth. (From Jackler RN. The surgical anatomy of cholesteatoma. *Otolaryngol Clin North Am* 1989;22:883–892, with permission.)

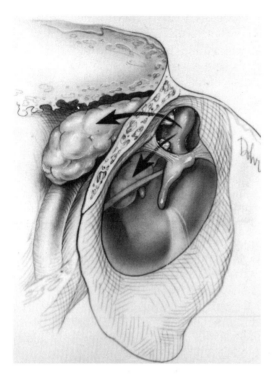

FIG. 30. Routes of extension of posterior epitympanic cholesteatoma (*arrows*). (From Jackler RN. The surgical anatomy of cholesteatoma. *Otolaryngol Clin North Am* 1989;22: 883–892, with permission.)

(102). The anterior pouch of von Tröltsch is a very small space between the pars tensa and the anterior malleolar fold (Fig. 29B).

Posterior Mesotympanic Cholesteatomas

The posterior superior aspect of the pars tensa is frequently the site of a retraction pocket that follows the loss of fibrous support, persistent negative pressure, and the formation of adhesions between the medial surface of the eardrum and the middle ear walls and ossicular elements. These pockets initially are limited superiorly by the posterior malleal ligament, medially by the posterior malleal fold, the long process of the incus and the stapes and stapedial muscle, and inferiorly (usually) by the chorda tympani nerve. The annular rim limits them posteriorly and the long process of the malleus (to some extent) anteriorly (Fig. 32). Cholesteatomas of this region are second in frequency and develop from retraction pockets or marginal perforations of the pars tensa. Extension takes place through the posterior tympanic isthmus, along the sinus tympani and retrofacial recess, thereafter progressing medially to the body of the incus to invade the mastoid (Figs. 33 and 34).

History and Physical Findings of Acquired Cholesteatoma

The history of acquired cholesteatoma is similar to that of COM. Intermittent aural drainage and progressive

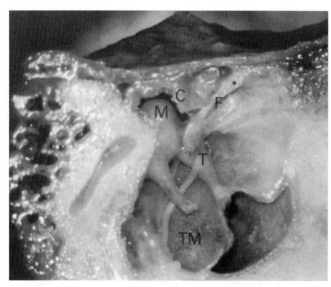

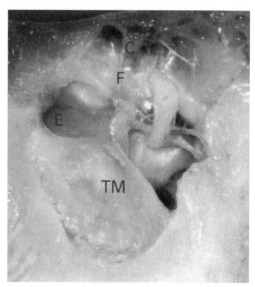

A

B

FIG. 31. A: Medial view of the left temporal bone. The supratubal ridge and tensor tympanic fold separate the type I anterior epitympanic space into two cavities. *Asterisk* indicates supratubal ridge. *C*, cog; *F*, tensor tympani fold; *M*, head of malleus; *T*, tensor tympanic tendon; *TM*, tympanic membrane. **B:** Lateral view of the left temporal bone. This type II anterior epitympanic space is made up of one cavity in front of the cog (*C*) that is continuous with the eustachian tube orifice (*E*). *F*, tensor tympani fold; *TM*, tympanic membrane. (From Onal K, Van Haastert RM, Grote JJ. Structural variations of the supratubal recess: the anterior epitympanic space. *Am J Otol* 1997;18:317–321, with permission.)

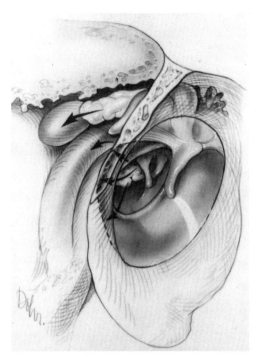

FIG. 32. Posterior mesotympanic cholesteatoma. This sac forms because of retraction of the posterior portion of the pars tensa and frequently involves the sinus tympani and facial nerves (*lower three arrows*). Extension to the mastoid occurs medial to the ossicle heads (*upper two arrows*). (From Jackler RN. The surgical anatomy of cholesteatoma. *Otolaryngol Clin North Am* 1989;22:883–892, with permission.)

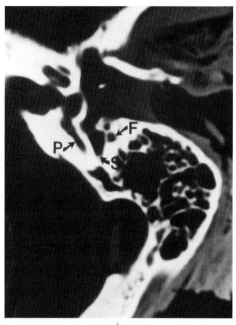

FIG. 34. Computed tomography of temporal bone specimen, showing a deep sinus tympani (*S*). *F*, facial nerve; *P*, posterior semicircular canal. (From Pickett BP, Cail WS, Lambert PR. Sinus tympani: anatomic considerations, computed tomography, and a discussion of the retrofacial approach for removal of disease. *Am J Otolaryngol* 1995;16:741–750, with permission.)

hearing loss are prominent complaints. At examination, findings vary depending on cholesteatoma location. In *pars flaccida lesions*, retraction of this portion of the eardrum with or without a perforation is seen. The bone of the surrounding ear canal may be eroded and a variable amount of squamous debris is present (Fig. 35: see color

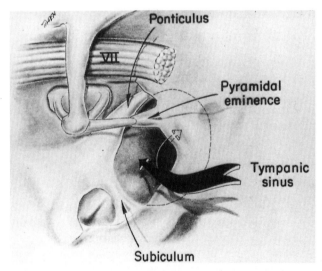

FIG. 33. Lateral view of the middle ear showing the entrance of the sinus tympani and its relation to neighboring structures. (From Schuknecht HF, Gulya AJ. The middle ear spaces. In: Sade J, ed. *Surgical anatomy of the ear and temporal bone*. Philadelphia: Lea & Febiger, 1986:3–34, with permission.)

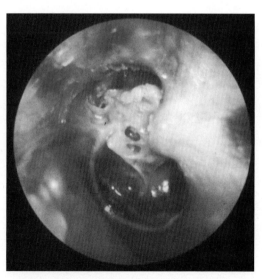

FIG. 35. Cholesteatoma (left ear). Extensive posterior superior retraction pocket with peripheral bone erosion (self-performed atticotomy). (Courtesy of Dr. Armando Lenis.)

plate 22 following page 484). A dry keratinaceous ball may form within the retracted area and be adherent to the underlying structures obscuring the true extent of the disease. Removal of this plug under the surgical microscope may be difficult without anesthesia and may need to be delayed until the time of definitive treatment. When cleared, portions of the malleal head and incus, normally covered by the missing scutum, may be seen. On occasion it is possible to identify the entire extent of a large, intact retraction pocket, a condition termed *self-performed atticotomy*. More frequently, the limits of a retraction pocket are unclear, and it is evident that the thinned lining of the pars flaccida has broken through.

Posterior mesotympanic cholesteatomas will exhibit similar findings except for their different location and the structures uncovered or damaged by their growth. Frequently the stapes (or a stapedial remnant), long process of the incus, and chorda tympani nerve can be identified with the cholesteatoma matrix draping over them.

In more advanced cases, especially when medical intervention has been lacking, the destruction caused by the cholesteatoma is more significant, with extensive breakdown of the tympanic membrane, marked mucosal changes, granulation tissue, and often abundant keratinaceous debris. Once the ear is cleaned, the cholesteatoma matrix may be noted to line the middle ear cleft to a variable extent. It may be limited to the area of prevalence (epitympanum and/or posterior superior quadrant of the pars flaccida) or extend to the entire middle ear cleft. Depending on the degree of erosion, several middle ear structures (intact or partially destroyed) may be seen, such as the chorda tympani, stapes, incudostapedial joint, malleus, promontory, and round window.

Occasionally, acquired cholesteatoma may be present behind an *intact tympanic membrane* (Figs. 36 and 37: see

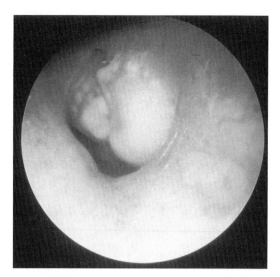

FIG. 37. Cholesteatoma (left ear). Extensive cholesteatoma behind an intact tympanic membrane. (Courtesy of Dr. Armando Lenis.)

color plates 23 and 24 following page 484). This condition is most frequently encountered following incomplete surgical removal and tympanoplasty. It also may be seen in congenital disease or in acquired cholesteatomas where spontaneous repair of the tympanic membrane has entrapped the lesion. These cholesteatomas appear as white masses sometimes difficult to differentiate from tympanosclerotic plaques. They often are more evident at pneumatoscopy. On displacement of the tympanic membrane by positive pressure, this structure may be made to drape over the mass, thereby enhancing its visualization.

Cholesteatomas appearing behind an intact tympanic membrane may be confused with cholesteatomas primarily involving this structure. *Tympanic membrane cholesteatomas* are rare. They are usually iatrogenic or secondary to trauma, and they present as indistinct whitish masses within the drum. Hearing loss usually is mild. When iatrogenic, they follow myringoplasty and entrapment of squamous cells from the lateral layer of the tympanic membrane medial to the graft. They also may develop (rarely) from untreated epithelial cysts secondary to the use of pressure equalization tubes.

Audiologic Examination

Tuning fork tests will document a conductive component in most cases, with Weber's test indicating lateralization to the affected (or more affected) ear and Rinne's test showing bone conduction to be better than air conduction. Audiometric studies will vary according to the location and extent of the disease. In advanced cases, a mixed hearing loss with a 40- to 50-dB conductive component and a high-frequency sensorineural loss is frequent. In cases where the disease is limited to the epitympanum, a conductive loss usually is seen, although it

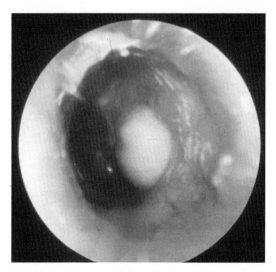

FIG. 36. Cholesteatoma (left ear). Posterior mesotympanic cholesteatoma behind an intact tympanic membrane. (Courtesy of Dr. Armando Lenis.)

is not rare to document only minimal changes. A mild low-frequency air–bone gap (secondary to increased stiffness) may be the sole finding.

Occasionally, in advanced cases with ossicular erosion, only a mild conductive loss is present because the cholesteatoma may be serving as a bridge to maintain ossicular continuity. This is an important feature of the disease. It must be discussed with the patient prior to surgical intervention, because cholesteatoma removal without ossicular reconstruction will result in increased conductive loss. Tympanometry does not add any significant information in the evaluation of cholesteatomas.

Radiographic Evaluation

Thin-section (2-mm) CT scans without contrast, taken in the coronal and axial projections, may be of value in the preoperative assessment of cholesteatomas. It must be emphasized that radiographs generally are not diagnostic of the disease, although several alterations of temporal bone anatomy frequently are associated with it. Among these, erosion of the scutum and expansion of the antrum within areas of air cell breakdown and soft tissue density are characteristic. Other features may include ossicular destruction and erosion of the otic capsule, especially over the horizontal semicircular canal, facial canal, and mastoid tegmen (see Chapter 18).

Routine CT scanning is not advocated for cholesteatoma diagnosis, but it is important in complicated disease (see Chapter 18) and in the evaluation of cholesteatomas and other masses behind an intact tympanic membrane, or when the clinical history correlates poorly with physical findings.

Medical Management of Cholesteatomas

The treatment of cholesteatoma is by surgical excision or exteriorization (see Chapter 18). However, in cases where the patient's general state of health prevents an operation, the disease may be controlled for some time by repeated cleansing under the surgical microscope. This may require topical anesthesia. Care must be taken to remove all impacted keratin debris. It must be emphasized that this type of manipulation requires experience and sophisticated knowledge of the anatomy of the middle ear under normal and pathologic conditions. Consequently, it should always be performed under adequate magnification by an otolaryngologist competent in the management of complex ear disease. Hypertrophic granulation tissue may be controlled with a low-concentration solution of trichloroacetic acid carefully applied with a fine probe. Topical ear drops containing antibiotics and corticosteroids are used, and systemic antibiotics, based on culture results, occasionally may be necessary.

Cholesteatoma in Children

Although the clinical characteristics of childhood cholesteatoma are similar to those of the disease in adults, there is considerable controversy regarding their pathogenesis, classification, natural behavior, and treatment (103–108).

The mean age of pediatric cholesteatoma at presentation is approximately 10 years. The disease is infrequent before age 4 and has a peak incidence in the early teens (13 to 15 years). It is slightly more frequent in males. The majority of cases (70% to 80%) develop in the epitympanum and present with hearing loss, intermittent purulent discharge, and a posterosuperior retraction pocket. The disease most frequently is unilateral, although COM often is present in the opposite ear (103–105).

Diagnosis and assessment of the extent of childhood cholesteatoma may be difficult because of lack of patient cooperation, small ear canal and meatus, and sometimes equivocal audiometric findings. CT scanning may be useful in establishing the limits of the cholesteatoma, but usually a precise assessment is achieved only by surgical exploration. There appears to be an increased incidence of residual and recurrent childhood cholesteatoma after surgical removal, when compared to adult disease (103, 104,109–112). The hypothesis that the biology of pediatric cholesteatomas may be different (i.e., more aggressive) has been proposed to explain these observations. The activity of growth factors normally elaborated in childhood and absent in adult may play a role. Alternatively it is possible that the intrinsic process is similar to that of adults but with associated factors leading to a more recalcitrant nature. For example, a sclerotic temporal bone secondary to childhood infections frequently is found in adults with cholesteatoma, whereas children often have a well-pneumatized temporal bone with deep air cell tracks, complicating disease removal. Other contributing factors include poor eustachian tube function that predisposes to tympanic membrane retractions (recurrent cholesteatoma) and frequent otitis media with secondary cholesteatoma infection.

Congenital Cholesteatoma

The existence of a congenital form of cholesteatoma remained controversial until 1965, when Derlacki and Clemis (113) presented a study of ten cases of middle ear cholesteatoma without previous history of otitis and occurring behind an intact tympanic membrane. These authors established strict guidelines for the diagnosis of congenital cholesteatomas and presented a classification based on site of origin: petrosal, mastoid, and middle ear. Prior to their report, there had been several cases where the lack of previous ear disease and integrity of the drum led to the clinical impression of congenital disease. Of special interest is the case of a small isolated middle ear lesion reported by Cawthorne (114) that first focused attention on this problem.

The pathogenesis of congenital cholesteatomas is unclear. In a review of the development of the epibranchial organs, Teed (115) noted an ectodermal epithelial thickening that developed in proximity of the geniculate ganglion, medial to the neck of the malleus. This mass of epithelial cells soon undergoes involution to become mature middle ear lining. Teed believed that if involution failed to take place, this formation could be the source of a congenital cholesteatoma. In pursuit of this theory, Michaels (116,117) undertook a review of fetal human temporal bones and identified a squamous cell tuft present from 10 to 33 weeks of gestation in 37 of 68 specimens studied. He termed this structure the *epidermoid formation* and noted it to be located in the anterosuperior wall of the developing middle ear cleft (Fig. 38). Failure of the epidermoid formation to involute could be the basis for the development of cholesteatomas in the anterior mesotympanum. Michaels also proposed that congenital cholesteatomas of the posterior cleft could result from migration of this tissue during ear development (117,118). This opinion is shared by Parisier and Weiss (119), whereas Sade et al. (80) support metaplasia of the middle ear mucosa as the genesis of congenital cholesteatomas.

Congenital cholesteatomas occur more frequently in males; the mean age of presentation varies somewhat with location. For example, posterior and mesotympanic lesions are usually detected at about 12 years, whereas anterior cholesteatomas (perhaps because they are more readily seen by the pediatrician during "well-child" visits) present at about age 4 years. Bilateral lesions are rare, with an overall incidence of 3% to 5% (120). Zappia and Wiet (121) recently reported on a congenital cholesteatoma presenting in a 30-year-old man with a posteriorly located lesion.

The patterns of extension for congenital cholesteatomas vary according to the site of origin. Anterior and anterosuperior lesions tend to grow toward the eustachian tube and produce middle ear effusion (Fig. 39: see color plate 25 following page 484). Inferior and posterior extensions are also frequent, as growth toward the attic tends to be limited by the middle ear diaphragm. Ossicular erosion is not frequent, but it is more common in posterior lesions and lesions with posterior extension (119,120).

The criteria for the diagnosis of a congenital cholesteatoma are well established. The diagnosis is considered in patients without a previous history of ear disease, in the presence of a normal, intact tympanic membrane through which a pearly white mass can be seen. Occasionally, the diagnosis is unsuspected until myringotomy or posterior tympanometry for an unexplained conductive hearing loss is performed. In general, the diagnosis of congenital cholesteatoma would appear more tenable in anterior, superior mesotympanic lesions where their development from remnants of the epidermoid formation is better understood. Furthermore, such lesions tend to extend medial to the malleus and are not attached to the tympanic membrane, suggesting an origin independent from this structure. When CT studies are done, the temporal bone pneumatization should be normal. Cases associated with congenital stenosis/atresia of the external ear canal should be excluded.

Petromastoid cholesteatomas are different lesions, closely related to the geniculate ganglion. Teed (115) described an epithelial mass, hypothetically a derivative

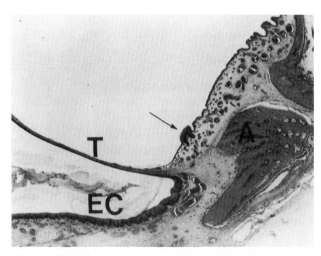

FIG. 38. Epidermoid formation (*arrow*) in the middle ear of a fetus. Note that the protympanum is aligned at an angle to the tympanic membrane (*T*) so that a congenital cholesteatoma arising from it would be visible at an early stage from the external canal (*EC*). The anterior limb of the bony annulus (*A*) is near the epidermoid formation (hematoxylin and eosin, original magnification × 44). (From Levenson MJ, Michaels L, Parisier SC. Congenital cholesteatomas of the middle ear in children. *Otolaryngol Clin North Am* 1989;22:941–954, with permission.)

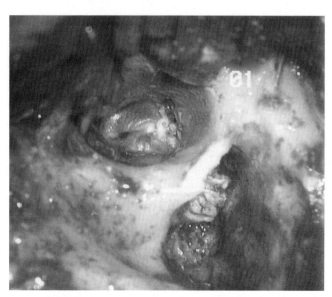

FIG. 39. Cholesteatoma (left ear). The mastoid has been opened surgically, and extension of the attic cholesteatoma into the antrum is evident.

of the first epibranchial placode, which could be responsible for the development of these cholesteatomas. However, other authors have speculated that at least some of these petrosal lesions may have a mesotympanic origin and that their mode of presentation reflects a different growth pattern rather than a separate embryonal rest origin (122,123). Because of their close relationship to the geniculate ganglion, facial nerve paralysis is a common presenting sign in these cases.

SUMMARY POINTS

- *P. aeruginosa* and *S. aureus* are the predominant organisms in COM; however, a mixed culture of aerobic and anaerobic bacteria usually can be obtained.
- COM causes changes to the tympanic membrane (e.g., perforation, collapse, tympanosclerosis), the ossicles (e.g., erosion, fixation), and the inner ear (e.g., labyrinthitis with SNHL and/or dizziness).
- Otalgia is uncommon in COM; if present, one must consider central nervous system involvement (e.g., epidural or brain abscess) or cancer.
- COM without cholesteatoma usually will respond to medical therapy consisting of cleaning and topical otic preparations; however, recurrence of the otorrhea is common, especially if a tympanic membrane perforation is present.
- Although uncommon, microbacteria infections and Wegener's granulomatosis can cause COM and should be considered in an ear refractory to standard treatments.
- Acquired cholesteatoma can result from a retraction pocket, squamous epithelial migration, and/or squamous metaplasia.
- Cholesteatomas may cause bone destruction by pressure (expanding keratin mass), release of biochemical factors (e.g., bacterial endotoxins, collagenases, cytokines), and/or induced osteoclastic activity.
- The majority of cholesteatomas are present in the epitympanum (pars flaccida) and posterosuperior portion of the mesotympanum.
- Compared with adults, pediatric cholesteatomas may be more difficult to remove surgically because of a more aggressive biology (secondary to the activity of childhood growth factors), frequent middle ear infection from eustachian tube dysfunction, and/or more extensive pneumatization of the temporal bone.
- The etiology of congenital cholesteatomas is unclear. Both squamous metaplasia and persistence of the epidermoid formulation have been implicated in their pathogenesis.

REFERENCES

1. John SK, Paparella MM, Kim CS, et al. Pathogenesis of otitis media. *Ann Otol Rhinol Laryngol* 1977;86:481–492.
2. Acosta-Bandek G. Histopathology of transudatory secretory otitis media. *Arch Otolaryngol* 1963;78:33–38.
3. Tos M, Bak-Pedersen K. The pathogenesis of chronic secretory otitis media. *Arch Otolaryngol* 1972;95:511–521.
4. Sade J. The biopathology of secretory otitis media. *Ann Otol Rhinol Laryngol* 1974;83[Suppl 11]:59–70.
5. McCabe BF. The etiology of chronic otitis media. *Clin Otolaryngol* 1977;3:243–248.
6. Smyth GDL. Tympanomastoid disease. In: Gibb AG, Smith MFW, eds. *Otology.* London: Butterworths, 1982:3–6.
7. Meyerhoff WL, Paparella MM, Kim CS. Pathology of chronic otitis media. *Ann Otol Rhinol Laryngol* 1978;87:749–760.
8. Smyth GDL. *Chronic ear disease.* New York: Churchill Livingstone, 1980.
9. Palva T, Palva A, Dammert K. Middle ear mucosa and chronic ear disease, II. Enzymes studies. *Arch Otolaryngol* 1970;91:50–56.
10. Palva T, Pekka K, Pala A, Karja J. Middle ear mucosa and chronic ear disease, IV. Enzyme studies of thick non-cholesteatomatous epithelium. *Arch Otolaryngol* 1975;101:380–384.
11. Abramson M, Huang C. Localization of collagenase in human middle ear cholesteatoma. *Laryngoscope* 1977; 87:777–785.
12. Widemar L, Hallstorm S, Stenfors LE. Different structural changes in membrana shrapnelli in serous and purulent otitis media. *Acta Otolaryngol (Stockh)* 1986;266–273.
13. Grote JJ, Bakker D, Hesseling SC, Van Blitterswijk CA. Tympanic membrane structure during a staphylococcus aureus induced middle ear infection. *Acta Otolaryngol (Stockh)* 1989;107:225–234.
14. Richardson GS. Aditus block. *Ann Otol Rhinol Laryngol* 1963;72:223–236.
15. Brook I. Bacteriology and treatment of chronic otitis media. *Laryngoscope* 1979;89:1129–1134.
16. Bluestone CD, Kenna MA. Chronic suppurative otitis media: antimicrobial therapy or surgery. *Pediatr Ann* 1984;13:417–422.
17. Erkan M, Aslan T, Seruk E, Guney E. Bacteriology of chronic suppurative otitis media. *Ann Otol Rhinol Laryngol* 1994;103:771–774.
18. Brook I, Yocum P. Quantitative cultures and beta lactamase activity in chronic suppurative otitis media. *Ann Otol Rhinol Laryngol* 1989;98:293–297.
19. daCosta SS, Paparella MM, Schachern PA, Yoon TH, Kimberly BP. Temporal bone histopathology in chronic infected ears with intact and perforated tympanic membranes. *Laryngoscope* 1992;102:1229–1236.
20. Sade J, Halevy A. The aetiology of bone destruction in chronic otitis media. *J Laryngol Otol* 1974;88:139–143.
21. Mayerhoff WL. Pathology of chronic suppurative otitis media. *Ann Otol Rhinol Laryngol* 1988;97[Suppl 131]:21–24.
22. Sade J. Atelectatic tympanic membrane: histologic study. *Ann Otol Rhinol Laryngol* 1993;102:712–716.
23. Sade J. The atelectatic ear. In: Sade J, ed. *Secretory otitis media and its sequelae.* New York: Churchill Livingstone, 1979:64–84.
24. Igarashi M, Korishi S, Alford BR, Guilford FR. The pathology of tympanosclerosis. *Laryngoscope* 1970;80:223–243.
25. Morgan WC. Tympanosclerosis. *Laryngoscope* 1977;87:1821–1825.
26. Bhaye MM, Schachern PA, Morizono T, Paparella MM. Pathogenesis of tympanosclerosis. *Otolaryngol Head Neck Surg* 1993;109:413–420.
27. Druss J. Labyrinthitis secondary to meningococcic meningitis: a clinical and histopathologic study. *Arch Otolaryngol* 1936;24:19–28.
28. Perlman HB, Lindsay JR. Relations of the internal ear spaces to the meninges. *Arch Otolaryngol* 1939;29:12–23.
29. Paparella MM, Sugiuva S. The pathology of suppurative labyrinthitis. *Ann Otol Rhinol Laryngol* 1967;76:554–586.
30. Dodge PR, Davis H, Feigin RD, et al. Prospective evaluation of hearing impairment as a sequela of acute bacterial meningitis. *N Engl J Med* 1984;311:869–874.
31. Brodie HA, Thompson TC, Vassilian L, Lee BN. Induction of labyrinthitis ossificans after pneumococcal meningitis: an animal model. *Otolaryngol Head Neck Surg* 1998;118:15–21.
32. Friedmann I. Epidermoid cholesteatoma and cholesterol granuloma of the ear. *Lancet* 1957;1:639–646.
33. Friedmann I. Epidermoid cholesteatoma and cholesterol granuloma. *Ann Otol Rhinol Laryngol* 1959;69:57–79.
34. Dota T, Nakamura K, Saheki M, Sasaki Y. Cholesterol granuloma.

Experimental observations. *Ann Otol Rhinol Laryngol* 1963;72: 346–356.

35. Paparella MM, Lim DJ. Pathogenesis and pathology of "idiopathic" blue ear drum. *Arch Otolaryngol* 1967;85:249–258.

36. Sheehy JL, Linthicum FH Jr. Chronic serous mastoiditis, idiopathic hemotympanum and cholesterol granuloma of the mastoid. *Laryngoscope* 1969;79:1189–1217.

37. Paparella MM, Oda M, Hiraide F, Brady D. Pathology of sensorineural hearing loss in otitis media. *Ann Otol Rhinol Laryngol* 1972;81: 632–647.

38. Paparella MM. Quiet labyrinthine complications from otitis media. *J Laryngol Otol* 1983;8[Suppl]:53–58.

39. Paparella MM, Morizono T, Le CT, et al. Sensorineural hearing loss in otitis media. *Ann Otol Rhinol Laryngol* 1984;93:623–629.

40. Parella MM, Coycoolea MC, Schachern PA, Sajjadi H. Current clinical and pathological features of round window diseases. *Laryngoscope* 1987;97:1151–1160.

41. Paparella MM, Brady DR. Sensorineural hearing loss in chronic otitis media and mastoiditis. *Trans Am Acad Ophthalmol Otolaryngol* 1970; 74:108–115.

42. Levine BA, Shelton C, Berliner KI, Sheehey JL. Sensorineural loss in chronic otitis media. Is it clinically significant? *Arch Otolaryngol Head Neck Surg* 1989;115:814–816.

43. Noordzij JP, Dobson EE, Ruth RA, Arts AA, Lambert PR. Chronic otitis media and sensorineural hearing loss: is there a clinically significant relation? *Am J Otol* 1995;16:420–423.

44. Walby AP, Barrera A, Schuknecht HF. Cochlear pathology in chronic suppurative otitis media. *Ann Otol Rhinol Laryngol* 1983;92[Suppl]: 13–15.

45. Lundman L, Santi PA, Morizono T, Harada T, Juhn SK, Bagger-Sjoback D. Inner ear damage and passage through the round window membrane of pseudomonas aeruginosa exotoxin A in a chinchilla model. *Ann Otol Rhinol Laryngol* 1992;101:437–444.

46. Leyden JJ, Kligman AM. Contact dermatitis to neomycin sulfate. *JAMA* 1979;242:1276–1278.

47. Brummett RE, Harris RF, Lingren JA. Detection of ototoxicity from drugs applied topically to the middle ear space. *Laryngoscope* 1976; 86:1177–1187.

48. Wright CG, Meyerhoff WL, Halama AR. Ototoxicity of neomycin and polymyxin B following middle ear application in the chinchilla and baboon. *Am J Otol* 1987;8:495–499.

49. Wright CG, Salama AR, Meyerhoff WL. Ototoxicity of an ototopical preparation in a primate. *Am J Otol* 1987;8:56–60.

50. Lundy LB, Graham MD. Ototoxicity and ototopical medications: a survey of otolaryngologists. *Am J Otol* 1993;14:141–146.

51. Sahni RS, Paparella MM, Schachern PA, Coycoolea MV, Le CT. Thickness of the human round window membrane in different forms of otitis media. *Arch Otolaryngol Head Neck Surg* 1987;110:630–634.

52. Schachern PA, Paparella MM, Duvall AJ III, Choo YB. The human round window. *Arch Otolaryngol* 1984;110:15–21.

53. John SK, Hamaguchi Y, Coycoolea M. Review of round window membrane permeability. *Acta Otolaryngol Suppl (Stockh)* 1988;457: 43–48.

54. Palva T, Palva A, Karja T. Tuberculous otitis media. *J Laryngol Otol* 1973;87:253–256.

55. Samuel J, Fernandes CMC. Tuberculous mastoiditis. *Am Otol Rhinol Laryngol* 1986;95:264–266.

56. Friedmann I. *Pathology of the ear.* Oxford, UK: Blackwell Scientific Publications, 1974:55–59.

57. Austin WK, Lockey MW. Mycobacterium fortuitum mastoiditis. *Arch Otolaryngol* 1976;102:558–560.

58. Neitch SM, Sydnor JB, Schleupner CJ. Mycobacterium fortuitum as a cause of mastoiditis and wound infection. *Arch Otolaryngol* 1982; 108:11–14.

59. Wardrop PA, Pillsbury HC III. Mycobacterium avium acute mastoiditis. *Arch Otolaryngol* 1984;110:686–687.

60. Lowry PW, Jarvis WR, Oberle AD, et al. Mycobacterium chelonae causing otitis media in an ear-nose-and-throat practice. *N Engl J Med* 1988;319:978–982.

61. Franklin DJ, Starke JR, Brady MT, Brown BA, Wallace RJ Jr. Chronic otitis media after tympanostomy tube placement caused by mycobacterium abscessus. A new clinical entity. *Am J Otol* 1994;15:313–320.

62. Swenson JM, Wallace RJ Jr, Silcox VA, Thornsberry C. Antimicrobial susceptibility of five subgroups of mycobacterium fortuitum and

mycobacterium chelonae. *Antimicrob Agents Chemother* 1985;28: 807–811.

63. Bradley PJ. Wegener's granulomatosis of the ear. *J Laryngol Otol* 1983;97:623–626.

64. Illum P, Thorling K. Otologic manifestations of Wegener's granulomatosis. *Laryngoscope* 1982;92:801–804.

65. Nicklasson B, Stangeland N. Wegener's granulomatosis presenting as otitis media. *J Laryngol Otol* 1982;96:277–280.

66. Macias JD, Wackym PA, McCabe BF. Early diagnosis of otologic Wegener's granulomatosis using the serologic marker C-ANCA. *Ann Otol Rhinol Laryngol* 1993;102:337–341.

67. McCaffrey TV, McDonald TJ, Facer GW, DeRemee RA. Otologic manifestations of Wegener's granulomatosis. *Otolaryngol Head Neck Surg* 1980;88:586–593.

68. Dagum P, Roberson JB Jr. Otologic Wegener's granulomatosis with facial nerve palsy. *Ann Otol Rhinol Laryngol* 1998;107:555–559.

69. Kornblut AD, Wolff SM, Fauci AS. Ear disease in patients with Wegener's granulomatosis. *Laryngoscope* 1982;92:713–717.

70. Mousa J, Abou-Elhmd KA. Wegener's granulomatosis presenting as mastoiditis. *Ann Otol Rhinol Laryngol* 1998;107:560–563.

71. Luquamni R, Jubb R, Emery P, Reid A, Adu D. Inner ear deafness in Wegener's granulomatosis. *J Rheumatol* 1991;18:760–768.

72. Nishino H, Rubino FA, DeRemee RA, Swanson JW, Parisi JE. Neurologic involvement in Wegener's granulomatosis: an analysis of 324 consecutive patients at the Mayo Clinic. *Ann Neurol* 1993;33:4–9.

73. Kunn A. Das cholesteatom des Ohres. *Z Ohrenheilk* 1891;21: 231–251.

74. Goodhill V. Chronic otomastoiditis—diagnosis and management. In: Goodhill V, ed. *Ear diseases, deafness and dizziness.* Hagerstown, MD: Harper and Row Publishers, 1979:330–354.

75. Palva T, Karma P, Makinen J. The invasion theory in cholesteatoma and mastoid surgery. In: Sade J, ed. *Cholesteatoma and mastoid surgery.* Amsterdam: Kugler Publications, 1982:249–264.

76. Habermann J. Zur Entsehung des Cholesteatoms des Mittelohrs. *Arch Ohrenheilk* 1889;27:42–50.

77. Bezold F. Ueber das Cholesteatom des Mittelohres. *Z Ohrenheilk* 1890;21:252–271.

78. Ruedi L. Pathogenesis and treatment of cholesteatoma in chronic suppuration of the temporal bone. *Ann Otol Rhinol Laryngol* 1957;66: 283–296.

79. Van Blitterswik CA, Grote JJ. Cytokeratin in expression in cholesteatoma matrix, meatal epidermis, and middle ear epithelium: a preliminary report. *Acta Otolaryngol (Stockh)* 1988;105:529–532.

80. Sade J. Pathogenesis of attic cholesteatoma. *J R Soc Med* 1978;71: 716–732.

81. Sade J, Babiacki A, Pinkus G. The metaplastic and congenital origin of cholesteatoma. *Acta Otolaryngol* 1983;96:119–129.

82. Juers AL. Cholesteatoma genesis. *Arch Otolaryngol* 1965;81:5–8.

83. Draper WL. Secretory otitis media in children: a study of 540 children. *Laryngoscope* 1967;77:636–653.

84. Aberg B, Edstrom S, Bagger-Sjoback D, Kindblom LG. Morphologic development of experimental cholesteatoma. *Arch Otolaryngol Head Neck Surg* 1993;119:272–275.

85. El Seifi A. Sequelae of otitis media with effusion (OME). Incidence and management. In: Myers E, ed. *New dimension in otorhinolaryngology head and neck surgery, volume 3.* Amsterdam: Elsevier Science Publishers B.V., 1985:279–282.

86. Iwanaga M, Yamamoto E, Fukumoto M. Cathepsin activity in cholesteatoma. *Ann Otol Rhinol Laryngol* 1985;94:309–312.

87. Grote JJ, Bakker A, Hesseling SC, Van Blitterswick CA. Tympanic membrane structure during a staphylococcus aureus induced middle ear infection. *Acta Otolaryngol* 1984;107:225–234.

88. Yuasa R, Kaneko Y, Takasaka T, Imo Y, Tomioka S, Hanajima T. The significance of keratinization in the mechanism of bone destruction in cholesteatoma. In: Sade J, ed. *Cholesteatoma and mastoid surgery.* Amsterdam: Kugler Publications, 1982:419–427.

89. Thomsen J, Jogensen MB, Bretlaw P, Kristensen HK. Bone resorption in chronic otitis media. A histological and ultrastructural study. II Cholesteatoma. *J Laryngol Otol* 1974;88:932–992.

90. Kaneko Y, Yuasa R, Yukiko Y, Shinkawa H, Rokugo M, Tomioka S. Bone destruction due to the rupture of a cholesteatoma sac: a pathogenesis of bone destruction in aural cholesteatoma. *Laryngoscope* 1980;90:1865–1871.

91. Moriyama H, Honda Y, Huang CC, Abramson M. Bone resorption in

cholesteatoma: epithelial mesenchymal cell interaction and collagenase production. *Laryngoscope* 1987;97:854–859.

92. Chole RA, McGinn MD, Tinging SP. Pressure induced bone resorption in the middle ear. *Ann Otol Rhinol Laryngol* 1985;94:165–170.

93. Orisek BS, Chole RA. Pressure exerted by experimental cholesteatomas. *Arch Otolaryngol Head Neck Surg* 1987;113:386–391.

94. Macri J, Chole RA. Bone resorption in cholesteatoma: the effects of implanted barriers. *Otolaryngol Head Neck Surg* 1985;93:3–17.

95. Chole RA. Osteoclasts in chronic otitis media, cholesteatoma and otosclerosis. *Ann Otol Rhinol Laryngol* 1988;97:661–666.

96. Chole RA. Differential osteoclast activation in endochondral and intramembranous bone. *Ann Otol Rhinol Laryngol* 1993;102:616–619.

97. Chole RA. Cellular and subcellular events in human and experimental cholesteatomas: the role of osteoclasts. *Laryngoscope* 1984;94:76–95.

98. Thomsen J. Bone resorption in chronic otitis media: the role of cholesteatoma, a must or an adjunct? *Clin Otolaryngol* 1981;6:179–186.

99. Thomsen J, Tos M, Nielsen M, Balsler Jorgensen M. Bone destruction in inflammatory diseases of the ear. In: Sade J, ed. *Cholesteatoma and mastoid surgery. Proceedings of the Second International Conference.* Amsterdam: Kugler Publications, 1982:397–411.

100. Proctor B. The development of the middle ear spaces and their surgical significance. *J Laryngol Otol* 1964;78:631–648.

101. Onal K, Van Haastert RM, Grote JJ. Structural variations of the supratubal recess: the anterior epitympanic space. *Am J Otol* 1997;18:317–321.

102. Horn KL, Brackmann DE, Luxford WM. The supratubal recess in cholesteatoma surgery. *Ann Otol Rhinol Laryngol* 1986;95:12–15.

103. Glasscock ME, Dickins JRE, Wiet R. Cholesteatoma in children. *Laryngoscope* 1981;91:1743–1753.

104. Sheehy JL. Cholesteatoma surgery in children. *Am J Otol* 1985;6:170–172.

105. Eldestein DR, Parisier SC, Abuja GS, et al. Cholesteatoma in the pediatric age group. *Ann Otol Rhinol Laryngol* 1988;97:23–29.

106. Cruz OLM, Takenti M, Caldas Neto S, Minitia M. Clinical and surgical aspects of cholesteatomas in children. *ENT Monthly* 1990;69:530–536.

107. Stern SJ, Fazekas-May M. Cholesteatoma in the pediatric population: prognostic indicators for surgical decision making. *Laryngoscope* 1992;102:1349–1352.

108. Mutlu C, Krahaba A, Saleh E, et al. Surgical treatment of cholesteatoma in children. *Otolaryngol Head Neck Surg* 1995;113:56–60.

109. Sanna M, Zini C, Scandellari R, Jemmi G. Residual and recurrent cholesteatoma in closed tympanoplasty. *Am J Otol* 1984;5:277–282.

110. Kinney SE. Intact canal wall tympanoplasty with mastoidectomy for cholesteatoma: long term follow up. *Laryngoscope* 1988;98:1190–1194.

111. Schuring AG, Lippy WH, Rizer RM, Schuring LT. Staging for cholesteatoma in the child, adolescent and adult. *Ann Otol Rhinol Laryngol* 1990;99:256–260.

112. Brackmann DE. Tympanoplasty with mastoidectomy: canal wall up procedures. *Am J Otol* 1993;14:380–382.

113. Derlacki EL, Clemis JD. Congenital cholesteatoma of the middle ear and mastoid. *Ann Otol Rhinol Laryngol* 1965;74:706–727.

114. Cawthorne T. Congenital cholesteatoma. *Arch Otolaryngol* 1963;78:40–41.

115. Teed RW. Cholesteatoma verum tympani (its relationship to the first epibranchial placode). *Arch Otolaryngol* 1936;24:455–474.

116. Michaels L. An epidermoid formation in the development of the middle ear: possible source of cholesteatoma. *J Otolaryngol* 1986;15:169–174.

117. Michaels L. Origin of congenital cholesteatoma from a normally occurring epidermoid rest in the developing middle ear. *Int J Pediatr Otolaryngol* 1988;15:51–65.

118. Michaels L. Biology of cholesteatoma. *Otolaryngol Clin North Am* 1989;22:869–881.

119. Parisier SC, Weiss MH. Recidivism in congenital cholesteatoma surgery. *ENT J* 1991;70:362–364.

120. Friedberg J. Congenital cholesteatoma. *Laryngoscope* 1994;104[Suppl 104]:1–24.

121. Zappia JJ, Wiet RJ. Congenital cholesteatoma. *Arch Otolaryngol Head Neck Surg* 1995;121:19–22.

122. Nager GT. Epidermoids involving the temporal bone: clinical, radiological and pathological aspects. *Laryngoscope* 1975;85[Suppl 2]:1–22.

123. Fisch V. Congenital cholesteatoma of the supralabyrinthine region. *Clin Otolaryngol* 1978;3:369–376.

The Ear: Comprehensive Otology,
edited by R. F. Canalis and P. R. Lambert.
Lippincott Williams & Wilkins, Philadelphia © 2000.

CHAPTER 26

Complications of Chronic Otitis Media

George T. Hashisaki

Overview
   Extracranial and Extratemporal Complications
   Intratemporal Complications

Intracranial Complications
Summary

Chronic otitis media (COM) is a common otologic condition. Although it does not occur as frequently as acute otitis media (AOM), COM remains a persistent and perplexing medical problem.

COM describes a condition of chronic infection and otorrhea through a tympanic membrane perforation. According to the Otitis Media Panel on Definition and Classification (1), this chronicity distinguishes the condition from AOM, otitis media with effusion, and a dry tympanic membrane perforation without otorrhea. The chronic infection involves the mucosa of the middle ear and aerated spaces of the temporal bone.

It is a frustrating condition for the patient, given the frequent, often foul-smelling otorrhea, intermittent pain, and hearing loss. It is a frustrating condition for the physician as well, with the difficulty in achieving a cure, the risks associated with therapy, and the ever-present specter of a serious complication. These complications are the content of this chapter.

OVERVIEW

The development of a complication of COM is dependent on the concurrent interplay of several factors. Neely organized these factors into five categories: (a) bacteriology, (b) antimicrobial therapy, (c) host resistance, (d) anatomic barriers, and (e) drainage (2). The first two categories are intertwined by microbiology. The latter three categories are factors related to the host.

The bacteriology of COM differs from that of AOM in several respects. *Staphylococcus aureus* and *Pseudomonas*

aeruginosa are more common in COM, replacing the gram-positive *Streptococcus pneumoniae* and gram-negative *Haemophilus influenzae* and *Moraxella catarrhalis* of AOM (3). In addition, anaerobic bacteria are more common in COM. With careful technique, anaerobic species such as *Bacteroides, Peptococcus,* and *Peptostreptococcus* can be cultured from ears with COM (4). The microenvironment of low oxygen tension, fluid-filled spaces, and granulation tissue promotes the growth of anaerobic bacteria.

Antimicrobial therapy must address these differences in bacteriology. Multidrug therapy is necessary to provide coverage for the possible combinations of organisms. Tissue delivery of antimicrobials may be impaired in COM, and resisted by granulation tissue and fluid-filled air cells. The same factors that promote bacterial growth serve to restrict antimicrobial penetration.

Host-related factors of resistance to infection, anatomic barriers, and drainage of pneumatized spaces are important issues in COM. Host resistance to infection can be affected by chronic disease, malnutrition, impaired immune function, or medications. Diabetes mellitus is a classic example of impaired host resistance, with alterations in microcirculation and impaired immune function. The anatomy of the host temporal bone impacts the spread of infection. Variations in bone thickness, natural apertures, and vascular anatomy can create potential pathways for propagation of disease. Pneumatized spaces in the temporal bone also create physiologic "dead" space. If clearance of fluid or foreign substances is impaired, the air cells of the temporal bone can become the nidus of infection, resulting in multiple small abscesses.

Complications of COM can be divided into three categories on an anatomic basis: extratemporal extracranial, intratemporal, and intracranial. These three categories

G. T. Hashisaki: Department of Otolaryngology–Head and Neck Surgery, University of Virginia Medical Center, Charlottesville, Virginia 22908

will be addressed with regard to affecting conditions, diagnosis, and treatment.

Extracranial and Extratemporal Complications

- Bezold abscess
- Subperiosteal abscess.

Extracranial and extratemporal complications of COM are uncommon and usually represent a mastoid abscess that has escaped the confines of the temporal bone into the surrounding soft tissues. These conditions are seen more commonly as complications of AOM, but they may occur with COM.

Bezold Abscess

A Bezold abscess occurs when a purulent mastoiditis erodes the tip of the mastoid bone and infects the soft tissue of the neck, deep to the sternocleidomastoid muscle. The abscess presents as a bulge high in the neck, displacing the sternocleidomastoid muscle. Left uncontrolled, the abscess can extend inferiorly down to the carotid sheath.

Diagnosis

With an indolent ear infection, the presenting symptom may be the sudden presence of a mass in the neck. Usually, the neck mass will be accompanied by fever, neck discomfort or stiffness, and otorrhea. The mass high in the neck must be distinguished from lymphadenopathy, a parotid mass or abscess, or an infected neck cyst. Needle aspiration will often yield pus, corroborating the diagnosis of an abscess but not the exact cause.

A contrast-enhanced computed tomographic (CT) scan of the neck and mastoid will give clues. Loss of bony trabeculae in the mastoid as seen with coalescent mastoiditis may be present. The abscess mass itself will be obvious, with peripheral contrast enhancement. The overlying soft tissue of the neck will show edema. By imaging the mastoid tip region, one may find evidence of bone dehiscence adjacent to the abscess mass.

Treatment

As with other neck abscesses, the treatment is drainage. A cortical mastoidectomy is indicated, given the mastoid infection. From the mastoid, the dehiscence into the neck soft tissue can be found. The abscess cavity should be evacuated and an external drain placed in a dependent position, exiting via the neck. The mastoid antrum requires drainage also. The drainage path may be through the aditus and epitympanum to the middle ear or the facial recess to the posterior mesotympanum. Middle ear drainage can be accomplished with a tympanostomy tube or by the eustachian tube, if patent. Cultures obtained at the time of surgery can direct adjunctive antimicrobial therapy.

Subperiosteal Abscess

Another route of escape for a coalescent mastoiditis is through the cortex of the mastoid bone. Bone erosion, via osteitis or necrosis, leads to a dehiscence into the postauricular soft tissue. A mass behind the ear, displacing the auricle anteriorly, is the classic sign. Symptoms of fever, pain, and otorrhea may precede the appearance of the postauricular mass. The abscess can suppurate via the postauricular skin.

Diagnosis

The differential diagnosis includes lymphadenopathy, suppurative lymphadenitis, or an infected cyst. A prominent auricle, anteriorly displaced, is a sign visible from across the exam room. Coupled with a tender, fluctuant mass over the mastoid and surrounding erythematous skin, the diagnosis of subperiosteal abscess is almost certain.

A contrast-enhanced CT scan will show the dehiscence in the mastoid cortex and the abscess mass. In addition, loss of bony septation in the mastoid air cells can be demonstrated.

Treatment

The mastoid infection requires drainage. If the abscess has not suppurated, then a standard postauricular incision and cortical mastoidectomy are performed. If suppuration has occurred, then the postauricular incision may be modified to incorporate the site of suppuration. After achieving effective drainage of the mastoid infection, the site of suppuration can be addressed. The surrounding soft tissue may be necrotic and thus require debridement. Whether or not to suture close that portion of the incision is left to the discretion of the surgeon.

Intratemporal Complications

- Mastoiditis
- Labyrinthitis
- Sensorineural hearing loss
- Petrous apicitis (petrositis)
- Facial paralysis
- Cholesteatoma
- Labyrinthine fistula.

Mastoiditis

Mastoid infection as a complication of COM can take one of two forms—acute coalescent mastoiditis or chronic mastoiditis with osteitis. Acute coalescent mastoiditis is more commonly associated with AOM, but it can occur as a complication of COM. Coalescent mastoiditis occurs in a pneumatized or partially pneumatized mastoid.

Acute coalescent mastoiditis can occur in an ear with COM. Obstruction of the aditus with cholesteatoma, granulation tissue, or hypertrophic mucosa creates a sealed space in the mastoid antrum. Acute infection of fluid in this space, an acute mastoiditis, can lead to bone necrosis and erosion. Osteolysis of the septae of the mastoid air cells produces a cavity of purulent material. With further breakdown of bone, the potential exists for the infection to escape the confines of the temporal bone. Erosion superficially (or laterally) can produce a Bezold abscess or subperiosteal abscess. Erosion medially leads to an intracranial complication.

Chronic mastoiditis may result from an acute mastoiditis, AOM, or COM. Changes in the mucosal lining of the mastoid air cells, production of an exudate, migration of inflammatory cells, and alteration of bone may occur.

The mucosa of the middle ear and mastoid undergoes metaplasia, with increased numbers of goblet cells. Granulation tissue filled with inflammatory cells replaces the air spaces of the mastoid and middle ear. With alterations in vascular supply, differential activation of osteoclasts versus osteoblasts, and active host inflammatory responses, bone erosion occurs (5). Areas of osteitis and osteomyelitis can exist in close proximity.

Diagnosis

Coalescent mastoiditis can be diagnosed by CT scan, with loss of septation between air cells of the mastoid. Chronic mastoiditis may not have any significant CT abnormalities and is often a clinical diagnosis. As a clinical diagnosis, it is one easily overlooked (6). Magnetic resonance imaging (MRI) will show regions of nonspecific bright signal, consistent with inflammation. Other intracranial complications may be detected (Fig. 1).

Treatment

Mastoidectomy is the surgical treatment for both coalescent mastoiditis and chronic mastoiditis. Necrotic bone or areas of osteitis and osteomyelitis must be removed.

Labyrinthitis

Inflammation of the labyrinth produces vestibular and auditory symptoms. COM can progress to a suppurative labyrinthitis, a purulent infection of the labyrinth, or a serous labyrinthitis. A suppurative labyrinthitis occurs after bacteria infiltrate the fluid space of the labyrinth from the middle ear. Naturally occurring dehiscences, temporal bone fractures, or inflammatory fistulas provide the access to the labyrinthine fluids.

Suppurative labyrinthitis acutely produces vertigo and hearing loss. During the acute phase of inflammation, vertigo is a product of vestibular stimulation, but as the infection continues, vestibular end organ damage occurs. Unilateral vestibular weakness or loss results. During the phase of central compensation, imbalance or unsteadiness may be present. As central vestibular compensation

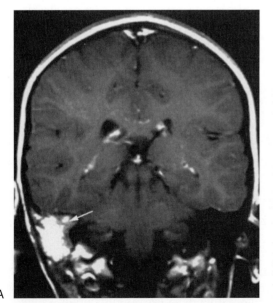 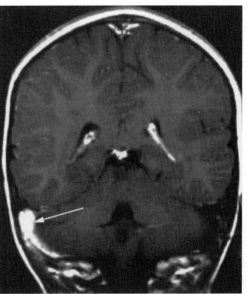

A   B

FIG. 1. A: Mastoiditis. A coronal T1-weighted magnetic resonance image, with gadolinium diethylene-triamine pentaacetic acid, shows high signal intensity in the mastoid air cells (*arrow*) on the right side. This finding may be seen with acute or chronic mastoiditis. **B:** Sigmoid sinus thrombosis in the same patient. The *arrow* indicates an area of high signal intensity in the sigmoid sinus on the right side. Normally, there should be an absence of signal in vascular structures, due to the rapid flow of blood. Sigmoid sinus thrombosis has occurred adjacent to the inflamed mastoid air cells.

occurs, the patient's balance usually recovers well. However, during severe perturbations of the vestibular system, such as with a rapid head rotation, patients will experience a brief sensation of vertigo.

The hearing loss associated with suppurative labyrinthitis usually is permanent. Damage to the organ of Corti produces a sensory hearing loss. Histologically, suppurative labyrinthitis causes varying degrees of damage, ranging from alterations in the stereocilia of hair cells to complete loss of the organ of Corti to labyrinthitis ossificans (7).

A serous labyrinthitis occurs from inflammation, rather than infection, in the labyrinth. Potential mediators of this response include bacterial toxins or inflammatory mediators. The inflammatory reaction in the labyrinth produces vertigo and sensory hearing loss. Inflammatory cells rather than bacteria are found in the labyrinthine fluids. The round window or oval window membranes are the presumed pathways for entry into the perilymph fluid.

Diagnosis

In the face of COM, there are no confirmatory tests that will establish a diagnosis of suppurative or serous labyrinthitis. The clinical picture of vertigo and sensorineural hearing loss is presumptive evidence for a labyrinthitis. A diagnosis of serous labyrinthitis can be made retrospectively if there is some recovery of hearing or vestibular function.

Treatment

During the acute phase of vertigo and hearing loss, supportive measures such as vestibular suppressants may relieve some of the dizziness and nausea. Intravenous antimicrobial therapy directed against the common pathogens seen in COM may limit the labyrinthine injury. Surgical therapy of the COM may be necessary.

Sensorineural Hearing Loss

Sensorineural hearing loss can occur as a secondary effect from serous or suppurative labyrinthitis, labyrinthine fistulas, or cholesteatoma invading the labyrinth.

Controversy exists as to whether or not COM alone, in the absence of any of the causes discussed, can produce a sensorineural hearing loss. Paparella et al. (8) noted greater than 10-dB sensorineural losses, especially in the higher frequencies in patients with COM. Other studies have not found a clinically significant correlation between sensorineural hearing loss and COM (9,10). Tos (11) found a 4% incidence of high-frequency hearing loss or anakusis in 229 cases of granulating otitis. It is likely that the chronic infection and inflammation associated with COM can lead to some sensory hearing loss; the question remains at to whether or not it is a clinically significant degree of loss.

Passage via the round window membrane is the proposed route of entry into the inner ear. Bacterial toxins or inflammatory mediators are potential causative agents of damage to the inner ear.

Diagnosis

Audiograms at regular intervals can detect changes in hearing thresholds. Bone conduction thresholds are imperative with adequate masking of the nontest ear.

Treatment

Other than addressing the problem of the underlying COM or cholesteatoma, there is no proven treatment for the sensory hearing loss. Prevention, thus, is the goal. Early and effective treatment of the cholesteatoma or COM will achieve this goal.

Petrous Apicitis

The petrous apex is the most medial and anterior portion of the temporal bone, positioned anterior to the otic capsule. The internal carotid artery is one of the prominent features of this region. In the 30% of temporal bones with pneumatization of the petrous apex, the carotid artery divides the air cell tracts into peritubal and apical portions. These air cells connect to the middle ear or mastoid spaces via narrow tracts adjacent to the otic capsule.

Infections of the middle ear and mastoid spaces can extend to and involve the petrous apex air cells. Given the central location of the petrous apex and its proximity to the posterior and middle cranial fossae, chronic petrositis or petrous apicitis often is associated with intracranial complications such as meningitis, epidural abscess, dural venous sinus thrombosis, or brain abscess.

The classic triad of deep ear or retroorbital pain, aural discharge, and ipsilateral abducens nerve palsy describes Gradenigo's syndrome. The aural discharge stems from the chronic ear infection, the deep pain arises from irritation of the trigeminal nerve at the gasserian ganglion, and the lateral rectus palsy originates from inflammation of the abducens nerve as it courses inferior to the petroclinoid ligament (Dorello's canal). The trigeminal nerve ganglion and the petroclinoid ligament are positioned immediately adjacent to the petrous apex.

Diagnosis

Deep pain in the distribution of the trigeminal nerve in the setting of COM is an important symptom. A lateral rectus palsy is rarely seen with petrous apicitis and is not pathognomonic for the condition. The clinical scenario and a temporal bone CT scan should enable one to make the diagnosis. In addition, a diligent search for an intracranial complication may require a lumbar puncture or MRI of the brain. As a clinical aside, persistent otorrhea following a mastoidectomy for COM can indicate an attendant petrous apicitis.

Treatment

Initial treatment consists of intravenous antimicrobials directed against the most likely pathogens. In COM, *S. aureus, Proteus* species, other gram-negative rods, and anaerobic bacteria predominate. Surgical drainage often is necessary, allowing cultures to be obtained.

If hearing is present in the affected ear, then the surgical approach should leave the otic capsule intact. Multiple approaches may be necessary to insure adequate postoperative drainage of the petrous apex. Retrolabyrinthine, infralabyrinthine, infracochlear, and subarcuate approaches can gain access to the petrous apex. None of these approaches affords particularly wide exposure to the air cells of the petrous apex, thus the potential need for more than one drainage path.

For cases with absent hearing in the affected ear, more direct approaches via a translabyrinthine or transcochlear route are possible. These two approaches have two disadvantages—loss of vestibular function in the affected ear and potential contamination of the cerebrospinal fluid (CSF) with bacteria. Otherwise, they can afford greater access to the petrous apex than the approaches preserving the otic capsule.

Facial Paralysis

Because of the long course of the fallopian canal through the temporal bone, the facial nerve is commonly affected by disease processes in the temporal bone. COM is no exception. The infection and inflammatory reaction associated with COM can affect the facial nerve, producing facial paresis or paralysis. This complication is more commonly seen in COM with cholesteatoma, but it can occur with COM alone.

Although protected by epineurium and the bone of the fallopian canal, the facial nerve fibers are subject to infection or inflammation with breaches in these defenses. Bony dehiscences in the fallopian occur naturally in 50% of ears. Erosion of the fallopian canal can occur with cholesteatoma or with reactive osteitis from COM. Presumably, the inflammatory process of cholesteatoma or COM extends to the nerve, inducing edema and nerve fiber compression. Facial paresis can result, with progression to facial paralysis.

Diagnosis

The onset of facial paresis or paralysis ipsilateral to an ear afflicted with COM or cholesteatoma gives an obvious diagnosis. However, the differential diagnoses for an acute facial palsy should be considered. A comprehensive head and neck examination is mandatory. Meanwhile, medical therapy consisting of intravenous antimicrobials directed against the pathogens of COM is instituted. Concurrent corticosteroids may be administered.

Treatment

Given no other confounding diagnoses, surgical treatment of the inflammatory process is indicated. A complete mastoidectomy with identification of the facial nerve is performed. The tympanic segment and second genu of the facial nerve are the most common regions involved by cholesteatoma (12,13). The fallopian canal is examined for evidence of overlying granulation tissue or bony dehiscence. Proximal and distal bone decompression of the facial nerve is performed. The epineurium is left intact. If infection has clearly penetrated the nerve, the epineurium is incised. In the rare event that the infectious process invades the nerve, accompanied by necrosis, the affected segment is resected. Nerve grafting should be delayed until the infection has been treated.

Cholesteatoma

Cholesteatoma as a complication of COM is addressed elsewhere in this textbook (see Chapters 25 and 27).

Labyrinthine Fistula

One of the more unsettling intratemporal complications of COM and cholesteatoma is a labyrinthine fistula. When auditory and vestibular functions are present in an ear with a labyrinthine fistula, the knowledge that only a few cell layers seal off the inner ear can be intimidating. The terminology of labyrinthine fistula includes the condition of bone erosion and exposure of the endosteal membrane of the inner ear, as well as a true fistula into the fluid compartment of the inner ear (Fig. 2).

Far and away, most labyrinthine fistulas are associated with cholesteatoma, but COM alone can lead to bone erosion (14). The granulomatous, inflammatory process associated with COM can produce resorption osteitis, with increased osteoclastic activity.

With cholesteatoma, labyrinthine fistulas occur in 5% to 10% of cases (11,15–17). The lateral semicircular canal is the most common location for fistulas (90%), but the cochlea may be eroded at the oval window or promontory in a small percentage of cases (16–20). Bone erosion can occur via two mechanisms: osteolysis or resorptive osteitis. With osteolysis, bone resorption is initiated by pressure from the cholesteatoma or by activated mediators from the cholesteatoma matrix. Resorptive osteitis occurs at the interface of active granulation tissue and underlying bone. There is an intense inflammatory response at this location leading to bone resorption (14).

Symptoms from labyrinthine fistulas depend, obviously, on the severity of the fistula. Bone erosion leading

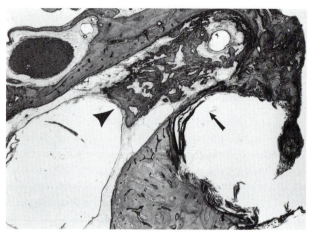

FIG. 2. Lateral semicircular canal fistula. This photomicrograph documents a fistula into the lateral semicircular canal (*arrow*). Squamous epithelial debris lines the margin of the cholesteatoma. This is likely an old fistula, as bone has formed within the lumen of the semicircular canal (*arrowhead*). Osteoneogenesis can occur in response to the inflammatory changes within the semicircular canals or cochlea, producing labyrinthitis ossificans.

to a "blue-lined" semicircular canal may be asymptomatic, except for occasional vertigo due to changes in air pressure or temperature. Exposure of the membranous labyrinth usually produces more symptoms of episodic vertigo and possibly hearing loss. With violation of the perilymph, a profound sensory hearing loss ensues, accompanied by severe vertigo. The hearing loss is not recoverable. With loss of vestibular function in the ear, symptoms of vertigo gradually abate as central vestibular compensation occurs.

Diagnosis

With symptoms of intermittent or constant vertigo in the setting of COM or cholesteatoma, suspicion for a labyrinthine fistula is high. In the absence of these symptoms, a fistula may not be suspected. The fistula test performed with a pneumatic otoscope in the office may be abnormal in only 50% of patients with labyrinthine fistula. Therefore, the dictum that every chronic ear surgery should be approached as if there were a fistula is sound advice.

A noncontrast-enhanced temporal bone CT scan may show evidence of a labyrinthine fistula, with loss of the otic capsule bone. Due to partial volume effects, a fistula may be erroneously diagnosed on the CT scan. Also, unless the scan sequence encompasses thin-section, overlapping images, small fistulas can be overlooked. With these caveats in mind, CT scanning can provide some useful information preoperatively. Some otologic surgeons believe, however, that unless an intracranial complication is suspected, a CT scan of the temporal bone is an unnecessary preoperative step. Their approach to

surgery would be unchanged by the results of the CT scan, unless an intracranial complication were found.

Treatment

Surgical intervention is the usual treatment for a labyrinthine fistula. The manner of surgical intervention depends on the experiences of the operator. There are controversies as to the optimal management of labyrinthine fistula due to COM or cholesteatoma.

Intraoperative management of a labyrinthine fistula can range from exteriorizing cholesteatoma matrix overlying a fistula to careful removal of cholesteatoma matrix. Performing a radical mastoidectomy or canal-wall-down mastoidectomy with tympanoplasty and leaving cholesteatoma matrix undisturbed on the horizontal semicircular canal is a prudent operation. Another surgical option is to perform the cholesteatoma removal in two stages. At the first operation, the cholesteatoma matrix is left in place overlying the fistula. If the anatomy is favorable, the canal wall may be left intact. At the second operation performed 9 to 12 months later, the cholesteatoma is often circumscribed in its extent and easily removed.

A third surgical option is to carefully remove the cholesteatoma matrix at the primary operation. The fistula can be closed with soft tissue, fibrin glue, or bone wax. Reports with limited numbers of patients have shown that this technique can preserve auditory function in a majority of cases. Rates of hearing preservation ranged from 58% to 100% (15–22).

Intracranial Complications

- Epidural abscess
- Lateral sinus thrombosis
- Otitic hydrocephalus
- Meningitis
- Brain abscess
- Subdural abscess.

Overview

Fortunately, intracranial complications of COM have become less common with improved access to medical care and medications. Broad spectrum antimicrobials have undoubtedly affected the nature of COM. In the pre-antibiotic era, intracranial complications occurred in 2% to 6% of COM cases (2,23). Although recent data are not available, a study published in 1962 documented that the incidence of intracranial complications decreased to 0.15% of cases during a period of antibiotics usage (24). Whether this reduction in the incidence rate is due solely to the advent of antibiotics is unclear, but it emphasizes the now rare occurrence of an intracranial complication.

The pathophysiology of intracranial complications of COM pertains to the complex interaction between microbiologic and host factors. With COM, the anatomic barriers to spread of infection are broken down. Periosteum, bone, blood vessels, the labyrinth, and dura can be penetrated by the inflammatory process. Virulent bacteria such as *Pseudomonas* and *Staphylococcus* can overwhelm host defenses once they gain access to the intracranial space.

Because direct extension of infection to intracranial structures may occur, bacteremia may not be present. Thus, circulating complement, one of the initial host defenses (25), is not able to activate the usual humoral cascade producing bacterial inactivation. Once bacteria gain access to intracranial structures, bacterial replication may proceed unimpeded until cell-mediated immunologic reactions are instituted. Exogenous cytokines such as interleukin 1β, interleukin 6, and tumor necrosis factor α induce a complex inflammatory response (26,27). The extent of disease will result from the complex interplay among bacterial virulence, host inflammatory response, anatomic barriers, and medical therapy.

Diagnosis

In treating COM, the possibility of an intracranial complication must be kept in mind. Symptoms and signs of an intracranial complication or impending crisis must be heeded. Changes from the usual symptoms of COM may herald one of these dreaded complications.

Intense otalgia, malodorous otorrhea, spiking fever, and headache are early symptoms and signs that may signal an intracranial complication. Altered mental status is a late sign, associated with an established intracranial complication (28). Other late signs or symptoms include seizures, aphasia, neck rigidity, and coma.

CT scans or MR images are critical in the evaluation of a potential intracranial complication. CT scans give accurate information regarding bony structures. With contrast enhancement, CT also demonstrates abnormalities such as abscesses, meningeal enhancement, and fluid collections. CT scanning units are widely available and scanning acquisition times are relatively short, making access for critical patients a minor problem. With short acquisition times, motion artifact is less likely to degrade image quality.

MR images are more sensitive in detecting extraaxial fluid collections, are better able to distinguish the extradural from subdural space, and are more sensitive in diagnosing parenchymal abnormalities (29). Venous magnetic resonance (MR) angiography has added a new dimension to the evaluation of blood flow in the dural sinuses, jugular bulb, cortical veins, and emissary veins (30). MR scans are free from bone artifact and have multiplanar imaging capability—issues that limit CT scans. However, MRI sequences have longer acquisition times and are subject to greater motion artifact than CT. Degradation of image quality due to patient movement is a per-

sisting problem, even as image acquisition times shorten with equipment improvements.

Epidural Abscess

Epidural abscesses from COM occur in proximity to the temporal bone. Chronic infection of the temporal bone produces an inflammatory process that extends via venous channels in the bone or by bone erosion to the epidural space. Reactive osteitis can result in bone erosion, even in the absence of cholesteatoma. The most common sites of extension are through the thin bone of the tegmen to the middle cranial fossa or through the bone adjacent to the sigmoid sinus and the posterior cranial fossa.

The epidural space is a potential space, created when the periosteum or outer dural layer is separated from the inner table of the cranial bone. The tough dura often will limit the spread of infection.

Not uncommonly, granulation tissue rather than pus occupies the epidural space. If the inflammatory process is interrupted with proper therapy, a purulent abscess may be averted.

Given the pathways of spread of COM to the intracranial spaces, other intracranial complications are frequently accompanied by a concomitant epidural abscess.

Diagnosis

Symptoms and signs are not specific to an epidural abscess. Symptoms arise from the underlying COM or an associated intracranial complication. A high index of suspicion is necessary to diagnosis an epidural abscess.

A contrast-enhanced CT scan or an MR image can diagnose an epidural abscess. MRI is more sensitive to early soft tissue changes associated with epidural disease (29). MRI with gadolinium can detect dural thickening and inflammation (31). Evidence of bone erosion can be detected with CT, utilizing axial and coronal scanning sequences. The area of the tegmen is best evaluated with the coronal images, and the sigmoid sinus and posterior fossa region with the axial images.

Treatment

Surgical exploration and drainage are necessary for adequate treatment. After completing a cortical mastoidectomy, the bone overlying the tegmen tympani, sigmoid sinus, and posterior fossa dura must be thinned, allowing visualization of the epidural space. Should granulation tissue or purulent fluid be discovered, bone removal should continue until noninflamed dura is encountered.

Lateral Sinus Thrombosis

The lateral and sigmoid sinuses are relatively unprotected structures situated adjacent to the inflammation of

COM. Direct extension of mastoid infection can occur secondary to bone erosion from osteitis or necrosis. Indirect extension can proceed via retrograde thrombophlebitis involving mastoid emissary veins. Infection in the perisinus tissue can induce the formation of a mural thrombus within the sinus lumen. Nonseptic or septic thrombophlebitis can propagate further intracranially along various dural venous sinuses or extracranially into the internal jugular vein.

Obstruction of venous drainage can produce elevated intracranial pressure and headache. Otitic hydrocephalus can complicate the course of lateral sinus thrombosis, leading to vision changes and abducens palsy. Septic emboli can disseminate the infectious process to distant body sites, and the constant bacteremia produces febrile episodes.

Retrograde thrombophlebitis can extend to the straight sinus and sagittal sinus via the confluens or torcula of Herophilus. The cavernous sinus can become involved via the superior or inferior petrosal sinuses (32).

The classic clinical picture—high, spiking fevers, headache, and active ear disease in a patient—is seldom encountered. The febrile course, modified by antibiotic therapy, may be more indolent. Neck stiffness or discomfort, especially near the insertion site of the ipsilateral sternocleidomastoid muscle, may be present. This symptom should be distinguished from the meningism producing Kernig's and Brudzinski's signs in bacterial meningitis.

Diagnosis

Clinical suspicion is the key element. As the symptoms and signs may be subtle, an inkling of concern should trigger further investigation. MRI and CT imaging can diagnose dural sinus thrombosis. Time-of-flight MR venography is a noninvasive and sensitive means of detecting sinus thrombosis (30,33). During the acute phase of thrombosis, the absence of flow signal produces a dramatic contrast to normal dural sinuses. In addition, after acquisition of MR venography images, routine spin-echo sequences can be obtained to assess for other intracranial complications (Figs. 3 and 4).

Contrast-enhanced CT scans can identify dural sinus thrombosis. A cross-sectional image of a dural sinus may exhibit the "delta" sign, a triangular rim of enhancement enclosing the low-intensity region of the thrombus. The absence of contrast material in a dural sinus is highly suggestive, but not diagnostic, of thrombosis (Fig. 5).

Treatment

Early institution of antibiotics and surgical exploration are the mainstays of therapy. A mastoidectomy is performed, exposing the sigmoid sinus. In a pediatric review, 53% of patients had epidural granulations or abscess, emphasizing the need for wide exploration (34). After

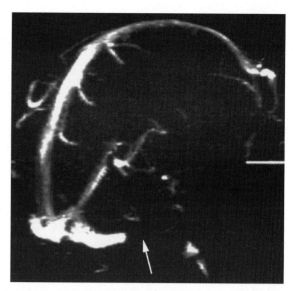

FIG. 3. Lateral sinus thrombosis. This magnetic resonance venogram (MRV) from a right oblique view demonstrates absent signal from the region of the right lateral sinus and adjoining sigmoid sinus, as indicated by the *arrow*. The confluens sinuum or torcular Herophili has a bright signal, abruptly ending at the site of lateral sinus thrombosis. Normally, vascular structures—in this case, the dural venous sinuses—have high signal intensity with magnetic resonance angiography or venography techniques.

exposing the sigmoid sinus, a needle may be used to aspirate the sinus. If free-flowing blood returns, then no additional surgery is needed. If no blood returns, then opening and draining the sinus are indicated. Several recent studies have shown good results with limited removal of blood clot and purulent material (35–38). Ligation of the internal jugular vein usually is not necessary. In the face

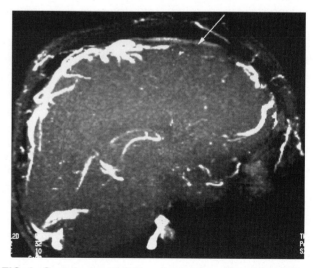

FIG. 4. Superior sagittal sinus thrombosis. On a lateral view, this magnetic resonance venogram has absent signal in the superior sagittal sinus (*arrow*), with collateral blood flow developing anterior and posterior to the site of thrombosis.

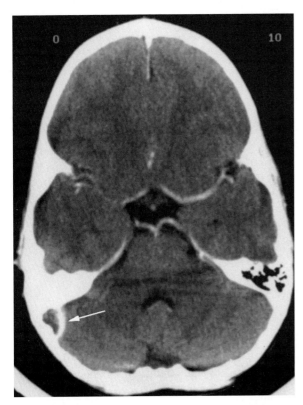

FIG. 5. Sigmoid sinus thrombosis. An axial computed tomographic scan with intravenous contrast finds the right mastoid is poorly aerated. The sigmoid sinus has modest enhancement, but the vessel wall shows remarkable enhancement, producing the "empty delta" sign (*arrow*). Enhancement in the triangular cross section of the dural sinus wall creates an outline of the delta symbol.

of ongoing septic pulmonary emboli, internal jugular vein ligation can be performed.

Intravenous antimicrobials are continued after surgery. Anticoagulation generally is not necessary, but it can be considered in individual cases, especially in the face of propagating thrombosis. Time-of-flight MR venography is a useful means of assessing progression or resolution of the thrombus.

Otitic Hydrocephalus

Otitic hydrocephalus or pseudotumor cerebri is a condition of elevated intracranial pressure with normal CSF parameters in conjunction with an otologic condition. COM and its associated complications can produce otitic hydrocephalus. Nonseptic lateral sinus thrombosis, in particular, is highly associated with otitic hydrocephalus.

The pathophysiology of otitic hydrocephalus is unknown. It is not truly hydrocephalus, because the ventricles are not enlarged; rather, the CSF pressure is elevated. Overproduction of CSF and reduced resorption of CSF are theoretical etiologies of the elevated CSF pressure. Obstruction of venous outflow, such as seen with

dural venous sinus thrombosis, also can produce elevated intracranial pressure. Lenz and McDonald (39) favored this second explanation over the theory of decreased resorption of CSF. In their review, 78% of 54 cases of otitic hydrocephalus had lateral sinus thrombosis, epidural abscess, or perisinus granulation tissue. Symonds (40) favored the theory of decreased resorption of CSF, which occurs when sagittal sinus thrombosis involves the arachnoid villi.

Symptoms and signs of otitic hydrocephalus are related to the elevated CSF pressure. Headache is a common symptom. Examination of the eyegrounds often will reveal papilledema. With persistently elevated CSF pressure, the optic nerve can be compressed at the cribriform area, producing optic atrophy and vision loss. Either traction effects from brainstem herniation or inflammation from involvement of the inferior or superior petrosal sinus can affect the abducens nerve, cranial nerve VI, as the nerve passes through Dorello's canal into the cavernous sinus. A lateral rectus palsy will follow. Fever is conspicuously absent.

The prognosis for recovery is very dependent on treatment. With timely intervention, otitic hydrocephalus usually resolves. Prevention of optic atrophy is a critical issue, to avoid a permanent change in vision.

Diagnosis

Otitic hydrocephalus is a diagnosis of exclusion. Lumbar puncture with normal CSF cell count and chemistries and negative culture effectively excludes a diagnosis of meningitis. An elevated CSF pressure is the only abnormality. A head CT or MRI will document the absence of other intracranial pathology. A careful ophthalmologic exam should detect any papilledema and will document visual function.

Treatment

After eradicating the infection and inflammation associated with the COM, efforts must be directed at reducing the elevated intracranial pressure. Acetazolamide and corticosteroids are useful in medical management. Serial lumbar punctures or placement of a lumbar drain can reduce intracranial pressure by removing CSF. Close observation is necessary at the initial stages of drainage procedures because of the small risk of transtentorial herniation. Long-term drainage, if necessary, can be accomplished with a lumboperitoneal shunt.

Meningitis

Among intracranial complications of COM, meningitis is one of the most common. In several series, meningitis accounted for 50% of the intracranial complications (41–43).

Meningitis remains a common infectious problem. Most cases of meningitis development from a distant infectious source with hematogenous seeding of the subarachnoid space and meninges. Otogenic and sinonasal infections are commonly implicated as the bacterial source. AOM, especially in children, is a much more frequent cause of otogenic meningitis than COM. Gower and McGuirt (43) noted 63 cases of meningitis due to AOM versus 13 cases due to COM over a 20-year period.

The pathophysiology of meningitis due to COM is poorly understood. In COM, bacterial contamination may occur via bone erosion with epidural abscess/granulation formation or retrograde thrombophlebitis of emissary veins. The dura is violated, as opposed to the blood–brain barrier (the pathway of hematogenous spread), to gain access to the subarachnoid space. This theory is supported indirectly by the frequent presentation of multiple simultaneous intracranial complications in conjunction with meningitis. Meningitis has an associated second intracranial complication in 16% to 33% of cases (6,42,44).

Diagnosis

With COM, fever accompanied by neck stiffness and altered mental status should trigger an immediate search for an intracranial complication. With intravenous contrast, either CT or MRI will document meningeal enhancement, often of a diffuse nature. In the absence of a mass lesion, lumbar puncture and examination of the CSF is mandatory. CSF leukocytosis is characteristic of meningitis, associated with low glucose and elevated levels of protein and lactate. Studies on the CSF should include gram stain, culture, and tests for bacterial antigens (Fig. 6).

Treatment

Urgent institution of broad spectrum intravenous antimicrobials is the treatment of choice. Given the bacterial spectrum of COM with and without cholesteatoma, therapy against aerobic and anaerobic bacteria is initiated. Culture and sensitivity reports from CSF samples can further direct antimicrobial therapy.

Adjunctive therapy may be useful in reducing the morbidity of successfully treated meningitis. Dexamethasone, a corticosteroid, has been shown to reduce the neurologic and auditory sequelae of bacterial meningitis in children (45,46). To be effective, corticosteroid therapy must be instituted very early in the treatment course (47).

Brain Abscess

Brain abscess ranks as the first or second most common intracranial complication of COM. Because of the high mortality and morbidity associated with this entity, it is a particularly dreaded complication. A study from Scotland

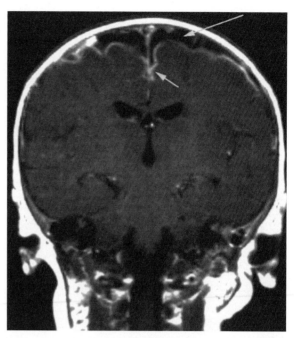

FIG. 6. Meningitis and subdural effusion. This patient with *Haemophilus influenzae* meningitis has meningeal enhancement (*short arrow*), as well as a subdural fluid collection (*long arrow*), on this coronal T1-weighted magnetic resonance image with gadolinium diethylenetriamine pentaacetic acid. Subdural effusions may be seen with *H. influenzae* meningitis, in particular. The effusion may become infected, producing a subdural empyema.

in 1990 determined the annual risk of developing a brain abscess for a patient with COM to be 1 in 12,467 (48). Data from a study from Thailand in 1993 gave a similar value of 1 in 11,905 (49). For a long, protracted duration of COM, the cumulative risk can become significant. As with other diseases possessing excessive mortality and morbidity, a policy of prevention has clear advantages over a policy of treating as complications arise.

Brain abscesses typically develop from hematogenous spread of bacteria. In cases of COM, direct extension along preformed pathways or perivascular channels is the more likely route of infection. This mechanism is supported by the preponderance of temporal lobe and cerebellar abscesses reported in large series of patients (42,44,48,50–55). From these series, 62% of abscesses were located in the temporal lobe and 34% in the cerebellum, for a total of 96% of brain abscesses.

The thin bone of the tegmen may be more easily violated than the bone overlying the posterior fossa dura, given the increased frequency of temporal lobe versus cerebellar abscesses. Once the dura is exposed, thrombophlebitis may spread infection to the cerebral or cerebellar parenchyma, or epidural infection may lead to contiguous involvement of adjacent brain tissue. Other than via thrombophlebitis, brain abscesses from COM uncommonly occur by hematogenous spread—frontal and parietal abscesses accounted for only 4% of cases in the those series (42,44,48,50–55).

The stages of development of a brain abscess were aptly described by Kornblut (56). Four phases can variably occur. The initial stage involves localized microfoci of cerebritis or encephalitis. Vascular inflammation occurs as well. In the second stage, fibrosis occurs in the region of hyperemia surrounding the necrotic tissue. The third stage is marked by expansion and secondary delineation of the abscess. The final phase is characterized by attempted repair with a dense fibroglial scar or rupture of the abscess. The capsule around the abscess forms in a period of 10 days to several weeks (56).

The bacteriology of brain abscesses related to chronic ear disease is considerably varied. Because no single organism predominates across reported series, culture of the abscess or at least the deep ear infection can be a critical step in determining optimal treatment. Clinical studies from various countries describe numerous bacteria (51,54,57,58). The more common organisms include *Proteus mirabilis, P. aeruginosa, S. aureus, Streptococcus* species, and *Staphylococcus epidermidis*. With careful technique, anaerobic bacteria were cultured in every series. *Bacteroides* and *Peptostreptococcus* were the most common anaerobic organisms, often present with mixed bacterial flora.

In addition to fever from the infectious process, symptoms and signs of brain abscess derive from both the overall mass effect of the abscess and specific effects peculiar to the abscess location. Headache, vomiting, and lethargy follow from increased intracranial pressure. Significant localizing signs include seizures, hemiparesis, cranial nerve palsies, and aphasia. However, both temporal lobe and cerebellar abscesses can exist with relatively few early localizing symptoms (52).

The morbidity and mortality associated with brain abscess continues to be a severe problem. Mortality rates from recent series with more than ten patients range from 6% to 42% (42,44,48,50,51,55,57,59). For survivors, cranial neuropathies, seizures, hemiparesis, or aphasia may persist.

Diagnosis

Given the suspicion for an intracranial complication of COM, a contrast-enhanced CT scan or MR image with paramagnetic contrast is indicated. Both techniques are excellent at detecting rim-enhancing parenchymal lesions of low attenuation. MRI may be more sensitive in defining areas of cerebritis.

Treatment

Multidrug antimicrobial therapy is clearly indicated for this serious condition. Metronidazole crosses the blood–brain barrier and is effective therapy for anaero-

bic bacteria. A combination of a third-generation cephalosporin or a penicillinase-resistant monolactam and an aminoglycoside can provide coverage for gram-positive and gram-negative aerobic bacteria (59). Corticosteroids often are administered as adjunctive therapy, to reduce brain swelling.

The role of surgical drainage requires close cooperation with neurosurgical colleagues. Craniotomy with drainage or excision of the abscess versus stereotactic aspiration are options that are determined on the basis of location and size of the abscess. Dominant versus nondominant hemisphere, posterior fossa versus supratentorial, superficial versus deep, and size less than or greater than 3.0 cm in diameter are important factors that will influence the neurosurgical approach.

Timing of the otologic surgery depends on the patient's clinical stability. In some cases, mastoid surgery can be accomplished at the time of the neurosurgical procedure. Otherwise, the otologic surgery can be delayed until the patient is more neurologically stable.

Subdural Abscess

Subdural abscesses are uncommon complications of COM. Intact dura provides an effective barrier to the spread of infection, and this may limit the number of subdural empyemas encountered from COM.

The subdural space is a potential space at the interface between the inner layer of the dura and the closely apposed arachnoid membrane. This potential space is separated from the CSF by the thin arachnoid membrane. The subdural space may derive from a splitting of dural layers rather than as a separation of dura and arachnoid (60).

Direct and indirect pathways from the temporal bone both may figure into the pathophysiology of subdural abscess. Direct extension of the infection of COM follows from bone erosion, dural exposure, and then dural penetration. Indirect involvement of the subdural space occurs when thrombophlebitis extends via dural perforating vessels.

Symptoms and signs from a subdural abscess are usually nonfocal and nonlocalizing. The small degree of mass effect is due to the spreading nature of the pus collection. Headache, nausea, fever, and meningism occur from cerebral inflammation and edema adjacent to the abscess.

Diagnosis

Imaging with CT or MRI is critical in diagnosing this complication. CT can demonstrate an extraaxial, hypodense layer. Contrast enhancement of the medial rim is highly suggestive of an infectious process (61). MRI may be more sensitive in detecting early lesions and can better distinguish among epidural, subdural, and brain abscess (29). In addition, subtle parenchymal abnormali-

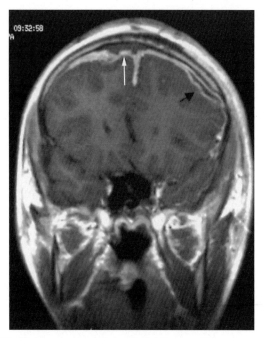

FIG. 7. Epidural and subdural abscesses. This coronal T1-weighted magnetic resonance image with gadolinium diethylenetriamine pentaacetic acid has two remarkable findings. An epidural abscess is indicated by the *white arrow.* Increased signal characteristics within the abscess help to distinguish it from the density of the cerebrospinal fluid. The *black arrow* highlights a subdural abscess over the left parietal cortex. The meningeal layers are thickened and enhance dramatically, with the subdural abscess confined, at this time, between the dura and pia mater. The subdural infection can easily spread over the surface of the cortex.

ties in the adjacent brain are more readily apparent on MR images (Fig. 7).

Treatment

A combination of immediate surgery and antibiotics is recommended for the treatment of subdural abscess. Neurosurgical drainage is necessary. There is some controversy as to whether craniotomy or burr hole drainage is more effective. Bok and Peter (62) reported a mortality rate of 7% using burr holes or burr holes and small craniectomies. In contrast, two studies reported significantly higher mortality rates using burr holes alone versus craniotomy surgery (48% vs. 8%, respectively) (63,64).

As with other intracranial complications of COM, multidrug antimicrobial therapy directed against gram-positive, gram-negative, and anaerobic organisms is indicated, until specific culture reports become available.

SUMMARY

There are a limited number of complications of COM. The possibility of one or more of these complications should be considered whenever the clinical scenario strays from the usual COM picture. Imaging studies, either CT or MRI, are of critical value in the evaluation process. However, these studies will not be performed unless someone thinks to order them.

Timely medical and surgical intervention are the major determinants in limiting the mortality and morbidity associated with these complications of COM.

SUMMARY POINTS

- Host-related factors, such as impaired resistance to disease or unfavorable anatomy, and microbiologic factors, such as bacterial invasiveness or degree of antimicrobial resistance, are intertwined in the pathophysiology of complications of COM.
- Labyrinthine fistulas can occur from COM, with or without associated cholesteatoma.
- Following a complete mastoidectomy for the treatment of COM, persistent suppuration or otorrhea may be an indication of a concomitant petrous apicitis.
- Intense otalgia is an uncommon symptom in COM and may indicate the onset of an intratemporal or intracranial complication of COM.
- It is not uncommon for more than one intracranial complication to occur simultaneously, such as lateral sinus thrombosis and epidural abscess, or meningitis and intracranial abscess.
- Multidrug antimicrobial therapy is indicated for the treatment of intracranial complications of COM. Metronidazole has excellent penetration into the central nervous system for anaerobic bacterial infections. Selective third-generation cephalosporins penetrate the blood–brain barrier and provide coverage against gram-positive and gram-negative organisms.
- CT scans and MR images are both efficacious in diagnosing an intracranial complication of COM. To be effective, these scans must be ordered whenever intracranial complications are a possibility.

REFERENCES

1. Paparella MM, Bluestone CD, Arnold W, et al. Definition and classification. *Ann Otol Rhinol Laryngol* 1985;94[Suppl 116]:8–9.
2. Neely JG. *Complications of suppurative otitis media. Part I: aural complications.* Rochester, MN: American Academy Otolaryngology Head Neck Surgery Foundation, 1989:7–59.
3. Kenna MA, Rosane BA, Bluestone CD. Medical management of chronic suppurative otitis media without cholesteatoma in children—update 1992. *Am J Otol* 1993;14:469–473.
4. Egelund E, Bak-Pedersen K. Suppurative labyrinthitis caused by anaerobic bacteria. *J Laryngol Otol* 1994;108:413–414.

5. Wright CG, Meyerhoff WL. Pathology of otitis media. *Ann Otol Rhinol Laryngol* 1994;103:24–26.
6. Holt GR, Gates GA. Masked mastoiditis. *Laryngoscope* 1983;93:1034–1037.
7. Schuknecht HF. *Pathology of the ear*, 2nd ed. Philadelphia: Lea & Febiger, 1993:212–216.
8. Paparella MM, Morizono T, Le CT. Sensorineural hearing loss in otitis media. *Ann Otol Rhinol Laryngol* 1984;93:623–629.
9. Levine BA, Shelton C, Berliner KI, Sheehy JL. Sensorineural loss in chronic otitis media. Is it clinically significant? *Arch Otolaryngol Head Neck Surg* 1989;115:814–816.
10. Noordzij JP, Dodson EE, Ruth RA, Arts HA, Lambert PR. Chronic otitis media and sensorineural hearing loss: is there a clinically significant relation? *Am J Otol* 1995;16:420–423.
11. Tos M. Sensorineural hearing loss in acute and chronic middle ear diseases. *Acta Otolaryngol (Stockh)* 1988;[Suppl 457]:87–93.
12. Antoli-Candela F, Stewart TJ. The pathophysiology of otologic facial paralysis. *Otolaryngol Clin North Am* 1974;7:309–330.
13. Savic DJ, Djeric DR. Facial paralysis in chronic suppurative otitis media. *Clin Otolaryngol* 1989;14:515–517.
14. Jang CH, Merchant SN. Histopathology of labyrinthine fistulae in chronic otitis media with clinical implications. *Am J Otol* 1997;18:15–25.
15. Pulec JL. Labyrinthine fistula from cholesteatoma: surgical management. *ENT J* 1996;75:143–148.
16. Ostri B, Bak-Pedersen K. Surgical management of labyrinthine fistulae in chronic otitis media with cholesteatoma by a one-stage closed technique. *ORL J Otorhinolaryngol Relat Spec* 1989;51:295–299.
17. Dornhoffer JL, Milewski C. Management of the open labyrinth. *Otolaryngol Head Neck Surg* 1995;112:410–414.
18. Canalis RF, Abemayor E, McClean P. Preservation of hearing in cholesteatomas with inner ear invasion. *J Otolaryngol* 1989;18:374–379.
19. Gamoletti R, Sanna M, Zini C, Taibah A-K, Pasanisi E, Vassalli L. Inner ear cholesteatoma and the preservation of cochlear function. *J Laryngol Otol* 1990;104:945–948.
20. Palva T, Ramsay H. Treatment of labyrinthine fistula. *Arch Otolaryngol Head Neck Surg* 1989;115:804–806.
21. Kobayashi T, Sato T, Toshima M, Ishidoya M, Suetake M, Takasaka T. Treatment of labyrinthine fistula with interruption of the semicircular canals. *Arch Otolaryngol Head Neck Surg* 1995;121:469–475.
22. Chao YH, Yun SH, Shin JO, Yoon JY, Lee DM. Cochlear fistula in chronic otitis media with cholesteatoma. *Am J Otol* 1996;17:15–18.
23. Kafka MM. Mortality of mastoiditis and cerebral complications with review of 3225 cases of mastoiditis with complications. *Laryngoscope* 1935;45:790–822.
24. Jeanes A. Otogenic intracranial suppuration. *J Laryngol Otol* 1962;76:388–402.
25. Quagliarello V, Scheld WM. Bacterial meningitis: pathogenesis, pathophysiology, and progress. *N Engl J Med* 1992;327:864–872.
26. Kornelisse RF, de Groot R, Neijens HJ. Bacterial meningitis: mechanisms of disease and therapy. *Eur J Pediatr* 1995;154:85–96.
27. Tunkel AR, Scheld WM. Pathogenesis and pathophysiology of bacterial meningitis. *Annu Rev Med* 1993;44:103–120.
28. Schwaber MK, Pensak ML, Bartels LJ. The early signs and symptoms of neurotologic complications of chronic suppurative otitis media. *Laryngoscope* 1989;99:373–375.
29. Weingarten K, Zimmerman RD, Becker RD, Heier LA, Haimes AB, Deck MDF. Subdural and epidural empyemas: MR imaging. *AJR* 1989;152:615–621.
30. Vogl TJ, Bergman C, Villringer A, Einhaupl K, Lissner J, Felix R. MR angiography of dural sinus thrombosis. *AJR* 1994;162:1191–1198.
31. Meltzer C, Fukui M, Kanal E, Smirniotopoulos J. MR imaging of the meninges. Part I. Normal anatomic features and nonneoplastic disease. *Radiology* 1996;201:297–308.
32. Doyle KJ, Jackler RK. Otogenic cavernous sinus thrombosis. *Otolaryngol Head Neck Surg* 1991;104:873–877.
33. Tsai FY, Wang A-M, Matovich VB, et al. MR staging of acute dural sinus thrombosis: correlation with venous pressure measurements and implications for treatment and prognosis. *AJNR* 1995;16:1021–1029.
34. Garcia RD, Baker A, Cunningham M, Weber A. Lateral sinus thrombosis associated with otitis media and mastoiditis in children. *Pediatr Infect Dis J* 1995;14:617–623.
35. Kelly KE, Jackler RK, Dillon WP. Diagnosis of septic sigmoid sinus thrombosis with magnetic resonance imaging. *Otolaryngol Head Neck Surg* 1991;105:617–624.
36. Singh B. The management of lateral sinus thrombosis. *J Laryngol Otol* 1993;107:803–808.
37. Teichgraeber JF, Per-Lee JH, Turner JS. Lateral sinus thrombosis: a modern perspective. *Laryngoscope* 1982;92:744–751.
38. Mathews TJ. Lateral sinus pathology. *J Laryngol Otol* 1988;102:118–120.
39. Lenz RP, McDonald GA. Otitic hydrocephalus. *Laryngoscope* 1984;94:1451–1454.
40. Symonds CP. Otitic hydrocephalus. *Neurology* 1956;6:681–685.
41. Wolfowitz BL. Otogenic intracranial complications. *Arch Otolaryngol* 1972;96:220–222.
42. Kangsanarak J, Navacharoen N, Fooanant S, Ruckphaopunt K. Intracranial complications of suppurative otitis media: 13 years' experience. *Am J Otol* 1995;16:104–109.
43. Gower D, McGuirt WF. Intracranial complications of acute and chronic infectious ear disease: a problem still with us. *Laryngoscope* 1983;93:1028–1033.
44. Singh B, Maharaj T. Radical mastoidectomy: its place in otitic intracranial complications. *J Laryngol Otol* 1993;107:1113–1118.
45. Lebel MH, Freij BJ, Syrogiannopoulos GA, Chrane DF, Hoyt MJ. Dexamethasone therapy for bacterial meningitis: results of two double-blind, placebo-controlled trials. *N Engl J Med* 1988;319:964–971.
46. Odio CM, Idis G, Paris M, et al. The beneficial effects of early dexazmethasone administration in infants and children with bacterial meningitis. *N Engl J Med* 1991;324:1525–1531.
47. Jafari HS, McCracken GH. Dexamethasone therapy in bacterial meningitis. *Pediatr Ann* 1994;23:82–88.
48. Nunez DA, Browning GG. Risks of developing an otogenic intracranial abscess. *J Laryngol Otol* 1990;104:468–472.
49. Kangsanarak J, Fooanant S, Ruckphaopunt K, Navacharoen N, Teotrakul S. Extracranial and intracranial complications of suppurative otitis media: report of 102 cases. *J Laryngol Otol* 1993;107:999–1004.
50. Bradley PJ, Manning KP, Shaw MDM. Brain abscess secondary to otitis media. *J Laryngol Otol* 1984;98:1185–1191.
51. Yen P-T, Chan S-T, Huang T-S. Brain abscess: with special reference to otolaryngologic sources of infection. *Otolaryngol Head Neck Surg* 1995;113:15–22.
52. Proctor CA. Intracranial complications of otitic origin. *Laryngoscope* 1966;76:288–308.
53. Brand B, Caparosa RJ, Lubic LG. Otorhinological brain abscess therapy—past and present. *Laryngoscope* 1984;94:483–437.
54. Lakshmi V, Rao RR, Dinakar I. Bacteriology of brain abscess—observations on 50 cases. *J Med Microbiol* 1993;38:187–190.
55. Samuel J, Fernandes CM, Steinberg J. Intracranial otogenic complications: a persisting problem. *Laryngoscope* 1986;96:272–278.
56. Kornblut AD. Cerebral abscess—a recurrent otologic problem. *Laryngoscope* 1972;82:1541–1556.
57. Ersahin Y, Mutluer S, Guzelbag E. Brain abscess in infants and children. *Child Nerv Syst* 1994;10:185–189.
58. Puthucheary SD, Parasakthi N. The bacteriology of brain abscess: a local experience in Malaysia. *Trans R Soc Trop Med Hyg* 1990;84:589–592.
59. Mamelak AN, Mampalam TJ, Obana WG, Rosenblum ML. Improved management of multiple brain abscesses: a combined surgical and medical approach. *Neurosurgery* 1995;36:76–85.
60. Haines D. On the question of a subdural space. *Anat Rec* 1991;230:3–21.
61. Weisberg L. Subdural empyema. Clinical and computed tomographic correlations. *Arch Neurol* 1986;43:497–500.
62. Bok APL, Peter JC. Subdural empyema: burr holes or craniotomy? *J Neurosurg* 1993;78:574–578.
63. Bannister G, Williams B, Smith S. Treatment of subdural empyema. *J Neurosurg* 1981;55:82–88.
64. Wackym PA, Canalis RF, Feuerman T. Subdural empyema of otorhinological origin. *J Laryngol Otol* 1990;104:118–122.

The Ear: Comprehensive Otology,
edited by R. F. Canalis and P. R. Lambert.
Lippincott Williams & Wilkins, Philadelphia © 2000.

CHAPTER 27

Surgical Treatment of Chronic Otitis Media and Cholesteatoma

Mark Kriskovich and Clough Shelton

Historically, the main indications for surgery of chronic otitis media were overwhelming infection or suppurative complications. With the advent of antibiotics, advances in anesthesia, and improved surgical techniques, it became possible to avoid wide resection or radical debridement, as well as many suppurative complications.

HISTORY

The introduction of the operating microscope and its subsequent improvements had a dramatic impact on otologic surgery (1,2). However, even today, disease eradication remains the most common indication for otologic surgery in chronic otitis media, but hearing restoration is also an important consideration. Although uncommon, the complications of chronic otitis media can be so devastating that, in many cases, patients with relatively innocuous symptoms require aggressive surgical therapy (see Chapter 26). Staging and prosthetic ossicular reconstruction are among the most recent advances against this surgical problem. Regardless of the specific technique or

materials used, the essence of successful surgery for chronic otitis media requires a systematic goal-oriented approach, while maintaining flexibility that is dependent on the pathology encountered for each patient.

Aims

The most important aims of surgery for chronic otitis media are the creation of safe, dry ear by elimination of disease and, if possible, restoration of middle ear function and the sound conducting mechanism. These goals include the prevention of recurrent disease and the avoidance of surgical complications. The importance of middle ear aeration also is emphasized. Cosmetic considerations including maintenance of normal anatomy and appearance are secondary. Concerns about anatomic contour primarily involve whether to use canal-wall-up (CWU) or canal-wall-down (CWD) mastoid surgery.

Terminology of Operations

Chronic otitis media surgery should be classified according to the American Academy of Otolaryngology–Head and Neck Surgery Standards to avoid confusion (Table 1) (3). This classification scheme was devel-

---

M. Kriskovich and C. Shelton: Department of Otolaryngology–Head and Neck Surgery, University of Utah School of Medicine, Salt Lake City, Utah 84132

TABLE 1. *Classification of the common operations performed in surgery for chronic ear infection*

A. Radical or modified radical mastoidectomy.
B. Mastoid obliteration operation—Any operation to eradicate disease when present and to obliterate a mastoid or fenestration cavity.
C. Myringoplasty—An operation in which the reconstructive procedure is limited to repair of a tympanic membrane perforation.
D. Tympanoplasty without mastoidectomy—An operation to eradicate disease in the middle ear and to reconstruct the hearing mechanism without mastoid surgery, with or without tympanic membrane grafting.
E. Tympanoplasty with mastoidectomy—An operation to eradicate disease in both the mastoid process and middle ear cavity and to reconstruct the middle ear conducting mechanism with or without tympanic membrane grafting.

From Committee on Conservation of Hearing of the American Academy of Ophthalmology and Otolaryngology. Standard classification for surgery of chronic ear infection. *Arch Otolaryngol* 1965;81:204–205.

oped to promote uniformity in description and to clarify communication regarding the operations for chronic otitis media. These include radical and modified radical mastoidectomy, mastoid obliteration, tympanoplasty with or without mastoidectomy, and myringoplasty.

The most common mastoid operations are tympanoplasty with mastoidectomy, either CWU or CWD. These will be covered in detail later in this chapter. Modified radical mastoidectomy occasionally is utilized; radical mastoidectomy only rarely. Modified radical mastoidectomy involves surgery to exteriorize cholesteatoma in the mastoid without surgery on the tympanic membrane or ossicles. Modified radical mastoidectomy is not synonymous with tympanoplasty and CWD mastoidectomy. Radical mastoidectomy is indicated when tympanoplasty would result in entrapment of cholesteatoma or in the presence of irreversible disease. Such an example would be middle ear cholesteatoma with fistula of the cochlear promontory; in this case, removal of cholesteatoma matrix would likely result in loss of cochlear function.

Although a logical and systematic approach is emphasized, each individual patient may not require the application of all techniques. Our discussion will focus on the individual components of surgery that can be used as clinically indicated. This will include tympanoplasty, ossicular chain reconstruction, staging tympanoplasty and use of plastic sheeting, and mastoidectomy.

Preoperative Assessment

Preoperative assessment, patient counseling, and surgical planning are multifactorial in patients with chronic otitis media. Considerations should include the degree of hearing impairment and the presence of otorrhea, pain, facial nerve dysfunction, or vertigo. The presence and type of perforation (whether total, marginal, central, pars tensa, or pars flaccida) and status of middle ear mucosa, eustachian tube, degree of mastoid pneumatization, and ossicles are assessed (4). The presence of an intact ossicular chain portends a better prognosis for hearing results. In the absence of an intact ossicular chain, the status and mobility of the stapes is particularly important. Tuning fork tests should accompany audiologic evaluation. Conductive hearing losses of 20 dB or less usually predict an intact ossicular chain when cholesteatoma is absent. Cholesteatoma itself may transmit sound through mass effect and may reduce the conductive deficit in the presence of ossicular chain discontinuity. An ossicular defect should be suspected with a conductive loss of greater than 30 dB (4).

Temporal bone or central nervous system complications may occur. Labyrinthine fistula, present in as many as 12% of chronic otitis media cases, is the most common temporal bone complication (5). The presence of fistulas is suggested by vertigo accompanying otorrhea and sensorineural hearing loss (6). The fistula test is present in approximately 40% of fistula cases, but its absence does not rule out its existence (5).

Assessment of the temporal bone may be accomplished by high-resolution computed tomographic (CT) scan preoperatively. There is controversy regarding the role of CT for routine evaluation of chronic otitis media. Leighton et al. (7) found the operative plan was altered in 50% of cases when preoperative imaging was utilized. Although routine imaging for chronic otitis media probably is not necessary, revisions or cases of suppurative complication or those surgeries in the only hearing ear are appropriate for preoperative imaging (8,9). Some believe that in children and the medically infirm, in limited tympanic membrane visualization on otoscopy, congenital cholesteatoma, former disease of the sinus tympani or facial recess, suspected labyrinthine fistula, or in a substantially better hearing ear, preoperative imaging may be useful (6,7,10).

CT is most helpful in identifying the extent of soft tissue disease and bone erosion, although it may be difficult to distinguish between mucosal disease and cholesteatoma. The position of the tegmen and sigmoid sinus, and the degree of mastoid sclerosis, are well delineated. Fistulas are identified with approximately 75% accuracy and 3.5% false-positive rate. Axial images are more helpful for this, although coronal images generally are better suited for temporal bone evaluation in chronic otitis media (10). Fistulas less than 2 mm are less likely to be detected (6).

Detection of ossicular abnormalities is limited. The malleus head and long process or body of the incus usually are well imaged, and the stapes superstructure often is seen as well. However, the most common ossicular abnormalities in chronic otitis media, erosion of the long process of incus or stapes superstructure, are difficult to identify accurately. Likewise, the manubrium is notable in only one third of cases (7). Facial nerve dehiscence and dural exposure are diagnosed much less accurately by CT (10).

We do not routinely image patients preoperatively. A temporal bone CT scan is obtained for those patients in whom a complication of chronic otitis media is suspected, or those who have cholesteatoma in an only hearing ear. Imaging should not be used to "diagnose" cholesteatoma. The diagnosis of cholesteatoma is based on clinical examination (binocular microscopy) rather than radiographic findings.

Prior to surgery, adjuvant therapies for concurrent or exacerbating conditions are implemented. Control of infection via cleaning and topical antibiotic and irrigant therapy is advocated. Although control of otorrhea is important, surgery is still appropriate if it persists. Some believe that sinonasal disease, allergy, immunodeficiency, and consideration of adenoidectomy should be included in preoperative assessment as predisposing factors for chronic otitis media (8), whereas others feel that these factors influence surgical results in a very small percentage of cases and should be addressed in treatment failures (5,11).

Preoperative patient counseling should include discussion of the probable outcomes regarding the aims of surgery, complications of untreated disease, potential for recurrence, and hearing loss. The possibility of, and rationale for, staging including examination for recurrence and better hearing results also are discussed. Risks of surgery are described, including bleeding, infection, hearing loss, tinnitus, dizziness, injury to the facial nerve, chorda tympani symptoms, cerebrospinal fluid leaks, and anesthesia risks.

Contraindications

Children less than 6 to 8 years of age generally are not candidates for tympanoplasty secondary to their susceptibility to recurrent otitis media. Ears with poor cochlear reserve may benefit from surgery to control infection, but not for hearing restoration.

Surgery on an only hearing ear should be avoided when possible, given the 2% risk of sensorineural hearing loss and higher risk in the presence of fistula (12). Progressive cholesteatoma is the most common indication for tympanoplasty in selected patients with only one hearing ear (13). In patients at risk for further hearing loss or suppurative complications because of persistent or uncontrolled disease, surgery may be carried out safely by experienced surgeons and with minimized risk of hearing loss (14). When hearing losses do occur, they are typically minor high-frequency losses secondary to drill-related trauma or ossicular manipulation. Rarely does a dead ear result and typically would involve those cases complicated by the presence of fistula.

Severe inflammatory disease of the external canal may affect the success of surgery; however, active middle ear infection and otorrhea are not contraindications. In some cases, the neovascularization may aid healing, although the thickened skin and mucosa may result in additional operative challenges and bleeding.

TYMPANOPLASTY

Tympanoplasty essentially involves grafting of the tympanic membrane, surgery of middle ear contents with removal of disease, and reconstruction of the ossicular chain with restoration of a middle ear space. Avoiding fibrosis and middle ear collapse while recreating a sound conducting connection between the tympanic membrane and cochlea are key elements to successful tympanoplasty. The aims of tympanoplasty surgery include an intact tympanic membrane, an air-containing middle ear space, and a secure connection between the eardrum and the cochlea (4).

During the 1950s, the development of tympanoplasty techniques furthered the goal of hearing restoration. Early success was limited by difficulties in maintaining a mucosalized, aerated middle ear cleft primarily due to the formation of adhesions between the tympanic membrane graft and the middle ear or promontory. Modifications and improvements in these techniques have resulted in the current state of the art.

In the 1870s, Kessel developed the early concepts of tympanoplasty, middle ear aeration, and ossicular reconstruction (15). However, in the 1950s Wullstein (16) and Zollner (17) ushered in the modern era of tympanic membrane grafting and tympanoplasty. Closure of the tympanic membrane to prevent infection with promotion of a vibratory surface were among their noteworthy goals.

Wullstein (16) initially described five types of tympanoplasty based on the relationship of the grafted tympanic membrane to the middle ear structures of sound conduction. His results showed a significant improvement in hearing, particularly when the stapes was present and functional. He also emphasized the work of Juers, Davis, and Walsh, who showed that the two major functions of the tympanic membrane are oval window sound pressure transformation and round window sound protection (2,15). Perforation eliminates sound protection for the round window in the presence of an intact conductive mechanism.

Early use of full- and split-thickness skin grafts was fraught with healing problems, eczema, and recurrent perforation. Canal skin was used but likewise abandoned due to graft problems that included perforation and a 40% failure rate (18). These difficulties eventually led to the progressive use of autogenous grafting materials, including vein, temporalis fascia, and tragal perichondrium. Storrs (19) described the use of temporalis fascia for the overlay technique in the early 1960s.

Current techniques primarily involve fascia, with success rates of greater than 90% for tympanic membrane grafting (5). Future techniques may involve use of growth factors to promote epithelialization, fibroblast proliferation, and wound healing organization (2,20). Studies of extracellular matrix substances such as the glycosaminoglycans and hyaluronic acid in perforations may yield additional therapeutic methods (21).

Homograft tympanic membranes have been used since their introduction in the late 1950s and early 1960s, but with somewhat less success. Some advocate its use in revision cases, although the material is rubbery and more difficult to manipulate than autogenous graft material (22). Concerns about transmission of infection, specifically human immunodeficiency virus (HIV) and Creutzfeldt-Jakob disease, have limited their use. Current fixation techniques do not inactivate Creutzfeldt-Jakob prions and incompletely permeate graft materials (23). HIV DNA was detected in the perichondrium but not the cartilage of tissues treated with fixatives including formaldehyde and cialit; however, these findings do not prove infectivity (24).

This history establishes the basis for the current principles of tympanoplasty. Whereas small central perforations with intact ossicular chains possibly may be closed with simple myringoplasty, tympanoplasty is used for more extensive perforation and disease. In myringoplasty, surgery is limited to the tympanic membrane and does not involve elevation of a tympanomeatal flap or entering the middle ear. Fat patch myringoplasty, which involves closure of a small perforation with a dumbbell of adipose tissue, is an example of this type of surgery.

Two methods dominate current tympanoplastic techniques. These include the overlay or lateral graft and the underlay or medial graft techniques. Controversy regarding which technique is superior can be summarized in the advantages and disadvantages of each as noted in Table 2. Both provide the prerequisites for successful reconstruction. When mastered, either gives high and comparable rates of success.

Transcanal or postauricular approaches may be used for the tympanoplasty. The transcanal approach is less invasive but has anterior exposure limits. Tragal perichondrium is easily within the surgical field for harvest. A postauricular approach provides superior visualization for anterior or subtotal perforations. It naturally allows for ready access to temporalis fascia. Because of the superior overall exposure, the grafting success rate is higher through a postauricular approach, and the authors perform all cases of tympanic membrane grafting through this approach.

The lateral surface or overlay technique has been our choice for tympanic membrane grafting. This technique essentially involves fascial placement along the lateral surface of the annulus but medial to the malleus. This technique may have more healing problems in less experienced hands, but it does have a very high graft take rate. Tympanic membrane closure occurs in 97% (5). Large perforations and the need for membrane remnant removal for disease elimination are particularly suitable for this method. This technique allows removal of all areas of avascular tympanosclerosis, as well as severely monomeric tympanic membrane remnants. Successful graft stabilization, particularly in the absence of manubrium or anterior remnant, is important to avoid anterior graft blunting or lateralization, which is the most significant healing problems in this technique. Blunting is secondary to anterior sulcus fibrous tissue. When minor or occurring with total ossicular replacement prostheses or partial ossicular replacement prostheses, it is a cosmetic problem only. When severe it can result in impairment of vibration of the tympanic membrane and a conductive hearing loss similar to the effects of significant lateralization. Tympanic membrane cysts and canal epithelial pearls, likely secondary to inadequate squamous remnant removal, are other less notable problems.

Both the overlay and underlay techniques work well for central perforations. The medial graft is best suited to posterior perforations, although the lateral technique also works well, particularly in the setting of significant anterior myringosclerosis. The graft take rate is not related to perforation size. Regardless of which technique is used, it is important to inspect and palpate the ossicles to ascertain if they are intact and mobile at the time of middle ear exploration.

Overlay Technique

This technique may be performed under general anesthesia. Although it is possible to perform the overlay grafting operation with the patient under local anesthesia, many patients are uncomfortable during the anterior canal drilling because it is very loud. The overlay technique is initiated with canal preparation. After injection of the ear canal with local anesthetic, the vascular strip becomes obvious. Vascular strip incisions are performed with a sickle knife. Starting at the 12 o'clock position adjacent to the short process of the malleus, the tympa-

TABLE 2. *Comparison of tympanic membrane grafting techniques*

Advantages	Disadvantages
Overlay grafting	
• Excellent exposure	• Requires precision
• High graft take rate	• Longer healing time (months vs. weeks)
• Applicable to all cases	• Possibility of blunting, lateralization, or epithelial pearls
Underlay grafting	
• Less blunting or lateralization	• Limited visualization
• High graft take rate	• Large, anterior perforation less suitable
• Simpler technique	• Difficult with small external auditory canal

nosquamous suture line is incised from the annular sulcus to the bony cartilaginous junction (Fig. 1A). An inferior incision at about the level of the chorda tympani and tympanomastoid suture line begins inferolaterally at the annulus to create a wide base posteriorly, thus preserving vascular supply. The vascular strip flap is back elevated using a lancet knife by sweeping laterally, continuing to maintain the knife on bone and taking care to avoid avulsing the malleus. An anterior canal incision is made using a small disposable scalpel blade (Beaver Co. no. 6400) at the bony–cartilaginous junction connecting the vascular strip incisions at their lateral extent (Fig. 1B).

A postauricular incision is made (Fig. 2). This incision is made 5 to 10 mm from the postauricular sulcus, taking care to avoid falling off the mastoid tip with resultant injury to the facial nerve. Placement of the incision behind the sulcus allows easier closure and provides better mastoid exposure than an incision in the sulcus. The inferior edge of the incision should be hidden by the lobule. The superior limb of the incision should allow for ready access to the temporalis fascia. The wide-based incision allows the ear to fall forward, and it is reflected using a self-retaining retractor with built-in suction with the handles toward the top of the patient's head and suction lines toward the surgeon.

Temporalis fascia is harvested by separating it from the underlying muscle by spreading with scissors. A larger piece of fascia generally is required for overlay techniques than for an underlay. Three times the surface area to be grafted usually is adequate. Some advocate the use of the overlying areolar tissue due to its tendency to heal

faster, with a resultant thinner tympanic membrane. This material is more difficult to manipulate and has less strength. However, its use does allow for future harvest of temporalis fascia should revision become necessary. Graft material then is placed on a polytetrafluoroethylene (Teflon) block to dry on the back table after removal of any muscle or unnecessary connective tissue.

A periosteal incision is made along the linea temporalis with a postauricular course toward the mastoid in the shape of a "7." Periosteum is elevated anteriorly toward the canal, with back elevation if mastoid surgery also is required. To prevent narrowing of the ear canal, a triangle of subcutaneous tissue abutting the superior external auditory canal often is excised.

Anterior canal skin is removed by elevating with a weapon on canal bone. Skin is lifted off the annulus. Care is taken to avoid perforations of the canal skin, as the medial elevation is performed primarily by feel. Likewise, all skin remnants are removed. The anterior canal wall bulge is removed using the drill equipped with cutting burs (Fig. 3). This enlarges the canal and facilitates graft placement through improved exposure of the tympanic sulcus. Canal enlargement also improves postoperative visualization of the tympanic membrane. Caution must be exercised to avoid excessive exposure of the temporomandibular joint or injury to the ossicular chain by the back side of the bur. Most injuries to the joint usually heal but should be avoided nonetheless. If tissue of the temporomandibular joint is exposed and prolapses into the ear canal, it can be cauterized with a bipolar cautery, which leads to retraction of the tissue. Starting inferiorly

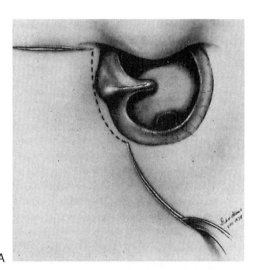
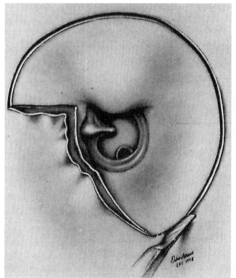

A   B

FIG. 1. A: The vascular strip becomes apparent after injection of the ear canal with local anesthesia. The incisions are made along the tympanosquamous and tympanomastoid suture lines. **B:** The anterior canal incision is made at the bony cartilaginous junction and connects the previously made vascular strip incisions. (From Sheehy JL. Surgery of chronic otitis media. In: English GE, ed. *Otolaryngology.* Philadelphia: JB Lippincott, 1986:1–86, with permission.)

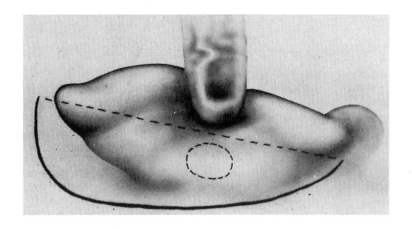

FIG. 2. The postauricular incision is placed 5 to 10 mm behind the postauricular sulcus, which allows for convenient skin closure. (From Sheehy JL. Surgery of chronic otitis media. In: English GE, ed. *Otolaryngology.* Philadelphia: JB Lippincott, 1986: 1–86, with permission.)

and working superiorly enables one to see the entire annulus without moving the microscope. When removal of the bone is complete, the risk of tympanic membrane blunting may be decreased by converting the usual acute angle of the anterior sulcus to an obtuse one. Also, by removing the anterior canal overhang, one can see the anterior annular sulcus and easily visualize the anterior graft placement.

The tympanic membrane remnant is completely deepithelialized. All monomeric portions, myringosclerotic segments, and avascular areas are removed. Because there is no change in graft take rate based on perforation size in the lateral graft technique, one should err on the side of removing too much remnant rather than too little. Cup forceps are utilized to remove any skin remnants to avoid epithelial pearls. When removing the remnant from the malleus, the dissection proceeds parallel to the axis of the handle to avoid excessive ossicular manipulation. There is a small cartilage cap at the tip of the short process of the malleus, and its removal allows access to a

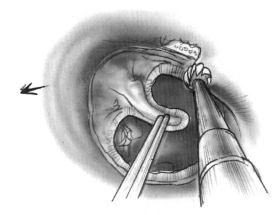

FIG. 3. After removal of the anterior canal skin, the overhang of the anterior canal wall is removed with a drill, which allows for complete visualization of the annulus. (From Sheehy JL. Tympanoplasty: outer surface grafting technique. In: Brackmann DE, Shelton C, Arriaga M, eds. *Otologic surgery.* Philadelphia: WB Saunders, 1994:121–132, with permission.)

subperiosteal plane along the handle. The tympanic membrane remnant is usually very adherent at the umbo and typically must be divided sharply. This area will be exterior to the tympanic membrane graft, so small squamous epithelial remnants do not pose a problem here. The middle ear is carefully inspected to identify mucosal disease, ossicular erosion, and the presence and extent of cholesteatoma. After addressing the middle ear disease, the decision is made regarding the necessity for a mastoidectomy. If the chorda tympani nerve is involved by cholesteatoma it is removed with the disease.

Several patterns may be found for middle ear cholesteatoma. Posterior perforations with cholesteatoma may result in annular or scutal erosions as well as local adhesions. Disease often is present between the chorda tympani and the long process of the incus and malleus head. The incudostapedial joint is divided, if necessary, and attention is paid to avoiding injury to a dehiscent facial nerve. Exploration should include inspection of the oval and round windows, sinus tympani, and facial recess. A round window reflex is elicited if there is doubt about the extent of ossicular mobility.

The middle ear including the eustachian tube then is carefully packed with Gelfoam soaked with antibiotic solution to prevent anterior failure or graft migration. Particularly in the presence of infection or significant edema or granulation, the use of Gelfoam soaked with antibiotic solution is recommended. In our experience, there have been no problems associated with the use of ototoxic antibiotics in the middle ear packing.

The fascia, which was dried on the back table, is cut and shaped as needed. Slits are cut in the fascia, allowing it to slide behind the manubrium with the fascial edges placed just lateral to the tympanic sulcus without significant extension onto the anterior canal wall (Fig. 4A). The graft should fit snugly within the anterior sulcus, and extra fascia should lie along the posterior canal wall (Fig. 4B). It often is helpful to place the graft under the manubrium first, then anteriorly onto the annular shelf. Extra fascia superiorly is folded down from above the malleus. In the absence of a malleus handle, a flap is

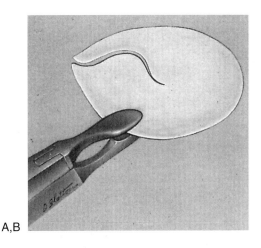
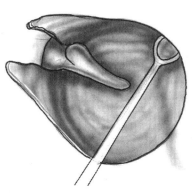

FIG. 4. A: The temporalis fascia graft is prepared so it will fit in the anterior annular sulcus, with a slit cut to allow placement under the malleus handle. (From Sheehy JL. Surgery of chronic otitis media. In: English GE, ed. *Otolaryngology.* Philadelphia: JB Lippincott, 1986:1–86, with permission.) B: The graft is shown in place, lateral to the annulus anteriorly and medial to the malleus handle. (From Sheehy JL. Tympanoplasty: outer surface grafting technique. In: Brackmann DE, Shelton C, Arriaga M, eds. *Otologic surgery.* Philadelphia: WB Saunders, 1994:121–132, with permission.)

made in the superior portion of the fascia and is placed medial to the scutum as an anchor (Fig. 5). Anterior canal skin is replaced and completely unfurled to coapt edges with the fascia, while avoiding significant overlap. Small pieces of Gelfoam are packed tightly at the anterior sulcus, and the vascular strip is replaced.

The ear is returned to its anatomic position, and the mastoid periosteum is closed with several interrupted absorbable sutures. Looking through the ear canal, the vascular strip is checked to ensure its position has not shifted, and the external canal is quickly packed with Gelfoam to avoid its filling with blood. A running subcuticular skin closure is performed and Steri-Strips applied lengthwise beginning inferiorly to allow for a single "zipper-like" removal at follow-up. A mastoid dressing is placed.

Underlay (Undersurface) Technique

An alternative grafting technique involves placement of the tympanic membrane graft medial to the annulus. The vascular strip and canal incisions are made and flaps are elevated (Fig. 6). A standard postauricular incision is

performed and the auricle retracted anteriorly. Temporalis fascia is harvested. The graft material is prepared and dried. If the anterior canal wall bulge is restricting the view of the anterior tympanic membrane, the bulge is removed with a small diamond bur after reflecting the canal skin medially. The mastoid periosteum is elevated. Next, the middle ear space and ossicles are examined, and the diseased drum remnant is removed. The margin of small perforations is "rimmed" with a Rosen needle to create a raw edge. The rationale for this lies in the finding that chronic perforations persist when a mucocutaneous junction is created between the epithelial and mucosal layers of the tympanic membrane, which is eliminated by rimming (21). After the canal skin flaps are raised, the sinus tympani, oval window region, and ossicles are examined. Disease is removed as previously described. Absorbable gelatin sponge (Gelfoam) then is placed into the middle ear and eustachian tube orifice. This will lay subjacent to the graft, supporting it in place medially as the graft abuts the annulus.

The fascia is trimmed, and a slit is made for the manubrium. The graft is placed medially under the

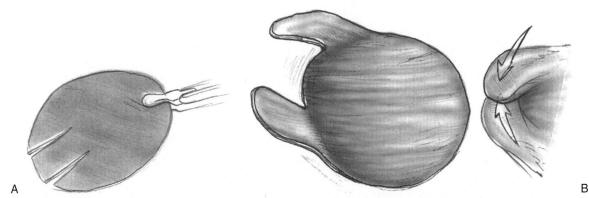

A

B

FIG. 5. A: In the absence of a malleus to secure the graft, a "tab" is cut in the superior portion of the graft. B: The tab is placed medial to the scutum, into the epitympanum. This tab anchors the fascia graft and prevents lateralization. (From Sheehy JL. Tympanoplasty: outer surface grafting technique. In: Brackmann DE, Shelton C, Arriaga M, eds. *Otologic surgery.* Philadelphia: WB Saunders, 1994:121–132, with permission.)

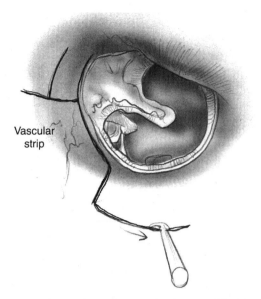

Vascular
strip

FIG. 6. For the undersurface graft, the canal incisions are shown, which includes the formation of a vascular strip flap. (From Glasscock ME, Strasnick B. Tympanoplasty: the undersurface graft technique—postauricular approach. In: Brackmann DE, Shelton C, Arriaga M, eds. *Otologic surgery.* Philadelphia: WB Saunders, 1994:141–152, with permission.)

malleus and then under the anterior annulus (Fig. 7A). The flaps surrounding the malleus are folded down and the remaining fascia laid against the posterior canal wall. If desired, cartilage may be placed posterosuperiorly below the graft to prevent retraction. Canal flaps and the vascular strip are replaced, holding the graft in place (Fig. 7B). The postauricular incision is closed with careful sub-

sequent verification of the graft position. The canal is packed with Gelfoam and a mastoid dressing is applied. This technique allows the graft to be placed under the drum remnant and does not have the potential for lateralization (22).

STAGING TYMPANOPLASTY

Although early graft failures and/or prosthesis extrusions were blamed for eustachian tube dysfunction, failure to obtain an adequately mucosalized middle ear space is the more likely cause. Removal of mucosal disease leaves bare promontory bone. If extensive, this can result in adhesions and fibrosis between the raw areas of the graft and promontory (Fig. 8). Adhesion formation has been experimentally shown to occur within days of injury and acute infection (25). Contracture, scar, and tympanic membrane atelectasis are all possible sequelae.

Techniques to prevent these outcomes include staging and the use of materials left within the middle ear space to decrease adhesions. Rambo (26) is credited with introducing the concept of two-stage tympanoplasty. He initially filled the middle ear space with paraffin, then later removed it at the second stage with subsequent performance of a fenestration for hearing improvement (26). Tabb in 1963 recommended a three-stage approach (27). Currently applied staging techniques are taken in great part from the work of Sheehy and Crabtree (28).

Plastic materials will be discussed later, but it is their use in the context of staging tympanoplasty that has led to better results. Placing customized small discs of plastic (or Gelfilm in less extensive cases) between these raw

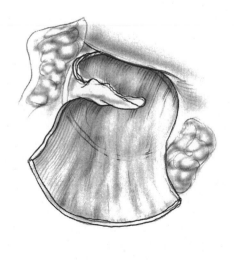

A

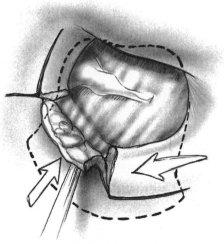

B

FIG. 7. A: Anteriorly, the temporalis fascial graft is placed medial to the annulus. It also is placed medial to the handle of the malleus and lays up the canal wall posteriorly. **B:** The canal skin flaps are replaced over the fascia graft. (From Glasscock ME, Strasnick B. Tympanoplasty: the undersurface graft technique—postauricular approach. In: Brackmann DE, Shelton C, Arriaga M, eds. *Otologic surgery.* Philadelphia: WB Saunders, 1994:141–152, with permission.)

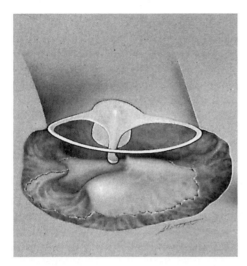

FIG. 8. Severe middle ear mucosal disease, which can lead to fibrous adhesions between the grafted tympanic membrane and the promontory. This middle ear fibrosis ultimately can lead to collapse of the tympanic membrane. (From Sheehy JL. Surgery of chronic otitis media. In: English GE, ed. *Otolaryngology.* Philadelphia: JB Lippincott, 1986:1–86, with permission.)

TABLE 3. *Plastic sheeting used for staging tympanoplasty*

Type	Thickness
Thin Silastic	0.005 inch
Reinforced Silastic	0.020 inch
Thick Silastic	0.040 inch
Supramid	0.3 mm

areas reduces the risk of adhesion and scarring. These materials may remain in place, or the plastic is removed at the second-look procedure, when the middle ear is inspected for residual or recurrent disease and ossicular reconstruction is accomplished.

Staging is a well-tested technique and previous descriptions recount early experiences (28). Chronic otitis media surgery that is staged allows for removal of recidivistic (residual or recurrent) cholesteatoma at second-look procedures, prevention of middle ear adhesions, and better opportunities for hearing reconstruction. Not all ears with chronic otitis media require staging. Failures may be committed to a total of three operations if a single stage is attempted in a highly diseased ear and fails (27).

Plastics

Various materials have been used to decrease the incidence of adhesions between the tympanic membrane and promontory and to restore a mucosa-lined middle ear space where mucosal disease or defects exist. Silastic was introduced in 1968, after studies showed a lack of tissue reactivity. Long-term studies on Silastic have validated its usage, showing no middle ear foreign body reaction, rejection, or chronic inflammation (29).

Plastic has been used in various thicknesses. Thin Silastic was used initially, but it failed in many cases secondary to being pushed aside or rolled up by advancing fibrous tissue (27). Later, stiffer plastics, such as Supramid, and thick Silastic were utilized with increased success. Currently, four thicknesses of plastic sheeting are commonly used (Table 3). In single-stage procedures, Gelfilm, which

resorbs, or thin Silastic, left permanently, may be used. For single-stage facial recess approaches, Gelfilm is used in many cases to decrease adhesions and potential retraction pockets or recurrent cholesteatoma, which otherwise could develop due to the presence of bare bone. The authors use Gelfilm to prevent adhesions in the presence of minor middle ear disease and "thick" Silastic sheeting (0.040-inch thickness) in cases of more extensive mucosal disease requiring a second-stage procedure.

In addition to decreasing the formation of adhesions, plastic sheeting may allow for an increased middle ear cleft depth in CWD cases. At the initial surgery, an appropriately sized piece is cut and placed on the promontory between exposed bone and the grafted tympanic membrane. The superior edge of the plastic is beveled where it covers the horizontal portion of the facial nerve and contacts the tympanic graft in CWD cases.

At second-stage surgery, the thick Silastic is removed with a right-angle hook via a transcanal approach. However, because of its stiffness, Supramid must be removed through a postauricular approach. In CWU procedures the plastic sheeting may be left indefinitely when residual cholesteatoma is not a concern and the resultant hearing is good. Plastic generally is removed before 2 years in CWD procedures, or extrusion may occur.

Indications

The three reasons to stage the operation are mucosal disease, ossicular fixation, and residual cholesteatoma. The extent of mucous membrane disease is the most common indication for staging. The absence of mucosa in the posterior half of the middle ear space and epitympanum is cited as one such indication (28). Staging has several potential advantages, including better hearing results, validation of complete cholesteatoma removal, and increased safety of oval window manipulation in a middle ear free of infection and granulation tissue.

In ears with chronic otitis media with or without cholesteatoma, the footplate may be fixed by tympanosclerosis or by coexisting otosclerosis. Stapes fixation in the presence of a perforated tympanic membrane is treated more safely using staging. Opening the oval window in the setting of active infection significantly increases the risk of labyrinthitis or a dead ear. In such cases, stapedectomy is best performed at a second stage, after the tympanic membrane has been repaired and the middle ear returned to a sterile space. Gradually progressive conductive hearing losses in the presence of inactive chronic otitis media are suggestive of coexisting tympanosclerosis or otosclerosis, and may require a second stage for stapedectomy (27).

The concern for residual cholesteatoma is the second most common reason for staging. Residual cholesteatoma in the middle ear occurs in about one third of cases following primary excision (5). More extensive cholesteatoma may be seen in well-pneumatized mastoids, and the possibility of residual disease must be considered in these cases as well. Severe granulation tissue and significant bleeding at the time of surgery increase the possibility of trapped epithelial matrix and formation of residual cholesteatoma.

Age less than 20 years and multiple sites of middle ear cleft cholesteatoma have been found to be predisposing factors for residual cholesteatoma (30). Compared with adults, children often are appropriate candidates for staging based on their increased incidence of recurrent disease, more advanced ossicular necrosis, and poorer hearing results (31–34). The more aggressive growth of residual disease in children may be related to their high rate of coexisting eustachian tube dysfunction and recurrent otitis media. It should be noted that some surgeons advocate CWD techniques with single-stage surgery due to the apparent aggressive nature of pediatric cholesteatoma and potential cost benefits (35).

The difference between recurrent and residual cholesteatoma must be emphasized. Findings of recurrent cholesteatoma are associated with tympanic membrane retractions typically involving the posterior superior pars flaccida with the reformation of a retraction pocket. This may be due to loss of tympanic membrane support as a result of scutal erosion, middle ear fibrosis, and retraction or persistent eustachian tube dysfunction. Recurrent cholesteatoma is more common in CWU than CWD surgery. In the majority of cases, residual disease is noted as small, easily removable, encapsulated squamous pearls from disease left behind at the previous operation. These pearls typically occur in middle ear areas that are difficult to reach for matrix removal, such as the sinus tympani.

Rates of residual cholesteatoma vary but are generally around 30% for CWU surgery that is staged for cholesteatoma (5,36). Sheehy and Crabtree (28) found residual disease to be present at the oval window in 38%, the middle ear in 31%, and tympanic recess in 12%. Residual or recurrent mastoid disease is easier to remove than that of the sinus tympani, facial recess, or middle ear space. Recurrent disease occurs in 15% or fewer cases (37) and may take years to become apparent. Recurrent disease may be prevented by reconstruction of the tympanic ring with cartilage or bone pate to reduce retraction pockets or by use of large cartilage battens placed over an ossicular prosthesis for support of the posterosuperior tympanic membrane (32).

Typically, second-look procedures are performed 6 to 12 months after initial surgery. Twelve months is recommended for cases of severe mucosal disease and cholesteatoma. For mucosal disease alone of a less severe nature, a second procedure at 9 months is appropriate; 6 months is advised for ossicular fixation cases.

OSSICULAR CHAIN RECONSTRUCTION

Chronic otitis media may affect the ossicular chain via mass effect, erosion, destruction, or adhesions. Incus necrosis is the most common ossicular defect, followed by erosion of the stapes superstructure. Austin (38) found the malleus and stapes intact in 59% of cases and the stapes superstructure absent in 23%. To restore hearing, the sound pressure transfer mechanism must connect the vibrating tympanic membrane with the cochlear fluids. This may be accomplished by sculpting and repositioning the patient's own ossicles or by using prosthetic material at either the initial or second-stage surgery.

Ossicular reconstruction materials can be divided into autografts or homografts (ossicles, cartilage, etc.) and alloplastic prosthetics. Ossicular transposition, primarily of the incus, and the use of autogenous materials, such as bone or cartilage, may lead to superior results in given situations. However, their utilization may require more intraoperative time if much sculpting is necessary. Incus interposition was first described by Guilford and advanced by Pennington (2). In this technique, a strut or crutch in the short process is created for the malleus, with a cup for the stapes capitulum. An intact tympanic membrane is required to maintain tension between the malleus and the prosthesis. Failures can occur due to displacement or fixation, ankylosis (bony or fibrous adhesions) to the promontory, facial ridge, or posterior medial canal wall. Care in sculpting the prosthesis, appropriate use of packing for support, and removal of all bone dust from the middle ear can diminish the chance of failure.

When using a strut reconstruction, such as a carved incus, it is crucial to access the relationship between the stapes capitulum (or footplate) and the malleus handle. The ideal relationship is approached as the anteroposterior distance between the malleus and stapes area becomes minimal. As the angle between these structures increases, the acoustic energy transmitted decreases due to a decrement in the applied force vector. The result is that less sound energy is transmitted to the inner ear and the risk of slippage increases. Packing should not be relied on to hold the strut in place. The prosthesis position should not be more than 30 degrees from the vertical and its length should be adequate to create tension to maintain its position.

Homograft ossicles are useful, although concerns about disease transmission, as noted for homograft tympanic membranes, recently have limited their application. Screening has been recommended for homograft donors

(23). However, Meylan et al. (39) postulated an extremely low possibility of infectivity based on low HIV concentrations in such homografts and the marked reduction of *in vitro* infectivity with current fixation techniques.

Autograft cartilage used as a strut eliminates problems with extrusion or rejection. Likewise, ankylosis found with ossicular or bone grafts does not occur with cartilage. Such materials are accessible from various sites, including the tragus. Disadvantages include time-consuming preparation and propensity for resorption. Longterm results show a gradual loss of tensile strength, with a tendency for hearing decline with time due to resorption. Infection may result in rapid reabsorption.

Because of the shortcomings of autograft techniques, the search for biocompatible reconstructive materials that were easy to manipulate resulted. Early prostheses included polyethylene and Teflon tubing or wire, all of which were prone to extrusion.

Plastipore, a high-density porous polyethylene used to fashion partial ossicular replacement prostheses and total ossicular replacement prostheses, initially was touted as being more biocompatible compared with polyethylene. This is due, in part, to the ingrowth of tissue within the porous prosthesis interstices and the material's limited tissue reactivity. However, not until cartilage was interposed between the tympanic membrane and prosthesis platform, as proposed by Coyle Shea, did extrusion rates decrease. Currently reported rates of extrusion approximate 5% (12).

Hydroxyapatite, a polycrystalline calcium phosphate ceramic, has been used extensively. An extrusion rate of 2.6% is reported by Goldenberg (40), although rates as high as 10% have been reported and overall are similar to Plastipore with cartilage. However, if placed next to the scutum, osseointegration can take place, with a resultant conductive hearing loss. Similarly, direct placement of a hydroxyapatite shaft to the oval window region can lead to fusion to bare bone in that region. Hybrid prostheses have been developed with Teflon or Plastipore shafts to prevent such occurrences. However, some of these hybrids are "top heavy," which can lead to later displacement.

Ceramic and inert glass materials, such as Bioglass and Ceravital, which were met with early excitement, generally are no longer used due to their brittle nature, extrusion problems, and lack of superior hearing results. Recently, a glass ionomer prosthesis has been introduced that is biocompatible, less brittle, and easier to manipulate than previous prosthetics (41). Likewise, a cartilage cap is not necessary for prosthesis extrusion concerns. Also, glass ionomeric bone cement may be used to bridge gaps between ossicular elements (42). Nonexothermic hardening occurs in minutes, allowing for malleability to customize repairs. Trials by the Food and Drug Administration are under way to evaluate the widespread utility of this material in ossicular reconstruction.

TABLE 4. *Typical trimmed prosthesis lengths*

	Canal-wall-up	Canal-wall-down
Total ossicular prosthesis	5 mm	3 mm
Partial ossicular prosthesis	3 mm	1 mm

Critical in the decision for ossicular chain reconstruction is the presence of a mobile stapes or footplate. Plastipore partial ossicular prostheses are placed between the stapes capitulum and tympanic membrane. Total ossicular prostheses are used when the stapes superstructure is absent. They are placed between the tympanic membrane and the stapes footplate. Both prostheses are used with a cartilage cap from the tragus to prevent extrusion. The size of these prosthesis platforms have decreased from 5 to 3 mm in diameter, which results in easier manipulation and decreased extrusion rate.

A key principle of ossicular chain reconstruction involves adequate tension between the tympanic membrane and stapes (or footplate) to maintain their position, while avoiding extrusion. Accurate preparation of prosthesis length is necessary for superior hearing results. Accurate length is critical. Typical lengths for prostheses are listed in Table 4.

Technique

Technical aspects of prostheses placement deserve mention (43–45). We prefer Plastipore total ossicular prostheses and partial ossicular prostheses with cartilage placed between the tympanic membrane and prosthesis for prevention of prosthesis extrusion and to provide broad contact with the tympanic membrane. The prosthesis is best trimmed on a saline-moistened tongue blade. The middle ear is packed with Gelfoam for prosthesis support. The prosthesis is most easily manipulated when it is moistened, held with a no. 3 suction, and guided into position onto the capitulum or footplate using a Rosen needle. The correct prosthesis length should result in the platform just touching the undersurface of the tympanic membrane without significant tension (Fig. 9).

A tragal cartilage disc, approximately 50% larger than the prosthesis platform, may be used to diminish the chance of extrusion. Advantages of tragal cartilage include its ready accessibility, adequate size, and attendant perichondrium, which may be useful as a grafting material in selected cases. For better cosmesis, the incision is made just posterior to the tragal edge. A portion of cartilage at least 5 mm × 5 mm is resected with its perichondrium. Larger portions may be removed for canal wall reconstruction and posterior quadrant tympanic membrane reinforcement to decrease retraction pockets as in cartilage tympanoplasty (22). The donor site is closed with absorbable sutures. The perichondrium is elevated and cartilage

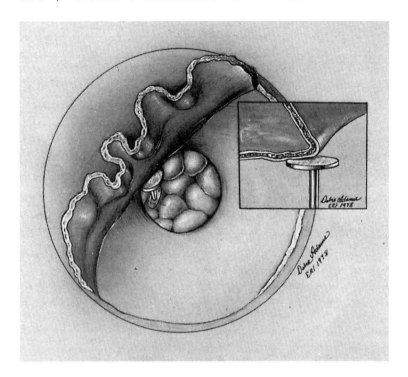

FIG. 9. A total ossicular prosthesis (TOP) in position on the stapes footplate, showing the proper prosthesis length. The prosthesis should just touch the undersurface of the tympanic membrane, without exerting tension on it. (From Sheehy JL. Surgery of chronic otitis media. In: English GE, ed. *Otolaryngology.* Philadelphia: JB Lippincott, 1986: 1–86, with permission.)

trimmed to size. The cartilage edges are beveled to expedite fitting under the scutum. Thinning and carving of the cartilage allows for the desired dome-shaped curvature.

To place the cartilage cap, the prosthesis is rotated slightly backward and the cartilage is slid along the medial surface of the tympanic membrane onto the prosthesis platform (Fig. 10). The cartilage provides the proper tension to hold the prosthesis in place. Tenting of

the tympanic membrane by the cartilage should occur (Fig. 11). The tympanic membrane flap is replaced and the canal packed with Gelfoam.

Results

The many variables involved in tympanoplasty surgery make it difficult to compare hearing results among sur-

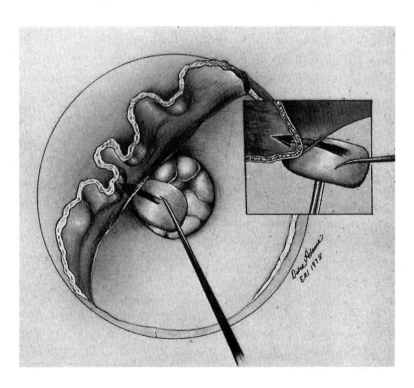

FIG. 10. The prosthesis is covered with tragal cartilage, which in turn is placed beneath the tympanic membrane and slightly under the bony external auditory canal margin. (From Sheehy JL. Surgery of chronic otitis media. In: English GE, ed. *Otolaryngology.* Philadelphia: JB Lippincott, 1986:1–86, with permission.)

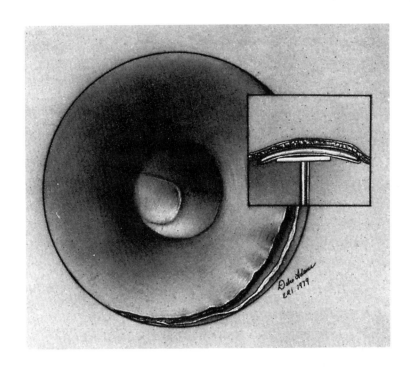

FIG. 11. The cartilage covering the prosthesis results in a slight tenting of the tympanic membrane, which is a sign of proper prosthesis length. The thickness of the cartilage adds tension to the assembly, which results in a secure connection. (From Sheehy JL. Surgery of chronic otitis media. In: English GE, ed. *Otolaryngology.* Philadelphia: JB Lippincott, 1986:1–86, with permission.)

geons or institutions. The variables include middle ear status (i.e., condition of muscosa, presence or absence of cholesteatoma), ossicular status (i.e., stapes present vs. footplate only), type of prosthesis used, and primary versus secondary (revision or staged) procedure. Postoperative hearing results typically are better following tympanoplasty versus tympanoplasty with mastoidectomy. Better hearing results are expected with use of partial ossicular prostheses compared with total ossicular prostheses, as the presence of a stapes superstructure results in more stable prosthesis position. A 15-dB gap for partial ossicular prostheses and 20-dB gap for total ossicular prostheses are considered by some to be good surgical results (43). Table 5 lists typical hearing results based on prosthesis type (12).

Two thirds of patients after tympanoplasty with mastoidectomy when staged will have closure to within 20 dB (5). Age correlates with hearing improvement, with teenagers having better results than children or adults

TABLE 5. *Hearing results by prosthesis type*

Postoperative hearing result (residual conductive deficit)	Partial ossicular prosthesis	Total ossicular prosthesis
≤10 dB	50%	40%
≤20 dB	75%	70%
≤30 dB	85%	80%

From Shelton C, Sheehy JL. TORPs and PORPs for ossicular reconstruction: the House Ear Clinic experience. In: Yanagihara N, Suzuki JI, eds. Proceedings of the second international symposium on transplants and implants in otology. Amsterdam: Kugler Publications, 1992:81–84.

(31). Long-term studies have shown that 5-year hearing levels generally are stable, although some gradual decline may occur over time. Extrusion rates approximate 5% and most typically occur within 2 years for Plastipore prostheses (5). Similar extrusion rates are observed with hydroxyapatite prostheses. Our experience suggests that tympanic membrane problems and eustachian tube dysfunction rather than biocompatibility are the most common causes of extrusion when the techniques of tympanoplasty and ossicular reconstruction are applied properly. If partial extrusion should occur (i.e., prosthesis platform exposed) without infection and with acceptable hearing, the patient is observed and maintained on water precautions (5).

MASTOIDECTOMY

Schwartze initially described the performance of, and indications for, standard mastoidectomy (15). Subsequently, techniques of radical and modified radical mastoidectomy developed to remove cholesteatoma and control chronic otitis media. From developments in tympanoplasty concepts, Jansen initially described CWU surgery and the facial recess approach was later applied and improved by others (2). Mastoid surgery may accompany tympanoplasty or less commonly is performed as an isolated procedure. The mastoid cavity may be exteriorized in a CWD procedure or isolated as in the CWU technique. The cavity may be obliterated. Radical, modified radical, and obliteration mastoidectomies are variations, as described in Table 1.

CWU and CWD mastoidectomies will be discussed in greater detail, as they are the most commonly performed in the setting of chronic otitis media surgery. The other techniques are applied more rarely. Modified radical mastoidectomy may be used in attic or pars flaccida cholesteatoma to exteriorize disease when cholesteatoma is present lateral to the ossicles with minimal conductive deficits. This technique also is applied in cases of an only hearing ear and as such is not staged.

Mastoid obliteration is used when hearing is not an issue and in the setting of extensive mastoidectomy. All squamous epithelium is removed from the cavity, the external auditory canal, and any tympanic membrane remnant. The cavity is obliterated with muscle and the external auditory canal sewn shut.

A well-performed mastoidectomy will help accomplish disease elimination and a dry ear. Creation of a healed, clean cavity without anatomic factors leading to residual or recurrent disease or hidden cholesteatoma is important.

Considerations

Controversy continues to exist with respect to the initial surgical approach for cholesteatoma removal and the use of either CWU or CWD techniques. Superiority is claimed by proponents of each, although proper application of either technique allows for success. Hearing results may be somewhat better with CWU surgery and the larger middle ear cleft provided. However, some suggest that rates of residual and recurrent disease are increased. CWD surgery has a longer healing period and requires regular cavity cleaning and water precautions.

Austin (46) found a significant difference in recidivism, with 4% for CWD and 39% for CWU, but somewhat better hearing results for the latter. He recommended CWD surgery in small sclerotic mastoids and when revision surgery was necessary because of recurrent disease. Although we use the CWU technique in the majority of primary cases, the CWD approach is used in cases of extensive posterior canal wall destruction or in contracted mastoids (low dural plate, forward sigmoid sinus).

Revision tympanoplasty with mastoidectomy may be required for recurrent cholesteatoma, persistent otorrhea, or poor hearing results. Recurrent infection is a common cause for revision surgery in CWD cases. Potential predisposing problems include an insufficient meatoplasty, high facial ridge, incomplete posterior canal wall removal, dependent mastoid tip cells, incomplete cell tract removal (commonly along the middle fossa dural plate), retained cholesteatoma, and excessive mucosal disease with granulation and debris (8).

Surgical Approaches

These operations usually are performed through a postauricular approach as used for tympanoplasty. Endaural mastoidectomy now is rarely taught and has limited visualization.

CWU Mastoidectomy

Advantages of this technique include the lack of need for cavity cleaning and water avoidance, faster healing, and possibly better hearing results (47). No canal distortion occurs, leading to better cosmesis and better accommodation of hearing aids, if necessary. Disadvantages include the technique itself, which may be difficult to perform because it usually requires a facial recess approach. Also, the risk of residual and recurrent cholesteatoma, as previously mentioned, is higher.

Using general anesthesia, the patient is prepped, draped, and secured. The postauricular and vascular strip/canal incisions are injected with 1% lidocaine with 1:100,000 epinephrine. Tympanoplasty canal skin incisions are performed as described previously. Next, a postauricular incision should be made 0.5 to 1 cm behind the sulcus from the superior insertion of the auricle to the mastoid tip, allowing for adequate forward retraction of the auricle and exposure of the temporalis fascia and eventually the external canal. Exposure of the mastoid cortex is accomplished with a "7"-shaped periosteal incision along the inferior border of the linea temporalis and at the zygomatic root perpendicular to the external canal. The mastoid periosteum is raised with subsequent anterior and inferior elevation. After periosteal elevation, temporalis fascia should be harvested. A superior triangle of muscle and soft tissue superior to the external auditory canal may be removed to prevent canal stenosis. Canal skin is removed, and the anterior canal wall bulge is drilled.

A self-retaining retractor is placed to maintain exposure. Bur cuts are made along the linea temporalis and tangential to the posterior external canal (Fig. 12). Deep to the juncture of these cuts lies the lateral semicircular canal. In drilling toward the antrum, the mastoid dissection should be kept high and forward along the dural plate and zygoma to avoid complications. Key landmarks are identified, including the middle fossa dural plate, which is skeletonized and followed medially. By staying "high" on the dural plate, one will remain superior to the lateral semicircular canal and facial nerve, enabling identification of the antrum. Using this technique, occasionally dura will be exposed while drilling, which causes no harm as long as it is not injured. The aditus is entered and the lateral canal identified (Fig. 13). This landmark allows for subsequent identification of the facial nerve as its tympanic segment abuts the lateral canal's inferior margin. Mastoidectomy is performed under continuous irrigation with exenteration of diseased air cells in the zygomatic arch, sinodural angle, sigmoid sinus, retrofacial region, and mastoid tip.

Removal of bony protrusions or edges is completed with saucerization of the cavity's cortical margin. Saucer-

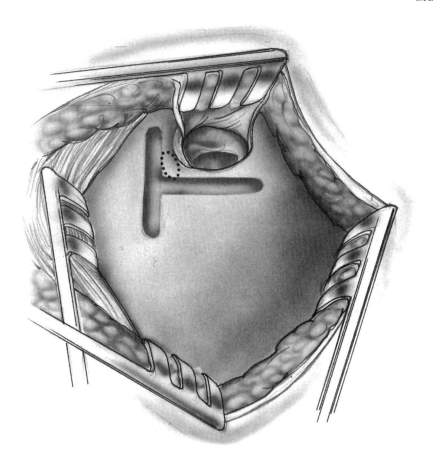

FIG. 12. When starting a mastoidectomy, the initial bur cuts are along the linea temporalis and tangential to the posterior external auditory canal. The *dotted oval* indicates the position of the lateral semicircular canal, within the depths of the mastoid. (From Sheehy JL. Mastoidectomy: the intact canal wall procedure. In: Brackmann DE, Shelton C, Arriaga M, eds. *Otologic surgery.* Philadelphia: WB Saunders, 1994:211–224, with permission.)

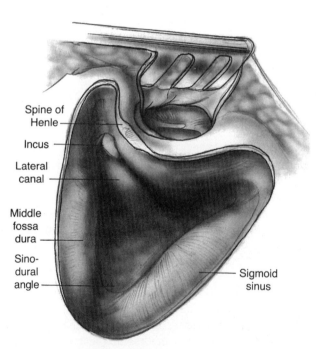

FIG. 13. A completed canal-wall-up mastoidectomy is shown. Note the wide saucerization along the middle fossa dural plate and the sigmoid sinus. The lateral canal and incus are the initial landmarks during this approach. (From Sheehy JL. Mastoidectomy: the intact canal wall procedure. In: Brackmann DE, Shelton C, Arriaga M, eds. *Otologic surgery.* Philadelphia: WB Saunders, 1994:211–224, with permission.)

ization is important to allow adequate visualization in the depth of the mastoid. Use of the largest bur possible is advocated; this is safest for uncovering structures without penetration. One should always consider possible damage to structures from the back side of the bur during drilling. Likewise, separation of the incudostapedial joint prior to mastoid work avoids sensorineural hearing loss from inadvertent trauma to the ossicular head (48).

Mastoid cholesteatoma and previously noted tympanic membrane and middle ear disease are removed. Adequate ventilation of the attic is necessary, and at times extensive disease will require removal of the incus, malleus head, and supporting connective tissue attachments. A lateral semicircular canal fistula should be suspected when elevating overlying matrix, particularly when the profile of the lateral canal is flattened or concave. The most conservative management of a fistula is to leave the medial wall of the cholesteatoma matrix intact. This is particularly true for large fistulas, with consideration given to removal at the second stage when less infection is present (49). Some advocate complete removal of matrix at the initial surgery with fistula coverage by fascia, bone wax, or muscle (6). A facial recess approach is drilled using the fossa incudis as the key landmark (Fig. 14A). This approach is critical in using CWU techniques as it allows removal of cholesteatoma and mucosal disease in that portion of the middle ear cleft that often is affected. The

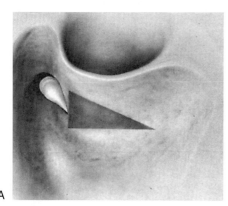
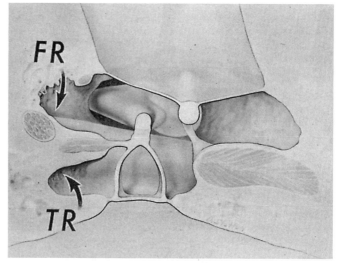

A

B

FIG. 14. A: The facial recess is shown by the *shaded triangle,* which is bordered by the chorda tympani, the vertical facial nerve, and the fossa incudis. B: The facial recess (*FR*) is shown between the cross section of the vertical facial nerve and the chorda tympani. The sinus tympani (*TR*) also is shown. (From Sheehy JL. Surgery of chronic otitis media. In: English GE, ed. *Otolaryngology.* Philadelphia: JB Lippincott, 1986:1–86, with permission.)

posterior external canal is thinned. Progressively smaller burs are used, stroking in the direction of the facial nerve until the middle ear is entered through the facial recess air cells located between the chorda tympani and facial nerve (Fig. 14B). Remaining between these two structures will help prevent undue resection of the posterior external auditory canal and maintenance of its buttressing properties (Fig. 15).

Removal of cholesteatoma from the oval window is completed with caution to prevent stapes subluxation. After use of appropriate instrumentation for removal of remaining disease within the middle ear, consideration is

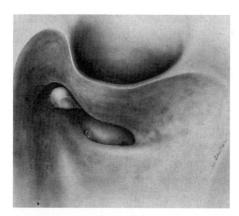

FIG. 15. A widely open facial recess allows access to the posterosuperior portion of the middle ear and all of the posterior epitympanum, the most common location for cholesteatoma. (From Sheehy JL. Surgery of chronic otitis media. In: English GE, ed. *Otolaryngology.* Philadelphia: JB Lippincott, 1986: 1–86, with permission.)

given to proceed with reconstruction or staging. If staging is chosen, Silastic sheeting is placed through the facial recess to the level of the tegmen. Gelfilm may be used similarly if the ear is not being staged. Ossicular chain reconstruction and tympanoplasty are performed as described previously.

The postauricular incision is closed with deep interrupted absorbable suture followed by a running subcuticular skin closure. Drains are not routinely used. A mastoid pressure dressing is applied for 24 hours.

CWD Mastoidectomy

This technique is primarily used in situations of revision surgery, lateral canal fistula to exteriorize cholesteatoma matrix, or cholesteatoma in an only hearing ear where limiting recurrence and minimizing hearing loss are paramount. Additional indications include a contracted, poorly aerated, sclerotic mastoid and a scutum or canal wall that has been severely eroded. Limitations of the CWD procedure include the narrowing of the middle ear space and less favorable hearing results (49).

Cavities created using this technique should be well rounded, with the floor of the mastoid cavity continuous with the floor of the external canal. A high facial ridge (posterior external auditory canal wall remnant) is the most common reason for the requirement of revision mastoid surgery in chronic otitis media and is affectionately known as a "beginner's hump." Avoidance of middle ear space narrowing and tympanostapediopexy are vital features in successful application of this technique (49). Staging may be useful for extensive disease and the indications are the same as for CWU surgery.

The technique is the same as that of CWU surgery until the performance of a facial recess approach, although the posterior canal wall can be removed simultaneously with execution of the mastoidectomy. A postauricular incision is used and a cortical mastoidectomy performed, with identification of landmarks and removal of air cell disease. The external auditory canal skin is elevated and the middle ear inspected. At this point the posterior canal wall is lowered to the level of the facial nerve, leaving a smooth rounded cavity without ledges or overhangs. Concern about injuring the facial nerve by inexperienced surgeons limits adequate removal of the facial ridge in many cases. Some advocate the use of facial nerve monitoring in this setting (8). As one approaches the nerve, the vasa nervorum will yield a pinkish hue, which aids in identification. In the setting of chronic disease and inflamed mucosa, identification of the facial nerve may be more difficult. A technique to identify the nerve in this setting involves use of a blunt instrument to palpate tissue of unsure origin. Nerve will bounce back rapidly, whereas mucosa will not. The chorda tympani should be sacrificed to enhance exposure and aid in disease removal. Some recommend sharp transection of the chorda to prevent retrograde facial nerve edema (8).

Mastoid tip air cells are removed if pneumatized, which prevents retention of collected debris postoperatively that is difficult to clean. The lateral tip is removed to the level of the digastric ridge (Fig. 16). The ridge is about the level of the stylomastoid foramen, but is not always an obvious landmark. Once the tip has been removed, the overlying soft tissue will fall in and obliterate this space.

Removal of disease and cholesteatoma of the middle ear space are performed as described previously. Adequate saucerization of cavity margins allows for settling of overlying soft tissue, resulting in a smaller cavity from autoobliteration. Additional techniques for cavity reduction include a Palva flap. This anteriorly based, postauricular subcutaneous flap can be placed into the mastoid posteriorly. Bone pate harvested early in the case from the cortical mastoidectomy also may be used to reduce the cavity size. A Palva-style flap or the use of bone pate in the inferior mastoid cavity can be used to create a less dependent, easier cleaning cavity. Tympanic membrane grafts should be large enough to cover the facial ridge.

Reconstruction of the scutum and posterior canal wall is advocated by some (50). Local flaps may be developed. Bone pate and autologous cartilage can recreate a buttress, as will hydroxyapatite implants. The benefits include those of CWU advantages, prevention of retraction, and better hearing possibilities, although the techniques are not always successful and require careful attention.

Meatoplasty

An enlarged meatus is essential in CWD surgery. Inadequate time and technique in performance of the meatoplasty can jeopardize an otherwise well-performed mastoidectomy due to diminished ventilation, retention of material, and cleaning difficulties. The meatoplasty should be wide, allowing for adequate aeration, prevention of accumulated moisture, and ease of cleaning and postoperative cavity examination. This

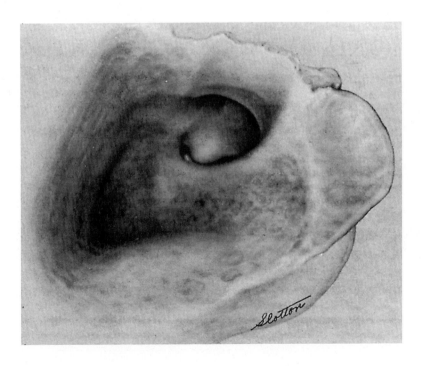

FIG. 16. A canal-wall-down mastoidectomy has been completed, showing saucerization along the middle fossa dural plate and the posterior margin of the cavity. In this case, the mastoid tip has been amputated to the level of the digastric ridge, allowing obliteration of this area with soft tissue. (From Sheehy JL. Surgery of chronic otitis media. In: English GE, ed. *Otolaryngology.* Philadelphia: JB Lippincott, 1986:1–86, with permission.)

portion of the procedure may be overlooked at the termination of the case, but it actually requires forethought and good technique. A no. 2 endaural incision is made through canal skin and the intratragal notch to the temporalis fascia (Fig. 17A). Periosteum and soft tissues are debulked posteriorly. A 1.5-cm crescent of conchal cartilage is excised. Due to circumferential contracture it is necessary to create an opening larger than that finally desired. When removing the conchal cartilage, an anteriorly based perichondrial flap is created, which can be sewn posteriorly to the periosteum with interrupted absorbable suture of adequate tension to create a generous meatus (Fig. 17B). Undue tension may result in rotation and undue prominence of the auricle. A meatus diameter large enough to accommodate the surgeon's thumb usually is adequate, as it will shrink with subsequent healing.

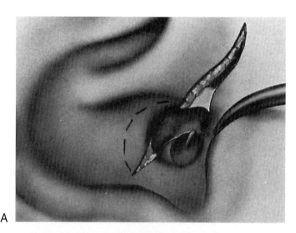

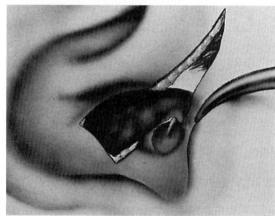

FIG. 17. A: For meatoplasty, the initial incision is a no. 2 endaural incision, with a second incision along the tympanomastoid suture line. A large crescent of conchal cartilage (*dotted line*) is removed to allow posterior retraction of the conchal skin. **B:** The conchal skin is sewn posteriorly, allowing enlargement of the resultant meatus. (From Sheehy JL. Surgery of chronic otitis media. In: English GE, ed. *Otolaryngology.* Philadelphia: JB Lippincott, 1986:1–86, with permission.)

Postoperative Care

Patients are instructed to remove their mastoid dressing on the first postoperative day and to maintain water avoidance for the ear. The initial visit is 1 week later. Removal of Steri-Strips from the postauricular incision and otoscopic examination to rule out infection are completed. Residual packing is removed at a second follow-up appointment 1 month postoperatively. To avoid fibrosis, care is taken to completely remove all external auditory canal packing. Drops are started 1 week prior to this appointment to loosen the remaining packing.

SUMMARY POINTS

- Successful surgery for chronic otitis media involves a systematic approach based on the primary aims of disease eradication, reconstruction of the middle ear and sound conducting mechanism, and prevention of cholesteatoma recurrence and surgical complication.
- Tympanoplasty should result in a healed membrane with a mucosalized, aerated middle ear cleft without adhesions for maximal ossicular reconstructive benefits.
- Overlay or underlay tympanoplasty techniques using fascia grafts result in reliable closure of tympanic membrane perforations.
- Adequate tension during ossicular chain reconstruction results in stable, long-term hearing results with prevention of extrusion.
- The decision to stage tympanoplasty is based on the degree of mucosal disease, presence of ossicular (stapes) fixation, and the possibilities of residual cholesteatoma.
- Hearing results from ossicular chain reconstruction are best with an intact stapes, rather than when only a stapes footplate is remaining.
- CWU techniques with a facial recess approach are applicable in most cases of severe disease and cholesteatoma and have the advantage of normal anatomic contour postoperatively.
- Children tend to have more aggressive cholesteatoma, although rates of recidivism and hearing results may be comparable to those of adults.
- The extrusion rates of hydroxyapatite and cartilage-covered Plastipore ossicular prostheses are similar.
- Important factors in creating a trouble-free CWD mastoid cavity include adequate lowering of the facial ridge, saucerization of the cavity margins, ample-sized meatus, and removal of mastoid tip, if pneumatized.

REFERENCES

1. Nylen CO. The microscope in aural surgery, its first use and later development. *Acta Otol Laryngol Suppl* 1954;116:226–240.
2. Briggs RJS, Luxford WM. Chronic ear surgery: a historical review. *Am J Otol* 1994;15:558–567.
3. Committee on Conservation of Hearing of the American Academy of Ophthalmology and Otolaryngology. Standard classification for surgery of chronic ear infection. *Arch Otolaryngol* 1965;81:204–205.
4. Sheehy JL. Surgery of chronic otitis media. In: English GE, ed. *Otolaryngology*. Philadelphia: JB Lippincott Co., 1986;1–86.
5. Shelton C, Sheehy JL. Tympanoplasty: review of 400 staged cases. *Laryngoscope* 1990;100:679–681.
6. Herzog JA, Smith PG, Kletzker GR, Maxwell KS. Management of labyrinthine fistula secondary to cholesteatoma. *Am J Otol* 1996;17:410–415.
7. Leighton SE, Robson AK, Anslow P, Milford CA. The role of CT imaging in the management of chronic suppurative otitis media. *Clin Otolaryngol* 1993;18:23–29.
8. Jackson CG, Schall DG, Glasscock ME, Macias JD, Widick MH, Touma BJ. A surgical solution for the difficult chronic ear. *Am J Otol* 1996;17:7–14.
9. Garber LZ, Dort JC. Cholesteatoma: diagnosis and staging by CT scan. *J Otolaryngol* 1994;23:121–124.
10. O'Reilly BJ, Chevretton EB, Wylie I, et al. The value of CT scanning in chronic suppurative otitis media. *J Laryngol Otol* 1991;105:990–994.
11. Sedwick J, Shelton C, Jackson CG. Preoperative treatment of allergy, nasal or sinus disease: does it affect the outcome of chronic ear surgery? *(submitted)*.
12. Shelton C, Sheehy JL. TORPs and PORPs for ossicular reconstruction: The House Ear Clinic experience. In: Yanagihara N, Suzuki JI, eds. *Proceedings of the Second International Symposium on Transplants and Implants in Otology*. Amsterdam: Kugler Publications, 1992:81–84.
13. Tos M, Falbe-Hansen J Jr. Tympanoplasty in only hearing ears. *J Laryngol Otol* 1975;89:1057–1064.
14. Perez de Tagle JRV, Fenton JE, Fagan PA. Mastoid surgery in the only hearing ear. *Laryngoscope* 1996;106:67–70.
15. Pappas DG. Otology through the ages. *Otolaryngol Head Neck Surg* 1996;114:173–196.
16. Wullstein H. Theory and practice of tympanoplasty. *Laryngoscope* 1956;66:1076–1093.
17. Zollner F. Principles of plastic surgery of the sound conducting apparatus. *J Laryngol Otol* 1955;69:637–652.
18. House WF, Sheehy JL. Myringoplasty: use of ear canal skin compared with other techniques. *Arch Otol Head Neck Surg* 1961;73:407–415.
19. Storrs LA. Myringoplasty with use of fascia graft. *Arch Otol Head Neck Surg* 1961;74:45–49.
20. Clymer MA, Schwaber MK, Davidson JM. The effects of keratinocyte growth factor on healing of tympanic membrane perforations. *Laryngoscope* 1996;106:280–285.
21. Spandow O, Hellstrom S, Dahlstrom M. Structural characterization of persistent tympanic membrane perforations in man. *Laryngoscope* 1996;106:346–352.
22. Glasscock ME, Jackson CG, Nissen AJ, Schwaber MK. Postauricular undersurface tympanic membrane grafting: a follow-up report. *Laryngoscope* 1982;92:718–727.
23. Glasscock ME, Jackson CG, Knox GW. Can acquired immunodeficiency syndrome and Creutzfeldt-Jakob disease be transmitted via otologic homografts? *Arch Otolaryngol Head Neck Surg* 1988;114:1252–1255.
24. Bujia J, Wilmes E, Kastenbauer E, Gurtler L. Influences of chemical allograft presentation procedures on the human immunodeficiency virus. *Laryngoscope* 1996;106:645–647.
25. Caye-Thomasen P, Hermansson A, Tos M, Prellner K. Pathogenesis of middle ear adhesions. *Laryngoscope* 1996;106:463–469.
26. Rambo JHT. Use of paraffin to create a middle ear space in musculoplasty. *Laryngoscope* 1961;71:612–619.
27. Sheehy JL, Shelton C. Tympanoplasty: to stage or not to stage. *Otolaryngol Head Neck Surg* 1991;104:399–407.
28. Sheehy JL, Crabtree JA. Tympanoplasty: staging the operation. *Laryngoscope* 1973;83:1594–1621.
29. Ng M, Linthicum FH. Long term effects of silastic sheeting in the middle ear. *Laryngoscope* 1992;102:1097–1102.
30. Gristwood RE, Venables WN. Factors influencing the probability of residual cholesteatoma. *Ann Otol Rhinol Laryngol* 1990;99:120–123.
31. Schuring AG, Lippy WH, Rizer FM, Schuring LT. Staging for cholesteatoma in the child, adolescent and adult. *Ann Otol Rhinol Laryngol* 1990;99:256–260.
32. Brackmann DE. Tympanoplasty with mastoidectomy: canal wall up procedures. *Am J Otol* 1993;14:380–382.
33. Smyth GDL, Hassard TH. Tympanoplasty in children. *Am J Otol* 1980;1:199–205.
34. Sheehy JL. Cholesteatoma surgery in children. *Am J Otol* 1985;6:170–172.
35. Parisier SC, Hanson MB, Han JC, Cohen AJ, Selkin BA. Pediatric cholesteatoma: an individualized single-stage approach. *Otolaryngol Head Neck Surg* 1996;115:107–114.
36. Gyo K, Sasaki Y, Hinohira Y, Yanagihara N. Residue of middle ear cholesteatoma after intact canal wall tympanoplasty: surgical findings at one year. *Ann Otol Rhinol Laryngol* 1996;105:615–619.
37. Glasscock ME, Miller GW. Intact canal wall tympanoplasty in the management of cholesteatoma. *Laryngoscope* 1976;86:1639–1657.
38. Austin DF. Ossicular reconstruction. *Arch Otol* 1971;94:525–535.
39. Meylan PRA, Duscher A, Mudry A, Monnier P. Risk of transmission of human immunodeficiency virus during tympano-ossicular homograft: an experimental study. *Laryngoscope* 1996;106:334–337.
40. Goldenberg RA. Hydroxyl apatite ossicular replacement prostheses: results in 157 consecutive cases. *Laryngoscope* 1992;102:1091–1096.
41. McElveen JT, Feghal JG, Barrs DM, et al. Ossiculplasty with polymaleinate ionomeric prosthesis. *Otolaryngol Head Neck Surg* 1985;113:420–426.
42. McElveen JT, Feghali JG, Barrs DM, et al. Bone cement reconstruction of the ossicular chain. *Laryngoscope* 1998;108:829–836.
43. Brackmann DE, Sheehy JL, Luxford WM. TORPs and PORPs in tympanoplasty: a review of 1042 operations. *Otolaryngol Head Neck Surg* 1984;92:32–37.
44. Daniels RL, Shelton C. Revision ossicular reconstruction. In: Pillsbury HC, Carrasco VN, eds. *Revision ossicular surgery*. New York: Thieme Medical Publishers, 1997:23–41.
45. Sheehy JL. Tympanoplasty: cartilage and porous polyethylene. In: Brackmann DE, Shelton C, Arriaga MA, eds. *Otologic surgery*. Philadelphia: WB Saunders, 1994:179–184.
46. Austin DF. Single-stage surgery for cholesteatoma: an actuarial analysis. *Am J Otol* 1989;10:419–425.
47. Brown JS. A ten year statistical follow-up of 1142 consecutive cases of cholesteatoma: the closed vs. the open technique. *Laryngoscope* 1982;92:390–396.
48. Palva T, Karja J, Palva A. High-tone sensorineural losses following chronic ear surgery. *Arch Otolaryngol* 1973;98:176–178.
49. Sheehy JL, Brackmann DE. Surgery of chronic ear disease: what we do and why we do it. In: *Otology, audiology, and neurotology instructional courses*, volume 6. St. Louis: Mosby, 1993:349–353.
50. Black B, Kelly S. Mastoidectomy reconstruction: management of the high facial ridge using hydroxyapatite implants. *Am J Otol* 1994;15:785–792.

The Ear: Comprehensive Otology,
edited by R. F. Canalis and P. R. Lambert.
Lippincott Williams & Wilkins, Philadelphia © 2000.

CHAPTER 28

Otosclerosis

Victor Goodhill, Irwin Harris, and Rinaldo F. Canalis

   I. Harris: Department of Surgery, Division of Head and Neck Surgery, University of California, Los Angeles, School of Medicine, Los Angeles, California 90095-6959
   R. F. Canalis: Department of Surgery, University of California, Los Angeles, School of Medicine, Los Angeles, California 90095-1624

DEFINITION

Otosclerosis is osteodystrophy limited to the temporal bone and primarily affecting the otic capsule. It usually results in stapes fixation but may also involve the cochlea and other parts of the labyrinth. This chapter focuses on the clinical features of otosclerosis. Other noninfectious entities characterized by conductive hearing loss are discussed briefly.

HISTORICAL PERSPECTIVE

Valsalva first described ankylosis of the stapes in 1704 during dissection of the ear of a cadaver of a man known to have been deaf for most of his life (1). Toynbee (2) in 1841 described fixation of the base of the stapes to the margins of the oval window and went on to find 136 similar cases during his dissections of more than 1,000 temporal bones (3). Politzer (4) first showed the histologic characteristics of the disease and established it as a primary disorder of the otic capsule that produced new abnormal bone.

EPIDEMIOLOGY

The exact incidence of clinical otosclerosis is unknown, but it is estimated at between 5% and 10% of the white population (5,6). Otosclerosis has been described histologically in fetuses, young children, and adults of all ages (7,8). In a classic study, Guild (7) found histologic otosclerosis in 8.3% of 518 temporal bones of white Americans and 1% of 482 African-Americans older than 5 years. The clinical disease appears to be more common among women (9,10); however, histologic studies have not shown a significant prevalence for either sex (7,8).

The genetic aspects of the disease were first discussed by Gapany-Gapanavicius (11) in a study that involved 974 patients. He concluded that otosclerosis is not inherited as a simple autosomal trait purely dominant or recessive but as a form of autosomal, dominant transmission with incomplete penetrance and variable expressivity. This view was supported by Donnell and Alfi (12), who reported that penetrance is less than 50% and the risk that a person with otosclerosis will have a child with the disorder is 1 in 4.

PATHOGENESIS

The causation and pathogenesis of otosclerosis are not clearly understood. Theories include traumatic, vascular, developmental, immunologic, and viral causes. Some theories have little or no experimental support and are only briefly mentioned here to provide a historical perspective. Mechanical stress–producing areas of breakdown and abnormal repair of the otic capsule were implicated by Mayer (13) and Sercer and Krmpotic (14). Mayer (15) and Mendoza and Ruis (16) believed that otosclerotic foci were present in areas of nonviable bone resulting from decreased blood supply. Wolff and Bellucci (17) related precursory bone changes to acidity of the perivascular tissue that produced decalcification of the osseous matrix and areas of abnormal repair.

Gussen (18,19) equated the changes in the otic capsule that led to otosclerosis to those of aging. These changes consist of obstruction of vascular canals that produces loss of osteocytes and mineralization of empty lacunae and canaliculi (micropetrosis). Gussen (20) also described aging changes in the stapediovestibular joint and showed their progression to degenerative arthritis and erosion of the articular cartilage and of the oval window rim. Repair by means of osteoneogenesis produces bone structurally identical to that of otosclerosis. Anson and Bast (21) first described the presence of embryonic cartilage rests in the otic capsule that they thought capable of producing abnormal bone similar to that of otosclerosis. Mann et al. (22) presented additional morphologic evidence supporting this concept, and Yoo et al. (23) found high levels of type II collagen (the prevalent or major collagen cartilage) in otosclerotic specimens. They proposed that otosclerosis derives from an autoimmune process against collagen molecules. Further support for this concept was advanced by Bujia et al. (24). These authors used an enzyme-linked immunosorbent assay to compare the sera of eight patients with otosclerosis with that of eight sex- and age-matched healthy donors. Levels of antibodies to collagen II and IX (a minor cartilage collagen) were significantly higher among persons with otosclerosis.

A possible viral cause of otosclerosis has been investigated by several authors (25,26) after acquisition of increasing evidence that a viral agent may be causative in Paget's disease of bone, which has similarities with dystrophy (27,28). Arnold and Friedman (25) first identified the presence of measles and rubella viruses around active otosclerotic foci. McKenna and Mills (26) used monoclonal antibody techniques to demonstrate specific reactivity for the measles virus in four temporal bone specimens of patients with otosclerosis. Reactions to other related paramyxoviruses were negative. Further evidence of the presence of the measles virus in areas of active otosclerosis was obtained by McKenna et al. (29) from 8 of 11 temporal bones by means of polymerase chain reaction aimed at identifying both the DNA and RNA sequences of the virus.

PATHOLOGY

The dystrophy of otosclerosis mainly involves the endochondral layer of the otic capsule. In the earliest stage otospongiosis occurs and is characterized by increased vascularity and bone resorption. This spongy vascular form is more frequent among children and young adults (Fig. 1). The more typical sclerotic form occurs among older patients, in whom vascular spaces are replaced by dense, mosaic-patterned immature bone with distinctive staining characteristics and architecture (Fig. 2). Combinations of both phases may be seen in the same specimen.

Schuknecht (30) described the morphologic features of the sequential changes of otosclerosis. The process starts with resorption of endochondral bone that is prob-

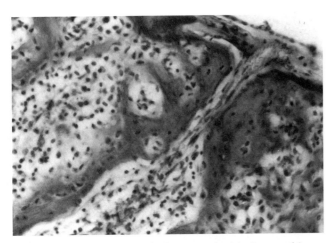

FIG. 1. Cellular otosclerosis (otospongiosis). Areas of bone resorption are filled with large numbers of osteoblasts and mononuclear cells surrounding capillaries (hematoxylin and eosin, original magnification × 420). (From Gussen R. Otosclerosis and vestibular degeneration. *Arch Otolaryngol* 1973; 97:484–487, with permission.)

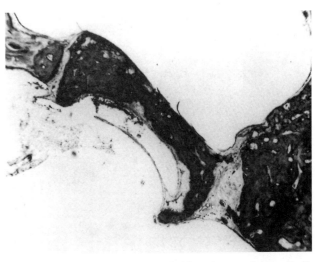

FIG. 3. Portion of normal stapedial footplate and crus. Cartilage lining is present along joint surface at right and along inner ear (vestibule) surface at bottom (hematoxylin and eosin, original magnification × 40). (From Gussen R. The ear. In: Coulson W, ed. *Surgical pathology*. Philadelphia: JB Lippincott, 1978, with permission.)

ably caused by the action of lysosomal hydrolases and osteoclasts. Thereafter osteoid is laid down within the collagen matrix and produces islands of immature basophilic bone called *blue mantles*. Finally the apposition of new mature, acidophilic and laminated bone leads to the emergence of the highly mineralized mosaic patterns typical of the disease.

Otosclerosis initially involves the anterior aspect of the oval window, the annular ligament of the stapes, and the root of the anterior crus (site of prevalence) (Figs. 3, 4). Otosclerotic lesions may remain limited to the footplate or extend to the promontory, facial canal (see Fig. 4), stapedial tendon and incudostapedial joint. Otosclerosis also may invade the vestibular (Fig. 5) and cochlear labyrinths (Fig. 6), round window niche (Fig. 7), and internal auditory canal. Schuknecht and Barber (31) found that 96% of patients with clinical otosclerosis had foci anterior to the oval window, and 49% had concomitant involvement of other areas. Otosclerosis of the stapes causes conductive hearing loss, and involvement of the labyrinth may cause sensorineural hearing deficits. The

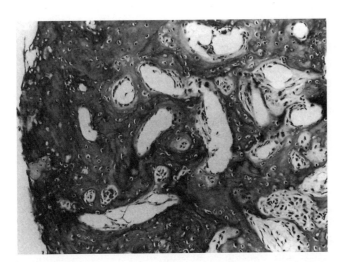

FIG. 2. Otosclerotic involvement of stapedial footplate. Cellular membrane bone has closely spaced osteocytes, considerable osteoblastic activity, and numerous vascular channels (hematoxylin and eosin, original magnification × 40). (From Gussen R. The ear. In: Coulson W, ed. *Surgical pathology*. Philadelphia: JB Lippincott, 1978, with permission.)

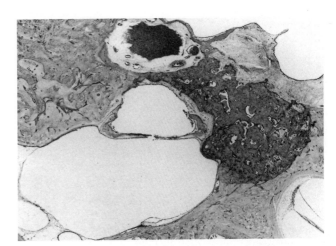

FIG. 4. Otosclerosis of oval window anterosuperiorly and partially lining facial nerve canal (hematoxylin and eosin, original magnification × 14). (From Gussen R. Otosclerosis and vestibular degeneration. *Arch Otolaryngol* 1973;97:484–487, with permission.)

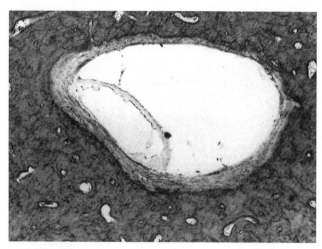

FIG. 5. Semicircular canal surrounded by otosclerotic bone. Collagenous endosteum is widened (uncovered) and bony surface is set farther back (hematoxylin and eosin, original magnification × 70). (From Gussen R. Otosclerosis and vestibular degeneration. *Arch Otolaryngol* 1973;97:484–487, with permission.)

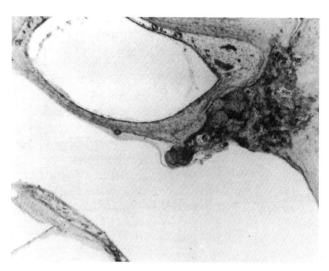

FIG. 7. Otosclerosis involving round window is direct continuation of nonankylosing otosclerosis of stapediovestibular joint. (From Goodhill V. Surgery for otosclerosis: stapedectomy, stapedioplasty and fenestration. In: English GM, ed. *Otolaryngology,* vol. II. Hagerstown, MD: Harper & Row, 1976:5, with permission.)

occurrence of otosclerosis limited to the cochlea and producing only sensorineural hearing loss has been under considerable scrutiny. In Schuknecht's large series, only two temporal bone specimens were found to have severe cochlear otosclerosis, which could be deemed the principal cause of the patient's deafness (32). A rare, rapidly progressive form of the disorder involving the oval and round windows, cochlea, and vestibular labyrinth is called *malignant otosclerosis.* It leads to severe or profound deafness (32).

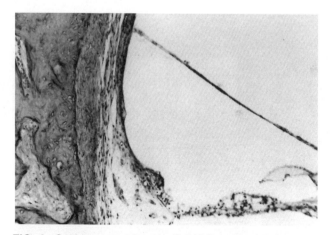

FIG. 6. Cochlear otosclerosis. Spiral ligament is abnormal. Fibrils are parallel and close together with marked loss of spaces. The eroded otosclerotic bone surface has a thickened collagenous endosteum (hematoxylin and eosin, original magnification × 75). (From Gussen R. Otosclerosis and vestibular degeneration. *Arch Otolaryngol* 1973;97:484–487, with permission.)

HISTORY AND PHYSICAL FINDINGS

The primary symptom of otosclerosis is conductive hearing loss. A positive family history is found among approximately 50% of patients (12). The clinical onset usually is in early- or mid-adult life, but the condition may present in childhood. Approximately 15% of patients treated with stapedectomy are reported to have had a hearing deficit before 18 years of age (33). The hearing impairment usually is progressive, reaching the maximum in the patient's forties. Thereafter the loss tends to remain stable, but the degree of eventual sensorineural deafness is unpredictable. Among women hearing loss frequently worsens during pregnancy (10,34). The rate of hearing deterioration tends to be asymmetric. A patient may have the impression that the loss of hearing is sudden after physical or emotional trauma or an acute illness. The importance of such apparently casual relations is unclear.

Otosclerosis is unilateral in only 15% of cases (5,6,10). When limited to the stapes, the hearing loss sometimes is associated with an unexplained phenomenon known as *paracusis of Willis* (better hearing ability in a noisy environment). Tinnitus is one of the most common symptoms of otosclerosis. It varies in intensity and may be unilateral or bilateral, continuous or fluctuating, and roaring or hissing in character. It is more common in the early stages and may abate as the disease matures. Vestibular disturbances are not infrequent, but vertigo, unsteadiness and other severe labyrinthine symptoms are rare and demand careful investigation to identify the origin (35,36). Otoscopic findings usually are normal. The tympanic membrane may have a transmitted red hue from the promontory (Schwartze's sign). This sign is presumably caused by increased vascularity of the otosclerotic focus.

AUDIOMETRY

Tuning Fork Tests

A negative Rinne test (256 and 512 Hz) response is common in early stapes fixation. Among patients with cochlear involvement, however, it may be difficult to demonstrate an air–bone gap with this test alone. Weber's test is confirmatory when it shows lateralization to the affected side in unilateral otosclerosis or to the poorer ear in bilateral disease.

Standard Audiometry

A progressive pattern may be seen in otosclerosis. The following stages occur among most patients:

1. Initial stiffening of the stapediovestibular joint that causes low-frequency stiffness tilt (37). A slight air–bone gap occurs on the audiogram (Fig. 8).
2. As the footplate becomes fixed, the air–bone gap widens and involves all frequencies (Fig. 9).
3. As frictional elements are added, the air conduction level drops throughout the audiometric range, and the air–bone gap widens. A cochlear lesion may

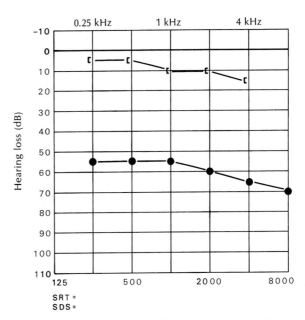

FIG. 9. Frictional component adds high-frequency tilt to both air conduction and bone conduction levels. •—•, Air conduction, unmasked, right ear; [—[, bone conduction, masked, right ear; speech reception threshold, 55%; speech discrimination score, 100%.

produce a high-frequency sensorineural hearing loss (Fig. 10) and a drop in speech discrimination score.
4. Cochlear loss progresses in severity and may reach a severe level of impairment.

The Carhart Notch

Patients with otosclerosis often show an apparent loss in bone conduction in the frequency region around 2,000 Hz (Fig. 11). This notch was first described by Carhart (38) in 1950. It is caused by stapedial fixation and reflects reduction of the middle ear component that contributes to the total bone conduction threshold. Carhart found that otosclerosis reduces bone conduction thresholds by 5 dB at 500 Hz, 10 dB at 1,000 Hz, 25 dB at 2,000 Hz, and 15 dB at 4,000 Hz. These observations are important in the assessment of surgical results because improvements in air conduction thresholds may exceed preoperative bone conduction thresholds by amounts that approximate the average magnitudes of the Carhart notch.

Acoustic Impedance

Tympanometric findings often are normal in otosclerosis, especially early cases. Impedance may increase in advanced cases because of severe fixation of the ossicular chain. The acoustic reflex almost always is absent.

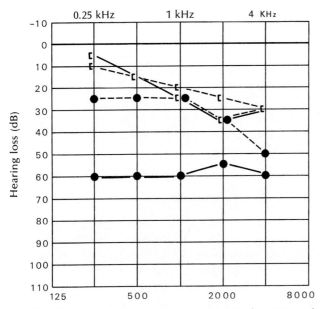

FIG. 8. Stiffness tilt in early otosclerosis. Low-frequency air conduction tilt with little change elsewhere. The 2-kHz bone conduction dip is attributable to the Carhart notch. •—•, Air conduction, unmasked, right ear; [—[, bone conduction, masked right ear.

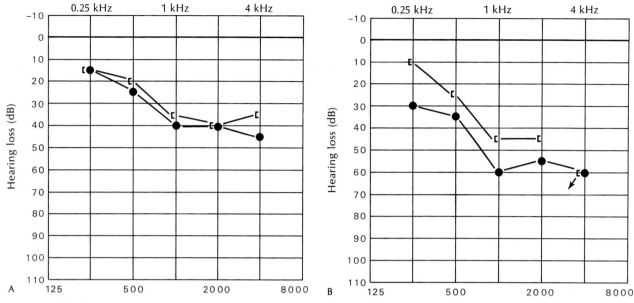

FIG. 10. A: Initial audiogram shows apparent sensorineural hearing loss, positive Rinne test responses, and high speech discrimination score. •—•, Air conduction, unmasked, right ear; [—[, bone conduction, masked, right ear; speech discrimination score, 98%. **B:** Audiogram 3 years later reveals drop in air conduction and an evolving diminishing air–bone gap. Negative Rinne test response at 256 Hz. The speech discrimination score (98%) remained unusually high. •—•, Air conduction, unmasked, right ear; [—[, bone conduction, masked, right ear; *arrow,* no response at maximum output.

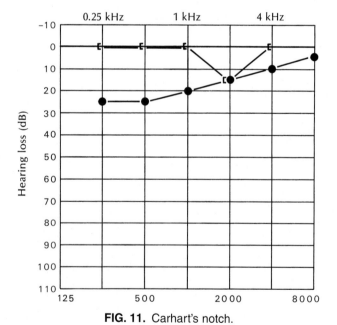

FIG. 11. Carhart's notch.

RADIOGRAPHIC STUDIES

Radiographic studies are not necessary in the routine evaluation of patients with otosclerosis. Computed tomography may be indicated in complex diagnostic problems, especially when structural anomalies or severe cochlear involvement is suspected.

DIFFERENTIAL DIAGNOSIS

The diagnosis of otosclerosis usually is made on the basis of conductive hearing loss, an intact and mobile tympanic membrane, patent eustachian tube, a negative Rinne test result, and absent stapedial reflex. The differential diagnosis includes secretory otitis media, chronic otitis media complicated by middle ear fibrosis, tympanosclerotic fixation of the ossicles, ossicular discontinuity, cholesteatoma behind an intact tympanic membrane, nonotosclerotic pathologic conditions involving the stapes, and congenital anomalies of the ossicles or labyrinthine windows. Most of these conditions are diagnosed at middle ear exploration, although ancillary tests such as computed tomography and myringotomy may help exclude otosclerosis when indicated on the basis of clinical evaluation.

MEDICAL MANAGEMENT

Medical therapies for otosclerosis have been attempted for more than 60 years. Phosphorous (39), thyroxine (40), and dicalcium phosphate (41) have been considered without success. The value of sodium fluoride in the management of active otospongiosis is controversial. Its potential clinical use was first considered when otosclerosis was found among cryolite miners (42) and when it was reported that the incidence of otosclerosis was higher in areas where the drinking water had a low fluoride content (43). It was then proposed that fluoride could inhibit resorbing enzymes present in otospongiotic bone and convert the bone to the inactive otosclerotic type (42). The immediate application of these observations would be to arrest the rapid cochlear deterioration that affects some patients with otosclerosis by preventing the release of damaging enzymes into the labyrinthine fluids from active endosteal foci adjacent to the spiral ligament (44). However, none of these theories has been proved or tested under controlled experimental conditions, and the use of fluoride remains based on clinical observations (45,46). The state of the controversy can be appreciated by the comments of several authorities recorded during a January 1984 conference on the state of the art in otosclerosis (47). At that conference, Shambaugh reported that his 24-year experience with sodium fluoride "demonstrated its value in arresting previously progressive sensorineural hearing loss." Linthicum stated that there were no undesirable side effects among 40,000 patients treated with sodium fluoride. McGee found that sodium fluoride did nothing for his patients. Hough described patients who received two different water supplies in neighboring geographic locations, one very high in fluoride and the other low. The incidence of otosclerosis was similar for both groups. Hough also referred to patients in India whose high intake of environmental fluorides produced toxic symptoms, yet the patients were found to have a high incidence of otosclerosis. Hough concluded that there is no evidence that fluorides help in otosclerosis. Schuknecht found no temporal bone evidence to support fluoride treatment and has never used it.

Research into drugs potentially effective in arresting otosclerosis continues to be focused on compounds to control the active, otospongiotic phase of the dystrophy. Some, such as etidronate disodium, have proved effective in the management of hearing loss associated with Paget's disease (48), have been tested in the management of otosclerosis with unclear results, and need additional study (49).

SURGICAL MANAGEMENT

The first attempt to manage otosclerosis surgically was by Kessel (50), who first mobilized a fixed stapes in 1878. Miot (51) in 1891 reported many successful results for more than 200 patients who underwent stapes mobilization. However, because of opposing views, surgical therapy for otosclerosis was abandoned until Passow (52) in 1897 fenestrated the cochlear promontory and Floderus (53) in 1899 suggested fenestration of the horizontal semicircular canal. This approach was further developed by Jenkins (54) in 1913, Holmgren (55) in 1923, and Sourdille (56) in 1930. Lempert (57) perfected a practical one-stage technique in 1938. In 1952 Rosen (58) reintroduced Miot's operation and established stapes mobilization as the primary therapy for otosclerosis. A year later Shea (59) described the technique of stapedectomy with a polyethylene strut prosthesis over a

vein graft to seal the oval window defect. Since then stapes surgery has become the primary therapy for otosclerosis. In this section the current surgical approaches to stapedial otosclerosis are discussed. Our modifications are included.

Candidate Selection

In general operations on the stapes are indicated for patients with otosclerosis regardless of age who have an average air–bone gap of at least 15 dB, speech discrimination scores of 60% or better, and no anatomic or medical contraindications to exploratory tympanotomy under local anesthesia. The aim of surgical treatment is restoration of available cochlear function, even though this may not always carry the possibility of unaided hearing. Exceptions include patients with a known history of otosclerosis with very poor speech discrimination scores and air conduction levels at the limit of the audiometer output.

Preoperative Management

The probability and definition of surgical success are carefully explained to the patient, and the alternative of hearing aid use is discussed. A detailed written explanation often is beneficial as part of the informed consent. As in any other surgical situation, the general medical condition of the patient is thoroughly evaluated.

SURGICAL TECHNIQUES

After sedation the patient is moved to an operating table capable of 20- to 25-degree lateral tilt. Local anesthesia is preferred by most American otologists. The help of a stand-by anesthesiologist to monitor deep sedation is favored. When general anesthesia is needed, careful infiltration of the surgical field with a local anesthetic (see later) is critical for bleeding control.

Anesthesia is obtained by means of injection of the ear canal with a solution of lidocaine 1% with epinephrine 1:200,000. An initial injection is made with a 27-gauge needle at the inferior apex of the helicotragal junction. Further circumferential injections are made at the osteocartilaginous junction. Approximately 2 mL is injected. The operation is performed through an ear speculum; an operating microscope is used for illumination and magnification.

Circumferential scalpels are used for the endomeatal incision. The incision in the posterior half of the canal skin is omega shaped. It is started at the inferior aspect of the annulus and ended above the short process of the malleus (Fig. 12). The posterior flap, consisting of skin and periosteum, is dissected from the bone. Elevation is facilitated by means of alternative sharp and blunt dissection with cotton pledgets impregnated with epinephrine (1:1,000). Elevation is carried medially to the poste-

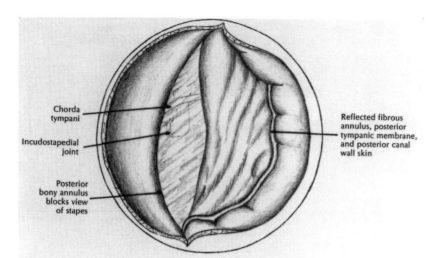

FIG. 12. Omega-shaped incision, elevation, and enucleation of tympanostomy flap.

rior margin of the annular sulcus. The endomeatal incision usually is adequate, but in some cases, such as in the presence of a narrow meatus, partial congenital canal atresia, or obstructive osteophytes, a modified Lempert endaural incision may be necessary. This approach provides a much wider field and is favored by many European surgeons. It has the added advantage of facilitating the use of both hands (60).

A curved pick is used to dislocate the fibrous annulus from the bony sulcus. This maneuver is best started at about the midpoint of the posterior margin. Entrance of the tympanic air space is accomplished by means of severing the mucosal lining between the chorda tympani nerve and the annulus fibrosus. Dislocation of the fibrous annulus is continued superiorly and inferiorly until expo-

sure of the posterior half of the middle ear is obtained. If clear visualization of the stapes is not accomplished, adequate exposure is obtained by means of removing enough annular bone with a curette to make this possible (Figs. 13, 14: see color plate 26 following page 484). The chorda tympani nerve is carefully preserved and displaced anteriorly.

The mobility of the incus is tested with a probe. If the incus is mobile, the integrity of the incudostapedial joint is assessed. Before direct manipulation of the stapes, pledgets of gelatin sponge, dipped in 1% lidocaine solution are placed close to the stapes for topical anesthesia of the tympanic plexus. The pledgets are left in place for a few minutes and then removed. The degree of stapes ankylosis is tested by means of palpating the

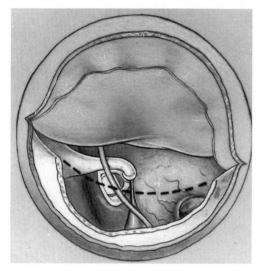

FIG. 13. Curettage of posterior-superior canal wall rim to allow complete visualization of incudostapedial joint and stapes.

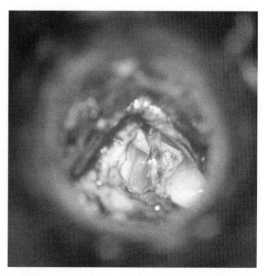

FIG. 14. Middle ear exploration of right ear. Chorda tympani nerve, incus, stapes, oval window, and facial nerve are visible.

capitulum. The surgeon occasionally encounters some degree of mobility. This may be real and should be followed by palpation of the footplate. If this structure is mobile and a round window reflex is elicited, the diagnosis of stapedial otosclerosis is incorrect, and the condition of the rest of the ossicular chain must be promptly reevaluated. After diagnosis of stapedial fixation a corrective technique is selected. The options are stapedioplasty, total or subtotal prosthetic stapedectomy, and stapedotomy.

Stapedioplasty

Stapedioplasty using the posterior arch (stapedial capitulum, neck, and posterior crus) does not require the use of a prosthesis but does involve adequate removal of the footplate. A control hole is made in the footplate with a needle to exclude a possible gusher (see later). The incudostapedial joint is sectioned with an angulated 0.5-mm knife, and the junction between posterior crus and footplate is scored to prepare a controlled fracture line (Fig. 15). The arch is fractured in a superior direction with pressure on the caudal surface of the posterior crus (Fig. 16). After fracturing the arch is lifted and rotated onto the promontory with the stapedial tendon intact. The anterior crus is amputated and removed (Fig. 17). Attention is directed at the footplate, and most of its posterior half is removed with a 90-degree hook and microalligator forceps (Fig. 18).

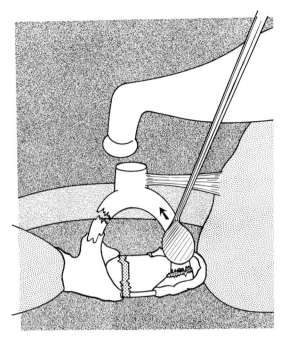

FIG. 16. Upward fracture of arch.

When an adequate oval window opening is achieved, it is sealed with an autologous graft, preferably tragal perichondrium. A canoe-shaped piece measuring 1.5 to 3.75 mm, on average, is obtained from the dome of the tragus. After placement of the graft (Fig. 19), the posterior arch

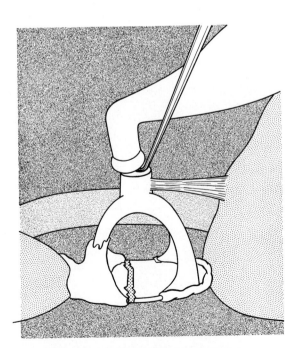

FIG. 15. Incudostapedial joint section.

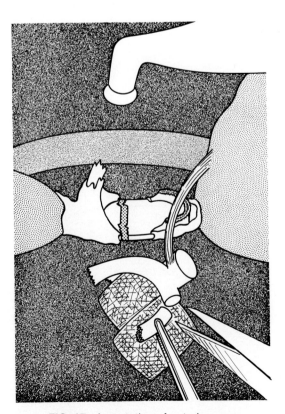

FIG. 17. Amputation of anterior crus.

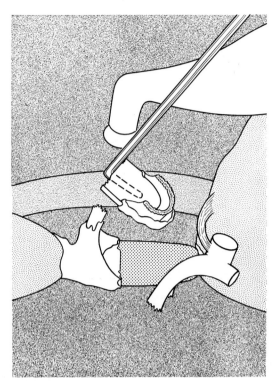

FIG. 18. Removal of posterior portion of footplate.

of the stapes is rotated gently back into the oval window niche. The posterior crus is directed medially into the concavity of the periochondrial graft. The incus is gently lifted to expedite approximation of the incudostapedial joint (Fig. 20).

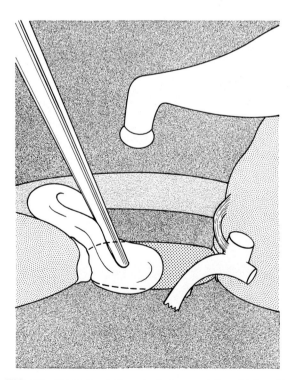

FIG. 19. Placement of oval window perichondrial graft.

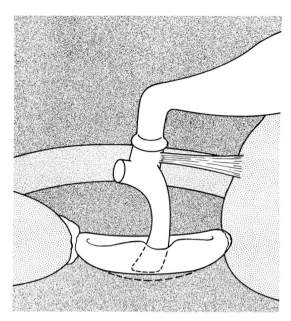

FIG. 20. Posterior arch readaptation to incus. Repositioned posterior arch in contact with concavity of perichondrial graft.

Stapedectomy

Many surgeons prefer to perform total removal of the stapes arch and all or part of the footplate. The operation follows the described steps, but after it is fractured the arch is removed from the footplate after section of the stapedius tendon. The posterior two thirds to three fourths of the footplate is removed. A perichondrial graft is used to seal the oval window, and a prosthesis is used for stapes replacement (Fig. 21). Many prostheses are available, but care should be taken in selecting one that is

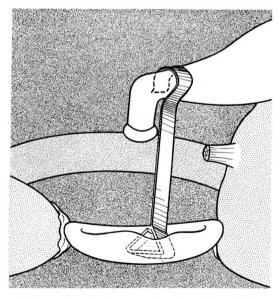

FIG. 21. Prosthesis in contact with perichondrial graft.

compatible with magnetic resonance imaging. Although essentially all currently produced prostheses are compatible, some older stainless steel units may still be in hospital storage.

Stapedotomy

Many otologic surgeons use a modified technique based on a small calibrated opening in the footplate (small fenestra technique) and introduction of a tantalum or platinum polytetrafluoroethylene (PTFE) piston surrounded by a mesodermal tissue graft (Fig. 22). A PTFE prosthesis is preferred so that the surgeon may modify its length as needed. Results of several studies (61–63) have implied lower risk for immediate and late cochlear loss with stapedotomy and better hearing results compared with traditional techniques. Cremers et al. (64), however, in 1991 evaluated the differences in hearing gain 1 year after stapedotomy or partial and total stapedectomy. The 311 patients were matched for age, sex, degree of otosclerosis, and type of prosthesis used. Hearing improvement was better for all frequencies regardless of the technique used. Glasscock et al. (65) conducted a similar comparison and found better results with stapedectomy than with stapedotomy.

Laser Stapedectomy

Perkins (66) introduced the argon laser to stapes surgery in 1980 to vaporize the stapes tendon and the posterior crus and to perform the initial footplate opening. Since then more surgeons have begun to use a laser

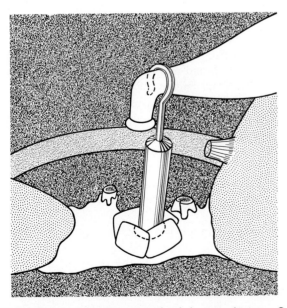

FIG. 22. Piston replacement prosthesis in stapedectomy. Seal is provided by soft tissue surrounding the footplate defect.

routinely (67). Silverstein et al. (68) reported delayed vestibular symptoms lasting from 1 to 3 weeks among 39% of patients when the footplate was opened with a laser (argon or potassium-titanyl-phosphate) and only a 12% incidence when it was opened with conventional methods. McGee (69) found no differences between patients undergoing traditional or laser stapedotomy in a review of 230 cases and recorded no adverse effects among more than 500 patients treated with laser otosurgical procedures.

Bilateral Stapedectomy

In the early years of surgery for otosclerosis, many surgeons refrained from bilateral operations because they preferred to avoid making two fenestration cavities that would require life-long care. After the popularization of stapes surgery, some authors advocated prudence before recommending bilateral procedures, because the long-term effects and incidence of complications were not defined (70). At present bilateral stapedectomy is favored; the second operation usually is performed 6 months to 1 year after the first.

Closure

Closure techniques are essentially the same regardless of how stapedial fixation was corrected. All blood is gently suctioned from the tympanic cavity. The posterior tympanotomy flap is replaced into position. Care is taken to ensure that the fibrous annulus is closely approximated to its sulcus. The canal is cleansed of blood and bone chips. Nylon gauze strips or gelatin foam pledgets are used to secure the skin margins. A cotton ball in the ear canal or light mastoid dressing is applied.

Postoperative Care

Stapedectomy usually is performed as an outpatient procedure. Straining, heavy lifting, and strenuous physical exercise are to be avoided for 3 weeks. At the first postoperative visit, 1 week after the operation, the flap usually is found to be well healed, and subjective hearing improvement frequently is found. Rinne test results usually are positive with 256 Hz and 512 Hz forks. Audiometry is deferred for 4 to 6 weeks unless complications are suspected. Patients should not travel by air for at least 2 weeks after the operation. Water in the external auditory canal should be avoided for 4 weeks. Swimming is allowed after complete healing, but diving is discouraged. The risks of barometric pressure changes, flying, mountain travel, and underwater swimming are explained in detail to the patient.

INTRAOPERATIVE PROBLEMS AND COMPLICATIONS

Intraoperative Vertigo

When the footplate is manipulated, some patients notice momentary dizziness. Care should be taken to avoid undue intravestibular manipulation. Suction should be maintained at a minimum close to and never directly on the open window.

Tympanic Membrane Perforation

The tympanic membrane occasionally is traumatized in the posterosuperior quadrant. Postoperative healing of the tear is spontaneous in most instances and can be hastened by filling in the defect with a small fibrous tissue graft.

Obliterative Otosclerosis

In some cases the footplate and medial crural regions are replaced by an amorphous mass of otosclerotic bone that completely fills the oval window niche (Fig. 23). The cause is unknown, but ethnic factors may be involved in some cases. Gristwood (71) and Willis (72) described a higher incidence of obliterative otosclerosis in Australia.

Management of obliterative otosclerosis is difficult and often is unsatisfactory. After removal of the arch, careful saucerization (Fig. 24) with cutting and diamond burs allows definition of the footplate region. Opening of the oval window is accomplished with a needle probe,

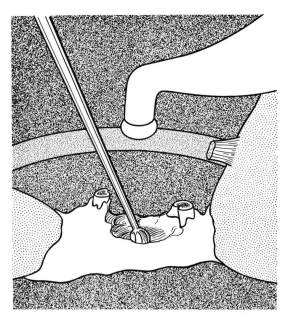

FIG. 24. Fenestra drilled through obliterative footplate lesion.

microchisel, or microdrill. A wire and PTFE piston is crimped to the long process of the incus, its medial end in contact with a tragal perichondrium graft. When an adequate opening can be achieved and a prosthesis introduced, a good immediate hearing result may be predicted. However, rapid regression is frequent. Cochlear losses are more frequent in drillouts. Revision rarely is effective and probably is contraindicated.

Cerebrospinal Fluid Otorrhea

Minor variations in perilymphatic pressure are not unusual, but cerebrospinal fluid otorrhea, a gusher, is rare. It usually is associated with a defect in the fundus of the internal auditory canal or wide cochlear aqueduct and may occur as soon as the footplate is opened. If a gusher occurs, a soft-tissue plug is placed over the footplate puncture, and absorbable gelatin is placed in the middle ear. The endomeatal flap is replaced and the external canal packed. A mastoid dressing applied. Fluid may continue to seep through the dressing for hours or, in some cases, a few days. The patient is maintained at bed rest with head elevated 35 degrees. Use of a subarachnoid catheter to relieve cerebrospinal fluid pressure is probably contraindicated. Excessive decompression may force air into the vestibule and cochlea and produce anacusis (73).

The use of prophylactic antibiotics is controversial. There is little discomfort other than mild vertigo, which may be controlled with a sedative. After the flow of cerebrospinal fluid stops, dressings can be removed. The endomeatal flap is inspected to assess its position and degree of healing. Audiometry may show a cochlear loss. Additional surgical intervention is contraindicated.

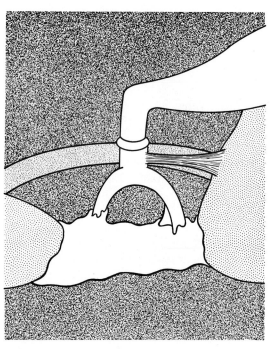

FIG. 23. Obliterative otosclerosis of the footplate.

Dehiscence of the Facial Nerve

Dehiscence of the facial nerve may occur in as many as 57% of cases. It is clinically significant among only 15% of patients when it is associated with displacement of the trunk so that the nerve abuts the stapedial crura (74). The condition is more dangerous when the nerve courses over the oval window (75) or inferior to it (76), because failure to recognize the anomaly causes avulsion of the nerve. Stapedectomy should not be attempted when the facial nerve obscures the oval window.

Floating Footplate

Floating footplate is among the most serious intraoperative complications of stapedectomy. If during the initial attempts at crural fracture the stapes appears to be mobilized, it is preferable to stop the procedure and close. Sometimes the hearing improvement resulting from this accident is similar to that obtained at purposeful mobilization. When the plate becomes loose after crurotomy, the steps to follow depend on the position of the footplate. Every move is aimed at preventing collapse of the footplate into the vestibule. If it has not been displaced from its anatomic position, the footplate probably retains some points of attachment at the annular ligament. It may then be best to place a perichondrial graft over the footplate and follow the graft with a prosthesis. Pressure on the plate should be carefully avoided. If a portion of the footplate dips into the vestibule, a 60- or 90-degree microhook may be used to retrieve it. Suction should be avoided and intravestibular manipulation kept to a minimum to prevent permanent and severe cochlear damage.

Subluxation of the Incus

Although some degree of increased mobility of the incudomalleal joint after removal of the stapes is common, dislocation is rare. If the subluxation is minor, repositioning the incus in its normal anatomic position with or without prosthesis placement is reasonable. If the incus has been severely displaced, it is removed and repositioned with its body against the malleus and the long process in contact with the oval window graft. The incus may have to be modified with a microdrill to achieve precise fitting. An alternative is a malleus to footplate prosthesis or a total ossicular replacement prosthesis.

POSTOPERATIVE COMPLICATIONS

Vertigo

Light postoperative vertigo usually is positional and lasts several hours to several days. More severe vertigo that necessitates bed rest and antivertigo drugs is uncommon. If vertigo is accompanied by nausea or vomiting (rare), 10 mg chlorpromazine is administered intramuscularly. The use of steroids is controversial. If vertigo persists and is accompanied by further hearing loss, distortion of sound, or tinnitus, prompt surgical reexploration may be necessary. Reexploration may reveal a fistula, an excessively long prosthesis, or vestibular granuloma.

Tinnitus

Among most patients the tinnitus that sometimes accompanies otosclerosis disappears as hearing improves. The cause of persistent tinnitus after hearing improvement is unclear. It may have a cochlear (possible otosclerosis) or central origin.

Cochlear Hearing Loss

Severe sensorineural hearing loss occurs among 1% to 2% patients who undergo surgical treatment of otosclerosis. In the absence of a fistula, prosthetic problems, or granuloma, it is difficult to explain this complication, which may be immediate or delayed.

Facial Paralysis

Facial dysfunction is uncommon and almost always is associated with dehiscence of the facial canal. Paresis is incomplete and short lasting when caused by diffusion of the anesthetic solution into the tympanic portion of the nerve. Persistent paralysis necessitates prompt surgical exploration. If instrumental damage has occurred, the prognosis depends on the expediency of decompression, degree of trauma, and quality of repair. Delayed facial paralysis is rare. It may be caused by an inflammatory process of the middle ear with secondary edema of a dehiscent nerve or by pressure on such a dehiscence by the surgical prosthesis. Oral steroids and possibly antibiotics are recommended. If spontaneous improvement does not occur within 5 to 7 days, surgical exploration may be indicated.

Otitis Media

Perioperative otitis media is uncommon and usually is caused by concomitant upper respiratory infection (77). The patient is aggressively treated with decongestants and intravenous antibiotics. Infection can cause disruption of the oval window repair, labyrinthitis, or meningitis (see later). Myringotomy is performed if initial conservative management fails.

Taste Disturbance and Oral Dryness

Unpleasant taste sensations and oral dryness occur when the chorda tympani nerve is manipulated or divided. These symptoms appear to be more pronounced when the nerve is avulsed rather than cut. In either case they tend nearly always to disappear or markedly improve in 1 to 3 months.

Perilymph Fistula

Persistent dizziness with a feeling of falling rather than subjective rotation suggests a perilymph fistula or an excessively long prosthesis (78). Symptoms occur early in the postoperative period and continue until they are surgically corrected or spontaneous healing occurs (in the case of a fistula). Nystagmus is common. Fluctuating conductive hearing loss may occur because a leaking vestibule can produce a coupling loss at the air-fluid interface (79). The mechanical deficit produced by the loss of vestibular perilymph may be small compared with the improved transmission that results from repair of the transducer mechanism. A marked gain in hearing and near closure of the air-bone gap do not necessarily exclude the presence of a small fistula.

Postoperative fistulas may be perioperative or delayed. Perioperative fistulas usually are technical. If the seal of the oval window defect is inadequate, perilymph pressure tends to prevent its closure. An effective seal occurs only with participation of viable cellular tissue from the surrounding mucoperiosteum, which ultimately envelopes the prosthesis and the repair graft. Secondary fistulas usually are caused by barotrauma; they were more frequent when polyethylene struts were used. Pressure changes such as those experienced in flight or scuba diving may drive the prosthesis through the graft, especially when equalization is impaired by poor eustachian tube function.

Treatment requires a high index of suspicion. A trial of antivertigo drugs and bed rest is advisable if symptoms are mild and there is no evidence of progressive cochlear damage. Mild but persistent disequilibrium and deterioration of speech discrimination scores call for prompt exploration. A sudden, marked loss of hearing with or without disequilibrium is a surgical emergency. At operation the prosthesis should be removed carefully but completely. After location of the fistula, the mucosal tract is removed and the defect closed with perichondrium or fascia. A cartilage autograft or prosthesis is used to maintain the new graft in position. Broad-spectrum antibiotics are used before and after the operation.

Prosthesis Discontinuity

In the early days when polyethylene struts were used, discontinuity was common. It now is infrequent. It may be caused by poor attachment, scar formation, incus necrosis, or extrusion of the prosthesis by recurrent otosclerosis.

Middle Ear Fibrosis

Middle ear fibrosis and prosthesis displacement may be caused by poor tolerance of plastic and wire prosthe-

ses or a reaction to gelatin sponge, rubber-glove powder, or retained bone chips. Middle ear fibrosis that fixes a prosthesis to the promontory may be managed by means of sharp dissection and prosthesis replacement without violating the oval window seal. Partial recovery of hearing may be expected. Fibrosis that fills the entire middle ear is rare but has a poor prognosis. Meticulous section of scars usually is quickly followed by recurrence. The role of laser probes in the management of this complex problem remains to be elucidated.

Granuloma

Poststapedectomy granuloma is an uncommon but serious problem (80). Granuloma was more frequent when gelatin film or fat was used as a window seal. Granuloma may represent an abnormal immunologic response or low-grade infection of the graft tissue. It may be limited to the middle ear or vestibule but can involve both (81). Granuloma is more frequent during the immediately postoperative period but can occur as late as 2 weeks after an operation. Tinnitus, ear pain, a decrease in hearing, and vertigo are common symptoms. Otoscopy demonstrates edema and erythema of the tympanic membrane. Surgical exploration is indicated. Prompt removal of a granuloma may eliminate it and allow substantial return of hearing but is a high-risk procedure. Intravestibular granuloma frequently is associated with a fistula. Reestablishing an oval window seal is critical.

Postoperative Labyrinthitis

Serous labyrinthitis is not common and may be associated with blood collection in the vestibule when this space is partially depleted of perilymph. The prognosis is favorable. Suppurative labyrinthitis is rare and may follow acute otitis media. It usually is manifested by marked loss of cochlear and vestibular functions. Prognosis for hearing preservation is poor. Management includes parenteral antibiotics, myringotomy, and lumbar puncture to rule out early meningitis.

Meningitis

Postoperative meningitis is rare and follows suppurative otitis media and labyrinthitis. It evolves rapidly, occurring within 36 to 48 hours after the onset of earache. Immediate hospitalization, lumbar puncture, myringotomy, and intravenous antibiotic therapy are mandatory as soon as this complication is suspected. After laboratory confirmation, if there is no prompt improvement, tympanotomy and surgical exploration should be performed.

Matz et al. (82) first reported the temporal bone findings in a case of meningitis following stapedectomy. A polyethylene strut had been used as a prosthesis. The infection spread to the vestibule and meninges. The pathways of infection followed two probable routes: along the vestibular nerve to the internal auditory canal or through the scala vestibuli to the modiolus and internal meatus. No definite evidence of a fistula was found. Palva et al. (83) described the case of a patient who contracted fatal meningitis after stapes surgery. Temporal bone studies showed that infection spread from an ear in which a polyethylene strut had been used. Retraction of the drum appeared to have drawn the prosthesis into the vestibule. The pathway to the meninges was through the cochlear aqueduct.

Recurrence

After stapedectomy new otosclerotic activity may invade footplate fragments and produce refixation. The most common origin is an anterior oval window focus, which may spread to close the entire fenestra. This type of capsular disease may extend much farther to progressively involve the entire otic capsule. In some cases of hearing regression, exploration reveals obliteration of the round window. This usually is associated with a bulging promontory, a sign of otic capsule otosclerosis. Drillouts of massive recurrences and round window otosclerosis are not successful.

EVALUATION OF THE RESULTS OF STAPES SURGERY

The degree of air–bone gap closure is a practical measure of the efficacy of stapes surgery. Goodhill (84) first proposed a uniform method to report surgical results. He advanced a formula whereby the difference between average preoperative and postoperative air conduction (the gain) is divided by the average preoperative air–bone gap (the maximum gain expected). The result is a percentage that indicates the degree to which the air–bone gap has been closed. Although this method and others introduced a degree of objectivity in assessing poststapedectomy results, they were handicapped by a lack of agreement regarding the frequencies to be averaged or whether it was preferable to use pre- or postoperative values when computing results. To create a single and uniform reporting method, the American Academy of Otolaryngology–Head and Neck Surgery committee on hearing and equilibrium (85) published a draft of the following guidelines: (a) the mean of thresholds at frequencies 0.5, 1, 2, and 3 kHz should be used to obtain a frequency pure tone average; (b) the air–bone gap should be reported for air and bone conduction levels obtained at the same time rather than comparing postoperative air conduction values with preoperative bone conduction thresholds; (c) four types of results assessed 12 months or more after the operation can be obtained (class A, 0 to 10 dB air–bone gap; class B, 11 to 20 dB gap; class C, 21 to 30 dB gap; class D, more than 30 dB gap).

With the guidelines as a reference Berliner et al. (86) used audiologic data from 240 patients who underwent stapes operations to generate and analyze the importance of a variety of outcome measures. The authors found that frequencies included in averaging made little difference in mean computed air–bone gaps, although the success rate was lower when 4 kHz rather than 3 kHz was used as part of a four-frequency average. The success rate was 2% higher when preoperative rather than postoperative bone conduction thresholds were used in computing the postoperative air–bone gap. When air conduction pure tone averages were selected as the outcome measure, patients with normal preoperative cochlear reserve had a 20% higher success rate than the general population of patients who underwent surgical treatment. The authors concluded that the greatest differences encountered were based on the success criteria chosen for computing. As such, success rates were higher when based on air–bone gap averages than when based on air conduction pure tone averages.

RESULTS OF PRIMARY STAPES SURGERY

Six to 12 months after stapedectomy approximately 90% of patients have a conductive deficit of 10 dB or less when measured against the best bone conduction average (pre- or postoperative). About 5% have an unsatisfactory result estimated at 15 dB or higher average air–bone gap (87–89). The degree of air–bone gap closure varies little through time (90–93). Among patients with bilateral otosclerosis who underwent an operation on only one ear, the treated ear remained the better. This finding supports the long-term beneficial results of the procedure (94). However, air conduction thresholds tend to deteriorate more rapidly than in control groups, the higher frequencies (2 to 4 kHz) being more commonly and severely affected. This long-term sensorineural hearing loss is believed to be caused by presbycusis alone or in association with cochlear otosclerosis. This tendency toward sensorineural hearing loss appears to be more prevalent among patients with unilateral otosclerosis. Willis (95) reported on a progressive, flat sensorineural hearing loss among some patients with unilateral disease. He attributed it to progressive otosclerotic involvement of the spiral ligament.

STAPEDECTOMY IN CHILDREN

The early and long-term results of stapedectomy among children and adolescents parallel the success of the procedure among adults (33,96–98). air–bone gap closures to within 10 dB in the speech frequencies have been reported to be between 80% and 100% in the early postoperative period (within 5 years) (96). Cole (98), however, reported a higher incidence of cochlear involvement in an analysis of 62 stapedectomies performed on 43 children. He attributed this to a higher number of cases with obliterative otosclerosis. Millman et al. (33) reviewed the available literature and discussed the results achieved by a population of 31 patients (40 stapedectomies) observed an average of 25 years. The authors concluded that stapedectomy is a safe and highly effective procedure for children and should be recommended. Obliterative otosclerosis and drillout procedures continue to be notable exceptions.

REVISION STAPEDECTOMY

Revision stapedectomy carries increased risk for cochlear loss. Selection of patients requires experience, good judgment, and conservative surgical technique. Crabtree et al. (99) reviewed the records of 35 patients who underwent revision stapedectomy. The two main causes of failure were displacement of the prosthesis and fibrous changes involving the middle ear and oval window. After revision, 46% of patients had hearing improvement, 34% were not improved, and 20% were made worse. Of the seven patients who had additional hearing loss, five were classified as having dead ears and were not candidates for hearing amplification. Similar findings were reported by Sheehy et al. (100) for a group of 258 patients who underwent revision stapedectomy. Displacement of the prosthesis to the inferior edge of the fenestra was the most common cause of failure with an incidence of 41%. Incus necrosis (17%) and fistula (16%) followed in frequency. After revision less than 50% of patients had a 10 dB air–bone gap or less, and 7% of patients had a sensorineural hearing loss, half of them a total loss.

FENESTRATION AND POSTFENESTRATION STAPEDECTOMY

No discussion of otosclerosis can be complete without consideration of Lempert's semicircular canal fenestration (57). Otologists must be familiar with the procedure, because many patients who underwent fenestration during the late 1950s still need care.

Canal-wall-down mastoidectomy sufficient to expose the dome of the horizontal semicircular canal is performed through an endaural incision. The canal wall skin is carefully preserved and a flap elevated to expose the posterior-superior position of the middle ear cleft and its contents. The incus is separated from the head of the malleus and removed. The neck of the malleus is divided and its head is removed. A tympanomeatal flap composed of the skin and periosteum that line the external auditory canal is developed. The flap is manipulated so that it closely adapts to the irregularities of the mastoid defect. The bony capsule over the dome of the horizontal semicircular canal is gradually worn down with a polishing bur. A bluish-gray cupola of endosteal bone is developed and removed under constant irrigation without disturbing the membranous labyrinth. The fenestra should be about 2 mm wide and 6 mm long (Fig. 25). The tympanomeatal

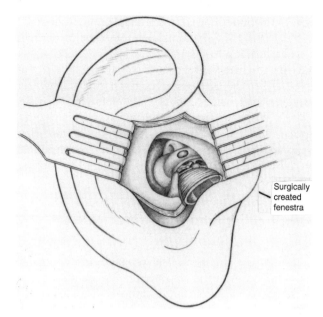

FIG. 25. Lempert fenestration of horizontal semicircular canal, prior to flap positioning.

Surgically created fenestra

flap is positioned so that its thinnest portion covers the new fenestra. The cavity is packed and the wound closed.

Regardless of the results of fenestration, patients may seek further hearing improvement. If audiometry indicates good cochlear function and a substantial air–bone gap, stapedectomy may be recommended. The operation may be performed under local anesthesia. The incision is made with great care to avoid damage to the fenestrated lateral semicircular canal and facial nerve. The middle ear is opened, and the remaining landmarks are identified. The distance between the oval window and the malleal manubrium is carefully measured, and an appropriate prosthesis is selected. After partial stapedectomy or stapedotomy, the prosthesis is placed from the long process of the malleus to the defect. The flap is then replaced and packed with gelatin sponge and gauze. The postoperative course is similar to that of ordinary stapedectomy.

NONOTOSCLEROTIC LESIONS OF THE STAPES

Paget's Disease

Paget's disease, or osteitis deformans, is progressive dyscrasia with primary involvement of the skull and long bones. The disease is common, affecting approximately 3% of persons older than 40 years (101). The skull and temporal bones are involved in about two thirds of patients. The disease may extend to the petrous pyramid, external canal, middle ear, and otic capsule (102). Hearing is impaired in approximately 50% of patients with temporal bone involvement, and vestibular function may be affected in about one fourth of cases. The hearing loss usually is mixed. The causes of the conductive component often are unclear, but they include fixation and resorption of the stapes (103). Fixation, however, is rare, having been reported only once (104). Stapedectomy and ossiculoplasty often are unsatisfactory (104–106).

Osteogenesis Imperfecta

Osteogenesis imperfecta, also known as *fragilitas ossium* or *van der Hoeve's syndrome,* is a genetic disorder of connective tissue caused by an error in type I collagen. It includes at least four major types (see Chapter 30) and is characterized by a history of multiple fractures with poor healing, blue sclerae, and conductive hearing loss in 25% to 60% of cases (107). Although otosclerosis may coexist, the disorder of lamellar bone formation affecting the stapes can produce atrophy, dehiscence, or separation of the crura from the footplate. If crural necrosis is present, tympanometry demonstrates abnormal tympanic membrane compliance and a positive stapedial reflex. Surgical correction of the conductive hearing loss may be possible with stapedectomy. The stapedial footplate may be thick, granular, and spongy. Additional procedures may be necessary to address associated ossicular deformities. Armstrong (108) reviewed the long-term outcome of stapedectomy for osteogenesis imperfecta (6 to 24 years). The results were excellent (air–bone gap closure) in 22 cases, good (closure within 15 dB) in 5 cases, and fair (closure within 20 dB or poorer) in 3 cases.

Tympanosclerosis

Tympanosclerosis of the middle ear is a rare sequela of chronic otitis media (see Chapter 25) and involves the stapes approximately 50% of the time (109). Treatment is controversial, ranging from amplification to stapedectomy and mobilization of the sclerotic focus. Overzealous plaque removal may result in inner ear damage and may not prevent recurrence (110). Giddings and House (111) reported their experience with 154 cases of stapedial tympanosclerosis managed with either mobilization or stapedectomy. They concluded that the procedures were safe and equally successful with marked improvement in most cases.

Degenerative Arthritis

Arthritic degeneration of the annular ligament and ossicular joints has been described and classified by Ethlom and Belal (112). The disease, which is uncommon, varies from fraying of the articular cartilage to atro-phy and various degrees of calcification and destruction of the capsule, articular cartilage, and articular disc. Fixation of the annular ligament is circumferential and diffuse. The incus, malleal, and incudostapedial joints undergo progressive ankylosis. Although surgical intervention can be considered for disease isolated to the stapes, there is no current information available to support its use.

OTHER CAUSES OF OSSICULAR FIXATION

Lateral Ossicular Fixation

Isolated lateral ossicular fixation is an infrequent cause of hearing loss first identified by Toynbee (3) more than a century ago. The lesion is idiopathic or acquired fusion of the head of the malleus to the tegmen with or without secondary fixation of the incus. Lateral ossicular fixation may be caused by chronic otitis media or tympanosclerosis. Ossification of the tensor tympani tendon and fusion of the malleus to the cochleariform process may occur in rare instances.

The patient usually presents with long-standing hearing loss and no signs of active ear disease. Audiometry reveals a moderate, low-frequency air–bone gap. The bone conduction curve frequently slopes downward in the higher frequencies, suggesting a cochlear lesion (Fig. 26). The acoustic reflex is absent. Speech discrimination is not affected. Restoration of ossicular mobility is best achieved with transection of the neck of the malleus. This necessitates removal of the lateral epitympanic wall (scutum) (Fig. 27) after division of the incudostapedial joint to prevent excessive mobilization of the stapes and cochlear damage (Fig. 28). The incudomalleal joint is divided (Fig. 29). The incus is removed and placed in a moist container for later use. The neck of the malleus is transected with a 1.5-mm cutting bur (Fig. 30). All tissue connections are divided to free the manubrium. The head of the malleus may be removed or partly drilled out with care not to injure the tegmen and overlying dura. The incus is made into a strut approximately 6.5 mm long and secured between the stapes capitulum and the mobile malleal handle (Fig. 31). A replacement prosthesis may be used.

Incus-Annulus Fusion

In long-standing middle ear fibrosis, osteogenic activity may produce bony fusion in several areas. On rare occasions this may result in attachment of the incus to the bony annulus, producing a secondary type of lateral ossicular fixation. Findings are similar to those of fixed malleus syndrome. Management is based on the principles of ossiculoplasty (see Chapter 27).

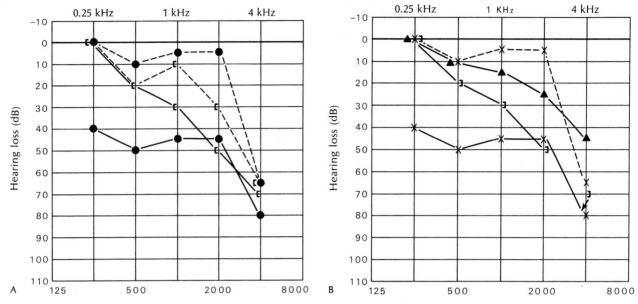

FIG. 26. A: Malleal fixation. Preoperative bone conduction level (mastoid placement) indicates probability of marked high-frequency hearing loss and only fair prognosis for hearing improvement with surgical treatment. Postoperative air conduction level reveals almost normal hearing. •—•, Air conduction, unmasked, right ear, before operation; [—[, bone conduction, masked, right ear, after operation. **B:** Audiogram of left ear of same patient as in **A**. Bone conduction by both mastoid and frontal placement. Substantial differences are present at at 500, 1,000, and 2,000 Hz. Postoperative air conduction level is in closer agreement with frontal bone conduction measurements. x––x, Air conduction, unmasked, left ear, before operation;]—], bone conduction, masked, left ear, before operation; ▲—▲, bone conduction, frontal, before operation; x—x, air conduction, unmasked, left ear, after operation; *arrow,* no response at maximum output.

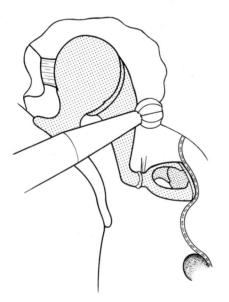

FIG. 27. Lateral atticotomy. Removal of a portion of the inferior aspect of the wall of the epitympanum to expose the incudomalleal joint.

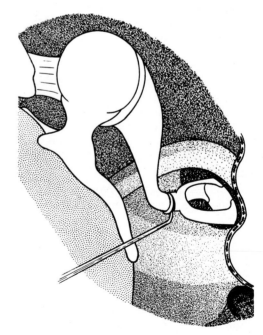

FIG. 28. Incudostapedial section protects the labyrinth from mechanical damage.

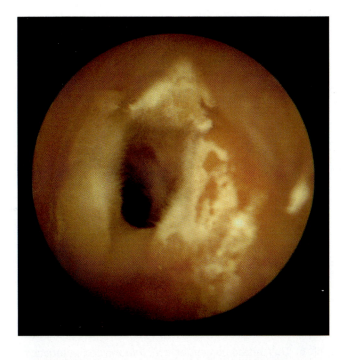

FIG. 1. Fungal otitis externa. (Courtesy of Dr. Armando Lenis.)

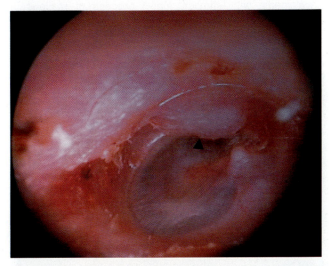

FIG. 2. Herniation of temporomandibular joint contents into the ear canal. With the patient's mouth closed this lesion is seen as an anterior soft-tissue mass (*arrow*).

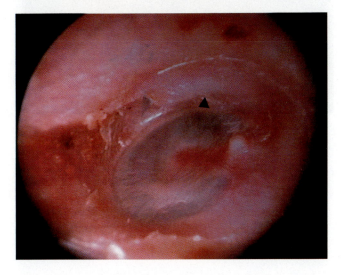

FIG. 3. With the patient's mouth open the temporomandibular joint contents are retracted back into the joint, leaving a slight depression in the wall of the ear canal (*arrow*).

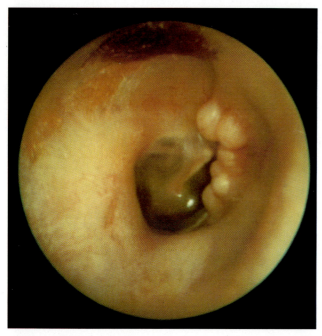

FIG. 4. Multiple osteomas involving the ear canal. (Courtesy of Dr. Armando Lenis.)

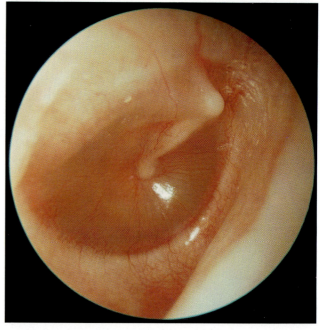

FIG. 5. Dull, retracted tympanic membrane characteristic of otitis media with effusion. Short process of malleus is prominent. (Courtesy of Dr. Armando Lenis.)

A

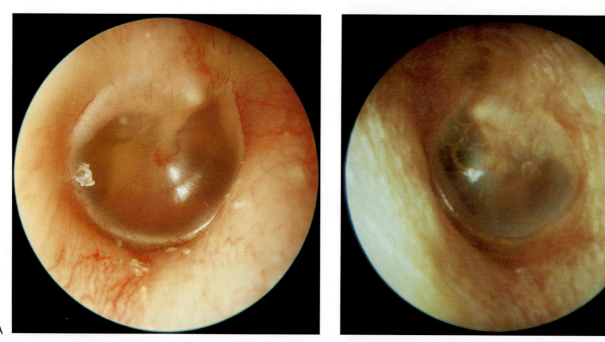

B

FIG. 6. Air-fluid level **(A)** or the presence of air bubbles **(B)** makes diagnosis of otitis media with effusion obvious. (Courtesy of Dr. Armando Lenis.)

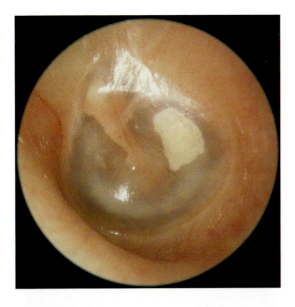

FIG. 7. Tympanosclerotic plaque in tympanic membrane.

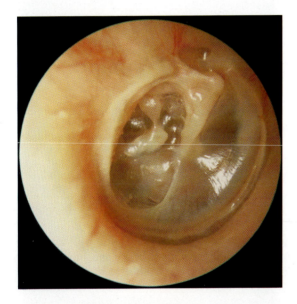

FIG. 8. Severe tympanic membrane retraction with erosion of incudo-stapedial joint. (Courtesy of Dr. Armando Lenis.)

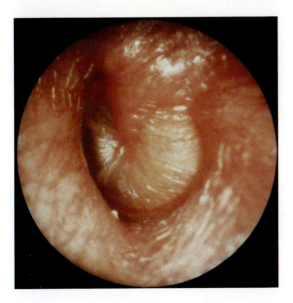

FIG. 9. Acute suppurative otitis media, early stage. Note erythema and bulging of tympanic membrane. The malleal short process and umbo are still visible. (Courtesy of Dr. Armando Lenis.)

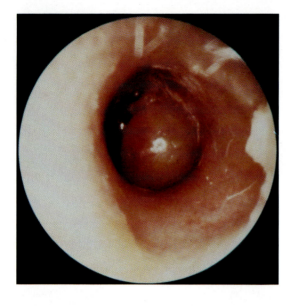

FIG. 10. Acute suppurative otitis media, advanced stage. Note severe bulging of tympanic membrane with loss of landmarks. (Courtesy of Dr. Armando Lenis.)

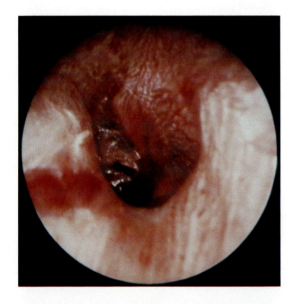

FIG. 11. Acute suppurative otitis media with spontaneous tympanic membrane rupture (anteroinferior quadrant). Note decompression of middle ear exudate with return of malleal landmarks. (Courtesy of Dr. Armando Lenis.)

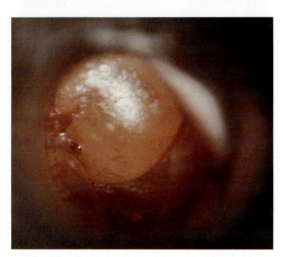

FIG. 12. Acute bullous myringitis. Note one large vesicle obscuring more than one half of the tympanic membrane. (Courtesy of Dr. Armando Lenis.)

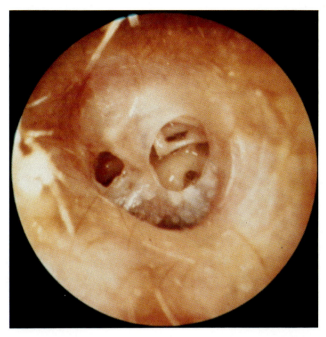

FIG. 13. Anterior and posterior tympanic membrane perforations (left ear). Note the incudostapedial joint, stapes, facial nerve, and round window. (Courtesy of Dr. Armando Lenis.)

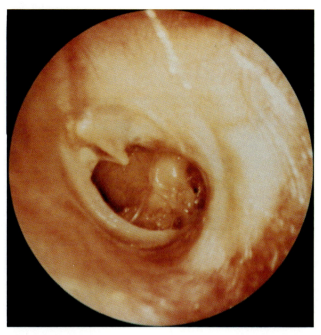

FIG. 14. Near-total perforation of the pars tensa (left ear). Note medial displacement of the malleus. (Courtesy of Dr. Armando Lenis.)

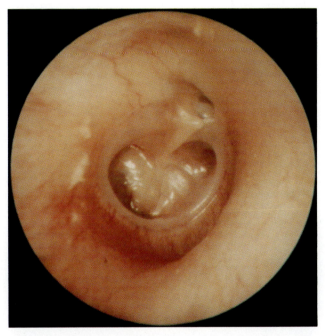

FIG. 15. Severe atelectasis of monomeric tympanic membrane (end-stage adhesive otitis media) of the right ear. (Courtesy of Dr. Armando Lenis.)

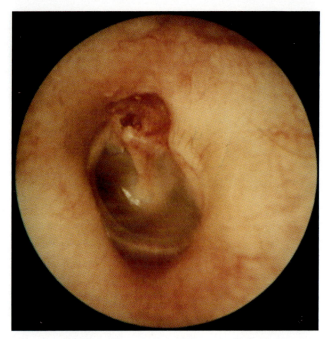

FIG. 16. Chronic otitis media (left ear). Early retraction pocket precursor of cholesteatoma. (Courtesy of Dr. Armando Lenis.)

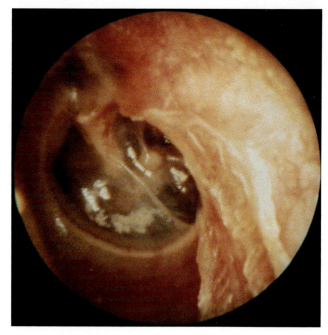

FIG. 17. Chronic otitis media (left ear). Note tympanosclerotic changes of the pars tensa and posterior mesotympanic collapse of the pars tensa over the stapes. A fibrous union at the incudostapedial joint and the stapedial tendon are noticeable. (Courtesy of Dr. Armando Lenis.)

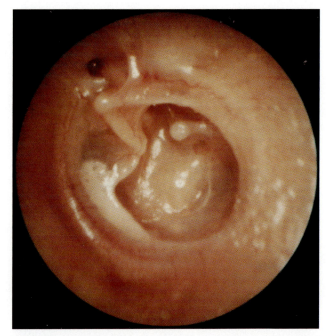

FIG. 18. Chronic otitis media (left ear). Note collapse of monomeric pars tensa, anterior tympanosclerotic plaque, anteromedially displaced malleal handle, absent (eroded) long process of the incus, and prominent head of the stapes. (Courtesy of Dr. Armando Lenis.)

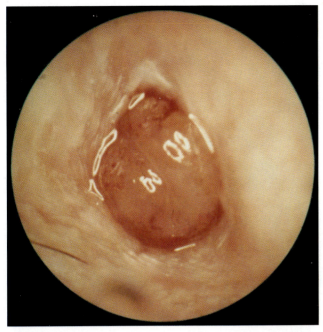

FIG. 19. Chronic otitis media. Note inflammatory polyp filling the external ear canal. (Courtesy of Dr. Armando Lenis.)

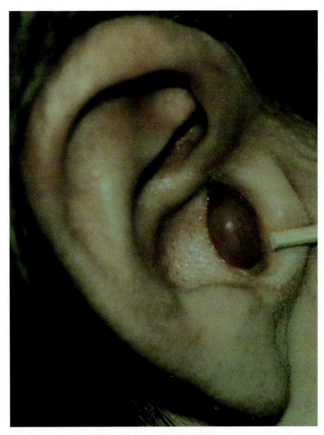

FIG. 20. Chronic otitis media. Note inflammatory polyp protruding through the external meatus.

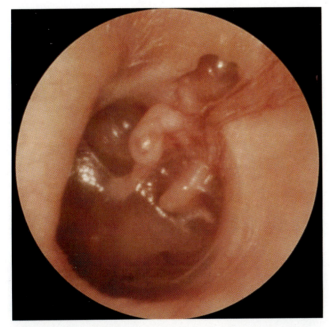

FIG. 21. Chronic otitis media (left ear). Note pars flaccida retraction pocket, partial collapse of the pars tensa with retraction pocket anterior to the malleus handle, exposure of incus long process, deformed malleus handle, and middle ear fluid. (Courtesy of Dr. Armando Lenis.)

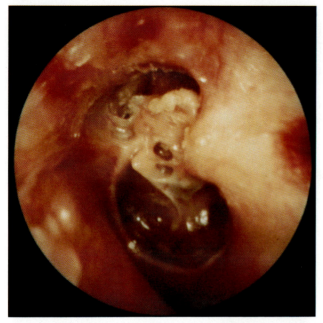

FIG. 22. Cholesteatoma (left ear). Extensive posterior superior retraction pocket with peripheral bone erosion (self-performed atticotomy). (Courtesy of Dr. Armando Lenis.)

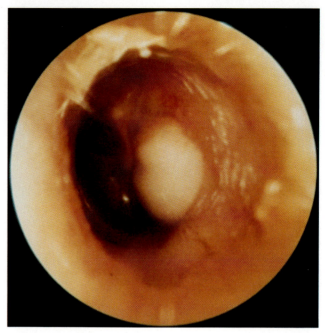

FIG. 23. Cholesteatoma (left ear). Posterior mesotympanic cholesteatoma behind an intact tympanic membrane. (Courtesy of Dr. Armando Lenis.)

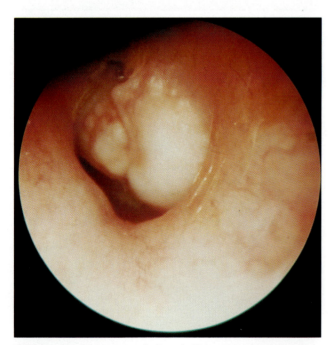

FIG. 24. Cholesteatoma (left ear). Extensive cholesteatoma behind an intact tympanic membrane. (Courtesy of Dr. Armando Lenis.)

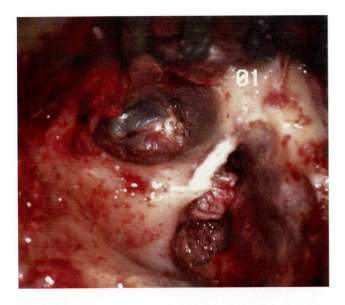

FIG. 25. Cholesteatoma (left ear). The mastoid has been opened surgically, and extension of the attic cholesteatoma into the antrum is evident.

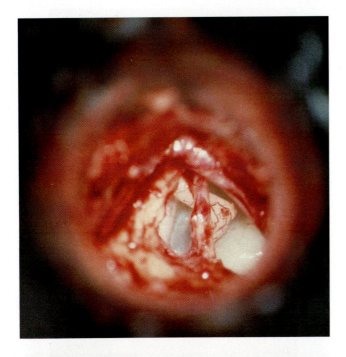

FIG. 26. Middle ear exploration of right ear. Chorda tympani nerve, incus, stapes, oval window, and facial nerve are visible.

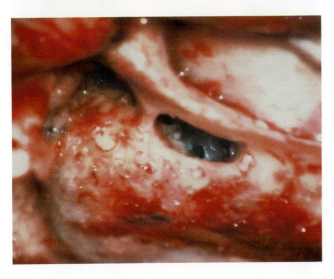

FIG. 27. Round window exposure through a facial recess approach, right ear.

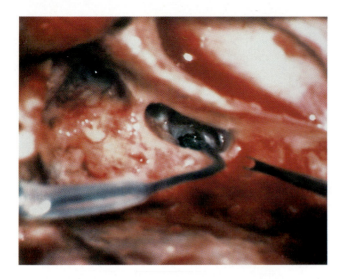

FIG. 28. Placement of a cochlear implant electrode through round window into scala tympani.

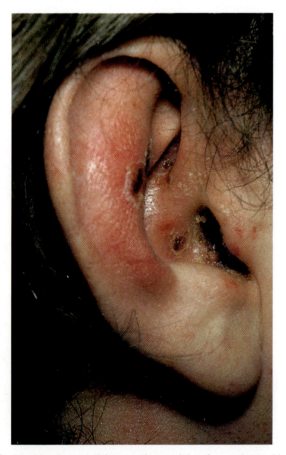

FIG. 29. Healing vesicles on the auricle of a patient with a facial paralysis secondary to Ramsay Hunt syndrome.

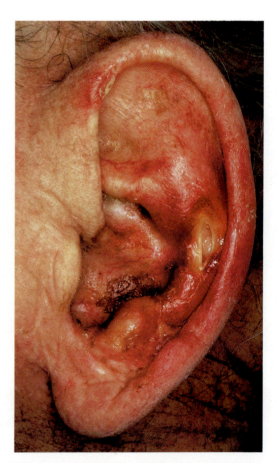

FIG. 30. Perichondritis after trauma to the pinna.

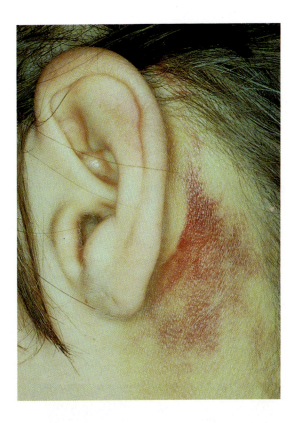

FIG. 31. Postauricular ecchymosis (Battle's sign) in a longitudinal temporal bone fracture.

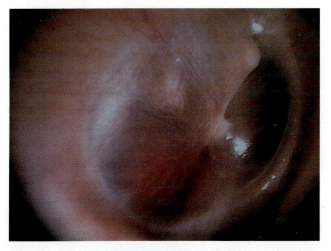

FIG. 32. Glomus tympanicum tumor of right ear involves posterior-inferior mesotympanum.

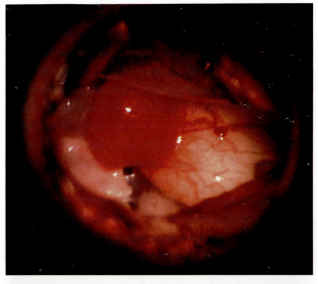

FIG. 33. Glomus tympanicum tumor of left ear attached to inferior promontory.

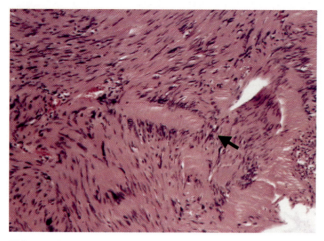

FIG. 34. Typical schwannoma. Note spindle cells distributed in alternating Antoni A areas (compact and more cellular) and Antoni B areas (loose and less cellular). Parallel rows of Schwann cells (*arrow*) known as Verocay bodies are highly characteristic of this tumor (hematoxylin and eosin, original magnification × 40). (Courtesy of Dr. Pier Luigi Di Patre.)

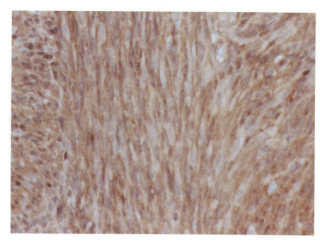

FIG. 35. Section of schwannoma immunostained for S100. Positivity for this marker is useful in the differential diagnosis with meningioma (original magnification × 60). (Courtesy of Dr. Pier Luigi Di Patre.)

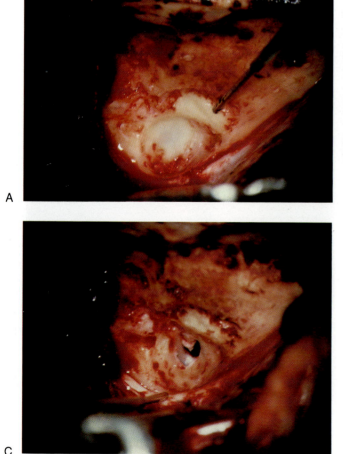

A

B

C

FIG. 36. Middle cranial fossa approach to acoustic tumors. **A:** Pointer is on the superior semicircular canal (SC); temporal lobe is retracted. **B:** SC is blue lined; geniculate ganglion is exposed; initial opening of the internal auditory canal (IAC). **C:** Dura of the IAC has been opened and tumor partially resected.

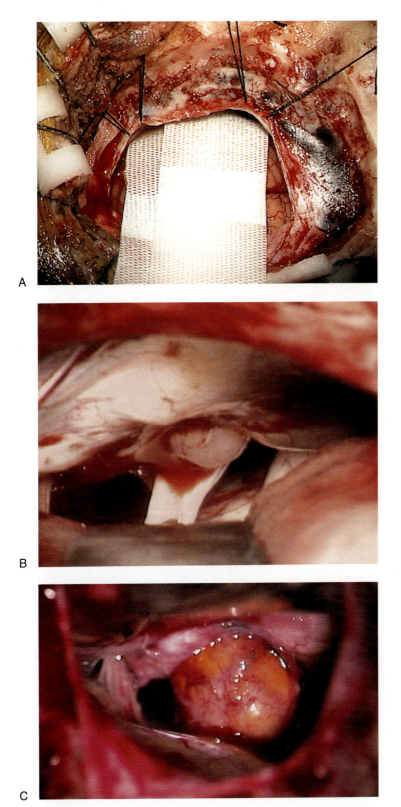

FIG. 37. Retrosigmoid approach to acoustic tumors. **A:** Retrosigmoid craniotomy/craniectomy is completed; sigmoid is exposed; initial dural opening. **B:** Small tumor extending just out of the internal auditory canal. Cranial nerve VIII bundle is clearly seen. **C:** Medium-size tumor. Branches of cranial nerves IX and X are seen to the left (inferior) of the tumor.

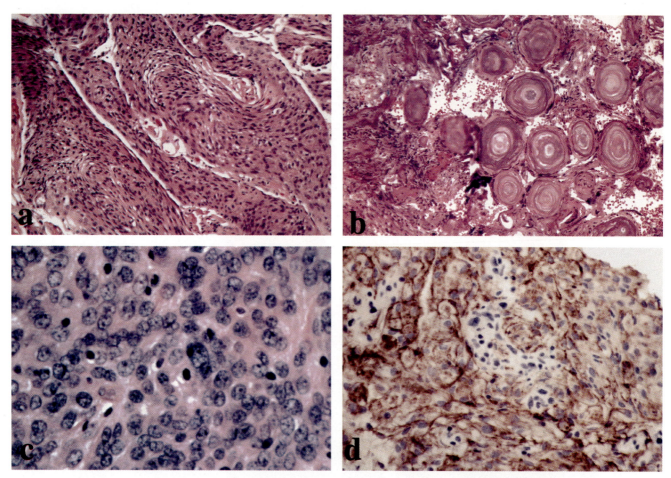

FIG. 38. A: Typical meningioma consisting of spindle-shaped cells arranged in fascicles and whorls (hematoxylin and eosin, original magnification × 40). **B:** Psammoma bodies are characteristic of meningiomas and may be abundant (original magnification × 60). **C:** Loss of whorling pattern and presence of mitotic activity characterize atypical anaplastic meningiomas (original magnification × 90). **D:** Section of meningioma immunostained for epithelial membrane antigen (EMA). Meningiomas are consistently immunoreactive for vimentin and EMA. (Courtesy of Dr. Pier Luigi Di Patre.)

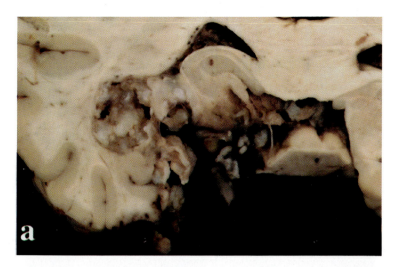

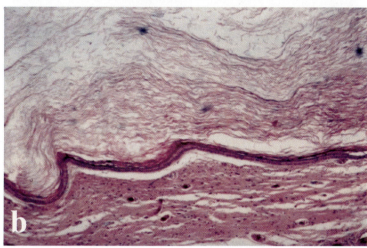

FIG. 39. Epidermoid tumor. **A:** Coronal slice of a brain from a patient with a large epidermoid tumor of the left cerebellopontine angle. The patient died of pulmonary thromboembolism after surgery. Residual tumor is present within the hippocampal fissure, compressing the hippocampus medially and the temporal lobe laterally. **B:** Photomicrograph of the epidermoid tumor. The cyst cavity is filled with keratin, and the wall consists of stratified squamous epithelium. Reactive gliosis is present in the surrounding brain (hematoxylin and eosin). (Courtesy of Dr. Pier Luigi Di Patre.)

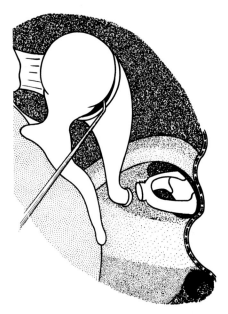

FIG. 29. Incudomalleal section immediately before removal of the incus.

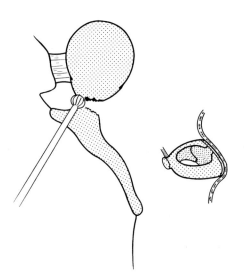

FIG. 30. Transection of the neck of the malleus.

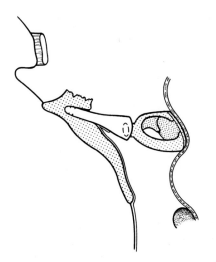

FIG. 31. Strut interposed between long process of malleus and stapes capitulum.

SUMMARY POINTS

- Otosclerosis is osteodystrophy limited to the temporal bone.
- The incidence of otosclerosis is estimated at 5% to 10% among whites. It is less frequent among African-Americans.
- Otosclerosis is inherited through autosomal dominant transmission with incomplete penetrance.
- The pathogenesis of otosclerosis includes traumatic vascular development, immunologic, and viral theories.
- The process involves mainly the otic capsule. Initially it is characterized by increased vascularity and bone resorption (otospongiosis). It later evolves into a sclerotic phase.
- The site of prevalence of otosclerosis is the root of the anterior crus of the stapes.
- The primary symptom of otosclerosis is conductive hearing loss; 85% of patients have bilateral disease.
- Otosclerosis may involve the cochlea, producing a sensorineural deficit.
- Audiometry in early otosclerosis confirms a conductive loss. A Carhart notch, an apparent bone conduction loss in the 2-kHz region, often is seen.
- The acoustic reflex is nearly always absent.
- The value of sodium fluoride in the management of otosclerosis is controversial.
- Current surgical procedures for otosclerosis include partial or total stapedectomy, stapedioplasty, and laser stapedectomy.
- In bilateral disease, surgical treatment of the second ear usually is recommended. The operation is performed 6 to 12 months after the first operation.
- Intraoperative problems include vertigo, laceration of the tympanic membrane, obliterative disease, perilymphatic gusher, floating footplate, dehiscent facial nerve, and subluxation of the incus.
- Postoperative complications are infrequent. They include vertigo, tinnitus, cochlear hearing loss (approximately 1%), facial weakness (rare), otitis media, dysgeusia, perilymphatic fistula, granuloma, labyrinthitis, meningitis, incus necrosis, and recurrence.
- After surgical treatment, approximately 90% of patients have a conductive deficit of 10 dB or less.
- Stapedectomy for children and adolescents parallels the success of the procedure among adults.
- Revision stapedectomy carries increased risk for cochlear loss. Improvement may be expected among 50% of patients.
- Nonotosclerotic lesions of the stapes include Paget's disease, osteogenesis imperfecta, tympanosclerosis, and degenerative arthritis.
- Causes of ossicular fixation include idiopathic fixation of the malleus, tympanosclerosis, and fixation of the incus to the annulus.

REFERENCES

1. Canalis RF. Valsalva's contribution to otology. *Am J Otolaryngol* 1990; 11:420–427.
2. Toynbee J. Pathological and surgical observations of the diseases of the ear. *Trans Med Chir Soc Lond* 1841;24:190–196.
3. Toynbee J. *The diseases of the ear: their nature, diagnosis and treatment.* London: HK Lewis, 1868.
4. Politzer A. Veber primare Erkankung der Knochernen Labyrinth Kapsel. *Ohrenheilkd* 1894;25:309–312.
5. Soifer N, Weaver K, Endahl GL, Holdsworth E. Otosclerosis: a review. *Acta Otolaryngol Suppl (Stockh)* 1970;269.
6. Levin G, Fabian P, Stable J. Incidence of otosclerosis. *Am J Otol* 1988; 9:299–307.
7. Guild SR. Histologic otosclerosis. *Ann Otol Rhinol Laryngol* 1944;53: 246–266.
8. Friedmann I. *Pathology of the ear.* Oxford, UK: Blackwell Scientific, 1974.
9. Shambaugh GE Jr. Fenestration operation for otosclerosis: experimental investigations and clinical observation in 2100 operations over a period of ten years. *Acta Otolaryngol Suppl (Stockh)* 1949;79:1–101.
10. Cawthorne T. Otosclerosis. *J Laryngol Otol* 1955;69:437–456.
11. Gapany-Gapanavicius B. *Otosclerosis: genetics and surgical rehabilitation.* New York: John Wiley & Sons, 1975:177–178.
12. Donnell GN, Alfi OS. Medical genetics for the otorhinolaryngologist. *Laryngoscope* 1980;9:40–46.
13. Mayer O. Untersuchungen uber die otosklerose. Vienna: Holder-Pichler-Tempsky, 1917.
14. Sercer A, Krmpotic J. Thirty years of otosclerosis studies. *Arch Otolaryngol* 1966;84:598–606.
15. Mayer O. Die Ursache der Knochen-neubildung bei der Otosklerose. *Acta Otolaryngol (Stockh)* 1931;15:35–41.
16. Mendoza D, Ruis M. Histology of the enchondral layer of the human otic capsule. *Acta Otolaryngol (Stockh)* 1966;62:93–102.
17. Wolff D, Bellucci RJ. Otosclerosis. *Arch Otolaryngol* 1964;79:571–582.
18. Gussen R. The labyrinthine capsule: normal structure and pathogenesis of otosclerosis. *Acta Otolaryngol Suppl (Stockh)* 1968;235:1–38.
19. Gussen R. Plugging of vascular canals in the otic capsule. *Ann Otol Rhinol Laryngol* 1969;78:1305–1316.
20. Gussen R. The stapediovestibular joint: normal structure and pathogenesis of otosclerosis. *Acta Otolaryngol (Stockh)* 1969;248:1–38.
21. Anson BJ, Bast TH. Development of the otic capsule in the human ear. *Q Bull Northwestern University Med School* 1959;32:157–172.
22. Mann W, Jonas I, Riede UN, Beck C. A contribution to the pathogenesis of otosclerosis. *Arch Otolaryngol Head Neck Surg* 1980;226:161–176.
23. Yoo TJ, Shea JJ Jr, Floyd RA. Enchondral cartilage rests collagen-induced autoimmunity: a possible pathogenetic mechanism of otosclerosis. *Am J Otolaryngol* 1987;8:317–324.
24. Bujia J, Alsalameh S, Jerez R, Sittinger M, Wilmes E, Burmeter G. Antibodies to the minor cartilage collagen type IX in otosclerosis. *Am J Otolaryngol* 1994;15:222–224.
25. Arnold W, Friedman I. Presence of viral specific agents (measles, rubella) around the active otosclerotic focus. *Ann Otol Rhinol Laryngol* 1987;66:167–171.
26. McKenna MS, Mills BG. Immunohistochemical evidence of measles virus antigens in active otosclerosis. *Otolaryngol Head Neck Surg* 1989; 101:415–421.
27. Mills BG, Singer FR. Nuclear inclusions in Paget's disease of bone. *Science* 1976;194:201–202.
28. Mills BG, Singer FR, Weiner LP, Suffin SC, Stabile E, Holst P. Evidence for both respiratory syncytial virus and measles virus antigens in the osteoclasts of patients with Paget's disease of bone. *Clin Orthop* 1984;183:303–311.
29. McKenna MJ, Kristiansen A, Haines J. Polymerase chain reacting amplification of a measles virus sequence from human temporal bone sections with active otosclerosis. *Trans Am Otol Soc* 1995:65.
30. Schuknecht H. *Pathology of the ear.* Cambridge, MA: Harvard University Press, 1974.
31. Schuknecht HF, Barber W. Histologic variants in otosclerosis. *Laryngoscope* 1985;95:1307–1317.
32. Schuknecht HF. Pathology of the ear, 2nd ed. Philadelphia: Lea & Febiger, 1993:378–379.
33. Millman B, Giddings NA, Cole JM. Long term follow up of stapedectomy in children and adolescents. *Otolaryngol Head Neck Surg* 1990; 115:78–81.
34. Gristwood RE, Venables WN. Pregnancy and otosclerosis. *Clin Otolaryngol* 1983;8:205–210.
35. Morales-Garcia C. Cochleovestibular involvement in otosclerosis. *Acta Otolaryngol (Stockh)* 1972;73:484–492.
36. Cody DTR, Baker HL Jr. Otosclerosis: vestibular symptoms and sensorineural hearing loss. *Am J Otol Rhinol laryngol* 1978;87:778–796.
37. Goodhill V. Moncur JP. The low-frequency air–bone gap. *Laryngoscope* 1863;73:850–867.
38. Carhart R. Clinical application of bone conduction audiometry. *Arch Otolaryngol* 1950;51:798–807.
39. Siebenmann F. Sur le traitement chirurgical de la sclerose otique. *Congr Int Med Sect d'otol* 1900;13:11–13.
40. Gray A. Otosclerosis treated by local application of thyroxine. *J Otolaryngol* 1935;50:729–733.
41. Guggenheim LK, Gunther L, Goodhill V et al. Reversal of halisteresis in the mammalian ear. *Arch Otolaryngol* 1941;34:501–522.
42. Kerr G, Hoffman GS. Fluoride therapy for otosclerosis. *Ear Nose Throat J* 1989;68:426–431.
43. Daniel HS III. Stapedial otosclerosis and fluoride in the drinking water. *Arch Otolaryngol* 1969;90:585–590.
44. Petrovic A, Stutzmann J. Effects of sodium fluoride, cholecalciferol and calcium gluconate on human normal and otospongiotic bone. In: Courvoisier B, Donath A, Baud CA, eds. *Fluoride and bone.* Bern: Huber, 1978:201–202.
45. Shambaugh GE Jr, Scott A. Sodium fluoride for the arrest of otosclerosis. *Arch Otolaryngol* 1964;80:263–274.
46. Shambaugh GE Jr. Therapy of cochlear otosclerosis. *Ann Otol Rhinol Laryngol* 1969;75:579–588.
47. State of the art in otosclerosis. Audio Digest Tape. Vol. 17, no. 19. 1984. Audio-Digest Foundation, Subsidiary of the California Medical Association, Glendale, California 91206.
48. Lando M, Hoover LA, Finderman G. Stabilization of hearing loss in Paget's disease with calcitonin and etidronate. *Arch Otolaryngol Head Neck Surg* 1988;114:891–894.
49. Kennedy DW, Hoffer ME, Holliday M. The effects of etidronate disodium on progressive hearing loss from otosclerosis. *Otolaryngol Head Neck Surg* 1993;109:461–467.
50. Kessel J. Uber das Mobilisieren des Steigbugels durch Ausschneiden des Trommelfelles, Hammers und Ambosses bei Undurchgangigkeit der tube. *Arch Ohrenheilkd* 1878;13:69–72.
51. Miot C. De la mobilisation de l'etrier. *Rev Laryngol* 1890;10:49–56.
52. Passow KA. Operative Anlegung einer offnug in die mediale paukenhohlenwand bei Stapesankylose. *Verh Dtsch Otol Ges* 1897;6:141–143.
53. Floderus B. Bidrag till stibgygelankylosens operativa Radikalbehandling. *Nord Med Ark* 1899;32:1–10.
54. Jenkins GJ. Otosclerosis: certain clinical features and experimental operative procedures. *Trans 17th Int Congr Med (Lond)* 1913;16:609–618.
55. Holmgren G. Some experiences in surgery of otosclerosis. *Acta Otolaryngol (Stockh)* 1923;5:460–472.
56. Sourdille M. Resultats primitifs et secondaires de quatorze cas de surdite par otospongiose operes. *Rev Laryngol* 1930;51:595–601.
57. Lempert J. Improvement of hearing in cases of otosclerosis: new one stage surgical technique. *Arch Otolaryngol* 1938;28:42–67.
58. Rosen S. Palpation of the stapes for fixation. *Arch Otolaryngol* 1952; 56:610–612.
59. Shea J. Fenestration of the oval window. *Ann Otol Rhinol Laryngol* 1958;67:932–951.
60. Fisch V. *Tympanoplasty and stapedectomy: a manual of techniques.* New York: Thieme–Stratton 1980:56–57.
61. Smyth GDL, Hassard TH. Eighteen years of experience in stapedectomy: the case for the small fenestra operation. *Ann Otol Rhinol Laryngol* 1978;87[Suppl 49]:3–36.
62. Fisch, U. Stapedectomie oder Stapedotomie? *HNO* 1979;27:361–372.
63. McGee TM. Comparison of small fenestra and total stapedectomy. *Ann Otol Rhinol Laryngol* 1981;90:633–636.
64. Cremers WRJ, Bensen JMH, Huygen PLM. Hearing gain after stapedotomy, partial platinectomy or total stapedectomy for otosclerosis. *Ann Otol Rhinol Laryngol* 1991;100:959–961.
65. Glasscock ME, Storper IS, Haynes DS, Bohrer PS. Twenty five years of experience with stapedectomy. *Laryngoscope* 1995;105:899–904.
66. Perkins RE. Laser stapedectomy for otosclerosis. *Laryngoscope* 1980; 90:228–240.
67. Gherini SG, Horn KL, Bowman CA, Griffin G. Small fenestra stapedotomy using a fiberoptic hand-held argon laser in obliterative otosclerosis. *Laryngoscope* 1990;100:1276–1282.

68. Silverstein H, Rosenberg S, Jones R. Small fenestra stapedotomies with and without KTP laser: a comparison. *Laryngoscope* 1989;99: 485–488.
69. McGee TM. The argon laser in surgery for chronic ear disease and otosclerosis. *Laryngoscope* 1983;93:1177–1182.
70. Pratt LL. Symposium of ear surgery, IV: postoperative complications associated with bilateral stapedectomy. *Laryngoscope* 1972;82: 1189–1198.
71. Gristwood RE. Obliterative otosclerosis. *J Otolaryngol Soc Aust* 1966; 2:4048–4060.
72. Willis R. The Teflon-wire piston in otosclerosis. *J Otolaryngol Soc Aust* 1967;2:2–8.
73. Andrews J, Canalis RF. Otogenic pneumocephalus. *Laryngoscope* 1986;96:521–528.
74. Baxter A. Dehiscence of the fallopian canal. *J Laryngol Otol* 1971;85: 587–594.
75. Welling DB, Glasscock ME, Ganz BJ. Avulsion of the anomalous facial nerve at stapedectomy. *Laryngoscope* 1992;102:729–733.
76. Mayers TG, Crabtree JA. The facial nerve coursing inferior to the oval window. *Arch Otolaryngol* 1976;102:744–746.
77. Pedersen CB, Felding JU. Stapes surgery: complications and airway infection. *Ann Otol Rhinol Laryngol* 1991;100:607–611.
78. Goodhill V. Variable oto-audiologic manifestations of perilymphatic fistulae. *Rev Panam Otorrinolaringol Broncoesofagol* 1967;1: 100–109.
79. Goodhill V. The conductive loss phenomenon in post-stapedectomy perilymphatic fistulae. *Laryngoscope* 1967;77:1179–1190.
80. Harris I, Weiss L. Granulomatous complications of oval window fat grafts. *Laryngoscope* 1962;72:870–885.
81. Kaufman RS, Schuknecht HF. Reparative granuloma following stapedectomy: a clinical entity. *Ann Otol Rhinol Laryngol* 1967;76: 1008–1017.
82. Matz GJ, Lockhart HB, Lindsay JR. Meningitis following stapedectomy. *Laryngoscope* 1968;78:56–63.
83. Palva T, Palva A, Karja J. Fatal meningitis in a case of otosclerosis operated bilaterally. *Arch Otolaryngol* 1992;96:130–137.
84. Goodhill V. Surgery for otosclerosis, stapedectomy, stapedioplasty and fenestration. In: English GM, ed. *Otolaryngology,* vol II. Hagerstown, MD: Harper & Row, 1976:107–112.
85. Monsell EM. Draft guidelines for the evaluation of results of treatment of conductive hearing loss. *AAO-HNS Bull* 1994;13:14–15.
86. Berliner KI, Doyle KJ, Goldenberg RA. Operative hearing results in stapes surgery: does choice of outcome measure make a difference? *Am J Otol* 1996;17:521–528.
87. Sheehy JL. Stapedectomy wire prosthesis for use with tissue grafts. *Trans Am Acad Ophthalmol* 1976;82:108–118.
88. Sheehy JL, Nelson RA, House HP. Stapes surgery at the Otologic Medical Group. *Am J Otol* 1979;1:22–26.
89. Ginsberg IA, Hoffman SR, Stinziano GD, White TP. Stapedectomy in depth analysis of 2405 cases. *Laryngoscope* 1978;88:1999–2016.
90. Shea JJ. Stapedectomy: a long term report. *Ann Otol Rhinol Laryngol* 1982;91:516–520.
91. Shea JJ. Thirty years of stapes surgery. *J Laryngol Otol* 1988;102: 14–19.
92. Langman AW, Jackler RN, Sooy FA. Stapedectomy: long term hearing results. *Laryngoscope* 1991;100:810–814.
93. Vartiainen E, Virtaniessi J, Kemppainen M, Karjalainen S. Hearing levels of patients with otosclerosis 10 years after stapedectomy. *Otolaryngol Head Neck Surg* 1993;108:251–255.
94. Willis R. The fate of the non-operated ear in otosclerosis. *Otolaryngol Head Neck Surg* 1989;100:224–226.
95. Willis R. Progressive flat sensorineural hearing loss occurring after initially successful stapedectomy. *J Otolaryngol Soc Aust* 1987;6: 27–28.
96. House JW, Sheehy JL, Antonez VC. Stapedectomy in children. *Laryngoscope* 1980;90:1804–1809.
97. Robinson M. Juvenile otosclerosis. *Ann Otol Rhinol Laryngol* 1983; 92:561–565.
98. Cole JM. Surgery for otosclerosis in children. *Laryngoscope* 1982;92: 859–861.
99. Crabtree JD, Britton BH, Powers WH. An evaluation of revision stapes surgery. *Laryngoscope* 1980;90:224–227.
100. Sheehy JL, Nelson RD, House HA. Revision stapedectomy: a review of 258 cases. *Laryngoscope* 1981;91:43–51.
101. Koller F. Uber die hereditat der ostitis deformans Paget. *Helv Med Acta* 1946;13:389–400.
102. Nager GT. Paget's disease of the temporal bone. *Ann Otol Rhinol Laryngol* 1975;84[Suppl 22]:1–32.
103. Khetarpal U, Schuknecht HF. In search of pathologic correlates for hearing loss and vertigo in Paget's disease: a clinical and histopathologic study of 26 temporal bones. *Ann Otol Rhinol Laryngol* 1990;99 [Suppl 145]:1–16.
104. Waltner JG. Stapedectomy in Paget's disease. *Arch Otolaryngol* 1968; 82;355–358.
105. Sparrow NL, Duvall AJ III. Hearing loss and Paget's disease. *J Laryngol Otol* 1967;81:601–611.
106. Harner SG, Rose DE, Facer GW. Paget's disease and hearing loss. *Otolaryngology* 1978;86:869–874.
107. Bergstrom LV. Osteogenesis imperfecta otologic and maxillofacial aspects. *Laryngoscope* 1977;87[Suppl 6]:1–42.
108. Armstrong BW. Stapes surgery in patients with osteogenesis imperfecta. *Ann Otol Rhinol Laryngol* 1984;3:634–636.
109. Austin DF. Reconstructive techniques in tympanosclerosis. *Ann Otol Rhinol Laryngol* 1988;97:670–674.
110. Smyth GDL. Tympanosclerosis. *Laryngoscope* 1978;87:1821–1825.
111. Giddings NA, House JW. Tympanosclerosis of the stapes: hearing results for various surgical treatments. *Otolaryngol Head Neck Surg* 1992;107:644–650.
112. Ethom B, Belal A Jr. Senile changes in the middle ear joints. *Ann Otol Rhinol Laryngol* 1974;83:49–54.

The Ear: Comprehensive Otology,
edited by R. F. Canalis and P. R. Lambert.
Lippincott Williams & Wilkins, Philadelphia © 2000.

CHAPTER 29

Nongenetic Sensorineural Hearing Loss in Children

Patrick E. Brookhouser

Evaluation of a Young Child with a Hearing Loss
  History and Physical Examination
  Laboratory Testing
  Audiometric Testing
Specific Causes of Nongenetic Sensorineural
    Hearing Loss
  Congenital and Early-onset Infections

Late-onset Infections
Ototoxic Drugs and Chemicals
Hyperbilirubinemia
Prematurity and Term Low Birth Weight
Ear and Head Trauma
Noise-induced Hearing Loss
Conclusions

The U.S. Department of Health and Human Services document *Healthy People 2000: National Health Promotion and Disease Prevention Objectives* (1) established a goal of reducing the average age for identification of significant hearing loss among infants from 24 to 30 months to no more than 12 months. The existence of a critical period in the first years of life for optimal acquisition of speech and language is supported by credible research. Without adequate auditory stimulation, the organizational development of an infant's central auditory pathway may be impeded. Longitudinal studies involving children with congenital or very-early-onset hearing loss have demonstrated an advantage in development of communicative skills over time among infants whose hearing losses are identified and intervention instituted before 6 months of age compared with infants of equal cognitive ability whose loss is identified later.

Congenital hearing loss often is an invisible disorder at birth. It may not be recognized until an infant does not achieve expected communicative milestones. Persistent congenital or early-onset sensorineural hearing loss (SNHL) in the moderate to profound range (41 to 100 dB) distorts a developing child's perception of his or her attempts at speech production and the speech of others. If

undetected, the impairment can impede acquisition of literacy skills, school achievement, and social and emotional development (2–5). Follow-up studies link even persistent unilateral SNHL in the moderate to profound range with poor academic performance, increased likelihood of repeating a grade, and school behavior problems (6,7). Children with unilateral SNHL can experience impaired speech perception when background noise is presented to the better ear.

In developed countries, 1.0 to 2.0 per 1,000 school-age children exhibit bilateral SNHL of 50 dB or worse, including 0.5 to 1.0 per 1,000 whose bilateral losses exceed 75 dB (8). Data from the United Kingdom indicate that 1 in 943 newborns monitored into elementary school were subsequently confirmed to have SNHL or mixed hearing loss (9). Neonatal intensive care unit (NICU) graduates experienced increased risk for hearing loss (1 in 174 NICU infants versus 1 in 1,278 non-NICU infants). The number of infants and children with lesser degrees of persistent hearing loss (hard of hearing versus deaf) is 5 to 10 greater than that with severe-to-profound losses (1,10). Unilateral SNHL of 45 dB or worse among U.S. school-age children has a prevalence of about 3/1,000, and 13/1,000 have unilateral SNHL worse than 26 dB. Prevalence data for unilateral SNHL among infants and preschoolers are scanty because most unilateral losses are discovered later in life than bilateral losses (mean age in one study 8.78 years) (7).

P. E. Brookhouser: Boys Town National Research Hospital; Department of Otolaryngology and Human Communication, Creighton University School of Medicine, Omaha, Nebraska 68131-2136

The 1993 National Institutes of Health consensus statement titled "Early Identification of Hearing Impairment in Infants and Young Children" (11) noted that the average age at diagnosis of congenital or early-onset hearing losses was 2½ years. The Joint Committee on Infant Hearing (established 1969) has written a series of position statements that enumerate risk indicators to aid in identifying a subset of infants who merit hearing screening. As many as 2% to 5% of neonates at high risk can be confirmed as having moderate-to-severe SNHL. Such focused screening programs, however, fail to identify as many as 50% of children with educationally significant hearing loss by elementary school age. Interest in universal hearing screening of the approximately 4,000,000 infants born annually in the United States has been sparked by the availability of reliable and cost-effective objective screening techniques that involve evoked otoacoustic emissions (EOAEs) and automated auditory brainstem responses (ABRs; see Chapter 13). The National Institutes of Health consensus statement recommends in-hospital hearing screening for all infants admitted to NICUs and screening of all other infants within the first 3 months of life. EOAE measures were recommended for initial screening followed by rescreening with ABR for all infants who do not pass EOAE screening. Infants who fail rescreening merit prompt referral for comprehensive audiologic evaluation.

The 1994 position statement of the Joint Committee on Infant Hearing (12) endorsed the goal of universal detection of hearing loss among infants as early as possible. The necessity of identifying SNHL acquired after 3 months of age also was emphasized. The Joint Committee advocates continued use of risk indicators in clinical settings where universal screening has not been implemented. The position statement includes an expanded list of indicators associated with SNHL and conductive hearing loss to help identify neonates in need of early hearing screening and to determine which infants should undergo rescreening or periodic monitoring of hearing. Indicators of delayed-onset SNHL include the following:

Family history of early-onset SNHL
Prenatal infection (e.g. cytomegalovirus [CMV] infection, rubella, syphilis, toxoplasmosis)
Neurofibromatosis type 2 and neurodegenerative disorders
Persistent pulmonary hypertension in the newborn period

Indicators of conductive hearing loss include the following:

Recurrent or persistent otitis media with effusion
Deformities and disorders that affect eustachian tube function
Neurodegenerative disorders

For a low-incidence disorder such as hearing loss, the sensitivity and specificity of universal newborn screening tests must be adequate to maintain the failure rate for initial screening at a manageable level and minimize unnecessary and expensive comprehensive audiologic evaluations. The Joint Committee on Infant Hearing statement identifies both EOAE and automated ABR as acceptable screening techniques. A multicenter clinical trial (13) has been funded by the National Institute on Deafness and other Communication Disorders to compare efficacy of the two methods. In carefully monitored programs the failure rate necessitating referral can be kept at about 3%.

EVALUATION OF A YOUNG CHILD WITH A HEARING LOSS

Comprehensive evaluation of a child with an educationally significant hearing loss is best accomplished by a team of specialists that includes an otolaryngologist with pediatric experience, a pediatric audiologic team competent in both behavioral and electrophysiologic testing, a pediatrician skilled in detecting subtle findings associated with hearing loss syndromes, a genetic counselor, a pediatric ophthalmologist with competence in electroretinography, a psychologist to assess the child's cognitive abilities, an educator of the deaf with expertise in early intervention, and a speech-language pathologist. Consultation in pediatric neurology and neuroradiology should be easily accessible.

History and Physical Examination

A thorough case history should comprise a detailed prenatal, birth, and postnatal history of the child and a complete family history for

Hearing loss
Speech and language disorders
Ear, nose, and throat disorders
Craniofacial deformities
Syndromic features such as the following:
  Kidney disorders
  Sudden death of a family member at a young age
  Thyroid disease
  Intracranial tumors
  Progressive blindness
  Café au lait spots
  Marital consanguinity

If a family history of hearing loss is identified, an exhaustive pedigree should be constructed that includes at least three generations. The physical examination must focus on subtle findings indicative of hearing loss syndromes such as the following:

Auricular displacement or subtle malformation
Preauricular or branchial pits
White forelock
Heterochromia irides
Blue sclerae

Dystopia canthorum
Facial asymmetry
Café au lait spots

Ophthalmologic evaluation is critical because of the enhanced developmental importance of the visual system in a child with impaired auditory acuity.

Laboratory Testing

An electrocardiogram should be obtained for all children with SNHL who do not have a documented nongenetic cause of the hearing loss. Basic laboratory studies should include complete blood cell count with differential and sickle cell preparation if indicated; basic blood studies, including chemistries, lipids, blood sugar, creatinine, blood urea nitrogen and thyroid studies; and urinalysis. If hematuria is present (red diaper for infants), additional renal studies such as ultrasonography should be undertaken. Serologic tests aimed at detecting congenital syphilis and toxoplasmosis, both of which are potentially treatable, may be indicated. Rubella vaccination status of the mother should be documented, particularly if she immigrated to the United States. Congenital CMV infection accounts for a large amount of childhood deafness, but confirmation of true congenital infection must be based on positive laboratory findings (e.g., viral isolation) within the first 2 or 3 weeks of life. After that, antibodies to perinatally or postnatally acquired CMV can obscure the diagnosis. It is unclear whether autoimmunity plays an etiologic role in progressive SNHL among children; a definitive test battery for use with this population has not been validated. Temporal bone imaging studies are used to assess profoundly deaf children for candidacy for cochlear implants and may also be used to detect such inner ear anomalies as Mondini dysplasia, which can have important prognostic and counseling implications.

Audiometric Testing

A pediatric audiologic evaluation must determine the type of hearing loss (conductive, sensorineural, or mixed),

degree of loss (mild, moderate, severe, profound, or anacusic), the audiometric configuration and symmetry of the impairment, and with serial assessment, the stability or progression of the loss. Vestibular dysfunction may coexist with hearing loss among some children with genetic deafness (e.g., Usher syndrome type I) and hearing loss attributable to such nongenetic causes as bacterial meningitis and exposure to ototoxic drugs and chemicals. Computerized rotational testing facilitates evaluation of the pediatric vestibular system and may help pinpoint an explanation for delayed development of gross motor skill, such as sitting unsupported, walking, and standing on one foot. Progressive and fluctuating SNHL with or without vertigo among children raises the specter of the presence of a perilymphatic fistula (PLF) or other treatable disorder. More extensive evaluation is indicated for these patients.

The serial auditory thresholds of children may be influenced by intrinsic and extrinsic factors that may not include a true change in auditory sensitivity over time. Hazardous sound exposure, including overamplification with hearing aids, may produce a temporary threshold shift. Young patients may improve in their ability to tune in more attentively to very soft sounds with resultant improvement in threshold responses. Criteria for grading a young child's conditioned response (e.g., head turn in visual reinforcement audiometry) to an auditory stimulus may vary across examiners. To avoid methodologic errors, the same audiologists should evaluate a particular child's hearing over time to ensure that any methodologic errors are consistent. Marked threshold changes at the four middle test frequencies (500, 1,000, 2,000, and 4,000 Hz) should trigger enhanced concern. Fluctuation or deterioration of thresholds without middle ear dysfunction at these frequencies by 15 dB or more should prompt careful reevaluation for a potentially treatable condition.

In one study among 230 ears with SNHL that had threshold variation over time (normal middle ear function), fluctuation with or without progressive deterioration was much more common than pure progressive loss (14) (Table 1). The probability of contralateral threshold fluctuation if one ear fluctuated was .91, whereas the probability of contralateral progressive threshold deterioration if one ear progressed was .67. A subset of these

TABLE 1. *Ears in the fluctuating progressive and progressive categories that demonstrated acuity loss of 15 dB or more at various standard audiometric test frequencies (n = 230)*

	Test frequency					
Progression	250 Hz	500 Hz	1,000 Hz	2,000 Hz	4,000 Hz	8,000 Hz
10 dB	175	179	178	188	184	173
15/20 dB	29	22	30	20	28	35
25/30 dB	11	11	8	11	7	14
35/40 dB	7	9	6	8	3	6
>40 dB	8	9	8	3	8	2

From Brookhouser PE, Worthington DW, Kelly WJ. Fluctuating and/or progressive sensorineural hearing loss in children. *Laryngoscope* 1994;104:958–964, with permission.

TABLE 2. *Mean range of fluctuation documented at each of the standard audiometric test frequencies in fluctuating nonprogressive ears (n = 135)*

Fluctuation	Test frequency					
	250 Hz	500 Hz	1,000 Hz	2,000 Hz	4,000 Hz	8,000 Hz
≤10 dB	45	50	60	58	63	72
15/20 dB	39	38	34	35	40	29
25/30 dB	21	20	22	17	10	19
35/40 dB	12	8	5	12	9	8
>40 dB	18	19	14	13	13	7

From Brookhouse PE, Worthington DW, Kelly WJ. Fluctuating and/or progressive sensorineural hearing loss in children. *Laryngoscope* 1994;104:958–964, with permission.

children experienced 20 dB or greater decrement in auditory acuity at one or more of the four frequencies (Table 2). Six months of follow-up evaluation after each 20-dB decrement demonstrated a significant tendency (approximately 50%) for spontaneous improvement of auditory acuity without treatment. Sixty-five of the 95 children (110 episodes) sustained 20 dB or greater deterioration of the three-frequency average (TFA) (500, 1,000, and 2,000 Hz thresholds). Improvement of 10 dB or more in the TFA without treatment was subsequently documented in 50% of these cases. The TFA remained stable in 45%, and a 10 dB or greater decline occurred among only 4% of children during 6 months of follow-up study.

Both genetic and nongenetic causes merit diagnostic consideration for children with fluctuating and progressive SNHL. These causes include a family history of nonsyndromic, hereditary, progressive SNHL. Syndromic features associated with fluctuating and progressive SNHL include anhidrosis, ataxia, branchial fistula, optic atrophy, piebald trait, and preauricular pits. Acoustic neuroma associated with neurofibromatosis, particularly neurofibromatosis type 2, can occur among younger patients. Inner ear anomalies such as Mondini dysplasia and enlarged vestibular aqueduct have strong association with fluctuating and progressive SNHL in children, often exacerbated by minimal head trauma. The differential diagnosis includes exposure to drugs and chemicals; noise trauma; ear and head trauma; mumps; and congenital infections such as rubella, CMV infection, toxoplasmosis, and syphilis; bacterial meningitis; hyperlipidemia, thyroid dysfunction, diabetes, and hypercoagulability state; sickle cell disease, leukemia, and autoimmune inner ear disease; and PLF.

The importance of PLF as a cause of fluctuating and progressive hearing loss among children has been debated. The lack of availability of a sensitive and specific diagnostic technique to confirm preoperatively the presence of a PLF necessitates surgical exploration when PLF is suspected. Even during a surgical procedure, confirmation of a PLF often is equivocal. This reemphasizes the need for perilymph-specific biochemical markers to differentiate perilymph from other clear middle ear fluids in the clinic or operating room. A positive fistula test may be helpful, but a negative result must be considered inconclusive on the basis of reported series. Temporal bone imaging studies are helpful in identifying middle ear anomalies in children with conductive or mixed losses. They also are helpful in the detection of inner ear or internal auditory canal anomalies or lesions associated with SNHL, which might predispose a child to fistula formation and progressive loss of hearing.

A diligent search for the etiologic factor in childhood SNHL even when state of the art techniques are used is inconclusive 30% to 40% of the time. Clinicians serving the needs of these families must be prepared to address concerns regarding lack of a definitive diagnosis as it affects risk for hearing loss among future offspring and the possibility of progression of the child's hearing loss.

SPECIFIC CAUSES OF NONGENETIC SENSORINEURAL HEARING LOSS

Pupil records at schools for the deaf have been the traditional source of data for estimates regarding the mix of causes of SNHL in childhood. About 50% of instances of childhood SNHL has been attributed to genetic factors and 20% to 25% to identifiable environmental causes occurring prenatally, perinatally, or postnatally. The remaining 25% to 30% are sporadic cases of uncertain causation, which no doubt include nonsyndromic genetic losses. These estimates vary depending on the specific population studied. Effective vaccines to prevent formerly common nongenetic infectious causes of SNHL should tilt future cohort studies in favor of genetic causes.

Congenital and Early-onset Infections

Viruses gain access to the inner ear from the bloodstream, middle ear, or cerebrospinal fluid (CSF). CMV has been isolated from human labyrinthine fluids. Seroconversion and virus isolation studies have confirmed an association between labyrinthitis and rubella, rubeola, mumps, influenza, varicella-zoster, Epstein-Barr virus infection, poliomyelitis variola, and adeno- and parainfluenza virus infections.

Viral studies on experimental animals confirm an inflammatory response in the cochlea within 48 hours of viral inoculation, but as inflammatory cells slowly clear from the cochlear duct a residual matrix may undergo calcification with obliteration of cochlear spaces. Histopathologic examination of the temporal bone in cases of prenatal rubella, mumps, rubeola, or CMV infection reveals evidence of endolymphatic labyrinthitis with pathologic changes limited to the cochlear duct, saccule, and utricle consistent with blood-borne spread of infection through vessels in the stria vascularis. Measles, mumps, and CMV infection may entail a meningoencephalitis, which facilitates direct spread along meningeal and neural structures into the perilymphatic spaces to produce inflammatory changes, which may progress to fibrosis. Davis and Johnson (15) observed selective vulnerability of inner ear structures of experimental animals to specific viruses. Influenza virus infected mesenchymal cells in the perilymphatic systems of newborn hamsters, whereas mumps virus infected principally endolymphatic structures. Rubeola and vaccinia viruses attacked both perilymphatic and endolymphatic cells, but herpes simplex involvement was essentially limited to the sensory cells of the labyrinth.

If congenital infection is suspected, it is important to perform serologic testing on both maternal and infant sera collected at the same time to facilitate accurate interpretation of the infant's antibody titer to such agents as herpes simplex virus (HSV) or *Toxoplasma gondii*. Maternal immunoglobulin G (IgG) antibodies, which are normally transmitted transplacentally to the fetus, gradually decline and disappear over the first 6 months of life. As a result, an infant IgG titer obtained in the first month of life that is equal to or less than maternal levels most likely represents passively transferred maternal antibodies. An infant titer equal to or more than four times higher than the mother's is highly suggestive of active infection. In contrast, immunoglobulin M (IgM) antibodies, which represent the early immune response of the neonate to infection, are not transferred transplacentally. Detection of neonatal IgM antibodies is an important step in confirming the presence of disorders such as congenital toxoplasmosis, rubella, and CMV infection.

Cytomegalovirus Infection

CMV, classified in the herpesvirus group, is prevalent among humans in both developed and undeveloped countries. Thirty to forty thousand infants are born each year in the United States with congenital CMV infection (approximately 1% of all newborns); 6,000 to 8,000 have or later experience CMV-related disabilities (15a). There are no known reservoirs or external vectors involved in the human transmission of CMV. Vertical (mother to child) or horizontal (person to person) transmission can occur. Primary infection gives rise to months or years of viral shedding in secretions, including saliva, urine,

semen, and cervical and vaginal fluids. Organ transplants, including blood transfusions from seropositive donors, can spread the virus to potentially immunocompromised patients. Reinfection with one of several antigenically distinct CMV strains is possible, especially among patients with compromised immunity. Maternal viremia enables transplacental passage of CMV to the fetus, where it spreads hematogenously to target organs such as the central nervous system (CNS), eyes, and liver. CMV affinity for eighth cranial nerve neurons and ependymal cells that line the ventricles of the brain has been documented. Congenital CMV infection can be transmitted to the fetus *in utero* during both primary maternal infection and after reactivation of latent virus in immune women. Transmission to the fetus can occur in the presence of maternal CMV antibodies, but the rate of transmission and severity of sequelae are reduced. The offspring of a mother with recurrent CMV infection are nine times less likely to have harmful congenital CMV infection than is true with primary maternal infection and few of these progeny have symptoms at birth.

About 45% of higher socioeconomic status (SES) women of childbearing age in the United States are susceptible to primary CMV infection, whereas 85% of lower SES women demonstrate immunity. About 1% to 4% of susceptible women experience primary CMV infection during pregnancy with a resultant fetal infection rate of 40%. Approximately 0.15% of the offspring of seropositive higher SES women deliver infants with congenital CMV infection, whereas the infection rate among offspring of immune lower SES mothers is 0.5% to 1.0%. The overall CMV infection rate in the United States is about 2% per year. The rate is higher among women being treated in sexually transmitted disease clinics and workers in day care centers for infants and preschoolers, where CMV infection is endemic. As many as 25% of children younger than 3 years in day care centers excrete CMV and can transmit the virus to their mothers during a subsequent pregnancy (16). In one population of seronegative mothers, 15% had children younger than 3 years who were CMV excreters, and 40% of these women became seropositive during a 1-year follow-up period. Child care workers experience an annual seroconversion rate of 11% compared with 2.2% in the general population. Sexually active adolescent women at sexually transmitted disease clinics seroconverted at a rate of 34% per year. The congenital CMV infection rate is particularly high (20% to 25%) among lower SES mothers younger than 20 years, most of whom are unmarried (80% in one study) (16a).

Congenital CMV infection is currently the most common cause of intrauterine infection, occurring in approximately 1% of all live births. Perinatal and postnatal transmission to an additional 4% to 10% of infants occurs through cervical virus shedding, virus in breast milk and blood transfusions. About 40% to 60% of seronegative infants who are breast fed for more than 1 month by a seropositive mother convert (16a). Perinatally infected infants may experience the following:

SNHL
Pneumonitis
Slow weight gain
Adenopathy
Rash
Jaundice
Anemia
Atypical lymphocytosis

All infants with congenital CMV infection shed the virus in high titers in bodily secretions. Definitive diagnosis can be confirmed by means of isolation of the virus from urine or saliva with polymerase chain reaction techniques within the first 2 weeks of life. Infants who acquire the infection perinatally typically begin excreting the virus at 3 to 12 weeks of age, making early viral isolation studies essential to the diagnosis of true congenital infection. Only 10% to 15% of infants with congenital infection have symptoms, 90% of whom have typical cytomegalic inclusion disease, characterized by involvement of the CNS and reticuloendothelial system, with hepatosplenomegaly, petechiae, and jaundice as common presenting findings. Microcephaly, intrauterine growth retardation, and prematurity also may be present, and the mortality rate approaches 30%. Severe mental and perceptual deficits by 2 years of age can be expected in nearly all infants with cytomegalic inclusion disease. Severe to profound SNHL and ocular abnormalities such as chorioretinitis and optic atrophy occur in 25% to 30% of cases.

Neonates with asymptomatic CMV infection, 90% of those with congenital infection, have an improved prognosis for normal neurologic development, but other sequelae can develop. SNHL ranging from mild to profound is the most common irreversible sequela of congenital CMV infection. The incidence is 30% to 50% among infants without symptoms, and SNHL eventually affects 10% to 15% of infants without symptoms. SNHL is bilateral in about 50% of cases and has varying degrees of severity (50 to 100 dB). Nearly 25% of patients have onset or increases in severity after the first year of life (17). Longitudinal hearing screening is an essential component of follow-up care of infants with congenital infection. Risk indicators for delayed-onset CMV hearing loss among infants without symptoms may include periventricular radiolucencies or calicifications on neonatal computed tomographic (CT) scans and significantly elevated maternal titers of envelope glycoprotein gB antibodies throughout the pregnancy, possibly reflecting prolonged antigenic stimulation.

In clinical trials, infants with symptomatic congenital CMV infection have been treated with ganciclovir, an acyclic nucleoside analogue of acyclovir, which acts to inhibit human herpesviruses. Preliminary reports confirming a decrease in viral excretion during treatment followed by a recurrence of excretion after drug withdrawal

have prompted recommendations for higher dosage schedules in an attempt to achieve greater benefit.

Development of a vaccine for CMV infection has been arduous. The Towne vaccine is an attenuated live-virus vaccine with demonstrated capability to induce both antibodies to CMV and cellular immunity but without sufficient immunogenicity to elicit lasting immunity in all test populations. The live viral component of the vaccine has evinced fears about latent infection and carcinogenicity. An alternative vaccine strategy entails noninfectious viral subunits, specifically a portion of the viral envelope that consists of glycoprotein gB. Early clinical trials of CMV gB protein vaccine confirmed that it can induce neutralizing antibody titers equivalent to those observed after exposure to wild-type virus. Epidemiologic data show that a program aimed at immunizing prepubertal girls could have substantial impact on the incidence of congenital CMV infection, which could achieve a significant decrease in the incidence of early-onset nongenetic SNHL.

Histopathologic examination of temporal bones from infants who died of cytomegalic inclusion disease has revealed characteristic inclusion bodies in superficial cells of the stria vascularis, Reissner's membrane, limbus spiralis, saccule, utricle, and semicircular canals. No inclusion-containing cells were found in the organ of Corti, cristae, or ganglia, but endolymphatic hydrops was found in at least a portion of each cochlear duct.

Rubella

Although rubella has been recognized as a distinct disease since the early nineteenth century, its viral causation was not confirmed until 1938. The rubella virus, isolated by Parkman et al. (18) and Weller and Neva (19) in 1962, is an enveloped RNA virus classified as a togavirus, which is most closely related to group A arboviruses, which cause eastern and western equine encephalitis. The rubella virus is transmitted by the respiratory route and undergoes initial replication in the nasopharynx and regional lymph nodes. It is during viremia 5 to 7 days after initial exposure that dissemination of the virus throughout the body and transplacental transmission of the virus to a developing fetus occur. Systemic symptoms in the expectant mother often are mild; 30% to 50% of cases are classified as subclinical.

During a rubella epidemic in Australia in 1941, the keen observations of Gregg (20) linked an array of congenital defects in infants with a history of maternal rubella during pregnancy. Swan et al. (21) were first to describe deafness as a component of the rubella triad, along with congenital cataracts and heart defects. The last major rubella epidemic in the United States occurred in 1964–1965, during which an estimated 12.5 million cases occurred, resulting in an estimated 11,250 abortions (spontaneous or surgical), 2,100 deaths during the neonatal period, and as many as 20,000 cases of congenital rubella syndrome (CRS). The estimated burden of disabilities attributable to CRS in this cohort included deafness for 11,800 children, blindness for 3,580, and mental retardation for about 1,800. As many as 90% of infants who acquire prenatal rubella during the first 11 weeks of pregnancy have some sequelae. As many as 50% of infants may acquire rubella as a result of maternal infection during the eleventh through twentieth weeks of gestation, but only one fourth to one half of these manifest sequelae, primarily hearing loss. Although third-trimester maternal rubella may infect a fetus, defects are rarely observed if the infection occurs after the twentieth week of gestation. The formal clinical case definition of CRS includes the following primary signs and symptoms:

Cataracts or congenital glaucoma
Congenital heart disease (typically patent ductus arteriosus or peripheral pulmonary arterial stenosis)
Hearing loss
Pigmentary retinopathy

Associated findings can include the following (22):

Purpura
Jaundice
Microcephaly
Splenomegaly
Mental retardation
Meningoencephalitis
Radiologic evidence of long-bone lucencies

Hearing loss is the most pervasive disability in CRS and may be the only sequela among infants infected after the fourth month of gestation. Infants with congenital rubella generally shed large quantities of virus in body secretions during the first year of life. They may serve as a source of infection for susceptible health care personnel.

Definitive diagnosis of acute rubella infection depends on a positive viral culture, the presence of rubella-specific IgM antibody, or demonstration of a marked rise in IgG antibody in paired acute (within 7 to 10 days of onset) and convalescent sera (preferably 2 to 3 weeks later). The virus has been isolated from cultures of nasal secretions, the throat, blood, urine, and CSF of patients with acute rubella and those with CRS. A number of serologic techniques have been used with rubella, but most current methods are based on an enzyme-linked immunosorbent assay (ELISA).

A rubella vaccine was first licensed in the United States in 1969, when three different vaccines were approved. These vaccines were superseded in 1979 by a safer and more immunogenic strain developed on human fibroblast diploid cultures (RA 27/3 Meruvax II), which is currently in use as a component of the measles-mumps-rubella (MMR) vaccine. In the prevaccine era, rubella epidemics recurred in a 6 to 9 year cycle with as many as 50% to 90% of susceptible persons contracting the illness during the height of the epidemic. The incidence of rubella in the United States fell from 57,686 cases (58 per 100,000 population) in 1969, the year the vaccine was introduced, to fewer than 1,000 cases (less than 0.5 cases per 100,000 population) in 1983. Outbreaks since then have been limited to populations who have not been immunized, such as recent immigrants and religious groups opposed to vaccination of their children. About three fourths of reported cases of rubella occurred among persons 15 to 44 years of age.

Most infants with congenital rubella that is asymptomatic at birth have sequelae within the first 5 years of life. Among 165 laboratory-documented cases of maternal rubella in one study (23), 49% were clinically apparent, and 51% were subclinical. Although first-trimester rubella was associated with the greatest range of congenital disabilities, some infants of mothers with second-trimester infection also had deafness, microcephaly, cataracts, and mental-motor retardation. Infants with only one or two components of the rubella triad were confirmed by means of laboratory studies to have congenital rubella infection. Hearing loss was the single most common problem and the only sequela identified in 22% of cases. About 30% of babies born of mothers with subclinical but laboratory confirmed infection had hearing loss. The hearing loss was typically sensorineural in character, ranging in severity with some asymmetry in degree and configuration. The most common audiometric curves were of the "cookie-bite" type with greatest loss in the middle frequencies, between 500 and 2,000 Hz. Audiologic follow-up evaluation documented a progressive decrease in auditory acuity in 25% of cases. Postmortem studies found a general miniaturization of organs from rubella-infected fetuses with histopathologic evidence of hypocellularity. Highly specialized cells, such as fiber cells in the lens of the eye, demonstrated increasing susceptibility to the effects of intracellular virus with increasing cellular specialization. As a consequence, gradual progression in cataract formation was found in the postnatal period.

Histopathologic examination of temporal bones from infants with congenital rubella revealed Scheibe-type cochleosaccular changes, whereas the utricle, semicircular canals, and spiral ganglion were relatively unaffected (23). Partial collapse of Reissner's membrane with adherence to the stria vascularis and organ of Corti was found, and the tectorial membrane was found to be rolled and lying in the internal sulcus in some sections. Saccular collapse with histologic evidence of recent acute inflammation was found in some cases. The organ of Corti per se was relatively unaffected, but the stria vascularis often was normal and cystic dilatation was found at the junction of Reissner's membrane and the spiral ligament.

Herpes Simplex Encephalitis

The HSV has two serotypes, HSV-1 and HSV-2, the latter being responsible for most recurrent cases of genital herpes, which affects an estimated 45 million persons in the United States. Genital herpes can be transmitted by a sex partner who is unaware he or she has the infection and has no symptoms at the time of transmission. Antiviral agents such as acyclovir, valacyclovir (a valine ester of acyclovir), and famciclovir (a prodrug of penciclovir) have been successful in suppressing signs and symptoms of some genital herpes episodes, but they do not eradicate the virus. The safety of systemic acyclovir and valacyclovir therapy has not been established for pregnant women, but the Centers for Disease Control and Prevention (CDC) recommends that an initial clinical episode of genital herpes during pregnancy be managed with oral acyclovir but that recurrent episodes of infection during pregnancy not be treated. Mothers giving birth to infants with neonatal herpes may be totally unaware they have genital herpes. Whereas the risk for transmission from an infected mother to her neonate is high among women who initially acquire herpes near the time of delivery (30% to 50%), the risk is low among women who have a history of recurrent herpes at term or who had primary HSV infection during the first half of pregnancy (3%). A substantial percentage of neonates with HSV infection are born prematurely of young, typically nulliparous mothers. Prevention strategies should be aimed at preventing maternal acquisition of infection from HSV-carrying partners late in pregnancy. Delivery by cesarean section may be recommended to minimize the infant's exposure to HSV if the mother has symptomatic infection.

Herpes simplex encephalitis is uncommon, but 25% to 30% of cases involve the pediatric age group. The reported neonatal HSV infection rate varies from 1:2,500 to 1:20,000 live births in published reports. Intrapartum or postpartum exposure is more common than intrauterine transmission, which accounts for only 5% of neonatal infections. Neonatal patients with HSV infection may have mucocutaneous involvement or disseminated infection; one fourth to one third of the infants also have meningoencephalitis. In contrast, as many as 20% of newborns with HSV infection never have cutaneous involvement. Among the postulated routes by which HSV might enter the CNS are hematogenous dissemination, direct spread from the nasopharynx through the cribriform plate, and retrograde spread from infected ganglia. The temporal and frontal areas of the brain are most commonly affected.

With an incubation period as long as 4 weeks, neonatal herpes simplex meningoencephalitis generally occurs during the second or third postpartum week. Only 50% of neonatal HSV infections can be related to a definite history of maternal or paternal infection, so the absence of a positive history does not exclude the disease. Nonspecific clinical findings, including fever and an altered mental state, are accompanied by abnormal CSF findings in more than 90% of patients. Electroencephalography, CT scanning, and magnetic resonance imaging are of benefit in detecting focal meningoencephalitis. The only definitive diagnostic study is brain biopsy, which has positive findings in 33% to 55% of cases of herpes simplex encephalitis.

Currently recommended therapy for all infants who have evidence of neonatal herpes is systemic acyclovir 30 to 60 mg/kg a day for 10 to 21 days. In the care of children with focal encephalitis of uncertain causation, clinicians are advised to institute broad-spectrum antibiotics in addition to acyclovir until a definitive diagnosis has been reached. A child with herpes simplex encephalitis should be treated by a team that includes neurologists, neurosurgeons, and pulmonary medicine, critical care, and infectious disease specialists.

Congenital Toxoplasmosis

T. gondii, a protozoan parasite, is most commonly spread to humans through ingestion of oocysts on food contaminated by cat feces or consumption of tissue cysts in undercooked meat products. Persons in some cultures traditionally consume undercooked meat, such as beef tartar, and are more likely to become infested. *Toxoplasma* infestation can be congenitally transmitted or spread in infested donor organs used in transplantation. The cat serves as natural host for *T. gondii,* excreting about 10 million oocysts a day during active infestation. The likelihood that various components of the U.S. meat supply contain *T. gondii* tissue cysts varies from 25% to 40% for pork to about 20% for lamb, with beef least involved. The oocyst sporulates about 1 to 5 days after excretion into sporozoites, the infesting form. Ingested by humans the organisms invade the intestinal mucosa and spread throughout the body. The infestation may cause cyst formation in all tissues of the body, including the placenta as a route for fetal infestation.

Except when a dormant infestation is reactivated in immunocompromised expectant mothers, primary maternal infestation during pregnancy is the most common source of congenital infestation. The rate of infestation varies with the stage of pregnancy at which maternal infestation occurs, from about 15% in the first trimester to 30% during the second trimester and 60% during the third trimester. Transmission to the fetus becomes highly probable if maternal infestation occurs a short time before delivery. In contrast with the increased risk for fetal infestation in late pregnancy, the greatest likelihood of severe congenital disease occurs early in gestation. Taking all these factors into account, it has been estimated that the highest risk for severe congenital toxoplasmosis is associated with primary maternal infestation during weeks 10 to 24 of pregnancy. Approximately three fourths of infants with congenital infestation have no symptoms at birth (90% in one study); another 15% manifest only ocular lesions, and the remaining 10% are severely involved (23a). The classic clinical triad heralding congenital toxoplasmosis includes chorioretinitis, hydrocephalus, and intracranial calcifications. Other findings may include the following:

Microphthalmia
Cataracts
Microcephaly
Thrombocytopenia
Hepatosplenomegaly
Jaundice

Careful clinical studies have documented a neurologically dominant type of involvement that is more common than a disseminated variant that affects multiple organ systems with a very poor prognosis for normal development. It is essential to detect subclinical infestation because untreated infants are at high risk for later chorioretinitis with decreasing visual acuity (as high as 85% by the age of 20 years), progressive CNS involvement with decreased intellectual function, deafness, and precocious puberty. Although 90% of babies found to have congenital toxoplasmosis in the New England Newborn Screening Program were thought to be clinically normal at discharge, targeted diagnostic studies (cranial CT scanning, CSF examination, ophthalmologic examination, including retinoscopy) showed evidence of CNS involvement among 40% of these infants (23a).

Acute toxoplasmosis in an expectant mother can be asymptomatic or produce only minimal findings, such as lymphadenopathy and fatigue, headache, sore throat, and myalgia. Compulsory testing for *Toxoplasma* seropositivity early in pregnancy has been implemented in France (24–27). Maternal infestation is confirmed with the presence of specific IgG in a previously seronegative patient or rising IgG titer after 3 weeks or more. The recommended treatment protocol includes a combination of pyrimethamine and sulfonamide of the sulfapyrimidine type (sulfadoxine or sulfadiazine), which decreases the likelihood of transmission to the fetus and mitigates the sequelae if fetal infestation occurs. French clinicians have administered spiramycin to infested mothers during pregnancy, markedly reducing the rate of transplacental transmission. Samples of amniotic fluid obtained through amniocentesis or fetal umbilical cord blood can be used for diagnostic studies such as mouse inoculation, IgM immunosorbent assays, and quantitative maternal and fetal IgG studies to document the presence of fetal infestation. Recent advances in the use of polymerase chain reaction techniques to detect traces of *T. gondii* organism from amniotic fluid are leading to safer fetal screening methods.

Results from French studies involving prenatal treatment of infested mothers reveal a 0.6% fetal infestation rate with maternal infestation before conception or in early pregnancy, a 3.7% infestation rate from maternal infestation during the sixth to sixteenth weeks of gestation, and a 20% rate after maternal infestation during the

sixteenth through twenty-fifth weeks. The incidence of fetal infestation among women in the sixteenth to twenty-fifth weeks of pregnancy was 70% less than found in previous studies. This finding confirmed the efficacy of aggressive management of primary maternal infestation during pregnancy. Infants with confirmed maternal infestation should be treated for up to 1 year with alternating courses of pyrimethamine and sulfonamide (sulfadiazine), coupled with folinic acid to prevent pyrimethamine complications. Careful follow-up evaluation should include CT scans to assess CNS status, ophthalmologic examination for chorioretinitis and audiologic evaluation to detect delayed-onset hearing loss. Outcome studies indicate that treatment of infants with congenital infestation begun at birth can reduce the frequency of chorioretinitis from 60% to 10%. Encysted forms of *Toxoplasma* are less responsive to medical therapy and delayed-onset chorioretinitis has been observed in treated cases. A Chicago-based study of treated infants with longitudinal ABR and behavioral audiologic tests found no hearing loss among 57 infested infants (28). Histopathologic examination of temporal bones from two infested infants revealed calcified scars, predominantly in the stria vascularis, comparable with those found in the CNS.

Estimated incidence figures for congenital toxoplasmosis in the United States range from 1:1,000 to 1:8,000 live births, yielding about 3,000 infants a year with *Toxoplasma* infestation. From 15% to 25% of inadequately treated infants with congenital infestation eventually have SNHL. Epidemiologic studies confirm that 85% to 90% of U.S. women of childbearing age are seronegative and susceptible to primary infestation during pregnancy. Prevention strategies have been aimed at prevention of maternal infestation through careful personal hygiene, cleaning of fruits and vegetables before ingestion, and thorough cooking of meat products. The cleaning of cat litter boxes is best left to nonpregnant family members. Development of an anti-*Toxoplasma* vaccine for administration to feline carriers shows promise as a control measure.

Syphilis

Congenital syphilis, resulting from transplacental transmission of *Treponema pallidum*, a spirochete that cannot be cultured *in vitro,* may be manifest at birth or may be inapparent until as late as the fifth decade of life (see Chapter 36). Infection of the fetus may occur during any stage of maternal disease, although it is most likely during primary syphilis (70% to 100%) and least likely (30%) in the late stage of the disease. The number of reported cases of syphilis rose from 30.5 per 100,000 population to 54.5 in 1990 (29). After 1990 the incidence declined to 26.2 per 100,000 in 1995. The reported incidence of congenital syphilis mirrored this pattern, increasing from 277 reported cases in 1980 to a high of 3,865 cases in 1990 followed by a decline to 1,549 in 1995. A 1997 report documented a direct relation between maternal illicit drug use (cocaine addiction) and congenital syphilis among their infants (30). Concurrent human immunodeficiency virus infection among patients with acquired syphilis may increase the likelihood of early progression to neurosyphilis and decrease responsiveness to penicillin therapy. Although SNHL has been reported among patients with primary, secondary, and later acquired syphilis, the primary concern among children is congenital infection.

Of all pregnant women with untreated syphilis, it is estimated that only 20% deliver a term healthy infant (31). Fetal death occurs in about 25% of cases; another 10% to 20% of these infants may die perinatally. A careful follow-up study of women who had maternal syphilis during a pregnancy that ended in the delivery of an infant with congenital syphilis revealed that if they had a subsequent pregnancy, 40% delivered a second infant with congenital infection. Forty-two percent of the patients in the study who delivered an infant without congenital syphilis with the first pregnancy delivered an infant with congenital syphilis with a subsequent pregnancy. Continued cocaine use was the most important risk factor for delivering a second infant with congenital syphilis (32). The manifestations of congenital syphilis are variable; about one third of surviving neonates with congenital syphilis manifest some findings at birth. This early-onset form, which generally presents itself within the first 3 months of life, is associated with maternal infection early in pregnancy. The infants often are of low birth weight and have hepatosplenomegaly and mucocutaneous involvement, which may include rhinitis (snuffles) and a diffuse, maculopapular, desquamating skin rash, characteristically involving the palms and soles of the feet. The classic stigmata of congenital syphilis, which may manifest themselves over the first several years of life, include the following:

SNHL
Interstitial keratitis
Hutchinson's teeth (notched incisors)
Mulberry molars
Clutton's joints (bilateral painless knee effusions)
Nasal septal perforation and saddle deformity
Frontal bossing
Skeletal deformities

Skeletal findings include osteochondritis and periostitis of the long bones that lead to saber shin deformity with radiographic evidence, particularly in the humerus and femur, of symmetric changes such as serrated metaphyseal ends, thickened periosteum, and metaphyseal defects of the upper medial tibia. These radiographic findings may be the sole presenting sign among as many as 20% of cases of early-onset congenital syphilis.

Transplacental transfer of nontreponemal and treponemal maternal IgG antibodies to the fetus can complicate the early diagnosis of congenital syphilis. Routine screening of umbilical cord blood is not recommended because it might yield a false-positive result through contamination with maternal blood. Infants born to seroreactive mothers should be carefully examined for signs of congenital syphilis. Histopathologic examination of the placenta or umbilical cord should be performed with specific fluorescent treponemal antibody (FTA) staining techniques. Careful examination of suspicious lesions or body fluids such as nasal drainage with FTA staining also may be helpful. Symptom-free infants should be presumed to have congenital syphilis and be treated if the mother had not been treated or been inadequately treated for syphilis at the time of delivery or showed evidence of relapse or reinfection after treatment, such as a fourfold or greater increase in nontreponemal antibody. Even if maternal syphilis was managed with an apparently adequate regimen, the infant should be treated unless a fourfold decrease in nontreponemal maternal antibody is documented. For evaluating CSF in these presumed cases, the CDC has defined the criteria for diagnosis of congenital syphilis as the presence of a positive nontreponemal test (Venereal Disease Research Laboratory) and a leukocyte count of 5 mm^3 or more or a CSF protein concentration of 100 mg/dL or more (33). The latest CDC treatment recommendations for congenital syphilis in a newborn should be consulted before therapy is instituted. Careful follow-up evaluation to document the effectiveness of treatment is essential.

Prevalence estimates of hearing loss among patients with congenital syphilis range from 3% to 38%. About 37% of cases become apparent before the age of 10 years, 51% between 25 and 35 years of age, and 12% even later in life. Few affected infants have SNHL during the neonatal period, so longitudinal audiologic screening is mandatory, and in some instances SNHL may be the only presenting symptom. A commonly reported audiometric configuration is bilateral, flat SNHL, which may become apparent among children as sudden, bilateral, profound impairment, usually without vertigo. In late congenital syphilis, the hearing loss may be sudden, asymmetric, fluctuating or progressive, and in many cases accompanied by episodic tinnitus and vertigo. Speech discrimination scores are typically poorer than predicted with the audiometric configuration, loudness recruitment is severe, and caloric responses are weak to absent. A positive labyrinthine fistula test result (Hennebert's sign) and disequilibrium in response to loud sounds (Tullio phenomenon) may be reported.

In cases of suspected otosyphilis, dark-field examination of perilymph for *T. pallidum* presents an unacceptable risk for additional hearing loss, so serologic methods present the best alternative diagnostic approach. *T. pallidum* infection evokes both nonspecific reagin antibody and specific antitreponemal antibodies. Whereas nonspecific tests are used for screening large numbers of patients from low-incidence populations, a reported prevalence of 570/100,000 of presumed otosyphilis among otologic referrals justifies use of more expensive *Treponema*-specific procedures. The FTA absorption test (FTA-ABS) has a high sensitivity in all stages of syphilis and a specificity (few false positives) that approaches 98% in large studies. Most false-positive results occur among patients with autoimmune or drug-induced collagen vascular diseases, such as systemic lupus erythematosus. *Treponema*-specific tests used to confirm FTA-ABS results are the microhemagglutination assay for *T. pallidum* and the *T. pallidum* inhibition test, a complex and expensive but highly specific (99%), procedure.

To help clarify the status of treated patients whose *Treponema*-specific test results may remain positive after adequate treatment, Birdsall et al. (34) introduced a western blot assay for antitreponemal antibody isotypes. In the presence of active infection, both antitreponemal IgM and IgG antibodies are present. Only IgG antibodies should remain after successful treatment. Careful follow-up testing of offspring of seropositive mothers with nontreponemal antibody tests should be conducted at 1, 2, 4, 6, and 12 months of age. Stable or rising titers by 6 months of age should prompt reevaluation and treatment. Infants with neurologic involvement should undergo serial lumbar punctures with CSF examination at 6-month intervals until the spinal fluid is normal.

The treatment of choice for all patients with a presumptive diagnosis of otosyphilis who are not allergic to penicillin is high-dose parenteral penicillin. The dosage level and duration must be sufficient to overcome potential limits on penicillin diffusion posed by the blood-CSF and blood-perilymph barriers. The discovery that treponemes may lie dormant for as long as 90 days between replications in late congenital syphilis dictates the necessity for longer treatment schedules for some patients. Current CDC treatment recommendations should be consulted before therapy is initiated. Desensitization to penicillin, rather than alternative therapy for patients with penicillin allergy, may be indicated in some instances.

Systemically administered corticosteroids (generally oral prednisone) as an adjunct to antimicrobial therapy have demonstrated effectiveness in stabilizing or improving hearing among approximately 50% of patients with syphilitic deafness. Speech discrimination scores may show greater improvement than pure tone thresholds. The mechanism of action of steroids in these cases may involve nonspecific reduction of vasculitis, suppression of immune reaction to spirochetal antigens, or enhancement of penicillin diffusion into the perilymph. Relative contraindications to steroid therapy include lack of immunity to varicella, recent vaccination, hypertension, diabetes mellitus, glaucoma, pregnancy, and peptic ulcer disease. Initially administered in a gradually tapered dosage regimen, steroids are usually discontinued after 4 to 8 weeks if hearing does not improve. Long-term maintenance therapy may be indicated to sustain hearing improvement. Alternate-day dosage appears to reduce the risk for sequelae, such as cataract formation, bone growth disturbance, and adrenal suppression. The risks and benefits of extended steroid therapy for all patients, particularly children, must be weighed carefully before an extended treatment regimen is begun.

Histopathologic findings in the temporal bones of patients with congenital otosyphilis include obliterative endarteritis, mononuclear cell infiltrates, osteitis of the otic capsule, and varying degrees of tissue necrosis. Early congenital syphilis may involve the labyrinthine structures and the eighth cranial nerve with round cell infiltration but can present itself as meningolabyrinthitis. Temporal bone osteitis with related involvement of the membranous labyrinth also can be found in late congenital otosyphilis. Atrophy of the organ of Corti and involvement of the stria vascularis, spiral ganglion, and eighth-nerve fibers have been found. Gummatous changes can affect all bones of the ear including the ossicles, converting SNHL to a mixed loss.

Neonatal Sepsis

The important etiologic role of infection with group B streptococci (GBS) in neonatal sepsis was first appreciated in the 1970s. By 1990 50% of approximately 15,000 reported cases of GBS disease involved neonates. Almost 80% of cases of GBS disease reported during the first week of life begin on the first day. Apart from neonatal mortality, disabilities attributable to GBS include hearing loss, vision problems, and developmental delay. Meningitis is a common outcome of bacteremia among patients with neonatal sepsis, and uncommon organisms such as *Listeria monocytogenes* may play a role in such cases. Postmeningitic hearing loss should be ruled out through age-appropriate evaluation, such as ABR testing of all survivors of neonatal meningitis.

The source of infection for most neonates is mother-to-infant transmission in the course of labor and delivery resulting from asymptomatic GBS colonization of the mother's genital and gastrointestinal tracts. About 98% of colonized infants have no symptoms, and the others have early-onset disease that includes sepsis, pneumonia, or meningitis. The risk increases as a result of prolonged labor with early membrane rupture, preterm delivery (before 37 weeks), and maternal intrapartum fever. The American Academy of Pediatrics (35) and the CDC (36) have advocated preventive strategies that include maternal vaginal and rectal cultures within 5 weeks of expected delivery (typically 35 to 37 weeks' gestation) and intrapartum administration of antibiotics to mothers with positive culture results and all who deliver preterm. Any mother who has delivered a previous infant with GBS infection or has experienced GBS bacteriuria during pregnancy should receive antibiotics. Data indicate that as many as 80% of cases of neonatal GBS disease can be prevented with a well-designed proactive program of diagnosis and intervention.

Late-onset Infections

Measles and Mumps

The parotitis and orchitis associated with mumps were described by Hippocrates in the fifth century B.C., but it was not until 1934 that Johnson and Goodpasture (37) demonstrated that mumps is caused by a filtrable agent present in saliva; the agent was isolated as a virus in 1945. An RNA paramyxovirus, the mumps virus is related to viruses that cause influenza, parainfluenza, and Newcastle disease. Spread by respiratory droplets, the virus undergoes initial replication in the nasopharynx and regional nodes, leading to a 3- to 5-day period of viremia sometime between day 12 and day 25. Viremic spread to multiple tissues can occur, including salivary glands and meninges. As many as 20% of cases of mumps are asymptomatic; an additional 40% to 50% are limited to primarily respiratory symptoms. About 30% to 40% of patients experience typical parotitis, which may be unilateral or bilateral. Aseptic meningitis, asymptomatic in 50% to 60% of cases, can present with headache and stiff neck, which generally resolve spontaneously in 3 to 10 days. Encephalitis occurs among fewer than 2 per 100,000 mumps patients, but permanent sequelae affect about 25% of survivors. Hearing loss affects about 5 of 10,000 mumps patients and is typically sudden in onset and may be accompanied by tinnitus, vertigo, nausea, and vomiting. Eighty percent of cases are unilateral.

The mumps virus can be isolated from saliva, urine, and CSF specimens collected during the initial 5 days of illness. Useful serologic tests include enzyme immunoassay and radial hemolysis antibody tests. The currently used Jeryl Lynn strain of live attenuated mumps virus vaccine was initially licensed in late 1967. With its use the number of cases of mumps in the United States declined from an estimated 212,000 in 1964 to about 3,000 (1.3 per 100,000 population) in 1983. After a transient resurgence of mumps to a peak level of 12,000 cases in 1987, there has been a steady drop to an all-time low of 658 reported cases in 1996, occurring mostly among adolescents (Fig. 1). The mumps component of the MMR vaccine has proved safe; the incidence of CNS complications, which includes hearing loss, is 1:1,000,000 doses of antigen.

Although the existence of measles as an acute viral infectious disease has been known since antiquity, the virus was finally isolated in human and monkey kidney tissue culture by Enders (38) and Peebles (39) in 1954. Classified as a paramyxovirus with a core of single-stranded RNA, the measles virus, which has a single antigenic type, is related to the canine distemper viruses. The initial site of infection is the respiratory epithelium of the

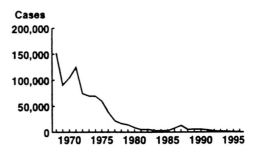

FIG. 1. Impact of immunization on reported cases of mumps in the United States.

nasopharynx, which gives rise to primary viremia 2 to 3 days after exposure, spreading the virus to the reticuloendothelial system, where further replication takes place. A second viremia occurs 5 to 7 days after initial infection and leads to involvement of other organs. One or more complications of measles occur in nearly 30% of reported cases, most commonly among patients younger than 5 years and older than 20 years. Acute encephalitis is reported in about 0.1% of cases; the mean time of onset is 6 days (range 1 to 15 days) after appearance of the characteristic rash. These patients can experience fever, headache, vomiting, nuchal stiffness and other signs of meningeal irritation, lethargy, seizures, and coma. The overall fatality rate approaches 15%. As many as 25% of survivors have neurologic sequelae, including SNHL.

Although not recommended for routine diagnostic purposes, measles virus can be isolated from urine, nasopharyngeal aspirates, heparinized blood, or throat swabs. The most widely used serologic methods are ELISA or enzyme immunoassay. In a single serum sample a positive ELISA result for IgM antibody, which is elevated in the early stages of infection, is diagnostic. Serologic diagnosis with IgG antibody levels requires acquisition of serial samples to demonstrate a rising antibody titer.

Before licensure of the first live attenuated measles vaccine in 1963, about 500,000 new cases, including approximately 500 measles-related deaths, were reported each year to U.S. public health authorities (Fig. 2) (39a). Accounting for unreported episodes, the true number of cases occurring annually was estimated at 3 to 4 million. Epidemics typically occurred in 2- to 3-year cycles, almost 50% of cases being among children 5 to 9 years of age. Widespread use of the vaccine caused a decline of more than 98% in the incidence of the disease, which has remained low except for a resurgence in 1989–1991, which was attributable to inadequate immunization coverage. Intensive vaccination efforts have decreased the number of cases of measles reported annually to fewer than 1,000 since 1993. The only vaccine currently available in the United States is the live attenuated viral strain introduced in 1986 and administered as part of the MMR

Measles - United States, 1950-1996

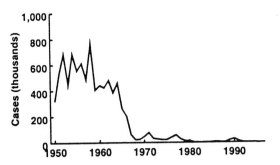

FIG. 2. Impact of immunization on reported cases of measles in the United States.

series. Adults born in 1957 or later who do not have a medical contraindication should receive at least one dose of MMR vaccine or present other acceptable evidence of immunity to these three diseases. All health care personnel should present evidence of immunity to measles and rubella.

Two different pathophysiologic mechanisms have been implicated in SNHL as a sequela of measles or mumps. If SNHL occurs without concurrent meningoencephalitis, the virus appears to enter the inner ear through the stria vascularis during viremia. Sluggish strial circulation and an intraepithelial capillary network predispose to inflammatory changes in this structure that may be followed by degeneration and scarring. Biochemical and volumetric changes in the endolymph are thought to promote degeneration of the stria vascularis, the organ of Corti, the tectorial membrane, and peripheral cochlear neurons. The changes proceed from the cochlear base to the apex. Collapse of Reissner's membrane with adherence to underlying structures has been found. The perilymphatic system, vestibular end organs, and content of the internal auditory canal generally remain intact. These histopathologic changes are compatible with findings among patients with SNHL caused by congenital rubella (40).

Temporal bone findings among patients who have had mumps or measles meningoencephalitis are highly suggestive of meningogenic bacterial labyrinthitis. Direct extension of the viral inflammatory process occurs along nerves and vessels in the internal auditory meatus into the inner ear. A finding compatible with such a transmeatal route of infection is severe degeneration of neural elements in the modiolus, which is contrasted to lesser degrees of involvement of neural structures in the cochlear duct. Temporal bones from infants who died during the acute stage of meningoencephalitis demonstrate lymphocytic infiltration along nerves and vessels in the internal auditory canal without concurrent involvement of the stria vascularis. Intralabyrinthine fibrosis and osteoneogenesis in perilymphatic spaces have been found in patients who survive the acute disease.

Bacterial Meningitis and Vaccine Development

Although *Escherichia coli* and GBS are the most common bacterial causes of meningitis among neonates, three pathogens historically have been responsible for about 80% of cases of bacterial meningitis throughout the world: *Haemophilus influenzae* type B (Hib), *Neisseria meningitidis,* and *Streptococcus pneumoniae* (41). All three have encapsulated forms that colonize the upper respiratory tract and can cause both bacteremia and invasive disease. The introduction of effective antimicrobial agents reduced the mortality rate for bacterial meningitis among young children from more than 90% to 2% to 3% for patients older than 1 month (42–44). Disappointing was that these life-saving antibiotics did not ameliorate such feared sequelae as postmeningitis SNHL. The emergence of bacterial strains resistant to a wide array of antibiotics has refocused the attention of public health authorities on prevention.

Preventive strategies for bacterial meningitis have traditionally been three pronged (41). First, use of hyperimmune globulin for passive immunization during epidemic periods has been effective but expensive. Second, treatment of patients at high risk and their contacts with prophylactic antibiotics has proved effective for limited periods of time. Last, active immunization through vaccine development in the past quarter century has witnessed productive efforts that began with purification of bacterial capsular polysaccharides for use in immunizing against capsulated bacteria, such as meningococci, pneumococci, and Hib.

Haemophilus influenzae

Unencapsulated strains of *H. influenzae* are etiologically involved in mucosal infections such as otitis media and sinusitis. Of the six capsular types (a through f) of Hib, only type b is virulent enough to cause bacteremia and meningitis. Epidemiologic studies have confirmed a striking pattern of age-dependent susceptibility to invasive Hib disease, the peak incidence of meningitis being 7 to 12 months of age, which is after the gradual disappearance of transplacentally transferred bactericidal, maternal Hib antibodies. Approximately 60% of invasive Hib disease occurs before 12 months of age. In the prevaccine era, most children had acquired natural immunity to Hib by 5 to 6 years of age through asymptomatic Hib exposure, so older children accounted for only 10% of the reported infections. Overall, 1 in 250 children would typically experience invasive Hib disease. Nearly 50% of these would be meningitis, which accounts for about 70% of all cases of meningitis among children younger than 5 years (44a).

The specific antigenic component of the capsule that elicits a host immune response is a polysaccharide, a heteropolymer of ribosyribitol phosphate. A pure capsular polysaccharide (CP) Hib vaccine licensed in 1985 successfully elicited protective antibody levels in adults and children 18 months and older but not in infants at highest risk for Hib disease. To develop a vaccine with enhanced immunogenicity, especially in infancy, Robbins et al. (45) adopted a strategy based on early observations that covalent linkage of CP to a protein carrier (conjugation) in a vaccine increased its immunogenic potential in infants by converting the CP from a T lymphocyte–independent to a T cell–dependent antigen. These Hib conjugate vaccines have had considerable effect on the incidence of invasive Hib disease, such as meningitis, epiglottitis, osteomyelitis, and septic arthritis. As a consequence of widespread administration of the Hib conjugate vaccine, licensed in 1989 for children 15 months and older and after 1990 approved for an initial dose at 2 months of age, the incidence of Hib invasive disease has decreased by 98%. More than 95% of infants have protective antibody levels after a two- to three-dose immunization series. From an estimated U.S. Hib infection occurrence rate of 20,000 cases (40 to 50 cases per 100,000 population) annually in the United States in the 1980s, the incidence of invasive Hib disease rapidly declined among both vaccinated and unvaccinated children, a phenomenon called *herd immunity*. It has been demonstrated that serum Hib-CP IgG antibody achieves inactivation of Hib on respiratory epithelium with consequent reduction in exposure of non-immune individuals.

Before the Hib vaccine became available, Hib infection was the leading cause of bacterial meningitis among infants and children 4 years and younger (70%). It accounted for approximately 12,000 cases per year with a case fatality rate of about 5%. An additional 15% to 30% of survivors could be expected to have an array of neurologic sequelae, including SNHL. By 1994–1995, infants 5 months of age or younger, who had not yet completed the primary Hib vaccination series, experienced the highest incidence of Hib invasive disease of all age groups (2.2 per 100,000). Strategies to promote strict compliance with the recommended immunization schedule are being advocated to ameliorate this problem. Administration of a resistant Hib conjugate vaccine to an infant younger than 6 weeks is contraindicated because it may induce immunologic tolerance, which renders the child unable to respond to subsequent doses. Because of the success of the Hib conjugate vaccine, this approach is being used to enhance the immunogenicity of CP for vaccines against pneumococci, meningococci, GBS, and *E. coli*.

Neisseria meningitidis

Before the Hib vaccine became available, *N. meningitidis* accounted for about 20% of all cases of meningitis reported annually to the CDC National Bacterial Meningitis Reporting System (46). Infants in the first year of life have the greatest susceptibility and mortality across all age groups (about 10%). Unlike other encapsulated bacteria, meningococci can cause epidemics, and the risk for infection extends from infancy through early adulthood. Of the 12 meningococcal serotypes (A, B, C, H, I, K, L, X, Y, Z, 29E, and W135) characterized with CP antigens, types B (50%) and C (20%) are responsible for most cases of meningococcal meningitis in the United States (41). Polysaccharide-based vaccines against group A have demonstrated efficacy among children as young as 3 months, but the effectiveness declines markedly over several years, particularly among children younger than 4 years. Similar group C vaccines proved even less immunogenic among young infants. Clinical trials are underway with polyvalent protein conjugate vaccines, which evoke antibodies against both group A and group C meningococcus and *E. coli* K1. Group B presents a unique challenge because the capsular antigen is not immunogenic among humans, and other noncapsular antigens have formed the basis for group B vaccines, which are moderately effective among older children and adults and are now undergoing trials. Recommendations regarding potential general use of the vaccine among young children must await the results of large clinical trials.

Streptococcus pneumoniae

S. pneumoniae has historically accounted for about 13% of cases of bacterial meningitis in the United States. Children younger than 2 years have greater susceptibility to the infection. The overall reported mortality rate for pneumonococcal meningitis is as high as 25%. In some studies, a high incidence of sequelae of meningitis, particularly SNHL, has been found among survivors of pneumococcal meningitis (47–49). The pneumococcus also plays an important etiologic role in otitis media and pneumonia. The alarming emergence of multiantibiotic-resistant stains of pneumococci has spurred development of effective vaccines with an aim of limiting antibiotic use.

S. pneumoniae serotypes are defined on the basis of antigenic specificity of CPs, which evoke type-specific protective antibodies in adults and children older than 2 years. Immune systems of children younger than 2 years process polysaccharide antigens as immunogens that are not T lymphocyte dependent, and the resultant antibodies are weak and short-lived. If conjugate vaccine techniques are used to link the CP to protein carriers, a much stronger and long-lasting immune response can be evoked, even in infants. Of the 84 known pneumococcal serotypes, types 4, 6, 14, 18, 19, and 23 most commonly affect children in the United States. All but type 6D are contained in a currently available 23 valent nonconjugated vaccine. A conjugate vaccine that links pneumococcal polysaccharide with tetanus toxoid and provides increased immunogenicity among children 2 to 5 years of age has been developed. Unfortunately, each serotype must be conjugated individually, limiting the number that can be included in a single vaccine. Recommendations for general use should be forthcoming as clinical trials are completed.

The effectiveness of the Hib conjugate vaccine in reducing the incidence of invasive Hib disease represents one of the signal public health success stories of the past several decades. A study of bacterial meningitis in the United States in 1995 (50) showed a notable shift in etiologic patterns from pre–Hib vaccine studies. The most common pathogen in the neonatal period was still GBS, but among infants 1 to 23 months of age, 78% of cases of bacterial meningitis were attributable to *S. pneumoniae* (47%) and *N. meningitidis* (31%). Among those in the 2- to 18-year age bracket, *N. meningitidis* caused 59% and *S. pneumoniae* 62% of cases among persons older than 19 years. Only 31% of cases of bacterial meningitis caused by these main pathogens occurred among children younger than 5 years. The study's most dramatic finding was a shift in the median age of patients with bacterial meningitis from 15 months in 1986 to 25 years in 1995. Two thirds of patients with bacterial meningitis in 1986 were between 1 month and 5 years of age. By 1995 the number of reported cases of meningitis in this age group had dropped 87%, and there was a 55% decrease in all cases of meningitis. These findings should have important implications for meningitis-related hearing loss, particularly among the prelingual age group.

Postmeningitic Hearing Loss

From 28% to 40% of patients with meningitis experience seizures before or during their hospital stay. Later CT scans often reveal evidence of brain infarction, arterial occlusion, and brain or spinal cord necrosis among meningitis survivors with long-term sequelae. Approximately 57% of survivors of pneumococcal meningitis and 14.5% of those with *H. influenzae* meningitis manifest one or more detectable disabilities 12 months after hospital discharge. In addition to SNHL these sequelae may include seizure disorders, motor abnormalities (e.g., cerebral palsy, hemiparesis, diplegia, quadriplegia), hydrocephalus, vestibular deficits, speech and language disorders, attention deficit disorder, visual impairment, and learning disabilities. These additional disabilities can complicate diagnostic and rehabilitative procedures in the care of children with postmeningitic hearing loss.

The reported incidence of postmeningitic SNHL is generally in the 15% to 20% range. Most losses are permanent, bilateral, and severe. In one series of 64 children with postmeningitic SNHL, 38% had bilateral, asymmetric SNHL, and 11% exhibited unilateral losses (51). Meningitis-related hearing loss has its onset early in the course of the disease, and the incidence has not been decreased with any specific antibiotic regimen. Richardson et al. in England (52) conducted an intensive study with 124 children (0.1 to 15.6 years of age; median 2.1

years) with meningitis. The evaluation, a combination of EOAE, ABR testing, and tympanometry, was performed within 6 hours of diagnosis and was repeated 6 to 12, 12 to 24, and 36 to 48 hours after diagnosis and at discharge. All children in the study who had hearing loss at any time during the study had abnormal EOAE findings at the time of the first evaluation. Three of these children had persistent SNHL, which appeared to be cochlear in origin according to EOAE results. Nine of 13 additional children with abnormal EOAEs at their first evaluation had evidence of normal hearing within 48 hours. The hearing of all 13 children, who initially had absent EOAEs with a normal tympanogram, indicating a cochlear site of the lesion, returned to normal within 5 days of diagnosis.

The explanation for rapidly reversible SNHL early in the course of meningitis in about 10% of cases is not yet clear. Richardson et al. (52) postulated possible disruption of the endocochlear potential caused by bacterial toxins, inflammatory mediators, or low glucose levels in the CSF. The etiologic agent was identified as *N. meningitidis* in 74% of study patients, a marked contrast with earlier studies in which Hib predominated, which may partially explain the lower observed incidence of permanent SNHL in this study. Earlier studies confirmed that a child with meningitis with a normal ABR after the first few days of inpatient antibiotic therapy is unlikely to have SNHL later (51). A few patients with documented mild to moderate losses after discharge have shown some improvement over time, whereas more severe losses among some children have fluctuated for as long as 1 year after hospital discharge (51). Well-documented late progression of postmeningitic SNHL after years of stability has been reported in a few cases (51).

Pathophysiologic studies of meningitic involvement of the inner ear show that direct spread of infection from otitis media through labyrinthine windows to the perilymph and CSF is uncommon. A more likely route is penetration of bacteria and bacterial toxins through the cochlear aqueduct or internal auditory canal that gives rise to perineuritis or neuritis of the cochleovestibular nerve or to suppurative labyrinthitis. Other pathophysiologic mechanisms that lead to hearing loss may include serous or toxic labyrinthitis, thrombophlebitis or embolization of labyrinthine vessels, and hypoxia or anoxia of the eighth cranial nerve and central auditory pathways (53). Direct bacterial action on nervous tissue and the host's inflammatory response evoked by bacterial disintegration caused by antibiotics may be operative in producing postmeningitic sequelae (54). In animal studies, bacterial surface components, including endotoxin and cell wall constituents, produced symptoms and signs of meningitis in the absence of viable bacteria. Hib lipooligosaccharide is solely responsible for the induction of meningeal inflammation, brain edema, and elevated intracranial pressure (55). The rapid inflammatory response with inflammatory exudate observed among neonates and young children after the initiation of antibiotic therapy is not thought to be critical for containment of the infection and may actually be harmful.

At the molecular level, interleukin-1β and tumor necrosis factor from astroglia trigger an inflammatory response, which is inhibited in animal models by the administration of dexamethasone. Corticosteroids inhibit the activity of phospholipase with a consequent decrease in prostaglandin E, thromboxane, and leukotriene formation. In placebo-controlled human trials, administration of corticosteroid (dexamethasone) initially yielded promising results, including a decrease in indices of meningeal inflammation at 24 hours and fewer neurologic sequelae than observed among placebo-treated controls (56). The effectiveness of this regimen in decreasing the incidence of postmeningitic hearing loss has not been conclusively demonstrated. Results suggesting a beneficial effect were limited for the most part to cases of Hib meningitis, which is rapidly declining in importance. A study of 122 infants and children in Finland compared the efficacy of oral glycerol (an osmotic diuretic) with that of dexamethasone in preventing neurologic and auditory sequelae among meningitis survivors (57). Only 7% of glycerol-treated patients had sequelae compared with 19% of those receiving dexamethasone.

Temporal bone histopathologic findings for 41 patients who died of acute bacterial meningitis revealed suppurative labyrinthitis in 49% of specimens (58). Although cochlear involvement (most often the perilymphatic spaces) was documented in all cases, the vestibular labyrinth, principally the lateral semicircular canal, was affected only 50% of the time. In contrast, a pattern of eosinophilic staining in the absence of inflammatory cells, a probable pathologic correlate of serous labyrinthitis, affected primarily the vestibular components, including the superior (100%) and posterior (86%) semicircular canals. The cochlea was involved in only 40% of these specimens. Both the cochlear aqueduct and modiolus were documented as routes by which the infection accessed the inner ear; perivascular and perineural channels in the modiolus were most often involved. When modiolar spread occurred, neural damage preceded hair cell involvement; the converse was observed with aqueductal spread. Sensory and neural structures were found to be intact in most bones with suppurative and serous-type changes, a finding that suggested preventive intervention to mitigate SNHL may be feasible. Severe degeneration of spiral ganglion cells was found in 12% of temporal bones, a finding that confirmed this subset of patients would be less likely to benefit from cochlear implantation.

Ototoxic Drugs and Chemicals

Federal reporting requirements have helped identify a growing number of potentially ototoxic drugs and chem-

TABLE 3. *Drugs and chemicals with ototoxic potential*

Antibiotics	Loop diuretics
Streptomycin	Ethacrynic acid
Dihydrostreptomycin	Furosemide
Neomycin	Other drugs
Gentamycin	Cisplatin
Kanamycin	Quinine
Vancomycin	Chloroquine
Polymyxin B	Salicylates
Erythromycin	Hexadimethrine (Polybrene)
Chemicals	Nitrogen mustard
Carbon monoxide	Thalidomide
Mercury	
Gold	
Lead	
Arsenic	
Aniline dyes	

icals (see Chapter 35). Exposure to medications such as thalidomide early in pregnancy produces severe embryopathic effects, including external, middle, and inner ear deformities and SNHL. Other ototoxic drugs and chemicals are more damaging to the differentiating sensory end organs of the inner ear if exposure occurs later in pregnancy. Table 3 is a partial list of drugs and chemicals with ototoxic potential.

Aminoglycosides

Aminoglycosides, which are bactericidal, are administered parenterally to overcome poor absorption from the gastrointestinal tract. The serum half-life averages 2 hours in patients with normal renal function. These antibiotics are not metabolized in the body and are excreted almost entirely through glomerular filtration, so patients with impaired renal function may experience urinary concentrations approaching 100 times serum levels. Hemodialysis and peritoneal dialysis can effectively lower serum levels in these patients. Inner ear levels never rise above serum levels, even when renal function is compromised, and there is no evidence that tissue level in cochlear and vestibular tissues correlates with differential damage to various subcomponents (59). Aminoglycosides are transmitted into hair cells by means of an energy-dependent process that entails binding to the phospholipid phosphatidylinositol biphosphate. The binding affinity of a particular aminoglycoside appears to be related to its ototoxic potential. Exploring the mechanism of ototoxicity, Brownell et al. (60) found that very high concentrations of gentamicin do not damage outer hair cells unless the drug has been has been pretreated enzymatically. The existence of a cytotoxic gentamicin metabolite (gentatoxin) was confirmed by Schacht (59). Attempts to block the toxicity of gentatoxin initially centered on glutathione, which as an antioxidant protects isolated outer hair cells against cytotoxicity when exposed to activated gentamicin. Gentamicin also serves as a chelator to promote production of free radicals in the presence of iron salts. The efficacy of competitive, less toxic iron chelators (e.g., deferoxamine) in reducing the ototoxicity of gentamicin without impeding its antimicrobial properties is being explored.

In cases of aminoglycoside ototoxicity, histopathologic studies have confirmed injury to the stria vascularis, suprastrial spiral ligament, pericapillary tissues in the spiral prominence, outer sulcus, and Reissner's membrane. Proceeding from the basilar turn toward the apex, damage is initially confined to the inner row of outer hair cells. Eventual destruction of the remaining outer hair cells may occur, but inner hair cells are typically spared. Type I vestibular hair cells of the crista ampullaris generally sustain greater damage from streptomycin, kanamycin, and gentamicin than do type II cells; supporting cells are largely spared.

The range of toxicity of specific aminoglycosides varies across studies. Neomycin shows the greatest ototoxicity, whereas netilmicin and sisomicin demonstrate significantly less toxicity. Streptomycin, gentamicin, and tobramycin are primarily vestibulotoxic, whereas kanamycin and amikacin are principally cochleotoxic. Gentamicin has greater vestibulotoxicity than tobramycin, and the toxic effect is potentiated by high hematocrit, elevated creatinine clearance, criticality of illness, and duration of therapy beyond 10 days (61). Careful monitoring of peak serum levels (30 minutes after intravenous administration) and trough levels (immediately before the next intravenous dose) is an important step in preventing ototoxicity. Appropriate dosage adjustments must be made if a child's renal function is compromised. Coexisting factors thought to increase risk for aminoglycoside ototoxicity include preexisting hearing loss, concurrent noise exposure, age, duration of therapy, previous aminoglycoside use, nutritional status, and concomitant use of other ototoxic drugs, such as other aminoglycosides or loop diuretics (e.g., ethacrynic acid and furosemide). If an aminoglycoside is administered before a loop diuretic, the ototoxic risk is greater than if the order of administration were reversed.

Aminoglycosides can pass transplacentally from mother to fetus, but the degree of ototoxicity that results is unclear. Even among neonates, the risk to hearing and balance function posed by aminoglycoside administration has been a matter of debate. Finitzo-Hieber et al. (62) reported that aminoglycosides at appropriate dosage levels pose minimal ototoxic risk among children. Eviatar and Eviatar (63) longitudinally evaluated factors such as acquisition of head control and nystagmus induced by position change, perrotatory stimulation with a torsion swing, and caloric irrigation among infants who received aminoglycosides for neonatal sepsis. Vestibular abnormalities and delay in acquisition of head control were documented among about 10% of these children. Serial high-frequency (more than 12,000 Hz) audiometric screening and vestibular evaluation may provide early warning of impending damage.

Widespread use of aminoglycosides in China facilitated identification of a subset of families with a point mutation at 1555 A-G in the mitochondrial 12S ribosomal RNA who are exquisitely sensitive to the ototoxic effects even at presumably safe dosage levels (63a,63b). Another study found that 17% of unrelated, ethnically diverse U.S. patients and families with hearing loss after aminoglycoside exposure demonstrated the nucleotide 1555 A-G mitochondrial mutation (63c). Screening for this predisposing mutation may become the standard of care before institution of aminoglycoside therapy.

Loop Diuretics

Loop diuretics such as ethacrynic acid and furosemide have demonstrated ototoxic potential (incidence 0.7% with ethacrynic acid; 6.4% with furosemide), which is greatest when the diuretic is administered concurrently with "safe" levels of aminoglycosides (64). Considerable hair cell loss and changes in the stria vascularis have been found in animal studies. Histopathologic examination of temporal bones from animals treated with toxic levels of these drugs reveals changes in the stria vascularis and marked hair cell loss. Rybak et al. (65) postulated that furosemide and ethacrynic acid have different mechanisms of action on the cochlea. Because of the repeatedly documented synergy between the ototoxic effects of loop diuretics and aminoglycosides, the respective dosages of these medications should be carefully adjusted when they are administered concurrently. The order of administration should be adjusted to minimize risk.

Erythromycin

Bilateral SNHL, typically associated with tinnitus and vertigo, has been described among adults, particularly those with concomitant renal or hepatic failure, who received erythromycin doses of 2 g per day. Ototoxicity was most likely with doses greater than 63 mg/L. On the basis of animal studies, a transient effect on the stria vascularis has been postulated.

Salicylates

Reversible hearing loss and tinnitus have long been associated with high therapeutic doses of salicylates (levels exceeding 20 mg/dL). Salicylates in the perilymph promote a reduction in levels of transaminases and cochlear adenosine triphosphate and cochlear blood flow. A salicylate-mediated increase in the membrane conductance of outer hair cells has been postulated as responsible for alterations in cochlear function. Animal studies have linked salicylate toxicity with lower than normal perilymphatic prostaglandins and elevated leukotrienes, which might be ameliorated with corticosteroid therapy.

Vancomycin

Nephrotoxicity and ototoxicity are likely among patients whose vancomycin blood levels exceed 45 mg/L. Adults have experienced tinnitus at slightly lower serum levels. Matz (64) found that premature infants were more susceptible to vancomycin ototoxicity than term infants because of the increased half-life of the drug in these neonates.

Cisplatin

The antineoplastic agent cisplatin (cis-diaminedichloroplatinum) can produce both cochleotoxic and vestibulotoxic effects. Inter- and intrastrand cross linking of DNA are the mechanisms by which the drug exerts its clinically desirable cytotoxicity. Undesirable side effects include myelosuppression, neurotoxicity, and nephrotoxicity, but it is the attendant ototoxicity that effectively imposes dosage limits in clinical practice. Cisplatin-associated hearing loss usually begins in the 10,000 to 18,000 Hz range with progressive involvement of frequencies below 8,000 Hz if treatment at potentially ototoxic doses continues. Audiometric screening at 12,000 and 14,000 Hz can provide early evidence of ototoxicity. Cochlear pathophysiologic processes involve drug-mediated blockade of outer hair cell transduction channels with a concurrent decrease in adenylate cyclase. Histopathologic examination shows initial outer hair cell loss in the basal turn of the cochlea that usually is followed by gradual involvement of inner hair cells that proceeds from the base to the apex of the cochlea. Strial atrophy and collapse of Reissner's membrane have been observed.

Risk estimates for ototoxicity vary across audiometric frequencies. Dreschler et al. (66) examined thresholds in treated patients from 8,000 to 20,000 Hz for deterioration of 20 dB or more at one frequency, 15 dB at two frequencies, or 10 dB at four frequencies. They found that 46% to 83% of patients in various study groups demonstrated some degree of loss, principally at higher frequencies. Eighty percent of the losses were bilateral. Dosage levels exceeding 3 to 4 mg/kg of body weight entailed definite risk for ototoxicity. Cisplatin is widely used to manage solid tumors in children, and high-frequency hearing loss (40 dB or greater at 1,000 Hz and above) has been documented in about one half of all children treated with a standard therapeutic dose (60 to 100 mg/m^2 per course). Permanent bilateral high-frequency SNHL occurred among 88% of children receiving cisplatin doses greater than 450 mg/m^2. Cochlear damage, directly related to cumulative doses exceeding 279 mg/m^2, was inversely related to the child's age. Synergy has been demonstrated in animal studies between the oto-toxic effects of hazardous noise exposure (85 dB SPL or greater) and cisplatin. Although conclusive evidence of such a synergistic effect in humans is not yet available, prudence would dictate avoidance of exposure to potentially damaging sound levels (e.g., amplified music at high volume) during cisplatin therapy.

Quinine and Chloroquine

The antimalarial agents quinine and chloroquine phosphate, a synthetic quinoline derivative, have demonstrated ototoxic potential. Administration of quinine to expectant mothers has been associated with varying degrees of severe to profound hearing impairment among their infants. Maternal chloroquine administration during pregnancy has been linked to both retinopathy and hearing loss among infants. Both drugs appear to produce vasculitis and ischemia in the inner ear with related degenerative changes in the stria vascularis, organ of Corti, and neuronal elements.

Retinoids

Systemic administration of retinoids (e.g., isotretinoin) to a pregnant woman can be associated with spontaneous abortion or severe malformations, including CNS, cardiovascular, and respiratory anomalies; cleft lip; cleft palate; and external ear defects, which may include canal agenesis.

Anoxia or Hypoxia

Perinatal anoxia or hypoxia related to factors such as cord compression and neonatal seizures is statistically correlated with subsequent SNHL among affected infants. A clinical history that suggests perinatal anoxia or hypoxia might include meconium staining, primary apnea, resuscitation at birth, low Apgar scores at 1 and 5 minutes, postnatal apneic episodes, and prolonged postnatal ventilatory assistance. Histopathologic damage to the brainstem reticular formation and cochlear nuclei due to anoxia can include decreased cell volume and numbers in direct relation to the duration and severity of oxygen deprivation. Other potential causes of SNHL may play a role among these high-risk infants. Neonates with chronic hypoxemia related to persistent fetal circulation experience a 20% incidence of SNHL, three-fourths of which is in the moderate to severe range and one fourth of which is profound.

Hyperbilirubinemia

Kernicterus occurs when bilirubin crossing the blood-brain barrier is deposited in a neonate's basal ganglia, particularly the ventrocochlear nucleus, and produces neurologic sequelae, including SNHL, the site of the lesion being central rather than cochlear. Elevation of neonatal bilirubin levels can result from inadequate bilirubin conjugation, impaired albumin binding, or increased unconjugated bilirubin production. With the availability of Rh immunoglobulin, exchange transfusions and phototherapy have decreased the incidence of kernicterus detected at autopsy, but reversible ABR changes (absence of the wave IV–V complex) documented among about one third of neonates with bilirubin levels in the 15 to 25 mg/dL range suggest transient encephalopathy. About 50% or more of infants have neonatal jaundice, and approximately 6% experience serum bilirubin concentrations exceeding 12.9 mg/dL. Among infants with actual kernicterus, about half die, and survivors may have cerebral palsy, mental retardation, and hearing loss. Measurement of exhaled carbon monoxide levels can aid in ascertaining which infants with hemolysis-related hyperbilirubinemia need more aggressive preventive intervention. Heme oxygenase inhibitors (e.g., tin-mesoporphyrin), which can bind heme oxygenase more aggressively than heme itself, appear able to impede access of the natural substrate to the binding site with a resultant decrease in heme degradation and bilirubin production.

Prematurity and Term Low Birth Weight

Although known risk factors for SNHL, such as perinatal hypoxia, sepsis, and kernicterus, may coexist among premature and dysmature neonates, prematurity itself constitutes an important risk indicator for hearing loss. NICU outcome studies indicate that premature infants are approximately 20 times as likely to have severe hearing loss than term, normal-weight infants. About 2% of all infants with birth weights of 3 pounds (1.35 kg) or less have marked SNHL.

Ear and Head Trauma

Middle ear and inner ear trauma can be traced to such antecedent events as a slap in the ear, insertion of a foreign body (e.g., cotton swab) in the external canal, or skull trauma, including temporal bone fracture in some instances. An infant's foreshortened ear canal predisposes the child to transcanal injury. Linguistically immature children may not be able to report symptoms such as acute pain, hearing loss, tinnitus, or vertigo. Mild to moderate conductive hearing loss is the most common trauma-related audiometric finding, but intralabyrinthine injury can produce SNHL that initially affects the high frequencies in most cases. Substantial conductive impairment points to possible ossicular damage, and disruption of the labyrinthine membrane, including perilymphatic fistula, and may manifest itself as fluctuating or progressive SNHL. Minimal head trauma may cause fluctuation or progression of SNHL among children with certain inner ear anomalies, such as Mondini malformation and enlarged vestibular aqueduct.

Motor vehicle accidents, mishaps involving bicycles, skateboards, or roller skates, and falls are among the common causes of temporal bone fractures among children and adolescents. Temporal bone fractures have been reported to occur among 7% of children who need hospital care after a head injury; about 13% of these children sustain SNHL. In a study population of 324 children and adolescents with unilateral SNHL, 10.8% of losses were attributed to head trauma, which in 35% of cases had been sustained at or before 6 years of age (7).

Noise-induced Hearing Loss

Sounds of sufficient loudness and duration produce ear damage that causes temporary or permanent hearing loss, often accompanied by tinnitus (see Chapter 48). Irreversible inner ear damage from loud sounds is cumulative over time. Typical noise-induced hearing loss impairs discrimination of speech sounds, which can affect classroom performance. Exposure to potentially harmful noise sources at home, on farms, and in recreational environments has placed increasing numbers of unsuspecting children and adolescents at risk. Noise-induced hearing loss is entirely preventable except in rare cases of accidental exposure.

Regulations issued by the U.S. Department of Labor establish the boundary between acceptable and damaging noise in the workplace at 85 dB (A) for continuous exposure during a full workday. *A* refers to a type of filter in the sound level meter that can be used to measure both continuous loud noise, as produced by amplified music, and intermittent, short-duration noises with very loud peak components, such as gunfire or firecrackers.

Ear damage resulting from hazardous noise exposure is classified as either acoustic trauma or noise-induced hearing loss. The pattern of damage resulting from a specific episode of exposure to a particular sound source depends on the frequency content, intensity (loudness), duration, and scheduling (continuous or intermittent) of the exposure and the susceptibility of the involved ear. Intense sounds (more than 140 dB [A]) of short duration, such as gunfire or an explosion, can produce immediate, severe, and permanent hearing loss, which is called *acoustic trauma.* The direct mechanical trauma resulting from such an event can disrupt virtually any structure in the ear, from the tympanic membrane and ossicles to the organ of Corti. Moderate exposure to less intense but potentially damaging sounds may cause a temporary threshold shift (TTS). Additional exposure can cause permanent noise-induced hearing loss. Initial involvement typically is in the 3,000 to 6,000 Hz range with a characteristically notched audiometric configuration.

Outer hair cells are the inner ear structures most vulnerable to noise damage. Electron microscopic examination of these cells has documented disruption of intracellular organelles, including endoplasmic reticulum, lysosomes, nucleus, and mitochondria together with disorganization, fusion and loss of stereocilia. Degeneration of damaged hair cells may lead to eventual loss of auditory nerve fibers with resultant alterations in auditory areas of the CNS. The subtle histopathologic changes in the inner ear during a TTS may be limited to swelling of hair cells and underlying afferent nerve fiber terminals that is reversible during a rest period away from loud sounds. Suggested pathophysiologic mechanisms involved in TTS include changes in stereocilia rootlets with resultant alterations in cochlear micromechanics and vascular spasm and metabolic exhaustion.

Impulse noises of short duration, such as the discharge of a large-caliber rifle or shotgun, produce very high sound intensity (132 to 170 dB [A] during the initial acoustic pulse of a typical gun discharge). Sound levels produced by toy weapons measured at a distance of 50 cm show mean peak values of 143 to 153 dB (A), and firecrackers produce peak levels measured at 3 m of 125 to 156 dB. Less readily apparent are other potentially damaging environmental sound sources. Average sound levels in a discotheque approximate 95 dB (A), but rock concerts often produce exposure to amplified sound as loud as 105 to 115 dB (A), well above the discomfort level for most people and likely to elicit a TTS, often accompanied by tinnitus, among most exposed individuals.

Personal cassette players can produce sound levels in excess of 110 to 115 dB (A) at the ear, and a child may unwittingly compensate for a TTS by increasing the volume to even more hazardous levels. Studies of personal cassette player (PCP) use among children in the mideelementary school age group found that 80% of the children owned personal cassette players and 5% to 10% listened at potentially hazardous volume levels for extended periods (67–68). If a child experiences aural fullness, muffled hearing, or tinnitus after noise exposure, counseling regarding safe listening habits should be provided and followed by audiologic evaluation if symptoms persist.

CONCLUSIONS

Diagnostic and therapeutic advances, particularly improved infant screening techniques, development of conjugate vaccine, and the availability of better hearing aids and cochlear implants, have had considerable impact on the identification and management of SNHL among children. The remarkable decline in childhood meningitis that followed introduction of the conjugate Hib vaccine may be a harbinger of what can be expected from effective preventive intervention directed against such pathogens as the pneumococcus and CMV. Increased understanding of the important interplay between genetic factors, such as mitochondrial mutations, and nongenetic causes, such as aminoglycoside exposure, may further decrease the role of nongenetic causes in future cohorts of children with SNHL.

SUMMARY POINTS

- Persistent, bilateral congenital or early-onset hearing loss in the moderate to profound range (41 to 100 dB) distorts the speech perception of a developing child. Studies link persistent unilateral SNHL in the moderate to profound range with poor school performance.

- In developed countries, 1 to 2 per 1,000 school-aged children exhibit a bilateral SNHL of 50 dB or worse, including 0.5 to 1.0 per 1,000 whose bilateral losses exceed 75 dB, with lesser degrees of loss (hard of hearing versus deaf) being 5 to 10 times more common than severe-to-profound losses.

- Interest in universal newborn hearing screening has been sparked by the availability of reliable and cost effective-objective screening techniques involving EOAE and automated ABR measures.

- Comprehensive evaluation of a child with educationally significant hearing impairment is best accomplished by a team of specialists. Both history and physical examination should address subtle findings associated with hearing loss syndromes. Ophthalmologic evaluation is essential. A diligent search for the cause of SNHL may prove inconclusive in 30% to 40% of cases.

- Serial auditory thresholds in children may be influenced by intrinsic and extrinsic factors and may not include a true change in auditory sensitivity over time. Marked threshold deterioration (e.g., 15 dB) at one or more of the four middle test frequencies (500, 1,000, 2,000, and 4,000 Hz) without middle ear dysfunction should prompt careful reevaluation.

- The development of effective vaccines to prevent such common childhood disorders as rubella, measles, mumps, and Hib meningitis has affected the current mix of new diagnoses of SNHL among infants and children. Effective treatment regimens for congenital toxoplasmosis and syphilis also have had an impact.

- The synergistic relation between genetic mutations (e.g., 1555 A-G in the mitochondrial genome) and aminoglycoside ototoxicity holds promise for future preventive and therapeutic strategies. Pharmaceutical agents designed to rescue ears exposed to ototoxic drugs or noise are being tested.

- Rehabilitative advances such as cochlear implants and improved hearing aid technology have improved the prospects for children with marked SNHL.

REFERENCES

1. U.S. Department of Health and Human Services, Public Health Service. Healthy People 2000: National Health Promotion and Disease Prevention Objectives. Washington, DC: U.S. Government Printing Office, 1990.
2. Bess FH, Paradise JL. Universal screening for infant hearing impairment: not simple, not risk-free, not necessarily beneficial, and not presently justified. *Pediatrics* 1994;93:330–334.
3. Mochizuki T, Lemmink HH, Mariyama M, et al. Identification of mutations in the alpha 3 (III) and alpha 4 (IV) collagen genes in autosomal recessive Alport syndrome. *Nat Genet* 1994;8:77–81.
4. Deleted in proof.
5. Greenberg MT. Family stress and child competence: the effects of early intervention. *Am Ann Deaf* 1983;128:407–417.
6. Bess FH, Klee T, Culbertson JL. Identification, assessment and management of children with unilateral sensorineural hearing loss. *Ear Hear* 1986;7:43–51.
7. Brookhouser PE, Worthington DW, Kelly WJ. Unilateral hearing loss in children. *Laryngoscope* 1991;101:1264–1272.
8. Brookhouser PE. Incidence and prevalence. Presented at National Institutes of Health Consensus Development Conference on Early Identification of Hearing Impairment in Infants and Young Children; March 1–3, 1993; Bethesda, MD.
9. Davis A, Wood S. The epidemiology of childhood hearing impairment: factors relevant to planning of services. *Br J Audiol* 1992;26:77–90.
10. White KR, Maxon AB. Universal screening for infant hearing impairment: simple, beneficial, and presently justified. *Int J Pediatr Otorhinolaryngol* 1995;32:201–211.
11. National Institutes of Health Consens. Early Identification of Hearing Impairment in Infants and Young Children. Statement March 1–3; 1993; 11(1):1–24 Bethesda, MD.
12. Joint Committee on Infant Hearing. 1994 position statement. *ASHA* 1994;36:38–41.
13. Otolaryngology Clinical Trials Cooperative Group. Grant 1 U01 DCO 3209-01, NIH-NIDCD, 4/15/97–3/31/02.
14. Brookhouser PE, Worthington DW, Kelly WJ. Fluctuating and/or progressive sensorineural hearing loss in children. *Laryngoscope* 1994;104:958–964.
15. Davis LE, Johnson RT. Experimental viral infections of the inner ear, I: acute infections of the newborn hamster labyrinth. *Lab Invest* 1976;34:349–356.
15a. Stagno S, Pass RF, Alford CA. Perinatal infections and maldevelopment. *Birth Defects* 1981;17(1):31–50.
16. Adler SP. Cytomegalovirus transmission and child day care. *Adv Pediatr Infect Dis* 1992;7:109–102.
16a. Hagay ZJ, Biran G, Ornoy A, Reece EA. Congenital cytomegalovirus infection: a long-standing problem still seeking a solution. *Am J Obstet Gynecol* 1996;174(1):241–245.
17. Stagno S, Pass RF, Dworsky ME, et al. Congenital cytomegalovirus infection: the relative importance of primary and recurrent maternal infection. *N Engl J Med* 1982;306:945–949.
18. Parkman PD, Buescher RL, Artenstein MS. Recovery of rubella virus from army recruits. *Proc Soc Exp Biol Med* 1962;111:225–230.
19. Weller TH, Neva FA. Propagation in tissue culture of cytopathic agents from patients with rubella-like illness. *Proc Soc Exp Biol Med* 1962;3:215–225.
20. Gregg NM. Congenital cataract following German measles in the mother. *Ophthal Cos Aust* 1941;3:35–46.
21. Swan C, Tostevin AL, Moore B, et al. Congenital defects in infants following infectious diseases during pregnancy with special reference to relationship between German measles and cataracts, deaf-mutism, heart disease and microcephaly and to period of pregnancy in which occurrence of rubella is followed by congenital abnormalities. *Med J Aust* 1943;2:201–210.
22. Bordley JE, Brookhouser PE, Hardy WG. Prenatal rubella. *Acta Otolaryngol (Stockh)* 1968;66:1–9.
23. Brookhouser PE, Bordley JE. Congenital rubella deafness. *Arch Otolaryngol* 1973;98:252–257.
23a. Hsu HW, Grady GF, Macuire JH, Weiblen BJ, Hoff R. Newborn screening for congenital toxoplasma infection: 5 years experience in Massachusetts, USA. *Scan J Infect Dis* [Suppl] 1992;84:59–64.
24. Desmonts G, Couvreur J. Congenital toxoplasmosis: a prospective study of 378 pregnancies. *N Engl J Med* 1974;290:1110–1116.
25. Daffos F, Forestier F, Capella-Pavlovsky M, et al. Prenatal management of 746 pregnancies at risk for congenital toxoplasmosis. *N Engl J Med* 1988;318:271–275.
26. Decoster A, Darcy F, Caron A, Capron A. IgA antibodies against P30 as markers of congenital and acute toxoplasmosis. *Lancet* 1988;2:1104–1106.
27. Stepick-Biek P, Thulliez P, Araujo FG, Remington JS. IgA antibodies for diagnosis of acute congenital and acquired toxoplasmosis. *J Infect Dis* 1990;162:270–273.
28. Stein LK, Boyer KM. Progress in the prevention of hearing loss in infants. *Ear Hear* 1994;15:116–125.
29. Sung L, MacDonald NE. Syphilis: a pediatric perspective. *Pediatr Rev* 1998;19:17–22.
30. Sison CG, Ostrea EM, Reyes MP, Salari V. The resurgence of congenital syphilis: a cocaine-related problem. *J Pediatr* 1997;130:289–292.
31. Ray JG. Lues-lues: maternal and fetal considerations of syphilis. *Obstet Gynecol Surv* 1995;50:845–850.
32. McFarlin BL, Bottoms SF. Maternal syphilis: the next pregnancy. *Am J Perinatol* 1996;13:513–518.
33. Centers for Disease Control. 1993 sexually transmitted diseases treatment guidelines. *MMWR Morb Mortal Wkly Rep* 1993;42:40–44.
34. Birdsall HH, Baughn RE, Jenkins HA. The diagnostic dilemma of otosyphilis: a new western blot assay. *Arch Otolaryngol Head Neck Surg* 1990;116:617–621.
35. American Academy of Pediatrics Committee on Infectious Diseases and Committee on Fetus and Newborn. Guidelines for prevention of group B streptococcal (GBS) infection by chemoprophylaxis. *Pediatrics* 1992;90:775.
36. Centers for Disease Control and Prevention. Prevention of group B-streptococcal disease: a public health perspective. *Federal Register* 1994;59:64764–64773.
37. Johnson CD, Goodpasture EW. Investigation of etiology of mumps. *J Exp Med* 1934;59:1–19.
38. Enders JF. Cytopathology of virus infections (particular reference to tissue culture studies). *Ann Rev Microbiol* 1954;8:473–502.
39. Peebles TC. Propagation in tissue cultures of cytopathogenic agents from patients with measles. *Proc Soc Exp Biol Med* 1954;86:277–286.
39a. Department of Health and Human Services, Public Health Service. Epidemiology and prevention of vaccine-preventable disease—"The Pink Book," *Measles,* 4th ed., 1997:117–137.
40. Bordley JE, Kapur YP. Histopathologic changes in the temporal bone resulting from measles infection. *Arch Otolaryngol* 1977;103:162–168.
41. Lieberman JM, Greenberg DP, Ward JI. Prevention of bacterial meningitis: vaccines and chemoprophylaxis. *Infect Dis Clin North Am* 1990;4:703–729.
42. Crook WG, Clanton BR, Hodes HL. Hemophilus influenza meningitis: observations on the treatment of 110 cases. *Pediatrics* 1949;4:643–658.
43. Koch R, Carson MJ. Management of *Haemophilus influenzae,* type B meningitis: analysis of 128 cases. *J Pediatr* 1955;46:18–29.
44. Dodge PR. Sequelae of bacterial meningitis. *Pediatr Infect Dis J* 1986;5:618–620.
44a. Department of Health and Human Services, Public Health Service. Epidemiology and prevention of vaccine-preventable disease—"The Pink Book," *Haemophilus influenza type B,* 4th ed., 1997:102–115.
45. Robbins JB, Schneerson R, Anderson P, Smith DH. Prevention of systemic infections, especially meningitis, caused by *Haemophilus influenzae* type b: impact on public health and implications for other polysaccharide-based vaccines. *JAMA* 1996;276:1181–1185.
46. Schlech WF, Ward JI, Band JD, Hightower A, Fraser DW, Broome CV. Bacterial meningitis in the United States 1978 through 1981: the National Bacterial Meningitis Surveillance Study. *JAMA* 1985;253:1749–1754.
47. Baraff LJ, Lee SI, Schriger DL. Outcomes of bacterial meningitis in children: a meta-analysis. *Pediatr Infect Dis J* 1993;12:389–394.
48. Pikis A, Kavaliotis J, Tsikoulas J, Andrianopopoulos P, Venzon D, Manios S. Long-term sequelae of pneumococcal meningitis in children. *Clin Pediatr* 1996;35:72–78.

49. Kaplan SL. Commentary: prevention of hearing loss from meningitis. *Lancet* 1997;350:158–159.

50. Schuchat A, Robinson K, Wenger JD, et al. Bacterial meningitis in the United States in 1995: active surveillance team. *N Engl J Med* 1997; 337:970–976.

51. Brookhouser PE, Auslander MC, Meskan ME. The pattern and stability of post-meningitic hearing loss in children. *Laryngoscope* 1988; 98:940–948.

52. Richardson MP, Reid A, Tarlow MJ, Rudd PT. Hearing loss during bacterial meningitis. *Arch Dis Child* 1997;76:134–138.

53. Nadol JB Jr. Medical progress: hearing loss [review article]. *N Engl J Med* 1993;329:1092–1102.

54. Mustafa MM, Ramilo O, Saez-Llorens X, Olsen KD, Magness RR, McCracken GH. Cerebrospinal fluid prostaglandins, interleukin 1B and tumor necrosis factor in bacterial meningitis. *Am J Dis Child* 1990;144:833–887.

55. National Institutes of Health, The Developmental Biology, Genetics and Teratology Branch Report to the National Advisory Child Health and Human Development Council; January, 1994; Bethesda, MD.

56. Schaad UB, Lips U, Gnehm HE, Blumberg A, Heinzer I, Wedgwood J. Dexamethasone therapy for bacterial meningitis in children: Swiss Meningitis Study Group. *Lancet* 1993;342:457–461.

57. Kilpi T, Peltola H, Jauhiainen T, Kallio MJ. Oral glycerol and intravenous dexamethasone in preventing neurologic and audiologic sequelae of childhood bacterial meningitis: the Finnish study group. *Pediatr Infect Dis J* 1995;14:270–278.

58. Merchant SN, Gopen Q. A human temporal bone study of acute bacterial meningogenic labyrinthitis. *Am J Otol* 1996;17:375–385.

59. Schacht J. Molecular mechanisms of drug-induced hearing loss. *Hear Res* 1986;48:297–304.

60. Brownell WE, Bader CR, Bertrand D, et al. Evoked mechanical responses of isolated cochlear outer hair cells. *Science* 1996;227:194–196.

61. Fee WE. Aminoglycoside ototoxicity in the human. *Laryngoscope* 1980;90[Suppl 24]:1–19.

62. Finitzo-Hieber T, McCracken GH Jr, Brown KC. Prospective controlled evaluation of auditory function in neonates given netilmicin or amikacin. *J Pediatr* 1985;106:129–136.

63. Eviatar L, Eviatar A. Development of head control and vestibular responses in infants treated with aminoglycosides. *Dev Med Child Neurol* 1982;24:372–379.

63a. Prezant TR, Agapian JV, Bohlman C, et al. Mitochondrial ribosomal RNA mutation associated with both antibiotic-induced and nonsyndromic deafness. *Nat Genet* 1993;4:289–294.

63b. Fischel-Ghodsian N, Prezant TR, Xiangdong B, Oztas S. Mitochondrial ribosomal RNA in a patient with sporadic aminoglycoside ototoxicity. *Am J Otolaryng* 1993;14(6):399–403.

63c. Fischel-Ghodsian N, Prezant TR, Chaltrow WE, et al. Mitochondrial gene mutation is a significant predisposing factor in aminoglycoside ototoxicity. *Am J Otolaryngol* 1997;18(3):173–178.

64. Matz GJ. Clinical perspectives on ototoxic drugs. *Ann Otol Rhinol Laryngol* 1990;99:39–41.

65. Rybak LP, Whitworth C, Morris C. Effect of ebelsen on cisplatin ototoxicity. Proceedings of the Association for Research in Otolaryngology, St. Petersburg, Florida; February 1996:31 (abstr).

66. Dreschler WA, Hulst RJAM, Tange RA. The role of high-frequency audiometry in early detection of ototoxicity. *Audiology* 1985;24:387–395.

67. Clark WW. Noise exposure and hearing loss from leisure activities. NIH Consensus Development Conference, Jan 22–24, 1990, [abst] 55–58.

68. Axelsson A. Noise exposure in adolescents and young adults. NIH Consensus Development Conference, Jan 22–24, 1990, [abst] 77–82.

The Ear: Comprehensive Otology,
edited by R. F. Canalis and P. R. Lambert.
Lippincott Williams & Wilkins, Philadelphia © 2000.

CHAPTER 30

Genetic Hearing Impairment in Children

Gary D. Josephson and Kenneth M. Grundfast

genetics the science concerned with the chemical and physical nature of genes and the mechanism by which they control the development and maintenance of the organism.
—*Dorland's Illustrated Medical Dictionary* (1)

Childhood hearing impairment can be either congenital, meaning present at birth, or noncongenital, often referred to as acquired. Not long ago, neonatal sepsis, meningitis, mumps, and administration of ototoxic medications were the leading causes of childhood acquired hearing loss. However, with improved neonatal care, close monitoring of peak and trough levels when administering ototoxic agents to infants, and the advent of the measles-mumps-rubella vaccine, the relative proportion of childhood hearing loss that is acquired has diminished while the relative incidence of hereditary hearing loss has increased.

   G. D. Josephson: Department of Otolaryngology and Pediatrics, University of Miami; Division of Pediatric Otolaryngology–Head and Neck Surgery, University of Miami, Jacksonville Hospital, Miami, Florida 33136
   K. M. Grundfast: Department of Otolaryngology–Head and Neck Surgery, Georgetown University School of Medicine, Washington, D.C. 20007

The notion that hereditary factors can cause human biologic disease has long been accepted. Advances in molecular genetics have enabled scientists to study and understand the human genome. As a result of gene mapping, the genetic cause of some disorders, including various types of hearing loss, have been found even though the precise biologic mechanisms that cause the genetic hearing loss are not known (2). Identifying the defective genes in diseases such as cystic fibrosis (3), von Recklinghausen's neurofibromatosis (4), and Duchenne's muscular dystrophy (5) was the first step toward understanding the fundamental aspects of these diseases. With information derived from gene mapping, researchers have the possibility to develop new methods of treatment, prevention, or reversal of genetic disorders. Applying these principles of understanding human genetic disease to inherited syndromes involving deafness offers a greater understanding of the cause of genetic hearing loss. This had been applied to several inherited syndromes involving hearing loss for which successful mapping and identification has been achieved (2). Scientific investigators now are attempting to isolate, identify, and locate genes that cause hereditary hearing loss.

Practicing otolaryngologists can play a role in the identification and further study of hereditary hearing loss. They detect and evaluate head and neck dysmorphology, even milder forms, that suggest many genetic disorders. Identifying these chromosomal abnormalities in persons with otolaryngologic disorders will further enhance our understanding, prompt additional information about head and neck embryogenesis and development, and help identify other genetic disorders and their gene locations (6). An otolaryngologist who might be consulted about an infant who is deaf or has a severe hearing loss can detect subtle dysmorphic features and recognize that the infant may have a syndrome. An otolaryngologist who is an astute diagnostician can be the physician who first raises suspicion that an infant's hearing loss may represent one component of a constellation of abnormalities recognizable as a syndrome. Of course, not all syndromes are the result of a single gene defect or multiple gene defects. For example, Goldenhar's syndrome, a common cause of childhood unilateral conductive hearing loss, has sporadic inheritance, meaning that this syndrome is probably not caused by a single gene abnormality.

RECOGNIZING HEREDITARY CAUSES OF HEARING LOSS

To provide quality care of patients with ear and hearing disorders, physicians need to have a basic understanding of relevant aspects of genetics and keep in mind the possibility that any observed condition might have a hereditary cause. Making the diagnosis of hereditary hearing loss depends mostly on an accurate, detailed family history and the detection at physical examination of subtle abnormalities that can reveal the patient has an inherited syndrome. When the only phenotypic expression of a gene defect is hearing loss, the disorder is called *nonsyndromic hereditary hearing loss*. When the gene defect that causes hearing loss also causes other phenotypic abnormalities recognizable as a syndrome, the disorder is known as *syndromic hereditary hearing loss*. Even though the genes for many types of nonsyndromic and syndromic hearing loss have been identified and cloned, there is no readily available method for determining the presence or absence of a specific gene defect and there is no gene test panel for screening patients for the many different kinds of genetic hearing loss. Therefore it is helpful to have a working knowledge of how genes that cause hearing loss are expressed and how these genes are being located and cloned.

Gene Penetrance versus Gene Expression

Many clinicians confuse *gene penetrance* with *gene expression*. *Penetrance* is the term used to state whether there is identifiable evidence that a gene has been expressed in the patient being examined. If a person has in his or her genome a particular gene but there is no evidence that the gene has been expressed, the gene is said to be *nonpenetrant* in that person. However, if there is any evidence of gene expression, the gene is described as being *penetrant* in the person. Penetrance is an all-or-none phenomenon; either a gene is penetrant or it is not penetrant. The gene for otosclerosis is autosomal dominant with approximately 50% penetrance. This means that a child has the 50% chance typical of autosomal dominant inheritance of receiving the gene for otosclerosis from one parent. Even if the child has inherited the gene from one parent, the child has a 50% chance of having the stapes fixation characteristic of otosclerosis, because the gene for otosclerosis is expressed only 50% of the time when it is present in a person's genome.

Unlike penetrance, gene expression is not an all-or-none phenomenon. The term *expression* describes the phenotypic manifestation of the gene effect. Some genes can be fully expressed, so a person who has the gene manifests all characteristics related to the effect of the gene. Many genes that cause hearing loss are said to have highly variable expression. This means that one person with the gene may have many identifiable characteristics whereas another with the same gene defect may manifest few of the characteristic abnormalities. For example, Waardenburg's syndrome is 95% penetrant with highly variable gene expression. This means that 95% of persons with the gene for Waardenburg's syndrome manifest at least some characteristic traits, although the abnormalities may be very subtle and almost imperceptible. One patient may have a white forelock, one blue eye and one brown eye with an abnormally wide space (dystopia canthorum) between the eyes, and bilateral profound sensorineural hearing loss (SNHL). This deaf patient would be described as having high or severe gene expression. A sibling or parent of this patient with Waardenburg's syndrome might have a much milder type of gene expression with normal hair and eye color and only unilateral moderate SNHL.

Finding the Genes That Cause Hearing Loss

The method most commonly used to locate genes that cause hereditary hearing loss is called *linkage analysis*. In this method, linkage is determined by means of assessing whether a genetic marker and a putative disease locus do or do not segregate independently after meiotic crossover. Analysis of coinheritance of the marker and disease trait makes possible determination of the physical proximity of linkage to each other. The statistical probability of linkage is expressed in terms of a logarithm of odds (LOD) score. The more frequently two markers are seen to cosegregate, the higher is the LOD score. Two markers are considered to be linked with a confidence level of 95% when the LOD score reaches 3.0, which means the odds in favor of linkage are 1,000 to 1.

The feasibility of using linkage analysis to locate hearing loss genes depends on the fact that many parts of the human genome are *polymorphic*, meaning that the DNA sequences are not the same for all individuals but may be similar among family members. The greater the polymorphism of a genetic marker being used in linkage analysis, the more likely it is that an individual will be heterozygous for the marker being followed relative to the hearing loss gene defect. To find genes through linkage analysis, investigators need to identify large families with a relatively clear pattern of transmission. The more severe the deafness in a family, the more difficult it can be to use the family for linkage analysis. This unusual phenomenon can be explained by the relatively frequent occurrence of marriages between two deaf persons. The affected spouses in these marriages are likely to have more than one gene causing the deafness, and this makes linkage analysis difficult or impossible. A way to circumvent this problem is to study large families who live in isolated areas where the gene pool of the entire population has been relatively stable for decades or centuries. Scientific investigators seeking to map genes for nonsyndromic hereditary hearing loss have searched the world looking for isolated geographic areas where there are large families that include multiple deaf persons. In 1992, the gene for an autosomal dominant from of nonsyndromic hearing loss was mapped to 5q31 in a large family living in Costa Rica, to the 1p32 locus in an extended family in Indonesia, and to 13q12 in a family in France (7).

Genes That Have Been Located

During the past decade, the genes that cause approximately 30 different kinds of syndromic hereditary hearing loss have been identified. Nonsyndromic forms of hereditary hearing loss are collectively referred to as DFN for the X-linked forms, DFNA for the autosomal dominant forms, and DFNB for the autosomal recessive forms. The autosomal recessive forms of hereditary hearing loss usually are the most severe and constitute most instances of congenital profound deafness. In contrast, the most common mode of inheritance of delayed onset (postlingual) hereditary hearing loss is autosomal dominant or maternally inherited and caused by mutations within mitochondrial DNA. The genes have been mapped for 20 DFNB, 14 DFNA, and 4 DFN loci. However, identification of these loci does not explain the pattern of inheritance for all of the families studied, suggesting that there remain a large number of unidentified loci that must be involved with isolated forms of hereditary hearing loss.

Applying Gene Identification to Patient Care

As more genes for nonsyndromic hereditary hearing loss are identified, it will become possible to correlate the findings in each clinical case with a gene defect that is likely to be causing the hearing loss in the patient. That is, once a gene for a particular type of hereditary hearing loss is identified, patients with a specific gene defect can be tentatively diagnosed if the patient has an audiometric pattern, time of onset of the hearing loss, and progression of hearing loss similar to those of persons known to have the gene defect that has been identified.

Two genes recently identified are likely to be the cause of many cases of nonsyndromic hereditary deafness. The CX26 gene, which contains a single coding exon, making the search for mutations easy, has been shown to account for as many as 50% of cases of prelingual autosomal recessive hearing loss. The discovery that mutations in the CX26 gene account for a huge proportion of isolated forms of deafness is helpful in genetic counseling because a genetic cause of deafness can be ruled in or out quickly in families with a single affected child. The 12S ribosomal RNA gene A1555G has been shown to be the cause of a unique form of deafness introduced during treatment with aminoglycosides (8). Discovery of a mutation in the A1555G gene probably means that a person is susceptible to hearing loss with administration of an aminoglycoside. The knowledge that has been gained about genetic causes of hearing loss has not resulted in development of any new therapies or cures for hereditary hearing loss.

HISTORICAL PERSPECTIVE

In the mid-nineteenth century, the work of two investigators, Wilheim Kramer and William Wilde, helped to distinguish otology as a separate entity in clinical medicine. Although Kramer and Wilde were influential in gaining acceptance for the field of otology, they both had very different views about heredity as a cause of hearing loss. Kramer did not believe genetics played a role in hearing loss; Wilde identified pedigrees and strongly supported the idea that hereditary transmission could be the cause of hearing loss among some persons. Because he further substantiated his hypothesis with the Irish census of 1857, Wilde is acknowledged as the first otologist to recognize that heredity is a cause of hearing loss in humans.

Despite Wilde's early observations, the notion that some hearing loss can be inherited was not widely accepted until 1882, when Adam Politzer published his observations on hereditary hearing loss. Politzer's assertion that hearing loss can be inherited was based largely on the report by Hartmann of his work at the Berlin School for the Deaf. Today we recognize that approximately 50% of congenital hearing loss is genetic and that more than 200 known syndromes include hearing loss (9–11).

INCIDENCE AND PREVALENCE

About half of cases of childhood hearing loss are believed to be inherited (12,13). The prevalence has been calculated at approximately 1 per 2,000 population (14). Two thirds of cases of hereditary hearing loss are nonsyndromic and have no recognizable associated features. One third of cases have recognizable characteristics and are considered part of syndromic hearing loss. Hereditary deafness may be caused by a single gene defect or by interaction of multiple genes. The most common mode of inheritance, accounting for 60% to 70% of cases of genetic hearing loss is autosomal recessive. Twenty to twenty-five percent of cases are autosomal dominant. Two percent to three percent of cases are X-linked

TABLE 1. *Types of genetic deafness*

Type of genetic deafness	Percentage of population
Autosomal recessive	60–70
Autosomal dominant	20–25
X-linked recessive	2–3
Mitochondrial	<1
Multifactorial	<1

recessive. Mitochondrial inheritance and multifactorial cases make up the remaining 1% of cases (Table 1).

INHERITANCE PATTERNS

The three most common inheritance patterns are described and shown in Figure 1.

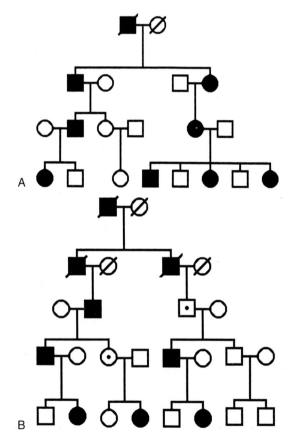

FIG. 1. A: Pedigree pattern shows transmission of autosomal dominant trait. The autosomal dominant trait is transmitted from affected parent to offspring, who have 50% probability of inheriting the disease allele. All carriers of the mutant gene express the disease trait, indicating complete penetrance of the mutant allele. **B:** Pedigree pattern shows transmission of autosomal dominant trait with incomplete penetrance. Not all carriers of the mutant gene are affected, indicating incomplete penetrance of the mutant allele. (From Lalwani AK, Lynch E, Mhatre AN. Molecular genetics: a brief overview. In: Lalwani AK, Grundfast KG, eds. *Pediatric otology and neurotology*. Philadelphia: Lippincott–Raven, 1998, with permission.)

Autosomal Dominant

Autosomal dominant inheritance is the ability of an allele to be expressed whether a single or pair of alleles is present. It is autosomal because the allele is on one of the 23 autosomes and is not encoded on the X or Y sex chromosome. It is dominant because the presence of a single allele reveals phenotypic expression. When a person has an abnormal gene, 50% of the offspring are affected. A vertical inheritance pattern can be clearly recognized in analysis of a family pedigree.

Autosomal Recessive

In an autosomal recessive disorder, the gene is not on the X or Y sex chromosome, and the gene expression of phenotype is seen only if there are two identical genes on the chromosome—one from each parent. In the case of hereditary hearing loss, neither parent may have hearing loss, but both parents carry the gene for the hearing loss and thus each passes the gene along. Subsequent offspring may have the impairment, so genetic recognition and counseling are important. Twenty-five percent of offspring of an affected individual inherit the disorder. The inheritance pattern is horizontal, meaning persons from prior generations may not be affected, but siblings or relatives in the same generation may have the trait.

X-linked

X-linked inheritance means the gene causing the disorder is located on the X chromosome. Most disorders on the X chromosome are recessive. There have to be two identical genes for expression of impairment. However, in male offspring, because the genetic makeup is XY, the presence of a single abnormal allele on the X chromosome is expressed. Female offspring must have a pair of alleles for expression of the disorder. A single allele encodes a woman as a carrier. Although less common, an X-linked dominant inheritance pattern is different because even in a female offspring, a single gene that encodes the impairment is expressed. If a woman has an X-linked dominant hearing loss, she experiences the hearing loss, and both her sons and daughters have a 50% chance of inheriting the disorder.

PATIENT EVALUATION

History

In obtaining the history from a patient or the parent of a patient who may have hereditary hearing loss, the clinician should focus on specific areas. A good first question is, Do you have any family members younger than 30 years who have a hearing loss or wear a hearing aid? Additional questions should be carefully prepared to elicit information that may lead to the diagnosis of nonsyndromic or syndromic hereditary hearing loss (Table 2). It is important to remember that each member of a family with a hereditary syndromic disorder does not

TABLE 2. *History questions suggestive of hereditary hearing impairment*

1. Have any family members been diagnosed with hearing impairment at birth or before 30 years of age?
2. Has any family member needed a hearing aid before the age of 30 years?
3. Do any family members have pigmentary abnormalities such as prematurely gray hair, white forelock, eyes of different colors, eyes spaced widely apart, broad-based nasal dorsum, hypopigmented areas of skin (Waardenburg's syndrome)?
4. Do any family members have hematuria, proteinuria, or kidney disorders (branchiootorenal syndrome, Alport's syndrome)?
5. Have any family members experienced blindness (Usher's syndrome)?
6. Are there any syncopal episodes or cardiac arrythmias (Jervell and Lange-Nielsen syndrome)?

TABLE 3. *Physical examination of children with hereditary hearing impairment*

Ears: shape and location of pinnae, size of external auditory canals, appearance of tympanic membrane, shape of malleus, presence of preauricular pits or tags
Eyes: eyebrow confluence, distance between the eyes, color of irides, extraocular movement, fundus, retinal pigmentation
Face: shape, symmetry
Skin: texture, pigmentation
Extremities: shape of fingers and toes, carrying angle of arms

TABLE 4. *Syndrome diagnosis scoring system*

Finding	A	B	C	D	G	J	P	S	T	U	W	X
Prematurely gray hair, white forelock											2	
Branchial cleft cyst		2										
Unilateral mandibular hypoplasia					3							
Bilateral mandibular hypoplasia									1		1	
Macrostomia					1				1			
Goiter (large thyroid)							4					
Pigmentary changes, vitiligo, depigmentation											1	
Skeletal abnormalities, enlargement of ankles, knees, wrists								3				
Pain or still joints								1				
Vertebral dysplasia					2							
ECG abnormalities, prolonged QT, interval fainting spells						4						
Stapes surgery, perilymph gusher												4
Chronic nephritis or renal insufficiency	1											
Hematuria	3											
Renal dysplasia or abnormally shaped kidneys	2	2										
Downward-sloping palpebral fissures									2			
Stapes fixation					1				1			2
Marfanoid habitus								1				
Mental retardation										1		
SNHL without findings listed above			1	1								
Congenital SNHL		1	4			1	1	1		2	1	
Mixed hearing loss		1							1	1		1
Congenital hearing loss		1			1				1	1		1
Progressive hearing loss	1			4								
Vestibular hypofunction										1	1	1
Preauricular pits		2			1							
Deformed external ear, microtia		1			1				3			
Atretic canal					1				1			
Retinitis pigmentosa										3		
Lenticonus, splenophakia, cortical cataracts	1							1				
Widely spaced medial canthorum, dystopia canthorum											1	
Confluent eyebrows (synophrys)											1	
Heterochromia											1	
Congenital, progressive myopia								2				
Retinal detachment								1				
Glaucoma, cataracts	1							1				
Coloboma					1					2		
Lateral cilia deficient to coloboma										1		
Flat midface, broad nasal root									1	1	1	
Unilateral facial paralysis					1							
Cleft lip or palate, high arch									1	1	1	
Patient's total score												

A, Alport's; *B*, branchiootorenal; *C*, dominant congenital; *D*, autosomal dominant–nonsyndromic; *G*, Goldenhar's; *J*, Jervell and Lange-Nielsen; *P*, Pendreds, *S*, Stickler, *T*, Treacher Collins; *U*, Usher's; *W*, Waardenburg's; *X*, X-linked mixed hearing loss with stapes gusher.
SNHL, sensorineural hearing loss.

have to have hearing loss. For example, the uncle of a child who is born deaf might have different-colored eyes. This suggests Waardenburg's syndrome, but the uncle may not be deaf, because the heterochromia irides might be the only manifestation of gene expression in the uncle, who has the autosomal dominant gene.

It also is important to remember that some components of syndromes that include hearing loss may not be present at birth or in early childhood. For example, developmental delay can be part of a syndrome, and this only becomes manifest over time. Loss of vision is a component of Usher's syndrome, but a person with this syndrome might be born with normal vision, so diagnosis of the autosomal recessive syndrome does not become apparent until after the loss of vision is reported or detected during a comprehensive evaluation.

Physical Examination

A comprehensive physical examination may identify even subtle findings that may lead to the diagnosis of hereditary hearing loss. The examination should not be limited to the head and neck. Depigmented areas of skin on the torso or extremities suggest Waardenburg's syndrome, and abnormalities of the hair or skin help to diagnose ectodermal dysplasia. An astute clinician performing an extensive examination in an orderly manner can identify abnormal findings that may lead to a diagnosis previously unrecognized (Tables 3, 4). To use Table 4, circle numerical values next to the findings present in the patient. The total sum is tallied at the bottom of each column. The column with the highest total numerical value predicts the likelihood of the patient having that particular syndrome.

TYPES OF HEREDITARY HEARING LOSS

More than 200 syndromes that include hearing loss have been described (15). The following are some of the more commonly recognized syndromes and their typical recognizable features.

Goldenhar's Syndrome

Goldenhar's syndrome, sometimes called *hemifacial microsomy* or *facioauriculovertebral dysplasia,* is a relatively common cause of congenital unilateral conductive hearing loss. Although there have been reports of autosomal dominant transmission of Goldenhar's syndrome, this

TABLE 5. *Typical features of Goldenhar's syndrome*

Facial asymmetry with unilateral mandibular
  underdevelopment
Preauricular skin tags
Microtia or abnormalities of the pinnae
Conductive hearing loss
Cervical vertebral dysplasia
Coloboma
Epibulbar dermoids

TABLE 6. *Typical features of Apert's syndrome*

Syndactyly
Stapes fixation causing flat conductive hearing loss
Craniofacial dysostosis
Proptosis
Hypoplastic maxilla
Saddle nose deformity
High arched palate
Frontal prominence
Exophthalmos
Spina bifida
Patent cochlear aqueduct

disorder usually is sporadic in origin, meaning there is no discernible mode of gene transmission in most cases (16). The incidence has been reported to range from 1 in 5,600 (17) to 1 in 26,500 (18) in the general population. The male to female ratio is 3:2. The ratio of right ear to left ear involvement also is 3:2. Diagnostic criteria for Goldenhar's syndrome include the presence but not necessarily all of the features listed in Table 5. Extreme variability of expression is possible (see Fig. 1). When a family member is affected, genetic inheritance is highly probable; however, multifactorial causes, including intrauterine insult, also are likely.

Apert's Syndrome

Apert's syndrome occurs in about 1 in 150,00 live births (19). It is autosomal dominant; however, the gene location has not been identified. At physical examination, the typical finding of syndactyly with one or more of the features listed in Table 6 makes the diagnosis clear (Figs. 2, 3).

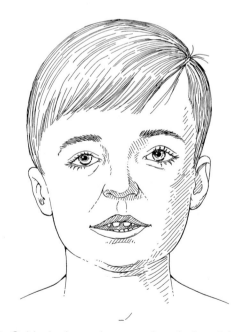

FIG. 2. Goldenhar's syndrome oculoauriculovertebral spectrum. Face is asymmetric, and hypoplasia of the mandible is present. (From Grundfast KG, Toriello H. Syndromic hereditary hearing impairment. In: Lalwani AK, Grundfast KG, eds. *Pediatric otology and neurotology.* Philadelphia: Lippincott–Raven, 1998, with permission.)

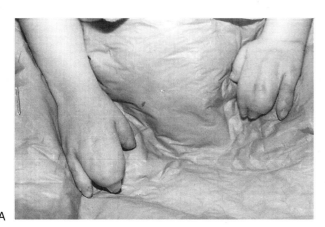
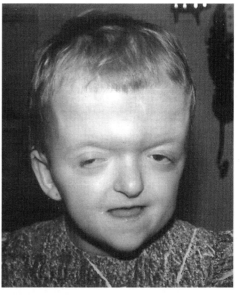

A
B

FIG. 3. A: Apert's syndrome has the additional feature of syndactyly. **B:** Apert's and Crouzon's syndromes both are characterized by craniosynostosis, hypertelorism, maxillary hypoplasia, and mandibular prognathism. (From Manaligod JM, Smith RJH. The syndromal child. In: Bailey BJ, ed. *Head & neck surgery–otolaryngology,* 2nd ed. Philadelphia: Lippincott–Raven, 1998, with permission.)

Crouzon's Syndrome

Crouzon's syndrome, also known as *craniofacial dysostosis,* is a congenital disorder that occurs among 15 to 16 per 1 million live births. The gene has been identified at the 10q locus of the chromosome (20). Several typical features may be present (Table 7), including a conductive or mixed hearing loss in one third of cases.

Treacher Collins Syndrome

Treacher Collins syndrome is an autosomal dominant disorder caused by a gene that has been found to be mapped to chromosome 5q31–34 (21); however, the syndrome is often a result of a spontaneous mutation, and the parents are not affected. Typical features are listed in Table 8 (Fig. 4).

Usher's Syndrome

Described by Charles Usher in 1914, Usher's syndrome is an autosomal recessive disease in which the patient has SNHL and retinitis pigmentosa (22). There are four types of Usher's syndrome; each has been identified on a different gene locus with a variable constellation of symptoms (Table 9). Electroretinography and electronystagmography may be helpful in establishing the diagnosis.

Pendred's Syndrome

Pendred's syndrome is an autosomal recessive disorder first described by Pendred in 1896. Profound SNHL and nontoxic goiter are the usual findings. About 50% of affected individuals have normal thyroid function, and 50% have hypothyroidism (23); therefore thyroid function tests are not always useful in making a diagnosis. The perchlorate test, which demonstrates a defect in the

TABLE 7. *Typical features of Crouzon's syndrome*

Cranial synostosis
Exophthalmos with divergent squint
Parrot-beaked nose
Short upper lip
Mandibular prognathism
Small maxilla
Hypertelorism
Premature closure of suture lines with resultant mental
   retardation

TABLE 8. *Typical features of Treacher Collins syndrome*

Antimongoloid palpebral fissures with notched lower lids
Malformation of ossicles with the stapes usually spared
Auricular deformities
Canal atresia
Mandibular and malar hypoplasia
Cleft lip and palate
Fish mouth
Normal intelligence

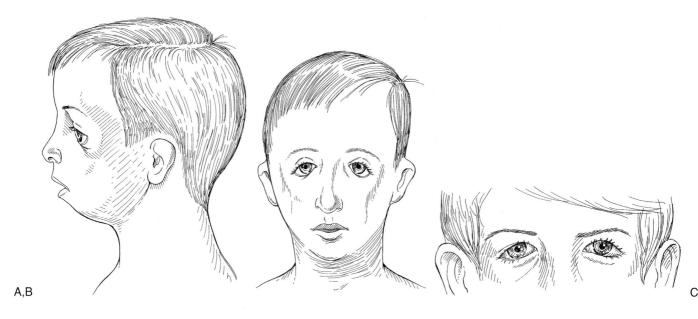

A,B

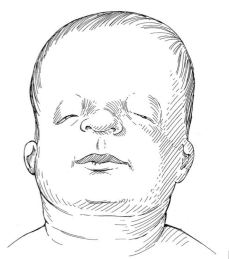

C

D

FIG. 4. Treacher Collins syndrome (mandibulofacial dysostosis). Patient has antimongoloid, down-sloping palpebral fissures, constricted midface, cup-shaped pinnae. **A:** Lateral view. **B:** Frontal view. **C:** Subtle antimongoloid slant of the eyes of a child with mild Treacher Collins syndrome. **D:** Infant with Treacher Collins syndrome. **E:** Mother of a child severely affected with Treacher Collins syndrome. Subtle findings of the autosomal dominant syndrome are present. Gene expression in this woman consists only of mild sensorineural hearing loss and antimongoloid, down-sloping palpebral fissures. **F:** Close-up view of subtle, down-sloping palpebral fissures. (From Grundfast KG, Toriello H. Syndromic hereditary hearing impairment. In: Lalwani AK, Grundfast KG, eds. *Pediatric otology and neurotology*. Philadelphia: Lippincott–Raven, 1998, with permission.)

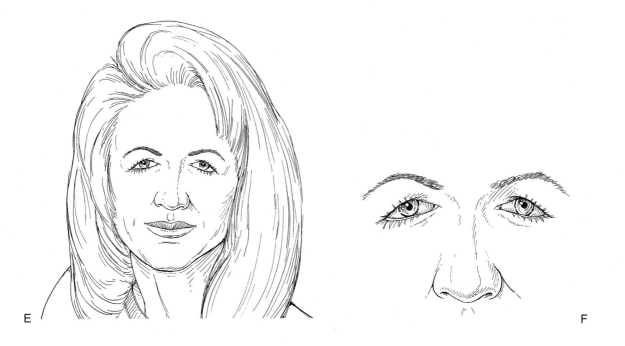

E

F

TABLE 9. *Four types of Usher's syndrome*

Type	Gene location	Hearing loss	Vestibular response
Type 1		Profound congenital	Absent
1A	14q		
1B	11q13		
1C	11p13		
Type 2	1q41	Moderate to severe congenital	Normal or decreased
Type 3	3q	Progressive	Absent
Type 4	X linked	Moderate to severe congenital	Normal or decreased

TABLE 11. *Different types of Alport's syndrome*

Type	Heredity	End-stage renal disease	Hearing loss
Type I	Autosomal dominant	Juvenile	Yes
Type II	X linked	Juvenile	Yes
Type III	X linked	Adult	Yes
Type IV	X linked	Adult	No
Type V	Autosomal dominant	Adult	Yes
Type VI	Autosomal dominant	Juvenile	Yes

organic binding of iodine, is diagnostic. An association between Pendred's syndrome and the Mondini inner ear deformity has been recognized, but the frequency of this association has not been clearly defined. The gene for Pendred's syndrome has been tentatively located at chromosome 8q24 (24).

Jervell and Lange-Nielsen Syndrome

Jervell and Lange-Nielsen syndrome is an autosomal recessive syndrome of congenital profound SNHL and the electrocardiographic abnormality of prolonged QT interval; it has been mapped to chromosome 11 (25). This disorder is characterized by repeated episodes of syncope and sudden lapses of consciousness beginning at 3 to 5 years of age. It once was believed that this syndrome may have been the cause of some of the unexplained deaths among children residing in schools for the deaf. At one time, half of affected individuals with Jervell and Lange-Nielsen syndrome died by 15 years of age. With the advent of β-adrenergic blocking agents, fatal arrhythmias are better controlled, and the mortality rate has decreased to less than 6% (26,27).

Stickler Syndrome

Stickler syndrome is an autosomal dominant disorder that may include hearing loss of the conductive (28), sensorineural (29), or mixed type. Typical features include those listed in Table 10. Gene mapping has identified the locus as 12q and 6p.

TABLE 10. *Typical features of Stickler syndrome*

Marfanoid habitus
Juvenile-onset arthritis
Severe myopia
Retinal detachment
Cataracts
Prominent ankle, knee, and wrist joints
Pierre Robin sequence
Midfacial hypoplasia

Alport's Syndrome

Alport's syndrome includes progressive glomerulonephritis and SNHL. The six types of Alport's syndrome have been identified as autosomal dominant or X-linked dominant in inheritance pattern (Table 11). A diagnosis of Alport's syndrome can be confirmed with the presence of three of the following criteria (30):

1. Family history of hematuria with or without renal failure
2. Electron microscopic evidence of glomerulonephritis at renal biopsy
3. Characteristic ophthalmologic signs
4. High-frequency SNHL, which usually begins during childhood and is progressive

Ocular anomalies may be present in types I, II, and VI Alport's syndrome. Macrothrombocytopenia may be found in type V.

Waardenburg's Syndrome

Waardenburg's syndrome is an autosomal dominant syndrome that has almost complete penetrance and variable expressivity. The syndrome has been subdivided into two types differentiated on the basis of presence of dystopia canthorum (lateral displacement of the medial canthi) as in type I, or absence of dystopia canthorum, as in type II. The gene for type I has been mapped to chromosome 2p; type II has been mapped to chromosome 3p. Estimates of prevalence suggest that Waardenburg's syndrome may affect 2% to 5% of all infants with congenital deafness (31,32). SNHL occurs in 20% of cases. Common findings are listed in Table 12.

TABLE 12. *Typical features of Waardenburg's syndrome*

Dystopia canthorum
Flat nasal root
Confluent eyebrows
Heterochromic irides
White forelock
Pigmentary abnormalities
Diminished vestibular function
Cleft lip and palate
Sensorineural hearing loss

Branchiootorenal Syndrome

First named by Melnickin in 1975, branchiootorenal syndrome includes branchial cleft fistula or cysts, otologic anomalies including malformed pinnae, preauricular pits or sinuses, hearing loss, and renal abnormalities. The inheritance is autosomal dominant, and the gene has been mapped to chromosome 8q (33).

X-linked Recessive Mixed Deafness with Perilymphatic Gusher

X-linked recessive mixed deafness with perilymphatic gusher is a nonsyndromic hereditary hearing loss. The hearing loss is characteristical of the mixed type; it is present at birth and becomes progressively worse. The conductive component of the hearing loss is greater at the lower frequencies (34) and may be a result of greater than normal perilymph pressure against the inner surface of the stapes footplate, which dampens its movement. Unless there is a family history of this disorder, it may not be clinically apparent. An otologic surgeon who attempts an operation on the stapes should be cautioned that a *sudden gush of perilymph fluid when the stapes footplate is entered can result in complete SNHL.* Computed tomography may be helpful in identifying the disorder. The lateral aspect of the internal auditory canal may be bulbous, and there may be incomplete bony separation from the base of the modiolus to the extent that a weak area can break through with an increase in cerebrospinal fluid pressure.

Autosomal Dominant Delayed-onset Progressive Sensorineural Hearing Loss

Autosomal dominant delayed-onset progressive sensorineural hearing loss is a relatively common nonsyndromic loss that usually manifests in the second or third decade of life and often progresses to bilateral, profound SNHL. The gene for this hereditary hearing loss is located on chromosome 5 (35).

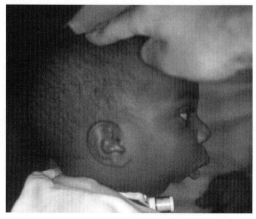

FIG. 5. Pierre Robin sequence. Lateral view shows severe micrognathia of mandible. Patient also has a cleft palate.

Pierre Robin Sequence

Pierre Robin is a sequence (see Glossary) not a syndrome. Patients with the sequence have been described as having hearing loss of a sensorineural or conductive type. The mode of inheritance has been suggested to be autosomal dominant (36). The classic findings in the sequence include micrognathia, glossoptosis, and cleft palate. Often the sequence is part of a syndrome such as Stickler syndrome (Fig. 5).

GENETIC COUNSELING

Physicians interested in hereditary hearing loss must be sensitive to the ethical and cultural issues present in embarking on research or attempting a search for cure. Many deaf persons identify deafness not as a disease but as a cultural difference. Deafness imparts a sense of belonging to a group who uses sign language as the primary means of communication. Common experiences often are shared, giving a deaf person a sense of unity with the group. Many deaf persons are concerned about the potentially adverse effect on the viability of deaf culture if research leads to prevention of hereditary hearing loss (37).

The importance of genetic counseling of deaf persons was first recognized by Nance (38,39). Genetic counseling offers an opportunity to ascertain large groups of deaf persons through schools and programs for the deaf. With the high rate of assortive mating among deaf persons, even those with environmental deafness would benefit from genetic counseling. Ninety percent of deaf persons marry another deaf person (40). If the investigator or clinician is sensitive to cultural and linguistic differences, deaf persons usually are enthusiastic about participating in genetic counseling (41).

Genetic counseling provides information and many supportive services to the affected person and his or her family (Table 13). Team members involved in counseling include clinical geneticists, genetic counselors, nurses, and social workers. Using a nondirective approach, a genetic counselor offers emotional support and assists in decision making without giving direct advice. This approach provides couples and families with the information they need to make their own educated decisions about what is best suited for their own personal needs. Genetic counseling is a process that should be empathic to societal pressures on the deaf population and promote individual needs rather than societal goals.

TABLE 13. *Indications for genetic counseling*

Comprehend medical facts
    Diagnosis
    Course of impairment
    Management
Guide course of action for patient and family
Identify childbearing issues (risk for transmission)
Educate unaffected family members
Afford assistance for placement in special schools if desired
Establish database for research and clinical studies

SUMMARY POINTS

- Genetics as a cause of hearing loss was first recognized by the otologist William Wilde. Since that time, heredity is believed to be the cause of as much as 50% of cases of hearing loss among children.
- Two thirds of cases of genetic hearing loss are nonsyndromic. One third of cases have recognizable characteristic findings and are considered part of a syndrome.
- A complete history and physical examination are of primary importance in the assessment of hearing loss believed to be of genetic origin. The otolaryngologist may be the first to detect subtleties that suggest a hearing loss is of genetic origin. An otolaryngologist can detect even mild dysmorphology in the head and neck region, which is associated with many hearing loss syndromes.
- Obtaining the diagnosis that hearing loss is of genetic origin is a systematic approach in which the history and physical examination guide the physician toward ordering additional radiologic and laboratory tests. The physician should be wary of an attempt to obtain a diagnosis by ordering a large battery of tests without sufficient reason.
- Although the medical community considers deafness a disease, many deaf persons believe it is a cultural difference. Many deaf individuals prefer to marry other deaf persons.
- Nance was were the first to identify and recommend genetic counseling for the deaf. Genetic counseling offers multiple opportunities and support mechanisms, from information about childbearing to community activities that cater to the deaf.
- Genetic counseling is beneficial even for patients with hearing loss of environmental origin because of the high rate of assortive mating among these persons.
- Additional resources are available for clinicians interested in new and updated information on hereditary hearing loss. A Web site contains updated information on newly located genes (http://dnalab/ww.uia.ac.be/dnalab/hhh/index:html).

GLOSSARY

allele   The alternative forms of a gene. Each person has two complete copies of DNA in every cell. One copy is obtained from each parent. The DNA sequence codes for a particular trait. Although a DNA sequence for two different traits may be present, the dominant trait is the one expressed. The other form is the allele.

autosomal dominant inheritance   The ability of an allele to be expressed whether a single or pair of alleles exists. The allele is on one of the 23 pairs of autosomes and is not encoded on one of the sex chromosomes.

autosomal recessive inheritance   The ability of an allele to be expressed only if a pair of alleles is present.

blotting   Transfer of DNA or RNA from an agar gel to filter paper. Hybridization with different probes is then performed.

congenital   Present at birth. Any disease whether genetic, infectious, or of other causation if present at birth is called a congenital disorder.

cryptogenic   Unknown. When the cause of a hearing loss is unknown or unfounded, it is often referred to as cryptogenic.

DNA   Deoxyribonucleic acid. The substance in the nucleus of all human cells except blood cells that contains all the genetic information for cell function and homeostasis.

dot blot   Hybridization of a labeled probe to DNA. These are spotted on filter paper.

genetic linkage studies   Following inheritance patterns of a particular trait over several generations with the hope of identifying the part of the chromosome responsible for the trait.

genome   All the genetic material present in the chromosomes of an individual. In humans there are approximately 6×10^9 base pairs.

genotype   The collection of alleles in an individual. The allele may or may not be expressed or seen physically.

heterozygous   Indicating the presence of two different alleles, one from each parent, for which a gene will be expressed. The dominant allele is phenotypically expressed although both alleles are present.

homozygous   Indicating the presence of two identical alleles, one from each parent, for which a gene is expressed.

inherited   Passage of a gene or trait to an offspring; synonymous with *genetic*.

locus   A position on a chromosome—the allele, the gene, or the entire segment of chromosome.

nonsyndromic   Autonomous; not usually found with other anomalies.

phenotype   The expression or physical characteristic determined by a genotype.

sequence   An anomaly directly caused by another anomaly.

Southern blot   Hybridization of labeled probe to DNA fragments separated by size in an agar gel. The fragments are blotted to filter paper.

sporadic occurrence   An anomaly that does not fit into the classic mendelian inheritance patterns and has no identifiable genetic origin.

syndrome   A constellation of congenital findings that occur together.

X-linked   The gene causing the disorder is located on the X chromosome.

REFERENCES

1. *Dorland's illustrated medical dictionary,* 27th ed. Philadelphia: WB Saunders, 1988.
2. Leppert MF, Lewis RA. Human genetic mapping and inherited deafness syndromes. *Ann N Y Acad Sci* 1991;630:38–48.
3. Riordan JJ, Rommens B, Kerem N, et al. Identification of the cystic fibrosis gene: cloning and characterization of complementary DNA. *Science* 1989;245:1066–1073.
4. Wallace MD, Marchuk AL, Anderson R, et al. Type 1 neurofibromatosis gene: identification of a large transcript interrupted in three NFI patients. *Science* 1990;249:181–186.
5. Monaco AR, Neve C, Colletti-Feener C, et al. Isolation of candidate cDNAs for portions of the Duchenne muscular dystrophy gene. *Nature* 1986;323;646–650.
6. Lalwani AK, Grundfast GM. A role for the otolaryngologist in identification and discovery of genetic disorders and chromosomal abnormalities. *Arch Otolaryngol Head Neck Surg* 1993;119:1074–1080.
7. Lalwani AK, Lunch E, Mhatre AN. Molecular genetics: a brief overview. In: Lalwani AK, Grundfast KM, eds. *Pediatric otology and neurotology.* Philadelphia: Lippincott–Raven, 1998.
8. Kalatzis V, Petit C. The fundamental and medical impacts of recent progress in research on hereditary hearing loss. *Hum Mol Genet* 1998;7:1589–1597.
9. Cremers CWRJ, Rijn PM, Hageman MJ. Prevention of serious hearing impairment or deafness in the young child. *Proc R Soc Med* 1989;82:483–486.
10. Fraser GR. *The causes of profound deafness in childhood.* Baltimore: Johns Hopkins University Press, 1976.
11. Konigsmark BW, Gorlin RJ. *Genetic and metabolic deafness.* Philadelphia: WB Saunders, 1976.
12. Reardon W. Genetics and deafness: clinical aspects. *Br J Hosp Med* 1992;47:507–511.
13. Chan KH. Sensorineural hearing loss in children: classification and evaluation. *Otolaryngol Clin North Am* 1994;27:473–486.
14. Reardon W. Genetic deafness. *J Med Genet* 1992;29:521–526.
15. Gorlin RJ, Cohen MM, Levin LS. *Syndromes of the head and neck.* New York: Oxford University Press, 1990.
16. Shokeir MHK. The Goldenhar syndrome: a natural history. *Birth Defects* 1977;13:67–83.
17. Grabb WC. The first and second branchial arch syndrome. *Plast Reconstr Surg* 1965;36:485–508.
18. Melnick M. The etiology of external ear malformation and its relation to abnormalities of the middle ear, inner ear and other organ systems. *Birth Defects* 1980;16:303–331.
19. Hanieh A, David DJ. Apert's syndrome. *Childs Nerv Syst* 1993;95:289–291.
20. Carinci F, Avantagiato A, Curioni C. Crouzon syndrome: cephalometric analysis and evaluation of pathogenesis. *Cleft Palate Craniofac J* 1994;31:201–209.
21. Leon PE, Raventos H, Lynch E, Morrow J, King MC. The gene for an inherited form of deafness maps to chromosome 5q31. *Proc Natl Acad Sci USA* 1992;89:5181–5184.
22. Smith RJH, et al. Clinical diagnosis of the Usher syndromes. *Am J Med Genet* 1994;50:32–38.
23. Johnson T, et al. Pendred's syndrome: acoustic, vestibular and radiologic findings in 17 unrelated patients. *J Laryngol Otol* 1987;101:1187–1192.
24. Grundfast KM. Hereditary hearing impairment in children. *Adv Otolaryngol Head Neck Surg* 1993;7:29–40.
25. Wang Q, et al. Positional cloning of a novel potassium channel gene KVLQT1 mutations cause cardiac arrhythmias. *Nature Genet* 1996;12:17–23.
26. Schwartz PJ, Periti M, Malliani A. The long Q-T syndrome. *Am Heart J* 1975;89:378–390.
27. Keating M, Atkinson D, Dunn C, et al. Linkage of cardiac arrhythmia, the long QT syndrome, and the Harvey *ras*-1 gene. *Science* 1991;252:704–706.
28. Gorlin RJ, Toriello HV, Cohen MM. *Hereditary hearing loss and its syndromes.* New York: Oxford University Press, 1995.
29. Temple IK. Stickler's syndrome. *J Med Genet* 1989;26:119–126.
30. Grundfast KM, Josephson GD. Hereditary hearing loss. In: Hughes G, Pensak M, eds. *Clinical otology.* New York: Thieme, 1997.
31. de Saxe M, Kromberg JG, Jenkins T. Waardenburg syndrome in South Africa: part 1: an evaluation of the clinical findings in 11 families. *S Afr Med J* 1984;66(7):256–261.
32. DiGeorge AM, Olmstead RW, Harley RD. Waardenburg syndrome. *J Pediatr* 1960;57:649–660.
33. Smith RJ, Coppage KB, Ankerstjerne JK, et al. Localization of the gene for branchiootorenal syndrome to chromosome 8q. *Genomics* 1992;14:841–844.
34. Cremers CWRJ. Audiologic features of the X-linked progressive mixed deafness syndrome with perilymphatic gusher during stapes surgery. *Am J Otolaryngol* 1985;6:243–246.
35. Leon PE, King MC. Gene mapped for inherited hearing loss. *Sci News* 1991;140:253.
36. Grundfast KM. Hearing loss. In: Bluestone C, Stool S, Kenna M. *Textbook of pediatric otolaryngology,* 3rd ed. Philadelphia: WB Saunders, 1996;239–283.
37. Grundfast KM, Rosen J. Ethical and cultural considerations in research on hereditary deafness. *Otolaryngol Clin North Am* 1992;25:973–978.
38. Nance WE. Genetic counseling for the hearing impaired. *Audiology* 1971;10:222–233.
39. Nance WE. Genetic counseling of hereditary deafness: an unmet need. In: Bess FH, ed. *Childhood deafness: causation assessment and management.* New York: Grune & Stratton, 1977:211–216.
40. Schein JD. *At home among strangers.* Washington, DC: Gallaudet University Press, 1989.
41. Arnos KS, Israel J, Cunningham M. Genetic counseling of the deaf, medical and cultural considerations. *Ann N Y Acad Sci* 1991;630:212–222.

The Ear: Comprehensive Otology,
edited by R. F. Canalis and P. R. Lambert.
Lippincott Williams & Wilkins, Philadelphia © 2000.

CHAPTER 31

Sudden Sensorineural Hearing Loss

George A. Gates

Differential Diagnosis
Pathophysiology
   Viral Causes of Idiopathic Sudden Sensorineural
      Hearing Loss
   Vascular Causes of Idiopathic Sudden Sensorineural
      Hearing Loss
   Membrane Breaks and Perilymphatic Fistula
Evaluation
   Audiometry
   Vestibular Testing

   Blood Studies
   Imaging Studies
Prognosis
Therapy
   Antiviral Therapy
   Antiinflammatory Therapy
   Rheologic Therapy
   Other Drugs
   Surgery
Results

Sudden sensorineural hearing loss (SNHL) is a common clinical syndrome that frequently poses a diagnostic and therapeutic dilemma because of uncertainty about causation, appropriate treatment, and prognosis in most instances. Sudden SNHL generally is depicted as unilateral, sudden-onset loss of hearing of 30 dB or more in three contiguous test frequencies. Persons of all ages may be affected, and there is no sex predilection. Bilateral cases are uncommon and are more likely to be associated with serious systemic disease. Recurrent sudden SNHL is infrequent and suggests the presence of another syndrome, such as endolymphatic hydrops, and the need for additional diagnostic information. Sudden worsening of preexisting hearing loss is not considered a part of the sudden SNHL syndrome.

The clinical patterns of sudden SNHL are quite variable. The hearing loss may vary from total loss to partial loss at one portion of the auditory spectrum. The vestibular system is involved in 30% to 40% of cases. Partial or complete spontaneous recovery occurs in one half to two thirds of cases depending on criteria for recovery. Extended evaluation may reveal occult underlying disease (acoustic neuroma, infectious disease) in 10% of cases.

Specific causes of sudden SNHL, such as trauma, systemic infectious diseases, and neoplasia, are well described in the older literature. Recent reports have expanded the list of possible causes in the categories of infectious disease, autoimmune disease, and neurodegenerative disorders. Many of these conditions initially become apparent as idiopathic sudden SNHL and necessitate active investigation to uncover a specific cause. In most instances of idiopathic sudden SNHL, however, no specific agent is found, and polytherapy is used in an effort to manage the most likely causes. Patient and physician alike often are uncertain about the most appropriate therapy. With the expanding national focus on cost containment in medicine, there is growing concern that many patients may receive limited evaluation and minimal treatment without evidence of efficacy in randomized clinical trials. Although existing studies have shown efficacy of medical therapy, there is considerable need for continuing research to further assess the value of treatment and search for better identification of the underlying pathophysiologic mechanism.

This chapter reviews the known causes of sudden SNHL, discusses putative causes of idiopathic sudden SNHL, describes the clinical evaluation, and evaluates what is known about the various treatment modalities. *Sudden SNHL* is used as a generic term to indicate acute, substantial, cochlear-retrocochlear hearing loss of any cause. *Idiopathic sudden SNHL* specifically indicates

   G. A. Gates: Department of Otolaryngology–Head and Neck Surgery, University of Washington; Virginia Merrill Bloedel Hearing Research Center, Seattle, Washington 98195-7923

sudden SNHL in which clinical assessment fails to reveal a cause. Most of the review that follows applies to unilateral cases and provides specific notes in regard to bilateral cases.

DIFFERENTIAL DIAGNOSIS

Sudden SNHL is a syndrome not a disease, and the list of disorders associated with sudden SNHL is long. A nosologic problem occurs when sudden SNHL develops in a patient with a known medical condition. Can one logically ascribe the hearing loss to the underlying condition, or should one assume no relation? Whereas each case has to be judged on its own merits, it is prudent to continue with a full evaluation to be as certain as possible one is not overlooking a second condition. For example, sudden deafness was found in an elderly patient with diabetes (1) who also had a pontine lesion that probably caused the sudden SNHL. Although it is likely the diabetic vascular disease contributed to the pontine infarction, it might be overly reductionistic to ascribe the sudden SNHL to diabetes per se. Wilson et al. (2) found slightly poorer recovery in a group of patients with diabetes and sudden SNHL as opposed to a group without diabetes who had sudden SNHL. The investigators found that the group with diabetes was older, which in and of itself might explain the poorer recovery. We tread on difficult ground when we make pathophysiologic assumptions on the basis of clinical associations that might be no more than chance occurrences.

Infection due to a wide spectrum of viruses (3) heads the differential diagnosis list, which includes mumps (4), influenza, rubella, rubeola, cytomegalovirus infection, Lassa fever (5), herpes zoster (6–9), herpes simplex (6, 10,11), hepatitis A (12), spumavirus infection (13), chicken pox (14), and Epstein-Barr virus infection (15, 16). These diseases have been implicated by direct and indirect evidence in cases of sudden SNHL. Patients with human immunodeficiency virus infection appear to have sudden SNHL only after the acquired immunodeficiency syndrome is manifested by systemic infections such as cryptococcosis (17–20). Other infectious disorders associated with sudden SNHL are Lyme disease (21,22) and toxoplasmosis (23). Treponemal infection has long been associated with hearing loss and may present itself as sudden SNHL (24–26).

A neoplasm in the temporal bone, internal auditory canal, or posterior fossa should always be considered as a possibility. Acoustic neuroma, brain tumor (27,28), metastatic lesions (29–31), leukemia (32), and myeloma (33) have been reported. Of special interest is acoustic neuroma (vestibular schwannoma), which is accompanied by SNHL in about 10% to 22% of cases (34–39); many patients exhibit reversible hearing loss with corticosteroid therapy (34,40,41). Some acoustic neuromas associated with sudden SNHL tend to be larger than 2 cm

(42). However, only 1% to 2% of cases of sudden SNHL are caused by acoustic neuroma (43).

Vascular disturbances include occlusion caused by embolism or thrombosis, reduced blood flow due to sludging, hyperviscosity, coagulopathy, and intracochlear hemorrhage. Many cases of sudden SNHL have been reported after open heart (44–47) and other operations (48) and are presumed to be the result of microembolization. Sudden SNHL has been found in a patient with unstable angina (49); the hearing improved after cardiac bypass surgery. Hypercoagulability has been suspected as a precursor to sudden SNHL (50). Waldenström's macroglobulinemia (51,52), leukemia (32,53), and carcinomatosis (54) may cause sudden SNHL from intracochlear hemorrhage. Buerger's disease (55), polyarteritis nodosa (56,57), temporal arteritis (58), and sickle cell disease (59–61) have been associated with sudden SNHL.

Systemic diseases detected among patients with sudden SNHL include lupus erythematosus (62–64), sarcoidosis (65,66), diabetes mellitus (2,67), ulcerative colitis (68), polyarteritis nodosa (56,57), Behçet's syndrome (69), Cogan's syndrome (70,71), sickle cell disease (59–61), thyrotoxicosis (72), aplastic anemia (73), polychondritis (74), paraneoplastic syndrome (75), and rheumatoid arthritis (76). Autoimmune inner ear disorders (64,77–81) have been increasingly recognized as a cause of sudden SNHL. In many cases there is no evidence of a systemic autoimmune syndrome, but in others there is an association with systemic disorders (79) and thus overlap with some of the foregoing systemic disorders. Sudden SNHL following vaccination (82,83) and administration of antithymocyte antiglobulin (84) has been ascribed to a hypersensitivity reaction.

Neurologic conditions known to be associated with sudden SNHL include meningitis (usually bilateral), multiple sclerosis lesions involving the eighth cranial nerve or root entry zone (85–90), pontine ischemia (1,91,92), neurosarcoidosis (66), carcinomatous encephalopathy (75), bilateral temporal lobe lesions (93), aneurysm (94), and migraine (95). Functional hearing loss should be considered in the differential diagnosis (96).

Exposure to ototoxic agents such as gentamicin (97), furosemide (98), cis-platinum (single dose) (99), vincristine (100), naproxen (101), interferon (102), dantrolene (103), oral contraceptives (104), and insecticides (105) has been cited as a cause of sudden SNHL.

PATHOPHYSIOLOGY

The three most commonly cited putative causes of idiopathic sudden SNHL are viral infection, circulatory disturbance, and membrane breaks. The literature contains evidence to support each theory in specific cases. However, it is clear that none of these theories adequately explains the clinical course of all or even a majority of cases of idiopathic sudden SNHL. Therefore, the reader should keep an open mind to the possibility that idiopathic sudden SNHL syndrome probably is caused by a variety of disorders that act singly or in combination. Lack of a clear-cut marker for each possibility has hampered the study of idiopathic sudden SNHL syndrome. Each patient with the idiopathic sudden SNHL syndrome should be evaluated in light of all possible causes.

Viral Causes of Idiopathic Sudden Sensorineural Hearing Loss

Many patients with idiopathic sudden SNHL report symptoms of a generalized antecedent viral infection, such as an upper respiratory tract infection. The low specificity of such symptoms detracts from the rationale of basing a diagnosis on those symptoms. Viral infections with localizing findings, such as mumps parotitis, provide more compelling clinical evidence. Nonetheless, there is considerable support for the prevalence of viral infection as the cause of a substantial proportion of cases of idiopathic sudden SNHL, particularly cases with severe to profound loss of hearing, vertigo, and other clinical evidence of infection, such as an elevated erythrocyte sedimentation rate (ESR). The most common model is viral cochleitis or labyrinthitis as the site of infection. Viral infection is estimated to be the cause of sudden SNHL in about one third of cases (106).

Why only one ear is attacked in most instances remains a mystery. Schuknecht and Donovan (107) concluded from their study of human temporal bones that the histopathologic findings in idiopathic sudden SNHL were most compatible with viral cochleitis rather than vascular disturbances or membrane breaks. However, all but one of their patients had long-standing hearing loss, and the one patient whose hearing returned to normal had no histologic abnormalities. The viral theory supports the findings in cases in which hearing is not recovered but does not account for the cases in which hearing returns. Wilson et al. (108) found a significantly higher seroconversion rate to mumps, rubeola, varicella zoster, cytomegalovirus infection, and influenza B among patients with idiopathic sudden SNHL than among controls. The presence or absence of seroconversion, however, bore no relation to degree of loss or recovery, which may reflect the temporal relation between seroconversion and the hearing loss. Laurikainen et al. (109) found no relation between seroconversion to common viral antigens and sudden SNHL. The association between sudden SNHL and recent infection with other viruses such as the herpesvirus family (6), spumavirus (70), and subclinical mumps (110) supports the infectious nature of many cases of sudden SNHL. Rapid onset, severe loss of hearing and vestibular function, and absence of spontaneous recovery suggest an infectious cause. However, some infectious agents are known to cause treatable, reversible sudden SNHL. These include syphilis (25) and Lyme disease (21). Khetarpal et

al. (111) commented that virus-induced structural alteration may not adequately explain all cases of idiopathic sudden SNHL.

Another model of viral pathogenesis exists, namely, Bell's palsy. In this condition, temporary loss of function occurs, often caused by reversible alteration in neural conduction. One possible pathophysiologic mechanism for this phenomenon is capillary endothelialitis, which causes leakage of plasma into the endoneurial spaces (112). Thus current knowledge of viral pathophysiologic mechanisms is compatible with retrocochlear neuritis as a theoretic cause of idiopathic sudden SNHL. A similar mechanism is postulated as the cause of vestibular neuronitis, in which return of function occurs in about 50% of cases (113). Sudden SNHL and vertigo are recognized components of Ramsay Hunt syndrome (7), in which facial paralysis caused by varicella-zoster virus is the dominant clinical feature. Although fluid accumulation in the facial nerve has been seen among some patients with Bell's palsy (114), we did not find inflammatory changes in the eighth cranial nerve on noncontrast T2-weighted magnetic resonance (MR) images of a small number of patients with idiopathic sudden SNHL (115). Gadolinium enhancement of the cochlea and eighth nerve on MR images of a patient with mumps and sudden SNHL is of interest; this suggests both neural and cochlear involvement (116).

Herpes zoster oticus (Ramsay Hunt syndrome) does cause sudden SNHL among a small proportion of patients (7,9). Given that the virus is known to attack ganglion cells, the hearing loss in herpes zoster oticus may indeed be neural rather than cochlear. However, proof of this assumption is lacking because of the small number of patients with herpes zoster oticus in general and the even smaller number with sudden SNHL. The available evidence is inconclusive in delineating labyrinthine as opposed to neural infection as the source of hearing loss in idiopathic sudden SNHL. Because of the availability of antiviral agents, the distinction is not just academic.

Vascular Causes of Idiopathic Sudden Sensorineural Hearing Loss

The vascular disease theories of idiopathic sudden SNHL describe a spectrum of putative pathophysiologic alterations at the capillary and microvascular levels. They include embolism, blood sludging, hypercoagulability, vasospasm, arteriosclerosis, systemic vascular disease, and connective tissue disorders. Each theory has been presented with a variable amount of supporting clinical and laboratory evidence. Schuknecht (117) refuted vascular dysfunction as a cause of sudden SNHL but did not propose a theory to explain reversible sudden SNHL. To better understand the possible role of vascular disorders in idiopathic sudden SNHL it is worthwhile to examine the evidence of the role of these conditions in idiopathic sudden SNHL within the several categories.

Vascular Occlusion and Blood Flow

Occlusion of the cochlear artery causes immediate loss of hearing that becomes irreversible within minutes. Because the cochlear artery is an end artery without collateral vessels, obstruction has dramatic results. *Cochlear apoplexy* is an old term used to describe such an event, which fortunately is rare. Hearing loss is uncommon in transient ischemic events involving the posterior fossa circulation but usually occurs after thrombosis of the anterior inferior cerebellar artery. Isolated hearing loss without any of the stigmata of occlusion of the anterior inferior cerebellar artery or lateral medullary syndrome is not characteristic of vascular thrombosis, although hearing loss is not a common manifestation of transient ischemic events involving the vertebrobasilar system. Watanabe et al. (118), however, described two cases of iatrogenic vertebrobasilar insufficiency associated with sudden SNHL and vertigo but not with any other neurologic deficit.

Some form of vascular dysfunction is the theoretic clinical model for many forms of idiopathic sudden SNHL. Because there is no direct method of assessing cochlear blood flow, indirect means have been used. Nagahara et al. (119) recorded perilymph oxygen tension in patients with idiopathic sudden SNHL. They consistently found reduced oxygen levels, in marked contrast to levels in patients with slowly progressive SNHL whose oxygen levels were normal. Although the mechanism for the hypoxia was not elaborated, the results of that study indicated significant interference with the delivery of oxygen to the cochlear tissues of some patients with idiopathic sudden SNHL.

Ohinata et al. (120) measured blood flow with Doppler ultrasound in the carotid and vertebral systems of 14 male patients with idiopathic sudden SNHL. Although there was no significant difference in blood flow between subjects and controls, there was a significant reduction in flow among the patients with hearing worse than 50 dB hearing level (HL) than among the patients with lesser hearing losses. Flow also varied inversely with blood viscosity. Daily stellate ganglion blocks improved blood flow on the ipsilateral side, but the effect diminished with age. A polytherapy regimen was associated with improved hearing in 13 of 14 patients, but the relation between blood flow and outcome was not described. Atherosclerosis in an anomalous carotid artery produced sudden SNHL that did not resolve after endarterectomy (121).

Vasospasm has been considered a factor in idiopathic sudden SNHL, although the cause of the spasm remains ill defined (122). A specific form of vasospasm related to migraine was associated with sudden SNHL by Viirre and Baloh (95), who described 13 patients with sudden SNHL associated with other vasospastic neurologic phenomena. Lipkin et al. (123) described a single case of recurrent sudden SNHL, which they ascribed to migraine.

Capillary Dysfunction

Given that most patients with sudden SNHL are younger than those with classic peripheral vascular disease, functional disturbances of the microcirculation rather than fixed lesions of the macrocirculation may play a greater role in sudden SNHL. Lawrence (124) described an animal model of reversible vascular occlusion at the capillary level following administration of quinine, which causes endothelial swelling and cessation of blood flow in the vas spirale. This was accompanied by loss of cochlear microphonics. With time there is spontaneous restoration of blood flow to the organ of Corti and recovery of microphonics. This recovery is not affected by calcium channel blockers (125). It is possible, but unproved, that reversible idiopathic sudden SNHL might be the result of virus-induced capillary inflammation in these vessels. Thus there is reason to suspect hematogenous viral infection of the cochlea as a possible cause in some cases of idiopathic sudden SNHL, in particular those in which recovery of auditory function occurs. This model combines the infectious and vascular theories and accounts for both the signs of viral illness and reversible loss of hearing. Of course, if the virus causes structural damage to the organ of Corti, recovery is not likely. These observations have provided a conceptual basis for including a vasoactive regimen in the management of idiopathic sudden SNHL. Another element of viral infection is decreased red blood cell deformability (126). It may be the case that viral infection can affect hearing in a reversible manner through the pathophysiologic mechanism of induced capillary dysfunction.

Coagulation Defects

Many types of hypercoagulability have been detected among persons with idiopathic sudden SNHL (50, 127–130). Zajtchuk et al. (50) reported that 8 of 14 patients with sudden SNHL had laboratory evidence of a hypercoagulable state manifest as abnormal thrombin generation, increased antithrombin III levels, or increased platelet count. Owen et al. (128) found abnormally high levels of antithrombin III in one case of inherited coagulation defect. Increased platelet aggregability was found among patients with sudden SNHL and vertigo (131). Decreased fibrinolytic activity has been found among patients with sudden SNHL (127). Einer et al. (132) compared 32 patients with sudden SNHL with 28 healthy controls matched for age, sex, and body mass. Twenty-five of the patients had isolated abnormalities in coagulation profiles, increased primarily plasminogen activation inhibitor, or increased fibrin degeneration products (older patients). However, the investigators concluded that pathologic hemostasis did not seem to play a role in the pathogenesis of sudden SNHL. Defibrinogenation has been found to be useful in the treatment of a small number of patients with idiopathic sudden SNHL (133). Increased blood viscosity has been found in association with sudden SNHL; there was positive correlation between hearing recovery and changes in viscosity with treatment (134).

Hemorrhage

Intracochlear hemorrhage is seen in a variety of disorders, including Waldenström's macroglobulinemia (51, 52), leukemia (32,53), and carcinomatosis (54). Recovery from hemorrhagic lesions is poor because of fibrosis and osteoneogenesis.

Membrane Breaks and Perilymphatic Fistula

Acute sudden SNHL occurring in chronologic relation to an abrupt change in barometric pressure, such as an airplane flight, or events that raise intracranial pressure, such as sneezing or coughing, are properly suspected as possible intracochlear membrane breaks, some of which may be associated with perilymphatic fistula (PLF). The prevalence of PLF among patients with sudden SNHL in Japan is less than 1% (135).

Simmons (136) introduced the concept of membrane breaks as a cause of sudden SNHL in 1968, the same year PLF was described by Fee (137). Goodhill (138) in 1971 associated sudden SNHL with rupture of the round window membrane. Goodhill et al. later extended those observations to include oval window fistulas (139). They contrasted implosive and explosive fistulas as resulting from external forces in the former and internal forces (e.g., straining) in the latter. Simmons (140) described multiple membrane breaks in 1978 and pointed out the difficulty in ascribing symptoms to rupture of Reissner's membrane as opposed to rupture of the oval or round window. For example, rupture of Reissner's membrane causes perilymphatic intoxication of endolymph and subsequent hearing loss (in the general area of the tear), which should recover as the membrane heals and the ionic composition of the respective fluids is restored. Failure of healing might result in incomplete recovery. Although loss of perilymph has been suspected as the cause of hearing loss and vertigo in explosive fistulas, the pathophysiologic mechanism of that assumption has received little attention.

Yanagihara and Nisioka (141) found release of air bubbles that had become trapped in the labyrinth in three cases of implosive fistula. They then made a laboratory model of pneumolabyrinth (142) in which the effects of a simulated explosive fistula were reproduced by means of aspiration of perilymph, which did not produce a shift in hearing parameters. When air was injected into the labyrinth, a significant decrease in auditory function occurred and was reversed by means of removal of the air bubbles. The investigators concluded that pneumolabyrinth affected hearing by mechanically preventing normal conduction of sound vibration along the basilar membrane. Thus there is evidence that pneumolabyrinth may cause reversible hearing loss in membrane breaks, particularly of the implosive type. Other investigators have reported this phenomenon (143–145). This model makes good clinical sense when one examines the success of surgical patches placed on the outside of the labyrinth, where outward flow of fluid would tend to displace the patch but inward air pressure would tend to hold it in place.

Patients with idiopathic sudden SNHL in whom membrane breaks or fistulas are expected on the basis of a history of a pressure event generally recover with bed rest and elevation of the head. Few patients need middle ear exploration. Most of these procedures are performed to control vertigo.

EVALUATION

The clinical challenge in the care of a patient with sudden SNHL is to uncover a specific cause of the hearing loss. In most cases there is no obvious cause, and few clues arise from the history, physical examination, and audiometric testing, which are the minimal elements of the basic clinical assessment. Common conditions such as acute otitis media, external meatal obstruction from severe wax impaction, or trauma usually can be excluded without delay. By definition, patients with sudden SNHL have normal otoscopic findings.

The most common causes of a sudden decrease in hearing are local conditions in the outer or middle ear. Wax impaction caused by sudden swelling of a cerumen accumulation after water exposure (e.g., swimming, shower) is a frequent problem. Removal is both diagnostic and therapeutic. Acute effusion from infection, allergy, or barotrauma is common. Therapy for the underlying disorder usually is straightforward and effective. Temporal bone trauma, including acute perforation or fracture, is suggested by a history of recent events and confirmed with typical physical findings of altered structure, traumatic effusion, and hemorrhage.

The right and left ears are affected equally in sudden SNHL. Most patients report rapid onset of symptoms or the presence of the hearing loss on awakening from a night's sleep. Others describe a progressive loss over several hours or days. Some patients are unable to pinpoint the onset but report with precision the onset of tinnitus, which invariably accompanies the hearing loss. The history should document the time and date of onset, subsequent change in hearing, and the presence or absence of tinnitus and dizziness or vertigo. The events related to the onset should be discussed with emphasis on activity that might acutely alter intracranial and intralabyrinthine pressure such as coughing, sneezing, straining, scuba diving, or rapid airplane descent. A history of hearing loss and vertigo should be sought. The history should include a thorough review of systems to find clues to possible infectious disease, neurologic syndromes including migraine, cancer, use of medications, and exposure to industrial noise or chemicals.

Audiometry

Estimation of pure tone air and bone thresholds and word recognition at comfortable loudness are the key audiometric tests. The severity and the shape of the audiogram define the basic clinical entity. Clinical hearing testing is not adequate for this purpose. Mattox and Simmons (146) emphasized the importance of limiting acoustic trauma to an acutely disturbed ear and recommended not establishing thresholds in excess of 90 dB HL. There is little to be gained in knowing the precise thresholds of a severe loss, even though tradition would urge a complete study. Patients with an upsloping audiometric threshold profile (more low-frequency loss) tend to have greater recovery and those with downsloping loss tend to have poorer recovery (146). Examination of the acoustic reflex threshold, reflex decay, and performance-intensity function of speech discrimination (PI-PB) should be added when a retrocochlear lesion is suspected.

Measurement of distortion product otoacoustic emissions (DPOE) has been used in the study of sudden SNHL (147). If the lesion affects the hair cells or the source of the endocochlear potential, DPOE should be reduced or absent. If DPOE are retained and hearing is impaired, the lesion may be retrocochlear (28). In our limited study of sudden SNHL (115), DPOE were abnormal in all instances.

Auditory brainstem response (ABR) testing should be performed if a retrocochlear site of lesion is suspected. However, in the usual case of idiopathic sudden SNHL, ABRs are absent with severe hearing loss and attenuated with lesser degrees. Portmann et al. (148) found evidence of retrocochlear pathologic conditions among 19 of 61 patients with sudden SNHL who underwent ABR testing. Among some patients with multiple sclerosis, sudden SNHL may be the initial presenting symptom, and ABR desynchronization aids in the diagnostic evaluation (149).

Vestibular Testing

As many as 40% of patients with sudden SNHL experience vertigo and disequilibrium at the time of onset (109) or later (150). Logic would label such cases labyrinthitis. These patients have a poor prognosis in general (151). Vestibular testing in the acute situation should include a clinical neurotologic examination with assess-ment of nystagmus and eye motor control and balance. Caloric stimulation of the labyrinth should be performed when a patient reports dizziness or vertigo and when there are oculomotor findings. Laird and Wilson (152) found more information with electronystagmography (ENG) than through a history and included abnormal ENG findings a risk factor for poor outcome regardless of history. Patients with abnormal ENG results had poorer recovery of hearing than those with normal ENG results (109). None of the patients described by Mattox and Simmons (146) who had a down-sloping audiogram, vertigo, and a hypoactive caloric response had recovery.

Blood Studies

A complete blood cell count with ESR always should be done because sudden SNHL may be a manifestation of anemia, leukemia, or generalized infection, all of which may be reflected in the blood examination. An elevated ESR carries a poor prognosis for hearing recovery (146). A host of studies have been examined in the literature. Because it is impractical to cast a wide laboratory net for every patient, selective use of screening tests based on clinical assessment is warranted.

If abnormal coagulation is suspected, a coagulation profile may be performed. A screening examination might include prothrombin and partial thromboplastin times and a platelet examination. Depending on the laboratory and the clinical signs and symptoms, a fuller examination might include partial thromboplastin activation times, thrombin generation, platelet count and platelet aggregation index, fibrinogen activation and consumption, factor VIII, serum antithrombin III, and serum plasminogen activation inhibitor. Consultation with a hematologist should be considered when a coagulation disorder is suspected on the basis of the history or screening tests.

Studies of thyroid metabolism have not been productive in the care of persons with no clinical indications for testing. A fasting blood sugar or glycosolated hemoglobin should be assessed to exclude the rare case of undiagnosed diabetes mellitus (67). Serum lipids have been shown not to be a factor in sudden SNHL (153).

A serologic test for syphilis should be considered in most instances even though only 1% to 2% of persons with sudden SNHL have syphilis. Western blot detection of antibodies to *Treponema pallidum* should increase the specificity of testing. Virus titers are not obtained routinely but may be in the presence of a severe or specific infectious syndrome. None of 80 patients studied in Finland had a change in their postconvalescence antibody titers to common viral antigens (109).

If immune-mediated inner ear disease is suspected, serum studies for cochlear antigen and heat shock protein may be obtained by means of Western blot examination. These examinations have been available as part of research protocols at the Massachusetts Eye and Ear Infirmary and the University of California at San Diego. The Western blot examination is now commercially available. Autoimmune inner ear disorder is being suspected more frequently as awareness of this condition has become more widespread. In general these patients have bilateral fluctuating hearing loss and dizziness, so the typical presentation is different from that of most cases of sudden SNHL. The first instance of autoimmune inner ear disorder often meets the criteria for sudden SNHL. Other serum tests for immune-mediated disease include antinuclear antibody, rheumatoid factor, anticardiolipin antibody (64), anti-parietal cell antibody, anti-mitochondrial antibody, and anti-smooth muscle antibody, which had highest positive rate in sudden SNHL in one study (81).

Imaging Studies

MR imaging should be done routinely to exclude possible retrocochlear disease, such as neoplasia and small strokes. Weber et al. (154) found three cases of specific, treatable neurologic disorders among 16 patients with sudden SNHL (multiple sclerosis, acoustic neuroma, meningioma). Acoustic neuroma often becomes apparent as sudden SNHL (10% of cases). I treated a young woman with sudden SNHL whose hearing thresholds, word recognition, and acoustic reflexes returned to normal after corticosteroid therapy and whose MR images showed a 4-cm acoustic neuroma. The high prevalence of occult disorders mandates imaging in sudden SNHL. Other lesions seen include multiple sclerosis, meningioma, and small strokes (92).

Recent developments in MR technology have greatly expanded the role of imaging in the evaluation of patients with otologic disorders (155). Two-dimensional fast spin echo imaging facilitates signal acquisition through increased signal-to-noise ratios while preserving image contrast, thus increasing scan efficiency. Use of phased-array external coils further improves signal-to-noise ratio and provides greater detail and magnification of images (156). This technology has been applied to MR neurography and has shown to be useful in the management of trauma and disorders such as carpal tunnel syndrome in which disruption of axonal transport from ischemia or compression produces bright T2-weighted signals in the nerve (157). My colleagues and I used phased-array coils to examine a small number of patients with sudden SNHL in the acute phase and found no evidence of auditory or vestibular nerve abnormality (gadolinium was not used). All these patients had audiometric evidence of cochlear dysfunction based on the absence of DPOE (115).

Early studies in which MR imaging was used in the diagnosis of idiopathic sudden SNHL were not performed during the acute phase (158). Recent MR studies with gadolinium have shown enhancement of the labyrinth in patients with acute sudden SNHL (159). The recovery rate was less among the patients with cochlear fluid enhancement (118). By comparison, in the acute stage of Bell's palsy, gadolinium enhancement of the facial nerve is a common finding that disappears with time or recovery (114). MR enhancement of the cochlea and eighth nerve has been found among patients with adult-onset mumps (116). As imaging technology continues to improve, there undoubtedly will be additional applications and benefit for patients with idiopathic sudden SNHL. Thin-section computed tomography of the cochlea may reveal a pneumolabyrinth and should be performed when PLF is suspected.

PROGNOSIS

The natural history of idiopathic sudden SNHL indicates spontaneous recovery in a substantial proportion of cases. Normal hearing is reached by about half of patients (160) and improvement to serviceable levels by two thirds (overall) (146). The criteria for improvement vary enough among studies that it is difficult to make direct comparisons. The landmark study of Mattox and Simmons (146) found prognosis is worsened by an elevated ESR, which suggests viral infection or systemic illness, the presence of vertigo, a downsloping audiogram, and longer duration of loss. Byl (160) found no correlation between ESR and outcome. Bilaterality and evidence of autoimmunity also adversely affect prognosis. Time between onset and start of therapy (160,161) and younger age have been found to be predictors of better outcome (162). Other studies have shown no effect of age (163). The age group most frequently affected is 50 to 59 years (164).

Investigators in Japan found that hearing loss that begins when the patient is awake has a better prognosis than that with onset during sleep (165); the opposite was found by in Sweden (166). Bilateral cases are uncommon (less than 2%) (167). In general, bilateral cases have a worse prognosis because severe or systemic disease often is implicated.

Wilson (168) related the pattern of loss to recovery profile. All his patients with mild, midfrequency losses recovered fully in contrast to none with profound, flat losses. Other investigators (169) did not find a relation between overall recovery and initial audiometric profile. Kallinen et al. (170) found that persons with an upsloping audiogram responded better to anticoagulant therapy, whereas patients with a downsloping audiogram responded better to carbogen treatment.

Vertigo accompanies hearing loss in 30% to 40% of cases. In general, the presence of vertigo worsens the prognosis for recovery of hearing (171). The pathophysiologic basis for this observation rests in the likelihood that the entire labyrinth is involved in an inflammatory process, which is apt to be nonreversible, rather than a transient ischemic event. Laird and Wilson (152) found that persons with vertigo and evidence of vestibular injury at ENG had the poorest recovery (30%), those with vertigo and normal ENG results did better (45% recovered), and those with normal ENG results and no vertigo had a 70% recovery rate.

Bilateral cases of sudden SNHL are uncommon and in general have a poor prognosis for hearing recovery. Because the prevalence of serious systemic disease is higher in association with bilateral sudden SNHL, great diligence should be taken to uncover a specific cause. Examples are carcinomatosis (29,54,172,173), lymphoma, intracranial aneurysm (94), Cogan's syndrome (70,174), meningitis (18,175), cerebrovascular disease (48,92), multiple myeloma (33), human immunodeficiency virus infection (19,176), collagen vascular disease (57,63), toxoplasmosis (23), sickle cell disease (60), and autoimmune inner ear disease (167).

THERAPY

Therapy for specific causes of sudden SNHL should follow the guidelines and therapeutic principles established for each particular cause. Space does not allow a detailed discussion of management of all the causes of sudden SNHL in the differential diagnosis. The discussion that follows reviews the treatment of patients with idiopathic sudden SNHL, that is, sudden SNHL for which no obvious cause is determined at initial evaluation. Patients with bilateral idiopathic sudden SNHL should receive comprehensive treatment as soon as possible to exclude serious underlying systemic disease.

Treatment selection ideally should be based on the cause (163). For the present, however, the best that can be done is to classify patients according to prognostic risk factors. These are the severity and type of hearing loss (low-frequency upsloping loss, flat loss, or high-frequency downsloping loss) and the presence or absence of vertigo and ENG abnormalities. Kallinen et al. (170) found, for example, that carbogen was more effective in the treatment of patients with high-frequency losses and that anticoagulant therapy was more effective in treating those with low-frequency losses. Laird and Wilson (152) also found a relation between hearing status and outcome. Patients with mild, midfrequency losses recovered spontaneously, and those with severe flat losses did poorly. Treatment with corticosteroids helped those with moderate to moderately severe losses. Laird and Wilson (152) also found that ENG abnormalities were associated with poorer outcome. These observations may be useful for prognostication, but their validity as criteria for patient selection has not been established.

Most studies have involved a multimodality treatment strategy based on the assumption that one or more medications or techniques will reverse the pathophysiologic changes in the auditory system. This empiric strategy is a rational approach to patient care, but it makes assessment of the efficacy of any single agent difficult. An emerging trend in health care is emphasizing value of therapy above cost effectiveness per se. Without broadly based, nationwide studies, it is becoming increasingly difficult to define the value of polytherapy for idiopathic sudden SNHL. Nonetheless, physicians continue to seek to provide the best scientifically based treatment possible. The following section reviews the efficacy of the most widely used therapies for idiopathic sudden SNHL.

Antiviral Therapy

Given the presumed high prevalence of viral infection associated with sudden SNHL, it is remarkable that antiviral therapy has received little use. Interferon alpha has been used to manage sudden SNHL; 64% of patients (27/42) had full recovery (176a). The prevalence of herpesvirus infection in sudden SNHL suggests that acyclovir would be effective in a proportion of cases. The combination of prednisone and acyclovir has shown benefit for hearing and facial paralysis in the management of Ramsay Hunt syndrome with an advantage for those receiving early treatment (177).

Antiinflammatory Therapy

Corticosteroid treatment has received the greatest attention and has been found effective in two studies. Wilson et al. (178) conducted a landmark prospective study. They reported the outcome for 119 patients with idiopathic sudden SNHL who were randomly assigned at either one of two institutions to receive prednisone or placebo within 10 days of the onset of the loss. Evaluations were double blind. The drug was administered in divided doses at the rate of 80 mg/day for 4 days with a rapid taper over 8 days. The investigators found no treatment effect at the extremes of hearing loss. There was poor recovery among persons with severe loss in both the treatment and control groups and excellent recovery in both groups with mild losses. The subjects with moderate hearing losses had a treatment benefit: the response rate was 38% in the placebo group and 78% in the treated group. In a study by Moskowitz et al. (179) 36 patients were treated nonrandomly and evaluated openly in a private practice setting over a 10-year period. Twenty-seven patients received 0.75 mg dexamethasone (Decadron) four times a day for 3 days with a slow, 9-day taper. The investigators found a recovery of at least 50% of the hearing loss in 89% of the corticosteroid group as opposed to 44% in the untreated group. They also found vertigo to affect prognosis adversely but found no relation between audiogram shape and outcome, except that patients with severe losses, which are generally of a flat profile, did poorly.

Corticosteroid therapy has become the standard of therapy for idiopathic sudden SNHL (169). A short course of a corticosteroid generally is well tolerated even though insomnia and restlessness can occur (179). Caution should be exercised in the care of patients with diabetes mellitus, pregnancy, and systemic infection. The corticosteroid appears to suppress inflammatory changes that might otherwise cause cellular infiltration and tissue edema. Limitation of the inflammatory response is presumed to increase tissue perfusion. Corticosteroid treatment was associated with return of normal hearing in one patient with temporal arteritis with sudden SNHL (58).

Rheologic Therapy

Given the many observations about circulatory disturbances as a factor in idiopathic sudden SNHL and the likelihood that viral illnesses may affect hearing by impairing the microcirculation, it is prudent to consider therapy to enhance blood flow through the cochlea. Unfortunately, there are no data to confirm the efficacy of rheologic therapy or to suggest which form might achieve the greatest benefit in addition to corticosteroid therapy.

Oral vasodilators, such as papaverine or nicotinic acid, produce facial flushing and headache, but there is no evidence that cochlear blood flow is increased (180). Because of autoregulation of cochlear blood flow, the local circulation is maintained within narrow limits to counter fluctuations in the systemic circulation. Intravenously administered histamine has been advocated in the past to increase cochlear circulation through a presumed antivasospastic effect (181). This therapy has not been listed as an indication by the manufacturer and has generally been discarded. The rare possibility of hypertensive crises from occult pheochromocytoma adds to the risk of its use. Mattox and Simmons (146) reported poorer outcomes among patients treated with intravenously administered histamine.

Carbogen is a mixture of 95% oxygen and 5% carbon dioxide that has been used widely to increase cochlear oxygenation through a presumed vasodilative effect on cochlear blood flow (170,182–185). Fisch (182), in a prospective randomized study involving subjects with idiopathic sudden SNHL, found significantly better outcomes among patients treated with carbogen inhalation than among those treated with orally administered papaverine and low-molecular-weight dextran. Edamatsu et al. (186) compared the hearing results among 86 patients treated with a polytherapy regimen, of whom 51 received carbogen and 35 did not, and found no difference in outcome. Kallinen et al. (170) evaluated the outcomes of 186 patients with sudden SNHL assigned to one of three treatment groups: anticoagulant, anticoagulant plus carbogen, and carbogen only. There was interaction between type of sudden SNHL and therapeutic outcome. Patients with low-frequency losses had more recovery with anticoagulation, whereas those with flat or high-frequency losses improved more with carbogen. None of the

patients had abnormalities in partial thromboplastin or activated partial thromboplastin times.

Carbogen treatment is given for periods of 15 to 30 minutes four to six times per day. It could be used as for outpatient or home therapy except for logistic difficulties. Given the nonuniform results from carbogen therapy, it is difficult to advise patients that expensive hospitalization for carbogen treatment is a cost-effective treatment. Given its safety, however, it should be made more widely available for home treatment.

Low-molecular-weight dextran has been used intravenously as a volume expander to decrease vascular sludging. (*Sludging* is an ill-defined term used to indicate any disorder in which blood flow decreases because of hyperviscosity, increased cellular adherence, or the presence of circulating fibrin products.) Hultcrantz et al. (166) reported their experience in Sweden with 112 patients over 10 years with 68% recovery rate and no serious complications. A death was reported (187) in conjunction with the use of low-molecular-weight dextran in the management of sudden SNHL. Because of the risk for allergy and the need to administer the material intravenously, this treatment has not received wide use in the United States.

First introduced by Dauman et al. (188), hemodilution is a less risky alternative method to dextran administration for decreasing intravascular sludging. In normovolemic hemodilution a single unit of blood is removed and replaced with a standard surgical plasma volume expander. This drops the hematocrit slightly and lowers blood viscosity and presumably decreases the tendency toward cellular sludging. Hypervolemic hemodilution was achieved by means of transfusion of hydroxyethyl starch plus pentoxifylline (189), but the results were similar to those for a control group that received saline infusion. Pentoxifylline is used to further reduce red blood cell adhesiveness and facilitate microcirculatory flow. The value of pentoxifylline in the acute situation is not established because of the long time required for an effect. Defibrination therapy with batroxobin and low-molecular-weight dextran has been explored in Japan (190) with apparently encouraging results among patients with severe flat hearing losses.

Use of anticoagulant therapy was reported by Donaldson (191). The results were not different from those among historical controls with recovery in 70%. Heparin therapy has been complicated by priapism (192) and is no longer used routinely in the United States. Many physicians recommend a daily, low-dose aspirin tablet to reduce platelet function, as is recommended for many cardiac patients.

Other Drugs

The possible value of intravenous contrast agents, reported by Morimitsu in 1977, was discovered accidentally after a patient with sudden SNHL noticed the return of hearing after an arteriogram (193). Emmett et al. (194) reported an 80% rate of return to normal hearing with the use of diatrizoate meglumine (Hypaque). This encouraging result has generally been replicated (194–197). However, most of the patients in these reports underwent polytherapy. No results of controlled clinical trial show the efficacy of intravenous contrast agents. The mechanism of effect is unknown, but theories have suggested an effect on the stria vascularis. Most studies of use of diatrizoate meglumine have included a variety of other agents, which obscures the effect of any single component. The investigators found better results among patients with some residual hearing and without vertigo who were treated within the first 30 days after onset. Allergic reactions to contrast agents, some fatal, raise concern about use of these substances. The following agents have been assessed in clinical studies and found to not have a measurable effect on outcome: calcium channel blockers (198), prostaglandin E_1 infusion (199), and ethacrynic acid (200).

Surgery

Exploratory tympanotomy has been used to treat patients with sudden SNHL who have a history of a discrete pressure event and who do not recover after 10 to 14 days of rest (201). Preoperative testing has largely been ineffective at identifying fistulas (202). Harris (201) reported a fistula detection rate of 89% among 157 patients with sudden SNHL who underwent exploratory tympanotomy but a hearing recovery rate of only 20%. Surgical treatment is clearly indicated in the care of persons with recurrent meningitis to prevent further infection and may be indicated in the care of persons with persistent vertigo and evidence of a fistula. The simultaneous presence of double membrane breaks may well account for the low effectiveness of surgical therapy for sudden SNHL (140). The method of Black et al. (203) for sealing a fistula incorporates autologous fibrin adhesive.

RESULTS

There are two problems in interpreting the results of studies reported in the literature. First, one must rely chiefly on historical controls because few of the reports include a comparison group. This presents an additional problem: the lack of validated clinical criteria for judging the comparability of the subjects or the nature of the illness among the various studies. In other words, one cannot be assured that the causes of sudden SNHL in study A were similar to those in study B because we lack reliable markers of causation. The recovery rates published in the literature vary widely. Assuming that these rates might just reflect the natural history of the disease, which is not at all clear, one might ask, "Which is the true rate?"

We cannot know whether the variations are caused by a different mix of causes each with its own prognosis, by yearly variations in the virulence of the agent, or by variations in host susceptibilities. Even though we have results of a few randomized clinical trials of therapy for sudden SNHL, we must rely heavily on these results for guidance because they provide concurrent controls.

The second problem is the cognitive dissonance that resounds in the literature. The untreated recovery rate to serviceable hearing cited by Mattox (163) was 63% in one report. In a later report, the recovery rate after intensive "shotgun" treatment was 52% of 33 patients receiving the full treatment and 54% of 76 cases who received most of the regimen (183). Byl (160) found a 45% rate of recovery to normal levels among 225 treated patients. Taken literally, these results might be construed as suggesting that therapy is harmful because the rate with treatment is lower than that among historical controls; in all likelihood, however, the historical controls differed from the treated patients in undetected ways. The authors of these three studies suggested that treatment was probably ineffective and the outcomes probably reflected the natural history of the disorder. Such statements are opinions and interpretations. Because they are not based on the outcomes among a placebo-treated control group, the results should be applied with caution.

Consider the natural history response rate in the placebo group in the study by Wilson et al. (178), which was 32% for the group randomly assigned to receive placebo and 58% for a group of 52 patients who refused randomization but received no treatment. Grandis et al. (185), in noting that only 54% of their patients had improvement of 10 dB or more, may have concluded with undue pessimism that their treatment regimen failed because the improvement rate was lower than the "natural history rate." Had they compared their results with the 32% recovery rate among the placebo group in the study by Wilson et al. (178), Grandis et al. might have concluded their treatment did have an effect. There is simply no way to know whether these results were not significantly different, including the possibility they may have been worse, from those due to natural history simply because there was no control group that would have been likely to account for variation in causation and case mix from earlier studies. If the cases of hearing loss in the study by Grandis et al. were more severe, the true treatment efficacy might have been better than the natural history results. Future studies of idiopathic sudden SNHL should plan for a concurrent randomly assigned control group.

There is a pressing need for clarification of the dilemmas posed by the relative lack of knowledge of the clinical pathologic process of sudden SNHL. Clarification can best be gained through the classic approach to biomedical science—a combination of fundamental and applied research. As our understanding of cochlear function has expanded, it should be possible to develop better methods of assessment of the normal and abnormal physiologic processes of the labyrinth such that reliable indices of function can be developed at the systems, cellular, and molecular levels. This research should allow us to properly identify and categorize the nature of the pathophysiologic perturbations in each patient. Once we can accurately classify and stage the disease, we can direct therapeutic approaches to the proper patients. We will then have a chance at determining the true value of the many options available now and in the future for the treatment of patients with idiopathic sudden SNHL.

SUMMARY POINTS

- Sudden SNHL is a common disorder of uncertain causation that causes an abrupt decrease in auditory function, often with vertigo, due to cochlear dysfunction.
- The hearing loss begins suddenly and has a variable prognosis, with full recovery in some cases and partial recovery in most.
- The cause is presumed to be viral and may be mediated by vascular involvement.
- Evaluation is directed at excluding treatable causes such as tumor or specific infection.
- Poor prognosis is indicated by severity of hearing loss, shape of loss on an audiogram (downsloping is worse), presence of vertigo, and evidence of systemic infection (elevated ESR).
- Treatment often is multimodal, although corticosteroids are the only agents shown to be effective and only for intermediate loss.
- Recurrent hearing loss or involvement of the opposite ear is uncommon and suggests a systemic disorder.
- Research into the causation and pathogenesis of sudden SNHL is vitally needed.

REFERENCES

1. Kam Hansen S, Sorensen H. Selective impairment of hearing and vestibular function in a brain stem lesion. *J Laryngol Otol* 1978;92:505–510.
2. Wilson WR, Laird N, Moo Young G, Soeldner JS, Kavesh DA, MacMeel JW. The relationship of idiopathic sudden hearing loss to diabetes mellitus. *Laryngoscope* 1982;92:155–160.
3. Veltri RW, Wilson WR, Sprinkle PM, Rodman SM, Kavesh DA. The implication of viruses in idiopathic sudden hearing loss: primary infection or reactivation of latent viruses? *Otolaryngol Head Neck Surg* 1981;89:137–141.
4. Nomura Y, Harada T, Sakata H, Sugiura A. Sudden deafness and asymptomatic mumps. *Acta Otolaryngol Suppl Stockh* 1988;456:9–11.
5. Liao BS, Byl FM, Adour KK. Audiometric comparison of Lassa fever hearing loss and idiopathic sudden hearing loss: evidence for viral cause [Comment]. *Otolaryngol Head Neck Surg* 1992;106:226–229.
6. Wilson WR. The relationship of the herpesvirus family to sudden hearing loss: a prospective clinical study and literature review. *Laryngoscope* 1986;96:870–877.
7. Hiraide F, Kakoi H, Miyoshi S, Morita M. Acute profound deafness in Ramsay Hunt syndrome: two case reports. *Acta Otolaryngol Suppl Stockh* 1988;456:49–54.
8. Scott MJS, Scott MJ Jr. Ipsilateral deafness and herpes zoster ophthalmicus. *Arch Dermatol* 1983;119:235–236.
9. Wayman DM, Pham HN, Byl FM, Adour KK. Audiological manifestations of Ramsay Hunt syndrome. *J Laryngol Otol* 1990;104:104–108.
10. Fukuda S, Furuta Y, Takasu T, Suzuki S, Inuyama Y, Nagashima K. The significance of herpes viral latency in the spiral ganglia. *Acta Otolaryngol Suppl Stockh* 1994;514:108–110.
11. Koide J, Yanagita N, Hondo R, Kurata T. Serological and clinical study of herpes simplex virus infection in patients with sudden deafness. *Acta Otolaryngol Suppl Stockh* 1988;456:21–26.
12. Urban GE Jr. Severe sensorineural hearing loss associated with viral hepatitis. *South Med J* 1978;71:724–725.
13. Pyykko I, Vesanen M, Asikainen K, Koskiniemi M, Airaksinen L, Vaheri A. Human spumaretrovirus in the etiology of sudden hearing loss. *Acta Otolaryngol Stockh* 1993;113:109–112.
14. Bhandari R, Steinman GS. Sudden deafness in chickenpox: a case report [Letter]. *Ann Neurol* 1983;13:347.
15. Williams LL, Lowery HW, Glaser R. Sudden hearing loss following infectious mononucleosis: possible effect of altered immunoregulation. *Pediatrics* 1985;75:1020–1027.
16. Shian WJ, Chi CS. Sudden hearing loss caused by Epstein-Barr virus. *Pediatr Infect Dis J* 1994;13:756–758.
17. Real R, Thomas M, Gerwin JM. Sudden hearing loss and acquired immunodeficiency syndrome. *Otolaryngol Head Neck Surg* 1987;97:409–412.
18. Timon CI, Walsh MA. Sudden sensorineural hearing loss as a presentation of HIV infection. *J Laryngol Otol* 1989;103:1071–1072.
19. Rarey KE. Otologic pathophysiology in patients with human immunodeficiency virus. *Am J Otolaryngol* 1990;11:366–369.
20. Kwartler JA, Linthicum FH, Jahn AF, Hawke M. Sudden hearing loss due to AIDS-related cryptococcal meningitis: a temporal bone study. *Otolaryngol Head Neck Surg* 1991;104:265–269.
21. Hanner P, Rosenhall U, Edstrom S, Kaijser B. Hearing impairment in patients with antibody production against *Borrelia burgdorferi* antigen. *Lancet* 1989;1:13–15.
22. Hyden D, Roberg M, Odkvist L. Borreliosis as a cause of sudden deafness and vestibular neuritis in Sweden. *Acta Otolaryngol Suppl Stockh* 1995;520:320–322.
23. Katholm M, Johnsen NJ, Siim C, Willumsen L. Bilateral sudden deafness and acute acquired toxoplasmosis. *J Laryngol Otol* 1991;105:115–118.
24. Nadol JB Jr. Hearing loss of acquired syphilis: diagnosis confirmed by incudectomy. *Laryngoscope* 1975;85:1888–1897.
25. Balkany TJ, Dans PE. Reversible sudden deafness in early acquired syphilis. *Arch Otolaryngol* 1978;104:66–68.
26. Linstrom CJ, Gleich LL. Otosyphilis: diagnostic and therapeutic update. *J Otolaryngol* 1993;22:401–408.
27. Merino GE, Hellin Meseguer D, Garcia Ortega F, Mondejar JM. Sudden deafness and cerebellar tumour. *J Laryngol Otol* 1994;108:584–586.
28. Monroe JA, Krauth L, Arenberg IK, Prenger E, Philpott P. Normal evoked otoacoustic emissions with a profound hearing loss due to a juvenile pilocytic astrocytoma. *Am J Otol* 1996;17:639–642.
29. Igarashi M, Card GG, Johnson PE, Alford BR. Bilateral sudden hearing loss and metastatic pancreatic adenocarcinoma. *Arch Otolaryngol* 1979;105:196–199.
30. Moloy PJ, del Junco R, Porter RW, Brackmann DE. Metastasis from an unknown primary presenting as a tumor in the internal auditory meatus. *Am J Otol* 1989;10:297–300.
31. Pringle MB, Jefferis AF, Barrett GS. Sensorineural hearing loss caused by metastatic prostatic carcinoma: a case report. *J Laryngol Otol* 1993;107:933–934.
32. Nageris B, Or R, Hardan I, Polliack A. Sudden onset deafness as a presenting manifestation of chronic lymphocytic leukemia. *Leuk Lymphoma* 1993;9:269–271.
33. Keay D. Total bilateral hearing loss as a complication of myeloma. *J Laryngol Otol* 1988;102:357–358.
34. Berg HM, Cohen NL, Hammerschlag PE, Waltzman SB. Acoustic neuroma presenting as sudden hearing loss with recovery. *Otolaryngol Head Neck Surg* 1986;94:15–22.

35. Pensak ML, Glasscock ME III, Josey AF, Jackson CG, Gulya AJ. Sudden hearing loss and cerebellopontine angle tumors. *Laryngoscope* 1985;95:1188–1193.

36. Sataloff RT, Davies B, Myers DL. Acoustic neuromas presenting as sudden deafness. *Am J Otol* 1985;6:349–352.

37. Ogawa K, Kanzaki J, Ogawa S, Tsuchihashi N, Inoue Y. Acoustic neuromas presenting as sudden hearing loss. *Acta Otolaryngol Suppl Stockh* 1991;487:138–143.

38. Yanagihara N, Asai M. Sudden hearing loss induced by acoustic neuroma: significance of small tumors. *Laryngoscope* 1993;103:308–311.

39. Moffat DA, Baguley DM, von Blumenthal H, Irving RM, Hardy DG. Sudden deafness in vestibular schwannoma. *J Laryngol Otol* 1994;108:116–119.

40. Mineta H, Nozue M, Ito H, Nozawa O, Nanba T. Acoustic tumor with hearing loss of sudden onset and recovery. *Auris Nasus Larynx* 1986;13[Suppl 2]:S123–S129.

41. Berenholz LP, Eriksen C, Hirsh FA. Recovery from repeated sudden hearing loss with corticosteroid use in the presence of an acoustic neuroma. *Ann Otol Rhinol Laryngol* 1992;101:827–831.

42. Yoshimoto Y. Clinico-statistical study on acoustic tumors with sudden hearing loss. *Auris Nasus Larynx* 1988;15:165–171.

43. Saunders JE, Luxford WM, Devgan KK, Fetterman BL. Sudden hearing loss in acoustic neuroma patients. *Otolaryngol Head Neck Surg* 1995;113:23–31.

44. Millen SJ, Toohill RJ, Lehman RH. Sudden sensorineural hearing loss: operative complication in non-otologic surgery. *Laryngoscope* 1982;92:613–617.

45. Plasse HM, Mittleman M, Frost JO. Unilateral sudden hearing loss after open heart surgery: a detailed study of seven cases. *Laryngoscope* 1981;91:101–109.

46. Young IM, Mehta GK, Lowry LD. Unilateral sudden hearing loss with complete recovery following cardiopulmonary bypass surgery. *Yonsei Med J* 1987;28:152–156.

47. Ness JA, Stankiewicz JA, Kaniff T, Pifarre R, Allegretti J. Sensorineural hearing loss associated with aortocoronary bypass surgery: a prospective analysis. *Laryngoscope* 1993;103:589–593.

48. Evan KE, Tavill MA, Goldberg AN, Silverstein H. Sudden sensorineural hearing loss after general anesthesia for nonotologic surgery. *Laryngoscope* 1997;107:747–752.

49. Judkins RF, Rubin AM. Sudden hearing loss and unstable angina pectoris. *Ear Nose Throat J* 1995;74:96–99.

50. Zajtchuk JT, Falor WH Jr, Rhodes MF. Hypercoagulability as a cause of sudden neurosensory hearing loss. *Otolaryngol Head Neck Surg* 1979;87:268–273.

51. Wells M, Michaels L, Wells DG. Otolaryngological disturbances in Waldenstrom's macroglobulinaemia. *Clin Otolaryngol* 1977;2:327–338.

52. Platia EV, Saral R. Deafness and Waldenstrom's macroglobulinemia. *South Med J* 1979;72:1495–1496.

53. Sando I, Egami T. Inner ear hemorrhage and endolymphatic hydrops in a leukemic patient with sudden hearing loss. *Ann Otol Rhinol Laryngol* 1977;86:518–524.

54. Johnson A, Hawke M, Berger G. Sudden deafness and vertigo due to inner ear hemorrhage: a temporal bone case report. *J Otolaryngol* 1984;13:201–207.

55. Kirikae I, Nomura Y, Shitara T. Sudden deafness due to Buerger's disease. *Arch Otolaryngol* 1962;75:502–505.

56. Jenkins HA, Pollack AM, Fisch U. Polyarteritis nodosa as a cause of sudden deafness. *Am J Otolaryngol* 1981;2:99–107.

57. Rowe Jones JM, Macallan DC, Sorooshian M. Polyarteritis nodosa presenting as bilateral sudden onset cochleo-vestibular failure in a young woman. *J Laryngol Otol* 1990;104:562–564.

58. Wolfovitz E, Levy Y, Brook JG. Sudden deafness in a patient with temporal arteritis. *J Rheumatol* 1987;14:384–385.

59. Orchik DJ, Dunn JW. Sickle cell anemia and sudden deafness. *Arch Otolaryngol* 1977;103:369–370.

60. O'Keeffe LJ, Maw AR. Sudden total deafness in sickle cell disease. *J Laryngol Otol* 1991;105:653–655.

61. Schreibstein JM, MacDonald CB, Cox LC, McMahon L, Bloom DL. Sudden hearing loss in sickle cell disease: a case report. *Otolaryngol Head Neck Surg* 1997;116:541–544.

62. Bowman CA, Linthicum FH Jr, Nelson RA, Mikami K, Quismorio F. Sensorineural hearing loss associated with systemic lupus erythematosus. *Otolaryngol Head Neck Surg* 1986;94:197–204.

63. Caldarelli DD, Rejowski JE, Corey JP. Sensorineural hearing loss in lupus erythematosus. *Am J Otol* 1986;7:210–213.

64. Hisashi K, Komune S, Taira T, Uemura T, Sadoshima S, Tsuda H. Anticardiolipin antibody–induced sudden profound sensorineural hearing loss. *Am J Otolaryngol* 1993;14:275–277.

65. Hybels RL, Rice DH. Neuro-otologic manifestations of sarcoidosis. *Laryngoscope* 1976;86:1873–1878.

66. Souliere CR Jr, Kava CR, Barrs DM, Bell AF. Sudden hearing loss as the sole manifestation of neurosarcoidosis. *Otolaryngol Head Neck Surg* 1991;105:376–381.

67. Ravi KV, Henderson A. Sudden deafness as the sole presenting symptom of diabetes mellitus: a case report. *J Laryngol Otol* 1996;110:59–61.

68. Hollanders D. Sensorineural deafness: a new complication of ulcerative colitis? *Postgrad Med J* 1986;62:753–755.

69. Gemignani G, Berrettini S, Bruschini P, et al. Hearing and vestibular disturbances in Behcet's syndrome. *Ann Otol Rhinol Laryngol* 1991;100:459–463.

70. Cote DN, Molony TB, Waxman J, Parsa D. Cogan's syndrome manifesting as sudden bilateral deafness: diagnosis and management. *South Med J* 1993;86:1056–1060.

71. Haynes BF, Pikus A, Kaiser Kupfer M, Fauci AS. Successful treatment of sudden hearing loss in Cogan's syndrome with corticosteroids. *Arthritis Rheum* 1981;24:501–503.

72. Moriyama K, Nozaki M, Kudo J, Takita A, Tatewaki E, Yasuda K. Sudden deafness in a man with thyrotoxic hypokalemic periodic paralysis. *Jpn J Med* 1988;27:329–332.

73. Ogawa K, Kanzaki J. Aplastic anemia and sudden sensorineural hearing loss. *Acta Otolaryngol Suppl Stockh* 1994;514:85–88.

74. Hoshino T, Ishii T, Kodama A, Kato I. Temporal bone findings in a case of sudden deafness and relapsing polychondritis. *Acta Otolaryngol Stockh* 1980;90:257–261.

75. McGill T. Carcinomatous encephalomyelitis with auditory and vestibular manifestations. *Ann Otol Rhinol Laryngol* 1976;85:120–126.

76. Kremer D, Hood WG, Nuki G. Sudden deafness with serosanguinous middle ear effusions in a patient with rheumatoid arthritis. *Br J Clin Pract* 1975;29:347–348.

77. Brookes GB. Immune complex–associated deafness: preliminary communication. *J R Soc Med* 1985;78:47–55.

78. Kanzaki J. Immune-mediated sensorineural hearing loss. *Acta Otolaryngol Suppl Stockh* 1994;514:70–72.

79. Veldman JE. Cochlear and retrocochlear immune-mediated inner ear disorders. Pathogenetic mechanisms and diagnostic tools. *Ann Otol Rhinol Laryngol* 1986;95:535–540.

80. Mayot D, Bene MC, Dron K, Perrin C, Faure GC. Immunologic alterations in patients with sensorineural hearing disorders. *Clin Immunol Immunopathol* 1993;68:41–45.

81. Yoshida Y, Yamauchi S, Shinkawa A, Horiuchi M, Sakai M. Immunological and virological study of sudden deafness. *Auris Nasus Larynx* 1996;23:63–68.

82. Mair IW, Elverland HH. Sudden deafness and vaccination. *J Laryngol Otol* 1977;91:323–329.

83. Hulbert TV, Larsen RA, Davis CL, et al. Bilateral hearing loss after measles and rubella vaccination in an adult. *N Engl J Med* 1991;325:134–135.

84. Vural A, Onder T, Tanboga H. A case of sudden deafness probably due to antithymocyte globulin treatment [Letter]. *Nephron* 1995;69:345.

85. Jabbari B, Marsh EE, Gunderson CH. The site of the lesion in acute deafness of multiple sclerosis: contribution of the brain stem auditory evoked potential test. *Clin Electroencephalogr* 1982;13:241–244.

86. Fischer C, Mauguiere F, Ibanez V, Confavreux C, Chazot G. The acute deafness of definite multiple sclerosis: BAEP patterns. *Electroencephalogr Clin Neurophysiol* 1985;61:7–15.

87. Shea JJ III, Brackmann DE. Multiple sclerosis manifesting as sudden hearing loss. *Otolaryngol Head Neck Surg* 1987;97:335–338.

88. Franklin DJ, Coker NJ, Jenkins HA. Sudden sensorineural hearing loss as a presentation of multiple sclerosis. *Arch Otolaryngol Head Neck Surg* 1989;115:41–45.

89. Furman JM, Durrant JD, Hirsch WL. Eighth nerve signs in a case of multiple sclerosis. *Am J Otolaryngol* 1989;10:376–381.

90. Schweitzer VG, Shepard N. Sudden hearing loss: an uncommon manifestation of multiple sclerosis. *Otolaryngol Head Neck Surg* 1989;100:327–332.

91. Biavati MJ, Gross JD, Wilson WR, Dina TS. Magnetic resonance

imaging evidence of a focal pontine ischemia in sudden hearing loss and seventh nerve paralysis. *Am J Otol* 1994;15:250–253.

92. Huang MH, Huang CC, Ryu SJ, Chu NS. Sudden bilateral hearing impairment in vertebrobasilar occlusive disease. *Stroke* 1993;24:132–137.

93. Ho KJ, Kileny P, Paccioretti D, McLean DR. Neurologic, audiologic, and electrophysiologic sequelae of bilateral temporal lobe lesions. *Arch Neurol* 1987;44:982–987.

94. Colclasure JB, Graham SS. Intracranial aneurysm occurring as sensorineural hearing loss. *Otolaryngol Head Neck Surg* 1981;89:283–287.

95. Viirre ES, Baloh RW. Migraine as a cause of sudden hearing loss. *Headache* 1996;36:24–28.

96. Gelfand SA, Silman S. Functional hearing loss and its relationship to resolved hearing levels. *Ear Hear* 1985;6:151–158.

97. Moffat DA, Ramsden RT. Profound bilateral sensorineural hearing loss during gentamicin therapy. *J Laryngol Otol* 1977;91:511–516.

98. Arnold W, Nadol JB Jr, Weidauer H. Ultrastructural histopathology in a case of human ototoxicity due to loop diuretics. *Acta Otolaryngol Stockh* 1981;91:399–414.

99. Buhrer C, Weinel P, Sauter S, Reiter A, Riehm H, Laszig R. Acute onset deafness in a 4-year-old girl after a single infusion of cis-platinum. *Pediatr Hematol Oncol* 1990;7:145–148.

100. Darlow BA, Horwood LJ, Mogridge N, Clemett RS. Prospective study of New Zealand very low birthweight infants: outcome at 7-8 years. *J Paediatr Child Health* 1997;33:47–51.

101. Chapman P. Naproxen and sudden hearing loss. *J Laryngol Otol* 1982;96:163–166.

102. Kanda Y, Shigeno K, Matsuo H, Yano M, Yamada N, Kumagami H. Interferon-induced sudden hearing loss. *Audiology* 1995;34:98–102.

103. Pace Balzan A, Ramsden RT. Sudden bilateral sensorineural hearing loss during treatment with dantrolene sodium (Dantrium). *J Laryngol Otol* 1988;102:57–58.

104. Hanna GS. Sudden deafness and the contraceptive pill. *J Laryngol Otol* 1986;100:701–706.

105. Harell M, Shea JJ, Emmett JR. Bilateral sudden deafness following combined insecticide poisoning. *Laryngoscope* 1978;88:348–351.

106. Jaffe BF. Viral causes of sudden inner ear deafness. *Otolaryngol Clin North Am* 1978;11:63–69.

107. Schuknecht HF, Donovan ED. The pathology of idiopathic sudden sensorineural hearing loss. *Arch Otorhinolaryngol* 1986;243:1–15.

108. Wilson WR, Veltri RW, Laird N, Sprinkle PM. Viral and epidemiologic studies of idiopathic sudden hearing loss. *Otolaryngol Head Neck Surg* 1983;91:653–658.

109. Laurikainen E, Aantaa E, Kallinen J. Electronystagmographic findings and recovery of cochlear and vestibular function in patients suffering from sudden deafness with a special reference to the effect of anticoagulation. *Audiology* 1989;28:262–267.

110. Okamoto M, Shitara T, Nakayama M, et al. Sudden deafness accompanied by asymptomatic mumps. *Acta Otolaryngol Suppl Stockh* 1994;514:45–48.

111. Khetarpal U, Nadol JB Jr, Glynn RJ. Idiopathic sudden sensorineural hearing loss and postnatal viral labyrinthitis: a statistical comparison of temporal bone findings. *Ann Otol Rhinol Laryngol* 1990;99:969–976.

112. Gates GA, Mikiten TM. Idiopathic facial paralyses (Bell's palsies). In: Graham M, House W, eds. *Disorders of the facial nerve.* New York: Raven Press, 1982:279–285.

113. Schuknecht HF, Kitamura K. Vestibular neuronitis. *Ann Otol Rhinol Laryngol* 1981;90:1–19.

114. Murphy TP, Teller DC. Magnetic resonance imaging of the facial nerve during Bell's palsy. *Otolaryngol Head Neck Surg* 1991;105:667–674.

115. Richards TL, Gates GA, Gardner JC, et al. Functional MR spectroscopy of the auditory cortex in healthy subjects and patients with sudden hearing loss [see comments]. *AJNR Am J Neuroradiol* 1997;18:611–620.

116. Comacchio F, D'Eredita R, Marchiori C. MRI evidence of labyrinthine and eighth-nerve bundle involvement in mumps virus sudden deafness and vertigo. *ORL J Otorhinolaryngol Relat Spec* 1996;58:295–297.

117. Schuknecht HF. Myths in neurotology [Comments]. *Am J Otol* 1992;13:124–126.

118. Kano K, Tono T, Ushisako Y, Morimitsu T, Suzuki Y, Kodama T. Magnetic resonance imaging in patients with sudden deafness. *Acta Otolaryngol Suppl Stockh* 1994;514:32–36.

119. Nagahara K, Fisch U, Yagi N. Perilymph oxygenation in sudden and progressive sensorineural hearing loss. *Acta Otolaryngol Stockh* 1983;96:57–68.

120. Ohinata Y, Makimoto K, Kawakami M, Haginomori S, Araki M, Takahashi H. Blood flow in common carotid and vertebral arteries in patients with sudden deafness. *Ann Otol Rhinol Laryngol* 1997;106:27–32.

121. Snyder SO Jr. Unilateral sudden hearing loss as a result of anomalous carotid anatomy. *J Vasc Surg* 1990;12:341–344.

122. Singleton GT. Cervical sympathetic chain block in sudden deafness. *Laryngoscope* 1971;81:734–736.

123. Lipkin AF, Jenkins HA, Coker NJ. Migraine and sudden sensorineural hearing loss. *Arch Otolaryngol Head Neck Surg* 1987;113:325–326.

124. Lawrence M. The function of the spiral capillaries. *Laryngoscope* 1971;81:1314–1322.

125. Jager W, Idrizbegovic E, Karlsson KK, Alvan G. Quinine-induced hearing loss in the guinea pig is not affected by the Ca2-channel antagonist verapamil. *Acta Otolaryngol Stockh* 1997;117:46–48.

126. Hall SJ, McGuigan JA, Rocks MJ. Red blood cell deformability in sudden sensorineural deafness: another aetiology? *Clin Otolaryngol* 1991;16:3–7.

127. Bomholt A, Bak Pedersen K, Gormsen J. Fibrinolytic activity in patients with sudden sensorineural hearing loss. *Acta Otolaryngol Suppl Stockh* 1979;360:184–186.

128. Owen MC, Borg JY, Soria C, Soria J, Caen J, Carrell RW. Heparin binding defect in a new antithrombin III variant: Rouen, 47 Arg to His. *Blood* 1987;69:1275–1279.

129. Jaffe BF. Hypercoagulation and other causes of sudden hearing loss. *Otolaryngol Clin North Am* 1975;8:395–403.

130. Gold S, Kamerer DB, Hirsch BE, Cass SP. Hypercoagulability in otologic patients. *Am J Otolaryngol* 1993;14:327–331.

131. Asakura M, Kato I, Takahashi K, et al. Increased platelet aggregability in patients with vertigo, sudden deafness and facial palsy. *Acta Otolaryngol Suppl Stockh* 1995;520:399–400.

132. Einer H, Tengborn L, Axelsson A, Edstrom S. Sudden sensorineural hearing loss and hemostatic mechanisms. *Arch Otolaryngol Head Neck Surg* 1994;120:536–540.

133. Shiraishi T, Kubo T, Matsunaga T. Chronological study of recovery of sudden deafness treated with defibrinogenation and steroid therapies. *Acta Otolaryngol Stockh* 1991;111:867–871.

134. Ohinata Y, Makimoto K, Kawakami M, Haginomori S, Araki M, Takahashi H. Blood viscosity and plasma viscosity in patients with sudden deafness. *Acta Otolaryngol Stockh* 1994;114:601–607.

135. Kanzaki J, Nomura Y. Incidence and prognosis of acute profound deafness in Japan. *Auris Nasus Larynx* 1986;13:71–77.

136. Simmons FB. Theory of membrane breaks in sudden hearing loss. *Arch Otolaryngol* 1968;88:41–48.

137. Fee GA. Traumatic perilymphatic fistulas. *Arch Otolaryngol* 1968;88:477–480.

138. Goodhill V. Sudden deafness and round window rupture. *Laryngoscope* 1971;81:1462–1474.

139. Goodhill V, Brockman SJ, Harris I, Hantz O. Sudden deafness and labyrinthine window ruptures: audio-vestibular observations. *Ann Otol Rhinol Laryngol* 1973;82:2–12.

140. Simmons FB. The double-membrane break syndrome in sudden hearing loss. *Laryngoscope* 1979;89:59–66.

141. Yanagihara N, Nishioka I. Pneumolabyrinth in perilymphatic fistula: report of three cases. *Am J Otol* 1997;8:313–318.

142. Nishioka I, Yanagihara N. Role of air bubbles in the perilymph as a cause of sudden deafness. *Am J Otol* 1986;7:430–442.

143. Mafee MF, Valvassori GE, Kumar A, Yannias DA, Marcus RE. Pneumolabyrinth: a new radiologic sign for fracture of the stapes footplate. *Am J Otol* 1984;5:374–375.

144. Grundfast KM, Bluestone CD. Sudden or fluctuating hearing loss and vertigo in children due to perilymph fisutla. *Ann Otol Rhinol Laryngol* 1978;87:761–771.

145. Axelsson A, Miller J, Silverman M. Anatomical effects of sudden middle ear pressure changes. *Ann Otol Rhinol Laryngol* 1997;88:368–376.

146. Mattox DE, Simmons FB. Natural history of sudden sensorineural hearing loss. *Ann Otol Rhinol Laryngol* 1977;86:463–480.

147. Ohlms LA, Lonsbury Martin BL, Martin GK. The clinical application of acoustic distortion products. *Otolaryngol Head Neck Surg* 1990;103:52–59.

148. Portmann M, Dauman R, Aran JM. Audiometric and electrophysiological correlations in sudden deafness. *Acta Otolaryngol Stockh* 1985;99:363–368.

149. Gstoettner W, Swoboda H, Muller C, Burian M. Preclinical detection

of initial vestibulocochlear abnormalities in a patient with multiple sclerosis. *Eur Arch Otorhinolaryngol* 1993;250:40–43.

150. Nadol JB Jr, Weiss AD, Parker SW. Vertigo of delayed onset after sudden deafness. *Ann Otol Rhinol Laryngol* 1975;84:841–846.

151. Watanabe Y, Aso S, Ohi H, Ishikawa M, Mizukoshi K. Vestibular nerve disorder in patients suffering from sudden deafness with vertigo and/or vestibular dysfunction. *Acta Otolaryngol Suppl Stockh* 1993;504: 109–111.

152. Laird N, Wilson WR. Predicting recovery from idiopathic sudden hearing loss. *Am J Otolaryngol* 1983;4:161–164.

153. Ullrich D, Aurbach G, Drobik C. A prospective study of hyperlipidemia as a pathogenic factor in sudden hearing loss. *Eur Arch Otorhinolaryngol* 1992;249:273–276.

154. Weber PC, Zbar RI, Gantz BJ. Appropriateness of magnetic resonance imaging in sudden sensorineural hearing loss. *Otolaryngol Head Neck Surg* 1997;116:153–156.

155. Shelton C, Harnsberger HR, Allen R, King B. Fast spin echo magnetic resonance imaging: clinical application in screening for acoustic neuroma. *Otolaryngol Head Neck Surg* 1996;114:71–76.

156. Hayes C, Tsuruda J, Mathis C. Temporal lobes: surface MR coil phased array imaging. *Radiology* 1993;189:918–920.

157. Filler AG, Kliot M, Howe FA, et al. Application of magnetic resonance neurography in the evaluation of patients with peripheral nerve pathology. *J Neurosurg* 1996;85:299–309.

158. Albers FW, Demuynck KM, Casselman JW. Three-dimensional magnetic resonance imaging of the inner ear in idiopathic sudden sensorineural hearing loss. *ORL J Otorhinolaryngol Relat Spec* 1994;56: 1–4.

159. Mark AS, Seltzer S, Nelson Drake J, Chapman JC, Fitzgerald DC, Gulya AJ. Labyrinthine enhancement on gadolinium-enhanced magnetic resonance imaging in sudden deafness and vertigo: correlation with audiologic and electronystagmographic studies. *Ann Otol Rhinol Laryngol* 1992;101:459–464.

160. Byl FM Jr. Sudden hearing loss: eight years' experience and suggested prognostic table. *Laryngoscope* 1984;94:647–661.

161. Simmons FB. Sudden idiopathic sensorineural hearing loss: some observations. *Laryngoscope* 1973;83:1221–1227.

162. Megighian D, Bolzan M, Barion U, Nicolai P. Epidemiological considerations in sudden hearing loss: a study of 183 cases. *Arch Otorhinolaryngol* 1986;243:250–253.

163. Mattox DE. Medical management of sudden hearing loss. *Otolaryngol Head Neck Surg* 1980;88:111–113.

164. Nakashima T, Yanagita N, Ohno Y, Kanzaki J, Shitara T. Comparative study on sudden deafness by two nationwide epidemiological surveys in Japan. *Acta Otolaryngol Suppl Stockh* 1994;514:14–16.

165. Murai K, Tsuiki T, Shishido K, Hori A. Clinical study of sudden deafness with special reference to onset. *Acta Otolaryngol Suppl Stockh* 1988;456:15–20.

166. Hultcrantz E, Stenquist M, Lyttkens L. Sudden deafness: a retrospective evaluation of dextran therapy. *ORL J Otorhinolaryngol Relat Spec* 1994;56:137–142.

167. Fetterman BL, Luxford WM, Saunders JE. Sudden bilateral sensorineural hearing loss. *Laryngoscope* 1996;106:1347–1350.

168. Wilson WR. Why treat sudden hearing loss. *Am J Otol* 1984;5:481–483.

169. Fetterman BL, Saunders JE, Luxford WM. Prognosis and treatment of sudden sensorineural hearing loss. *Am J Otol* 1996;17:529–536.

170. Kallinen J, Laurikainen E, Laippala P, Grenman R. Sudden deafness: a comparison of anticoagulant therapy and carbogen inhalation therapy. *Ann Otol Rhinol Laryngol* 1997;106:22–26.

171. Nakashima T, Yanagita N. Outcome of sudden deafness with and without vertigo. *Laryngoscope* 1993;103:1145–1149.

172. Civantos F, Choi YS, Applebaum EL. Meningeal carcinomatosis producing bilateral sudden hearing loss: a case report. *Am J Otol* 1992;13: 369–371.

173. Houck JR, Murphy K. Sudden bilateral profound hearing loss resulting from meningeal carcinomatosis. *Otolaryngol Head Neck Surg* 1992; 106:92–97.

174. Bellucci RJ, Grobeisen B, Sah BC. Bilateral sudden deafness in Cogan's syndrome. *Bull NY Acad Med* 1974;50:672–681.

175. Maslan MJ, Graham MD, Flood LM. Cryptococcal meningitis: presentation as sudden deafness. *Am J Otol* 1985;6:435–437.

176. Grimaldi LM, Luzi L, Martino GV, et al. Bilateral eighth cranial nerve neuropathy in human immunodeficiency virus infection. *J Neurol* 1993; 240:363–366.

176a. Kanemaru S, Fukushima H, Nakamura H, Tamaki H, Fukuyama Y, Tamura Y. Alpha-interferon for the treatment of idiopathic sudden sensorineural hearing loss. *Eur Arch Otorhinolaryngol* 1997;254: 158–162.

177. Murakami S, Hato N, Horiuchi J, Honda N, Gyo K, Yanagihara N. Treatment of Ramsay Hunt syndrome with acyclovir-prednisone: significance of early diagnosis and treatment. *Ann Neurol* 1997;41: 353–357.

178. Wilson WR, Byl FM, Laird N. The efficacy of steroids in the treatment of idiopathic sudden hearing loss: a double-blind clinical study. *Arch Otolaryngol* 1980;106:772–776.

179. Moskowitz D, Lee KJ, Smith HW. Steroid use in idiopathic sudden sensorineural hearing loss. *Laryngoscope* 1984;94:664–666.

180. Fisch U, Murata K, Hossli G. Measurement of oxygen tension in human perilymph. *Acta Otolaryngol Stockh* 1976;81:278–282.

181. Sheehy JL, Robinson JV, Bush JE. Intravenous histamine in otologic practice: side effects in 2,347 administrations. *Arch Otolaryngol* 1980; 106:159–160.

182. Fisch U. Management of sudden deafness. *Otolaryngol Head Neck Surg* 1983;91:3–8.

183. Wilkins SA Jr, Mattox DE, Lyles A. Evaluation of a "shotgun" regimen for sudden hearing loss. *Otolaryngol Head Neck Surg* 1987;97: 474–480.

184. Cole RR, Jahrsdoerfer RA. Sudden hearing loss: an update. *Am J Otol* 1988;9:211–215.

185. Grandis JR, Hirsch BE, Wagener MM. Treatment of idiopathic sudden sensorineural hearing loss. *Am J Otol* 1993;14:183–185.

186. Edamatsu H, Hasegawa M, Oku T, Nigauri T, Kurita N, Watanabe I. Treatment of sudden deafness: carbon dioxide and oxygen inhalation and steroids. *Clin Otolaryngol* 1985;10:69–72.

187. Zaytoun GM, Schuknecht HF, Farmer HS. Fatality following the use of low molecular weight dextran in the treatment of sudden deafness. *Adv Otorhinolaryngol* 1983;31:240–246.

188. Dauman R, Cros AM, Mehsen M, Cazals Y. Hemodilution in sudden deafness: first results. *Arch Otorhinolaryngol* 1983;238:97–102.

189. Desloovere C, Lorz M, Klima A. Sudden sensorineural hearing loss influence of hemodynamical and hemorheological factors on spontaneous recovery and therapy results. *Acta Otorhinolaryngol Belg* 1989; 43:31–37.

190. Shiraishi T, Kubo T, Okumura S, et al. Hearing recovery in sudden deafness patients using a modified defibrinogenation therapy. *Acta Otolaryngol Suppl Stockh* 1993;501:46–50.

191. Donaldson JA. Heparin therapy for sudden sensorineural hearing loss. *Arch Otolaryngol* 1979;105:351–354.

192. Clark SK, Tremann JA, Sennewald FR, Donaldson JA. Priapism: an unusual complication of heparin therapy for sudden deafness. *Am J Otolaryngol* 1981;2:69–72.

193. Ushisako Y, Morimitsu T. Studies on amidotrizoate therapy in sudden deafness (1978–1987). *Acta Otolaryngol Suppl Stockh* 1988;456: 37–42.

194. Emmett JR, Shea JJ. Diatrizoate meglumine (Hypaque) treatment for sudden hearing loss. *Laryngoscope* 1979;89:1229–1238.

195. Hirashima N. Treatment of sudden deafness with sodium salts of triiodobenzoic acid derivatives. *Ann Otol Rhinol Laryngol* 1978;87: 29–31.

196. Huang TS, Chan ST, Ho TL, Su JL, Lee FP. Hypaque and steroids in the treatment of sudden sensorineural hearing loss. *Clin Otolaryngol* 1989;14:45–51.

197. Redleaf MI, Bauer CA, Gantz BJ, Hoffman HT, McCabe BF. Diatrizoate and dextran treatment of sudden sensorineural hearing loss. *Am J Otol* 1995;16:295–303.

198. Mann W, Beck C. Calcium antagonists in the treatment of sudden deafness. *Arch Otorhinolaryngol* 1986;243:170–173.

199. Nakashima T, Kuno K, Yanagita N. Evaluation of prostaglandin E1 therapy for sudden deafness. *Laryngoscope* 1989;99:542–546.

200. Konishi K, Nakai Y, Yamane H. The efficacy of Lasix-vitamin therapy (L-V therapy) for sudden deafness and other sensorineural hearing loss. *Acta Otolaryngol Suppl Stockh* 1991;486:78–91.

201. Harris I. Sudden hearing loss: membrane rupture. *Am J Otol* 1984;5: 484–487.

202. Shepard NT, Telian SA, Niparko JK, et al. Platform pressure test in identification of perilymphatic fistula. *Am J Otol* 1992;13:49–54.

203. Black FO, Pesznecker S, Norton T, et al. Surgical management of perilymphatic fistulas: a Portland experience. *Am J Otol* 1992;13:254–262.

The Ear: Comprehensive Otology,
edited by R. F. Canalis and P. R. Lambert.
Lippincott Williams & Wilkins, Philadelphia © 2000.

CHAPTER 32

Autoimmune Inner Ear Disease

Bruce L. Fetterman and Lucy Shih

Rapidly progressive, bilateral sensorineural hearing loss (SNHL) is a devastating condition that often defies aggressive diagnostic measures. Although many causes of SNHL have been identified, few effective or promising treatments exist (1). Advances in otoimmunology have opened a new venue of treatment possibilities. In 1979, McCabe (2) described a small group of patients with a treatable form of SNHL. On the basis of the hypothesized cause, he proposed the new diagnostic entity *autoimmune SNHL*. Since then, many patients worldwide have been found to have an autoimmune form of SNHL (3–8).

Many terms have been used to describe this disorder, including *autoimmune SNHL, immune-mediated inner ear disease or disorder, immune-mediated SNHL,* and *steroid-responsive SNHL* (9–12). However, the most accurate term to characterize this disorder is *autoimmune inner ear disease (AIED)* (6,13,14). In AIED, both cochlear and vestibular dysfunction may occur, and the response to immunosuppressive therapy usually is favorable. The underlying immunopathologic process of AIED is discussed in this chapter. Diagnostic and therapeutic guidelines are presented to assist the clinician in the management of this unusual but treatable disorder of the inner ear.

BACKGROUND

In his original report, McCabe described a type of SNHL among young adults that was typically bilateral,

B. L. Fetterman: Department of Otolaryngology–Head and Neck Surgery, University of Tennessee, Memphis, Tennessee; Shea Ear Clinic, Memphis, Tennessee 38119
L. Shih: Department of Otolaryngology, University of Southern California School of Medicine, Los Angeles, California 90033

asymmetric, and progressive over a period of weeks to months. It was commonly associated with vestibular dysfunction and occasionally with facial paralysis or tissue destruction within the middle ear or mastoid. McCabe found that this unique group of patients responded favorably to immunosuppressive agents and had abnormalities in immunologic tests in which inner ear antigen was used. On the basis of these observations, McCabe concluded the cause was an autoimmune process involving the inner ear (2).

As more cases of AIED are being identified, more variability in clinical presentation is being found than originally described. AIED has been classified into primary and secondary forms. The primary form is an immunologic disorder that begins within the inner ear. The secondary form originates outside the ear (15). The secondary form includes systemic disorders that exert a direct or indirect effect on the function of the inner ear through the presence of circulating immune complexes, systemic vasculitis, or other processes.

GENERAL IMMUNOLOGIC PRINCIPLES

The immune system has two divisions—the nonspecific (innate) response and the specific (adaptive) response. The nonspecific response is the body's first line of defense against infection. Table 1 lists the components of this system. This form of immune response prevents foreign microorganisms from entering the body. If microorganisms gain access, the nonspecific response destroys the invading organisms locally with phagocytic cells that act in concert with nonspecific humoral ele-

TABLE 1. *The nonspecific immune system*

Skin and mucosal membranes (includes cilia)
Enzymes and other substances produced by skin and
  mucosa (e.g., lysozymes, sebaceous gland secretions,
  stomach acid, mucus)
Phagocytes (neutrophils, monocytes, Kupffer cells)
Natural killer cells
Acute phase proteins (e.g., C-reactive protein)
Complement system (via the alternative pathway)
Interferons

ments, such as complement. If the nonspecific immune response fails, the body must rely on its specific response, which consists of humoral (B cell) and cellular (T cell) mediated systems (16,17).

Lymphocytes differentiate from a lymphoid stem cell, the lymphoblast, in the bone marrow. The B lymphocytes complete their maturation in the bone marrow. After stimulation by an antigen, the B cells proliferate and mature into plasma cells. These cells produce specific antibodies directed against one antigen (the antigen that stimulated them). Antibodies constitute about 20% of the total plasma proteins. The hallmark of this system is a high degree of specificity and a built-in memory for foreign substances that have previously stimulated the immune system. The T lymphocytes differentiate under the influence of various hormones in the thymus, regulate the immune response, and control the cell-mediated response. The different subsets of T cells include the helper, suppressor, cytotoxic, delayed hypersensitivity, and amplifier T cells (16,17). After maturation, the different lymphocytes are dispersed into the circulatory system, where they compose 20% to 30% of the leukocytes.

THEORIES OF AUTOIMMUNITY

Autoimmune diseases constitute a condition under which immunoglobulins or T cells display a specificity for self-antigens. Tolerance to self-antigens exists because of processes that occur during fetal development. Potential antigens arise in the fetus before the immune system has matured, and these antigens induce tolerance in the lymphoid cells as they mature and differentiate. The persistence of these antigens enables self-tolerance to continue. If something alters this process, self-antigens can elicit an immune response as if they were exogenous antigens (18,19). For autoimmunity to develop, either the state of tolerance is disrupted or an auto-antigen is produced. Autoimmune responses are not as rare as once thought and not all autoimmune responses cause disease. For example, the idiotype–antiidiotype reaction that regulates antibody production, the immune response to cell

membrane antigens transcribed from the major histocompatibility complex, and phagocytosis of senescent cells are normal processes of the mature immune system (19). The focus of this discussion is on autoimmune processes that cause functional or structural damage.

Five theories have been offered to explain development of an abnormal autoimmune response (18–22). First, there is a response to an antigen that usually does not circulate in the bloodstream (a sequestered antigen). Antigens commonly recognized as being sequestered include milk casein, ocular lens proteins, and certain reproductive system proteins. A potential problem with classifying an antigen as sequestered is that available assays may not have sufficient sensitivity for detection of low levels of a suspected antigen. If such an antigen is not "found" in the blood, it is mistakenly assumed to be noncirculating. Another potential problem is not accounting for the normal degradation and elimination of circulating proteins. An antigen may not be detectable because it is degraded rapidly or cleared from the system quickly.

A second theory to explain autoimmunity is that the immune system reacts to an altered antigen. Antigens can be altered through biologic, chemical, or physical mechanisms. Biologic methods include mutations that produce new antigens that may not be recognized as "self" and can initiate an immune response. These can arise spontaneously or can be induced by processes such as viral infection. Chemical methods are exemplified by the coupling of haptens with normal self-antigens, which cause a response that may later develop into a response against the self-antigen carrier protein only. Physical methods include protein denaturation, ultraviolet and infrared radiation damage, and the effects of temperature on proteins within the body with production of obviously altered antigens capable of initiating an immune response. Inherent with this theory, in which it is assumed that an altered antigen initiates the immune response, is that a reaction against normal antigens would require that the body "confuse" the altered antigens with the normal antigens. A suspected autoimmune response may actually be a "true" immune response in that the body is reacting against the biologically, chemically, or physically altered antigens, and this response inadvertently leads to damage of a normal part of the body.

A third mechanism is a response to nonself-antigens that cross react with self-antigens. It is theoretically possible for a foreign antigen to share a structure or chemical sequence with a self-antigen. If an immune response is directed against the shared portion, these antibodies might initiate an immune response against the foreign antigens and the self-antigens.

Another method involves various genetic mutations that can arise anywhere along the immunologic pathway,

TABLE 2. *Gell and Coombs reactions*

Type	Mediator	Example
I immediate hypersensitivity (allergy)	IgE	Allergic rhinitis, anaphylactic shock
II cytotoxic	IgG, possibly IgM	Hemolytic anemia, Rh disease
III immune complex	IgG, IgM	Arthrus reaction, glomerulonephritis
IV delayed hypersensitivity (cell mediated)	T-cell dependent	Contact dermatitis, tuberculosis

from tolerance induction defects to lymphocyte or lymphocyte product defects, such as immunoglobulins and regulatory proteins. This might allow immunocompetent cells to react with self-antigens.

The last explanation involves a loss of regulation by helper or suppressor T cells, which actually is the loss of self-tolerance. Without immunoregulation, there would be an augmented response against all antigens, both non-self and self.

Damage to a tissue or organ can be caused by either a direct cytotoxic effect initiated by autoantibodies (Gell and Coombs hypersensitivity reaction type II), from deposition of antigen-antibody immune complexes (type III), or from activation of cytotoxic T cells (type IV) (23,24). Table 2 describes the different types of hypersensitivity reactions as classified by Gell and Coombs.

For an immune response to accurately be established as the cause of a disease, Witebsky's postulates should be met (18).

1. The disease must be routinely associated with the autoimmune response.
2. An animal model for the disease must be available.
3. The immunologic and pathologic changes seen in the natural and in the experimental disease should be similar.
4. It should be possible to induce the autoimmune disease in normal recipients by transferring serum or lymphocytes from the subjects with the disease.

For many conditions believed to be caused by autoantibodies, these criteria are not met, and the only conclusion that can be made is that autoantibodies exist and are associated with the disease. In these cases, detection of autoantibodies can help diagnose the disease even though a true cause and effect relation cannot be proved.

INNER EAR IMMUNOLOGY

Much has been learned about the local immune processes of the inner ear, but the specific details of this system are still being worked out. It has been shown that the fluids of the inner ear are protected from extracellular fluids and that the composition of the ear fluids is regulated by several barrier systems—the blood-labyrinth barrier, the cerebrospinal fluid (CSF)–labyrinth barrier, and the middle ear–labyrinth barrier (25). These systems act by means of selective permeability to protect the integrity and function of the inner ear from changes in the surrounding fluids (blood, CSF, and middle ear fluid). This is analogous to the function of the blood-brain barrier in maintaining homeostasis within the central nervous system.

Despite the presence of these barriers, it has been shown that the inner ear is not necessarily an immunoprivileged site because immunoglobulins (Ig) have been detected within the inner ear (26,27). These immunoglobulins, usually IgG but also IgM or IgA, either pass directly through the blood-perilymph barrier or are produced locally within the inner ear (26–30). The concentration of immunoglobulins in perilymph is about 7/1,000 the concentration found in serum and two to four times the concentration found in CSF (26–28). Harris et al. (27,29–32) demonstrated that after exposure to antigen, the inner ear can produce a localized immune response that is independent of CSF and serum, can induce a systemic response, and is stronger after a second exposure.

Many experiments have demonstrated the histologic changes that occur after inner ear and systemic inoculation of inner ear antigens (23,31,33). After the first inner ear antigenic challenge (primary), a localized fibromyxoid reaction with some plasma cells is seen beneath the basilar membrane of the basal cochlear turn. In contrast, after a repeat exposure to inner ear antigen (secondary), a greater immunologic response is seen throughout the membranous labyrinth with plasma cell infiltration of the scala tympani, perilabyrinthine fibrosis, degeneration of spiral ganglion cells and the organ of Corti, and hemorrhage. Primarily immunized animals demonstrate a small elevation in hearing threshold, whereas secondarily immunized animals show a much larger change (31).

When inner ear antigen is given systemically, the immunologic response is similar to the response after direct inner ear challenge (23,33). Antibodies against inner ear antigen were found in serum and perilymph. Lymphocytes and polymorphonuclear leukocytes were seen in the cochlea, endolymphatic sac, and round window membrane, and cochlear neuron loss, perivascular infiltration of plasma cells, edema, and hemorrhage were demonstrated. An elevation in hearing thresholds was found. Many animals had only unilateral losses, and several animals underwent spontaneous remission of experimental autoimmune labyrinthitis, but not complete recovery (23,33). The apparent portal of entry into the inner ear for inflammatory cells is the spiral modiolar vein with its collecting venules. This finding corresponds with the finding of inflammatory cells within the scala tympani, the "venous" side of the inner ear (30,34).

For inner ear inflammatory reactions to occur, an intact endolymphatic sac (ES) is necessary (23,35). The ES contains lymphocytes and macrophages and has a rich surrounding network of lymphatic vessels (36). IgG and IgA have been identified within the ES, whereas no immunocompetent cells have been demonstrated outside the ES in normal ears (7,23). After immune stimulation, there is an increase in the number of plasma cells within the ES and in the connective tissue surrounding the ES (35). These findings suggest that the ES may play a role in the systemic and local immune response to inner ear antigen.

Hearing loss has been demonstrated in animals immunized with type II collagen, a major constituent of the inner ear (37–39). In these animals antibodies to type II collagen developed in both serum and perilymph. When serum from collagen-immunized animals was injected into nonimmunized animals, hearing loss occurred. Histologic changes included perivasculitis with mononuclear infiltrates and fibrosis of the cochlear artery, cochlear neuron degeneration, and inflammation of the organ of Corti and stria vascularis. However, other experiments demonstrating type II collagen antibodies with associated autoimmune arthritis did not show hearing loss or histologic lesions in the temporal bone; this lack of consistency may be due to differences in the animal models used (40). It has been shown that type II collagen generates a strong response in the lymphocyte transformation test (LTT) in about 50% of patients with AIED (41). Other investigators have found antibodies to type II collagen in about 44% of patients with bilateral progressive SNHL and have shown that the detection of collagen antibodies may help identify patients who respond to corticosteroids (42). The results of these studies suggest that in certain cases, type II collagen may be the antigen giving positive results when inner ear extract is used in tests such as leukocyte migration inhibition test (LMIT) or LTT. Thus type II collagen may be important in the development of AIED (43–45).

DIAGNOSTIC EVALUATION

In the evaluation of AIED, a complete medical history is important to help make the diagnosis. The hearing loss should be characterized with emphasis on onset, duration, fluctuation, and progression. The qualities of tinnitus, if present, should be documented. The course of hearing loss in AIED is characteristic and helps to differentiate it from other types of SNHL. Patients with AIED typically have bilateral, progressive SNHL. When present, vestibular symptoms may be similar to those of Meniere's disease; however, rather than being free from symptoms between episodes, patients characteristically have ataxia, especially in the dark (2,46). Many patients with AIED have an associated systemic disorder, so a careful review of systems should be performed to check for rheumatologic or immunosuppressive disorders.

The physical examination findings of the ears typically are normal, although an increase in vascularity of the tympanic membrane has been described (2). The findings of a head and neck examination also may be normal. The visible tissue destruction originally described with this disorder may have been caused by other systemic disorders (2). A thorough neurotologic evaluation must be performed to find abnormalities of the vestibular system and other cranial nerves.

Audiometric test results often vary with the severity and duration of the condition. Hearing loss always is sensorineural, typically bilateral, and often asymmetric. Speech discrimination score varies with the severity of hearing loss. The appropriate use of imaging studies such as computed tomography or magnetic resonance imaging is important to rule out other causes of asymmetric SNHL. If there is systemic involvement, biopsies of other involved sites can be helpful, because tissue biopsy of the inner ear is not possible. A radionuclide scan with gallium which binds to leukocytes, is an effective method to detect inflammation and direct potential biopsy sites (5).

Laboratory studies are determined by the history and need to check for other systemic disorders. The standard screening tests include a complete blood cell count with differential, urinalysis, erythrocyte sedimentation rate (ESR), fluorescent treponemal antibody absorption (FTA-ABS) test, rheumatoid factor, antinuclear antibody (ANA), and a quantitative immunoglobulin analysis of IgG, IgM, and IgA. Not everyone agrees on which are the best tests to screen for an autoimmune abnormality, but the minimum should include ESR, FTA-ABS, and ANA. For more indicative results, these tests should be obtained when the patient has symptoms and before immunosuppressive treatment is begun. If abnormalities are found in the screening tests, additional immunologic studies are performed that include either antigen-specific or antigen-nonspecific tests (10,47). Antigen-specific tests include the LMIT, the LTT, the Western blot assay, indirect immunofluorescence (IIF), and enzyme-linked immunosorbent assay (ELISA). These tests detect immunologic reactivity to inner ear antigens by the presence of a specific cellular or humoral response. Antigen-nonspecific studies include measurements of the complement system (e.g., C3, C4, and CH50), circulating immune complexes (e.g., C1q-binding assay, anti-C3 antibody assay, and Raji cell assay), and cryoglobulins (48). Abnormal results are indirect evidence of altered or enhanced immune processes.

With both the LMIT and LTT it is assumed that the patient's lymphocytes recognize and respond to the inner ear antigen *in vitro* and that the immunologic response is an antigen-antibody response. The inner ear antigen is prepared from intact human membranous labyrinth tissue removed during labyrinthectomy for other diseases (e.g., translabyrinthine craniotomy). This unrefined tissue presumably contains the putative antigen involved with AIED (2,6,10). Because the inner ear antigen mixture contains various components, the specificity of the test results is questionable, especially with the LMIT (5,10,11). However, with suspected AIED, the LTT is considered to have a predictive value of 70%, sensitivity of 70% to 80%, and specificity of 93% (10,47).

The Western blot assay is performed with serum from the test subject and fresh inner ear antigen. Patients with progressive SNHL and animals with hearing loss following immunization with inner ear antigen demonstrate specific banding patterns at the 68 kd region. This appears to represent an autoantibody directed against inner ear antigen (8,49). The target of this autoantibody appears to be a member of the heat shock protein 70 family (50,51). The presence of this antibody has been correlated with activity of the disease and with response to steroids (52). For IIF thinly sliced sections from human or animal temporal bones are incubated with the patient's serum and fluorescein-labeled antibody against human immunoglobulin is added. The specimen is examined with a fluorescence microscope to see whether labeled antibody is present (i.e., attached to human immunoglobulin that is bound to inner ear antigenic sites in the temporal bone). Several investigators have identified inner ear autoantibodies in patients with AIED, and correlation with the LTT has been demonstrated (7,53–55). In ELISA, the patient's serum is added to plates containing extract protein, which is incubated with enzyme-labeled antibody against human immunoglobulin. After unbound antibody is rinsed away, enzyme substrate is added. The resultant color change is measured with a spectrophotometer and compared with controls (10).

THERAPY

The use of immunosuppressive agents has been the foundation of therapy, because AIED represents one of the few causes of sensorineural dysfunction responsive to medical treatment. The realistic expectations of therapy

for this condition are not necessarily to achieve normal hearing but to stabilize the progressive nature of the hearing loss, possibly improve hearing level, and maintain long-term hearing stability.

McCabe emphasized the importance of using cyclophosphamide (CTX) and prednisone as an effective method to test immunoresponsiveness and achieve long-term benefit. He recommended a 4-week trial of 60 mg CTX (2 mg/kg) every 12 hours and 30 mg prednisone every other day. If audiometric test results improve by 15 dB in any three frequencies or by more than 20% in speech discrimination score, the test result is considered positive, and treatment is continued with these two drugs at the same dosage for 3 months (56). After 3 months, CTX is discontinued, and the prednisone is continued for an additional 2 weeks. If hearing does not worsen during this interval, the prednisone is tapered and discontinued. If hearing declines, the two-drug treatment regimen is repeated for an additional 3 months. This regimen can be repeated as needed in 3-month cycles (56). Other regimens with CTX and steroids have been described (2,14).

Adverse reactions to CTX include nausea and vomiting, alopecia (usually reversible), infertility, hemorrhagic cystitis, bladder carcinoma (with long-term use), and bone marrow suppression (leukopenia, thrombocytopenia) with resultant increased susceptibility to infection (57). White blood cell count should be determined once a week; if it falls below 5,000/µL CTX should be discontinued until the count recovers to more than 5,000/µL (56). Complications involving the bladder can be reduced by maintaining full hydration and by emptying the bladder before going to sleep. Alternatives to CTX include methotrexate and azathioprine, which may be less toxic (58–60).

Some authors do not use CTX if hearing returns during 7 to 14 days of treatment with corticosteroids and remains stable after steroids are stopped (61). Regimens with prednisone only have been developed, and cytotoxic drugs are reserved for refractory cases. Hughes et al. (10, 62) recommended a 4-week course of 1 mg/kg per day prednisone. If hearing improves or stabilizes, a maintenance dose of 10 mg every other day is used for several months (i.e., as long as required to maintain hearing). An alternative is tapering the dosage. If hearing declines, prednisone should be increased to the amount used previously to maintain hearing and continued at this higher level for 1 month. Then maintenance therapy can be titrated to maintain hearing.

Contraindications to long-term use of steroids include pregnancy, peptic ulcer disease, tuberculosis, hypertension, diabetes, glaucoma, and recent vaccination. Side effects of steroids include gastrointestinal reactions, edema, hypokalemia, osteoporosis, central nervous system effects (e.g., euphoria, mood swings, and insomnia), myopathy, osteonecrosis, ocular effects (e.g., cataracts), and suppression of the hypothalamic-pituitary-adrenal axis (63). Some of these side effects can be alleviated with dosing once a morning or every other day. Patients receiving large doses for a prolonged period should be gradually withdrawn from corticosteroids.

An alternative method of treatment is plasmapheresis, a technique in which immune complexes, free antigen, and inflammatory mediators are removed from plasma (64,65). This technique is recommended when progressive hearing loss shows initial response to immunosuppressive agents with subsequent failure or when these medications cannot be used. The results have been encouraging in that 50% to 75% patients show improvement in hearing and some patients no longer need other treatment modalities (64,65).

OTHER RELATED CONDITIONS

In approximately 25% to 50% of cases of AIED, other autoimmune disorders, including Cogan's syndrome, rheumatoid arthritis, systemic lupus erythematosus, and ulcerative colitis, develop over time (29,56,62). Many systemic immunologic disorders are associated with SNHL. These include Cogan's syndrome, Wegener's granulomatosis, relapsing polychondritis, systemic lupus erythematosus, rheumatoid arthritis, ulcerative colitis, polyarteritis nodosa, and scleroderma (66–73).

Cogan's Syndrome

One of the secondary types of AIED is Cogan's syndrome, a rare disorder characterized by acute nonsyphilitic interstitial keratitis and audiovestibular symptoms (74). If untreated, Cogan's syndrome usually progresses to profound bilateral SNHL over several months; however, it rarely results in permanent visual impairment (75,76). Cogan's syndrome has been divided into two types—typical and atypical. With typical Cogan's syndrome, interstitial keratitis occurs suddenly with photophobia, ocular pain, and eye redness. These symptoms are associated with fluctuating and progressive bilateral SNHL, tinnitus, vertigo, and loss of vestibular function. The audiovestibular dysfunction usually occurs just before the interstitial keratitis, but it may occur up to 6 months before or after the interstitial keratitis (75). With atypical Cogan's syndrome, audiovestibular symptoms occur with ocular disease other than interstitial keratitis, such as uveitis, iritis, scleritis, and conjunctivitis. There may be a wide range of systemic findings, including vasculitis, aortic insufficiency,

arthritis or arthralgia, rashes, auricular pain, polychondritis, gastrointestinal hemorrhage, renal disease, and myalgia (76).

Therapy for Cogan's syndrome consists of corticosteroid eye drops for the ocular symptoms and high-dose corticosteroids for the hearing loss. Other immunosuppressive agents, such as CTX and azathioprine have been used (77). Patients with measurable hearing who start steroid therapy quickly often have a return of auditory function; however, if no measurable hearing exists, steroids are of little benefit (76).

Because of its associated systemic symptoms, response to immunosuppressive therapy, and autoimmune reactivity against corneal and inner ear antigen, many investigators consider Cogan's syndrome to be the prototype of immune-mediated inner ear disease (15,67,78). The temporal bone pathologic findings of Cogan's syndrome are similar to those of other autoimmune diseases. They include severe bilateral degeneration of the cochlea and vestibular labyrinth (including loss of all hair cells and atrophy of ganglion cells), endolymphatic hydrops, and a fibroosseous reaction within the cochlea and vestibular labyrinth. These pathologic findings suggest that the cause is an inflammatory reaction involving the membranous labyrinth (79–82). The distinctive features of Cogan's syndrome are thought to result from an immune response directed against membranous labyrinth proteins that occurs concurrently with an autoimmune disorder involving the eye and, with atypical Cogan's syndrome, other organs (82).

Wegener's Granulomatosis

Wegener's granulomatosis is an uncommon disorder characterized by necrotizing granulomatous vasculitis of the upper and lower respiratory tract and kidney. Untreated, Wegener's granulomatosis has a mortality rate of 90% at 2 years, mainly from renal failure and sepsis (83,84). Otologic involvement occurs in 19% to 61% of cases, serous otitis media being the most common manifestation (83–86). McDonald et al. (83) found that 9 of 108 patients with Wegener's granulomatosis had SNHL, Five of these patients had total or partial recovery with treatment. The SNHL may be caused by vasculitis involving the labyrinthine vessels or endolymphatic sac (87,88). The use of CTX and corticosteroids has led to long-term remissions among many patients and has reversed the conductive hearing loss and SNHL (83,84). If Wegener's granulomatosis is suspected, testing with a serologic marker, antineutrophil cytoplasmic autoantibody–cytoplasmic pattern (C-ANCA), can help make an early diagnosis (89). Confirmation of the diagnosis, however, requires tissue biopsy; the lung is most likely to show the typical histologic changes (84).

SUMMARY POINTS

- In 1979, McCabe described a group of patients with rapidly progressive, bilateral, asymmetric SNHL that responded favorably to immunosuppressive therapy. He called this disorder *autoimmune SNHL*.
- A more accurate term for this entity is *autoimmune inner ear disease* (AIED), which can be primary (immunologic disorder that begins within the inner ear) or secondary (originates outside the ear).
- Theories of autoimmunity include sequestered antigens, altered antigens, cross-reacting antigens, genetic mutations of the immunologic pathway, and loss of regulation by helper or suppressor cells.
- Despite the blood-labyrinth barrier, the CSF-labyrinth barrier, and the middle ear–labyrinth barrier, the inner ear is not an immunoprivileged site. For inner ear inflammatory reactions to occur, an intact endolymphatic sac is needed.
- Patients with AIED typically have a history of asymmetric, bilateral SNHL that progresses over several weeks to months with a normal appearing ear. At a minimum, screening laboratory tests should include ESR, FTA-ABS, and ANA.
- Antigen-specific studies include the LMIT, LTT, Western blot assay, IIF, and ELISA. Antigen-non-specific studies include measurements of the complement system, circulating immune complexes, and cryoglobulins.
- A 68-kd antigen has been found with Western blot assays. This antigen may represent an autoantibody against inner ear antigen and appears to be related to heat shock protein 70.
- When AIED is suspected, aggressive treatment should be started that consists of long-term use of high-dose immunosuppressive agents (corticosteroids, CTX, methotrexate, azathioprine) as both a test for suspected cases and actual therapy for the disorder.
- The prognosis generally is considered favorable; most patients with active disease show stabilization or improvement in hearing with appropriate treatment.

REFERENCES

1. Schorn K. Differential diagnosis of hearing disorders. In: Naumann HH, ed. *Differential diagnosis in otorhinolaryngology.* New York: Thieme Medical Publishers, 1993:55–96.
2. McCabe BF. Autoimmune sensorineural hearing loss. *Ann Otol Rhinol Laryngol* 1979;88:585–589.
3. Kanzaki J, O-Uchi T. Steroid-responsive bilateral sensorineural hearing loss and immune complexes. *Arch Otorhinolaryngol* 1981;230:5–9.
4. Kanzaki J, O-Uchi T. Circulating immune complexes in steroid-responsive sensorineural hearing loss and the long-term observation. *Acta Otolaryngol Suppl (Stockh)* 1983;393:77–84.
5. Veldman JE, Roord JJ, O'Connor AF, Shea JJ. Autoimmunity and inner ear disorders: an immune-complex mediated sensorineural hearing loss. *Laryngoscope* 1984;94:501–507.
6. Hughes GB, Kinney SE, Barna BP, Calabrese LH. Practical versus theoretical management of autoimmune inner ear disease. *Laryngoscope* 1984;94:758–767.
7. Arnold W, Pfaltz R, Altermatt HJ. Evidence of serum antibodies against inner ear tissues in the blood of patients with certain sensorineural hearing disorders. *Acta Otolaryngol (Stockh)* 1985;99:437–444.
8. Harris JP, Sharp PA. Inner ear autoantibodies in patients with rapidly progressive sensorineural hearing loss. *Laryngoscope* 1990;100:516–524.
9. Discussion. *Adv Otorhinolaryngol* 1991;46:93–96.
10. Hughes GH, Barna BP. Autoimmune inner ear disease: fact or fantasy?. *Adv Otorhinolaryngol* 1991;46:82–91.
11. Soliman AM. Immune-mediated inner ear disease. *Am J Otol* 1992;13:575–579.
12. O-Uchi T, Kanzaki J, Tsuchihashi N. Clinical analysis of steroid-responsive sensorineural hearing loss. *Auris Nasus Larynx* 1993;20:79–93.
13. Harris JP, Ryan AF. Immunobiology of the inner ear. *Am J Otolaryngol* 1984;5:418–425.
14. McCabe BF. Autoimmune inner ear disease. In: Bernstein J, Ogra P, eds. *Immunology of the ear.* New York: Raven Press, 1987:427–435.
15. Hughes GB, Barna BP, Calabrese LH, Koo A. Immunologic disorders of the inner ear. In: Bailey BJ, ed. *Head and neck surgery–otolaryngology.* Philadelphia: JB Lippincott, 1993:1833–1842.
16. Barrett JT. *Textbook of immunology: an introduction to immunochemistry and immunobiology,* 4th ed. St. Louis: Mosby, 1983:77–94.
17. Baroody FM, Naclerio RM. An overview of immunology. *Otolaryngol Clin North Am* 1993;26:571–591.
18. Barrett JT. *Textbook of immunology: an introduction to immunochemistry and immunobiology,* 4th ed. St. Louis: Mosby, 1983:402–407.
19. Bernstein JM. The immunobiology of autoimmune disease of the inner ear. In: Bernstein J, Ogra P, eds. *Immunology of the ear.* New York: Raven Press, 1987:419–426.
20. Bauman GP, Hurtubise P. Anti-idiotypes and autoimmune disease. *Clin Lab Med* 1988;8:399–407.
21. Veldman JE. Immunology of hearing: experiments of nature. *Am J Otol* 1989;10:183–187.
22. Melchers F. Immunity and autoimmunity with special reference to inner ear diseases. *Adv Otorhinolaryngol* 1991;46:17–25.
23. Harris JP. Experimental autoimmune sensorineural hearing loss. *Laryngoscope* 1987;97:63–76.
24. Gudat F. Immunopathology and autoimmunity: the view of an immunopathologist. *Adv Otorhinolaryngol* 1991;46:9–16.
25. Juhn SK. Barrier systems in the inner ear. *Acta Otolaryngol Suppl (Stockh)* 1988;458:79–83.
26. Mogi G, Lim DJ, Watanabe N. Immunologic study on the inner ear: immunoglobulins in perilymph. *Arch Otolaryngol* 1982;108:270–275.
27. Harris JP. Immunology of the inner ear: response of the inner ear to antigen challenge. *Otolaryngol Head Neck Surg* 1983;91:18–23.
28. Palva T, Raunio V. Disc electrophoretic studies of human perilymph. *Ann Otol Rhinol Laryngol* 1967;76:23–36.
29. Harris JP. Immunology of the inner ear: evidence of local antibody production. *Ann Otol Rhinol Laryngol* 1984;93:157–162.
30. Harris JP, Fukuda S, Keithley EM. Spiral modiolar vein: its importance in inner ear inflammation. *Acta Otolaryngol (Stockh)* 1990;110:357–365.
31. Woolf NK, Harris JP. Cochlear pathophysiology associated with inner ear immune responses. *Acta Otolaryngol (Stockh)* 1986;102:353–364.
32. Harris JP. Experimental immunology of the inner ear. *Adv Otorhinolaryngol* 1991;46:26–33.
33. Yamanobe S, Harris JP. Spontaneous remission in experimental autoimmune labyrinthitis. *Ann Otol Rhinol Laryngol* 1992;101:1007–1014.
34. Fukuda S, Harris JP, Keithley EM, Ishikawa K, Kucuk B, Inuyama Y.

Spiral modiolar vein: its importance in viral load of the inner ear. *Ann Otol Rhinol Laryngol* 1992;101[Suppl 157]:67–71.

35. Tomiyama S, Harris JP. The endolymphatic sac: its importance in inner ear immune responses. *Laryngoscope* 1986;96:685–691.

36. Rask-Anderson H, Stahle J. Immunodefense of the inner ear? Lymphocyte-macrophage interaction in the endolymphatic sac. *Acta Otolaryngol (Stockh)* 1980;89:283–294.

37. Yoo TJ, Tomoda K, Stuart JM, Cremer MA, Townes AS, Kang AH. Type II collagen–induced autoimmune sensorineural hearing loss and vestibular dysfunction in rats. *Ann Otol Rhinol Laryngol* 1983;92:267–271.

38. Yoo TJ, Tomoda K, Hernandez AD. Type II collagen–induced autoimmune inner ear lesions in guinea pigs. *Ann Otol Rhinol Laryngol* 1984; 93[Suppl 113]:3–5.

39. Yoo TJ, Yazawa Y, Floyd R, Tomoda K. Antibody activity in perilymph from rats with type II collagen–induced autoimmune inner ear disease. *Ann Otol Rhinol Laryngol* 1984;93[Suppl 113]:1–2.

40. Harris JP, Woolf NK, Ryan AF. A re-examination of experimental type II collagen autoimmunity: middle and inner ear morphology and function. *Ann Otol Rhinol Laryngol* 1986;95:176–180.

41. Berger P, Hillman M, Tabak M, Vollrath M. The lymphocyte transformation test with type II collagen as a diagnostic tool of autoimmune sensorineural hearing loss. *Laryngoscope* 1991;101:895–899.

42. Helfgott SM, Mosciscki RA, Martin JS, et al. Correlation between antibodies to type II collagen and treatment outcome in bilateral progressive sensorineural hearing loss. *Lancet* 1991;337:387–389.

43. Yoo TJ, Floyd RA, Sudo N, et al. Factors influencing collagen-induced autoimmune ear disease. *Am J Otolaryngol* 1985;6:209–216.

44. Yoo TJ, Floyd R, Ishibe T, Shea JJ, Bowman C. Immunologic testing of certain diseases. *Am J Otol* 1985;6:96–101.

45. Yoo TJ, Floyd RA, Kitano H. Animal model of autoimmune ear disease. In: Bernstein J, Ogra P, eds. *Immunology of the ear*. New York: Raven Press, 1987:463–480.

46. Hughes GB, Kinney SE, Hamid MA, Barna BP, Calabrese LH. Autoimmune vestibular dysfunction: preliminary report. *Laryngoscope* 1985; 95:893–897.

47. Hughes GB, Barna BP, Kinney SE, Calabrese LH, Nalepa NL. Predictive value of laboratory tests in "autoimmune" inner ear disease: preliminary report. *Laryngoscope* 1986;96:502–505.

48. Suzuki M, Kitahara M. Immunologic abnormality in Meniere's disease. *Otolaryngol Head Neck Surg* 1992;107:57–62.

49. Gottschlich S, Billings PB, Keithley EM, Weisman MH, Harris JP. Assessment of serum antibodies in patients with rapidly progressive sensorineural hearing loss and Meniere's disease. *Laryngoscope* 1995; 105:1347–1352.

50. Billings PB, Keithley EM, Harris JP. Evidence linking the 68 kilodalton antigen identified in progressive sensorineural hearing loss patient sera with heat shock protein 70. *Ann Otol Rhinol Laryngol* 1995;104: 181–188.

51. Bloch DB, San Martin JE, Rauch SD, Moscicki RA, Bloch KJ. Serum antibodies to heat shock protein 70 in sensorineural hearing loss. *Arch Otolaryngol Head Neck Surg* 1995;121:1167–1171.

52. Moscicki RA, San Martin JE, Quintero CH, Rauch SD, Nadol JB Jr, Bloch KJ. Serum antibody to inner ear proteins in patients with progressive hearing loss: correlation with disease activity and response to corticosteroid treatment. *JAMA* 1994;272:611–616.

53. Salomon P, Charachon R, Lejeune JM. Indirect immunofluorescence in the investigation of rapidly progressive sensorineural hearing loss and Meniere's disease. *Acta Otolaryngol (Stockh)* 1993;113:318–320.

54. Arnold W, Pfaltz CR. Critical evaluation of the immunofluorescence microscopic test for identification of serum antibodies against human inner ear tissue. *Acta Otolaryngol (Stockh)* 1987;103:373–378.

55. Plester D, Soliman AM. Autoimmune hearing loss. *Am J Otol* 1989;10: 188–192.

56. McCabe BF. Autoimmune inner ear disease: results of therapy. *Adv Otorhinolaryngol* 1991;46:78–81.

57. Immunomodulators. In: *Drug evaluations*, 6th ed. Chicago: American Medical Association, 1986:1147–1165.

58. Sismanis A, Thompson T, Willis HE. Methotrexate therapy for autoimmune hearing loss: a preliminary report. *Laryngoscope* 1994;104: 932–934.

59. Sismanis A, Wise CM, Johnson GD. Methotrexate management of immune-mediated cochleovestibular disorders. *Otolaryngol Head Neck Surg* 1997;116:146–152.

60. Saracaydin A, Katircioglu S, Katircioglu S, Karatay MC. Azathioprine

in combination with steroids in the treatment of autoimmune inner-ear disease. *J Int Med Res* 1993;21:192–196.

61. Veldman JE. Immune-mediated inner ear disorders: an otoimmunologist's view. *Adv Otorhinolaryngol* 1991;46:71–77.

62. Hughes GB, Barna BP, Kinney SE, Calabrese LH, Nalepa NJ. Clinical diagnosis of immune inner-ear disease. *Laryngoscope* 1988;98:251–253.

63. Adrenal corticosteroids in nonendocrine disease. In: *Drug evaluations*, 6th ed. Chicago: American Medical Association, 1986:1089–1104.

64. Brookes GB, Newland AC. Plasma exchange in the treatment of immune complex–associated sensorineural deafness. *J Laryngol Otol* 1986;100:25–33.

65. Luetje CM. Theoretical and practical implications for plasmapheresis in autoimmune inner ear disease. *Laryngoscope* 1989;99:1137–1146.

66. Barna BP, Hughes GB. Autoimmunity and otologic disease: clinical and experimental aspects. *Clin Lab Med* 1988;8:385–398.

67. Hughes GB, Kinney SE, Barna BP, Tomsak RL, Calabrese LH. Autoimmune reactivity in Cogan's syndrome: a preliminary report. *Otolaryngol Head Neck Surg* 1983;91:24–32.

68. Peeters GJ, Cremers CW, Pinckers AJ, Hoefnagels WH. Atypical Cogan's syndrome: an autoimmune disease? *Ann Otol Rhinol Laryngol* 1986;95:173–175.

69. Bowman CA, Linthicum FH, Nelson RA, Mikami K, Quismorio F. Sensorineural hearing loss associated with systemic lupus erythematosus. *Otolaryngol Head Neck Surg* 1986;94:197–204.

70. Nores JM, Bonfils P. Rheumatoid arthritis and autoimmune hearing loss: a case study. *Clin Rheumatol* 1988;7:520–521.

71. Weber RS, Jenkins HA, Coker NJ. Sensorineural hearing loss associated with ulcerative colitis. *Arch Otolaryngol* 1984;110:810–812.

72. Jenkins HA, Pollack AM, Fisch U. Polyarteritis nodosa as a cause of sudden deafness: a human temporal bone study. *Am J Otolaryngol* 1981;2: 99–107.

73. Abou-taleb A, Linthicum FH. Scleroderma and hearing loss: histopathology of a case. *J Laryngol Otol* 1987;101:656–662.

74. Cogan DG. Syndrome of nonsyphilitic interstitial keratitis and vestibuloauditory symptoms. *Arch Ophthalmol* 1945;33:144–149.

75. Haynes BF, Kaiser-Kupfer MI, Mason P, Fauci AS. Cogan syndrome: studies in 13 patients, long-term follow-up and a review of the literature. *Medicine (Baltimore)* 1980;59:426–441.

76. Vollertsen RS, McDonald TJ, Younge BR, Banks PM, Stanson AW, Istrup DM. Cogan's syndrome: 18 cases and a review of the literature. *Mayo Clin Proc* 1986;61:344–361.

77. McDonald TJ, Vollertsen RS, Younge BR. Cogan's syndrome: audiovestibular involvement and prognosis in 18 patients. *Laryngoscope* 1985;95:650–654.

78. Majoor MHJM, Albers FWJ, Van der Gaag R, Gmelig-Meyling F, Huizing EH. Corneal autoimmunity in Cogan's syndrome? report of two cases. *Ann Otol Rhinol Laryngol* 1992;101:679–684.

79. Fisher ER, Hellstrom HR. Cogan's syndrome and systemic vascular disease: analysis of pathologic features with reference to its relationship to thromboangiitis obliterans (Buerger). *Arch Pathol* 1961;72: 572–592.

80. Wolff D, Bernhard WG, Tsutsumi S, Ross IS, Nussbaum HE. The pathology of Cogan's syndrome causing profound deafness. *Ann Otol Rhinol Laryngol* 1965;74:507–520.

81. Rarey KE, Bicknell JM, Davis LE. Intralabyrinthine osteogenesis in Cogan's syndrome. *Am J Otolaryngol* 1986;7:387–390.

82. Schuknecht HF, Nadol JB. Temporal bone pathology in a case of Cogan's syndrome. *Laryngoscope* 1994;104:1135–1142.

83. McDonald TJ, DeRemee RA. Wegener's granulomatosis. *Laryngoscope* 1983;93:220–231.

84. Campbell SM, Montanaro A, Bardana EJ. Head and neck manifestations of autoimmune disease. *Am J Otolaryngol* 1983;4:187–216.

85. Kornblut AD, Wolff SM, Fauci AS. Ear disease in patients with Wegener's granulomatosis. *Laryngoscope* 1982;92:713–717.

86. Murty GE. Wegener's granulomatosis: otorhinolaryngological manifestations. *Clin Otolaryngol* 1990;15:385–393.

87. Karmody CS. Wegener's granulomatosis: presentation as an otologic problem. *Otolaryngol Head Neck Surg* 1978;86:573–584.

88. Leone CA, Feghali JG, Linthicum FH. Endolymphatic sac: possible role in autoimmune sensorineural hearing loss. *Ann Otol Rhinol Laryngol* 1984;93:208–209.

89. Macias JD, Wackym PA, McCabe BF. Early diagnosis of otologic Wegener's granulomatosis using the serologic marker C-ANCA. *Ann Otol Rhinol Laryngol* 1993;102:337–341.

The Ear: Comprehensive Otology,
edited by R. F. Canalis and P. R. Lambert.
Lippincott Williams & Wilkins, Philadelphia © 2000.

CHAPTER 33

Presbycusis

Hamed Sajjadi, Michael M. Paparella, and Rinaldo F. Canalis

DEFINITION

Presbycusis is a form of hearing loss associated with aging that was first recognized by Zwaardenhaer at the end of the nineteenth century (1). The typical patient affected by this process is an elderly person who complains of progressive hearing loss and increasing difficulty in communicating effectively, especially in a noisy environment (Table 1). Audiometry will reveal various patterns of sensorineural hearing loss (SNHL).

EPIDEMIOLOGY

Presbycusis is the most common form of SNHL encountered in industrialized nations. In the United States, it affects approximately 40% of the population older than 75 years of age (2–4). It is more prevalent and severe in men, who also experience a hearing deterioration rate that is more than twice that experienced by

women. Declines in hearing sensitivity may be detected in all frequencies in men by age 30, whereas women show a later onset of auditory impairment (5,6). Thereafter, the degree of hearing loss continues to increase with age and tends to be greater in the high frequencies (Fig. 1). Once the impairment is clinically detectable, women tend to have better hearing than men at frequencies above 1,000 Hz, whereas men have better hearing than women at lower frequencies (6).

ETIOLOGY

The precise mechanisms by which aging results in presbycusis are not known, but noise, heredity, and systemic degenerative changes appear to contribute to its development.

Noise

Rosen et al. (7) evaluated hearing levels in an isolated Sudanese tribe whose members (the Mabaans) live in a relatively noise-free environment. These authors found significant hearing preservation in this community when compared with individuals living in an industrialized environment grouped by corresponding age and sex. There were no gender differences. Other pathologies noted to be absent in the Mabaans and possibly related to

H. Sajjadi: Minnesota Ear, Head, and Neck Clinic, Minneapolis, Minnesota 55454

M. M. Paparella: Otopathology Laboratory, Department of Otolaryngology, University of Minnesota, Minneapolis; Minnesota Ear, Head, and Neck Clinic, Minneapolis, Minnesota 55454

R. F. Canalis: Department of Surgery, University of California, Los Angeles School of Medicine, Los Angeles, California, 90095-1624

TABLE 1. *Clinical characteristics of presbycusis*

Insidious onset
Symmetric sensorineural hearing loss
Progressive loss with age
No other otologic diseases
Normal ear examination

a low-stress environment were hypertension, coronary artery disease, allergies, duodenal ulcers, and bronchial asthma. Another study addressing the effects of industrialization on hearing decline was done by Goycolea et al. (8). These authors studied median hearing thresholds in a statistically significant number of natives from Easter Island. Three groups of islanders were studied, and their auditory thresholds were compared with those of citizens from the United States grouped by corresponding sex and age. Group 1 consisted of subjects who had always lived on the island; group 2 consisted of islanders who had lived in an industrialized environment for 3 to 5 years; and group 3 consisted of individuals who had lived in an industrialized environment for more than 5 years. The results indicated a progressive deterioration of hearing as a function of the number of years spent in civilization. In addition, the median hearing thresholds of group 1, which was made up of almost equal numbers of males and females, were similar to those of American females for corresponding ages.

Results of several studies performed in military personnel (9) and industrial workers (10) support the additivity of noise and age in the development of presbycusis,

whereas a few others found no interaction. Among the latter, in a cross-sectional study of 80 workers aged 30 to 59 years exposed to industrial noise for 5 to 10 years, Norotny (11) found that all age groups showed similar hearing levels for equal levels of exposure.

Heredity

A genetic basis may play a role in as many as 50% of adult patients who present with symmetric SNHL (12). Paparella et al. (13) demonstrated findings similar to those of presbycusis, including atrophy of the organ of Corti and loss of ganglion cells in the basal turn of the cochlea and degeneration of the stria vascularis in several adult temporal bone specimens of individuals with genetic SNHL.

Degenerative Changes

Other factors that may contribute to SNHL of aging are peripheral and central ischemia (14,15), cochlear nerve compression by hyperostosis (16), neurochemical changes producing a decrease of essential neurotransmitters (17), intracellular accumulation of catabolites (18), and mitochondrial DNA deletions (19). The histologic evidence implicating these changes as possibly related to presbycusis is addressed in detail later in this chapter.

CLINICAL AND PATHOLOGIC OBSERVATIONS

SNHL of aging has been characterized primarily by cochlear changes, but the middle ear and central auditory system also can be affected. Great variations occur in the degree and chronology of these changes and in individual differences, making the attempts to define the parameters of presbycusis difficult. Age-related hearing loss results in a variety of auditory patterns, although most patients have involvement limited to the mid to high frequencies, with relatively good speech discrimination scores (Fig. 2).

Schuknecht's Classification

Classification of presbycusis must take into account several variables that may not allow precise correlation between pathologic and clinical findings. The most commonly used classification is the one by Schuknecht, who attempted to correlate the audiometric patterns of SNHL in the elderly with potentially significant pathophysiologic mechanisms. He proposed six types of presbycusis (Table 2) (20,21).

Sensory Presbycusis

This type of SNHL is characterized by progressive atrophy of the organ of Corti at the extreme basal end of

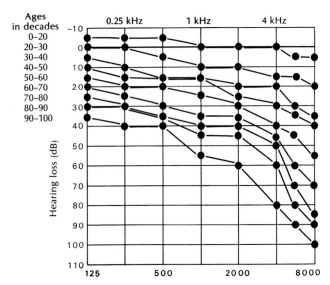

FIG. 1. Decade audiogram illustrating the progression of hearing loss due to the aging process. Audiometric patterns encountered in an urban otologic practice. (From Goodhill V. *Ear diseases, deafness and dizziness.* New York: Harper & Row, 1979:727.)

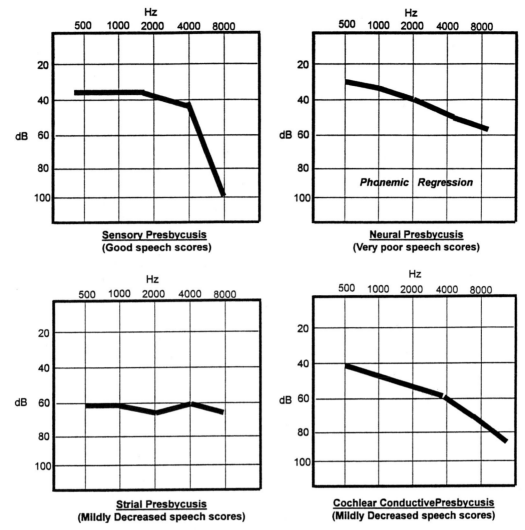

FIG. 2. Pure tone audiometric patterns in classic presbycusis (normal conductive mechanism, no air–bone gap).

the cochlea (Fig. 3). The organ of Corti initially undergoes distortion and flattening, which is followed by gradual disappearance of hair and supporting cells. In later stages it loses all recognizable elements and becomes barely identifiable; it may disappear. At the onset, these changes are associated with progressive degeneration of sensory cells, which is particularly pronounced in the outer hair cells (22,23).

Audiometrically, the speech frequencies are rarely involved during the early phases of sensory presbycusis. Thus, the initial impairment is an abrupt, symmetric, high-tone hearing loss in the region of 6 to 8 kHz, with relatively good speech discrimination scores (Fig. 2). Eventually the hearing loss accentuates, and the audiogram shows involvement of the mid frequencies and decreased speech discrimination ability (Fig. 4).

TABLE 2. *Schuknecht's classification of presbycusis*

Type	Site of lesion	Hearing loss	Speech
Sensory	Atrophy of the organ of Corti	Abrupt high frequency	Good
Neural	Atrophy of spiral ganglion and neurons	Mild sloping loss	Very poor (phonemic regression)
Strial (metabolic)	Atrophy of stria vascularis	Flat loss	Mild loss
Cochlear conductive (mechanical)	Thickened basal membrane	Linear and gradual high frequency	Mild loss
Mixed	Any combination of above	Any combination of above	Mild loss
Indeterminate	No distinct lesions seen	Flat or abrupt high frequency	Mild loss

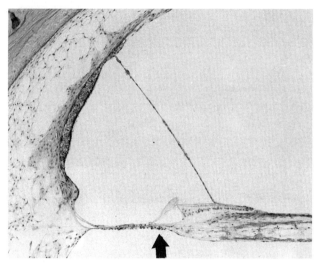

FIG. 3. Sensory presbycusis. *Arrow* points to atrophy of the organ of Corti.

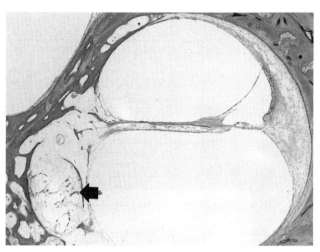

FIG. 5. Neural presbycusis. *Arrow* points to a severe loss of spiral ganglion cells.

Neural Presbycusis

The most common form of degeneration seen in the aging cochlea is atrophy and death of cochlear neurons (spiral ganglion cells) (Fig. 5) and possibly of neurons in the central auditory pathways (Fig. 6) (24). Sensory cells undergo total degeneration including axon, stroma, and dendritic fibers, a condition termed "primary neuronal degeneration." Otte et al. (25) counted the population of neurons in 100 temporal bones of hearing subjects, who ranged in age from the first to the tenth decade of life.

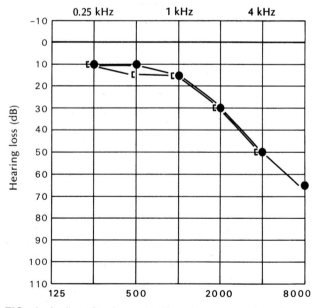

FIG. 4. Audiogram demonstrating the progression of sensory presbycusis. Speech reception threshold (SRT) at 15 dB reflecting normal low-frequency hearing and mild drop in speech discrimination (70% at 45 dB [+30]; 82% at 55 dB [+40]). ●—●, Air conduction unmasked; [- [, bone conduction masked. (From Goodhill V. *Ear diseases, deafness and dizziness.* Harper & Row, 1979:727.)

They found a progressive loss of about 2,100 neurons per decade, ranging from a high of 36,918 in the youngest subjects to a low of 18,626 in the oldest individuals. Arensen (26) measured the total number of neurons in the temporal bone of six elderly subjects (76 to 89 years) and detected a 50% or more loss of cochlear neurons compared to the mean for normal neonatal ears. The most significant consequence of the loss of cochlear neurons is the inability to understand words, but losses of up to 50% are still compatible with normal or near-normal speech discrimination. Pauler et al. (27) studied neuronal counts from the base to the apex of four regions of the cochlea. They determined that loss of cochlear neurons in the 15- to 22-mm region (the locus for speech frequencies) correlated positively with a loss of word discrimination scores. Approximately 90% of cochlear neurons must be lost before pure tone thresholds are affected (24).

The characteristic audiometric finding in neural presbycusis is a progressive drop in word discrimination scores with preservation of relatively normal pure tone thresholds (Fig. 2). This phenomenon has been labeled "phonemic regression" by Gaeth (28). Patients with neural presbycusis often suffer from other degenerative changes of the central nervous system manifested by lack of coordination, weakness of the extremities, tremors, irritability, intellectual deterioration, and memory loss. It has been hypothesized that the rate of neuronal atrophy in neural presbycusis may be a genetically determined phenomenon (29).

Strial (Metabolic) Presbycusis

The stria vascularis is important in the production of the endocochlear potential, a positive 80-mV direct-current potential in the scala media (30–32), and is thought to be the source of endolymph formation (33). It contains oxidizing enzymes that are required for the metabolism of glucose, which is the essential element for energy transport in cochlear function (34). Consequently, strial atrophy (Fig. 7) may result in alterations in the endo-

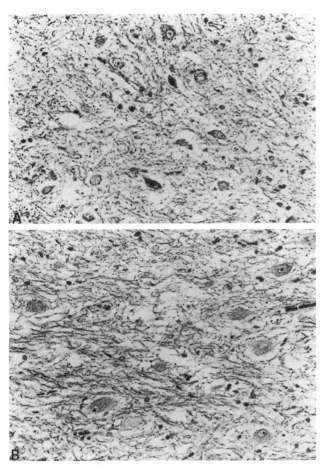

FIG. 6. Photomicrograph of superior ventral cochlear nucleus. **A:** At 4-kHz level, loss of spheroid cells is estimated at 90% to 95%. **B:** At the 500-Hz level, loss of spheroid cells is estimated at 65%. (From Dublin WB. The combined correlated audiohistogram: incorporation of the superior vestibular nucleus. *Ann Otol Rhinol Laryngol* 1976;85:813–819, with permission.)

cochlear potential, endolymph formation, and/or glucose metabolism. Electron microscopic studies of temporal bones in subjects over the age of 60 years have shown that the stria undergoes two forms of atrophy: a patchy type, which predominantly affects the marginal cells and is most severe in the apical and middle turns (Fig. 4) (29); and a diffuse type, which is characterized by widening of the intracellular spaces, a feature that is undetectable by light microscopy (35).

It has been demonstrated that a 30% loss of strial tissue results in hearing loss (35). The audiologic features of strial presbycusis are a flat, slightly sloping, symmetric SNHL and good speech discrimination scores (Figs. 2 and 8). Hearing deterioration has a gradual onset in the fourth to sixth decades of life, and usually it progresses slowly.

Cochlear Conductive (Mechanical) Presbycusis

This type of presbycusis lacks a definitive histologic correlate. Patients present in middle age with a symmetric SNHL that gradually increases in severity from low to

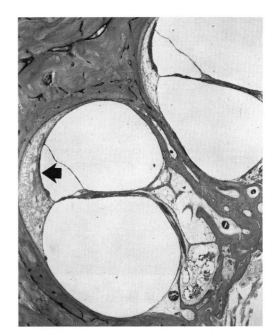

FIG. 7. Strial (metabolic) presbycusis. *Arrow* points to atrophy of the stria vascularis.

high frequencies (Fig. 2). Word discrimination scores remain good. Temporal bone studies have shown normal hair cells, cochlear neurons, and stria vascularis. Given the lack of obvious cochlear pathology, Schuknecht (20,21) postulated a mechanical alteration of cochlear function. Because the hearing loss increments show a linear relationship to sound frequencies, he hypothesized that they are caused by changes in the resonance fre-

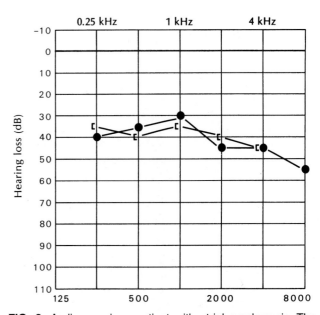

FIG. 8. Audiogram in a patient with strial presbycusis. The speech reception threshold (35 dB) is consistent with the pure tone average. Discrimination ability is high (88% at 65 dB [–30]). ●—●, Unmasked air conduction threshold; [–[, marked bone conduction threshold. (From Goodhill V. *Ear diseases, deafness and dizziness.* New York: Harper & Row, 1979:727.)

quency of the cochlear duct, which determines the distribution of sound frequency. The apparent site for such alterations is the basilar membrane, which features a linear increase in width and decrease in elasticity from base to apex (36,37). Therefore, it is assumed that the linearity of the descending audiogram seen in cochlear mechanical presbycusis is related to a loss of compliance in the cochlear duct, possibly due to stiffening of the basilar membrane (38). This is supported by Glorig and Davis (39), who demonstrated a lack of loudness recruitment in these patients.

Mixed Presbycusis

Although most patients present with one of the preceding types of presbycusis, some show a mixed pattern. Patients with both sensory and strial presbycusis may present with an abrupt high-tone hearing loss superimposed on a flat audiogram, whereas those with a sensory and cochlear conductive presbycusis combination would have an audiogram demonstrating an abrupt high-tone loss superimposed on a descending, sloping SNHL.

Indeterminate Presbycusis

Approximately 25% of patients with presbycusis may present with audiometric patterns similar to those for strial or sensory presbycusis but without a histopathologic correlate. Potential etiologies include impaired cellular metabolism, diminished synaptic function, and/or chemical alterations of the endolymph. Dysfunction in the central auditory pathways also may explain symptoms in patients with indeterminate presbycusis (39). Some patients may have atrophy of the spiral ligament, a persistent finding in aging animal models, predominantly affecting the apical half of the cochlea (40).

Other Classifications

Lowell and Paparella (41) reviewed 400 patients with bilateral symmetric SNHL and an otherwise negative otologic history. They described four different patterns of SNHL: (a) flat, (b) basin shaped that (c) over time becomes downward sloping, and (d) downward sloping involving only the high frequencies. Three patient groups were identified in this study: (a) *presbycusis,* including patients over age 65 years with no discernible etiology for their hearing loss; (b) *familial presbycusis,* including patients over age 65 years without a specific etiologic basis for hearing loss, but who had one or more family members with a similar hearing loss pattern; and (c) *familial hearing loss,* including patients younger than age 65 years with a clear family history of hearing loss. Patients with presbycusis showed a gradually or abruptly descending SNHL; those with familial presbycusis

showed a flat, gradually declining SNHL with an occasional basin-shaped configuration and speech discrimination scores in the range from 70% to 80%; and patients with familial hearing loss showed a flat or basin-shaped audiometric curve with good speech discrimination scores. The authors concluded that a flat audiometric configuration and good speech discrimination were suggestive of a familial predisposition and proposed the term "genetic presbycusis" for this group.

OTHER LIGHT MICROSCOPIC FINDINGS IN THE AGING EAR

Cochlear

The pathology of presbycusis has been under intense scrutiny for more than 60 years. In 1937, von Fleandt and Saxen (42) first reported on age-related temporal bone changes. They studied 33 specimens of individuals aged 50 years or older and described spiral ganglion atrophy and degeneration of the epithelial elements of the cochlear duct. More recently, Suga and Lindsay (43) studied the temporal bones of 17 elderly individuals with SNHL. The primary finding was a decrease in the population of spiral ganglion cells; however, in many cases there was also diffuse atrophy of the organ of Corti and stria vascularis. No correlation was found between the degree of arteriosclerosis and the degree of cochlear degeneration, and no consistent correlation between a given type of audiometric curve and the pathologic changes encountered could be established.

Johnsson and Hawkins (44) documented the sensory and neural changes associated with aging in multiple comparative studies of the human inner ear. Their most consistent findings were severe degeneration of the myelinated radial nerve fibers in the lower half of the basal turn along with degeneration of the organ of Corti (Fig. 9).

An interesting finding seen in the aging process of the ear is atrophy of Reissner's membrane (45,46), which is characterized by the presence of vacuoles and blebs in the epithelial cell layer along with diffuse structural thinning. Atrophy may lead to rupture of Reissner's membrane and its collapse over the organ of Corti and the tectorial membrane. These changes can occur independently from a significant hair cell loss, but they do interfere with the mechanics of the organ of Corti, leading to SNHL similar to that seen in sensory presbycusis.

Wright and Schuknecht (40) showed degenerative changes of the spiral ligament that, when extreme, may result in flattening of the cochlear duct. The audiometric changes produced by atrophy of the spiral ligament are unknown, but they are more noticeable in ears with a sensory type of presbycusis.

Crowe et al. (22) reported that atrophy of the organ of Corti in the basal turn of the cochlea was the most com-

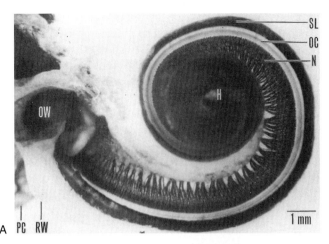

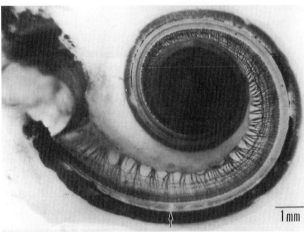

FIG. 9. A: Normal-appearing cochlea from a 25-year-old woman; right ear, strangulation suicide. Fixation in osmium tetroxide approximately 23 hours postmortem. *H,* helicotrema; *N,* network of myelinated radial and intralaminar spiral nerve fibers; *OC,* organ of Corti seen as a dark band on the translucent basilar membrane, representing inner and outer hair cells separated by the tunnel; *OW,* oval window; *PC,* posterior canal and ampulla; *RW,* round window; *SL,* spiral ligament, mostly dissected away. **B:** Cochlea from a 92-year-old female; right ear, burn patient. Fixation with osmium tetroxide 11 hours postmortem. Note degeneration of myelinated radical nerve fibers in the lower half of the basal turn. Intralaminar spiral fibers are clearly seen in the basal turn. There is some patchy degeneration *(arrow)* of the organ of Corti. (From Johnsson LG, Hawkins JE. Sensory and neural degeneration with aging or seen in microdirections of the human inner ear. *Ann Otol Rhinol Laryngol* 1972;81: 179–193, with permission.)

mon finding in presbycusis, followed by partial atrophy of the cochlear nerve supplying the basal turn. Saxen (47) agreed with those findings, but noted that, in some patients, high-frequency hearing loss had no obvious histopathologic correlates.

Makishima (48) demonstrated atrophy of the spiral ganglion and stria vascularis with depletion of hair cells in elderly patients with high-frequency SNHL. Makishima (49) also found arteriosclerotic narrowing of the internal auditory artery. Felder and Schrott-Fischer (50), studying human temporal bones of patients with high-frequency SNHL, demonstrated a loss of neural fibers in the spiral lamina along the entire length of the cochlea. This loss of nerve fibers was found to be age related, with reductions in the 30% to 40% range when compared with normal middle-aged persons. There was an 80% reduction in the outer hair cells noted mainly in apical parts of the cochlea. No significant loss of inner hair cells was observed, as also noted by Spoendlin and Schrott-Fischer (51).

Central

Central auditory system pathology may be responsible for hearing loss in subjects with normal inner ear findings. Kirikae (52) and Kirikae et al. (53) found in elderly patients several signs of central auditory degeneration, including cellular atrophy, nuclear pyknosis, and the appearance of ghostlike, indistinct ganglion cells. Dublin (54) described changes in the ventral cochlear nucleus, including a tendency toward dorsal (high-frequency) involvement, characterized by loss of spheroid cells and reparative gliosis (Fig. 6). In the inferior colliculus, there is loss of neuronal elements, nerve cell deterioration, and glial increase. Cellular degeneration also occurs in the medial geniculate body and in the auditory cortex.

Vascular

Degenerative changes of the internal auditory artery and its branches begin during the first decade of life. Gussen (55) described plugging of vascular canals in the otic capsule as part of the ear's aging process. Fisch et al. (14) reported progressive thickening of the tunica adventitia of the internal auditory artery associated with an increase of collagenous tissue. The increasing compactness of the adventitial layer results in reduced blood supply to the cochlea and loss of sensory elements.

Graton et al. (15) suggested that atrophy of the stria vascularis seen in some temporal bones specimens from elderly subjects was not a primary event but secondary to partial or complete vascular occlusion. This hypothesis is supported by Igarishi et al. (56), who demonstrated a segmental pattern of strial atrophy in experimental animals following obstruction of inner ear vessels with polymeric beads.

Osseous

Krmpotic-Nemanic et al. (16) described increased apposition of bone in the otic capsule with advancing age. Hyperostosis of the lamina cribrosa in the internal auditory canal may lead to compression of the nerve bundles originating primarily at the basal turn of the cochlea.

ULTRASTRUCTURAL FINDINGS

For the most part, electron microscopic studies have corroborated light microscopic findings. A marked loss of outer hair cells and a mild loss of inner hair cells in the organ of Corti, especially in the basal coil, are the most common observations. Surviving cells may show significant structural alterations characterized by marked cellular elongation and thickening, termed "giant sterociliary degeneration" by Soucek et al. (18). Thickening results from the adherence of adjacent hair cells to each other. This change may be found in the inner hair cells throughout the cochlea, but it severely affects the outer cells only in the apical and middle turns.

Fused or modified stereocilia in the inner and outer hair cells also were found by Engstrom et al. (57), who used both scanning and transmission electron microscopy in temporal bone studies of elderly subjects (Figs. 10A and 10B). These authors also noted, in all specimens studied, a clustering of osmophilic structures of lysosomes and lipofuscin (Figs. 10C and 10D). Lipofuscin, also called the pigment of aging, is found primarily in the

upper portion of the cells of the organ of Corti and stria vascularis (Fig. 11) and to a lesser degree in the upper portion of border and pillar cells. When the pigment is abundant, it may fill the entire cell. Of interest, in familial lipofuscinoses there is early deterioration of sensory organs and dementia, which suggests that the accumulation of lipofuscin seen in aging may play a role in hearing deterioration (58).

NEUROCHEMICAL CHANGES IN PRESBYCUSIS

Kaspary et al. (17) postulated a neurochemical basis for the central auditory dysfunction of aging. Neurotransmitters such as γ-aminobutyric acid (GABA) play a significant role in the temporal, spectral, and spatial coding of sound processing mechanisms in the central nucleus of the inferior colliculus. Working with an aging animal model, these investigators demonstrated a significant decrease in the number of GABA immunoreactive neurons, abnormalities in the GABA receptor binding sites, and an overall

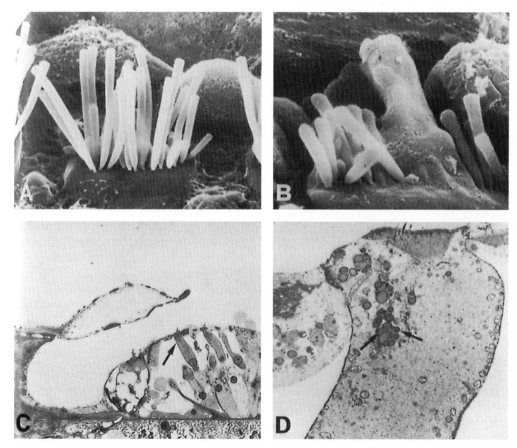

FIG. 10. A: Scanning electron microscopic photograph of an inner hair cell with normal appearance in the apical turn from a 64-year-old woman. **B:** Scanning electron microscopic photograph of an inner hair cell with fused cilia from the basal turn of a male. **C:** Light microscopic photograph of the organ of Corti, middle turn. *Arrow* indicates lipofuscin in the apical portion of an outer hair cell. **D:** Transmission electron microscopic photograph of the upper portion of an outer hair cell. *Arrows* indicate lipofuscin. (From Engstrom B, Hillerdal M, Laurel L, Bagger-Sjoback D. Selected pathological findings in the human cochlea. *Acta Otolaryngol (Stockh)* 1987;96[Suppl 436]:110–116, with permission.)

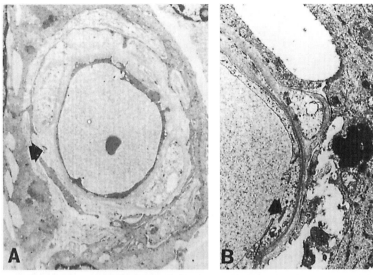

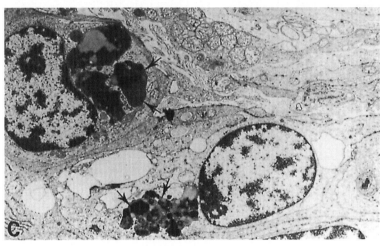

FIG. 11. A: Transition electron microscopic photograph of a capillary in the stria vascularis of a 72-year-old man who had hypertension for many years. *Arrows* point to the thick wall of a vessel. **B:** Transition electron microscopic photograph of a capillary in the stria vascularis with a normal appearance. *Arrow* points to the wall of the capillary. **C:** Transition electron microscopic photograph of stria vascularis. *Arrows* point to lipofuscin inclusions. (From Engstrom B, Hillerdal M, Laurel L, Bagger-Sjoback D. Selected pathological findings in the human cochlea. *Acta Otolaryngol (Stockh)* 1987;96[Suppl 436]:110–116, with permission.)

decrease in the concentration of GABA. These findings suggest that age-related hearing loss may be due to altered function of this neurotransmitter. Other investigators demonstrated that the ability to determine accurately the direction of sound is, in part, dependent on GABA-mediated neural inhibition in the central nucleus of the inferior colliculus (59–62). In addition, age-related alterations in morphology relative to auditory brainstem responses and middle latency responses have been noted in elderly patients, suggesting central auditory dysfunction (63–65).

PRESBYCUSIS AT THE MOLECULAR LEVEL

The aging process is defined as the progressive accumulation of metabolic and physiologic changes occurring through time and determining an increasing susceptibility to illness. Although there are several hypotheses, there are two that currently are favored to explain the degenerative changes of aging. The *dys-differentiation theory* proposes a preprogrammed activation of genes noxious to cells (66), whereas the *membrane theory* is based on the progressive accumulation of oxidative damage due to the activity of reactive oxygen metabolites produced in

increasing amounts as the body grows old. In addition, there is a drop in the level of enzymes, such as glutathione and superoxide dismutase, which normally protect the cell from reactive oxygen species (67,68).

Regardless of the mechanism, mitochondrial genomic mutations are currently viewed as very important in the development of disease. Mitochondria have their own DNA (mtDNA) and enzymatic complexes that act as vehicles for the transcription and translation of genetic information into proteins. Mitochondrial DNA deletions and their progressive life-long enhancement are known to contribute to aging. SNHL has been shown to be associated with mtDNA deletions in some patients with encephalomyopathy and in some with maternally transmitted diabetes (69,70).

Bai et al. (19) recently studied the cochlear mtDNA in 17 normal human temporal bones and in 17 with presbycusis (19). The specimens with presbycusis showed a 4,977 base pair deletion in the mtDNA genome that is known to be associated with aging. Concurrent studies in rodents demonstrated an age-dependent increase in mtDNA deletion, further suggesting that the 4,977 base pair deletion may, among many others, contribute to presbycusis.

EVALUATION AND DIFFERENTIAL DIAGNOSIS

A serious dilemma in the differential diagnosis of elderly patients with SNHL is posed by the variability of factors that may contribute to it. The fundamental question is as follows: Is the loss due to (a) true aging phenomena? (b) environmental noise? and/or (c) undiagnosed cochlear lesions that may have nothing to do with age or noise? Bearing these variables in mind, the most important step in the evaluation of presbycusis is a detailed otologic history with special attention to noise exposure and familial patterns of hearing loss. Specific questions regarding recreational (hunting, target practice, loud music), industrial, and home (chain saws, lawn mowers, and power tools) noise exposure need to be included. The history also should address questions regarding childhood otitis media, ear operations, head trauma, and exposure to ototoxic medications. Some elderly patients may have had ear infections at a time when antibiotic or surgical therapy was not available, and they may have sustained significant inner ear damage. Inflammation enhances transmission of macromolecules across the semipermeable round window membrane, producing sensory cell damage and end organ dysfunction at the basal turn that initially is silent but ultimately involves the lower frequencies with clinically detectable hearing loss (71–76). As the patient ages, the inflammatory process may abate, but the SNHL persists, thus suggesting presbycusis.

The role of heredity may be difficult to identify. Approximately 30% of patients with congenital deafness have associated anomalies that tend to separate them from patients with presbycusis (12,13). In their absence, adult patients with genetic SNHL may be more difficult to diagnose, because most hereditary SNHLs are recessive and have a negative family history. If hearing loss is present in a family member(s), audiograms of those individuals should be compared with the patient's audiometric pattern. Some cases of genetic hearing loss can be distinguished on the basis of mode of transmission, age of onset, and severity of deafness, as well as the audiometric pattern.

The role of advanced vascular disease may be important in hearing loss. Transient ischemic attacks and related brainstem ischemia may compromise blood flow. Therefore, in some patients an evaluation of cerebrovascular integrity may be indicated, including Doppler studies of the carotid artery and magnetic resonance imaging. Imaging may show diffuse microinfarctions of the cerebellum suggestive of alterations in the posterior cerebellar circulation, which may include the internal auditory artery.

Other factors to exclude in the evaluation of presbycusis are ototoxic drug exposure (see Chapter 35), radiation to the temporal bone, and metabolic disorders such as vitamin D deficiency. As with ototoxic agents, the predominant cochlear lesion with vitamin D deficiency is a loss of outer hair cells (77–79). Other debilitating neurologic disorders, such as muscular dystrophy and multiple sclerosis, have been associated with progressive bilateral symmetric SNHL (80) and need to be excluded in complex cases.

Audiometry should include pure tone (air and bone) thresholds and tympanometry. If asymmetric hearing loss is found, auditory brainstem response and/or magnetic resonance imaging should be performed. If dizziness, vertigo, light-headedness, or imbalance are present, electronystagmography may be necessary. Once a detailed history is obtained and diagnostic workup is completed, elderly individuals with symmetric, high-frequency SNHL, in whom an etiologic factor cannot be identified, are classified as having presbycusis, bearing in mind that coexisting otopathologies are common (81).

PREVENTION AND TREATMENT

Presbycusis is a growing problem in our constantly aging society. Contributing factors such as industrial, urban, and recreational noise that may lead to a high-frequency hearing loss can be prevented. Counseling is especially important for young patients with genetic or familial patterns of hearing loss. Annual or biennial audiograms in high-risk patients can lead to early diagnosis of a progressive SNHL that may be favorably influenced by career or lifestyle changes.

Current experience indicates that there is no effective medical or surgical treatment for presbycusis. However, management of elderly patients with SNHL requires experience, good judgment, and close interaction with a competent audiologist. Although many elderly patients with presbycusis benefit greatly from hearing aids, others with relatively mild SNHL or complex audiometric configurations may not be candidates for amplification. Unnecessary or poorly fitted hearing aids not only confuse and upset these patients, but they may contribute to the general notion that the devices are worthless. For most patients with mild presbycusis, there is usually no need for anything other than the use of a telephone buzzer and amplifier, a loud door buzzer instead of a bell, radio and television earphone attachments, and, above all, an understanding by the patient's family of the social aspects of SNHL. A thorough discussion on hearing aids indications and fitting is given in Chapter 37.

PROGNOSIS

Although the majority of patients with presbycusis will exhibit a slow deterioration of hearing, those with neural presbycusis, phonemic regression, and poor discrimination scores may worsen more rapidly and ultimately be profoundly deaf. The rehabilitation of these patients and others with moderate-to-severe SNHL requires close and frequent audiologic intervention, including precise hearing aid fitting, hearing aid modifications, periodic otologic examinations, lip reading classes, counseling, and possibly cochlear implantation.

CURRENT AND FUTURE AREAS OF INVESTIGATION

Much research is needed to improve our understanding of the etiology and pathogenesis of presbycusis and of those factors that may be susceptible to prevention and/or treatment. Little is known of the influence that demographics and socioeconomic conditions may have on the age of onset of presbycusis and the rate of hearing decline. Similarly, the contribution of dietary habits, tobacco use, alcohol consumption, and common diseases such as diabetes or hypertension has received only sporadic attention, producing few practical results but considerable controversy. The following abbreviated survey of some of the most salient studies fueling this controversy gives a perspective of our rudimentary understanding of these issues. Lowry and Issacson (82) found no differences in cholesterol levels among 100 elderly men with or without presbycusis, whereas Rosen et al. (83) noted better hearing preservation in individuals on a fat-restricted diet when compared with those on a diet high in saturated fats. Although animal experiments support the association of SNHL and hyperlipidemia (84,85), no relation was noted between hearing loss and those factors in 1,000, 50-year-old Scandinavian men studied by Drettner et al. (86). These factors were analyzed further by Gates et al. (87) in a carefully structured study of the possible relation of presbycusis to cardiovascular disease. They assessed the hearing status of 1,662 elderly men and women compared with their 30-year prevalence of cardiovascular disease. Many risk factors, including hypertension, blood glucose level, tobacco use, and cholesterol levels, were included in the study. The authors concluded that there was a small but statistically significant association of cardiovascular disease with hearing levels in the elderly, particularly in women, and more in the low than in the high frequencies. They further concluded, and we agree, that further research in this area, coupled with observations in animal models, is critical if we are to provide some concrete answers to the many unresolved issues fostering and complicating the development of SNHL in the elderly.

SUMMARY POINTS

- Age-associated SNHL in the high frequencies, in the absence of known otologic disorders, appears to be extremely common in the United States and other industrialized nations.
- Schuknecht's study performed in 1955 and the later revision performed in 1964 have been the gold standard in understanding the pathophysiology of presbycusis. His classification of the four different types of presbycusis remains a landmark study.
- Sensory presbycusis is associated with atrophy of the organ of Corti and the auditory nerve. Patients present with abrupt high-frequency SNHL and good speech discrimination scores. This pattern starts when patients are in their middle age years and progresses slowly.
- Neural presbycusis results from loss of neurons in the auditory pathways of the cochlea. Patients present with a relatively normal pure tone audiometry in comparison to very poor speech discrimination scores that fall abruptly as patients get older.
- Metabolic presbycusis is believed to be due to defects in physical and chemical processes of energy production in the sensory organs, resulting in a flat audiogram. The underlying pathologic condition is suspected to be atrophy of stria vascularis affecting all frequencies, leading to a flat audiogram.
- Mechanical presbycusis is associated with disorders of the mechanics of the cochlear duct, with relatively good cell populations in the stria vascularis and neurons. Basilar membrane thickening in the basal turn of the cochlea results in high-frequency hearing loss as seen in patients with mechanical presbycusis.
- A mixed pattern of the four different types of presbycusis can be seen in some patients. Therefore, patients may present with varying combinations of audiometric patterns, as described by the four classic types of presbycusis.
- Neurotransmitters such as GABA play a significant role in the function of the inferior colliculus in auditory processing. Kaspary et al. in 1995 postulated a neurochemical basis for the central auditory dysfunction in aging.
- Once the true importance of neurotransmitters, such as GABA, in deformities of central auditory processing is discovered, there is always the possibility that pharmacologic agents could become available that would reverse such defects, leading to improvement in hearing.
- Patients presenting with high-frequency SNHL deserve a properly directed diagnostic workup, regardless of their age. Rehabilitation continues to be with amplification devices, and patients should be encouraged to use these highly efficient units, despite the continuing stigmata associated with wearing hearing aids.

REFERENCES

1. Hinojosa R, Naunton RF. Presbycusis. In: Paparella MM, Shumrick DA, Meyerhoff WL, Gluckman J, eds. *Otolaryngology,* 3rd ed. Philadelphia: WB Saunders, 1990:1629–1637.

2. Gloric A, Wheeler D, Quiggle R, Grings W, Sommerfield A. Some medical implications of the 1954 Wisconsin State Fair hearing survey. *Trans Am Acad Ophthal Otolaryngol* 1957;61:160–171.

3. Hinchcliffe R. Threshold of hearing as a function of age. *Acoustica* 1959;9:303–313.

4. Hinchcliffe R. The threshold of hearing of a random sampled rural population. *Acta Otolaryngol (Stockh)* 1959;50:411–430.

5. Hinchcliffe R. Aging and sensory threshold. *J Gerontol* 1962;17:45–61.

6. Peterson JD, Morrell CH, Salent SG, et al. Gender differences in a longitudinal study of age associated hearing loss. *J Acoust Soc Am* 1995;97:1196–1205.

7. Rosen F, Bergman M, Plester D, El Mufti A, Sati MH. Presbycusis: study of a relatively noise free population in the Sudan. *Ann Otol* 1962;71:727–743.

8. Goycolea HV, Goycolea HG, Farfan C, Rodrigues L, Martinez GC, Vidal R. Effect of life in industrialized societies of hearing in natives of Eastern Island. *Laryngoscope* 1986;96:1391–1396.

9. Macrae JH. Noise induced hearing loss and presbycusis. *Audiology* 1971;10:323–333.

10. Wellenschik B, Raber A. Einfluss von Expositions Zeit und Alter anf den Irmbedingsten Horverlust. Boebachtungen an 25,544 industrierarbeitern. *Laryngol Rhinol Otol (Stugg)* 1978;57:1037–1048.

11. Norotny Z. Development of occupational deafness after entering a noisy job at an advanced age. *Cask Otolaryngol* 1975;24:151–154.

12. Sank D, Kallman RJ. The role of heredity in total deafness. *Volta Rev* 1963;68:461–470.

13. Paparella MM, Hanson DG, Rao KN, Olvestad R. Genetic sensorineural deafness in adults. *Ann Otol Rhinol Laryngol* 1975;84:459–472.

14. Fisch U, Dobozi M, Greig D. Degenerative changes of the arterial vessels of the internal auditory meatus during the process of aging. *Acta Otolaryngol (Stockh)* 1972;73:259–266.

15. Graton MA, Schmiedt RA, Schulte BA. Age-related decreases in endocochlear potential are associated with vascular abnormalities. *Hearing Res* 1996;94:116–124.

16. Krmpotic-Nemanic J, Nemanic C, Kostovic I. Macroscopical and microscopical changes in the bottom of the internal auditory meatus. *Acta Otolaryngol (Stockh)* 1972;73:254–258.

17. Kaspary DH, Millbrandt JC, Helfert RH. Central auditory aging: GABA changes in the inferior colliculus. *Exp Gerontol* 1995;30:349–360.

18. Soucek S, Michaels L, Frolich A. Pathological changes in the organ of corti in presbycusis as revealed by microslicing and straining. *Acta Otolaryngol Suppl* 1987;436:93–102.

19. Bai U, Seidman MD, Hinojosa R, Quirk WS. Mitochondrial DNA deletions associated with aging and possibly presbycusis: a human archival temporal bone study. *Am J Otol* 1997;18:449–453.

20. Schuknecht HF. Presbycusis. *Laryngoscope* 1955;65:402–419.

21. Schuknecht HF: Further observations of presbycusis. *Arch Otolaryngol* 1964;80:369–382.

22. Crowe SJ, Guild ST, Polugg LM. Observations of the pathology of high tone deafness. *Bull Johns Hopkins Hosp* 1934;54:315–379.

23. Schuknecht HF, Gacik MR. Cochlear pathology in presbycusis. *Ann Otol Laryngol Rhinol* 1993;102:1–16.

24. Schuknecht HF, Woellner RC. Hearing losses following partial section of the cochlear nerve. *Laryngoscope* 1953;63:441–465.

25. Otte J, Schuknecht HG, Kerr AG. Ganglion cell populations in normal and pathological human cochleae: implications for cochlear implantation. *Laryngoscope* 1978;88:1231–1246.

26. Arensen AR. Presbycusis: loss of neurons in the human cochlear nuclei. *J Laryngol Otol* 1982;96:503–511.

27. Pauler N, Schuknecht H, Thornton AL. Correlative studies of cochlear neuronal loss with speech discrimination and pure tone thresholds. *Arch Otolaryngol* 1986;243:200–206.

28. Gaeth JH. *Study of phonemic regression in relation to hearing loss.* Thesis. Chicago, IL: Northwestern University, Chicago, 1948.

29. Schuknecht HF. *Pathology of the ear.* Cambridge, MA: Harvard University Press, 1974.

30. Takahashi T. The ultrastructure of the pathological stria vascularis and spiral prominence in man. *Ann Otol Laryngol* 1971;80:721–735.

31. Takaski I, Spyropoulos CS. Stria vascularis as source of endocochlear potential. *J Neurophysiol* 1959;22:149–155.

32. Misrahy GA, DeJonge BR, Shinabarger EW, Arnold JE. Effect of localized hypoxia on electrophysiological activity of cochleae of the guinea pig. *J Acoust Soc Am* 1958;30:705–709.

33. Nachlas NE, Lurie MH. Stria vascularis: review and observations. *Laryngoscope* 1951;61:989–1003.

34. Vosteen KH. Neue Aspekte zur Biologie und Pathologie des Innenohres. *Arch Ohren Nasen Kehikopfheilk* 1961;178:1–104.

35. Davis H, Deatherage BH, Rosenblut B, Fernandez C, Kimura R, Smith CA. Modification of cochlear potentials produced by streptomycin poisoning and by extensive venous obstruction. *Laryngoscope* 1958;68:596–627.

36. Lever EG. The width of the basilar membrane in man. *Ann Otol Rhinol Laryngol* 1938;47:37–47.

37. von Bekesy G. On the elasticity of the cochlear partition. *J Acoust Soc Am* 1948;20:227–241.

38. Minor O. Das Anatomische Substrat der Alterschwerhorigkeit. *Arch Ohren Nasen Kehikopfheilk* 1919;105:1–13.

39. Glorig A, Davis H. Age, noise and hearing loss. *Ann Otol Rhinol Laryngol* 1961;70:556–571.

40. Wright JL, Schuknecht HF. Atrophy of the spiral ligament. *Arch Otolaryngol* 1972;96:16–21.

41. Lowell SH, Paparella MM. Presbycusis: what is it? *Laryngoscope* 1977;87:1710–1717.

42. von Fleandt H, Saxen A. Pathologic und Klinik der alters schwerhorigkeit. *Acta Otolaryngol Suppl* 1937;27[Suppl 23]:85–102.

43. Suga F, Lindsay J. Histopathological observations of presbycusis. *Ann Otol Rhinol Laryngol* 1976;85:169–184.

44. Johnsson LG, Hawkins JE. Sensory and neural degeneration with aging or seen in microdirections of the human inner ear. *Ann Otol Rhinol Laryngol* 1972;81:179–193.

45. Johnsson LG. Reissner's membrane in the human cochlea. *Ann Otol Rhinol Laryngol* 1971;80:425–438.

46. Watanuki K, Sato N, Kaku Y, et al. Reissner's membrane in human ears. *Acta Otolaryngol (Stockh)* 1981;91:65–74.

47. Saxen A. Pathologie und Klinik der Auterscherberhorkeit. In: Paparella MM, Shumrick DA, Meyerhoff WL, Gluckman J, eds. *Otolaryngology,* 3rd ed. Philadelphia: WB Saunders, 1990;2:1629–1637.

48. Makishima K. Clinical pathological studies in presbycusis. *Otol Fukuoka* 1967;13[Suppl 3]:333–350.

49. Makishima K. Clinical pathological studies in presbycusis: central and cochlear findings. *Otol Fukuoka* 1967;13[Suppl 1]:183–211.

50. Felder E, Schrott-Fischer A. Quantitative evaluation of myelinated nerve fibers and hair cells in cochleae of humans with age related high tone hearing loss. *Hearing Res* 1995;91:19–32.

51. Spoendlin H, Schrott-Fischer A. Quantitative evaluation of the human cochlear nerve. *Acta Otolaryngol (Stockh)* 1990;98[Suppl 470]:61–70.

52. Kirikae I. Auditory function in advanced age with reference to histological changes in the central auditory system. *Int Audiol* 1969;8:221–248.

53. Kirikae I, Sato T, Shitarat T. Study of hearing in advanced age. *Laryngoscope* 1964;74:205–230.

54. Dublin WB. *Fundamentals of sensorineural auditory pathology.* Springfield, IL: Charles C. Thomas Publisher, 1976:173–183.

55. Gussen R. Plugging of vascular canals in the otic capsule. *Ann Otol Rhinol Laryngol* 1969;78:1305–1315.

56. Igarishi M, Alfred BR, Konishi S, Shaver EF, Gielford FR. Functional and histopathological correlations after microembolism of the peripheral labyrinthine artery in the dog. *Laryngoscope* 1969;79:603–623.

57. Engstrom B, Hillerdal M, Laurel L, Bagger-Sjoback D. Selected pathological findings in the human cochlea. *Acta Otolaryngol (Stockh)* 1987;96[Suppl 436]:110–116.

58. Ishii T, Murakami Y, Kimura R, Baloh K. Electron microscopic and histochemical identification of lipofuscin in the human ear. *Acta Otolaryngol (Stockh)* 1967;64:17–29.

59. Faingold CL, Gehlbach G, Kaspary DN. On the role of GABA as an inhibitory neurotransmitter in inferior colliculus neurons: iontophoretic studies. *Brain Res* 1989;500:302–312.

60. Fujita I, Konishi N. The role of GABAergic inhibition in processing of interaural time difference in the owl's auditory system. *J Neurosci* 1991;11(3):722–739.

61. Park TJ, Pollak JD. GABA shapes sensitivity to interaural intensity disparities in the mustache bat's inferior colliculus: implications for encoding sound location. *J Neurosci* 1993;13:2050–2067.
62. Pollak JD, Park TJ. The effects of GABAergic inhibition on monaural response properties of neurons in mustache bats' inferior colliculus. *Hearing Res* 1993;65:99–117.
63. Funikawa FM, Weber DA. Effects of increased stimulus rate on brainstem electric response (BER) audiometry as a function of age. *J Am Audiol Soc* 1977;3:147–150.
64. Rowe NJ. Normal variability of the brainstem auditory evoked response in young and old adult subjects. *Electroencephalogr Clin Neurophysiol* 1978;44:459–470.
65. Maurizi M, Altissimi G, Ottaviani F, Paludetti G, Bambini M. Auditory brainstem response (ABR) in the aged. *Scand Audiol* 1982;11:213–221.
66. Sohal RS, Allen RG. Relationship between metabolic rate free radicals, differentiation and aging: a unified theory. In: Wooghead A, Blacket AD, Hollander A, eds. *Molecular biology of aging. Brook Haven Symposium, volume 35.* New York: Plenum Press, 1985:75–104.
67. Semsei I, Szeszek F, Nagy I. In vivo studies of age dependent decrease of the rates of total and mRNA synthesis in the brain cortex of rats. *Arch Gerontol Geriatr* 1982;1:29–42.
68. Richardson A, Butler JA, Rutherford MS, et al. Effects of age and dietary restrictions on the expression of alpha-2-8 microglobulin. *J Biol Chem* 1987;262:605–613.
69. Lindane AW, Marzuki S, Ozawa T, et al. Mitochondrial DNA mutations as an important contributor to aging and degenerative diseases. *Lancet* 1985;1:642–645.
70. DiMauro S, Bonilla E, Lombes A, et al. Mitochondrial encephalomyopathies. *Neurol Clin* 1990;8:483–506.
71. Paparella MM, Schachern PA, Yoon TH. Survey of interactions of middle ear and inner ear. *Acta Otolaryngol (Stockh)* 1988;97[Suppl 467]:9–24.
72. Paparella MM. Insidious labyrinthine changes of otitis media. *Acta Otolaryngol (Stockh)* 1981;92:513–520.
73. Paparella MM, Goycoolea MV, Shea D, Meyerhoff WL. Endolymphatic hydrops in otitis media. *Laryngoscope* 1979;81:43–54.
74. Paparella MM, Sajjadi H. Current clinical and pathological features of round window disease. *Laryngoscope* 1986;97:1151–1160.
75. Kawabata I, Paparella MM. Fine structures of the round window membrane. *Ann Otol Rhinol Laryngol* 1971;80:13–26.
76. Meyerhoff WL, Paparella MM, Kim CS. Pathology of chronic otitis media. *Ann Otol Rhinol Laryngol* 1978;86:481–502.
77. Brooks GD, Morrison AW. Vitamin D deficiency and deafness. *Br Med J* 1981;278:442–443.
78. Brooks GD. Vitamin D deficiency: a new cause of cochlear deafness. *J Laryngol Otol* 1983;97:405–420.
79. Brooks GD. Vitamin D deficiency and deafness: 1984 update. *Am J Otol* 1985;6:102–107.
80. Huygen P, Verhagen W, Noten J. Auditory abnormalities include precocious presbycusis in myotonic dystrophy. *Audiology* 1994;33:73–84.
81. Paparella MM, Schachern PA, Goycoolea MV. Multiple otopathological disorders. *Ann Otol Rhinol Laryngol* 1988;97:14–18.
82. Lowry LD, Issacson SR. Study of 100 patients with bilateral sensorineural hearing loss for lipid abnormalities. *Ann Otol Rhinol Laryngol* 1978;87:404–408.
83. Rosen S, Olin P, Rosen HV. Dietary prevention of hearing loss. *Acta Otolaryngol* 1970;70:242–247.
84. Morizono T, Paparella M. Hypercholesterolemia and auditory dysfunction. *Ann Otol Rhinol Laryngol* 1978;87:804–814.
85. Pillsbury HC. Hypertension, hyperlipoproteinemia, chronic noise exposure: is there synergism in cochlear pathology? *Laryngoscope* 1986;96:1112–1138.
86. Drettner B, Hedstrad H, Klockhoff I, Svedberg A. Cardiovascular risk factors and hearing loss (a study of 1000, 50 year old men). *Acta Otolaryngol (Stockh)* 1975;79:366–371.
87. Gates GA, Cobb JL, D'Agostino RB, Wolff PA. The relation of hearing in the elderly to the presence of cardiovascular disease and cardiovascular risk factors. *Arch Otolaryngol* 1993;119:56–161.

The Ear: Comprehensive Otology,
edited by R. F. Canalis and P. R. Lambert.
Lippincott Williams & Wilkins, Philadelphia © 2000.

CHAPTER 34

Tinnitus

Gregory A. Ator, Paul R. Lambert, and Rinaldo F. Canalis

DEFINITION

Tinnitus is a frequently presenting complaint best defined as a noise or sound arising in the head of the affected individual. Although the term (from the Latin *tinnere*: ringing) most often is applied to buzzing, ringing, or roaring sounds, it also includes pulsatile beats, clicks, and other abnormal noises that may or may not have an ear source. Therefore, tinnitus is not a disease or a syndrome, but only a symptom that may result from any one of a number of lesions.

All ear sounds are not pathologic. When placed in an anechoic chamber, the healthy person with no otologic abnormalities will hear a variety of sounds generated by the body at work. Examples include breathing, heart contraction, and blood circulation. Circumstances conducive to hearing these physiologic sounds are rarely present, as even in a quiet bedroom at night there is sufficient mask-

ing from the ambient noise level of 25 to 30 dB. Tinnitus becomes a symptom when such sounds have a higher intensity level than the masking environmental noise.

The history of otology has many interesting anecdotes of early attempts to treat and understand this vexing symptom. Two merit special mention. The first is the tragic death of Joseph Toynbee (1866) while experimenting with chloroform and hydrocyanic acid for tinnitus control, and the second is the striking description by Ludwig Von Beethoven of his increasing hearing loss. In a letter to his good friend Wegeler in 1801, he had these words to say about his symptoms: "only my ears whistle and buzz continuously day and night. I can say I am living a wretched life." Many tinnitus sufferers today would voice similar sentiments about this very bothersome and distracting malady.

PREVALENCE

Tinnitus is common, especially in middle and older age groups. According to the National Center for Health Statistics, approximately 32% of adults report tinnitus at some time in their lives; of these 32%, 6% characterize it as severe enough to be debilitating (1).

Recent studies showed that 17% of the British population have a problem with tinnitus (2). Of those ques-

G. A. Ator: Department of Otolaryngology, The University of Kansas Medical Center, Kansas City, Kansas 66160

P. R. Lambert: Department of Otolaryngology–Head and Neck Surgery, University of Virginia Health Sciences Center, Charlottesville, Virginia 22908-0430

R. F. Canalis: Department of Surgery, University of California, Los Angeles, School of Medicine, Los Angeles, California 90095-1624

tioned, about 1% had tinnitus producing severe annoyance, and 0.5% had such intense tinnitus that they were unable to lead a normal life. A current European survey found that 14% of adults suffered from tinnitus often or always, and 2.4% considered it severe (3). In this study, as in many others, tinnitus was associated with hearing loss (3). The prevalence of tinnitus has been noted to increase with age up to about 70 years and thereafter decline in frequency (4). An analysis of these statistics indicates that tinnitus is a major problem in industrialized societies, and it is likely to become even more significant in the future, given the increasing exposure to high ambient noise levels inherent to urban living.

PATHOGENESIS

The events responsible for the development of tinnitus vary according to its source and, for the most part, are addressed under each individual type later in this chapter. In this section we briefly discuss tinnitus theory as it pertains to the sensorineural structures of the auditory system.

Attempts have been made to identify cochlear correlates of tinnitus, as many conditions that cause peripheral damage to the auditory system result in this symptom. However, no definite histopathologic or physiologic alteration has been documented that implicates the end organ as solely responsible for this symptom (5). Jastreboff (6) showed that all levels of the auditory system may be involved in the activity responsible for the perception of abnormal noise. Furthermore, it is common for patients with a nonfunctioning cochlea to have severe tinnitus. Currently, abnormal neural excitation is thought to be responsible for the development of tinnitus. Two mechanisms appear plausible: (a) ephaptic excitation of one nerve by a neighboring nerve leading to synchronization of discharges, as might occur in an acoustic neuroma; and (b) spontaneous excess influx of potassium and calcium into sensory hair cells causing a synchronous release at all their synapses, which could occur in noise trauma and ototoxicity (7). Support for abnormal excitation theories may be found in such diverse conditions as hemifacial spasm and trigeminal neuralgia. In these cases, a vascular loop surrounding the involved cranial nerve (VII and V, respectively) is frequently found. Relief of symptoms following surgical decompression suggests that such loops may stimulate excessive neural discharges while preserving some features from the normal function of the nerve (8). Using this concept, tinnitus may be interpreted as an abnormal perception of the auditory nerve that is synchronously discharging.

Otoacoustic emissions are recently described phenomena that are thought to be related to spontaneous and evoked instabilities of the filtering system of outer hair cells. Recent work on cochlear emissions by Kemp (9) showed that some ears emit extremely low-intensity sounds that can be recorded in the external ear canal but may or may not be heard by the patient or the observer. In a comprehensive review, Norton et al. (10) found that spontaneous otoacoustic emissions were more likely to be the source of tinnitus when the subject had residual hearing. Nevertheless, these authors concluded that spontaneous emissions are the cause of tinnitus only in a small percentage of patients. This opinion was substantiated by Penner (11), who found the incidence to be 4.2%. The tinnitus associated with spontaneous emissions may be suppressed with aspirin, which raises the possibility of effective symptom control in this small group of patients. Studies with evoked otoacoustic emissions have shown that cochlear mechanical injury, such as that caused by noise, may produce prolonged oscillating emissions and be accompanied by tinnitus. The emission, however, is not the source of the tinnitus (10).

DIAGNOSIS

Patients who present with tinnitus should have a thorough history taken and head and neck examination focusing on the auditory system. Important points to consider are the duration, location, extent, and nature of the noise and whether or not it is synchronous with the heartbeat. Other details regard positions or maneuvers that improve or worsen the tinnitus, prior episodes, and history of ear disease or ear surgery. Exposure to ototoxic agents, intense noise, or ear trauma also are important.

Otoscopy should be undertaken under the microscope. If pulsatile tinnitus is present, auscultation of the ear, temporal region, and neck should be performed, preferably in an auditory booth. Auscultation of the external auditory canal is performed using a Toynbee tube (see following and Chapter 7). Audiometry is essential in the evaluation of all forms of tinnitus. Unless a specific cause is readily found (e.g., presbycusis, noise-induced hearing loss, Meniere's disease), magnetic resonance imaging (MRI) studies with gadolinium contrast is indicated, especially if the tinnitus is unilateral. Although unusual, some retrocochlear lesions may present without significant audiometric findings and with tinnitus as their sole symptom. In cases of temporal bone trauma or middle ear disease, computerized axial tomography (CT) with or without contrast may be indicated. The evaluation of vascular tinnitus is described in detail later in this chapter.

CLASSIFICATION

Many schemes have been proposed to classify tinnitus, a fact that emphasizes its diverse causes. Traditional classifications are based on site of origin and on whether or not the tinnitus can be perceived by the observer. Tinnitus heard by the observer is known as *objective,* whereas tin-

TABLE 1. *Etiologic classification of tinnitus*

Vascular
    Arterial
    Venous
Muscular
    Palatal myoclonus
    Tensor tympani or stapedial myoclonus
Internal auditory canal lesions
    Eighth cranial nerve tumors
    Vascular loops
Cochlear disorders
    Noise trauma
    Temporal bone trauma
    Meniere's disease
    Presbycusis
    Sudden sensorineural hearing loss
    Otoacoustic emissions
Ototoxicity
    Aspirin
    Quinine
    Aminoglycosides
Middle ear pathology
    Effusions
    Otosclerosis
    Patulous eustachian tube
Miscellaneous
    Cerumen impaction
    Foreign bodies

TABLE 2. *Vascular etiologies of pulsatile tinnitus*

Extracranial arterial disease
    Atheroscleroses
    Fibromuscular dysplasia
    Dissection
    Tortuosity
Intratemporal arterial anomalies
Arteriovenous lesions
    Dural arteriovenous fistula
    Extracranial arteriovenous fistula
    Pial arteriovenous malformation
Increased intracranial pressure
    Benign intracranial hypertension
    Dural sinus thrombosis
    Hydrocephalus
Glomus tumors
Venous anomalies
    Jugular anomalies
    Abnormal emissary veins
    Transverse sinus stenosis
Hyperdynamic vascular states
    Pregnancy
    Hyperthyroidism
    Anemia

nitus heard only by the patient is termed *subjective.* In general, objective tinnitus is believed to have an identifiable acoustic (vibratory) source, whereas subjective tinnitus is thought to originate in the peripheral and/or central auditory pathways. Tinnitus also can be classified as *pulsatile* or *nonpulsatile*, the former usually indicating a vascular etiology; pulsatile tinnitus may be objective or subjective. In many cases, tinnitus is more complex than suggested by classification schemes. We believe that it is more accurate to classify tinnitus according to its probable source of origin and have used this concept in the organization of this chapter (Table 1).

VASCULAR LESIONS

Vascular tumors (e.g., glomus tympanicum or jugulare, hemangioma) and vascular abnormalities (e.g., arteriovenous malformations, aneurysms, stenosis of the carotid artery, transmitted cardiac murmurs, transverse sinus stenosis, venous hums) can cause turbulent blood flow resulting in a pulsatile "murmur" heard by the patient (12–15). In addition to these specific lesions, conditions that cause a hyperdynamic vascular state, such as anemia, pregnancy, or hyperthyroidism, can produce a functional murmur that is transmitted to the ear and heard as a pulsating sound (Table 2).

In most vessels, blood flow is laminar and inaudible. When blood flow loses its laminar quality and assumes a random pattern, its kinetic energy is increased. This energy is released, in part, by vibration of the vessel wall, producing a murmur or hum that usually is in the audible frequency range. Whether blood flow would be laminar or turbulent can be predicted by Reynold's number (R):

$$R = \frac{v \cdot d}{\frac{\eta}{\rho}}$$

where d is the vessel diameter, v is the velocity of blood flow, η is the blood viscosity, and ρ is the density of the blood. The larger this number, the greater the tendency for turbulent flow. Thus, turbulence is directly related to vessel size and blood velocity and indirectly related to blood viscosity. The likelihood of turbulence is especially high in areas where there are abrupt changes in vessel size or contour.

The first turn of the petrosal carotid artery passes within a few millimeters of the basal turn of the cochlea, but this is rarely the source of tinnitus. In the presence of a conductive hearing loss, carotid blood flow may produce a pulsatile "body noise" audible by the patient but not by the examiner. Infrequently, tympanic membrane movements synchronous with the patient's pulse may be noted. The possibility of a dehiscence of the carotid plate or an anomalous carotid artery (Figs. 1 and 2) must be excluded. Myringotomy is contraindicated until radiographic (CT) documentation of a normal carotid is documented.

A *venous hum* is produced by flow disturbances in the high-velocity veins in the region of the ear. A cervical

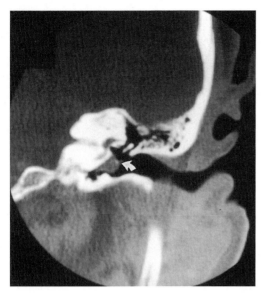

FIG. 1. Coronal computerized tomographic scan showing a mass *(arrow)* on the left promontory in a patient with pulsatile tinnitus.

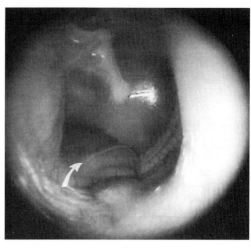

FIG. 3. Otoscopic view of the right ear of a patient complaining of pulsatile tinnitus. A bluish mass representing a large, dehiscent jugular bulb was apparent in the posterior mesotympanum, extending several millimeters lateral to the annulus *(arrow)*.

venous hum is a well-described phenomenon in children (16,17). In that setting, it is almost always a normal finding and asymptomatic. The cause or location of the turbulent blood flow in adults causing a venous hum is uncertain, although in most cases it appears to arise within the internal jugular vein–jugular bulb–sigmoid sinus system. Partial compression of the internal jugular

vein by impingement from the second vertical vertebrae has been hypothesized (18). In our experience, identification of an obstructing lesion is seldom found, and the jugular vein usually has a normal angiographic appearance. It is noteworthy, however, that most patients with venous hum tinnitus have an enlarged jugular bulb on the

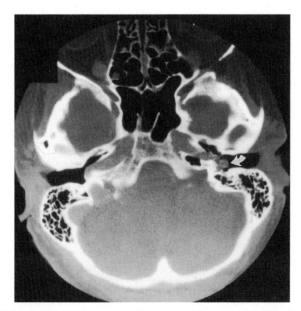

FIG. 2. Axial computerized tomographic scan showing that the "mass" in Fig. 1 was an aberrant internal carotid artery. (Note the same aberrancy on the right side.) This "mass" has been biopsied, resulting in a pseudoaneurysm of the internal carotid artery *(arrow)*.

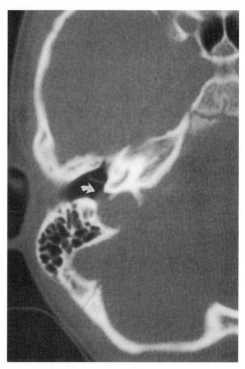

FIG. 4. Axial computed tomographic scan showing a dehiscent jugular bulb in a patient with a bluish mass in the hypotympanum and pulsatile tinnitus *(arrow)*.

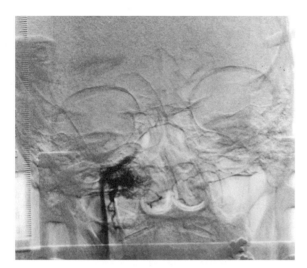

FIG. 5. Selective right ascending pharyngeal arterial injection showing an arteriovenous malformation involving the jugular bulb.

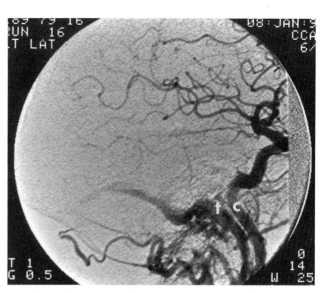

FIG. 7. Carotid arteriogram. Internal carotid artery injection showing a dural arteriovenous fistula involving the transverse sinus *(t)* and the petrosal portion of the internal carotid artery *(c)*.

affected side (19). Given that turbulence is encouraged by abrupt changes in vessel size or contour, the sigmoid sinus–jugular bulb or jugular bulb–internal jugular vein interfaces may be the site of origin of the venous hum. A diverticulum or dehiscence of the jugular bulb has also been associated with a venous hum (Figs. 3 and 4). Also

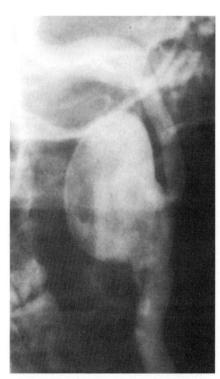

FIG. 6. Carotid arteriogram. Left internal carotid artery injection showing a 4- × 2-cm aneurysm of that vessel at the skull base.

of note is the predilection for this condition to occur in mildly obese women in the third to fifth decade of life.

Benign intracranial hypertension (BIH) has been associated with a venous hum (20). This idiopathic increase in intracranial pressure usually presents with headache and visual changes, such as transient visual obscurations, blurred vision, and a loss of visual field or acuity (21,22). Thus, a venous hum associated with any of the aforementioned symptoms should raise the possibility of benign intracanial hypertension.

High-pressure arterial sources typically produce a sound that varies with the heart rate and generally is due to an *arteriovenous malformation* (AVM) in proximity to the temporal bone (Fig. 5). The most common type of AVM is between branches of the occipital artery and the transverse sinus (23). Trauma to the temporal bone can also result in an *arteriovenous shunt*, which can enlarge and produce a bruit that progresses in intensity over time. Trauma to the neck or skull base also can produce an aneurysm of the internal carotid artery (Fig. 6). Dural arteriovenous fistulas may present in the absence of trauma and produce tinnitus (Fig. 7).

Physical Examination

Physical examination frequently will disclose the correct diagnosis in patients complaining of pulsatile tinnitus. The synchrony of the patient's tinnitus with the pulse should be evaluated. Auscultation over the neck and cranium adjacent to the ear is important in revealing a carotid bruit or AVM. A venous hum can often be heard by the examiner if a Toynbee tube is placed in the external ear canal. Glomus tumors or other middle ear vascular masses usually can be seen by otomicroscopy. In most cases of venous hum, light compression of the lateral neck that is sufficient to occlude the jugular vein but not the carotid artery will reduce the tinnitus. This finding will not be the case for most arterial sources of pulsatile tinnitus. Some patients with a venous hum will report that turning their head either toward or away from the affected side will diminish the sound. The Valsalva maneuver, which increases intrathoracic pressure and decreases venous return to the heart, is effective in reducing tinnitus of venous origin, but should have little effect on tinnitus of arterial sources.

Audiometric and Radiographic Studies

Results of audiometric studies in most patients with vascular tinnitus are normal. An obvious exception is the conductive hearing loss caused by a glomus tumor involving the ossicular chain. Occasionally, an apparent low-frequency sensorineural hearing loss is present secondary to the masking effect of the tinnitus found in cases of venous hums (24). Abolishing the tinnitus in such cases will return bone conduction thresholds to their true level. Rhythmic compliance changes on tympanometry may be present with carotid abnormalities or with middle ear vascular tumors.

Most patients with pulsatile tinnitus should undergo an imaging study to exclude the presence of a vascular or neoplastic lesion (Fig. 8). An exception would be the older individual with atherosclerotic vascular disease who notes bilateral tinnitus. Some patients will require conventional cerebral angiography, which remains the test of choice for the identification of complex vascular lesions associated with this symptom. Magnetic resonance angiography (MRA) is an excellent initial imaging study in most cases; however, it is possible for MRA to miss a small glomus tympanicum tumor or small dural AVM. In the former case, CT scan is preferable and phys-

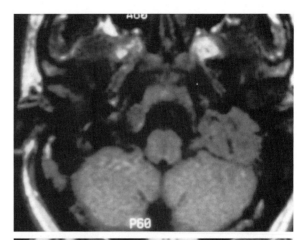

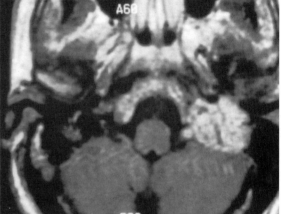

FIG. 8. Axial T_1-weighted magnetic resonance image showing a large left glomus jugulare tumor. The *bottom panel* demonstrates tumor enhancement following gadolinium infusion. Note the flow voids representing vascular channels within the tumor.

ical examination of the ear will usually disclose the lesion. A cerebral angiogram may be necessary for definitive diagnosis of a small dural AVM. Figure 9 shows flow diagrams for radiographic evaluation depending on otoscopic findings.

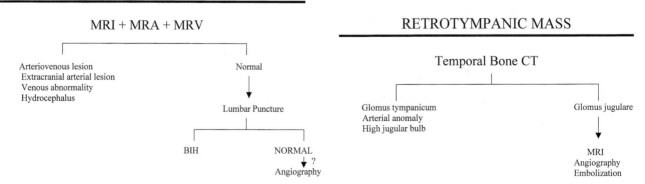

FIG. 9. Radiographic evaluation of pulsatile tinnitus.

Treatment

Tinnitus associated with vascular lesions such as AVMs or aneurysms is uncommon. However, when present, embolization of an AVM usually is associated with reduction or elimination of tinnitus. For suspected venous hums, management first involves exclusion of other vascular lesions and identification of an adequate alternate venous drainage by angiographic studies as just described. Ligation of the internal jugular vein frequently produces permanent control of the venous hum. Obliteration of the sigmoid sinus may be considered, but risk to the superficial cerebral veins (especially if surgery is being performed on the dominant side) must be carefully assessed if such surgery is contemplated.

MUSCULAR LESIONS

Muscular sources of tinnitus are associated with abnormal rhythmic activity of muscles adjacent to the auditory system. The most common example is *palatal myoclonus* (or *palatal tremor*). Patients with this condition have an intermittent tinnitus that correlates temporally with intermittent contractions of the soft palate and other oropharyngeal muscles. These movements can usually be observed transorally or transnasally. Documentation of this disorder by tympanometry is easily done by observing rhythmic variability in the tracing that corresponds to the patient's involuntary muscle activity.

Patients with palatal myoclonus should have an MRI scan to evaluate potential brainstem pathology. Lesions that have been associated with this entity include multiple sclerosis, small vessel disease, tumor, and degenerative neurologic diseases. Procedures such as sectioning of the palatal muscles and medical therapy with carbamazepine have been used with limited success (25). Significant side effects from carbamazepine, such as hepatic toxicity, may limit its usefulness in routine cases (26).

Tensor tympani or *stapedius muscle myoclonus* can occur in association with palatal myoclonus, or it can occur as an isolated finding. Movements of the tympanic membrane are not necessarily rhythmic in these cases, and the tinnitus may resolve spontaneously. Sectioning of the tensor tympani tendon and/or the stapedius tendon can be curative for persistent cases.

AUDITORY NERVE LESIONS

Acoustic Neuroma

Auditory nerve lesions of various types can produce tinnitus. The most common mass in the cerebellopontine angle is the *acoustic neuroma* (see Chapter 53). These tumors arise from the vestibular portion of the eighth cranial nerve and slowly compress adjacent structures. Tinnitus can occur in isolation or in combination with hearing loss. The onset can be sudden or progressive, but it is nearly always unilateral. Auditory brainstem response testing or MRI is required to evaluate for possible retrocochlear lesions in all patients with unilateral tinnitus. Neuromas arising from the facial nerve also can produce tinnitus (27).

Vascular Loops

A vascular loop compressing the auditory nerve has been implicated in the etiology of tinnitus (1,28,29). The pathophysiology of this type of tinnitus is not understood. It is hypothesized that the auditory nerve experiences an "irritation" from a vessel that is in close contact with it. Brainstem auditory nuclei may be secondarily affected by changes in the auditory nerve and be the actual generator site(s) for the tinnitus. This scenario is consistent with auditory brainstem response data that has suggested central, rather than auditory nerve, abnormalities in patients with presumed vascular compression as the etiology for their tinnitus (30).

Other cranial nerves can be affected by a vascular loop and result in sensory or motor dysfunction. Examples are hemifacial spasm and trigeminal neuralgia from compression of the facial and trigeminal nerves, respectively. In both these conditions, brainstem abnormalities (facial motor nucleus and trigeminal sensory nucleus) appear to result from cranial nerve compression, thus supporting the tinnitus hypothesis discussed earlier (31,32). Vascular loops can be difficult to diagnosis, but they are best demonstrated by MRI/MRA.

Microvascular decompression has been successful in alleviating trigeminal neuralgia and hemifacial spasm. Moller et al. (33) reviewed their experience with this surgical modality in the management of incapacitating tinnitus. In a series of 72 patients, 18% experienced total relief and 22% had marked symptomatic improvement. The majority of these patients had suffered from tinnitus for less than 3 years. Choice of surgery was predominantly based on history and, to a lesser extent, on audiometric data, but the authors acknowledge that precise patient selection is difficult.

COCHLEAR LESIONS

Various processes that inflict damage on the cochlea can produce bothersome tinnitus. The most common, *presbycusis,* is a sensorineural hearing impairment usually presenting in the fifth to sixth decade of life (see Chapter 33). Patients usually complain of bilateral high-pitched tinnitus. Another frequent source of damage to the cochlea leading to tinnitus is *noise trauma* (see Chapter 48). The association of tinnitus with this disorder is stronger than for presbycusis. Nearly all patients with a significant sensorineural hearing loss at 4 to 6 kHz will complain of tinnitus. Again, it is typically constant, bilateral, and high frequency.

Meniere's disease is frequently accompanied by tinnitus, a symptom originally proposed by Prosper Meniere as part of the diagnostic triad of the disease (see Chapter 40). The tinnitus is noted by the patient to be louder during acute attacks and usually is associated with low-frequency sensorineural hearing loss, vertigo, and aural fullness. In contrast to the high-pitched tinnitus characteristic for presbycusis, the tinnitus of Meniere's disease typically is described as a low-pitched roaring sound. Treatment with diuretics and dietary elimination of salt, caffeine, and other stimulants may be helpful in controlling these symptoms.

PHARMACOLOGIC FACTORS

Drugs are a common cause of tinnitus, with *aspirin* and *quinine* being the most frequent offenders. Tinnitus induced by large doses of aspirin is usually high frequency (7 to 9 kHz), tonal in nature, and frequently accompanied by a temporary threshold shift (34). These effects resolve spontaneously with withdrawal of the drug, but the mechanism of action is controversial and may involve alteration of the cochlear mechanics of the outer hair cells (35). Quinine, as well as other antimalarial drugs, also is associated with reversible tinnitus as a side effect (36). Essentially any ototoxic agent acting on the auditory or vestibular system may cause transient or permanent tinnitus. *Chemotherapeutic* drugs (e.g., cisplatinum) and *aminoglycoside* antibiotics are especially significant (see Chapter 35).

MIDDLE EAR LESIONS

Miscellaneous causes of tinnitus include middle ear pathology, most frequently *otosclerosis,* and other causes of conductive hearing loss, such as middle ear *effusions* and less frequently *tumors.* Many of these disorders cause tinnitus by producing a conductive hearing loss that masks out environmental noise and allows the background "body noise" to become manifest. Elimination of the conductive hearing loss will usually cause the tinnitus to improve or disappear.

Patulous Eustachian Tube

Under normal conditions, the eustachian tube is maintained in a closed position by virtue of the pliability of its cartilage and extraluminal factors such as the peritubal fat pad. A patulous eustachian tube occasionally is seen in patients experiencing rapid weight loss, mucosal atrophy (as occurs after radiotherapy), or muscular dysfunc-

tion. This abnormality allows for a to-and-fro movement of the tympanic membrane, synchronous with nasal respiration, which in turn results in an annoying and distracting noise of varying severity. Patients usually complain of their voice reverberating in their ear, especially with nasal sounds (e.g., "m" and "n"), and aural fullness or "stuffiness." This disorder usually is seen in adult patients. Recumbency may relieve the symptom because of increased venous stasis and passive compression of the tube. Nasal congestion from an upper respiratory tract infection also may alleviate the problem. At otoscopy the tympanic membrane is noted to move medially on inspiration and laterally on expiration. This finding can be exaggerated by forced respiration with mouth closed and the contralateral nostril occluded. Tympanometry may be of help in the diagnosis by showing fluctuations in the tympanometric tracing that are coincident with the patient's breathing.

Treatment

A saturated solution of potassium iodine (SSKI) or conjugated estrogen (Premarin) nose drops can be effective in the management of the noise associated with a patulous eustachian tube. By increasing mucus secretion, SSKI causes congestion around the eustachian tube orifice with improved tubal closure. The dose is 10 drops of the liquid in a glass of juice three times per day. A potential side effect is parotid swelling and/or pain caused by enhanced secretory activity within the gland. If this occurs, the medication dose should be halved (or discontinued if symptoms persist). Premarin nose drops consist of 25 mg of Premarin in a 30-cc normal saline solution. The dosage is three drops in the affected side nostril given three times a day (37).

Surgical control of the noise generated by nasal breathing and tympanic membrane movements noted in patulous eustachian tube disorders may be difficult. Insertion of a pressure equalization tube may be tried, but in the authors' experience the results are equivocal. Cauterization of the eustachian tube meatus has been reported with occasional success. Polytetrafluoroethylene (Teflon) injection has proved effective, although it may migrate and its use is restricted. Of necessity, most obstructive procedures of the eustachian tube meatus tend to produce permanent dysfunction requiring life-long use of pressure equalization tubes; therefore, patients should be selected with extreme care. Bluestone and Cantekin (38) described a reversible procedure that involves gaining access to the middle ear and the eustachian tube via an anterior tympanostomy flap. An angiocath then is introduced into the tube after fashioning it for each individual case. Hammulotomy or transposition of the tensor veli palatini muscle to restrict opening of the eustachian tube had been attempted by Stroud et al. (39) with some degree of improvement; however, the efficacy of this operation lacks confirmation.

GENERAL MANAGEMENT

Drug Therapy

Drug therapy has been in the forefront of tinnitus research for many years, but a medication that is consistently effective in the long-term treatment of this symptom has not yet been identified. Several agents currently under investigation show some promise for the treatment of tinnitus.

Niacin and its derivatives, such as *nicotinamide*, are vasodilators that have been widely used empirically in the treatment of cochlear disorders. Early work by Flottorp and Willie (40) indicated that most patients with Meniere's disease would receive some benefit from long-term niacin (as nicotinic acid) administration. However, recent work using nicotinamide has not been as encouraging (41).

Trimetazidine, an antiischemic drug with antioxidant properties, was evaluated by Coyas and Annales (42) in a double-blind, placebo-controlled study of 45 tinnitus patients. They found that although objective audiometric findings remained unchanged, there was a statistically significant subjective improvement in patients treated with this drug. In another multicenter controlled study, Pech (43) confirmed the value of this agent, particularly for patients with tinnitus of recent onset (less than 2 years) and tinnitus presumably related to ischemic disease (43).

Vitamin A given in high doses has been reported to improve thresholds and inhibit tinnitus (44). However, toxicity is a real concern that limits its practical use.

Intravenous *lidocaine,* an amide local anesthetic with central nervous system actions, has been widely reported to be beneficial for tinnitus control. The mechanism of action of lidocaine in the relief of tinnitus is not known. Martin and Coleman (45) used a double-blind, cross-over design in a study that showed reduction of tinnitus frequency and intensity following lidocaine treatment (45). Overall, a 31% improvement in the matched intensity of tinnitus was recorded by these authors; subjectively, however, up to 72% of patients noted symptomatic improvement after treatment. More recently, Yamanaka et al. (46) treated 149 patients with weekly injections of lidocaine. They noted long-term relief in 61% of cases. Treatment appeared to be more beneficial for low-pitched tinnitus and in older patients. Because clinical responses often were noted to increase after eight treatments, they recommended long-term trials before assessing efficacy. The intravenous mode of delivery limits lidocaine usefulness in the routine management of tinnitus.

Tocainide is an oral derivative of lidocaine with a long half-life. Emmet and Shea (47) used tocainide in individuals who had experienced improvement with intravenous lidocaine and noted a 60% reduction in tinnitus severity in 36 patients who took the drug four times a day. It appears, however, that tocainide is less effective than lidocaine. Lenarz (48) reported that only 25% of patients responded to this drug. Several drugs currently used in the treatment of trigeminal neuralgia have been found to be of some benefit for tinnitus control. Melding and Goodey (49) gave both *lidocaine* and *carbamazepine* to patients with severe tinnitus. After 2 to 3 months on the drug, 60% of patients noted elimination or reduction of tinnitus to about 30% of pretreatment levels based on subjective measures. In general, only patients who responded favorably to lidocaine noted relief with carbamazepine.

The effect of antidepressants on tinnitus was studied by Mihail et al. (50), who evaluated the tricyclic *trimipramine* in a double-blind, placebo-controlled study. Although they found several patients reporting improvement and even elimination of tinnitus, they could not conclude that the results were medication related. Other investigators found a positive effect with nortriptyline and other antidepressants, but they attributed this to mood elevation and improved coping ability (51,52).

Surgery

Surgery plays a role in tinnitus management when it can be applied to the correction of the disorder producing the symptom. House (53) reported that of 109 patients undergoing stapedectomy for otosclerosis, 37% noted elimination of their tinnitus, 39% said it was improved, and 20% experienced no change. Only 4% noted that the tinnitus was worse.

Cochlear implants have been shown to have some effect on tinnitus. In a recent survey by Tyler and Kelsay (54), 81% of subjects with cochlear implants indicated that the device had a positive effect on their tinnitus, while 2% thought the tinnitus was made worse. Other investigators reported similar results (55). Although a single-channel cochlear prosthesis presenting sinusoidal waveform signals has been reported effective in the long-term suppression of tinnitus, this approach has not been investigated in large clinical trials (56).

Cochlear Nerve Section

Although intuitively attractive, cochlear nerve section for tinnitus remains controversial, primarily because results are unpredictable. More than a half century ago, Dandy (57) noted that approximately 50% of 40 patients experienced a decrease in tinnitus following cochlear nerve section for Meniere's disease. This experience parallels more recent results following translabyrinthine acoustic neuroma resection (58). Several authors, including Fisch (59) and Barrs and Brackmann (60), investigated tinnitus improvement in patients with Meniere's disease treated by either a vestibular nerve section or a cochlear vestibular nerve section. The improvement rate was increased 10% to 15% with the addition of the cochlear neurectomy, although these differences were not statistically significant. Other authors, however, have not demonstrated any numerical difference in tinnitus relief between these two procedures (61). Pulec (62) and Silverstein et al. (63) reported series with very high rates of tinnitus cure or improvement following vestibular nerve section (67% and 76%, respectively). It should be noted that in the latter report involving patients undergoing surgery for Meniere's disease, an endolymphatic sac procedure also resulted in tinnitus relief or improvement in 66% of patients. Most recently, Wazen et al. (64) reported improvement in two patients who underwent a retrosigmoid or retrolabyrinthine selective cochlear nerve section for debilitating tinnitus. The potential advantage of this approach is preservation of vestibular function in those patients who still have an intact labyrinth.

In general, sectioning of the cochlear nerve (with or without labyrinthectomy or vestibular nerve section) does not reliably improve tinnitus. The possibility of worsening the symptom with surgery, which has been reported in approximately 10% of cases, must be considered (60,61).

Masking

The use of masking relies on the principle that application of an acoustic tone of the same characteristics as the tinnitus will make the offending noise inaudible. A trial of this type of device is indicated for patients with intractable tinnitus. Masking can be applied by several devices, including some specifically designed to look like conventional hearing aids but lacking a microphone. In general, a *masker* produces a band of nose that can be tailored to match the patient's tinnitus frequency and intensity measurements. Some patients, however, are not able to precisely match the pitch of the tinnitus to an externally applied sound. In such cases, a series of noise bands are presented to the patient in an attempt to select the one that best masks the tinnitus. Patients who successfully use maskers may have a variable period of residual inhibition that continues after the device is removed (65,66).

A simple alternative to maskers is to tune an FM radio to a frequency between stations and play this sound at a low level during the night when scant ambient noise intensifies tinnitus awareness. A wideband white noise results, which can be helpful in reducing tinnitus audibility. This form of masking also can be supplied by a personal stereo with headphones to avoid exposing others to this continuous noise.

Many patients with a hearing loss requiring amplification find that *hearing aid(s)* act as a masking device by increasing ambient noise. This approach is the initial one recommended for patients with tinnitus and an aidable sensorineural hearing loss. *Tinnitus instruments,* which combine a hearing aid and masker in one device, also can be tried.

Electrical Suppression

Electrical stimulation applied to the area of the temporal bone and the tympanic membrane has met with varying levels of success in tinnitus reduction. It is apparent that the closer the stimulation site is to the cochlea and eighth cranial nerve, the more effective the treatment will be. Kuk et al. (67) noted reduction in tinnitus annoyance and loudness in 5 of 10 patients who had electrical stimulation of the tympanic membrane. However, externally applied electrical stimulation has been less effective. Two controlled studies using a specific device have noted success rates on the order of 5% to 7% in patients with tinnitus of peripheral origin (68,69). This is in marked contrast to an initial report by Shulman (70) of a 62% success rate.

Miscellaneous Treatments

Dietary modification, biofeedback, acupuncture, and hyperbaric oxygen have been suggested for tinnitus control (71–74). These treatments have sometimes been successful and may be tried when more conventional therapies fail. Acupuncture has not been successful in producing long-term relief. Biofeedback is a well-documented means to identify and reduce stress and may be of value in some cases (75). The majority of these treatment programs do not alter the intensity of the perceived noise, but they are effective in controlling the psychological symptoms associated with severe tinnitus. In this way they reduce stress and improve the patient's ability to cope with the disorder.

Psychosocial Aspects

Psychiatric illness may complicate the management of individuals with debilitating tinnitus. Sullivan et al. (76) showed a high incidence of major depression in tinnitus sufferers. Simpson et al. (77) noted that 63% had a psychiatric disorder, most commonly a mood disturbance. Briner et al. (78) noted a significant incidence of personality disorders and severe anxiety in a similar study group. The high incidence of psychiatric disorders in patients with incapacitating tinnitus emphasizes the need to assess these patients for psychiatric disease and initiate treatment or referral as needed.

SUMMARY POINTS

- Tinnitus can be classified as pulsatile/nonpulsatile and objective/subjective.
- Most patients with tinnitus experience a subjective, nonpulsatile noise that results, at least initially, from cochlear pathology (e.g., nose trauma, presbycusis).
- Evaluation of subjective, nonpulsatile tinnitus includes audiometric testing and, if unilateral, retrocochlear testing (auditory brainstem response and/or MRI) to rule out an acoustic tumor or other lesion affecting the eighth cranial nerve.
- Pulsatile tinnitus (subjective or objective) usually has a definable cause, such as neoplasm, vascular anomaly, or muscular dysfunction.
- The most common neoplasm causing pulsatile tinnitus is a glomus tumor (tympanicum or jugulare).
- Venous hums, AVMs, and transmitted cardiac or carotid sounds are common vascular abnormalities causing pulsatile tinnitus.
- Turbulent flow within the sigmoid sinus, jugular bulb, and/or internal jugular vein is thought to be responsible for a venous hum. This condition may be associated with benign intracranial hypertension.
- If no middle ear mass is evident otoscopically, unilateral pulsatile tinnitus should be evaluated by MRI/MRA/MRV (magnetic resonance venography); if a mass is seen, CT is the preferred imaging modality.
- Treatment of tinnitus is difficult. Although intravenous lidocaine appears to have transient benefit, no oral pharmacologic agent provides consistent relief. Likewise, the results of surgery (e.g., cochlear nerve section) are unpredictable.
- It is possible to "mask" a patient's tinnitus. This masking sound can be provided by amplifying ambient noise with a hearing aid or by introducing noise with a masking device.

REFERENCES

1. National Center for Health Statistics. *Hearing Status Among Adults, United States, 1960–1962.* U.S. Department of Health, Education and Welfare, 1968.
2. Institute of Hearing Research. Epidemiology of tinnitus. *Ciba Found Symp* 1981;85:204–216.
3. Axelsson A, Ringdahl A. Tinnitus—a study of its prevalence and characteristics. *Br J Audiol* 1989;3:53–62.
4. Reed GF. An audiometric study of two hundred cases of subjective tinnitus. *Arch Otolaryngol* 1960;71:94–104.
5. Oliveira CA, Schuknecht HD, Glynn RJ. In search of cochlear morphologic correlates for tinnitus. *Arch Otolaryngol Head Neck Surg* 1990;116:937–939.
6. Jastreboff PJ. Phantom auditory perception (tinnitus): mechanisms of generation and perception. *Neurosci Res* 1990;8:221–254.
7. Eggermont JJ. On the pathophysiology of tinnitus: a review and a peripheral model. *Hear Res* 1990;48:111–123.
8. Moller AR. Pathophysiology of tinnitus. *Ann Otol Rhinol Laryngol* 1984;93:39–44.
9. Kemp DT. Stimulated acoustic emissions from within the human auditory system. *J Acoust Soc Am* 1978;64:1386–1391.
10. Norton SJ, Schmidt AR, Stover LJ. Tinnitus and otoacoustic emissions: is there a link? *Ear Hear* 1990;11:159–166.
11. Penner MJ. Aspirin abolishes tinnitus caused by spontaneous otoacoustic emissions. A case study. *Arch Otolaryngol Head Neck Surg* 1989;115:871–875.
12. Penner MJ. An estimate of the prevalence of tinnitus caused by spontaneous otoacoustic emissions. *Arch Otolaryngol Head Neck Surg* 1990;116:418–423.
13. Arenberg IK, McCreary HS. Objective tinnitus aurium and dural arteriovenous malformations to the posterior fossa. *Ann Otol Rhinol Laryngol* 1972;80:111–120.
14. Courteney-Harris RG, Ford GR, Innes AJ, Colin JF. Pulsatile tinnitus: three cases of arteriovenous fistula treated by ligation of the occipital artery. *J Laryngol Otol* 1990;104:421–422.
15. Levine SB, Snow JB. Pulsatile tinnitus. *Laryngoscope* 1987;97:401–406.
16. Fowler NO, Gause R. Cervical venous hum. *Am Heart J* 1964;67:135–136.
17. Hardison JE. Cervical venous hum. *N Engl J Med* 1968;278:587–590.
18. Cutforth R, Wiseman J, Sutherland RD. The genesis of the cervical venous hum. *Am Heart J* 1970;80:488–492.
19. Buckwalter JA, Sasaki CT, Virapongse C, Kier EL, Bauman N. Pulsatile tinnitus arising from jugular megabulb deformity: a treatment rationale. *Laryngoscope* 1983;93:1534–1539.
20. Sismanis A. Otologic manifestations of benign intracranial hypertension syndrome: diagnosis and management. *Laryngoscope* 1987;97 [Suppl 42]:1–17.
21. Wall M. Idiopathic intracranial hypertension. *Neurol Clin* 1991;9:73–95.
22. Marcelis J, Silberstein SD. Idiopathic intracranial hypertension without papilledema. *Arch Neurol* 1991;48:392–399.
23. Arenberg IK, McCreary HS. Objective tinnitus aurium and dural arteriovenous malformations of the posterior fossa. *Ann Otol Rhinol Laryngol* 1972;80:111–120.
24. Chandler JR. Diagnosis and cure of venous hum tinnitus. *Laryngoscope* 1983;93:892–895.
25. Diehl GE, Wilmes E. Etiology and clinical aspects of palatal myoclonus. *Laryngorhinootologie* 1990;69:369–372.
26. Mardini MK. Ear-clicking "tinnitus" responding to carbamazepine. *N Engl J Med* 1987;317:1542.
27. O'Donoghue GM, Brackmann DE, House JW, Jackler RK. Neuromas of the facial nerve. *Am J Otol* 1989;10:49–54.
28. Jennetta PJ. Neurovascular compression in cranial nerve and systemic disease. *Ann Surg* 1981;192:518–525.
29. Meyerhoff WL, Mickey BE. Vascular decompression of the cochlear nerve in tinnitus sufferers. *Laryngoscope* 1988;98:602–604.
30. Moller AR, Moller MB, Jennetta PJ, Jho HS. Compound action potentials recorded from the exposed VIIIth nerve in patients with intractable tinnitus. *Laryngoscope* 1992;102:187–197.
31. Moller AR. A cranial nerve vascular compression syndrome: II. A review of pathophysiology. *Acta Neurochir (Wien)* 1991;113:24–30.
32. Moller AR, Jennetta PJ. On the origin of synkinesis in hemifacial spasm: results of intracranial recordings. *J Neurosurg* 1984;61:569–576.
33. Moller MB, Moller AR, Jennetta PJ, Hae DJ. Vascular decompression surgery for severe tinnitus: selection criteria and results. *Laryngoscope* 1993;103:421–427.
34. Boettcher FA, Salvi R. Salicylate ototoxicity: review and synthesis. *Am J Otolaryngol* 1991;12:33–47.
35. Stypulkowski PH. Mechanisms of salicylate ototoxicity. *Hear Res* 1990;46:113–146.

36. Dwivedi GS, Mehra YN. Ototoxicity of chloroquine phosphate. *J Laryngol Otol* 1978;92:701–703.

37. Dyer RK, McElveen JT. The patulous eustachian tube: management options. *Otolaryngol Head Neck Surg* 1991;105:832–835.

38. Bluestone CD, Cantekin EL. Management of the patulous eustachian tube. *Laryngoscope* 1981;91:149–152.

39. Stroud MH, Spector GJ, Maissel RH. Patulous eustachian tube syndrome: a preliminary report of the use of the tensor velopalatine transposition procedure. *Arch Otolaryngol* 1974;99:419–421.

40. Flottorp G, Willie C. Nicotinic acid treatment of tinnitus: a clinical-audiological examination. *Acta Otolaryngol* 1955;118:85–99.

41. Hulshof JH, Vermeij P. The effect of nicotinamide on tinnitus: a double-blind controlled study. *Clin Otolaryngol* 1987;12:211–214.

42. Coyas A, Annales D. The efficacy of trimetazidine in cochleovestibular disorders of ischemic origin. A crossover control versus placebo trial. *Ann Otolaryngol Chir Cervicofac* 1990;107[Suppl 1]:83–87.

43. Pech A. A multicenter double blind versus placebos study of trimetazidine in tinnitus. A clinical approach to tinnitus. *Ann Otolaryngol Chir Cervicofac* 1990;107[Suppl 1]:66–67.

44. Graham JT. Tinnitus aurium. *Acta Otolaryngol* 1965;201:1–32.

45. Martin FW, Coleman BH. Tinnitus: a double-blind crossover controlled trial to evaluate the use of lignocaine. *Clin Otolaryngol* 1980;5:3–11.

46. Yamanaka EK, Saiki T, Yanagihara N. The effect of intravenous administration of Xylocaine for the treatment of tinnitus. *Nippon Jibiinkoka Gakkai Kaiho* 1989;92:566–573.

47. Emmett JR, Shea JJ. Treatment of tinnitus with tocainide hydrochloride. *Otolaryngol Head Neck Surg* 1980;88:442–446.

48. Lenarz T. Treatment of tinnitus with lidocaine and tocainide. *Scand Audiol* 1986;88:442–446.

49. Melding PS, Goodey RJ. The treatment of tinnitus with oral anticonvulsants. *J Laryngol Otol* 1979;92:111–122.

50. Mihail RC, Crowley JM, Walden BE, Fishburne E Jr, Zajtchuk JT. The tricyclic trimipramine in the treatment of subjective tinnitus. *Ann Otol Rhinol Laryngol* 1988;97:120–123.

51. Sullivan MD, Katon W, Dobie R, et al. Disabling tinnitus. Association with affective disorder. *Gen Hosp Psychiatry* 1988;10:285–291.

52. Tandon R, Grunhaus L, Greden JF. Imipramine and tinnitus. *J Clin Psychiatry* 1987;48:109–111.

53. House JW. Therapies for tinnitus. *Am J Otolaryngol* 1989;10:163–165.

54. Tyler RS, Kelsay D. Advantages and disadvantages reported by some of the better cochlear-implant patients. *Am J Otol* 1990;11:282–289.

55. Battmer RD, Heerman R, Laszig R. Suppression of tinnitus by electric stimulation in cochlear implant patients. *Head Neck Otolaryngol* 1989;37:148–152.

56. Hazell JW, Meerton LJ, Conway MJ. Electrical tinnitus suppression (ETS) with a single channel cochlear implant. *J Laryngol Otol* 1989;18:39–44.

57. Dandy WE. Surgical treatment of Meniere's disease. *Surg Gynecol Obstet* 1941;72:421–425.

58. House JW, Brackmann DE. Tinnitus: surgical management. *Ciba Found Symp* 1981;85:204–216.

59. Fisch U. Surgical treatment of vertigo. *J Laryngol Otol* 1976;90:75–86.

60. Barrs DM, Brackmann DE. Translabyrinthine nerve section: effect on tinnitus. *J Laryngol Otol* 1984;[Suppl 9]:287–293.

61. Gardner G. Neurologic surgery and tinnitus. *J Laryngol Otol* 1984;[Suppl 9]:311–318.

62. Pulec JL. Cochlear nerve section for intractable tinnitus. Presented at the Western Section Meeting of the American Laryngological, Otological and Rhinological Society, January 1994.

63. Silverstein H, Haberkamp T, Smouha E. The state of tinnitus after inner ear surgery. *Otolaryngol Head Neck Surg* 1986;95:438–441.

64. Wazen JJ, Foyt D, Sisti M. Selective cochlear neurectomy for debilitating tinnitus. *Ann Otol Rhinol Laryngol* 1997;106:568–570.

65. Feldman H. Homolateral and contralateral masking of tinnitus by noise-bands and by pure tones. *Audiology* 1971;10:138–144.

66. Vernon JA, Schleuning AJ. Tinnitus: a new management. *Laryngoscope* 1978;85:413–419.

67. Kuk F, Tyler R, Rustad N, Harker L, Tye-Murray N. Alternating current at the ear drum for tinnitus reduction. *J Speech Hear Res* 1989;32:393–400.

68. Thedinger B, Karlsen E, Schack S. Treatment of tinnitus with electrical stimulation: an evaluation of the Audimax Theraband. *Laryngoscope* 1987;97:33–37.

69. Dobie RA, Hoberg KE, Rees TS. Electrical tinnitus suppression: a double-blind crossover study. *Otolaryngol Head Neck Surg* 1986;95:319–323.

70. Schulman A. External electrical stimulation in tinnitus control. *Am J Otolaryngol* 1985;6:110–115.

71. DeBartolo H Jr. Zinc and diet for tinnitus. *Am J Otolaryngol* 1989;10:256.

72. House JW. Management of the tinnitus patient. *Ann Otolaryngol Rhinol Laryngol* 1981;90:597–601.

73. Thomas M, Laurell G, Lundeberg T. Acupuncture for the alleviation of tinnitus. *Laryngoscope* 1988;98:664–667.

74. Schumann KJ, Lamm K, Hettich M. Effect and effectiveness of hyperbaric oxygen therapy in chronic hearing disorders. Report of 557 cases. *Head Neck Otolaryngol* 1990;38:408–411.

75. Landis B, Landis E. Is biofeedback effective for chronic tinnitus? An intensive study with seven patients. *Am J Otolaryngol* 1992;13:349–356.

76. Sullivan MD, Dobie RA, Sakai CS, Katon WJ. Treatment of depressed tinnitus patients with nortriptyline. *Ann Otol Rhinol Laryngol* 1989;98:867–878.

77. Simpson RB, Nedzelski JM, Barber HO, Thomas MR. Psychiatric diagnosis in patients with psychogenic dizziness of sever tinnitus. *J Otolaryngol* 1988;17:325–330.

78. Briner W, Risey J, Guth P, Norris C. Use of the Million Clinical Multiaxial Inventory in evaluating patients with severe tinnitus. *Am J Otol* 1990;11:334–337.

The Ear: Comprehensive Otology,
edited by R. F. Canalis and P. R. Lambert.
Lippincott Williams & Wilkins, Philadelphia © 2000.

CHAPTER 35

Cochlear and Vestibular Ototoxicity

Phillip A. Wackym, Ian S. Storper, and Anita N. Newman

For more than a century, the ability of certain pharmacologic agents to produce otologic effects has been recognized (1,2). Although these effects usually are detrimental to patient well-being, some of these medications have become used more frequently as therapeutic agents. As the choice of pharmacologic options has increased and with an increasingly complex medicolegal environment, it has become even more important for the clinician to understand the otologic effects of prescribed medications. Four commonly used classes of medications cause ototoxic effects. These are antibiotics, antineoplastic agents, loop diuretics, and analgesics/antipyretics and antimalarial drugs. The most commonly used agents in each group will be discussed in this chapter. Table 1 summarizes currently recognized drugs that have been associated with ototoxicity; the reader is referred to the references cited in Table 1 for additional information about specific, less frequently encountered, ototoxic agents should the clinical need arise.

P. A. Wackym: Department of Otolaryngology and Communication Sciences, Medical College of Wisconsin; Department of Otolaryngology–Head and Neck Surgery, Froedtert Memorial Lutheran Hospital, Milwaukee, Wisconsin 53226
I. S. Storper: Department of Otolaryngology–Head and Neck Surgery, College of Physicians and Surgeons, Columbia University; and Department of Otolaryngology/Head and Neck Surgery, Columbia University, New York, New York 10032
A. N. Newman: Department of Head and Neck Surgery, University of Southern California School of Medicine, and University Hospital, School of Medicine, Los Angeles, California 90020

As early as the 1800s, salicylates and quinine were recognized to produce loss of balance, loss of hearing, and tinnitus (3,4). In the early 1900s, the ototoxic effects of alcohols, arsenicals, nicotine, and heavy metals were recognized (5). The ototoxic effects of streptomycin, an aminoglycoside antibiotic, were recognized shortly after its introduction for tuberculosis treatment in 1944 (6). When other aminoglycosides were introduced in the 1960s, their otologic effects were recognized almost immediately, leading to extensive studies of their mechanisms of action (7). Other classes of antibiotics, including glycopeptides, have been reported to induce hearing loss, with vancomycin being a well-known agent (8). The ability of certain diuretics, such as furosemide, bumetanide, and ethacrynic acid to produce both temporary and permanent hearing loss was recognized since their introduction in the early 1960s and first reported by Maher and Schreiner in 1965 (9). Ototoxic effects have also been associated with antineoplastic agents, with platinum derivatives and nitrogen mustards being frequently implicated (10). Cisplatinum-induced hearing loss in humans was reported as early as 1974 by Piel et al. (11).

The most common symptoms of drug-induced ototoxicity are tinnitus, sensorineural hearing loss, and vestibular dysfunction. The vestibular dysfunction may occasionally be manifest as true vertigo; more often, it is characterized by disequilibrium and the patient may complain of dizziness or loss of balance. Nystagmus may or may not be present. Due to the typical global vestibular

TABLE 1. *Common agents associated with ototoxicity*

Antibiotics
  Aminoglycosides
    Gentamicin (27,28,38,56–58)
    Tobramycin (10,44)
    Amikacin (22,43,44)
    Streptomycin (6,19)
    Dihydrostreptomycin (10,48,50)
    Neomycin (37–40)
    Netilmicin (44)
    Kanamycin (44)
  Nonaminoglycosides
    Vancomycin/ristocetin (8,64,65)
    Erythromycin (62,63)
    Polymyxin B (66)
    Colistin (polymyxin E) (66)
    Minocycline (67)
    Chloramphenicol (10)
Diuretics
  Loop diuretics
    Furosemide (16,79,80)
    Bumetanide (16)
    Ethacrynic acid (78,81)
  Nonloop diuretics
    Mannitol (10)
    Acetazolamide (10)
Analgesics/antipyretics and antimalarial drugs
  Salicylates (84,87–89)
  Quinine (12)
  Chloroquine (10)
Antineoplastic drugs
  Cisplatinum (11,69,71)
  Carboplatinum (10,12)
  Nitrogen mustard (10,12)
  Vincristine
  Bleomycin
Miscellaneous
  Alcohol (12)
  Aniline dyes
  Arsenic (12)
  Atropine
  Barbiturates
  Caffeine
  Carbon monoxide (93)
  Chenopodium (90)
  Desferrioxamine (91,92)
  Ergot
  Gold (94)
  Hydrocyanide
  Lead (94)
  Lidocaine
  Mercury (94)
  Nicotine
  Strychnine

If no reference is cited, see Walker EM Jr, Fazekas-May MA, Bowen WR. Nephrotoxic and ototoxic agents. *Clin Lab Med* 1990;10:323.

Adapted from Shulman, *The ear*, 1st ed., and Walker EM, Fazekas-May MA, Bowen WR. Nephrotoxic and ototoxic agents. *Clin Lab Med* 1990;10:339.

dysfunction that may result from ototoxicity, patients become more dependent on visual and proprioceptive information to maintain orientation. Consequently, the clinical vestibular presentation of older patients with impaired visual and proprioceptive function may be more

severe. The tinnitus usually is high pitched, ranging from 4 to 6 kHz, and it often precedes or supersedes sensorineural hearing loss. Over time, as neural elements degenerate, the tinnitus may decrease in magnitude, although it rarely resolves completely (12).

Antibiotic-induced ototoxicity varies with the type of agent administered. Aminoglycoside ototoxic effects can be both cochleotoxic and vestibulotoxic, with differing degrees of toxicity for each individual drug (Table 2).

If a specific aminoglycoside antibiotic is cochleotoxic, the most frequent symptom is bilateral high-frequency sensorineural hearing loss. The hearing loss may progress to a profound degree in all frequencies. Vestibular toxicity is commonly characterized by ataxia and unsteadiness of gait or an inability to maintain visual fixation. Vancomycin ototoxicity is characterized by tinnitus and high-frequency hearing loss in patients at the extremes of age (10,13,14).

The ototoxicity of loop diuretics may be severe, particularly if infused intravenously. Symptoms include mild-to-severe, high-pitched tinnitus accompanied by sensorineural hearing loss that may be severe and permanent, especially in the case of ethacrynic acid. Although the precise incidence of loop diuretic ototoxicity is not known, reported rates are 0.7% for ethacrynic acid, 1.1% for bumetanide, and 6.4% for furosemide. Furosemide toxicity can be reduced by slow infusion over 15 minutes (15,16).

Ototoxicity caused by antineoplastic agents frequently begins as bilateral, high-frequency sensorineural hearing loss that progresses to hearing loss in all frequencies (17). Vestibular symptoms are not unusual.

Symptoms of salicylate and quinine ototoxicity are typically dose dependent and reversible; permanent hearing loss has not been documented. Generally, symptoms are characterized by severe tinnitus and mild-to-moderate sensorineural hearing loss, both resolving quickly after discontinuation of therapy. Usually, exceedingly high doses of aspirin are necessary to produce ototoxic effects, with blood levels of greater than 20 mg/dL. Symptoms generally are encountered only in patients with rheumatoid arthritis or other disorders requiring very high doses (10).

The toxicity of the four classes of drugs will be discussed here in greater detail.

TABLE 2. *Relative toxicity of aminoglycosides*

Drug	Cochlear toxicity	Vestibular toxicity
Dihydrostreptomycin	+++	+
Streptomycin	+	+++
Gentamicin	+	++
Kanamycin	++	+
Tobramycin	++	+
Amikacin	+	+/–
Neomycin	+	+/–

Adapted from Walker EM, Fazekas-May MA, Bowen WR. Nephrotoxic and ototoxic agents. *Clin Lab Med* 1990;10:341.

ANTIBIOTICS

Aminoglycosides

Aminoglycoside antibiotics have played an essential role in the treatment of gram-negative sepsis and resistant infections by interacting with the bacterial 30s ribosomal subunit, thereby inhibiting protein synthesis (17). The association of aminoglycoside therapy with ototoxicity was evident soon after the earliest clinical trials of streptomycin (18,19), when it was introduced to clinical medicine in 1944 by Hinshaw and Feldman (6). The introduction of streptomycin soon was followed by neomycin (1949), kanamycin (1957), gentamicin (1963), tobramycin (1967), and amikacin (1972). Netilmicin and sisomicin are among the latest aminoglycosides introduced for pharmacologic therapy.

Clinical Findings

With aminoglycoside therapy, the incidence of ototoxic side effects has been reported to be as high as 10% (20). As mentioned previously, the most common symptoms are tinnitus, sensorineural hearing loss, and vestibular dysfunction. Hearing loss most often is bilateral, most severe in the high frequencies, and characterized by decreased speech intelligibility. As toxicity becomes more severe, it also can involve the lower frequencies and result in profound, permanent deafness (7,10,12–14,18). Hearing loss usually becomes noticeable within 1 to 2 weeks of therapy initiation; it can, however, become evident as early as 1 day after initiation of therapy or as late as 2 to 6 months after discontinuation of therapy (21,22). In rare cases, some recovery of hearing has been reported (23–29). Vestibular effects are characterized by loss of balance, sensations of dizziness or disequilibrium, and failure of visual fixation. More disabling vestibular effects, such as ataxia and severe vertigo, are not unusual with certain drugs of this class (7,10,12).

The degree of cochleotoxicity and/or vestibulotoxicity depends on the specific aminoglycoside antibiotic that is administered (Table 2), along with renal function of the patient. Streptomycin is predominantly toxic to the vestibular system, in a more severe fashion than other aminoglycosides. This severe toxicity has limited the clinical usefulness of this drug in tuberculosis treatment; however, it has led to successful treatment of intractable Meniere's disease by functional vestibular ablation, when injected through the tympanic membrane (10,14,30–33), perfused into the endolymphatic compartment (34), or administered intramuscularly in cases of intractable bilateral Meniere's disease (30,31). The reduced state of streptomycin, dihydrostreptomycin, is strongly cochleotoxic (12). Ablation of peripheral vestibular function is discussed later in this chapter. Neomycin is also strongly cochleotoxic and, like dihydrostreptomycin, has been eliminated from parenteral therapy. Applied topically, however, neomycin has been found to exhibit little toxic-

ity. Neomycin therefore is used in oral preparation of the bowel prior to abdominal surgery, as absorption through gut mucosa is minimal, and in otic drops. The use of aminoglycoside-containing otic drops remains controversial (see Chapter 25). Whereas it generally is agreed that these drops are safe when there is no perforation in the tympanic membrane, numerous studies have documented sensorineural hearing loss following the topical administration of aminoglycoside-containing medications (Fig. 1) (35–40). It is clear that, in a noninfected ear, these drops can diffuse across the round window membrane and have ototoxic effects; however, McCabe and Schuknecht have both stated that, in an infected ear, damage caused by otic drops has not been encountered (13). Matz (13) suggests that this actual lack of damage may be attributed to the oblique orientation of the round window membrane and/or difficulty diffusing through infected middle ear mucosa. Due to these conflicting opinions, the administration of aminoglycoside-containing drops should be performed judiciously and appropriately by the clinician. Kanamycin, introduced in 1957, also frequently induces severe cochleotoxicity. On occasion, it may be unilateral. Due to this effect, it also has been discontinued from pharmacologic therapy (10).

More recently introduced to clinical use are gentamicin, tobramycin, and amikacin, which all have significant activity against gram-negative organisms. Gentamicin is predominantly vestibulotoxic, although usually to a much lesser degree than streptomycin. Hearing loss has been reported in 2% of patients receiving gentamicin (41). Tobramycin is predominantly cochleotoxic, but it can exert some vestibular effects. This drug has comparable efficacy to gentamicin, but comparable ototoxicity to kanamycin (42). Amikacin, introduced in 1972, has a lower incidence of cochleotoxicity than gentamicin, with minimal vestibular toxicity. Its antimicrobial spectrum is similar to that of gentamicin, but it is less susceptible to enzymatic degradation by resistant bacteria (43). Netilmicin is a new aminoglycoside antibiotic, which apparently has lower ototoxic effects than its predecessors (44).

Pharmacology

Aminoglycosides consist of two or more amino sugars bound to a central nucleus (aminocyclitol) by glycosidic linkages (44). Gentamicin, tobramycin, amikacin, and neomycin contain deoxystreptamine; streptomycin and dihydrostreptomycin contain streptidine. Variations in the structural configuration affect activity and ototoxicity. This polar, cationic configuration contributes to poor gastrointestinal absorption (less than 3% of an oral dose) and poor penetration across the blood–brain barrier, occasionally necessitating intrathecal administration (12). Serum levels vary greatly; concentration in the tissues is usually one third of the serum concentration. Temperature, pH, electrolyte content, hematocrit, and oxygen tension have

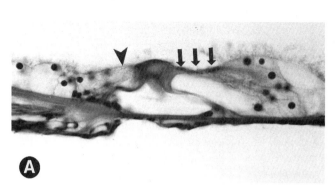
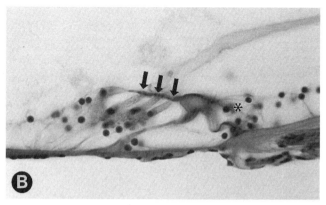

FIG. 1. Light micrographs showing the temporal bone pathology associated with the topical application of Cortisporin otic suspension (GlaxoWellcome), containing neomycin and polymyxin B, on the round window of the chinchilla. Fifty microliters of Ringer's solution was applied to the round window membranes of the left temporal bones (control side). Fifty microliters of Cortisporin otic suspension was applied to the round window membranes of the right temporal bones for 10 minutes and then rinsed away with Ringer's solution (experimental side). The animals had compound action potentials recorded at 1, 2, and 24 hours after treatment (see reference 40 for review). One month after treatment, these animals were perfused and their temporal bones decalcified, embedded in celloidin, sectioned at 20 μm, and stained with hematoxylin and eosin. (Courtesy of Dr. Tesuo Morizono, Otitis Media Research Center, Department of Otolaryngology, University of Minnesota, Minneapolis, Minnesota.) **A:** Experimental side, right organ of Corti. *Arrowhead* indicates absence of inner hair cell. *Arrows* indicate absence of all three rows of outer hair cells. **B:** Control side, left organ of Corti. *Asterisk* indicates normal inner hair cell. *Arrows* indicate three rows of normal outer hair cells.

all been shown to affect tissue levels. These drugs are excreted unmetabolized by the kidney. Because aminoglycoside concentration in perilymph has been shown to be proportional to ototoxicity, patients with poor renal function have higher incidences of aminoglycoside ototoxicity (45). A single dose of an aminoglycoside results in a peak serum level in 1 hour; within 6 hours this level will be almost completely eliminated. In perilymph, the peak level is reached in 6 hours; the time for complete elimination is 24 to 36 hours. The half-lives of gentamicin, tobramycin, and amikacin in perilymph are 12, 10, and 10 hours, respectively. For repeated doses, if the dosing interval is spaced improperly, these drugs have been shown to accumulate in perilymph (46). The half-life of kanamycin in perilymph is 15 hours, thereby predisposing it to an accumulation in perilymph. This may be an explanation for the increased ototoxicity of kanamycin over gentamicin, tobramycin, and amikacin (12). Because levels remain low in cerebrospinal fluid, aminoglycosides are believed to enter the inner ear via capillary beds (47). Specifically, these drugs can enter the perilymph through the vessels in the spiral ligament and thereby diffuse into the vestibular cristae, maculae, and the organ of Corti (48).

Histopathology

Whereas the histopathologic effects of aminoglycoside ototoxicity are becoming clearer at the ultrastructural level, the mechanisms of action of these drugs remain incompletely understood. Originally, it was proposed that the secretory and absorptive substances of the labyrinth

were injured, thereby damaging the hair cells as the result of a changed environment (49,50). It also has been proposed that hair cell loss occurs as a result of impaired aerobic metabolism in the stria (50). A two-step model has been proposed in which the aminoglycoside first blocks calcium-dependent potassium channels on the apical aspect of the hair cells, followed by eventual degeneration secondary to interference with cell membrane lipid metabolism. More recent studies suggest that aminoglycoside ototoxicity results from an alteration of phospholipid metabolism (51–53). In these experiments, guinea pigs were treated chronically with neomycin and found to have reduced labeling of phosphatidylinositol diphosphate in inner ear tissues when they were injected with a radioactive phosphorous tracer. Aminoglycoside effects on the cochlear microphonic tend to correlate with *in vitro* polyphosphoinositide films (51–53).

It has been known for at least 3 decades that aminoglycosides cause an unmistakable destruction of cochlear and vestibular neuroepithelium, primarily to the hair cells at the center of the crista, the saccule, and the utricle (Figs. 2 and 3) (54). In the cochlea, ototoxic effects are seen in the outer hair cells of the basal turn. With increased dosages, the toxicity progresses toward the upper turns and the inner hair cells (Fig. 1) (55).

Pathologic changes induced in the receptor cells were reported recently by Takumida et al. (56–58). In their experiments, 5 mg of gentamicin was infused directly into the middle ears of guinea pigs. Gentamicin is known to reach the inner ear by diffusion through the round window. Sections of the inner ear were studied with high-res-

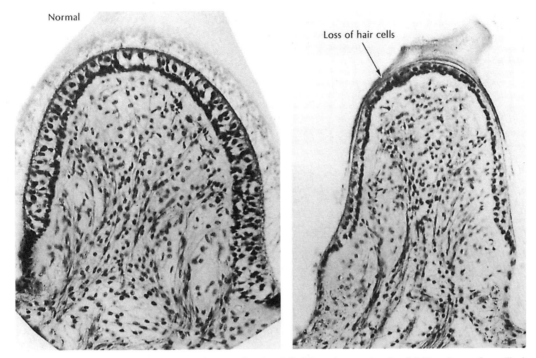

FIG. 2. Cristae of horizontal canals of normal animal **(left)** and an animal exhibiting loss of vestibular function caused by intramuscular administration of streptomycin sulfate, 200 mg/kg/d for 28 days **(right)**. In the treated ear the sensory epithelium is flattened, and about 50% of the hair cells are missing. The remaining hair cells appear shrunken and have pyknotic nuclei. Posttreatment survival time was 15 months. (From Schuknecht HF. *Pathology of the ear.* Cambridge, MA: Harvard University Press, 1974:277, with permission.)

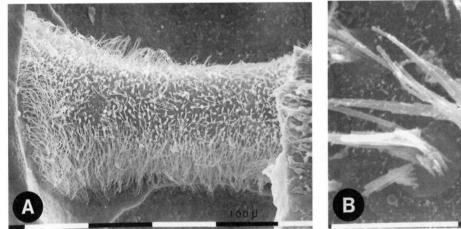
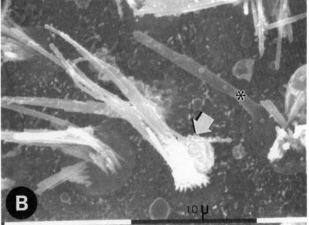

FIG. 3. A: Scanning electron micrograph of a guinea pig crista ampullaris 7 days after administration of gentamicin solution (0.1 mL of 50 mg gentamicin sulfate per milliliter) into the tympanic bulla. Early after gentamicin vestibular ototoxicity the central part of the crista has lost its sensory hair cell stereocilia bundles, but the periphery appears normal. **B:** Scanning electron micrograph of a guinea pig crista ampullaris 7 days after administration of gentamicin solution (0.1 mL of 50 mg gentamicin sulfate per milliliter) into the tympanic bulla. The least damaged stereocilia bundle shows fusion of the stereocilia and bulging of the cuticular plate *(arrow)*, whereas those that are more damaged show complete stereocilia fusion *(asterisk)* or disappearance. (From Takumida M, Bagger-Sjöbäck D, Harada Y, Lim D, Wersäll J. Sensory hair fusion and glycocalyx changes following gentamicin exposure in the guinea pig vestibular organs. *Acta Otolaryngol (Stockh)* 1989;107:39, with permission.)

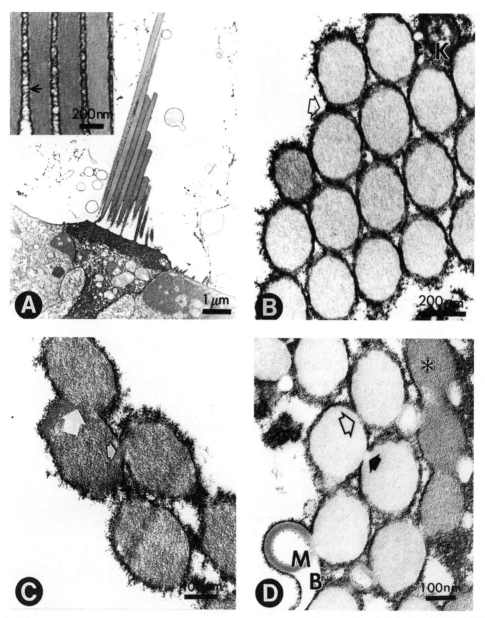

FIG. 4. Transmission electron micrographs of vestibular and cochlear hair cell glycocalyx and the effect of gentamicin intoxication on the glycocalyx and stereocilia (ruthenium red, uranyl acetate, and lead citrate stain). **A:** Utricular macula. The glycocalyx covers the entire surface of both the sensory and supporting cells. **Inset:** The glycocalyx is seen over the entire length of the stereocilia that are interconnected by thin filaments of glycocalyx *(arrow)*. **B:** Utricular macula. The glycocalyx emerges from the outer layer of the plasma membrane *(open arrow)* and forms the interconnection between the kinocilium *(K)* and the stereocilia, as well as between stereocilia themselves. **C:** Organ of Corti 7 days after gentamicin intoxication. The initial change in the stereocilia of outer hair cells is a loss of glycocalyx *(large arrow)* and subsequent plasma membrane fusion *(small arrow)* between the neighboring cilia. **D:** Crista ampullaris 7 days after gentamicin intoxication. Different stages of the sensory hair fusion process. *Open arrow* indicates decrease in glycocalyx and plasma membrane contact. *Arrow* indicates membrane fusion. *Asterisk* indicates protoplasmic contact between the sensory hairs. *B,* ballooning of the plasma membrane; *M,* myelinlike figure formation. (Courtesy of Dr. Masaya Takumida, Department of Otolaryngology, Hiroshima University School of Medicine, Hiroshima, Japan.)

olution scanning and transmission electron microscopy at successive intervals after aminoglycoside administration. The glycocalyx (Fig. 4) is described by Takumida and co-workers as a "fuzzy layer" that spreads over the entire surface of the apical plasma membrane, including receptor cells. This layer is believed to keep the cilia at fixed distances apart, thus preventing both excessive separation and excessive fusion.

"Tip links," or specialized types of stereocilia interconnections (Fig. 5), have been suggested to participate in the transduction mechanism by encouraging unified stereocilia motion. Treatment with gentamicin results in a smaller glycocalyx, which in turn results in complete fusion of hair cell stereocilia and elongation of tip links (Figs. 4C and 4D).

Seven days after gentamicin treatment, the sensory cells near the striola of the macula and the central portion of the crista showed even more severe changes, from fusion to loss of hair cell stereocilia, with greater changes in the type I than in the type II vestibular hair cells. Tip links disappeared by this time point. Peripheral regions appeared normal. At the final stage, destruction progressed in the direction of the peripheral regions, and stereocilia were lost in the central regions, leaving holes in the glycocalyx (Fig. 5C).

Prevention

Prevention of aminoglycoside ototoxicity can be accomplished by either performing tests that can detect

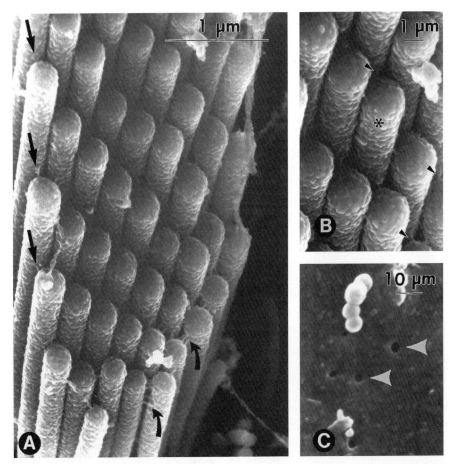

FIG. 5. Scanning electron micrographs of normal and gentamicin-treated guinea pig vestibular hair cell stereocilia. **A:** Normal appearing sensory bundle in the extreme periphery of the utricular macula shows the normal appearance of the glycocalyx and the stereocilia interconnections. The stereocilia are interconnected by numerous thin fibrillar structures *(curved arrows)*. At the tip of the stereocilium, the tip link stretches toward its taller neighbor where it connects to the shaft *(straight arrows)*. **B:** Higher power shows that the stereocilia membrane is rough in a regular way *(asterisk)*. The distances between neighboring stereocilia are quite regular, ranging from 10 to 40 nm. *Arrowheads* indicate tip links. **C:** Seven days after administration of gentamicin solution (0.1 mL of 50 mg gentamicin sulfate per milliliter) into the tympanic bulla. With gentamicin vestibular ototoxicity, at places where all stereocilia have disappeared, small holes *(arrowheads)* are observed in the cuticular plate. They have a uniform diameter of approximately 40 nm. (From Takumida M, Bagger-Sjöbäck D, Wersäll J, Harada Y. The effect of gentamicin on the glycocalyx and the ciliary interconnections in the vestibular sensory cells: a high resolution scanning electron microscopic investigation. *Hear Res* 1989;37:163, with permission.)

toxicity at the subclinical level, leading to early discontinuation of the drug from a patient's regimen, or prescribing an alternative medication. Renal function should be maximized via hydration and diuresis, if necessary. Serum levels should be monitored carefully, along with blood urea nitrogen and creatinine; dosage and interval should be adjusted appropriately. Daily audiometry (especially high-frequency testing) and, if possible, electronystagmography are recommended to detect toxicity while it is still reversible. Evoked otoacoustic emissions testing, which assesses outer hair cell function, may prove to be an excellent screening approach. Bedside tests of the vestibuloocular reflex, such as the head-shaking test or the dynamic visual acuity test, may provide an early indication of vestibular toxicity (see Chapter 9).

Alternative antibiotics often are available so as to avoid using the aminoglycosides. These alternatives include some of the third-generation cephalosporins, imipenem, ciprofloxacin, and aztreonam (59). Third-generation cephalosporins occasionally have strong enough gram-negative coverage to be adequate alternatives. Imipenem, a monobactam antibiotic, is currently active against all gram-positive and gram-negative organisms. Ciprofloxacin is a fluoroquinolone with broad gram-positive and gram-negative (including *Pseudomonas aeruginosa*) coverage. Aztreonam is a monobactam antibiotic active against all gram-negative organisms. Ceftazidime ototoxicity is extremely rare (60). Imipenem and aztreonam ototoxicity have not been reported.

Although a great deal has been learned in recent years about the histopathologic effects of aminoglycoside antibiotics on the cochlear and vestibular receptors, much controversy remains regarding their mechanism of action. Recently, Huang and Schacht (61) suggested that toxic metabolites of aminoglycosides may be the actual ototoxic agents, not the aminoglycosides themselves. If this is true, many of the current concepts of aminoglycoside ototoxicity will need to be reassessed.

Nonaminoglycosides

Erythromycin

Whereas the ototoxicity of aminoglycosides is well known, the effects on the human inner ear of other classes of antibiotics, including macrolides, glycopeptides, and antimycotics, also have been documented. Macrolide antibiotics are commonly prescribed. The most well-known macrolide antibiotic in the United States is erythromycin, which was discovered in 1952. The mechanism of action of this antibiotic is by binding to the bacterial 50s ribosomal subunit, thus inhibiting protein synthesis. Erythromycin is a bacteriostatic antibiotic, and its uses range from oral therapy for acute sinusitis, tonsillitis, gonorrhea, and syphilis in penicillin-allergic patients, to intravenous therapy for *Legionella* and endocarditis. It is prescribed as the antibiotic agent of choice for *Legionella* and *Mycoplasma* infections. The most common side effects of this antibiotic are gastrointestinal upset, fever, thrombophlebitis, and eosinophilia.

The first case of hearing loss secondary to erythromycin ototoxicity was reported in 1973 (62). At least 32 cases of bilateral sensorineural, mainly high-frequency, hearing loss have been reported in recent years for both oral and intravenous administration (63). Most patients are over 60 years of age, usually with hepatic or renal insufficiency. Accompanying the hearing loss are "blowing" tinnitus and, occasionally, vertigo. These symptoms can resolve within 2 weeks of discontinuation of therapy. In patients with renal failure, the following recommendations have been made to avoid toxicity: (a) daily audiograms with discontinuation of therapy if new hearing loss is recognized; (c) keeping daily dosage to less than 1.5 g; and (c) avoiding prescribing it in combination with other ototoxic drugs. The mechanism of toxicity, along with the precise histopathology of the end organs, remains unknown.

Vancomycin

Vancomycin is a glycopeptide antibiotic introduced in 1956. It only exerts systemic effects when it is administered intravenously. Its ototoxicity was first reported in 1958 (8). It is a narrow spectrum antibiotic, effective mainly against gram-positive organisms. Its use generally is reserved for methicillin-resistant *Staphylococcus aureus* infections or severe gram-positive infections in penicillin-allergic patients. It is prescribed for oral administration in *C. difficile* enterocolitis. This drug acts as an inhibitor of bacterial cell wall synthesis, specifically of peptidoglycan (64).

There have been 28 reported cases of vancomycin-induced hearing loss since 1958, usually for drug levels greater than 50 mg/L, but occasionally for levels as low as 30 mg/L. The hearing loss encountered begins as a bilateral high-frequency sensorineural hearing loss, which progresses to bilateral profound deafness in all frequencies. This toxicity generally is irreversible. Accompanying the hearing loss is high-pitched tinnitus. Vestibular dysfunction has rarely been reported. Strategies for avoiding toxicity include following serum levels, checking serial audiograms, and avoiding combinations with other ototoxic drugs. Once any degree of ototoxicity has been detected, administration should cease, if possible. As for erythromycin, the mechanism of action of vancomycin and the histopathologic changes it induces are unknown (65).

Antimycotic Drops

Antimycotic drops, containing propylene glycol and/or acetic acid, have recently been found to induce hair cell loss in guinea pigs, when injected into the middle ear. However, the authors believed that these results could not be extrapolated to clinical practice in human beings, as the round window membrane is considerably thicker and the concentration of these agents in the drops supplied commercially is much lower. They thought that it is necessary to follow carefully all patients to whom these medication are prescribed (66).

Other Antibiotics

Some semisynthetic tetracycline derivatives, such as minocycline (67), appear to produce vestibular toxicity. Nausea, vomiting, and ataxia without nystagmus have been documented. This toxicity is reported to be reversible (67). Viomycin and capreomycin, in high doses, cause irreversible cochleotoxicity and vestibulotoxicity (68). Ceftazidime has been associated with a reversible inflammatory reaction in the middle ear when applied topically to chinchillas (60).

ANTINEOPLASTIC DRUGS (CISPLATINUM)

Numerous antineoplastic agents have been associated with ototoxicity. The most commonly known drug in this category is cisplatinum. Other ototoxic agents in this group include nitrogen mustard, 5-fluorouracil, bleomycin, and vincristine (10). Nitrogen mustard, an alkylating agent, can cause hearing loss when used in total body perfusion therapy or regional infusion. Experimental studies demonstrate damage to the outer hair cells of the basal and middle turns of the cochlea, along with shrinkage of the organ of Corti (10).

Cisplatinum is a potent cytoreductive agent that is effective against a wide variety of tumors. Its mechanism of cytotoxic action is believed to occur via the formation of irreversible bonds to DNA, making intrastrand cross links between guanine residues. In time, frameshift and base substitution mutations are induced, thus decreasing neoplastic activity (69). This drug possesses numerous side effects, the most severe of which are nephrotoxicity and ototoxicity (70). It is disputed whether the ototoxic or nephrotoxic effect is dose limiting in prescribing this drug.

Cisplatinum-induced ototoxicity is most frequently manifest as tinnitus, hearing loss, and/or otalgia. Ototoxic effects usually occur within 2 days of initialization of therapy, but they can appear up to 7 days after discontinuation of therapy. The hearing loss is predominantly in the high frequencies, ranging from 6 to 8 kHz, but it also can involve the middle and low frequencies as the total dose increases. Most commonly, this hearing loss presents clinically as a sensation of hearing muffled voices, with a decreased speech discrimination score. When cochleotoxicity is mild, it usually is reversible. Once it has progressed to profound deafness, it is irreversible. Vestibular dysfunction also has been reported. The reported incidence of ototoxicity is extremely variable, ranging from 25%, with all cases subclinical and no loss exceeding 25 dB, to 90%, with all cases symptomatic (71). Ototoxicity has been found to correlate

with age, tumor site, cumulative dose administered, prior radiation exposure of the cranium, and brown eye color (72). To lower the probability of ototoxicity, sequential audiograms with immediate discontinuation of therapy, if possible, slow infusion, and intravenous hydration prior to administration have all been recommended (73). Schweitzer et al. (74) showed that when fosfomycin, an antibiotic that inhibits cell wall synthesis by inhibiting phosphoenolpyruvate transferase, is administered along with cisplatinum, ototoxicity is markedly reduced, with a 33% to 61% auditory brainstem response threshold lowering at 6 and 15 kHz. From current studies, this antibiotic does not limit tumoricidal activity (74).

Cisplatinum has complex pharmacokinetics and bioavailability that appear to vary from patient to patient. Critical cumulative doses of 3 to 4 mg/kg or 100 to 400

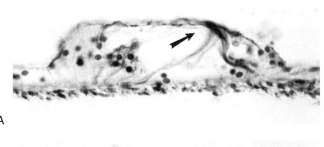

A

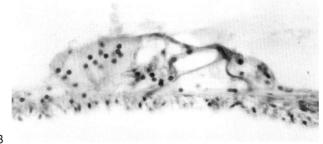

B

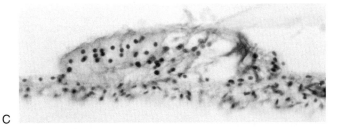

C

FIG. 6. Left temporal bone, organ of Corti from a 9-year-old with cisplatinum ototoxicity (hematoxylin and eosin, original magnification×400). **A:** Basal turn. Note loss of all outer hair cells *(arrow)*, pillar and Deiters' cells with fair preservation, and inner hair cell degeneration. **B:** Middle turn. There is a single remaining well-preserved outer hair cell. Inner hair cell, pillar cells, and Deiters' cells are present. **C:** Apical turn. Two remaining outer hair cells. Inner hair cell, pillar cells, and Deiters' cells are present. (From Strauss M, Towfighi J, Lord S, Lipton A, Harvey HA, Brown B. Cis-platinum ototoxicity: clinical experience and temporal bone histopathology. *Laryngoscope* 1983;93:1554, with permission.)

mg/m^2 have been proposed to avoid ototoxicity, but discrepancy is great between doses recommended by various studies (14,75,76).

At this time, very little is known about the mechanism responsible for the ototoxic effects of cisplatinum. Adenylate cyclase, ATPase, and membrane-bound phosphatases are all inhibited by this drug, but no direct link has been made to the molecular pathway responsible for the ototoxicity that results from its administration (69). The most commonly reported histopathologic change has been degeneration of the outer hair cells in the basal turn of the cochlea (Fig. 6) (71).

As toxicity progresses, inner hair cells and more apical receptor cells become involved. The stria vascularis, spiral ganglion, and cochlear nerve have also been shown to be affected (Fig. 7) (71). Fusion of individual hair cell stereocilia, disarray, and loss have all been reported, but not to the degree of the changes associated with aminoglycoside ototoxicity.

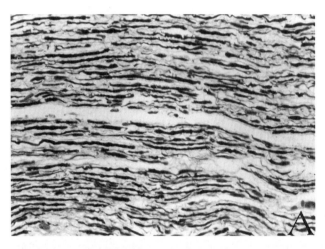

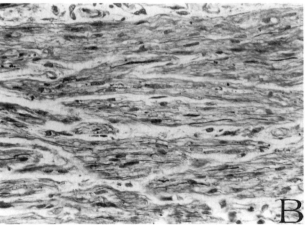

FIG. 7. Right eighth cranial nerve from a 9-year-old with cisplatinum ototoxicity, longitudinal section (modified Bielschowsky stain, original magnification×350). **A:** Vestibular nerve containing intact axons. **B:** Cochlear nerve containing degenerated axons. (From Strauss M, Towfighi J, Lord S, Lipton A, Harvey HA, Brown B. Cis-platinum ototoxicity: clinical experience and temporal bone histopathology. *Laryngoscope* 1983;93:1554, with permission.)

LOOP DIURETICS

The most frequent clinically used loop diuretics are furosemide, bumetanide, and ethacrynic acid. This designation was assigned to this group of diuretics because of their shared primary action at the level of the ascending limb of the loop of Henle in the nephron. Shortly after the introduction of furosemide and ethacrynic acid, hearing impairment of patients was noted and first reported in 1965 by Maher and Schreiner (9). Hearing loss was almost exclusively seen in patients with renal compromise, uremia, or high intravenous bolus doses approaching the therapeutic maximum. Hearing loss generally occurs in the range from 2 to 4 kHz and almost always is reversible. Rare incidents of permanent deafness have been reported, especially for intravenous doses of ethacrynic acid. Severe tinnitus, also reversible, may be present immediately following an intravenous bolus dose. Very rare reports of vestibular toxicity have been published regarding these agents (18). Bumetanide is a newer loop diuretic than furosemide and ethacrynic acid, and it has been reported to be less ototoxic than both. In a series of 179 patients treated with loop diuretics, the incidence of hearing loss was 1.1% in bumetanide-treated patients and 6.4% in furosemide-treated patients (16).

The mechanism of action of loop diuretics on the inner ear remains unclear. Due to the similarity of the secretory cells in the inner ear to the secretory cells in the nephron, it was assumed that loop diuretics function in the inner ear as they do in the nephron (12,14,77,78). In the nephron, the theory of Burg et al. (79) of inhibition of chloride transport in the ascending limb of the loop of Henle has been generally accepted. However, Hommerich (80) proved that chloride concentrations in the inner ear are not altered. In addition, the ability of these diuretics to inhibit the Na$^+$/K$^+$-ATPase pump in the nephron has been recognized and postulated to be similar in the inner ear. Hommerich (80) disproved this hypothesis by showing that ion concentrations in the inner ear do not change in the same manner that they do in the kidney. At this time, the mechanism of action in the inner ear remains unknown.

The primary site of injury to the inner ear induced by loop diuretics is the stria vascularis; a secondary effect is destruction of hair cells. This was first reported by Quick and Duvall (81) in 1970. Electron microscopy shows interstitial edema in the intermediate cells of the stria vascularis, with a concomitant hydrops of the marginal cells, after ethacrynic acid parenteral infusion (80). Similar changes were not seen in the vestibular system, which explains the unlikelihood of vestibular toxicity, although ethacrynic acid has been reported to reduce calorically induced nystagmus. Prevention of loop diuretic-induced ototoxicity is best accomplished by avoiding rapid intravenous push administration, especially for ethacrynic acid. It should be noted that, as the primary site of injury is the stria vascularis, loop diuretics can act synergistically with aminoglycosides to cause ototoxicity (82). Therefore, concomitant use should be avoided, if possible.

ANALGESICS/ANTIPYRETICS AND ANTIMALARIAL DRUGS

Aspirin and Nonsteroidal Antiinflammatory Drugs

The ototoxic effects of acetylsalicylic acid, or aspirin, were first reported in 1884 by Schwabach (3). This medication is an analgesic, antipyretic, and antiinflammatory drug. Whereas exceedingly high doses are necessary to produce ototoxic effects, often greater than 2,700 mg/d, many patients who suffer from rheumatoid arthritis or other collagen vascular disease require doses of this magnitude (83).

Classically, the ototoxic effects of aspirin include tinnitus and reversible high-frequency sensorineural hearing loss. These effects often occur with overdosage (salicylism), but they also have been reported to occur with therapeutic dosages. Hearing loss is recognized by the patient as poor speech discrimination, and it is not usually worse than 30 to 40 dB in the high frequencies. Recovery from these effects occurs within 2 to 3 days after termination of therapy (84). The incidence of ototoxicity of classic nonsteroidal antiinflammatory drugs (NSAIDs), including ibuprofen and piroxicam, is disputed, but believed by most to be very low (14,85).

Sodium salicylate selectively reduces the cochlear action potential response, which suggests that the cochlea is the site of action (12). Because aspirin blocks cyclooxygenase and thereby inhibits the synthesis of vasoactive prostaglandins, a vascular basis of toxicity has been proposed. This theory has been refuted for two reasons: first, NSAIDs also block cyclooxygenase and do not cause ototoxicity; and second, blood supply to the cochlea has been found to be autoregulated (14,86). The stria vascularis has been proposed as a possible site of toxicity, as autoradiographic studies have demonstrated aspirin in the strial vessels within minutes of systemic administration. Changes in membrane permeability have also been proposed as an alternative mechanism of toxicity. Much work remains to be done before these issues are resolved.

Electron microscopy has failed to demonstrate any morphologic lesion in the cochlea in animals treated with suprapharmacologic doses (87). Temporal bone sections of patients suffering from salicylism also have failed to demonstrate any damage (88,89).

Currently, it is believed that salicylates exert a temporary metabolic effect that is not strong enough to result in cytotoxicity. The moderate degree of hearing loss suggests that outer hair cell function may be impaired. Prevention of salicylate ototoxicity is accomplished by prescribing the minimal dose necessary to achieve therapeutic effect and switching to NSAIDs or alternative methods of therapy, if possible.

Antimalarials

Quinine and chloroquine are drugs that have been used extensively to treat malaria. Quinine is naturally occurring and is an alkaloid found on the bark of the cinchona tree. Deafness resulting from the use of this bark for analgesia was reported as early as 1696. With either of these drugs, small doses may cause tinnitus and reversible bilateral high-frequency sensorineural hearing loss. Larger doses can cause permanent sensorineural deafness; this effect is more likely to occur with chloroquine (4,10,12).

Quinine-induced deafness is most common in elderly people taking this medication chronically for leg cramps. Recent histopathologic studies show the most severe degenerative changes in the basal turn of the cochlea. Vasoconstriction is seen in the capillary beds of the spiral ligament, basilar membrane, and stria vascularis (12). Local narrowing of capillary lumens caused by endothelial cell swelling also is seen. Treatment for ototoxic effects is withdrawal of the drug.

MISCELLANEOUS DRUGS

There are many more drugs that have been associated with ototoxicity whose mechanisms of action and histopathologic influences are not well understood. In the eighteenth and nineteenth centuries, the *oil of chenopodium* was used in the treatment of nematode infections (1,2). The active ingredient in this toxin is 1,4-peroxido-p-methane, which can cause headaches, central nervous system depression, coma, and death. Ototoxic effects include ataxia, tinnitus, and permanent sensorineural deafness (1,90).

Desferrioxamine, a necessary iron chelator in thalassemic patients, has been linked to sensorineural hearing loss in patients receiving repeated exposure. In a series of 37 patients, Porter et al. (91) documented reversible sensorineural hearing loss in nine, tinnitus in two, and vestibular neuropathy in two. Sections of the inner ear studied by Shirane and Harrison (92) showed cytoplasmic protrusions of the hair cells at the base of the cochlea, which is consistent with hypoxic injury. It is believed that the chelator removes necessary trace elements of zinc and copper from the cochlea, thus preventing oxidative metabolism (92).

Carbon monoxide, carbon disulfide, carbon tetrachloride, arsenic, lead, mercury, potassium bromate, toluene, and benzole all have ototoxic effects. *Carbon monoxide* causes central hearing loss; discrete lesions are located in the reticular formation (93). *Potassium bromate* (found in home permanent wave kits) produces cochlear damage by an unknown mechanism when ingested orally (93). *Lead* is toxic to neural tissue, destroying brain cells and causing neuralgia in the central nervous system and peripheral axons, sometimes resulting in deafness. *Mercury* causes atrophy of cerebral and cerebellar cortices by an unknown mechanism (94). *Arsenicals* have been linked to sensorineural hearing loss in children. The site of insult appears to be the stria vascularis, with subsequent damage to the hair cells (93). *Toluene* has been shown in rats to cause selective damage to outer hair cells (95,96).

Other drugs that have occasionally been linked with ototoxicity include propranolol (93), quinidine (via a similar mechanism to that of quinine) (93), bromocriptine (97), pentobarbital (93), hexane (93), very high doses of chloramphenicol and ampicillin (10), methenamine mandelate (Mandelamine) (10), and horse serum tetanus antitoxin (12).

SUMMARY

In this chapter the ototoxicities of numerous drugs and chemical agents were reviewed. For the four most commonly recognized classes of ototoxic drugs—aminoglycoside antibiotics, loop diuretics, antineoplastic drugs, and analgesics/antipyretics and antimalarial drugs—possible mechanisms of action and histopathologic findings were discussed. It is important to recognize that, at present, molecular mechanisms of ototoxicity are only rarely understood. Histopathologic changes are only slightly better defined. For this reason, there are no pharmacologic countermeasures to ototoxic effects; one unusual exception is the use of fosfomycin in conjunction with cisplatinum. The best treatment of ototoxicity is avoidance of its occurrence by hydration, minimizing synergistically toxic combinations of drugs, and sequential serologic or physiologic testing of a subject during administration to recognize subclinical effects. If ototoxic effects occur, early withdrawal of the agent is recommended, if permitted by the patient's medical condition.

CLINICAL APPLICATIONS

Genetic Basis of Aminoglycoside Ototoxicity

Recent molecular genetic research has provided evidence that it is possible in some cases for individuals to have a predetermined sensitivity to aminoglycoside ototoxicity. A specific defect in the mitochondrial genome is responsible for this susceptibility; however, before discussing the specific mechanism, it is necessary to review the genetics of mitochondrial DNA (mtDNA) disorders. A maternal inheritance pattern is seen with mtDNA genetic disorders, because all mitochondria present in an individual is inherited exclusively from the mother. Because the mother's ovum contributes the mtDNA to both male and female offspring, mtDNA genetic disorders can affect both sexes. Each cell has hundreds of mitochondria, whose primary function is to synthesize ATP by oxidative phosphorylation. Each mitochondrion has several mtDNA chromosomes, which in humans are 16,569 base pair double-stranded circles. Replication, transcription, and translation of the mtDNA occur autonomously within each mitochondrion. The mtDNA encodes 13 mRNAs, the large and small ribosomal RNAs, and 22 transfer RNAs. The mRNAs are translated on mitochondrion-specific ribosomes, using a mitochondrion-specific genetic code into 13 proteins. These proteins interact with 60 nuclear-encoded proteins to form the five enzyme complexes required for oxidative phosphorylation (98).

Studies of families with maternal inheritance patterns have identified a mtDNA mutation in a form of nonsyndromic deafness. One pedigree in the Far East had familial aminoglycoside-induced deafness (99). The laboratory of Fischel-Ghodsian investigated the molecular basis for deafness in three Chinese pedigrees with aminoglycoside ototoxicity, as well as in the Arab–Israeli pedigree (100). Because the mitochondrial ribosome is structurally similar to the bacterial ribosome, the hypothesis tested by Fischel-Ghodsian was that the cochlear mitochondrial ribosome was the target of aminoglycoside ototoxicity. They sequenced the entire mitochondrial ribosomal RNA genes in two of the Chinese pedigrees, as well as in the Arab–Israeli pedigree. They identified a point mutation at position 1555, with adenosine substituted by guanosine (A-G) in the mitochondrial 12S ribosomal RNA gene, which was common to all three families with maternally inherited hypersensitivity to aminoglycoside ototoxicity and absent in nearly 300 control subjects (100). The application of polymerase chain reaction amplification of this mtDNA in temporal bone sections from patients with profound sensorineural hearing loss and bilateral vestibular paralysis following aminoglycoside administration would allow the molecular detection of specific genetic alterations and histologic correlation after studying the mounted sections with light microscopic techniques (101,102).

Ablation of Peripheral Vestibular Function

Interest in intratympanic administration of an aminoglycoside as an alternative to endolymphatic sac surgery and vestibular neurectomy has increased in recent years. Although it is a nonsurgical office procedure, intratympanic aminoglycoside therapy is difficult to control. In at least one current form of drug delivery, it appears to be associated with a 10% rate of deafness in the treated ear (103,104). Other protocols may be associated with a lower rate of deafness. This therapy has a place in the treatment of Meniere's disease, but the optimal treatment protocol and the boundaries of its exact role remain to be defined.

Recent studies are leading to an improved understanding of why vertigo may persist following chemical labyrinthectomy. The main causes are persistence of functional vestibular sensory tissue; recovery from the ototoxic effect, including vestibular hair cell regeneration (105,106); and delayed vertigo due to the treatment itself. Recent reports have suggested that the total cumulative dose is the main factor in the ototoxic effect of aminoglycosides (107). As intramuscular or intratympanic treatment is repeated, there is continuous accumulation of the drug in the perilymph. As the intracellular level of drug reaches some critical level, the hair cell ceases to function and may die. Depending on the number of hair cells, the patient can experience an attack of vertigo, which usually is perceived as different in character from the attacks that occur from Meniere's disease. This is one form of vertigo occcuring after aminoglycoside therapy. Vertigo also may occur from the underlying disease if the chemical ablation of hair cells is incomplete, or possibly if the hair cells regenerate and re-form functional neural connections with the central nervous system (105,106).

Damage to vestibular dark cells, which are thought to play a role in the production of endolymph, has been reported following administration of doses of aminoglycoside below the threshold for damage to hair cells. An attractive hypothesis is that the impaired function of dark cells would be beneficial in patients with Meniere's disease, because decreased production of endolymph would affect the fluid homeostasis of the inner ear (108,109).

Preparation of Gentamicin Solution

Gentamicin solution may be used either as a stock solution of 40 mg/mL with a pH of about 5.4, or the gentamicin solution may be buffered to a pH of 6.4 to reduce the discomfort associated with intratympanic injection. One method described by Monsell et al. (110) as well as Wackym and Monsell (111) is to prepare the buffered solution as follows: 1.5 mL of gentamicin solution (40 mg/mL) is injected into a sterile 5-mL vial. A 0.6 mol/L sodium bicarbonate per liter solution is prepared by combining 2 mL of 8.4% sodium bicarbonate and 1.36 mL of sterile water in a 5-mL sterile vial. Add 0.5 mL of the 0.6 mol/L sodium bicarbonate solution to the sterile vial containing 1.5 mL of gentamicin to form 2 mL of a solution of gentamicin (30 mg/mL, pH 6.4) ready for injection.

Injection Technique

The patient should be positioned comfortably in the standard otologic position for examination under the operating microscope, i.e., supine with the head turned away from the ear to be treated. In this position, the eustachian tube will be uppermost to avoid dependent drainage of the gentamicin solution out of the middle ear. This position is maintained for 30 minutes following the injection. The patient is instructed not to swallow or clear the middle ear during this period. Providing the patient with a cup for gentle expectoration during this period helps accomplish this goal. Topical application of phenol to a small injection site on the surface of the tympanic membrane provides anesthesia, and the gentamicin is injected in the middle ear using a tuberculin syringe and a 27- or 25-gauge spinal needle. Typically, about 0.5 mL of solution fills the middle ear.

Administration Protocols

Numerous administration protocols have been described. Nedzelski et al. (103) and Nedzelski and

Chiong (104) had patients administer gentamicin intratympanically three times a day via a tympanostomy tube and a small flexible tubing for 4 days. The protocol introduced by Beck and Schmidt (112) advocates a once-daily regimen until the earliest sign of ototoxicity is observed. With this schedule, 1 to 12 doses (mean 4 to 6) are given.

A number of other investigators (including one of the authors, P.A.W.) use a dosing regimen that titrates the administration of gentamicin using patient response measured by caloric response, audiometric function, and patient symptoms. The rationale is to reduce the risk of hearing loss while maintaining control of vertigo by giving less medication per dose and extending the time of treatment with repeated applications as necessary. A second injection of approximately 0.5 mL of gentamicin, 30 mg/mL, pH 6.4, is given 1 to 2 weeks after the first dose. Additional doses may be given if vertigo is not controlled or recurs. As more is learned about aminoglycoside vestibulotoxicity and delivery vehicles, it is anticipated that this therapy will become an important treatment method in managing patients with Meniere's disease.

SUMMARY POINTS

- The four most common classes of ototoxic agents are antibiotics; antineoplastic agents; loop diuretics; and analgesics/antipyretics and antimalarial drugs.
- The most common symptoms of drug-induced ototoxicity are tinnitus, sensorineural hearing loss, and vestibular dysfunction. Disequilibrium due to bilateral vestibular paresis is the most frequent type of vestibular dysfunction. True vertigo is rare.
- Gentamicin is more vestibulotoxic than cochleotoxic.
- Mitochondrial DNA defects can increase the susceptibility to ototoxic damage by aminoglycosides. These defects are passed on via a maternal inheritance pattern.
- Cochlear and vestibular neuroepithelia are injured by aminoglycosides.
- Cisplatinum-induced ototoxicity is most frequently manifest as tinnitus, hearing loss, and/or otalgia. These symptoms usually occur within 2 days of initiate of therapy, but they can appear up to 7 days after stopping therapy.
- Hearing loss due to loop diuretics almost always is reversible.
- Exceedingly high doses of acetylsalicylic acid (aspirin) are necessary to produce reversible high-frequency sensorineural hearing loss and tinnitus.

REFERENCES

1. North A. Two cases of poisoning by the oil of chenopodium. *Am J Otol* 1880;2:197.
2. Brown TR. Case of poisoning by the oil of chenopodium. *Maryland Med J* 1878;4:20.
3. Schwabach D. Uber bleibende Storungen im Gehororgan nach Chinin und Salicylgebrauch. *Dtsch Med Wschr* 1884;10:163.
4. Roosa DB, John ST. Experiments concerning the effects of quinine upon the ear. *Trans Am Otol Soc* 1875;2:93.
5. Werner CF. Das Labyrinth. *Bau, Funktion and Krankheiten des Innenohres von Standpunkte eines experimentellen und vergleichenden Pathologie.* Leipzig: Georg Thieme Verlag, 1940.
6. Hinshaw HL, Feldman WH. Streptomycin in the treatment of clinical tuberculosis: a preliminary report. *Proc Mayo Clin* 1945;20:313.
7. Lerner SA, Matz GJ, Hawkins JE Jr, eds. *Aminoglycoside ototoxicity.* Boston: Little, Brown & Company, 1981.
8. Geraci JE, Heilman FR, Nichols RD. Antibiotic therapy of bacterial endocarditis. VII. Vancomycin for acute microbial endocarditis. *Proc Staff Meet Mayo Clin* 1958;33:172.
9. Maher JF, Schreiner GE. Studies on ethacrynic acid on patients with refractory edema. *Ann Intern Med* 1965;62:15.
10. Walker EM Jr, Fazekas-May MA, Bowen WR. Nephrotoxic and ototoxic agents. *Clin Lab Med* 1990;10:323.
11. Piel IJ, Meyer D, Perlia CP. Effects of cis-diaminedichloroplatinum (NSC-119875) on hearing function in man. *Cancer Chemother Rep* 1974;58:871.
12. Stringer SP, Meyerhoff WL, Wright CG. Ototoxicity. In: Paparella MM, Shumrick DA, Gluckman JL, Meyerhoff WL, eds. *Otolaryngology*, 3rd ed. Philadelphia: WB Saunders, 1991:1653.
13. Matz GJ. Clinical perspectives on ototoxic drugs. *Ann Otol Rhinol Laryngol Suppl* 1990;148:39–41.
14. Huang MY, Schacht J. Drug-induced ototoxicity. Pathogenesis and prevention. *Med Toxicol Adverse Drug Exp* 1989;4:452–467.
15. Boston Collaborative Drug Surveillance Program. Drug-induced deafness. *JAMA* 1973;224:515–516.
16. Tuzel IH. Comparison of adverse effects to bumetanide and furosemide. *J Clin Pharmacol* 1981;21:615–619.
17. Benveniste R, Davies J. Structure-activity relationships among the aminoglycoside antibiotics: role of hydroxyl and amino groups. *Antimicrob Agents Chemother* 1973;4:402–409.
18. Rybak LP. Drug ototoxicity. *Ann Rev Pharmacol Toxicol* 1986;26:79–99.
19. Waksman SA. Streptomycin: background, isolation, properties and utilization. *Science* 1953;118:259.
20. Kahlmeter G, Dahlager JI. Aminoglycoside toxicity—a review of clinical studies published between 1975 and 1982. *J Antimicrob Chemother* 1984;13[Suppl A]:9–22.
21. Serles W. Streptomycinschaden im Elektronystagmogramm. *Wochenschr Ohrenkeilk* 1966;100:251.
22. Beaubien AR, Desjardins S, Ormsby E, Bayne A, Carrier K, Cauchy MJ. Delay in hearing loss following drug administration. A consistent feature of amikacin ototoxicity. *Acta Otolaryngol (Stockh)* 1990;109:345–352.
23. Tucci DL, Rubel EW. Physiologic status of regenerated hair cells in the avian inner ear following aminoglycoside ototoxicity. *Otolaryngol Head Neck Surg* 1990;103:443–450.
24. Cruz RM, Lambert PR, Rubel EW. Light microscopic evidence of hair cell regeneration after gentamicin toxicity in chick cochlea. *Arch Otolaryngol Head Neck Surg* 1987;113:1058–1062.
25. Girod DA, Tucci DL, Rubel EW. Anatomical correlates of functional recovery in the avian inner ear following aminoglycoside ototoxicity. *Laryngoscope* 1991;101:1139–1149.
26. McFadden EA, Saunders JC. Recovery of auditory function following intense sound exposure in the neonatal chick. *Hear Res* 1989;41:205–215.
27. Moffat DA, Ramsden RT. Profound bilateral sensorineural hearing loss during gentamicin therapy. *J Laryngol Otol* 1977;91:511–516.
28. Winkel O, Hansen MM, Kaaber K, Rozarth K. A prospective study of gentamicin ototoxicity. *Acta Otolaryngol* 1978;86:212–216.
29. Fee WE Jr. Aminoglycoside ototoxicity in the human. *Laryngoscope* 1980;90:1–19.
30. Schuknecht HF. Ablation therapy for the relief of Meniere's disease. *Laryngoscope* 1950;66:859.
31. Schuknecht HF. Ablation therapy in the management of Meniere's disease. *Acta Otolaryngol (Stockh)* 1957;[Suppl 132].
32. Wersäll J, Björkroth B, Flock Å, Lundquist PG. Experiments on ototoxic effects of antibiotics. *Adv Otorhinolaryngol* 1973;20:14–41.
33. Odkvist LM. Middle ear ototoxic treatment for inner ear disease. *Acta Otolaryngol (Stockh)* 1989;[Suppl 457]:83.
34. Shea JJ, Norris CH. Streptomycin perfusion of the labyrinth. In: Nadol JB Jr, ed. *Second international symposium on Ménière's disease.* Amsterdam: Kugler & Ghedini Publications, 1989:463.
35. Dumas G, Bessard G, Gavend M, Charachon R. Risque de surdite par instillations de gouttes auriculaires contenant des aminosides. *Therapie* 1980;35:357.
36. Nomura Y. Otological significance of the round window. *Adv Otorhinolaryngol* 1984;33:1.
37. Murphy KW. Deafness after topical neomycin. *Br Med J* 1970;2:114.
38. Smith BM, Myers MG. The penetration of gentamicin and neomycin into perilymph across the round window membrane. *Otolaryngol Head Neck Surg* 1979;87:888–891.
39. Ikeda K, Morizono T. Round window membrane permeability during experimental purulent otitis media: altered cortisporin ototoxicity. *Ann Otol Rhinol Laryngol Suppl* 1990;148:46–48.
40. Morizono T. Toxicity of ototopical drugs: animal modeling. *Ann Otol Rhinol Laryngol* 1990;99[Suppl 148]:42–45.
41. Jackson GG, Arcieri G. Ototoxicity of gentamicin in man: a survey and controlled analysis of clinical experience in the United States. *J Infect Dis* 1971;124[Suppl]:130.
42. Keene M, Hawke M. Pathogenesis and detection of aminoglycoside ototoxicity. *J Otolaryngol* 1981;10:228–236.
43. Lerner SA, Selighson R, Matz GJ. Comparative clinical studies of ototoxicity and nephrotoxicity of amikacin and gentamicin. *Am J Med* 1977;62:919–923.
44. Edson RS, Terrell CL. The aminoglycosides: streptomycin, kanamycin, gentamicin, tobramycin, amikacin, netilmicin, and sisomicin. *Mayo Clin Proc* 1987;62:916–920.
45. Kaye D, Levison ME, Labovitz ED. The unpredictability of serum concentrations of gentamicin: pharmacokinetics of gentamicin in patients with normal and abnormal renal function. *J Infect Dis* 1974;130:150–154.
46. Federspil P, Schatzle W, Tiesler E. Pharmacokinetics and ototoxicity of gentamicin, tobramycin, and amikacin. *J Infect Dis* 1976;134 [Suppl]:S200–S205.
47. Hawkins JE Jr, Boxer GE, Jeninek VC. Concentration of streptomycin in brain and other tissues of cats after acute and chronic intoxication. *Proc Soc Exp Biol* 1950;75:759.
48. Balogh K Jr, Hiraide F, Ishii D. Distribution of radioactive dihydrostreptomycin in the cochlea—an autoradiographic study. *Ann Otol Rhinol Laryngol* 1970;79:641–652.
49. Hawkins JE Jr. Ototoxic mechanisms: a working hypothesis. *Audiology* 1973;12:383.
50. Musebeck K, Schatzle W. Experimentelle Studies zur ototoxicat des Dihydrostreptomycins. *Arch Klin Exp Ohr Naskelkopfheilk* 1962;181:41.
51. Lim DJ. Effects of noise and ototoxic drugs at the cellular level in the cochlea: a review. *Am J Otolaryngol* 1986;7:73.
52. Schacht J. Molecular mechanisms of drug-induced hearing loss. *Hear Res* 1986;22:297.
53. Williams SE, Zenner HP, Schacht J. Three molecular steps of aminoglycoside ototoxicity demonstrated in outer hair cells. *Hear Res* 1987;30:11.
54. McGee TM, Olszewski J. Streptomycin sulfate and dihydrostreptomycin toxicity. Behavioral and histopathologic studies. *Arch Otolaryngol* 1962;75:295.
55. Huizing EH, de Groot JCMJ. Human cochlear pathology in aminoglycoside ototoxicity—a review. *Acta Otolaryngol (Stockh)* 1987;[Suppl 436]:117.
56. Takumida M, Wersäll J, Bagger-Sjöbäck D. Sensory hair fusion and glycocalyx changes after gentamicin exposure in the guinea pig. *Acta Otolaryngol (Stockh)* 1988;[Suppl 457]:78.
57. Takumida M, Bagger-Sjöbäck D, Harada Y, Lim D, Wersäll J. Sensory hair fusion and glycocalyx changes following gentamicin exposure in the guinea pig vestibular organs. *Acta Otolaryngol (Stockh)* 1989;107:39.
58. Takumida M, Bagger-Sjöbäck D, Wersäll J, Harada Y. The effect of gentamicin on the glycocalyx and the ciliary interconnections in the

vestibular sensory cells: a high resolution scanning electron microscopic investigation. *Hear Res* 1989;37:163.

59. Sobel JD. Imipenem and aztreonam. *Infect Dis Clin North Am* 1989; 3:613.

60. Brown OE, Wright CG, Edwards LB, Meyerhoff WL. The ototoxicity of ceftazidime in the chinchilla middle ear. *Arch Otolaryngol Head Neck Surg* 1989;115:940.

61. Huang MY, Schacht J. Formation of a cytotoxic metabolite from gentamicin by liver. *Biochem Pharmacol* 1990;40:R11.

62. Mintz U, Amir J, Pinkhas J. Transient perceptive deafness due to erythromycin lactobionate. *JAMA* 1973;225:1122.

63. Schweitzer VG, Olson NR. Ototoxic effect of erythromycin therapy. *Arch Otolaryngol* 1984;110:258.

64. Hermans PE, Wilhelm MP. Vancomycin. *Mayo Clin Proc* 1987; 62:901.

65. Bailie GR, Neal D. Vancomycin ototoxicity and nephrotoxicity: a review. *Med Toxicol* 1988;3:376.

66. Marsh RR, Tom LWC. Ototoxicity of antimycotics. *Otolaryngol Head Neck Surg* 1989;100:134.

67. Williams DN. Minocycline: possible vestibular side-effects. *Lancet* 1974;2:744.

68. Quick CA. Chemical and drug effects on the inner ear. In: Paparella MM, Shumrick DA, eds. *Otolaryngology*, 2nd ed. Philadelphia: WB Saunders, 1980:1804.

69. McAlpine D, Johnstone BM. The ototoxic mechanism of cisplatin. *Hear Res* 1990;47:191.

70. Laurell G, Skedinger M. Changes of stapedius reflex and hearing threshold in patients receiving high-dose cisplatin treatment. *Audiology* 1990;29:252.

71. Strauss M, Towfighi J, Lord S, Lipton A, Harvey HA, Brown B. Cisplatinum ototoxicity: clinical experience and temporal bone histopathology. *Laryngoscope* 1983;93:1554.

72. Barr-Hamilton RM, Matheson LM, Keay DG. Ototoxicity of cisplatinum and its relationship to eye colour. *J Laryngol Otol* 1991;105:7.

73. Higby DJ, Wallace H Jr, Albert D. Diaminedichloroplatinum in chemotherapy of testicular tumors. *J Urol* 1974;112:100.

74. Schweitzer VG, Dolan DF, Abrams GE, Davidson T, Snyder R. Amelioration of cisplatin-induced ototoxicity by fosfomycin. *Laryngoscope* 1986;96:948.

75. Murakami T, Inoue S, Sasaki K, Fujimoto T. Studies on age-dependent plasma platinum pharmacokinetics and ototoxicity of cisplatin. *Selective Cancer Ther* 1990;6:145.

76. Schaefer SD, Post JD, Close LG, Wright CG. Ototoxicity of low- and moderate-dose cisplatin. *Cancer* 1985;56:1934.

77. Benet LZ. Pharmacokinetics/pharmacodynamics of furosemide in man: a review. *J Pharmacokinet Biopharm* 1979;7:1.

78. Prazma J, Thomas WG, Fisher D. Ototoxicity of ethacrynic acid. *Arch Otolaryngol* 1972;95:448.

79. Burg M, Stoner L, Cardinal J, Green N. Furosemide effect on isolated perfused tubules. *Am J Physiol* 1973;225:119.

80. Hommerich CP. Ototoxicity of loop diuretics. Morphological and electrophysiological examinations in animal experiments. In: Pfaltz CR, ed. *Advances in otorhinolaryngology, volume 44*. Basal: Karger, 1990;92.

81. Quick CA, Duvall J. Early changes in the cochlear duct from ethacrynic acid: an electron microscopic evaluation. *Laryngoscope* 1970;80:954.

82. Konishi T. Some observations on negative endocochlear potential during anoxia. *Acta Otolaryngol* 1979;87:506.

83. Hinojosa R, Lindsay JR, Matz GJ. The inner ear. In: Riddell RH, ed. *Pathology of drug-induced and toxic diseases*. New York: Churchill Livingstone, 1982:155.

84. McCabe B, Dey F. The effect of aspirin upon auditory sensitivity. *Ann Otol Rhinol Laryngol* 1965;74:312.

85. Vernick DM, Kelly JH. Sudden hearing loss associated with piroxicam. *Am J Otol* 1986;7:97.

86. Quirk WS, Dengerink HA, Harding JW. Autoregulation of cochlear blood flow in normotensive and spontaneously hypertensive rats following intracerebroventricularly mediated adjustment of blood pressure. *Hear Res* 1989;38:119.

87. Deer BC, Hunter-Duvar I. Salicylate ototoxicity in the chinchilla: a behavioral and electron microscope study. *J Otolaryngol* 1982; 11:260.

88. Bernstein JM, Weiss AP. Further observations on salicylate ototoxicity. *J Laryngol Otol* 1967;81:915.

89. De Maura LFP, Hayden RE Jr. Salicylate ototoxicity: a human temporal bone report. *Arch Otolaryngol* 1968;87:60.

90. Roth DA. Some dangers of the chenopodium treatment. *South Med J* 1918;11:733.

91. Porter JB, Jawson MS, Huehns ER, East CA, Hazell JWP. Desferrioxamine ototoxicity: evaluation of risk factors in thalassemic patients and guidelines for safe dosage. *Br J Hematol* 1989;73:403.

92. Shirane M, Harrison RV. A study of deferoxamine in chinchilla. *J Otolaryngol* 1987;16:334.

93. Quick CA. Ototoxicity. In: English G, ed. *Otolaryngology*. New York: Harper & Row, 1984:1.

94. Meyerhoff WE, Liston S. Metabolic hearing loss. In: English G, ed. *Otolaryngology*. New York: Harper & Row, 1984:5.

95. Sullivan MJ, Rarey KE, Conolly RB. Ototoxicity of toluene in rats. *Neurotox Teratol* 1989;10:525.

96. Rebert CS, Matteucci MJ, Pryor GT. Multimodal effects of acute exposure to toluene evidenced by sensory-evoked potentials from Fischer-344 rats. *Pharmacol Biochem Behav* 1989;32:757.

97. Lanthier PL, Morgan MY, Ballantyne J. Bromocriptine-associated ototoxicity. *J Laryngol Otol* 1984;98:399.

98. Anderson A, Bankier AT, Barrell BG, et al. Sequence and organization of the human mitochondrial genome. *Nature* 1981;290:457.

99. Hu D-N, Qiu W-Q, Wu B-T, et al. Genetic aspects of antibiotic induced deafness: mitochondrial inheritance. *J Med Genet* 1991; 28:79.

100. Hutchin T, Haworth I, Higashi K, et al. A molecular basis for human hypersensitivity to aminoglycoside antibiotics. *Nucleic Acids Res* 1993;21:4174.

101. Wackym PA. Molecular temporal bone pathology: I. Historical foundation. *Laryngoscope* 1997;107:1156.

102. Wackym PA. Molecular temporal bone pathology: II. Ramsay Hunt syndrome (herpes zoster oticus). *Laryngoscope* 1997;107:1165.

103. Nedzelski J, Schessel D, Bryce G, Pfleiderer A. Chemical labyrinthectomy: local application for the treatment of unilateral Ménière's disease. *Am J Otol* 1992;13:18.

104. Nedzelski JM, Chiong CM. Intratympanic gentamicin instillation as treatment of unilateral Ménière's disease: update of an ongoing study. *Am J Otol* 1993;14:278.

105. Warchol ME, Lambert PR, Goldstein BJ, Forge A, Corwin JT. Regenerative proliferation in inner ear sensory epithelia from adult guinea pigs and humans. *Science* 1993;259:1619.

106. Lambert PR. Inner ear hair cell regeneration in a mammal: identification of a triggering factor. *Laryngoscope* 1994;104:701.

107. Monsell EM, Cass SP, Rybak LP. Pharmacologic labyrinthectomy for Ménière's disease. *Otolaryngol Clin North Am* 1993;26:737.

108. Park J, Cohen G. Vestibular ototoxicity in the chick: effects of streptomycin on equilibrium and on ampullary dark cells. *Am J Otolaryngol* 1982;6:117.

109. Pender D. Gentamicin tympanoclysis: effects on the vestibular secretory cells. *Am J Otolaryngol* 1985;6:358.

110. Monsell EM, Cass SP, Rybak LP. Chemical labyrinthectomy, methods and results. In: Brackmann DE, ed. *Otologic surgery*. Philadelphia: WB Saunders Co, 1994:509.

111. Wackym PA, Monsell EM. Revision vestibular surgery. In: Carrasco VN, Pillsbury HC III, eds. *Revision otologic surgery*. New York: Thieme Medical Publishers, 1997:109.

112. Beck C, Schmidt CL. Ten years of experience with intratympanically applied streptomycin (gentamicin) in the therapy of morbus Ménière. *Arch Otorhinolaryngol* 1978;221:149.

The Ear: Comprehensive Otology,
edited by R. F. Canalis and P. R. Lambert.
Lippincott Williams & Wilkins, Philadelphia © 2000.

CHAPTER 36

Otosyphilis and Otologic Manifestations of AIDS

Marshall E. Smith and Rinaldo F. Canalis

Syphilis, "the great imitator," has long been identified as an etiologic factor in otologic disease during the various stages of congenital and acquired infection. Although syphilis was particularly prevalent in the prepenicillin ear, its current role in ear pathology, particularly in sensorineural hearing loss, demands renewed attention for several reasons. First, the incidence of primary syphilis increased sharply during the 1980s (1,2). This ensures that delayed complications such as otosyphilis will be with us for some time to come. Second, the wide variety of presentations and manifestations of luetic involvement of the temporal bone requires constant vigilance and awareness on the part of the clinician. Third, otosyphilis is an eminently treatable form of hearing loss; therefore, prompt diagnosis and initiation of treatment may yield favorable results. Fourth, the subtleties of diagnosis and treatment of otosyphilis are not well known outside of our specialty. Primary care physicians, internists, neurologists, and infectious disease specialists, although well versed in the variety of other manifestations of syphilis, are less likely to identify the patient with luetic otitis than is the otolaryngologist.

M. E. Smith: Division of Otolaryngology–Head and Neck Surgery, University of Utah School of Medicine, Salt Lake City, Utah 84132

R. F. Canalis: Department of Surgery, University of California, Los Angeles, School of Medicine, Los Angeles, California 90095-1624

INCIDENCE

Epidemiologic studies show an increase in the incidence of both congenital and acquired syphilis in the United States during the late 1980s, peaking in 1990 (Fig. 1) (3,4). Between 1981 and 1990, the incidence of primary and secondary syphilis increased 43% (5). Total numbers of reported cases for all stages of syphilis reached 53.8 per 100,000 in 1990, but the numbers have gradually declined to levels below those seen in the early 1980s (3). Congenital syphilis also went through a sharp rise, peaking at 112 cases per 100,000 live births in 1991. It has since fallen to 34 per 100,000 live births, which is still well above the incidence level of the early 1950s when penicillin first became widely used against the infection (3). The data also show gender, racial, and regional trends. Although historically the incidence has been higher for men than for women, the numbers have converged in recent years and now are almost equal (3). The incidence for all races has declined, but the 1995 rate for African-Americans was still 60 times greater than the rate for Caucasians. States in the South, Southeast, and along the East Coast continue to report the highest incidences (3). Despite the overall decline observed during this decade, sporadic epidemic outbreaks of syphilis still have occurred (6,7). An association of these outbreaks with the abuse of crack cocaine and the practice of trading sex for drugs was documented. This problem probably was largely responsible for the generalized increase in syphilis during the 1980s.

SYPHILIS (primary and secondary) — by sex, United States, 1981–1995

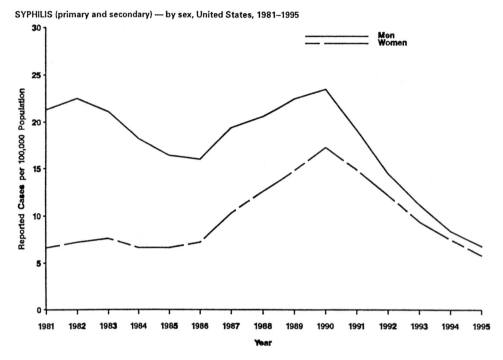

SYPHILIS (primary and secondary) — by race, United States, 1981–1995

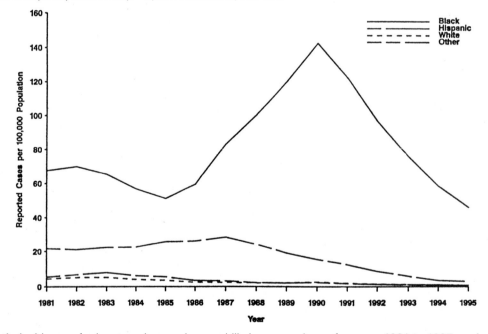

FIG. 1. Incidence of primary and secondary syphilis by sex and race for years 1981 to 1995, and congenital syphilis for years 1965 to 1995 reported by the Centers for Disease Control (3).

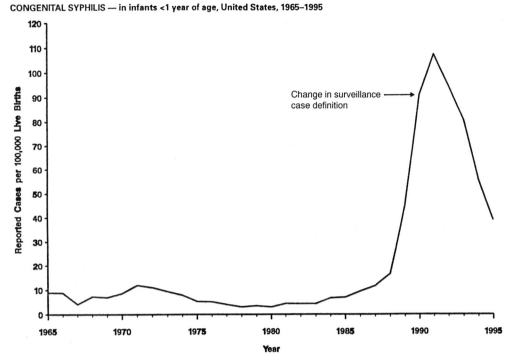

CONGENITAL SYPHILIS — in infants <1 year of age, United States, 1965–1995

FIG. 1. *Continued.*

PATHOLOGY

There appear to be two different pathologic processes affecting the vestibular and auditory structures that parallel the various stages of the congenital and acquired forms of syphilis (8). Basilar meningitis affecting directly the eighth cranial nerve complex occurs in early (infantile) syphilis and in the acute intracranial processes of secondary and possibly tertiary meningovascular neurosyphilis (8–10). In late (tardive) congenital and in late latent and tertiary forms of acquired otosyphilis, osteitis of the temporal bone is the predominant lesion with involvement of the membranous labyrinth. This temporal bone pathology has been well documented since the early histopathologic studies of Mayer and Fraser (11) and Goodhill (12). Findings include mononuclear lymphocytic infiltrate, rarefying osteitis of the otic capsule, obliterative endarteritis, and endolymphatic hydrops (Fig. 2). Areas of bone resorption, including the ossicles, are replaced by inflammatory fibrous infiltrate and eventually by marrow tissue (Fig. 3) (8,13). The hydropic swelling of Reissner's membrane may result from microgummatous infiltration and fibrous obliteration of the endolymphatic sac (14). These changes and progressive vascular occlusion from endarteritis lead to degeneration of the membranous labyrinth (Fig. 4) (8).

The pathologic changes seen are similar to those seen in other organ systems involving syphilis, namely, mononuclear lymphocytic infiltrate and obliterative endarteri-tis (8,15) However, the mechanisms underlying these pathologic changes are unclear. The route of initial infection to the temporal bone may be blood borne or by contaminated cerebrospinal fluid (CSF) through the cochlear aqueduct. In the temporal bone there has been only one study showing spirochetal-type organisms in the temporal bone of a patient with late congenital syphilis that was treated (16). This study has not been confirmed (17). The persistence of spirochetal organisms following penicillin treatment in the aqueous humor of the eye (18), lymph nodes (19), and CSF (20) has been observed, but the viability and virulence of these organisms are unknown (20). At present, any consideration of reactivation of temporal bone treponemes as a primary mechanism in the secondary and tertiary stages of the disease is speculative and controversial (21). The pathologic changes resulting from a prolonged immune response to, or previous, spirochetal infection provide a plausible explanation for the vestibular and auditory findings in otosyphilis (22).

CLINICAL FEATURES

Congenital syphilis is acquired prenatally or natally from maternal inoculation. It occurs in two forms. The early (infantile) type yields overwhelming multisystem involvement, and hearing is of secondary concern. Late (tardive) congenital syphilis shows great variation in age of onset and presentation of symptoms. In congenital syphilis, hearing loss occurs in 25% to 38% of patients

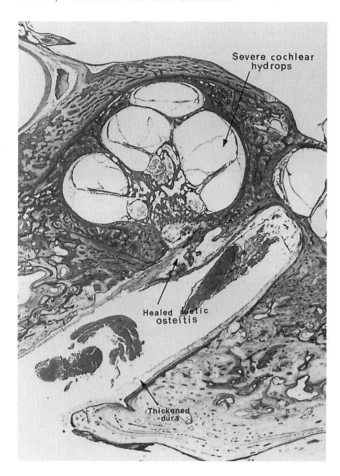

FIG. 2. Region of the right internal auditory canal showing syphilitic changes in the anterior wall. There is severe endolymphatic hydrops with degeneration of the organ of Corti and cochlear neurons. There is thickening of the dura mater lining the internal auditory canal. (From Belal A Jr, Linthicum FH Jr. Pathology of congenital syphilitic labyrinthitis. *Am J Otolaryngol* 1980;1:109–118, with permission.)

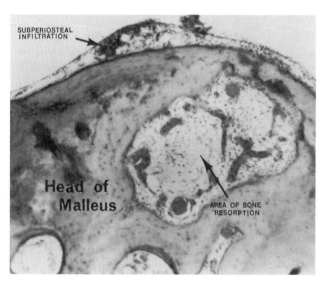

FIG. 3. Congenital syphilis of the temporal bone. The head of the malleus *(right)* shows areas of bone resorption containing fibrous tissue, lymphocytes, and plasma cells. (From Belal A Jr, Linthicum FH Jr. Pathology of congenital syphilitic labyrinthitis. *Am J Otolaryngol* 1980;1:109–118, with permission.)

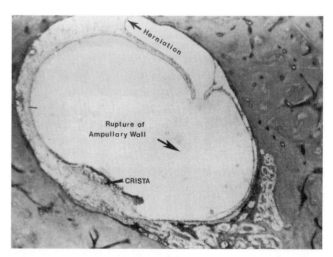

FIG. 4. Congenital syphilis of the temporal bone. There is rupture of the ampullary wall of the posterior semicircular canal, forming an otic-periotic fistula. The membranous wall of the canal has herniated into the perilymphatic space. The crista is shrunken and shows a nearly total loss of hair cells. (From Belal A Jr, Linthicum FH Jr. Pathology of congenital syphilitic labyrinthitis. *Am J Otolaryngol* 1980;1:109–118, with permission.)

(13,23). When it occurs before age 10 (37%), hearing loss usually is abrupt, bilateral, and unaccompanied by vestibular symptoms (13). Manifestations of hearing loss later in life, from adolescence through mid adulthood, are quite varied. Unilateral or asymmetric bilateral hearing loss, fluctuating hearing loss, and episodic vertigo similar to Meniere's disease may be present (24,25). Tinnitus may be a presenting symptom and is eventually present in most patients (25). These varied presentations are identical to the symptoms of late acquired otosyphilis. Other stigmata of congenital syphilis include interstitial keratitis, dental abnormalities with peglike teeth (Hutchinson's triad of congenital syphilis includes interstitial keratitis, peglike teeth, and sensorineural deafness), collapse of nasal cartilage framework (snuffles), and periostitis of cranial bones (bossing) and tibia (saber shins). Interstitial keratitis, although present in about 9% of congenital syphilitics without deafness (26), has been found to be present in 73% to 90% of those with congenital syphilitic hearing loss (25,27).

Otologic disease associated with acquired luetic infection may occur in the context of different stages of the disease. Again, the manifestations are varied. Secondary syphilis occurs 4 to 10 weeks after primary infection. It is characterized by headaches, stiff neck, diffuse bilateral symmetric papulosquamous skin rashes, lymphadenopathy, genital lesions (condyloma lata), and occasionally optic neuritis and cranial nerve palsies (including cranial nerve VIII). There are several case reports of hearing loss in early acquired (secondary) syphilis (9,10,28). The other systemic manifestations may be minimal to absent. It is usually abrupt in onset, bilateral, and rapidly progressive. In the majority of cases, CSF demonstrates a lymphocytic pleocytosis, elevated protein, and normal glucose.

After the untreated lesions of secondary syphilis resolve, a latent stage of the infection begins. "Early latent" syphilis is defined as duration less than 1 year and "late latent" syphilis is duration more than 1 year (29). Asymptomatic or minimally symptomatic, untreated patients are still regarded as infective, and results of serologic tests remain positive, although with normal CSF examination (20,30,31). Symptoms that develop years after the latent stage define "tertiary" syphilis (29). In this stage, patients may develop otologic symptoms in two clinical settings. The first clinical setting is in the context of neurosyphilis, which occurs in 7% of untreated adults and causes meningovascular syphilis, generalized paresis, or tabes dorsalis (29). The second, and more common, clinical setting is monosymptomatic otosyphilis. It usually occurs in patients 40 to 60 years old, but it may present as early as 25 years of age (21). Hearing loss may initially be unilateral, progressing to bilateral involvement. Vestibular symptoms may accompany or precede hearing loss, may present by themselves, or may present with other cranial neuropathies (usually seventh or third cranial nerve) (32). In a recent series, bilat-

eral sensorineural hearing loss was present in 82% of patients and unilateral in 18% of patients. Forty-two percent had episodic vertigo, and 24% had symptoms consistent with Meniere's disease (25). Becker (21) states that there is no consistent clinical or audiologic picture with either congenital or acquired otosyphilis.

In the clinical examination of a patient with suspected otosyphilis, some audiologic tests can be used. A positive result of the fistula test in the absence of middle ear disease is called Hennebert's sign. This phenomenon may be explained by fibrous bands between the footplate and membranous labyrinth (vestibulofibrosis) (33). The Tullio phenomenon describes the elicitation of vertigo and nystagmus with exposure to loud noise. The mechanism of this may be similar. Audiometry in congenital syphilis typically shows a flat sensorineural hearing loss. Early in the course of the disease, the loss may be greater in the low frequencies. Speech discrimination may be poor in relation to pure tone thresholds and may fluctuate over time. A middle ear component may be present. Vestibular function tests may show a decreased caloric response.

DIAGNOSIS

The organism *Treponema pallidum* cannot be cultured *in vitro*. However, syphilitic infection triggers a complex immune response involving both humoral and cell-mediated immune systems (34). The humoral response yields a variety of serologic tests that are divided into nontreponemal and treponemal categories (21). Nontreponemal tests include flocculation (Venereal Disease Research Laboratory [VDRL]) and complement-fixation (Kolmer) tests. They are reactive in most patients with primary syphilis and nearly all patients with secondary syphilis. They usually become nonreactive with effective treatment in the early stages, but they may stay reactive (become serofast). In untreated patients they may become nonreactive with time. False-positive results may occur in various conditions including malaria, systemic lupus erythematosus, viral infections, pregnancy, and intravenous drug abuse. Their use has limited specificity and unreliability in the late stages of syphilis during which otologic symptoms arise.

Treponeme specific tests assay for antibodies directed against the organism itself. The treponeme pallidum immobilization test was developed in 1949, and in 1963 the fluorescent treponemal antibody absorption (FTA-ABS) test appeared. The FTA-ABS test is reactive in 95% to 98% of patients with late syphilis, treatment notwithstanding, and it is the recommended test in diagnosis of otosyphilis (21,35). The degree of reaction is graded from 1 to 4+. Weakly positive tests may become nonreactive on repeat testing. They may represent false-positive results for various diseases (e.g., systemic lupus erythematosus, rheumatoid arthritis, autoimmune hemolytic anemia, alcoholic cirrhosis) or pregnancy, or they may give inconsistent results between different laboratories (36,37). These results should be investigated further before making the diagnosis of otosyphilis.

Another issue to be addressed in understanding the results of serologic tests involves their "predictive value." Hughes and Rutherford (38) discussed this issue in detail. The predictive value of a positive test result is the number of true-positive results divided by the number of true-positive plus false-positive results. The FTA-ABS test is, by definition, 100% sensitive but 98% specific due to the inherent false-positives. In a large population with a low prevalence of the disease, more positive test results are likely to be false-positives. Hughes and Rutherford state that for the population in Cleveland, Ohio, the prevalence-related predictive value of otosyphilis is 22%, that is, only 22% of FTA-ABS positive patients with suspected otosyphilis will actually have syphilis. In a patient population with a high incidence of syphilis, the predictive value of a positive test result will be greater (39).

Other diagnostic tests for otosyphilis have been investigated. The value of perilymph tap via stapedotomy was studied by Wiet and Milko (40) and Clemis (41). Each reported on one patient in whom perilymph treponemes in perilymph were demonstrated by dark-field microscopy and fluorescent antibody methods, despite prior penicillin therapy. Problems with treponeme identification using these methods have been addressed (42,43). Becker (21) performed stapedotomy and perilymph aspiration to confirm diagnosis of otosyphilis in four patients. Three of the specimens were examined by an experienced treponematologist, who found no treponemes but reported "fibrin extrusions" with brownian motion that could have been misinterpreted as motile spirochetes by an inexperienced observer. He discounted the prior case reports and did not recommend perilymph tap as a reliable diagnostic test. Nadol (15) performed incudectomy in one patient with a diagnosis of otosyphilis and found histologic evidence of otosyphilis with round cell infiltrate and reactive bone formation. Becker (21) repeated this procedure in one patient and found no pathologic changes. Thus, invasive otologic diagnostic procedures cannot be routinely recommended in the evaluation of suspected otosyphilis.

TREATMENT

The treatment of syphilis has undergone persistent review in the last decade (44–46). Several reports (47–49) and reviews (45,46,50,51) have discussed the development of various manifestations of neurosyphilis despite prior penicillin therapy. In the treatment of active neurosyphilis, the Centers for Disease Control recommends one of three alternative regimens, acknowledging that none has been adequately studied (52). The treatment of otosyphilis with penicillin has tended to follow the Centers for Disease Control recommendations for the

TABLE 1. *Centers for Disease Control treatment regimen for active neurosyphilis*

Aqueous crystalline penicillin G, 12 to 24 million units intravenously per day (2 to 4 million units every 4 hours) for 10 days, followed by benzathine penicillin G, 2.4 million units intramuscularly per week for three doses

or

Aqueous procaine penicillin G, 2.4 million units intramuscularly per day, plus probenecid 500 mg by mouth four times a day, both for 10 days, followed by benzathine penicillin G, 2.4 million units intramuscularly per week for three doses

or

Benzathine penicillin G, 2.4 million units intramuscularly per week for three doses

Data from Centers for Disease Control. STD treatment guidelines. *MMWR* 1985;34[Suppl]:94S–99S.

treatment of neurosyphilis (Table 1). Dobbin and Perkins (53) and Durham et al. (54) used penicillin G 10 million units intravenously every day for 2 weeks, followed by benzathine penicillin 2.4 million units intramuscularly every week for 3 weeks. Zoller et al. (22) used a three-month course of weekly benzathine penicillin intramuscular injections. Becker (21) recommended a minimum of 3 weeks of intramuscular benzathine penicillin and added that it "probably should be continued for several months longer." Recent recommendations on treatment of indolent or asymptomatic neurosyphilis have advised aqueous procaine penicillin G 2.4 million units intramuscularly on alternate days for 20 days, plus probenecid 500 mg four times daily during this time (46). Musher et al. (50) and Muser (51) argue that these dosages are inadequate in immunologically impaired patients. They advocate 12 to 24 million units of penicillin, with follow-up CSF examinations (50,51). A recent study by Gleich et al. (55) used these higher dosages of penicillin, combined with steroids, and followed by long-term amoxicillin. In their series of 18 patients, they achieved hearing improvement in 5 of 16 patients (31%), which is better than in most other series. In cases of severe penicillin allergy (which should be thoroughly investigated with verification by skin testing), tetracycline, erythromycin, chloramphenicol, and third-generation cephalosporins have been used, although efficacy is uncertain (30). Penicillin, or derivatives such as ampicillin, are believed to be inadequate as the sole therapy in arresting deterioration of hearing in the majority of cases (54).

The beneficial effect of prednisone as an adjuvant in the treatment of otosyphilis has been known for some time (56), and it has even been used alone in congenital luetic hearing loss (57). More recent studies with long-term follow-up have not been as promising (21,22,25,53). It has been difficult to predict which patients respond to steroid therapy. Another disappointing aspect has been the difficulty of maintaining a favorable response while tapering the steroid dose. Becker (21) recommended a trial of 40 to 60 mg/d for a minimum of 2 weeks and noted that those who benefited from steroids did so within a few days. Steckelberg and McDonald (25) recommended prednisone 40 to 60 mg every other day for a prolonged period. Zoller et al. (22) used a 3-month course of prednisone 80 mg every other day that was discontinued after 1 month if no improvement was seen. They reported hearing gains 1 year following treatment in only 8 ears of 29 patients (15%), and they found that prolonged steroid therapy was necessary to maintain improvement. This same regimen was also used by Gleich et al. (55). Dobbin and Perkins (53) treated otosyphilis in 13 patients with long-term penicillin and prednisone. They defined a response as a 15% improvement in speech discrimination or pure tone average on audiogram. In nine patients with acquired otosyphilis, an initial response was seen in 43% and a lasting response in 25%. No lasting responses were seen in those with congenital syphilis. Better results in maintaining hearing improvement in congenital syphilitic hearing loss were reported by Adams et al. (58) with the addition of periodic adrenocorticotropic hormone injections to ampicillin and prednisone therapy. Despite efforts to preserve or improve hearing with penicillin and steroids, a successful response is not commonly seen (21,22,25,53,55,59,60). Studies report an average 23% improvement, with speech discrimination slightly more responsive than speech reception thresholds. With their more aggressive regimen, Gleich et al. (55) reported that 31% (5 of 16 patients) experienced improvement in hearing; those with hearing loss of duration less than 5 years, fluctuating hearing loss, and age less than 60 years were more likely to respond (55).

Management of vestibular symptoms in otosyphilis is symptomatic, although improvement may occur following antibiotic treatment. In addition, in patients with symptoms of endolymphatic hydrops, dietary salt restriction and a diuretic may be used. The surgical treatment of vertiginous symptoms in patients with otosyphilis is controversial. Shih et al. (61) reported six patients treated with endolymphatic shunt surgery, from a chart review between 1974 and 1984 of patients treated at the House Ear Institute. The operation failed in four patients, based on patient report of vertigo symptoms at 6 months postoperatively. Histologic review of three temporal bone specimens with documented syphilis from the House Ear Institute collection revealed gummatous obliteration of the endolymphatic duct, at its origin in one specimen and at the junction of the duct and intracranial portion of the sac in another. A third specimen demonstrated obliteration of the region of the vestibular aqueduct with microgummata and fibrosis. This led Shih et al. to conclude that endolymphatic duct shunt surgery would not be expected to be successful in these patients. This study contradicts other clinical reports of success with sac

surgery in this population (62,63). Perilymph leak contributing to fluctuating hearing loss was reported by Goodhill (12). In his histopathologic studies of 16 luetic temporal bones one specimen revealed a fracture line between the hypotympanum and endolymphatic duct. He subsequently reported a case in which a perilymph fistula was found at surgical exploration of a patient with fluctuating hearing loss, vertigo, tinnitus, and positive syphilis serology. Closure of bony dehiscences inferior to the round window with perichondrium resulted in a 15-dB hearing improvement and 50% air–bone gap closure (64). In the audiologic rehabilitation of patients with otosyphilis, hearing amplification is essential. Cochlear implantation has been reported in a patient with profound unaidable luetic deafness (65,66).

In the last 15 years, the appearance of acquired immunodeficiency syndrome (AIDS) and the discovery of its causative agent, human immunodeficiency virus (HIV), have been associated with syphilis and its varied manifestations. Surveys have shown a history of syphilis in up to 63% of HIV seropositive patients (67–69), whereas treponemal markers have been found in up to 30% of homosexual males and 55% of HIV-infected patients (40,70,71). In a recent series, 18% of all documented HIV seroconversion cases seen in sexually transmitted disease clinic patients were attributable to syphilis infection (72). Infection with HIV has been associated with accelerated development of neurosyphilis (73,74) and with persistent CSF infection in patients treated for primary and secondary syphilis by conventional means (20). Cranial nerve dysfunction has been a common presenting finding in HIV patients who develop neurosyphilis (50). Otosyphilis in HIV-infected patients has been reported in several series (55,75,76), and an accelerated development of otosyphilis in HIV-infected patients has been postulated (75). Otosyphilis should be suspected in HIV seropositive patients presenting with otologic complaints. At this time it is recommended that prednisone be avoided in treatment of otosyphilis in these immunocompromised patients.

Several issues remain outstanding regarding otosyphilis, particularly its pathophysiology, accurate means of diagnosis, and effective treatment. The increasing incidence of syphilis and the onset of HIV with its reported interaction in the various stages of luetic infection have brought syphilis again to the forefront as one of the most challenging of infectious diseases.

OTOLOGIC MANIFESTATIONS IN HIV INFECTION AND AIDS

Background and Pathophysiology of HIV Infection

The medical community first became aware of AIDS with a report of *Pneumocystis carinii* pneumonia in five homosexual men in Los Angeles in 1981 (77). Since then, the occurrence of opportunistic infections and unusual neoplasms such as Kaposi's sarcoma were identified. Such cases arising in intravenous drug users and hemophiliacs suggested a blood-borne pathogen. The cause of this epidemic was found to be a retrovirus, now termed HIV-1. The virus has a very high mutation rate, which allows it to evade the host's immune system. It contains a diploid single-stranded RNA (ssRNA) genome and a unique DNA polymerase, termed reverse transcriptase (78). The reverse transcriptase uses the ssRNA within the viral particle as a template to synthesize a double-stranded DNA provirus with long terminal repeats, which facilitate control of the viral genes. The provirus inserts into the host genome, producing viral particles to infect additional cells (horizontal transmission) and is passed on to daughter cells when the infected cell replicates its DNA and divides (vertical transmission). The virus has a predilection for the CD4 helper lymphocyte, but it also can infect other cells, including macrophages, microglial cells, endothelial cells, and follicular dendritic cells.

Infection with the virus can be due to exchange of body fluids and tissues via sexual intercourse, blood product transfusion, intravenous drug use, organ donation, or vertical transmission to infants from an HIV-infected mother. After infection, an asymptomatic period exists during which the immune system battles the virus. Large numbers of CD4$^+$ cells are produced and killed. Through the high mutation rate of reverse transcriptase, viral strains eventually develop that are more cytotoxic and replicate faster, thus reducing the number of CD4$^+$ cells available to fight higher numbers of viral particles. The highly virulent strains of the 1980s caused much mortality. The increased survival times for HIV-infected individuals seen in the 1990s are a reflection that less virulent strains of HIV-1 are surviving longer in a more healthy host to ensure chances for transmission over an extended period.

As the host immune function declines with drop in CD4$^+$ cells, the patient becomes vulnerable to a variety of infections and neoplastic diseases as a result of the immunodeficiency. When these conditions develop, AIDS exists.

Temporal Bone Studies

Four studies examined temporal bone histopathology in patients who died of AIDS (78–81). A study from New York City examined ten temporal bones in five adult patients (78). Procurement and processing problems allowed the examination and reporting of findings in seven specimens. One patient had *P. carinii* mastoiditis and epidural abscess. The others had no otologic symptoms. Notable pathologic findings included severe petrositis and marrow replacement with inflammatory cells, as well as inflammatory changes in the mastoid and middle ear regions. Two specimens lacking such findings instead had fibrous granulation tissue, inflammatory response, or reactive mucosal edema. The semicircular canals were found to have an inflammatory endolymphatic infiltrate. Yet the organ of Corti was relatively spared, showing only hypocellularity of the spiral ligament and, in one case, the stria vascularis. A second study from the same institution examined the ultrastructural details of the vestibular end organs in six patients who died of AIDS (79). All patients were male and had received potentially ototoxic drugs. No predeath clinical information on vestibular complaints or evaluation was available. The utricle, saccule, and three ampullae were removed from the vestibule and examined using electron microscopy. A variety of abnormalities were seen, including inclusion bodies in hair cells, viral-like particles, and hair bundle malformations. These abnormalities were also seen in epithelial and connective tissue cells, and

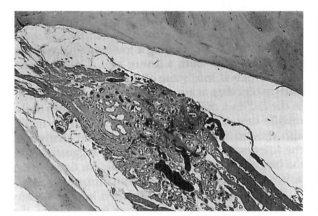 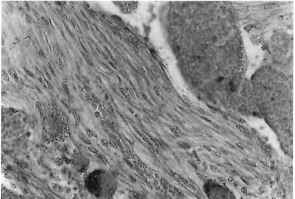

FIG. 5. Deposit of Kaposi's sarcoma in the eighth cranial nerve in the internal auditory canal. Note marked vascularity of tumor (hematoxylin and eosin stain, original magnification × 50). *Right:* Higher power magnification of Kaposi's sarcoma of previous figure (*left*). Note vacuolar spaces and spindle cells. The pigmented cells are ganglion cells of the vestibular ganglion (hematoxylin and eosin stain, original magnification × 800). (From Michaels L, Soucek S, Liang J. The ear in the acquired immunodeficiency syndrome: I. Temporal bone histopathologic study. *Am J Otolaryngol* 1994;15:515–522, with

they were believed to represent direct neuroepithelial infection with HIV.

A study from England examined 49 temporal bones in 25 adult patients (24 male) (80). A wider variety of otologic pathologies were observed. Eight specimens (five patients) had severe otitis media, and 27 specimens (15 patients) had low-grade otitis media. Cholesteatoma was observed in two specimens. In the inner ear, four temporal bones were found to have evidence of *Cryptococcosis*, and seven specimens had histologic changes and/or findings by *in situ* hybridization of cytomegalovirus in the cochlea, acoustic nerve, or endolabyrinthine organs. Kaposi's sarcoma deposit in the eighth cranial nerve was seen in one specimen (Fig. 5). The authors' technique of decalcification in acid was believed to result in negative stains for cytomegalovirus by immunohistochemistry, yet they attributed the frequent finding of middle ear effusions to the effects of cytomegalovirus infection. Unfortunately, no clinical correlation was reported of predeath otologic symptoms with these temporal bone findings.

A clinicopathologic study of temporal bones in 14 men who died of AIDS was reported in 1995 (81). All patients had bimonthly clinic visits prior to death, were regularly screened for hearing or balance complaints, and were examined by a neurologist. No patient complained of hearing loss; one patient had vertigo. Despite the paucity of otologic complaints, the temporal bone specimens in these patients showed a variety of pathologic findings of viral or bacterial middle or inner ear disease. Adenovirus type 6 and cytomegalovirus, alone or with herpes simplex virus type 1, were found in the inner ear in three patients. These viral infections, also found in other organs at autopsy, appeared to be generally asymptomatic and elicited little pathologic response, either due to low virulence or immunosuppression from AIDS.

Otologic Manifestations in HIV Infection

Otitis Media

The most commonly reported otologic problems in HIV infection involve otitis media and hearing loss (82–84). These conditions have particular relevance to the pediatric population with HIV, especially those in whom unresponsiveness to treatment for otitis media may be a sign of immunodeficiency (85,86). It would be expected that otitis media, a common pediatric infection, has greater prevalence in HIV-infected children. Barnett et al. (87) studied the incidence of acute otitis media in 28 HIV-infected children and compared the rate with that in 33 children who had seroreverted to HIV-antibody negative status. They found that, in the HIV-infected group, the number of acute otitis media episodes per year increased from 1.89 to 2.40. In the control group, the mean number of episodes decreased from 1.33 to 0.13. By 3 years, 80% of the HIV-positive children had experi-

enced six or more episodes of otitis media. Children with low CD4$^+$ lymphocyte counts had a threefold increased risk of recurrent otitis media compared with HIV-infected children with normal CD4$^+$ counts. Other uncontrolled studies also reported a high rate of acute otitis media in children with AIDS (88,89).

Whereas acute otitis media does not appear to occur more frequently in HIV-infected adults than in the normal population, serous otitis media is more common in the adult AIDS population (83). An association among adenoid hypertrophy, HIV seropositivity, and secretory otitis media has been reported in adults (90).

The bacterial organisms generally responsible for acute otitis media (*Streptococcus pneumoniae, Hemophilus influenzae,* group A β-hemolytic streptococcus) are found in similar prevalence among HIV-infected children and controls (91). However, *Staphylococcus aureus* or *Candida* may be found more frequently in immunocomprised patients with HIV (89,91). The treatment of otitis media in HIV-infected patients is generally similar to that of non-HIV patients. First-line antibiotics are used for uncomplicated cases, but for persistent cases a culture to guide treatment may be useful (92). Children with symptomatic HIV infection have more treatment failures of otitis media than controls (93) and a higher rate of pressure equalization tube placement (87). Adenoid biopsies in HIV patients show nonspecific lymphoid hyperplasia (90). Appropriate universal precautions in procuring specimens via tympanocentesis are required. HIV virus has been isolated from middle ear fluid specimens from patients with HIV (83,94).

Unusual Otologic Infections and HIV

Pneumocystis carinii infection of the ear has been reported in ten HIV-infected patients, all adult males, all with a history of homosexual activity or intravenous drug abuse (82,95–101). Each patient presented with an aural polyp arising from the middle ear or external ear canal (Fig. 6). *Pneumocystis carinii* aural polyp has been the initial manifestation of HIV infection (95,97). Even those patients with AIDS who are taking aerosolized pentamidine can have extrapulmonary spread of pneumocystis. Histologic examination of the specimen reveals an eosinophilic foamy or honeycombed exudate and granulation tissue. The organism is demonstrated on methenamine-silver stain (101). Treatment is with trimethoprim-sulfamethoxazole.

Another uncommon fungal otologic infection found in HIV-infected patients is aspergillus. Strauss and Fine (102) reported two cases of aspergillus otomastoiditis. One patient initially presented with otorrhea and otalgia as the initial symptom of HIV-related disease. She was later found to have HIV and to be severely immunocompromised. Slow progression of invasive aspergillus infection in the temporal bone led to intracranial thrombosis

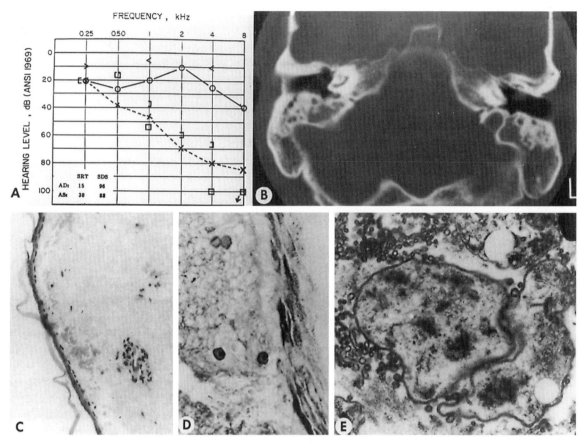

FIG. 6. Clinical and pathologic findings in *Pneumocystis carinii* involvement of the temporal bone. **A:** Pretreatment audiogram. **B:** Pretreatment computed tomogram of the temporal bone. An anteriorly based polyp can be seen in the left external auditory canal. **C:** Light microscopic examination shows typical perivascular appearance of *P. carinii* (hematoxylin and eosin stain, original magnification × 400). **D:** *Pneumocystis carinii* cysts (Grocott-Gomori methenamine silver nitrate stain, hematoxylin and eosin background, original magnification × 1,000). Squamous epithelium is seen on the *right*. **E:** Electron micrograph showing two trophozoites with characteristic curvilinear material adjacent (uranyl acetate-lead citrate stain, original magnification × 28,500). (From Breda SD, Hammerschlag PE, Gigliotti F, Schinella K. Pneumocystis carinii in the temporal bone as a primary manifestation of the acquired immunodeficiency syndrome. *Ann Otol Rhinol Laryngol* 1988;97:427–431, with permission.)

and death. The second patient with known HIV had a mild case of aspergillus infection that was treated successfully with antifungal medication. Ramsay Hunt syndrome, due to herpes zoster virus, has been reported to occur as an initial manifestation of immunocompromise in a high-risk patient found to be positive for HIV (103).

Hearing Loss

Estimates of hearing loss in HIV-seropositive and AIDS patients vary from 21% to 69% (104,105). A prospective study obtained audiograms in 69 patients with AIDS (105). Forty-three patients (69%) had thresholds below 20 dB at any frequency; 39% had losses in the low and high frequencies and were normal in the middle range. The composite audiogram of this group showed mild hearing loss with thresholds below 20 dB outside the speech frequencies, yet the authors state that significant numbers of their study group had more severe losses. Although most

patients with AIDS do not complain of hearing loss, it occasionally occurs. Sudden hearing loss (106), tinnitus (105), and vertigo (81,104,105) have all been reported.

The etiology of hearing loss in HIV is unknown. A variety of factors may be present, including neuropathic effects of the virus itself, from secondary infections and/or neoplastic diseases from immunosuppression, or ototoxic effects of drugs used to treat AIDS-related diseases. Findings from auditory brainstem response testing suggest both cochlear and retrocochlear involvement. Findings include increased wave I and wave V latencies (104,107), and elevated interpeak latencies (108). A study that compared patients with AIDS, HIV-seropositive patients, and controls found increased I–V and III–V interpeak intervals in AIDS patients compared with the other groups, which suggests upper brainstem impairment (108). Progressive increase in auditory brainstem response latencies has correlated with neurologic impairment in pediatric AIDS cases (109). A demyelinating process seen in AIDS may be responsible for these findings (110). Central auditory dysfunction is believed to be part of the pathophysiology of hearing loss in some of these patients (104).

The evaluation of hearing loss in HIV-seropositive and AIDS patients involves complete audiometric testing and other studies as needed. Computed tomographic scan is helpful to assess temporal bone and intracranial invasion of aggressive infections (111). Serologic testing for otosyphilis should be considered in this population, especially those with hydropic symptoms of vertigo and low-frequency hearing loss (75).

SUMMARY

HIV infection leads to otologic disease in a variety of ways. Mass lesions of the ear, infectious diseases of the temporal bone, and auditory and vestibular dysfunction are all possibilities. The virus has neurotropic tendency to invade the vestibulocochlear and central nervous system.

The immunosuppression from HIV leads to infectious or neoplastic diseases seen in AIDS. Common bacterial pathogens cause otitis media in these patients. Pathogens less common to otologic problems require the clinician to consider HIV when such pathogens are found in the ear, because occasionally otologic manifestations occur as the initial sign of underlying HIV infection.

SUMMARY POINTS

- Although the incidence of syphilis is now declining, it went through a peak in the late 1980s so that delayed manifestations, such as otosyphilis, may occur with increasing frequency into the twenty-first century.
- The pathology of cochlear and auditory effects in otosyphilis are due to (a) basilar meningitis affecting the eighth cranial nerve complex in early and secondary forms, and (b) obliterative endarteritis and mononuclear infiltrate of the temporal bone leading to osteitis and scarring in the late and tertiary stages of syphilis.
- Clinical features of otosyphilis include hearing loss, tinnitus, and dizziness in varying degrees. Hearing loss may fluctuate and disproportionately affect speech discrimination.
- Diagnosis of otosyphilis is based on clinical assessment, FTA-ABS serology, and CSF examination for VDRL, protein, or leukocytosis.
- Otosyphilis is treated with prolonged high-dose penicillin and prednisone. Prednisone may be withheld in immunocompromised patients. Despite treatment, hearing may not recover, although tinnitus and vestibular symptoms often improve.
- Patients with HIV may have antecedent or coincident syphilis infection. They may develop neurosyphilis or otosyphilis, which may occur at an accelerated rate. If HIV status is unknown, patients with suspected otosyphilis should be tested for HIV.

REFERENCES

1. Centers for Disease Control. Continuing increase in infectious syphilis—United States. *MMWR* 1988;37:35–38.
2. Centers for Disease Control. Syphilis and congenital syphilis—United States, 1985–88. *MMWR* 1988;37:486–489.
3. Centers for Disease Control. Summary of notifiable diseases, United States, 1995. *MMWR* 1996;44:1–96.
4. Centers for Disease Control. Congenital syphilis—New York City, 1986–88. *MMWR* 1989;38:825–829.
5. Rolfs RT, Nakashima AK. Epidemiology of primary and secondary syphilis in the United States, 1981 through 1989. *JAMA* 1990;264:1432–1437.
6. Centers for Disease Control. Epidemic early syphilis—Montgomery County, Alabama, 1990–1991. *MMWR* 1992;41:790–794.
7. Centers for Disease Control. Outbreak of primary and secondary syphilis—Baltimore City, Maryland, 1995. *MMWR* 1996;45:166–169.
8. Schuknecht HF. *Pathology of the ear*. Cambridge, MA: Harvard, 1974:262–266.
9. Vercoe GS. The effect of early syphilis on the inner ear and auditory nerves. *J Laryngol Otol* 1976;90:853–861.
10. Saltiel P, Melmed CA, Portnoy D. Sensorineural deafness in early acquired syphilis. *Can J Neurol Sci* 1983;10:114–116.
11. Mayer O, Fraser JS. Pathological changes in late congenital syphilis. *J Laryngol Otol* 1936;51:755–778.
12. Goodhill V. Syphilis of the ear: a histopathological study. *Ann Otol Rhinol Laryngol* 1939;48:676–777.
13. Karmody CS, Schuknecht HF. Deafness in congenital syphilis. *Arch Otolaryngol* 1966;83:18–27.
14. Belal A, Linthicum FH. Pathology of congenital syphilitic labyrinthitis. *Am J Otolaryngol* 1980;1:109–118.
15. Nadol JB. Hearing loss of acquired syphilis: diagnosis confirmed by incudectomy. *Laryngoscope* 1975;85:1888–1897.
16. Mack LW, Smith JL, Walter EK, et al. Temporal bone treponemes. *Arch Otolaryngol* 1969;90:37–40.
17. Griffin W, Silverstein H. Inner ear fluids in certain human otologic disorders. In: Paparella M, ed. *Biochemical mechanisms in hearing and deafness. Research Otology International Symposium.* Springfield, IL: Charles C. Thomas Publisher, 1970:309–321.
18. Smith JL, Israel CW. Spirochetes in the aqueous humor in seronegative ocular syphilis: persistence after penicillin therapy. *Arch Ophthalmol* 1967;77:474–477.
19. Collart P. Persistence of treponema pallidum in late syphilis in rabbits and humans, notwithstanding treatment. In: *Proceedings of the World Forum on Syphilis and other Treponematoses.* Washington, DC: US Government Printing Office, 1964:285.
20. Lukehart SA, Hook EW, Baker-Zander SA, et al. Invasion of the central nervous system by Treponema pallidum: implications for diagnosis and treatment. *Ann Intern Med* 1988;109:855–862.
21. Becker GD. Late syphilitic hearing loss: a diagnostic and therapeutic dilemma. *Laryngoscope* 1979;89:1273–1288.
22. Zoller M, Wilson WR, Nadol JB. Treatment of syphilitic hearing loss: combined penicillin and steroid therapy in 29 patients. *Ann Otol Rhinol Laryngol* 1979;88:160–165.
23. Dalsgaard-Neilson E. Correlation between syphilitic interstitial keratitis and deafness. *Acta Ophthalmol* 1938;16:635–647.
24. Kerr AG, Smyth GDL, Cinnamond MJ. Congenital syphilitic deafness. *J Laryngol Otol* 1973;87:1–12.
25. Steckelberg JM, McDonald TJ. Otologic involvement in late syphilis. *Laryngoscope* 1984;94:753–757.
26. Fiumara NJ, Lessell S. Manifestations of late congenital syphilis: an analysis of 271 patients. *Arch Dermatol* 1970;102:78–83.
27. Morrison AW. *Management of sensorineural deafness.* Boston: Butterworths, 1975.

28. Balkany TJ, Dans PE. Reversible sudden deafness in early acquired syphilis. *Arch Otolaryngol* 1978;104:66–68.

29. Knox JM, Guzick ND. The pathogenesis of syphilis and related tre-ponematoses. In: Johnson RC, ed. *The biology of parasitic spiro-chetes.* New York: Academic Press, 1976:327–337.

30. Musher DM. Syphilis. *Infect Dis Clin North Am* 1987;1:83–95.

31. Tamari M, Itkin P. Penicillin and syphilis of the ear. *Eye Ear Nose Throat Monthly* 1951;30:252–261,301–309,358–366.

32. Hungerbuhler JP, Regli F. Cochleovestibular involvement as the first sign of late syphilis. *J Neurol* 1978;219:199–204.

33. Nadol JB. Positive fistula sign with an intact tympanic membrane. *Arch Otolaryngol* 1974;100:273–278.

34. Musher DN, Schell RF. The immunology of syphilis. *Hosp Pract* 1975;10:45–50.

35. Zoller M, Wilson WR, Nadol JB, Girard KF. Detection of syphilitic hearing loss. *Arch Otolaryngol* 1978;104:63–65.

36. Becker GD. Late syphilis: otologic symptoms and results of the FTA-ABS test. *Arch Otolaryngol* 1976;102:729–731.

37. Miller JN. The value and limitations of non-treponemal and trepone-mal tests in the laboratory diagnosis of syphilis. *Clin Obstet Gynecol* 1975;18:191–203.

38. Hughes GB, Rutherford I. Predictive value of serologic tests for syphilis in otology. *Ann Otol Rhinol Laryngol* 1986;95:250–259.

39. Jaffe HW. The laboratory diagnosis of syphilis: new concepts. *Ann Intern Med* 1975;83:836–858.

40. Wiet RJ, Milko DM. Isolation of the spirochetes in the perilymph despite prior antisyphilitic therapy. *Arch Otolaryngol* 1975;101:104–106.

41. Clemis JD. Luetic labyrinthitis. *Tex Med* 1977;73:60–65.

42. Montenegro EN, Nicol WG, Smith JL. Treponemalike forms and arti-facts. *Am J Ophthalmol* 1969;68:196–205.

43. Yobs AR, Brown L, Hunter EF. Fluorescent antibody technique in early syphilis. *Arch Pathol* 1964;77:220–225.

44. Musher DM. How much penicillin cures early syphilis? *Ann Intern Med* 1988;109:849–851.

45. Simon RP. Neurosyphilis. *Arch Neurol* 1985;42:606–613.

46. Jordan KG. Modern neurosyphilis—a critical analysis. *West J Med* 1988;149:47–57.

47. Hooshmand H, Escobar MR, Kopf SW. Neurosyphilis: a study of 241 patients. *JAMA* 1972;219:726–730.

48. Joyce-Clark N, Molteno AC. Modified neurosyphilis in the Cape Peninsula. *S Afr Med J* 1978;53:10–14.

49. Luxon L, Lees AL, Greenwood RJ. Neurosyphilis today. *Lancet* 1979;1:90–93.

50. Musher DM, Hamill RJ, Baughn RE. Effect of human immunodefi-ciency virus infection on the course of syphilis and response to treat-ment. *Ann Intern Med* 1990;113:872–881.

51. Musher DM. Syphilis, neurosyphilis, and AIDS. *J Infect Dis* 1991;163:1201–1206.

52. Centers for Disease Control. STD treatment guidelines. *MMWR* 1985;34[Suppl]:94S–99S.

53. Dobbin JM, Perkins JH. Otosyphilis and hearing loss: response to penicillin and steroid therapy. *Laryngoscope* 1983;93:1540–1543.

54. Durham JS, Longridge NS, Smith JM, et al. Clinical manifestations of otological syphilis. *J Otolaryngol* 1984;13:175–179.

55. Gleich LL, Linstrom CJ, Kimmelman CP. Otosyphilis: a diagnostic and therapeutic dilemma. *Laryngoscope* 1992;102:1255–1259.

56. Patterson ME. Congenital luetic hearing impairment. *Arch Otolaryn-gol* 1968;87:378–382.

57. Morton RS. Cortisone therapy in congenital syphilitic nerve deafness. *J Laryngol Otol* 1957;71:850–852.

58. Adams DA, Kerr AG, Smyth GDL, Cinnamond MJ. Congenital syphilitic deafness—a further review. *J Laryngol Otol* 1983;97:399–404.

59. Wong RT, Lepore ML, Burch GR, Henderson RL. Luetic hearing loss. *Laryngoscope* 1977;87:1765–1769.

60. Pillsbury HC, Shea JJ. Luetic hydrops—diagnosis and therapy. *Laryn-goscope* 1979;89:1135–1144.

61. Shih L, McElveen JT, Linthicum FH. Management of vertigo in patients with syphilis: is endolymphatic shunt surgery appropriate? *Otolaryngol Head Neck Surg* 1988;99:574–577.

62. Huang TS, Lin CC. Endolymphatic sac surgery for refractory luetic vertigo. *Am J Otol* 1991;12:184–187.

63. Paparella MM, Kim CS, Shea DA. Sac decompression for refractory luetic vertigo. *Acta Otolaryngol* 1980;89:541–546.

64. Goodhill V. Leaking labyrinth lesions, deafness, tinnitus, and dizzi-ness. *Ann Otol Rhinol Laryngol* 1981;90:99–106.

65. Johnsson L-G, House WF, Linthicum FH. Bilateral cochlear implants: histological findings in a pair of temporal bones. *Laryngoscope* 1979;89:759–762.

66. Linthicum FH, Galey FR. Histologic evaluation of temporal bones with cochlear implants. *Ann Otol Rhinol Laryngol* 1983;92:610–613.

67. Sindrup JH, Weismann K, Wantzin GU. Syphilis in HTLV-III infected male homosexuals. *AIDS Res* 1986;2:285–288.

68. Quinn TC, Piot P, McCormick JB, et al. Serologic and immunologic studies in patients with AIDS in North America and Africa. The poten-tial role of infectious agents as cofactors in human immunodeficiency virus infection. *JAMA* 1987;257:2617–2621.

69. Moss AR, Osmond D, Bacchetti P, et al. Risk factors for AIDS and HIV seropositivity in homosexual men. *Am J Epidemiol* 1987;125:1035–1047.

70. Potterat JJ, Muth JB, Markwich GS. Serological markers as indicators of sexual orientation in AIDS-virus infected men. *JAMA* 1986;256:712.

71. Potterat JJ. Does syphilis facilitate sexual acquisition of HIV? *JAMA* 1987;258:473.

72. Otten MW Jr, Zaidi AA, Peterman TA, Rolfs RT, Witte JJ. High rate of HIV seroconversion among patients attending urban sexually trans-mitted disease clinics. *AIDS* 1994;8:549–553.

73. Johns DR, Tierney M, Felsenstein D. Alteration in the natural history of neurosyphilis by concurrent infection with the human immunode-ficiency virus. *N Engl J Med* 1987;316:1569–1572.

74. Berry CD, Hooton TM, Collier AC, et al. Neurologic relapse after benzathine penicillin therapy for secondary syphilis in a patient with HIV infection. *N Engl J Med* 1987;316:1587–1589.

75. Smith ME, Canalis RF. Otologic manifestations of AIDS: the oto-syphilis connection. *Laryngoscope* 1989;99:365–372.

76. Little JP, Gardner G, Acker JD, Land MA. Otosyphilis in a patient with human immunodeficiency virus: internal auditory canal gumma. *Otolaryngol Head Neck Surg* 1995;112:488–492.

77. Centers for Disease Control. Pneumocystis carinii pneumonia—Los Angeles. *MMWR* 1981;30:250–252.

78. Chadrasekhar SS, Siverls V, Chandrasekhar HK. Histopathological and ultrastructural changes in the temporal bones of HIV-infected human adults. *Am J Otol* 1992;13:207–214.

79. Pappas DG, Roland JT, Lim J, Lai A, Hillman DE. Ultrastructural findings in the vestibular end-organs of AIDS cases. *Am J Otol* 1995;16:140–145.

80. Michaels L, Soucek S, Liang J. The ear in the acquired immunodefi-ciency syndrome: I. Temporal bone histopathologic study. *Am J Otol* 1994:15:515–522.

81. Davis LE, Rarey KE, McLaren LC. Clinical viral infections and tem-poral bone histologic studies of patients with AIDS. *Otolaryngol Head Neck Surg* 1995;113:695–701.

82. Kohan D, Rothstein SG, Cohen NL. Otologic disease in patients with acquired immunodeficiency syndrome. *Ann Otol Rhinol Laryngol* 1988;97:636–640.

83. Sooy CD. The impact of AIDS on otolaryngology-head and neck surgery. *Adv Otolaryngol Head Neck Surg* 1987;1:1–28.

84. Poole MD, Postma D, Cohen MS. Pyogenic otorhinologic infections in acquired immunodeficiency syndrome. *Arch Otolaryngol Head Neck Surg* 1984;110:130–131.

85. Post JC, Ehrlich GD. Otologic disorders in the HIV-positive child. In: Lalwani AK, Grundfast KM, eds. *Pediatric otology and neurotology.* Philadelphia: Lippincott-Raven Publishers, 1998:479–485.

86. Sculerati N, Borkowsky W. Pediatric human immunodeficiency virus infection: an otolaryngologist's perspective. *J Otolaryngol* 1990;19:182–188.

87. Barnett ED, Klein JO, Pelton SI, Luginbuhl LM. Otitis media in chil-dren born to human immunodeficiency virus-infected mothers. *Pedi-atr Infect Dis J* 1992;11:360–364.

88. Church JA. Human immunodeficiency virus (HIV) infection at Chil-dren's Hospital of Los Angeles: recurrent otitis media or chronic sinusitis as the presenting process in pediatric AIDS. *Immunol Allergy Pract* 1987;9:25–32.

89. Williams MA. Head and neck findings in pediatric acquired immune deficiency syndrome. *Laryngoscope* 1987;97:713–716.

90. Desai SD. Seropositivity, adenoid hypertrophy, and secretory otitis media in adults—a recognized clinical entity. *Otolaryngol Head Neck Surg* 1992;107:755–757.

91. Marchisio P, Principi N, Sorella S, Sala E, Tornaghi R. Etiology of acute otitis media in human immunodeficiency virus-infected children. *Pediatr Infect Dis J* 1996;15:58–61.

92. Shar UK, McGuirt WF, Forsen J, Caradonna D, Jones D. Congenital and acquired immunodeficiency in the pediatric patient. *Curr Opin Otolaryngol Head Neck Surg* 1994;2:462–467.

93. Principi N, Marchisio P, Tornaghi R, Onorato J, Massironi E, Picco P. Acute otitis media in human immunodeficiency virus-infected children. *Pediatrics* 1991;88:566–571.

94. Liederman, EM, Post JC, Aul JJ, et al. Analysis of adult otitis media: polymerase chain reaction versus culture for bacteria and viruses. *Ann Otol Rhinol Laryngol* 1998;107:10–16.

95. Breda SD, Hammerschlag PE, Gigliotti F, Schinella K. Pneumocystis carinii in the temporal bone as a primary manifestation of the acquired immunodeficiency syndrome. *Ann Otol Rhinol Laryngol* 1988;97:427–431.

96. Smith MA, Hirschfield LS, Zahtz G, Siegal FP. Pneumocystis carinii otitis media. *Am J Med* 1988;85:745–746.

97. Gherman CR, Ward RR, Bassis ML. Pneumocystis carinii otitis media and mastoiditis as the initial manifestation of the acquired immunodeficiency syndrome. *Am J Med* 1988;85:250–252.

98. Sandler ED, Sandler JM, LeBoit PE, Wenig BM, Mortensen N. Pneumocystis carinii otitis media in AIDS: a case report and review of the literature regarding extrapulmonary pneumocystosis. *Otolaryngol Head Neck Surg* 1990;103:817–821.

99. Park SK, Wunderlich H, Goldenberg RA, Marshall M. Pneumocystis carinii infection in the middle ear. *Arch Otolaryngol Head Neck Surg* 1992;118:269–270.

100. Wasserman L, Haghighi P. Otic and ophthalmic pneumocystosis in acquired immunodeficiency syndrome. Report of a case and review of the literature. *Arch Pathol Lab Med* 1992;116:500–503.

101. Henneberry JM, Smith RLR, Hruban RH. Pathologic quiz case 2: Pneumocystis carinii infection of the external auditory canal. *Arch Otolaryngol Head Neck Surg* 1993;119:467–469.

102. Strauss M, Fine E. Aspergillus otomastoiditis in acquired immunodeficiency syndrome. *Am J Otol* 1991;12:49–53.

103. Mishell JH, Applebaum EL. Ramsay-Hunt syndrome in a patient with HIV infection. *Otolaryngol Head Neck Surg* 1990;102:177–179.

104. Lalwani AK, Sooy CD. Otologic and neurotologic manifestations of acquired immunodeficiency syndrome. *Otolaryngol Clin North Am* 1992;25:1183–1197.

105. Soucek S, Michaels L. The ear in the acquired immunodeficiency syndrome: II. Clinical and audiologic investigation. *Am J Otol* 1996;17:35–39.

106. Real R, Thomas M, Gerwin JM. Sudden hearing loss and acquired immunodeficiency syndrome. *Otolaryngol Head Neck Surg* 1987;97:409–412.

107. Frank Y, Vishnubhakat SM, Pahwa S. Brainstem auditory evoked responses in infants and children with AIDS. *Pediatr Neurol* 1992;8:262–266.

108. Pagano MA, Cahn PE, Garau ML, et al. Brain-stem auditory evoked potentials in human immunodeficiency virus-seropositive patients with and without acquired immunodeficiency syndrome. *Arch Neurol* 1992;49:166–169.

109. Frank Y, Pahwa S. Serial brainstem auditory evoked responses in infants and children with AIDS. *Clin Electroencephalogr* 1993;24:160–165.

110. Petito CK, Vavia BA, Cho ES, et al. Vacuolar myelopathy pathologically resembling subacute combined degeneration in patients with the acquired immunodeficiency syndrome. *N Engl J Med* 1985;312:874–879.

111. Kohan D, Hammerschlag PE, Holliday RA. Otologic disease in AIDS patients: CT correlation. *Laryngoscope* 1990;100:1326–1330.

The Ear: Comprehensive Otology,
edited by R. F. Canalis and P. R. Lambert.
Lippincott Williams & Wilkins, Philadelphia © 2000.

CHAPTER 37

Hearing Aids

Donald D. Dirks, Jayne B. Ahlstrom, and Laurie S. Eisenberg

For most adults with acquired hearing loss that does not yield to medical or surgical intervention, hearing aid amplification is usually an integral part of a more general treatment plan of auditory rehabilitation. In this chapter, the reader is provided with a broad overview of the theoretical, technical, and clinical aspects of hearing aid amplification. The chapter is intended to reflect current thoughts and practices in the fitting and measurement of performance of a hearing aid. The information is most relevant to air conduction hearing aids and generally applies to both adults and children; however, specific details regarding amplification among infants and children or issues relevant to cochlear implants are described in other chapters of this book.

HISTORICAL DEVELOPMENT

Although amplification devices such as acoustic horns, trumpets, or speaking tubes have been used for several

D. D. Dirks: Division of Head and Neck Surgery, University of California, Los Angeles, School of Medicine, Los Angeles, California 90095

J. B. Ahlstrom: Department of Otolaryngology and Communicative Sciences, Medical University of South Carolina, Charleston, South Carolina 29425

L. S. Eisenberg: Children's Auditory Research and Evaluation Center, House Ear Institute, Los Angeles, California 90057

centuries, progress in hearing aid technology has essentially paralleled advancements in electronic technology. Lybarger (1) divided the developments in hearing aid technology into four major time periods: first, an acoustic era (prior to 1900), during which horns and trumpets were utilized to amplify sound; second, the carbon hearing aid era (~1900–1925), during which telephone technology was adapted to hearing aids; third, the vacuum tube era (~1925–1950), leading to greater amplification, wider frequency response range, and reduced internal noise; and fourth, the transistor era (~1950), during which reduced battery size led to miniaturization, reduction in the cost of operation, and hearing aids in which the entire aid could be located at the ear of the patient. A fifth era should now be added to this time frame, a digital era in which digital signal processing (DSP) is incorporated in modern hearing aids and digital techniques are used to program an increasing variety of hearing aid features, such as multiple memories, frequency shaping, adaptive filtering, and nonlinear amplification.

As hearing aid technology developed, the size, construction, and circuitry of hearing aids have undergone dramatic changes. Some of these changes are illustrated in Figs. 1–5, which include hearing aids used during specific time periods of development. Figure 1 shows an ear

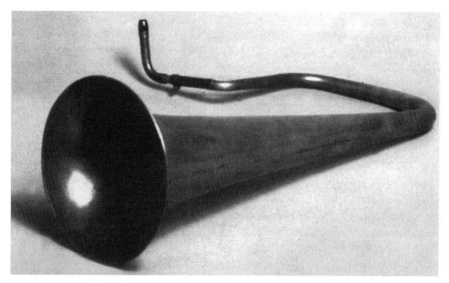

FIG. 1. Ear trumpet used as a mechanical hearing aid. (From Goldenberg RA. *Hearing aids: a manual for clinicians.* Philadelphia: Lippincott-Raven, 1996:142, with permission.)

trumpet used to amplify sound during the acoustic era. Most of the old-fashioned ear trumpets were more than simply scoops for collecting sound energy. They were often tuned broadly to frequencies in the speech range and sometime amplified sound within this range by 10 to 15 dB. A carbon hearing aid with two battery packs is illustrated in Fig. 2. These hearing aids were a distinct improvement over mechanical aids but obviously were not convenient to wear. The frequency range in the carbon hearing aids usually was limited, and distortion was a

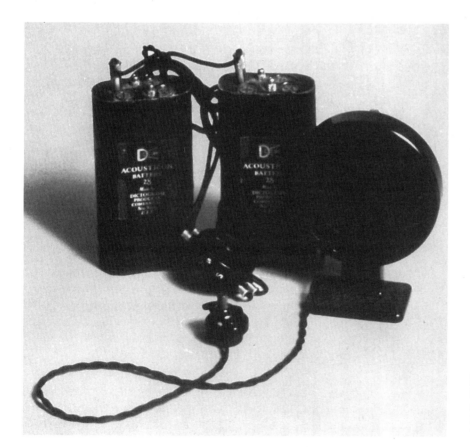

FIG. 2. Carbon hearing aid with two battery packs. (From Goldenberg RA. *Hearing aids: a manual for clinicians.* Philadelphia: Lippincott-Raven, 1996: 144, with permission.)

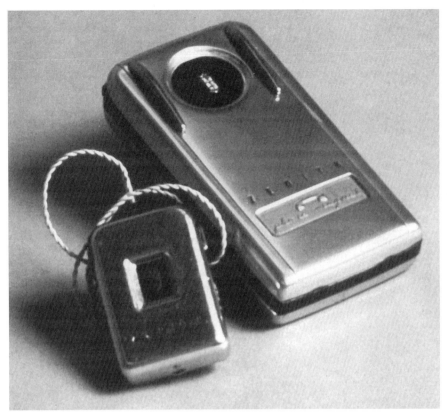

FIG. 3. Body-worn vacuum tube and transistor hearing aids. (From Goldenberg RA. *Hearing aids: a manual for clinicians.* Philadelphia: Lippincott-Raven, 1996:145, with permission.)

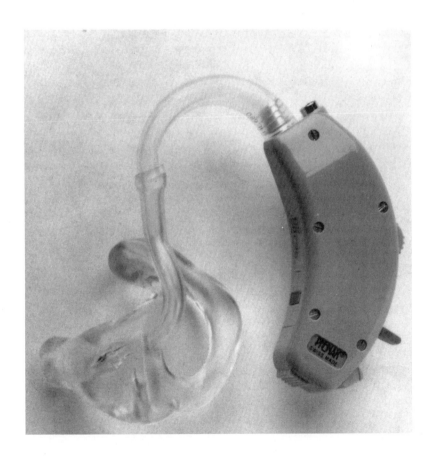

FIG. 4. Behind-the-ear (BTE) hearing aid and earmold. (From Goldenberg RA. *Hearing aids: a manual for clinicians.* Philadelphia: Lippincott-Raven, 1996:150, with permission.)

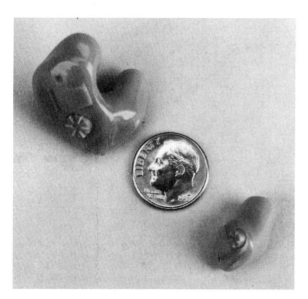

FIG. 5. In-the-ear (ITE) and in-the-canal (ITC) hearing aids. (From Goldenberg RA. *Hearing aids: a manual for clinicians.* Philadelphia: Lippincott-Raven, 1996:152, with permission.)

major problem. Following the pioneering development of transistor batteries by the Bell Telephone Laboratories, transistors were used to power hearing aids. Transistors were much more efficient than vacuum tubes, and only one transistor was required rather than the A and B batteries necessary for vacuum tube aids. The small size of the transistor eventually permitted the microphone, circuit, receiver, and battery to be housed in a single package and worn on the head. Most of the early transistor aids were body-style aids but were much reduced in size from the vacuum tube instruments. A comparison between the size of a body-worn transistor and vacuum tube hearing aid is shown in Fig. 3. With the advent of transistors, *behind-the-ear* (BTE) hearing aids worn entirely on the head eventually replaced most body-worn aids. A BTE hearing aid is illustrated in Fig. 4. Transistors also provided the means to house the hearing aid circuit and battery in a single small shell that was cosmetically more appealing than body-worn or BTE aids. Figure 5 provides examples of modern analog *in-the-canal* (ITC) and *in-the-ear* (ITE) aids that have became popular due to their reduced size and convenience. Hearing aids that process speech digitally are now available and are housed in instruments similar in shell style and size to conventional analog aids.

CURRENT STATUS

As the previous discussion suggests, a consistent trend in the development of hearing aids has been that of miniaturization. Cosmetic considerations or the desire to make the hearing aid less visible has been a dominating, although not exclusive, force directing this trend. Hearing aids have progressed through various stages of develop-

ment from tabletop electronic devices to the currently popular *completely in-the-canal* (CIC) aid (Fig. 6) in which the instrument is essentially invisible except during direct ear canal inspection.

A second, more recent trend in hearing aid development has been the rapid increase in signal processing capabilities. Progress toward more advanced signal processing capabilities has been greatly enhanced by the application of digital techniques to hearing aids. Major advances have occurred in the development of *digitally programmable hearing aids* that provide flexible control of numerous physical parameters used in fitting hearing aids. Specifically digital designs (a) allow for convenient and detailed control of the frequency response of the hearing aid, including phase response; (b) have the potential for providing more effective types of adaptive filtering so that frequency shaping can be changed by the level and spectral shape of the incoming audio signal; and (c) have almost unlimited capabilities for processing speech signals.

Digital and *programmable* are generic terms, and often their meaning with regard to hearing aids is not clearly distinguished. In conventional hearing aids, programming was usually achieved mechanically with screwdriver potentiometers and switches. Control functions in modern-day hearing aids are increasingly performed by digital circuitry. As a consequence, the terms programmable and digital are sometimes used synonymously in describing a hearing aid. Most programmable hearing aids, however, are hybrid analog/digital hearing aids. The audio pathway from microphone to output transducer in these aids consists of analog components (such as a microphone and output power amplifier), whereas the operating characteristics (such as gain, output limiting,

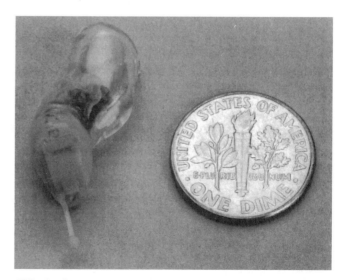

FIG. 6. Completely-in-the-canal (CIC) hearing aid. (From Goldenberg RA. *Hearing aids: a manual for clinicians.* Philadelphia: Lippincott-Raven, 1996:154, with permission.)

compression parameters) are controlled digitally. In addition, programmable hearing aids often have very useful features such as multiple memory, compression, or nonlinear amplification, and adaptive filtering used for noise reduction. They are, however, not true digital hearing aids in which the audio signal is digitally processed.

In addition to hybrid analog/digital instruments, there are several quasidigital hearing aids in use. In the quasidigital aid, the electrical signal that represents the audio waveform is sampled at regular intervals but the samples remain in analog form. These samples are not converted to strings of binary digits as in a digital computer or a "true digital hearing aid." The quasidigital instruments have all the features of the hybrid analog/digital hearing aid, such as programmability and memory, but additionally enable the audio signal to be amplified and filtered with great precision. True digital aids, of course, have all the advantages of the hybrid and quasidigital instruments and have ever expanding capabilities for advanced signal processing.

While we have really just entered the new digital era in hearing aid technology, the use of digital techniques in acoustic amplification was achieved more than a decade ago (2). The first digital aid was rack mounted and designed as a research tool for laboratory-based experiments. In 1987, the first commercial digital hearing aid, known as "Phoenix," became available. It was a body-worn device, and although it was not a commercial success, it paved the way for future applications of digital techniques to hearing aids. The most serious problems in applying digital technology to wearable hearing aids are the large physical size needed to house the hardware and the high power consumption. A major breakthrough in alleviating these problems came with the development of high-speed DSP chips. Today, true digital hearing aids are commercially available even in CIC models, and the number no doubt will grow as solutions to size and power consumption are achieved.

A serious limitation to successful applications of digital techniques to hearing aids is a fundamental lack in understanding of the optimal way to process speech to make it more intelligible to persons with sensorineural hearing loss (3). The potential to improve speech understanding in noise through digital processing is yet to be realized in the true digital hearing aid. Another problem of critical concern is the lack of valid and reliable methods for fitting the new programmable hearing aids with their many adjustable variables (e.g., different forms of compression amplification and other dynamic forms of amplification). In this new digital era, the hearing aid dispenser will be faced with an increasing number of flexible options and an increasing array of complex digital processing techniques. An immediate challenge is to develop methods of fitting necessary to deal with this flexibility and its great potential to meet the individual communication needs of persons with hearing impairment.

COMPONENTS AND TYPES OF HEARING AIDS

Hearing Aid Components

Hearing aids are electronic devices whose functions are to amplify sound and deliver it to the ear with as little distortion as possible. Figure 7 shows simplified diagrams of a conventional analog hearing aid (Fig. 7A) and a digital hearing aid (Fig. 7B). As illustrated in Fig. 7A, hearing aids consist of several basic components: microphone, volume control, amplifier, power supply (batteries), and receiver.

The microphone is an energy transducer that converts acoustic energy to an electrical signal. In analog instruments, the sound is usually filtered (to shape the spectrum of the sound) and amplified and then delivered to the receiver, which converts the electrical signal to an acoustic output. A volume control is provided to modify the output intensity of the sound to the desired level. The hearing aid is powered by a small transistor battery.

A block diagram of a DSP hearing aid is shown in Fig. 7B. The microphone in a digital hearing aid is the same type of microphone that is used in an analog instrument. The microphone output signal or the preamplified signal is connected directly to an analog-to-digital converter, which converts the analog signal to a digital form that represents the original sound. The microphone output is not processed in a continuous manner as in an analog hearing aid; rather, the output is sampled at discrete intervals in time (e.g., 16,000 samples per second). The DSP performs the mathematical operations on the digitized signals that define the signal processing algorithms and make it possible to create very complex and versatile functions, such as precise filtering and adaptive nonlinear amplification.

As indicated in Fig. 7B, the digitized signal is then converted back to an analog signal (digital-to-analog converter) and delivered to the ear via a receiver. The remaining blocks in Fig. 7B contain support circuitry that enables the converters and DSP to process the sound correctly. Memory is used to store the processing algorithms, which consist of a list of instructions that tell the DSP how to process the signal. A clock provides a series of periodic timing pulses that are used to synchronize the operation of all of the digital logic. Thus, the signal passed through the DSP is processed at the correct time and in the proper sequence. Logic performs miscellaneous digital housekeeping functions to control the sequence of operations. Finally, a battery is required to power the circuitry. Although not shown in Fig. 7B, fitting software and hardware (housed in a personal computer) are now routinely used to program digital and hybrid analog/digital hearing instruments. Fitting decisions, as a consequence, have become very versatile and often highly complex.

Hearing Aid Styles

Although there are many different circuits and shell styles available commercially, hearing aids can be broadly

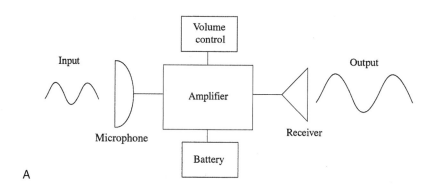

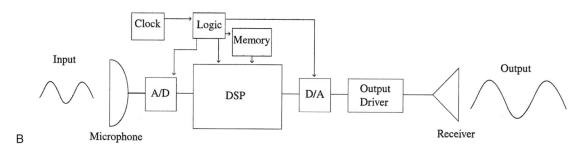

FIG. 7. Simplified block diagrams of the components of a conventional analog hearing aid **(A)** and a generic digital signal processing (DSP) hearing aid **(B)**.

classified as either air conduction or bone conduction hearing aids. Air conduction aids are coupled to the ear via an earmold, and the amplified sound is delivered acoustically to the eardrum. For bone conduction hearing aids, the amplified sound is transmitted via a vibrator most often coupled to the mastoid process or, in some instances, surgically implanted in the temporal bone (4).

BTE, ITE, ITC, and CIC Aids

As previously described, most air conduction hearing aids are worn behind or in the ear. The magnitude of an individual's hearing loss continues to be a general consideration in choosing the style of hearing aid. Older guidelines recommended that severe hearing losses be fitted with BTE aids, whereas moderate losses should be fitted with ITE aids. Only mild-to-moderate losses were recommended for ITC aids. These guidelines no longer necessarily apply, because increased power capacity is available in many styles of hearing aids. Although BTE aids continue to be the choice for persons with severe-to-profound hearing loss or for young children, ITE and CIC aids may be considered for patients with mild-to-severe

impairment. In addition to the magnitude of the hearing loss, the slope of the audiometric configuration is a consideration when choosing the style of hearing aid. With some styles it may be nearly impossible to provide enough gain in the high frequencies, especially if the slope is precipitous. In such instances, providing audibility for sounds in the frequency region where the thresholds are changing rapidly may be particularly important and more effectively achieved with an ITE aid than with a BTE aid. Fortunately today, programmable hearing aids with precise adjustable bands or channels can be used to shape the high-frequency output.

There are other practical considerations that may dictate a particular shell or earmold design. For example, persons with dexterity problems may have great difficulty inserting and removing ITE and CIC aids, so other larger shells would be more appropriate. If an individual is involved in physical activities or sports, a style should be chosen that is compatible with the level of the activity. Finally, a user's choice of style may be related to financial considerations. For example, CIC hearing aids and programmable instruments usually are substantially more costly than other hearing aids.

Contralateral and Bilateral Contralateral Routing of Signals

Typically, the microphone in an air conduction hearing aid is located at or near the pinna. However, other microphone locations can be selected for special purposes. In 1965, Harford and Barry (5) described fitting persons with a unilateral loss by locating the microphone of a hearing aid at the pinna on the side of the poor ear but transmitting the output electrically to a receiver coupled to an open unoccluding earmold on the normal hearing ear. This arrangement was known as contralateral routing of signals (CROS). Such an arrangement prevents head shadow effects by amplifying sound from the unaidable ear and delivering it, along with sound from the other side of the head, to the "aided normal hearing ear." Dodds and Harford (6) also noted that patients with predominately unilateral impairments were able to benefit from CROS fittings even when the better ear had a mild high-frequency loss. Wireless CROS aids, consisting of a microphone and FM transmitter on the side of the head and an FM receiver on the other side, are available. A modification of the CROS aid is the BICROS aid, which contains two microphones feeding a single amplifier and receiver mounted in a standard occluding earmold in the better ear. This arrangement is useful for patients with bilateral loss whose poorer ear is not suitable for amplification, so signals from both sides of the head are routed to the better ear and amplified.

Bone Conduction and Implantable Devices

Bone conduction hearing aids are recommended mainly for persons with conductive hearing loss who cannot wear an air conduction hearing aid, due to congenital causes or for medical reasons (such as persons with chronically draining ears). Because bone conduction is a much less efficient medium than air conduction for the conduction of sound waves to the cochlea, the bone conduction hearing aid requires substantial gain. Thus, a body or a BTE aid is often used to power the bone vibrator transducer. A representative example of a bone conduction hearing aid with the microphone input and power supplied by a BTE is shown in Fig. 8.

During the past decade, bone conduction aids consisting of a magnetic vibrator have been developed (7,8). These "implantable" hearing aids can be surgically applied directly to the skull bone and provide increased efficiency relative to the more conventional bone conduction aid with the vibrator coupled externally to the mastoid process. The implantable bone conduction aid bypasses the skin and is coupled directly to the skull, which reduces the impedance mismatch between the vibrator and skin. As a result, somewhat greater amplification is available to the patient. These implantable aids were designed for those patients who can benefit from conventional bone conduction aids but who find those

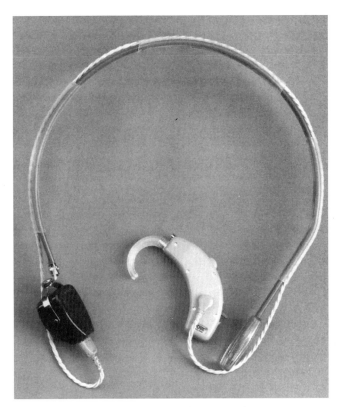

FIG. 8. Bone conduction hearing aid transducer powered by a behind-the-ear (BTE) aid and a headband. (From Goldenberg RA. *Hearing aids: a manual for clinicians.* Philadelphia: Lippincott-Raven, 1996:149, with permission.)

aids unacceptable due to the cosmetic affect of the vibrator or to the discomfort caused by the pressure of the vibrator on the head. In addition, patients with mild sensorineural impairment, together with a large conductive loss, may find that the implantable aid provides more adequate amplification than the conventional bone conduction hearing aid due to the increased efficiency from application of the vibrator directly in the skull.

In addition to bone-anchored hearing aids, other implantable devices that are directly coupled to the ossicular chain or the round window membrane are in various stages of development. Advocates for these implantable aids suggest that such devices have certain positive features not available in more conventional hearing aids. Theoretically, by directly driving the ossicular chain, a better impedance match can be provided with efficient sound transmission, less distortion than a conventional aid, and elimination of feedback. The status of middle and inner ear electronic implantable devices has been reviewed recently (9), and several devices have been approved by the Food and Drug Administration (FDA) to undergo clinical trials.

HEARING AID CIRCUITS

Although it has been conventional to classify hearing aids by type or shell style, any particular hearing aid may incorporate different circuitry components. Thus, hearing aids also can be classified by the circuit electronics or by the manner in which the circuit acts on the signal input level. The most common classification is *linear* versus *nonlinear amplification* systems. Figure 9 shows examples of the input-output response characteristics of two ITE hearing aids, one with linear amplification (Fig. 9A) and the second with nonlinear amplification (Fig. 9B). As indicated in Fig. 9A, for a linear amplification system, each 10-dB increase of input results in a 10-dB increase in the output level until the aid reaches saturation. Prior to the late 1980s or early 1990s, most hearing aids contained linear amplification systems and peak clipping was used to saturate the system.

Most modern, advanced hearing aids provide some form of nonlinear amplification (amplification where increments in input sound pressure level [SPL] cause smaller increments in output SPL). This type of amplification has been advocated for a wide variety of reasons, which will be detailed in a later section of this chapter. It is sufficient here to mention that some form of nonlinear amplification may have a theoretical advantage over linear amplification, because it reduces the normal dynamic range of the output signal so that a wide range of signal input levels can be positioned within the reduced dynamic range of an ear with sensorineural hearing loss. Recall that the dynamic range of useful hearing is often substantially reduced from the normal range in ears with sensorineural hearing loss.

The physical measurement of nonlinear amplification systems is somewhat more complex than for linear amplifiers, because the gain in the former varies as the input level increases. The gain of a nonlinear amplifier is often controlled automatically by a so-called *automatic gain*

control system. Automatic gain control action is achieved by a level detecting device located before the output receiver. This detector feeds back level information, which controls amplifier gain. This dynamic action is usually described as a process of *compression*, because a large range of output levels is compressed within a much smaller range. Figure 9B illustrates the input-output characteristics of a representative nonlinear compression system. The response curve of the hearing aid is shown for input levels from 40 to 90 dB. The compression system in Fig. 9B shows several distinct changes in the output function as input signal level increases. The output deviates from linearity once the compression threshold (input level where compression begins) is reached. For the hearing aid shown in Fig. 9B, the compression threshold was set at 60 dB. The degree to which the signal will be compressed is determined by the compression ratio (the ratio of an increment in input SPL to the corresponding increment in output SPL). The output response curves in Fig. 9B can be divided into three parts: (a) a linear output section (below the compression threshold), at low input levels from 40 to 60 dB (10-dB increase in output for each 10-dB increase in input); (b) a nonlinear output section with a compression ratio of 2:1 (5-dB increase in output for each 10-dB input increase) at moderate input levels from 60 to 90 dB; and (c) a second variation in the nonlinear function for input levels above 90 dB, in which the compression ratio is high (10:1) and used to limit or saturate the hearing aid output (1-dB increase for each 10-dB input signal increase). Because compression is accomplished by feedback circuitry, time lags are created as the system goes in and out of compression. "Attack time" refers to the length of time required for the circuit to set the new gain following a strong input signal level

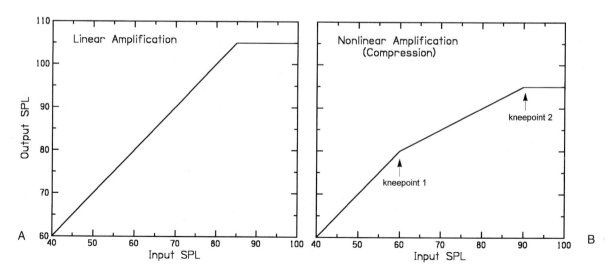

FIG. 9. Examples of output characteristics as a function of input signal level for a linear amplifier **(A)** and a nonlinear compression amplifier **(B)**. *Kneepoint 1* refers to the input level at which the output changes from linear to compression amplification and *kneepoint 2* indicates the input level at which compression ratio changes for limiting the output.

above the compression threshold. "Release time" is the length of time required for the compressed signal to return to normal amplification after the strong input signal is no longer present. Attack and release times vary depending on the application. For example, compression systems used for discomfort avoidance have a quick rise time (1 to 5 ms), so that high-level sounds are quickly attenuated before the loud signal reaches the ear. Release time is often kept relatively long (greater than 200 ms) to maintain a reduced optimal level of performance in conditions where party noise or babble is high and continuous.

There are many variations of the generalized compression curve shown in Fig. 9B. For example, some hearing aids contain two or three channels so that different compression characteristics can be implemented simultaneously in different frequency regions. Such systems are used to accommodate differences in suprathreshold loudness growth functions for persons with hearing loss that varies across the audible frequency range. The choice of compression nonlinear characteristics also is dependent on the rationale for using compression. These rationales were reviewed recently by Dillon (10) and include discomfort avoidance, loudness normalization, noise reduction, and signal dynamic range reduction. Currently, a wide variety of nonlinear circuits are available in hearing aids. More detailed descriptions of compression systems can be found in Dillon (11) and of nonlinear circuits in Staab and Lybarger (12).

HEARING AID CANDIDACY

Potentially any individual with a hearing impairment may be considered a candidate for a hearing aid. To determine the advisability of including hearing aid amplification as part of the aural rehabilitation program, it is critical to conduct a medical and audiologic assessment of the hearing disorder. The outcome of these examinations is used to determine whether medical or surgical treatment is an option and whether there are any contraindications to fitting a hearing aid (e.g., chronic ear infection). The audiologic assessment provides information regarding the magnitude and configuration of the hearing loss as well as the characteristics from which various physical options, such as hearing aid type and circuitry, may be inferred. There have been attempts to classify the expected benefits from amplification based on the degree of hearing loss, commonly using the threshold loss averaged for 500, 1,000, and 2,000 Hz (13). These classification systems, although useful, have at least two major weaknesses. First, categorization based on the speech reception threshold (using spondee words) or the pure tone average loss at 500, 1,000, and 2,000 Hz underestimates the importance of high-frequency hearing loss and its contribution to understanding speech in background noise. Second, there is a growing realization that psy-chosocial factors (e.g., motivation, expectations, physical and occupational status) play an important role in deciding whether or not an individual with hearing loss is a suitable candidate for a hearing aid.

It is recognized today that audiologic measurements do not provide complete characterization of the hearing status of an individual. The correlation between audiometric results and reported disability and handicap is moderate (14,15). In addition, audiometric data do not fully explain the benefit or satisfaction individuals gain from hearing aids (16). Thus, a comprehensive approach to determining hearing aid candidacy should include a thorough case history together with the audiologic and medical assessments. The case history and formal evaluations should address such topics as the physical status of the patient (motor skills and vision), occupational status (demands on hearing in the work environment), lifestyle (daily activities and situations that the patient particularly wants to hear), motivation (issues that prompted the patient to be tested), expectation (the patient's understanding of benefit from a hearing aid), and attitude (positive or negative attitude toward impact of hearing loss or acceptance of a hearing aid). A more complete discussion of evaluation procedures that might be used prior to determining hearing aid candidacy or other rehabilitation recommendations can be found in a recent review by Saunders (17).

PHYSICAL MEASUREMENT OF HEARING AID PERFORMANCE

The overall goal of performing physical measurements of the electroacoustic output of hearing aids is to provide data that are useful in selecting and adjusting a hearing aid for a particular patient. In addition, objective measurements of the physical performance of a hearing aid are conducted to permit accurate comparison of hearing aid characteristics among different clinics and/or laboratories and to provide a permanent record of the physical characteristics of a particular hearing aid at the time of purchase. Repeated measurements then may be made subsequent to purchase to determine if a patient's complaints about changes in hearing under amplification conditions are related to changes in the performance of the hearing aid or due to progressive hearing loss.

Standard Coupler Measurements

The physical performance of a hearing aid can be estimated objectively by measuring the hearing aid output in a standard coupler or by obtaining *in situ* measurements with the use of a real-ear probe microphone system. A description of standardized physical measurements of hearing aid performance in a standard coupler can be found in ANSI S3.22-1987 (18). In addition to providing operational definitions, the ANSI standard specifies the methods used for testing hearing aid performance in a coupler and provides allowable tolerances that suggest how closely hearing aid characteristics must adhere to specifications provided by a manufacturer. Although this document is not the only ANSI standard pertaining to hearing aids, it is probably the most well known and used since its guidelines and recommendations were adapted by the FDA to help ensure hearing aid quality and control. Under the "Medical Device Amendments of 1976," a hearing aid has been categorized by the FDA as a medical device (19).

Measurement Environment and Instrumentation

An ideal environment for measuring hearing aid performance is the sound field of an anechoic chamber. Because most clinics and laboratories cannot afford an anechoic chamber, several hearing aid analyzer systems are commercially available in which a free field test enclosure is contained within a large but portable *sound box*. The walls of these enclosures are highly absorbent and insulated to provide a quiet test space free of undesirable reflections. Figure 10 shows the inside of a hearing aid analyzer test box. In Fig. 10, a BTE hearing aid is coupled to a 2-cc coupler. The test instrument is positioned on a mesh support, below which is a loudspeaker that delivers the acoustic calibrated signal. The standard test signals are either pure tones swept across the audible frequency range or broadband speech-shaped noise. After setting the volume control of the hearing aid, according to specifications described in the ANSI standard, the amplified output of the hearing aid is transmitted to a coupler located in the sound box. The acoustic output of an air

conduction, hearing aid receiver is measured on a standard 2-cc coupler or an ear simulator. The amplified acoustic signal developed in the coupler is then transmitted via a microphone to an analysis system.

ANSI S3.7-1973, entitled "Methods for Coupler Calibration of Earphones," provides specifications for the use of several couplers, each designed to accommodate different hearing aid measurement arrangements (button receiver only, tubing and earmold, or shell for ITE) (20). The effective value of the standard coupler cavity is 2 cc. This coupler was initially described in 1942 by Romanow (21) and continues to be used today because it is simple in design, it is inexpensive to construct, and the results are highly reproducible. The 2-cc volume was originally intended to account for the compliance of the ear canal and middle ear system when the canal was occluded by a hearing aid shell or earmold. However, subsequent investigations and observations determined that the 2-cc coupler has a greater volume than an average adult ear that is occluded by an earmold. In addition, the impedance factors above 1,500 Hz, incorporated in the coupler, differ from the normal ear. Because the occluded ear canal volume in an adult is smaller than 2 cc, the SPL level measured in a hearing aid occluded ear is higher than the output of the same hearing aid measured in a 2-cc coupler. The average difference in SPL between the average occluded real ear and the 2-cc coupler is frequency dependent, varying from 2 to 3 dB for low frequencies to approximately 14 dB at 6,000 Hz (22).

An alternate coupler that more closely resembles the real ear was developed by Zwislocki (23,24). This so-called *ear simulator* takes into account the acoustic capacitance (volume), the inertance (mass), and the acoustic resistance of real ears. It contains an ear canal portion that duplicates the diameter and length of a median adult ear canal. Because the ear simulator clearly resembles a median adult real ear, it has been considered for replacement of the 2-cc coupler for hearing aid measurements. In the United States, the characteristics of an occluded ear simulator are specified in ANSI S3.25-1979 (25).

There has been reluctance to standardize hearing aid performance in terms of the ear simulator for several reasons. First, because of its more complicated construction, the ear simulator probably is not sufficiently rugged for inexpensive high-volume production. Second, a change from the standard 2-cc coupler to an ear simulator for determining the performance of a hearing aid would result in an immediate increase in the gain measured for existing hearing aids. This situation poses a serious problem for currently produced aids because their specifications would have to be republished. Fortunately, sufficient studies have demonstrated that frequency-dependent corrections can be applied to 2-cc coupler results to specify the hearing aid output levels as measured in an ear simulator or a real ear. The ANSI working group on hearing aid specifications currently remains committed to utilizing the 2-cc coupler

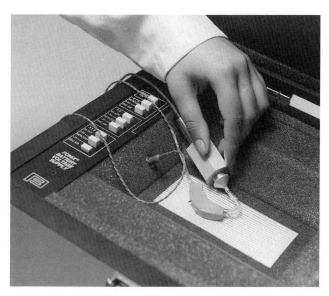

FIG. 10. Behind-the-ear (BTE) hearing aid coupled to a 2-cc coupler located in a hearing aid analyzer test chamber. (Courtesy of Frye Electronics, Inc., Tigard, Oregon.)

for measuring hearing aid performance, because it provides highly repeatable measurements on the same hearing aid across multiple laboratories and because of its simple construction and therefore lower cost (26).

The electroacoustic performance of a hearing aid also can be measured on the ear of an anthropometric mannequin such as the Knowles Electronics Mannequin for Acoustic Research (KEMAR) (27). Specifically the height and breath of KEMAR's head, neck diameter, shoulder, and chest width are within 4% of normal adults. The mannequin is fitted with ear simulators (described previously) located at the ends of ear canal extensions starting at the medial end of the concha. ANSI S3.35-1985 provides recommendations for use of the mannequin for estimating hearing aid performance (28). Currently, the mannequin has been used primarily for research purposes, but the results are especially informative when electroacoustic measurements are required that reflect acoustic behavior for hearing aids in simulated *in situ* working conditions.

Standard Electroacoustic Measurements

Among the various electroacoustic specifications for hearing aids recommended in ANSI S3.22-1987, three measurements are especially critical in describing the physical performance of any hearing aid: frequency response, gain, and saturation sound pressure level (SSPL). The top panel of Fig. 11A shows an example of the frequency response of a hearing aid coupled to a 2-cc coupler and measured in a hearing aid test box. The frequency response provides information concerning the SPL output of the aid at various frequencies within the bandpass of the instrument. When measuring hearing aid output, it is necessary to specify the position of the volume control, which is adjustable on many hearing aids. The volume control on the hearing aid is set to a "full-on" gain position for the initial measurements recommended in the standard. Full-on gain refers to the amount of gain provided by the hearing aid when its volume control is set at the highest available position. Additional measurements are performed at a specified reduced volume setting that more closely approximates the setting used by the wearer.

Figure 11B illustrates the corresponding gain of the instrument for a signal input level of 60 dB. Gain is defined as the difference in decibels between the amplified output SPL and the input SPL. The hearing aid illustrated in Fig. 11B provides the lowest output and gain in the low frequencies below about 700 Hz and the greatest output between 1,000 and 3,000 Hz. The shape of the gain curve will vary depending on the needs of the patient; however, the overall response curve shown in the example is typical for patients with moderate hearing loss who have greater loss in the high frequencies and thus usually require greater amplification in that frequency region.

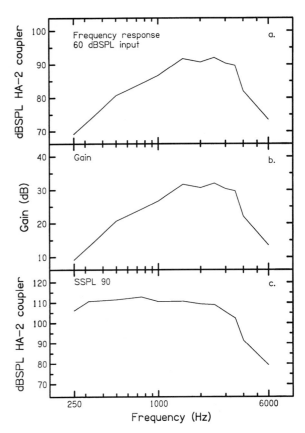

FIG. 11. Output characteristics of a hearing aid described in terms of frequency response **(A)**, acoustic gain **(B)**, and saturation sound pressure level (SSPL) **(C)**. Measurements were conducted in a 2-cc coupler with an input signal level of 60-dB SPL for the frequency response and gain measurements and 90-dB SPL for the SSPL measurements.

Response curves for a hearing aid are typically obtained at input levels of 60 and 90 dB. The former is a moderate intensity level signal that is usually considered comfortable for a normal hearing listener and a level corresponding to normal conversational speech, whereas the latter represents a high intensity level environmental sound and usually provides information about saturation characteristics of the hearing aid. Figure 11C shows the response for an input signal level of 90 dB, at which level the hearing aid output has become nonlinear and indicates that the amplifier is operating in saturation (notice the response curve has become more uniform throughout the entire frequency region). According to the standard, the SSPL is obtained by turning the aid's volume control to full-on and then presenting an input signal at the high intensity level of 90 dB. The resulting performance curve is designated as SSPL90, with the 90 referring to the input signal level. The measurement of SSPL90 is of importance because it provides a practical measure of the maximum capability of the hearing aid for a high-intensity input signal. In practice, the maximum power output level of the hearing aid for a 90-dB input level signal should not exceed the patient's perceived discomfort level. The discomfort listening level is a behavioral estimate of the point at which the input signal becomes uncomfortable and annoying and is often considered the upper limit of the useful dynamic range of hearing for a patient.

ANSI S3.22-1987 recommends that a hearing aid with a nonlinear automatic gain control system should be measured at input levels of 50 and 90 dB. The level of 50-dB input was chosen because many automatic gain control systems are already in compression at 60-dB input levels (the recommended level for hearing aids with linear amplifiers). Thus, the 50-dB input level would more likely provide frequency response information for the aid at low input levels below or near compression threshold. For a complete physical analysis of automatic gain control hearing aids, it is advisable to measure the frequency response curve at several signal presentation levels from soft to high, because the output gain varies as a function of input SPL.

Although frequency response, gain, and SSPL90 performance are routinely measured as part of the electroacoustic analysis for hearing aids, other performance measurements also are useful. These include the measurement of harmonic and intermodulation distortion, equivalent input (internal) noise level of the aid, and current battery drain. The details of these measurements also can be found in ANSI S3.22-1987.

Real-Ear Probe Microphone Measurements

Regardless of whether a 2-cc coupler or a Zwislocki ear simulator is used to measure hearing aid output, coupler measurements can only provide average response characteristics. They cannot adequately address normal variations in response imposed by variability among ear canals, the load impedance at the eardrum, and baffle effects produced by sound that is absorbed or reflected from the head, pinna, and torso. These sources of variability are generally small for low-frequency signals with long wavelengths, which tend to bend around objects and are only moderately affected by variations in ear canal length. However, the significant variability that exists among individuals' external ear canals and pinna results in large differences in high-frequency response among individuals who wear the same hearing aid.

To address these issues, real-ear probe tube microphone measures have become an attractive, objective method for measuring and verifying the performance of a hearing aid on an individual user. Commercially available systems, which are user friendly and affordable, can rapidly and efficiently measure the SPL present at a reference microphone location on the head (usually near the ear) and compare this SPL to that developed in the ear canal, close to the eardrum. Figure 12 shows a commercially available probe microphone inserted in the ear canal of the patient who is wearing an ITE hearing aid. The reference microphone is positioned directly above

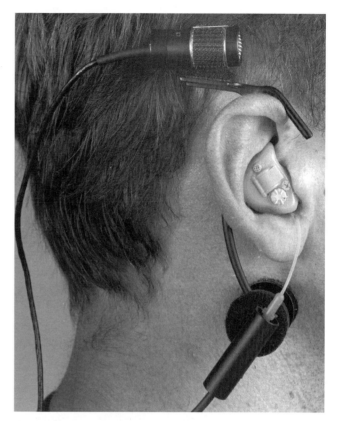

FIG. 12. Real-ear probe microphone system arranged for measurement of the performance of an in-the-ear (ITE) hearing aid *in situ*. Note the probe microphone tubing inserted in the ear canal between the hearing aid and the canal wall and the reference microphone located directly above the pinna. (Courtesy of Frye Electronics, Inc., Tigard, Oregon.)

the pinna. The probe tube is connected to a microphone located in the dark tubelike container near the bottom of the figure. A speech-shaped noise or pure tone swept stimulus is delivered via a loudspeaker, and the response characteristics of the hearing aid are measured by the probe microphone located near the eardrum. The response is stored on a computer and a hard copy is printed for a permanent record.

Although a variety of measurements can be made with a probe microphone system, an estimate of insertion gain is most commonly obtained. Insertion gain is the difference between the response of the unaided ear and the aided ear, or the real-ear gain of the hearing aid as worn by the individual patient. The top panel in Fig. 13 shows the real-ear unaided response together with the real-ear aided response from a patient wearing a hearing aid. The difference between these responses (the shaded area) is an estimate of the real-ear insertion gain of the hearing aid when coupled to the ear of the patient. The bottom panel in Fig. 13 also illustrates the acoustic gain of a hearing aid measured in a standard coupler as compared to the real-ear insertion gain, obtained with a probe microphone system for a patient wearing a hearing aid.

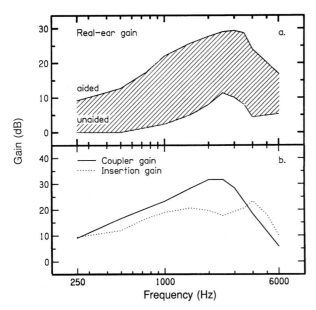

FIG. 13. Gain measured for a hearing aid using a real-ear probe microphone system. **Top panel:** Aided and unaided (open-ear) performance. The *shaded area* indicates the insertion gain. **Bottom panel:** Comparison between the acoustic gain of the hearing aid measured in a 2-cc coupler and the real-ear insertion gain (from top panel).

It is common to observe significant differences between the real-ear gain and the acoustic gain measured in a coupler. In the example shown in Fig. 13B, the largest difference between the two measurements of gain is found in the frequency region between 1,500 and 4,000 Hz, where the resonant characteristics of the unaided ear are most prominent. The resonance is shifted to a much higher frequency in the aided ear when compared to the unaided ear, because the earmold effectively reduces the length of the canal. In this example, the coupler gain overestimated the real gain of the hearing aid, because neither the individual open ear response nor the unique physical characteristics of the particular hearing aid user are incorporated in the coupler gain measurement. Real-ear probe tube measurements are not limited to insertion gain; they also can be used to measure changes in the overall output level for a compression system with input level increases or to estimate the output level in the ear when the aid is in saturation.

To minimize measurement error when conducting probe tube measurements, several important test variables must be controlled. Before initiating probe tube measurements, the ear canal should be inspected otoscopically to determine that the canal is free of cerumen. Cerumen can occlude the probe or interfere with the guidance of the probe tube along the canal to the eardrum. Other sources of error include an inability to maintain constant insertion depth of the probe tube during both unaided and aided measurements and from variations in the location of the reference microphone (29). In addition, the subject's head must remain stationary during the measurement, and the elevation and azimuth of the sound source must be constant for open and occluded ear measurements. Specific recommendations regarding real-ear test protocols and sources of error can be found in Mueller et al. (30), Tecca (31), and de Jonge (32).

Finally, it should be emphasized that probe microphone results provide an estimate of real-ear gain on an individual listener while wearing his or her own hearing aid. The real-ear probe measurement is therefore an important objective method for measuring the performance characteristics of a hearing aid on an individual listener. However, probe measurements provide no direct information about speech perception or other functional abilities, although the results may be used in interpreting perceptual performance. The results from the probe microphone measurements should be used in conjunction with other evaluation measures (speech recognition, sound quality judgments, etc.) as part of the total hearing aid selection, fitting, and verification procedure.

HEARING AID FITTING PROCEDURES

Preselection Measurements

The objective of most hearing aid fitting procedures is threefold: first, to make conversational speech audible through amplification; second, to shape the speech spectrum to accommodate changes in hearing threshold and suprathreshold loudness growth; and third, to maintain the intensity of amplified speech or environmental sounds below the level where sounds become uncomfortably loud. Prior to application of any hearing aid fitting algorithm, clinicians usually estimate the *dynamic range* of useful hearing by measuring the sound level that is just barely audible (threshold) and the level at which the sound becomes uncomfortably loud (ULL). The decibel difference between the ULL and threshold is considered the functional dynamic range for the individual patient. The dynamic range can be estimated for frequency-specific stimuli (e.g., pure tones, frequency-modulated tones, or narrowband noise) or more grossly with a broadband signal such as speech. In addition to determining the threshold and ULL, clinicians often obtain a measure of the most comfortable listening level (MCL), which lies between the threshold and the ULL. Most hearing-impaired listeners find that speech is most intelligible and of acceptable quality at SPLs near the MCL or within the range of comfortable loudness. As a result, a number of fitting strategies are designed to amplify and spectrally shape conversational level speech to MCL.

The dynamic range of hearing is substantially affected by the type of hearing loss. For listeners with normal hearing, the dynamic range of useful hearing is approximately 85 to 95 dB. The dynamic range for hearing may be normal or nearly normal for patients with pure conductive impairment, where the lesion simply attenuates the input signal. For individuals with cochlear impair-

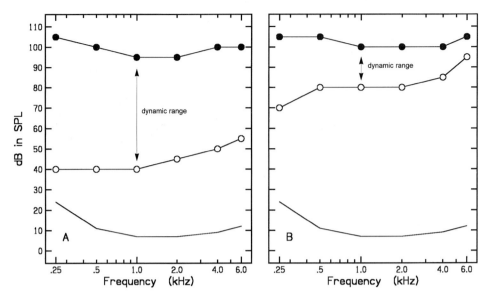

FIG. 14. Examples of the dynamic range of useful hearing as measured for patients with a moderate sensorineural hearing loss (*left panel*) and a severe sensorineural hearing loss (*right panel*). The dynamic range is estimated from the difference between the uncomfortably loud level (ULL; ●—●) and the threshold (○—○) of hearing at each test frequency. The threshold for normal hearing (—) is shown for reference.

ment, the dynamic range is reduced, often dramatically in frequency regions with severe hearing loss. The reduced dynamic range for listeners with cochlear impairment is primarily due to the threshold elevation, because the ULL remains nearly equivalent to that observed in the normal hearing listener. This result is a reflection of the presence of loudness recruitment or the rapid growth of loudness above threshold as the physical intensity of sound increases. Figure 14 illustrates the dynamic range of hearing for two individuals with cochlear hearing loss, one with a moderate hearing loss (Fig. 14, left panel) and the other with a severe hearing loss (Fig. 14, right panel). For reference, the average curve for auditory threshold and the ULLs for normal hearing listeners are shown (solid lines). For the listener with moderate hearing loss, the dynamic range is reduced from normal and approximates 50 dB. For the individual with a 75-dB hearing loss (Fig. 14, right panel), the dynamic range is severely restricted (less than 25 dB). Because soft to loud speech levels vary over a range of nearly 50 dB, it becomes extremely difficult to position the normal level variations in speech within the small dynamic range available, especially for the latter patient, and still maintain an audible level for soft speech and comfortable loudness for loud speech or sounds.

Development of Fitting Strategies

The hearing aid fitting process has been one of the more widely discussed and investigated topics in audiology. Numerous procedures have been advocated over the years. They can be classified into several basic approaches: (a)

frequency-selective procedures; (b) fixed frequency gain techniques; and (c) comparison methods.

Prescriptive methods, in which the frequency gain response and saturation level can be prescribed on the basis of audiometric data, are extremely popular today. Modern (frequency-selective) prescriptive methods originated as early as the 1930s, limited, of course, by the technology and audiometric equipment available at that time (33). Knudsen and Jones (33) suggested an audiogram-mirroring method, which compensated for the hearing loss by providing frequency-selective amplification based on audiometric thresholds. It was soon realized, however, that this method provided too much gain because of the rapid growth of loudness above threshold and the reduced dynamic range found among persons with sensorineural hearing loss. Watson and Knudsen (34) were among the first investigators to adjust the frequency response of the hearing aid to account for the reduced dynamic range in hearing. Although their procedure was very time consuming and required obtaining "most comfortable equal-loudness counter" data, this method was an early version of modern frequency-selective procedures.

In striking contrast to the method of selective amplification, the well-known Harvard Study recommended that a uniform frequency response characteristic, ranging between a "flat" and a 6-dB per octave rise, provided the most satisfactory performance for nearly all individuals with hearing impairment regardless of audiometric configuration (35). This recommendation also was supported by an independent study conducted in Great Britain and published as the Medresco Report (36). Results from these studies virtually eliminated the use of frequency-selective procedures for nearly 30 years.

Toward the end of World War II, the armed forces established comprehensive aural rehabilitation programs for personnel with hearing loss. These programs included hearing aid fittings and rehabilitation lasting from weeks to as much as 2 months. It was in this climate that Carhart (37) pioneered the comparative hearing aid evaluation procedures that were used extensively until the late 1970s. The basic purpose of this evaluation procedure was to compare results from speech perception tests obtained with several commercially available aids, and then select the best hearing aid. This procedure remained popular until research demonstrated that differences in speech recognition performance among preselected aids rarely were of sufficient magnitude to provide the clinician with high statistical confidence that such differences were real (38,39).

As the popularity of the Carhart procedure diminished, several theoretically and empirically based formulas for prescribing the gain and frequency response of a hearing aid were developed (40–45). Although each procedure varied in approach and detail, these frequency-selective procedures generally shared the common objective of amplifying conversational speech to optimize speech recognition. Technological advances, such as the development of high-speed, microprocessor-based computers, probe microphone measurement equipment, and programmable hearing aids have facilitated the strong resurgence of prescriptive methods. The desired prescription can be achieved with flexibility and precision using software that interfaces with programmable hearing aids, and the results can be verified objectively with real-ear probe microphone measurements. Until recently, prescriptive procedures were designed to be implemented with linear hearing aid amplification systems. For the linear hearing aid amplifier, the frequency response characteristic of the prescription remains the same regardless of signal input level until the aid saturates. With the increased popularity of nonlinear hearing aids, new prescriptive techniques are being developed to incorporate changes in the frequency gain response as signal input levels increase. The remaining discussion of prescriptive methods is divided into those that are designed for linear amplifiers and others that are advocated for nonlinear amplification.

Prescriptions for Linear Amplification

Current hearing aid prescription formulas prescribe the gain and, in some instances, the maximum output of a hearing aid at each audiometric frequency. In contrast to fixed gain methods, advocates of prescriptive procedures assume that a specific frequency gain function can be prescribed for each individual with hearing impairment. For most prescriptive procedures, the specific goal is to amplify speech to the MCL. Typically, a single represen-

tation of speech, such as the long-term average speech spectrum, is considered the input signal (46). The various gain algorithms can be divided into formulas that are threshold based and those that utilize suprathreshold audiometric data. As the name implies, threshold-based methods prescribe the frequency gain function based solely on audiometric thresholds. Suprathreshold methods usually provide prescriptions from suprathreshold loudness measures such as the MCL, ULL, or the upper limit of comfort loudness. The fundamental difference between the two approaches lies in the assumed or measured relationship between threshold and suprathreshold measures.

Consider, for example, a fitting procedure that aims to amplify conversational speech to MCL. If there is a strong relationship between threshold and MCL, then there is no need to conduct suprathreshold measurements. The clinician would simply measure threshold, estimate the MCL, and then amplify the speech accordingly. Advocates of suprathreshold-based methods, however, suggest that the relationship between threshold and suprathreshold loudness measures is too variable across hearing-impaired listeners to allow for an accurate estimate of MCL or other suprathreshold loudness measures. The data available are not entirely clear on this issue, but some results suggest that the relationship between threshold and suprathreshold is modest and suprathreshold characteristics (such as MCL and ULL) cannot be predicted from thresholds with great precision (47,48). Regardless, threshold-based procedures have become very popular. Humes and Halling (49) proposed several explanations to account for this popularity. First, threshold measurements can be obtained in less time than suprathreshold loudness measures; second, many manufacturers only require a patient's threshold at audiometric frequencies; third, suprathreshold loudness measures are not easily obtained from children or adults with diminished intellectual capacity; and fourth, the test-retest variability of suprathreshold loudness measures is higher than that for threshold measurements.

Currently there is no single prescriptive procedure that is universally accepted as the best approach for selecting a hearing aid. In addition, the frequency gain characteristics specified by the various methods do not lead to exactly the same prescription (49,50). Differences in outcome among the methods apparently are related to differences in the goals among the methods, the choice of audiometric data used for calculating the frequency gain characteristics (e.g., threshold or suprathreshold measurements), and design differences in the studies used to establish a particular method. However, a recent study by Van Buuren et al. (51) suggests that subtle variations in frequency gain response curves generally do not result in different speech recognition scores.

To illustrate the outcome of a prescription method, results from the National Acoustic Laboratory-Revised

(NAL-R) approach are shown in Fig. 15 for a patient with moderate hearing loss. The threshold-based NAL-R method was chosen because it is the most frequently used of the available prescription methods and its development was based on considerable research and verification data (43). The goals of the procedure are to shape a speech signal so that all frequency bands contribute equally to its loudness and provide adequate amplification so that the speech signal is sufficiently audible when the hearing aid volume control is set for comfort. Emphasis is placed on prescribing the appropriate frequency response characteristics, and minor adjustments for comfort are made with the volume control on the hearing aid.

Figure 15A illustrates the gain recommendations obtained from the NAL-R method for a patient with moderate hearing loss, somewhat greater in the high frequencies. In Fig. 15A, the long-term average peak levels of conversational speech have been converted to hearing levels so that they could be presented in audiogram form. Notice that the speech is barely audible above the elevated threshold only in the low frequencies. The gain prescribed by the NAL-R method is illustrated in Fig. 15B at the major audiometric test frequencies. This gain, if achieved, would increase the intensity level of the speech in the unaided ear so that the speech is clearly audible above the impaired threshold within the frequency region between 250 and 6,000 Hz. The gain prescribed by NAL-R is referred to as "insertion gain" and, as previously described, refers to the difference in decibels between the SPL measured near the eardrum in the open unaided ear and the same ear occluded by the hearing aid. The shape

of the speech signal amplified by the NAL-R prescription is shown in Fig. 15A. Sufficient gain has been prescribed so that the peaks of the speech are now audible above the elevated thresholds throughout the frequency region important for speech recognition.

Despite the popularity and overall positive results when using prescriptive procedures, there are several limitations regarding prescriptive procedures that need to be mentioned. First, as indicated previously, these methods generally assume that a single specific frequency gain characteristic is sufficient for each individual. However, available data suggest that there may be no one single set of hearing aid characteristics that will be optimal for an individual in all environmental settings (52,53). For example, the desired frequency gain characteristics may vary with the presence or absence or the type of background interference. For individuals who must accommodate to changes in the acoustic environment, more than one frequency gain characteristic may be required. This consideration is sometimes used as rationale for multiple-memory hearing aids, which provide different prescriptions according to the interfering acoustic environment. Second, the previously described prescription methods have been developed for hearing aids with linear amplifiers. It is assumed that one prescription is satisfactory for all signal input levels. However, rapid changes in the loudness growth function of listeners with sensorineural hearing loss suggest that the frequency gain response of the hearing aid may need to be varied as signal input levels increase. To accommodate changes in the slope of loudness growth functions, a hearing aid with a nonlinear

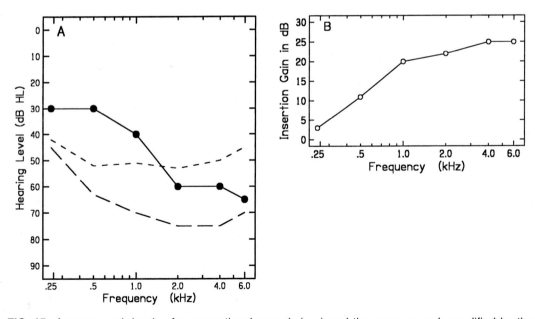

FIG. 15. Average peak levels of conversational speech (– –) and the same speech amplified by the National Acoustic Laboratory-Revised (NAL-R) prescription (— —) for a listener with a moderate hearing loss **(A)**. The speech levels have been converted to hearing level values for direct comparison with the audiogram. The insertion gain (difference between the two dashed curves) prescribed by NAL-R for patient in A are provided in **B**.

amplifier is required and the fitting procedure must necessarily prescribe a different frequency gain characteristic for soft, conversational, and loud signal input levels.

Prescribing Nonlinear Amplification

During the past decade, a significant number of new prescriptive methods has been developed to facilitate the fitting of modern programmable hearing aids. These hearing aids generally incorporate some form of nonlinear amplification achieved by compression. It has become typical to fit many of the new types of programmable hearing aids with manufacturer-specific fitting methods that often include proprietary formulas for calculating the amplification requirements as well as for adjusting the hearing aid. Alternatively, several prescriptive methods have been developed that are not specific to a particular manufacturer's hearing aid (54–57). The rationale for most nonlinear amplification prescriptions is based on normalizing the relationships between environmental sounds and loudness perception and is referred to as "loudness normalization." Because the Independent Hearing Aid Fitting Forum (IHAFF) and the desired sensation level, input-output (DSL I/O) approaches have received increasing research and clinical attention, and they present two potentially viable methods for prescribing nonlinear hearing aids, they are briefly described.

The primary goal of the IHAFF protocol is to provide amplification so that soft speech is perceived as soft, conversational level speech as comfortable, and loud speech as loud but not uncomfortable. Loudness growth is measured at selected frequencies using a scaling procedure such as category rating, and the software is designed to calculate the relationship between speech input levels (which correspond to soft, average, and loud) and the individuals' loudness judgments. From these calculations, the required compression ratios in different frequency bands are determined and a hearing aid is chosen that can be programmed accordingly. Although normalizing the relationship between speech sounds and loudness perception is theoretically appealing, Van Tasell (58) observed there is no conclusive evidence that loudness relationships among various frequency regions of speech are important for intelligibility, only that the speech must be sufficiently audible for intelligibility and not uncomfortably loud. Clinical experience, mostly anecdotal, has suggested that prescribing frequency response characteristics based on loudness normalization can provide acceptable speech recognition performance. Continued research is needed to determine if amplification systems adjusted for normal loudness sensations necessarily provide for optimal speech perception.

The DSL I/O method is a frequency-specific theoretical approach to linear or nonlinear amplification fitting (57). The DSL I/O fitting formula was developed from an earlier DSL formula in which linear gain only was pre-scribed. The general goal of the DSL I/O fitting formula is to map the acoustic region corresponding to the normal auditory dynamic range into the residual auditory areas of a hearing-impaired individual. The fitting target is derived from parameters including the sound field thresholds, the average sound field to ear canal transformation, the long-term average speech spectrum, and the upper limit of comfortable hearing.

Figure 16 contains representative input-output functions for two hearing aids based on DSL I/O calculations, linear gain amplification (Fig. 16A), and compression gain amplification (Fig. 16B). The hearing-impaired individual's threshold and the upper limit of comfortable listening are illustrated in Fig. 16, along with the threshold for normal hearing. The parameter is the output frequency response characteristics prescribed for the listener over a range of speech input levels. A target prescription is calculated, and the clinician chooses an aid that meets the theoretical target as closely as possible. The illustrations in Fig. 16 are additionally instructive because they depict the problem faced when fitting linear gain amplification systems, namely, the difficulty of providing adequate gain to achieve audibility for low input speech signals while not providing too much gain for conversational and high signal input levels. Note that, for the linear gain amplifier (Fig. 16A), the soft speech input signal (20 to 50 dB) is not sufficiently amplified above the elevated thresholds of the listener to achieve adequate speech recognition, i.e., much of the speech signal at low input levels is inaudible or heard at sensation levels above thresholds that are insufficient for adequate speech recognition. For the nonlinear gain system (Fig. 16B), a compression system is used to fit the entire input dynamic range into the residual auditory area of the listener. In this particular example, a fixed compression system was described, and the various signal input levels can be fit into the available residual auditory area of the individual hearing-impaired listener. As suggested previously, if linear gain amplification is chosen, the only way this hearing-impaired individual can maintain audibility and comfort is to raise or lower the volume control of the hearing aid depending on the signal input level. For compression amplification, the long-term level variations of speech are reduced, so that audibility is maintained for soft speech and comfort is achieved for high signal input levels. The DSL I/O formula is intended to define the theoretically ideal output for a given input level. The use of the DSL I/O formula still requires more complete empirical validation, a necessity for all nonlinear gain prescriptions that are still relatively new to researchers and dispensers.

As indicated previously, there has been a trend toward manufacturer-specific fitting systems that include proprietary formulas for calculating amplification requirements and methods for adjusting the hearing aid parameters. The consequence of the rapid growth in the number of proprietary nonlinear strategies is that ampli-

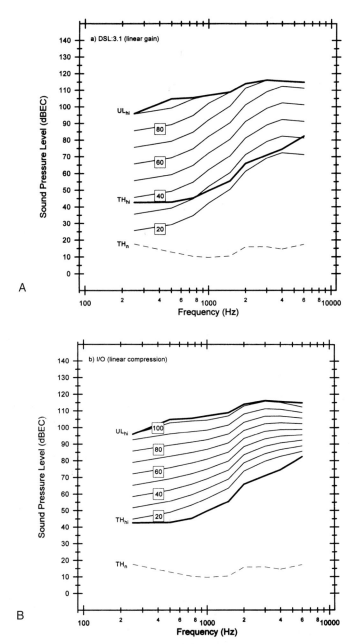

FIG. 16. Input-output (I/O) functions for desired sensation level (DSL) linear gain **(A)** and DSL I/O compression **(B)**. Hearing-impaired individual's threshold (THhi) of audibility and the upper limit (ULhi) of comfort are shown. The normal auditory threshold (THn) is plotted for reference. The specified output as a function of frequency is plotted for signal input levels from 20 to 100 dB. The output levels are references to decibels in the ear canal (dBEC). (From Cornelisse LE, Seewald RC, Jamison DG. The input-output formula: a theoretical approach to the fitting of personal amplification devices. *J Acoust Soc Am* 1995;97:1854–1865, with permission.)

fication may be prescribed by a wide variety of formulas, of which only a few, if any, are validated by published research (59). That there is currently such a large number of procedures available for fitting nonlinear hearing aids indicates that much research is still needed

to determine the optimal nonlinear system or systems for understanding speech.

ADDITIONAL HEARING AID FITTING CONSIDERATIONS

In the following section, several important considerations are addressed that may facilitate the hearing aid fitting and selection process. They include the use of omnidirectional or directional microphones, the choice of a binaural or a monaural hearing aid, and modification of the hearing aid output by choice of earmold. Preselection considerations regarding the use of directional microphones and binaural aids are important, because they represent two demonstrated methods for improving the understanding of speech in noise. The choice of earmold systems has a strong effect on the overall performance of a hearing aid and must be given careful consideration.

Directional Microphones

Most microphones used in hearing aids are omnidirectional, that is, they are equally sensitive to sounds arising from all directions. Some hearing aids (usually BTE models and a few ITE models) contain directional microphones or provide a switching network for the user to choose between omnidirectional or directional microphones. A directional microphone system provides an output level that varies with the amplitude and the direction of the sound source relative to the microphone. A logical application for the directional microphone in a hearing aid is the differentiation between a talker and background noise by proper orientation of the microphone with respect to the sound sources. For example, a listener at a cocktail party may wish to hear a person he is facing, while sounds from behind or at his extreme sides are unwanted or of little importance. For this application, a directional microphone would be effective in improving the signal-to-noise ratio at the output of the hearing aid. The pickup of the directional microphone would be maximum at 0-degree incidence and be reduced at the sides (±90 degrees) and from the rear (180 degrees). Considering this example, it may already be clear that the utilization of a directional microphone in a hearing aid is based on two assumptions: first, that the user will turn his or her head toward the main talker and second, that the interfering signals are located at the sides and back of the wearer. When these conditions exist, a hearing aid with a directional microphone should improve speech recognition in noise.

The effect of a directional microphone may be quite dramatic in an anechoic room where the directions of the sounds (talker from the front, noise from the back) at the head of the listener are clearly separated. Madison and Hawkins (60) found that the directional mode of a hearing aid gave 10.7-dB improvement in signal-to-noise ratio for monosyllabic words in an anechoic room. In a reverberant condition (more typical in day-to-day life environments because sound arrives with equal intensity from all directions, including the front of the listener), the improvement in speech perception was found to be approximately 3.0 dB (61). Although this latter result is less dramatic, it may be sufficient to make nearly unintelligible conversation understandable.

Some of the early research regarding hearing aids with directional microphones yielded mixed results (62,63). Recently, some manufacturers have introduced directional microphone as an option in both BTE and ITE instruments, and results have been positive (64). Because these modern hearing aids incorporate switch-selectable directional/omnidirectional modes of operation, the perceived benefit from selected listening situations where directional microphones are useful may provide a better frame of reference to judge their benefit. Currently, much experimental effort is being directed toward the implementation of multiple microphone systems to improve signal-to-noise ratio in real-life settings. The use of binaural hearing aids and directional microphones are two available strategies that can be used for noise reduction to improve, but not eliminate, the difficulties of understanding speech in noise among hearing-impaired listeners.

Binaural or Monaural Amplification

An important decision in the hearing selection process is whether to fit a binaural or a monaural amplification system. Prior to the 1950s, hearing aids were necessarily housed in cases that could not be worn at ear level. As a consequence, the older binaural hearing aid was really a body-worn aid with one microphone input and two outputs, one to each ear. Thus, the same signal was presented to both ears, and these binaural aids were a diotic (one input and two outputs) system. These body aids were insensitive to the interaural intensity and phase differences that occur at an individual's ear when listening to persons speaking at different locations in a room. Once ear level hearing aids were developed, it was theoretically possible to fit a true binaural hearing aid (a microphone pickup at each ear) that potentially preserved the conditions that prevail for normal, two-eared listening. Although some controversy still remains relative to the simulation of true binaural listening via hearing aid amplification systems, binaural amplification is an appropriate recommendation for most patients with hearing loss.

The major advantages of wearing binaural versus monoaural aids are as follows: (a) the elimination of the head shadow effect, which can result in a reduction in the level of the sound to the ear opposite the sound source due to the mass of the head (65); (b) binaural summation, which can increase the signal level by 3 to 5 dB, depending on the relationship of the signal source and the posi-

tion of the head (66); and (c) the improved ability to hear speech in noise at adverse signal-to-noise ratios (binaural squelch effect). The first of these attributes, the absence of the head shadow effect is not the result of true binaural processing between the ears. The improvements come from fitting two monaural aids, one at each ear. Regardless of whether the speaker is located on either side of the listener, one aided ear is always in a favorable acoustic location, which minimizes the need to rely on head movement to position a monaurally aided ear toward the sound. Binaural summation and the binaural advantage when listening to speech in noise are results of binaural processing of phase and intensity differences between the two ears for the signal and the noise. Although fitting binaural aids does not guarantee a complete recapturing of the normal binaural squelch effect (about 3 to 4 dB for speech in noise), there is evidence to suggest that hearing-impaired listeners perform somewhat better in noise when they are fit binaurally (67,68). It should be noted, however, that some hearing-impaired listeners may not perform binaurally as well as normal hearing listeners (61). Thus, it is useful during the hearing aid verification process to assess binaural and monaural hearing aid performance to ensure that binaural enhancement has been achieved. If improvements are not observed binaurally, further adjustments of one or the other hearing aid might be considered.

There are some patients who may not be candidates for binaural amplification. According to Markides (69), individuals who have a uniform or flat hearing loss configuration in one ear and a steeply sloping loss configuration in the other ear may not benefit from binaural hearing aids. Stach et al. (70) observed elderly patients with central auditory nerve disorders and poor binaural processing capabilities who also may be poor candidates for binaural amplification systems. In such cases, binaural performance decreases relative to that observed for the monoaural aided condition. In addition, the cost of the second hearing aid may be prohibitively expensive for some patients, and health and welfare agencies often support costs for only one hearing aid.

Earmolds

A successful hearing aid fitting depends greatly on the quality of the custom-molded portion of the complete amplification system that fits into the concha and ear canal. Because the earmold or the shell of an ITE makes physical contact with the ear canal and concha, it must be comfortable to wear, provide an adequate seal to prevent or minimize acoustic feedback, be cosmetically attractive, and be easy to clean. Dispensers have a wide range of materials and style options available for earmolds and custom-made shells. A large majority of hearing aid fittings today incorporate custom hearing aids (ITE, CIC). The final configuration for the shell of these units usually is determined by the hearing aid manufacturer and based on accommodation of circuitry, power supply, and the need to provide some degree of venting. Earmolds that deliver sound to the ear from a BTE require tubing that can drastically change the output of the hearing aid to suit the needs of the user.

There are a wide range of variations of earmold designs that may be chosen to meet the needs and comfort of the patient. Three of the major types of earmolds are shown in Fig. 17. They include a standard earmold (Fig. 17A), skeleton earmold (Fig. 17B), and a nonoccluding earmold (Fig. 17C). The *standard earmold* fills most of the concha and extends into the ear canal. In a body aid fitting, the external receiver of the aid snaps into a ring or sponge on the earmold. A shell earmold, similar to the standard earmold, also may be used with BTE aids. For these fittings, a tube extending from the BTE, via an earhook, is generally cemented into the bore of the earmold. The *skeleton earmold* is used with tubing and contains only the amount of material needed for comfort and provision of an adequate seal. The *nonoccluding earmold*, which is designed without a canal system, is also used with tubing that extends into the ear canal. The rationale for this type of earmold is to take advantage of the natural resonance of the ear canal, which may amplify by about 15 to 17 dB at 3,000 Hz. Low-frequency sounds are attenuated with this type of fitting; thus, the nonoccluding earmold is used to achieve maximum high-frequency gain. Because the canal is open with the nonoccluding earmold, considerable care is needed to avoid acoustic feedback. Additionally, nonoccluding earmolds often are used with a CROS fitting, as described earlier in this chapter. Variations of the major types of nonoccluding and occluding earmolds are described more comprehensively in Staab and Lybarger (12) and Valente et al. (71).

For the typical BTE fitting, the output from the hearing aid receiver is transmitted via an earhook and tubing to the earmold. In addition to the electroacoustic characteristics of the hearing aid, the output is modified by each of the delivery components. For instance, the high-frequency output from the receiver is reduced because of the length of the necessary tubing. To maintain the high-frequency output, earhooks, various types of tubing, and acoustically tuned earmolds are available (72). Unfortunately, some hearing aid tubing arrangements can cause sharp resonance peaks in the frequency response. When these resonances occur within the frequency range important for listening to speech or other environmental sounds, they degrade sound quality, introduce transients, and allow the output to exceed the loudness discomfort level of the patient. To avoid these problems, the user often reduces the gain of the aid and thus defeats the primary purpose of the hearing aid fitting. To maintain a smooth frequency response, damping material or modified earhooks and earmolds can be used to alleviate the problem. For ITE fittings with custom-made shells, the control of hearing aid characteristics through earmold modification is limited. Usually some type of venting is used to provide barometric equalization in the ear canal and often to reduce the low-frequency gain of the aid.

Acoustic Feedback

In addition to intentional venting of an earmold or shell, unintentional leaks exist with almost all earmolds and often produce poor acoustic isolation between the hearing receiver and microphone. As the gain of the hearing aid is increased, a certain amount of the acoustic signal escapes either around or through the earmold.

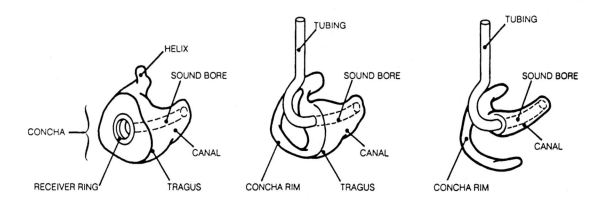

TYPICAL STANDARD MOLD   TYPICAL SKELETON MOLD   TYPICAL NON-OCCLUDING MOLD

FIG. 17. Three basic earmold types. (From Valente M, Valente MA, Potts L, Lybarger EH. Options: earhooks, tubing, and earmold. In: Valente M, ed. *Hearing aids: standards, options, and limitations.* New York: Thieme Medical Publishers, 1996:279, with permission.)

Some of this energy radiates to the hearing aid microphone and combines with the acoustic energy already present. As a consequence, the spectrum of the signal at the microphone begins to take on a more irregular shape and develops peaks and valleys. The spectrum of the signal becomes progressively irregular as the signal input level to the hearing aid increases. This acoustic feedback often is audible to the listener and is perceived as a "squeal" or "whistle." The spectrum of the signal at the microphone can become quite irregular, even before the feedback is audible (73). The physical characteristics of the peaks and valleys created by acoustic feedback are related to the magnitude of intentional (venting) or unintentional leaks, SPL of the hearing aid output signal, and the distance between the receiver and the microphone. The seal provided by the earmold or custom-made shell has become increasing important as the hearing aid microphone in the commonly used ITE or ITC fittings is located so close to the receiver. Interestingly, feedback may not be a problem for an individual with mild-to-moderate hearing loss fitted with a CIC hearing aid. The CIC instrument fits tightly, deep in the canal, and, thus, minimizes the possibility of the acoustic signal at the microphone interacting with the amplified signal at the receiver. However, in cases where the CIC is used for more severe loss or when mandibular movements break the seal, feedback may occur. Regardless of the choice of hearing aid, the problem of acoustic feedback can be minimized by taking an acceptable earmold impression of the ear, carefully considering the size of an intentional vent, and replacing earmolds that shrink due to age and wear.

ESTIMATING HEARING AID BENEFIT

Ultimately, the benefit from a hearing aid will not be completely determined in the clinic or laboratory. Information concerning the performance with a hearing aid in naturalistic or everyday settings will be the deciding factor for the individual hearing aid user. The benefit provided by hearing aids can be assessed by two general clinical methods: first, by measuring the increase in speech understanding while wearing a hearing aid and second, by questioning the user about the benefit he or she perceives in everyday life. Speech recognition tests have general face validity and known reliability, and they are readily available. However, such measures are poor predictors of speech recognition performance in everyday environmental settings and correlate only modestly with patient's self-reports of communication difficulties outside the clinic or laboratory. Thus, self-report methods that explore the user's assessment of benefit have become increasingly popular. These self-report inventories usually assess hearing aid benefit in a variety of listening situations to which users often are exposed. Dillon et al. (74) categorized self-report methods according to the manner in which the benefit measure is derived. In the approach referred to as subtraction of disability or handicap, the patient describes the difficulty encountered when listening over a range of situations and details the impact of these difficulties on lifestyle. An example is the Hearing Handicap Inventory for the Elderly (75). The benefit is calculated from the difference in scores obtained before and after using a hearing aid.

In other variations of the subtractive method, the patient is asked to rate separately the difficulty of communicating in a variety of situations with and without the hearing aid. The Profile of Hearing Aid Benefit and the Abbreviated Profile of Hearing Aid Benefit are examples of this approach (76). This type of self-report method has the advantage that the same response scales are used for the aided and unaided conditions; thus, the measurement errors are correlated. This lack of independence may be favorable, because the resulting difference scores are likely to contain less error than if the two scales are completed independently.

In an alternative approach to the subtractive method, the listener is asked to assess directly the aided benefit of a situation. For this method, called the direct differential approach, the user must mentally compare the difficulty of listening in a situation with and without a hearing aid. One example of this approach is the Hearing Aid Performance Inventory (77). All of the aforementioned approaches have the advantage of assessing receptive communication in a large number of representative everyday listening situations. A probable disadvantage is that the user is required to rate difficulty or handicap or benefit in some situations that are irrelevant because they are never or seldom experienced.

A departure from the described self-reports is the Client Oriented Scale of Improvement developed by Dillon et al. (74). In this method, the client essentially writes the self-report questionnaire by nominating up to five individualized listening situations in which help in hearing is personally important. After the hearing aid is used for a short time or the rehabilitation period is completed, the reduction in disability and the resulting ability to communicate in these relevant situations is quantified. An advantage of this approach for quantifying hearing aid benefit is the relevance of each listening situation assessed. A possible disadvantage is that results obtained with the Client Oriented Scale of Improvement from different users cannot be easily compared because each listener is rating different listening situations. According to Dillon et al. (74), clinicians who participated in the assessment of this method found it appealing because the test assessed only relevant problems described by the patient and measured the degree to which these problems were alleviated by the hearing aid. Of course, these are steps that a clinician would normally assess in a more informal manner, and so the extra effort provides documentation and quantification of the results. Regardless of the approach, self-report methods used to assess hearing aid benefit acknowledges the wide range of difficulties that hearing aid users experience under a variety of environmental situations. Moreover, such approaches take into consideration psychosocial factors as well as acoustic factors that influence the overall assessment of hearing aid benefit and satisfaction.

CONCLUSION

After reading this chapter, it should be evident that hearing aid technology and fitting strategies are in a continued state of development and evolution. Rapid technological progress in hearing aid design, especially the more recent advances made available by digital processing, does not always permit independent study of these new developments. With existing digital technology there are almost unlimited capabilities for processing speech. Much research is required to develop and evaluate the optimal method(s) of processing speech to alleviate the difficulties of listening to speech in noise, which is the most common unresolved difficulty reported by persons with hearing loss. Fortunately, hearing aid fitting and verification procedures have improved greatly over the past decade: first, by development of practical real-ear probe microphone methods; second, with increased options and flexibility for fitting and modifying hearing aid characteristics using programming software; and third, with the development of self-report methods that evaluate the benefit of a hearing aid in a potentially more comprehensive manner than possible with speech recognition tests. Advances in digital techniques confront many of the difficulties that have faced auditory researchers and clinicians in their efforts to maximize the use of residual hearing for hearing impaired individuals through amplification systems.

SUMMARY POINTS

- For individuals with acquired hearing loss that does not yield to medical or surgical intervention, hearing aid amplification is an integral part of a more general treatment plan of auditory rehabilitation.
- Progress in hearing aid technology has essentially paralleled advancements in electronic technology. These advancements in electronic technology have led to more efficient and reliable processing schemes for amplifying sound with minimum distortion.
- A consistent trend in the development of hearing aids has been the desire to reduce the size of the aid to make it less visible. Another more recent trend has been the rapid increase in signal processing capabilities, which have been enhanced by the application of digital techniques to hearing aids.
- Conventional hearing aids are analog instruments in which the electrical signal from the microphone usually is filtered, amplified, and delivered to the receiver. More recently developed digital hearing aids contain a DSP that samples the input sound at discrete intervals in time and performs mathematical operations in the digitized signal to create complex and versatile functions.
- Broadly defined, the input-output response characteristics of hearing aids incorporate a linear or nonlinear amplification system. A majority of modern hearing aids contain some form of nonlinear amplification, most often a compression amplifier that reduces the normal dynamic range of the output signal so that the wide range of signal input levels can be positioned within the reduced dynamic range of an ear with sensorineural hearing loss.
- The physical measurements of hearing aid performance are conducted objectively using a standard coupler or *in situ* using a real-ear probe microphone system.
- Although numerous hearing aid fitting strategies have been developed, prescriptive methods, in which the frequency gain response and saturation level can be prescribed on the basis of audiometric data, are currently very popular. These methods have been facilitated by the development of programmable hearing aids in which the operating characteristics can be controlled and varied rapidly using digital techniques.
- Because of the wide variety of naturalistic or everyday acoustic environments, the performance of a hearing aid in an individual listener cannot be determined completely by current clinical or laboratory tests. This has led to the development of self-report inventories that assess the benefit of a hearing aid by subjective ratings of performance in a variety of listening situations.
- Although modern hearing aids incorporate numerous technical advances in design, which have resulted in improved reliability, reduced noise levels, and less distortion, continued research is required to develop optimal methods of processing speech, especially to alleviate the difficulties of listening to speech in noise.

REFERENCES

1. Lybarger SF. A historical overview. In: Sandlin RE, ed. *Handbook of hearing aid amplification.* Boston: College Hill Press, 1988:1–30.
2. Levitt H, Neuman A, Mills R, Schwander T. A digital master hearing aid. *J Rehab Res Dev* 1986;23:79–87.
3. Levitt H. Digital hearing aids: past, present, and future. In: Tobin H, ed. *Practical hearing aid selection and fitting.* Baltimore, MD: Department of Veteran Affairs, Veterans Health Administration, 1997:xi–xxiii.
4. Fay T. Implantable auditory systems. In: Studebaker G, Bess F, Beck J, eds. *Vanderbilt hearing-aid report II.* Parkston, MD: York Press, 1991:101–122.
5. Harford ER, Barry JA. A rehabilitative approach to the problem of unilateral hearing impairment: contralateral routing of signals (CROS). *J Speech Hear Dis* 1965;30:121–138.
6. Dodds E, Harford E. Modified earpieces and CROS for high-frequency hearing losses. *J Speech Hear Res* 1968;11:204–217.
7. Hakansson B, Tjellstrom A, Rosenhall U, Carlson P. The bone-anchored hearing aid. *Acta Otolaryngol* 1985;100:229–239.
8. Haugh J, Hemelick T, Johnson B. Implantable bone conduction hearing device: audiant bone conductor. *Ann Otol Rhinol Laryngol* 1986;95:498–504.
9. Maniglia AJ. Middle and inner ear electronic implantable devices for partial hearing loss. *Otolaryngol Clin North Am* 1995;28:73–83.
10. Dillon H. Compression? Yes, but for low or high frequencies, for low or high intensities, and with what response times. *Ear Hear* 1996;17:287–308.
11. Dillon H. Compression in hearing aids. In: Sandlin R, ed. *Handbook of hearing aid amplification: volume 1, technical and theoretical considerations.* Boston: College Hill Press, 1988:121–146.
12. Staab WJ, Lybarger SF. Characteristics and use of hearing aids. In: Katz J, ed. *Handbook of clinical audiology.* New York: Williams & Wilkins, 1994:657–722.
13. Berger KW, Millin IP. Hearing aids. In: Rose DE, ed. *Audiologic assessment.* Englewood Cliffs, NJ: Prentice Hall, 1971:207–240.
14. Demorest ME, Walden BE. Psychometric principles in the selection, interpretation, and evaluation of communication self-assessment inventories. *J Speech Hear Dis* 1984;49:226–240.
15. Newman CW, Weinstein BE, Jacobson GP, Hug GA. The Hearing Handicap Inventory for Adults: psychometric adequacy and audiometric correlates. *Ear Hear* 1990;11:430–433.
16. Gatehouse S. Components and determinants of hearing aid benefit. *Ear Hear* 1994;15:30–49.
17. Saunders G. Other evaluative procedures. In: Tobin H, ed. *Practical hearing aid selection and fittings.* Baltimore, MD: Department of Veterans Affairs, Veterans Health Administration, Scientific and Technical Publications Section, 1997:103–120.
18. American National Standards Institute. Specifications of hearing aid characteristics (ANSI S3.22-1987). New York: Acoustical Society of America, 1987.
19. Medical Device Amendments of 1976, Publication L. *Federal Register* 1976:94–295.
20. American National Standards Institute. Methods for coupler calibration of earphones (ANSI S3.7-1973). New York: Acoustical Society of America, 1973.
21. Romanow FF. Methods for measuring the performance of hearing aids. *J Acoust Soc Am* 1942;13:294–304.
22. Sachs RM, Burkhard MD. *Zwislocki coupler evaluation with insert earphones.* Report No. 20022-1. Franklin Park, IL: Knowles Electronics, 1972.
23. Zwislocki FF. *An acoustic coupler for earphone calibration.* Report LSC-S-7. Syracuse, NY: Laboratory of Sensory Communication, Syracuse University, 1970.
24. Zwislocki FF. *An earlike coupler for earphone calibration.* Report LSC-S-9. Syracuse, NY: Laboratory of Sensory Communication, Syracuse University, 1971.
25. American National Standards Institute. Occluded ear simulator (ANSI S3.25-1979, R1989). New York: Acoustical Society of America, 1979.
26. Preves DA. Standardizing hearing aid measurements parameters and electroacoustic performance tests. In: Valente M, ed. *Hearing aids: standards, options and limitations.* New York: Thieme Medical Publishers, 1996:8–35.
27. Burkhard MD, Sachs RM. Anthropometric manikin for acoustic research. *J Acoust Soc Am* 1975;58:214–222.
28. American National Standards Institute. Methods of measurement of performance characteristic of hearing aids under simulated in-situ working conditions (ANSI S3.35-1985). New York: Acoustical Society of America, 1985.
29. Dirks DD, Kincaid GE. Basic acoustic considerations of ear canal probe measurements. *Ear Hear* 1987;8[Suppl]:60–67.
30. Mueller HG, Hawkins DB, Northern JL, eds. *Probe microphone measurements: hearing aid selection and assessment.* San Diego: Singular Publishing Group, 1992.
31. Tecca JE. Use of real-ear measurements to verify hearing aid fittings. In: Valente M, ed. *Strategies for selecting and verifying hearing aid fittings.* New York: Thieme Medical Publishers, 1994:88–107.
32. de Jonge R. Real-ear measures: individual variation and measurement error. In: Valente M, ed. *Hearing aids: standards, options, and limitations.* New York: Thieme Medical Publishers, 1996;61–91.
33. Knudsen VO, Jones IH. Artificial aids to hearing. *Laryngoscope* 1935;45:48–69.
34. Watson NA, Knudsen VO. Selective amplification in hearing aids. *J Acoust Soc Am* 1940;11:406–419.
35. Davis H, Stevens SS, Nichols RH, et al. *Hearing aids: an experimental study of design objectives.* Cambridge, MA: Harvard University Press, 1947.
36. Medical Research Council. *Hearing aids and audiometers.* Special Report Series 261. Report of the Committee on Electroacoustics. London: His Majesty's Stationery Office, 1947.
37. Carhart R. Tests for the selection of hearing aids. *Laryngoscope* 1946;56:780–794.
38. Walden BE, Schwartz PM, Williams DL. Test of the assumptions underlying comparative hearing aid evaluation. *J Speech Hear Dis* 1983;48:264–273.
39. Thornton AR, Raffin MJM. Speech-discrimination scores modeled as a binomial variable. *J Speech Hear Res* 1978;21:507–518.
40. Byrne D, Tonisson W. Selecting the gain of hearing aids for persons with sensorineural hearing impairments. *Scand Audiol* 1976;5:51–59.
41. McCandless GA, Lyregaard PE. Prescription of gain/output (POGO) for hearing aids. *Hear Instrum* 1983;1:16–17,19–21.
42. Seewald RC, Ross M, Spiro MK. Selecting amplification characteristics for young-hearing impaired children. *Ear Hear* 1985;6:48–53.
43. Byrne D, Dillon H. The National Acoustics Laboratories (NAL) new procedure for selecting the gain and frequency response of a hearing aid. *Ear Hear* 1986;7:257–265.
44. Cox RM. The MSUv3 hearing instrument prescription procedure. *Hear Instrum* 1988;39:6–10.
45. Skinner MW. Preselection of a hearing aid and earmold. In: Skinner M, ed. *Hearing aid evaluation.* Englewood Cliffs, NJ: Prentice Hall, 1988:69–90.
46. Cox RM, Moore JN. Composite speech spectrum for hearing aid gain prescriptions. *J Speech Hear Res* 1988;32:102–107.
47. Kamm C, Dirks DD, Mickey R. Effect of sensorineural hearing loss on loudness discomfort level. *J Speech Hear Res* 1978;21:668–681.
48. Cox RM, Bisset JD. Prediction of aided preferred listening levels for hearing aid gain prescription. *Ear Hear* 1982;3:66–71.
49. Humes LE, Halling DC. Overview, rationale, and comparison of suprathreshold-based gain prescription methods. In: Valente M, ed. *Strategies for selecting and verifying hearing aid fittings.* New York: Thieme Medical Publishers, 1994:19–37.
50. McCandless GA. Overview and rationale of threshold-based hearing aid selection procedures. In: Valente M, ed. *Strategies for selecting and verifying hearing aid fittings.* New York: Thieme Medical Publishers, 1994:1–18.
51. Van Buuren RA, Festen JM, Plomp R. Evaluation of a wide range of amplitude-frequency responses for the hearing impaired. *J Speech Hear Res* 1995;38:211–221.
52. Keidser G, Dillon H, Byrne D. Candidates for multiple frequency response characteristics. *Ear Hear* 1995;16:562–574.
53. Keidser G, Dillon H, Byrne D. Guidelines for fitting multiple memory hearing aids. *J Am Acad Audiol* 1996;16:406–418.
54. Independent Hearing Aid Fitting Forum (IHAFF). *A comprehensive hearing aid fitting protocol.* Distributed at Jackson Hole Rendezvous, Jackson Hole, Wyoming, 1994.
55. Cox RM. Using loudness data for hearing aid selection: the IHAFF approach. *Hear J* 1995;48:39–44.
56. Killion M. *FIG 6.* Distributed at Jackson Hole Rendezvous, Jackson Hole, Wyoming, 1994.

57. Cornelisse LE, Seewald RC, Jamison DG. The input-output formula: a theoretical approach to the fitting of personal amplification devices. *J Acoust Soc Am* 1995;97:1854–1865.

58. Van Tasell DJ. Hearing loss, speech, and hearing aids. *J Speech Hear Res* 1993;36:228–244.

59. Byrne D. Hearing aid selection for the 1990's: where to? *J Am Acad Audiol* 1996;7:377–395.

60. Madison TK, Hawkins DB. The signal-to-noise ratio advantage of directional microphones. *Hear Instrum* 1983;34:18–26.

61. Hawkins DB, Yacullo WS. Signal-to-noise advantage of binaural hearing aids and directional microphones under different levels of reverberation. *J Speech Hear Dis* 1984;49:278–286.

62. Frank T, Gooden R. The effect of hearing aid microphone types on speech discrimination scores in a background of multi-talker noise. *Maico Audiol Series* 1972;10:9–14.

63. Lentz W. A summary of research using directional and omnidirectional hearing aids. *J Audiol Technique* 1974;13:42–66.

64. Valente M, Fabry DA, Potts LG. Recognition of speech in noise with hearing aids using dual microphones. *J Am Acad Audiol* 1995;6:440–448.

65. Olsen WO, Carhart R. Development of test procedures for evaluation of binaural hearing aids. *Bull Prosthet Res* 1967;10:22–29.

66. Nordlund B, Fritzell O. The influence of azimuth on speech signals. *Acta Otolaryngol* 1963;56:132–146.

67. Byrne D. Binaural hearing aid fittings: research findings and clinical application. In: Libbey ER, ed. *Binaural hearing aids and amplification*. Chicago: Zenetron, 1980:23–74.

68. Balfour PB, Hawkins DB. A comparison of sound quality judgments for monaural and binaural hearing aid processed stimuli. *Ear Hear* 1992;13:331–339.

69. Markides A. Binaural hearing with amplification. In: Stephens SDG, ed. *Disorders of auditory function*. London: Academic Press, 1976:101–115.

70. Stach BA, Loiselle LH, Jerger JF. Special hearing aid considerations in elderly patients with auditory processing disorders. *Ear Hear* 1991;12:131–141.

71. Valente M, Valente MA, Potts L, Lybarger EH. Options: earhooks, tubing, and earmold. In: Valente M, ed. *Hearing aids: standards, options, and limitations*. New York: Thieme Medical Publishers, 1996:170–185.

72. Killion MC. Earmold options for wideband hearing aids. *J Speech Hear Res* 1981;46:10–20.

73. Cox R, Studebaker G. Problems in the recording and reproduction of hearing aid-processed signals. In: Studebaker G, Hochberg I, eds. *Acoustical factors affecting hearing aid performance*. Baltimore, MD: University Park Press, 1978:169–196.

74. Dillon H, Alison J, Ginis J. Client oriented scale of improvement (COSI) and its relationship to several other measures of benefit and satisfaction provided by hearing aids. *J Am Acad Audiol* 1997;8:27–43.

75. Ventry IM, Weinstein BE. The Hearing Handicap Inventory for the Elderly: a new tool. *Ear Hear* 1982;3:128–134.

76. Cox RM, Alexander GC. The abbreviated profile of hearing aid benefit. *Ear Hear* 1995;16:176–186.

77. Walden BE, Demorest ME, Helper EL. Self-report approach to assessing benefit derived from amplification. *J Speech Hear Res* 1984;27:49–56.

The Ear: Comprehensive Otology,
edited by R. F. Canalis and P. R. Lambert.
Lippincott Williams & Wilkins, Philadelphia © 2000.

CHAPTER 38

Education and Communication Choices for Children with Hearing Loss

Amy McConkey Robbins and Richard T. Miyamoto

The communication and educational methodologies used with deaf children have long been the subject of controversy within the professional community. In this chapter, we describe the various methodologies used in deaf education, and, where available, we cite studies that have documented the performance of children using these methodologies. We review the three categories of support services that may be provided to families: education, guidance, and counseling. We then present our recommendations for assisting families in choosing a methodology consistent with their philosophy and their child's abilities. Finally, we suggest the role that the otologist may play in assisting families with these decisions.

A controversy has been raging for more than 200 years regarding the most appropriate educational method for deaf children. Historically, there were two schools of thought on this issue. Educators who advocated the use of sign language for deaf children were known as "manualists." Those who advocated the use of speech and lipreading without signs were called "oralists." Until the last 30 years, almost all programs for the

deaf utilized one method or the other. In the early 1970s, a third methodology was introduced. Known as "total communication," this methodology advocated the use of multiple sources of input for deaf children, including lipreading, residual hearing, signing, and combinations of these methods.

When parents first learn that their child is deaf, they are often overwhelmed by the decisions that need to be made promptly, including the fitting of appropriate amplification and the selection of a communication methodology. The latter is a critical decision, because it affects not only the child but also the entire family, and it may mean a commitment to learning a foreign language. But as critical as this decision is, parents need time to process the mountains of new and sometimes conflicting information they receive from their otolaryngologist and from the audiologists, speech pathologists, and educators of the hearing impaired. Professionals often unwittingly put enormous pressure on families to make a decision when families need to explore for themselves and take ample time with what is a monumental task.

Northcott (1) identified three categories of support services that professionals can provide to families: *education,* where we teach the parents the facts about hearing loss and familiarize them with our professional "lingo"; *guidance,* where we assist the family in making

   A. McConkey Robbins: Communication Consulting Services, Indianapolis, Indiana 46260
   R. T. Miyamoto: Department of Otolaryngology–Head and Neck Surgery, Indiana University School of Medicine, Riley Hospital, Indianapolis, Indiana 46202

choices; and *counseling,* where we support parents as they experience the grieving process. A balanced combination of these three support services is appropriate for most families. An approach that focuses exclusively on educating the family about facts and ignores the guidance and counseling needs is a disservice to parents. In this chapter, we deal primarily with issues surrounding the first and second categories of services, education and guidance. These support services enable families to make important decisions regarding educational and communicative options for their child.

PREMISES WHEN SERVING FAMILIES

Three underlying premises should form the basis of dealing with newly diagnosed deaf children and their families:

1. Families deserve to receive information about *all* available methodologies and services along the continuum of deaf education. The optimum way for families to evaluate different methodologies is for them to visit different centers and to see the methods in practice as well as to hear an explanation of each method from those who actually practice it.

2. Given adequate information and ample time, we have confidence that families will choose the methodology that most closely fits their child's and family's need.

3. No communication method is right for all deaf children.

EDUCATING FAMILIES ABOUT COMMUNICATION METHODOLOGIES

What do parents expect of us as we advocate for them? Matkin (2) outlined three major areas of competence that parents have a right to expect from the professionals dealing with their child's hearing loss. These persons should be (a) technologically competent, (b) knowledgeable about the available resources within the community, and (c) willing to take time to listen. As noted previously, to educate families about the communication philosophies that are available, we provide information regarding these philosophies and encourage parents to visit and observe different programs. The communication methodologies widely in use may be grouped under three broad headings: (a) auditory-oral approaches, (b) the bilingual/bicultural approach, and (c) the total communication approach.

Auditory-Oral Approaches

Teaching methodologies that fall under this heading require children to use only spoken language for face-to-face communication and avoid the use of a formal sign language. For children who are hard of hearing and thus able to use audition as their primary modality for learning language, these approaches are overwhelmingly selected. Auditory-oral approaches also are chosen for children with severe-to-profound hearing losses, although the demographics of communication modes changed in the 1960s and 1970s. Over the last 30 years, oralism has been replaced by some form of manual communication in approximately two thirds of the educational programs in the United States, a trend that has been praised by some and criticized by others. The recent advent of pediatric cochlear implantation has added a new dimension to the choices about communication mode, as we shall discuss later.

Three auditory-oral approaches are most commonly used and will be described. These are multisensory, auditory-verbal, and cued speech.

The *multisensory method* is widely used within auditory-oral programs. Also known as "look and listen" or "auditory-global," this method requires children to use their residual hearing in combination with speechreading (previously called lipreading) to understand speech. Teachers in this method encourage the development of oral language through listening, speechreading, and kinesthetic and tactile cues, such as placing the child's hand on the teacher's face and neck.

Published studies documenting the performance of children using the multisensory method include several reports from the Central Institute for the Deaf (CID). In one such study, the EPIC project (experimental project in instructional concentration), a subgroup of students from CID, where the multisensory approach was used, received specific instructional attention and were evaluated longitudinally over a period of 21 months (3). The results suggested that the children involved in an intensive, multisensory oral program made greater progress in language and academics than did children in a matched control group from the same school. The control subjects followed the typical curriculum at CID, rather than an intensive one. In another investigation, a comparison was made between the English syntax skills of students educated in oral/aural and total communication programs across the country (4). Their results indicated that the oral/aural students scored substantially higher in their mastery of oral syntax forms and performed equally well on several other skills compared to their total communication counterparts.

The *auditory-verbal method* emphasizes the use of residual hearing as the primary modality for learning language, even in profoundly deaf children. Helen Beebe and other pioneers in this method, also known as acoupedic or unisensory, expressed concern that when combined visual and auditory inputs were offered to a deaf child, the unimpaired modality would be dominant. Therefore, auditory-verbal proponents encourage a dependence on listening by often depriving the child of speechreading cues, hoping to allow the child to use his or her aided hearing to its full potential. Also essential to this philosophy are the early integration of children with hearing loss into regular school and an "attitude of listening" that goes beyond structured auditory training.

Several reports are available in the literature documenting encouraging performance by children educated in the auditory-verbal method (5,6). There reports suggested that a substantial number of deaf children identified early and enrolled in intensive auditory-verbal programs were later able to be in regular educational environments and to compete with normal hearing peers.

A third method under the auditory-oral category is the *cued speech method*. Cued speech is a phonemically based hand supplement to speechreading. It uses handshapes to distinguish speech sounds that look alike on the lips, thereby disambiguating the spoken message. It is not considered a language because the manual cues are meaningless unless accompanied by spoken English. Developed by R. Orin Cornett in 1966, this method has gained popularity and has shown promising results. One disadvantage of the method for some children is that it is not widely available as an educational option in many areas of the United States. On the other hand, a number of public school systems have included cued speech programs among their educational options. Children who utilize cued speech should ideally be in a setting where there are many other users of this method, so as not to isolate the child and the child's family.

Bilingual/Bicultural Approach

This approach primarily uses American Sign Language (ASL), a manual language that is native to deaf people, with English taught secondarily through reading and writing. Supporters of the bilingual/bicultural or Bi/Bi approach argue that because ASL is a natural and complete language that is totally visual, it provides the deaf child with full access to language in a way that no other communication approach can. Once a foundation in language is established through ASL, English can be taught for the purpose of reading and academics. Many proponents of this approach align themselves with the Deaf community, which recognizes deafness as a cultural difference rather than a disability or handicap. The success of this approach would appear to hinge heavily on the ASL proficiency of those around the child, as this determines the complexity and richness of language modeling that the child receives. Given that ASL has a completely different grammatical structure than does English, the task of learning ASL for a normal hearing parent is not a small one. This is a significant issue, because 90% of deaf children are born to hearing parents.

The rationale behind the bilingual approach is the linguistic interdependence model (7,8). This model posits the existence of a universal proficiency underlying all languages. Proponents of the model argue that cognitive and academic skills learned in a first language (i.e., ASL) will generalize to the learning of related skills in a second language (i.e., English). Proponents use the example of deaf children of deaf parents who acquired ASL as a first language and who demonstrate higher academic achievement than deaf children of hearing parents. Other researchers have refuted the theoretical applicability of Cummins' model to deaf learners of English literacy (9). They argue that Cummins' model only applies to instances where literacy may be achieved *in the first language*. In the case of ASL this is impossible, as no written form of ASL exists.

A small number of research studies have recently appeared in the literature to document the proficiency of students in the Bi/Bi approach. Researchers evaluated the relationship between ASL skills and English literacy in 160 students who attended a residential school for the deaf (10). A comprehensive battery of tests in ASL and English literacy was administered. The results revealed a consistent and statistically significant relationship between ASL and English literacy skills. Subjects who demonstrated moderate-to-high proficiency in ASL also had the best English skills, regardless of parental hearing status. The authors concluded that deaf children's acquisition of even moderate fluency in ASL benefits English language acquisition.

Total Communication Approaches

Total communication approaches gained wide popularity in the 1970s. These methods advocate the use of all communication modalities appropriate for a given child, including speech, signs, gestures, fingerspelling, speechreading, reading, writing, and listening. The objective is the development of communication using whatever modalities maximize learning. Although the concept of total communication does not require simultaneous use of different communication modalities, by far the most common implementation of the total communication method is simultaneous speech and sign. Most programs using a total communication philosophy utilize a form of manually coded English as opposed to ASL. This is logical, because only a manual form of English can be used simultaneously with spoken English. In addition, advocates of total communication support the theory that hearing-impaired children exposed to such a combined code will develop competence in the English language in a more spontaneous and natural manner than could be provided through spoken English alone.

Several signing systems are available under the rubric of total communication. Seeing essential English, SEE-1, is a system that attempts to complement speech and is not signed in the concepts of ASL. It serves both an educational and a social need, with a goal of "giving comprehension of correct, colloquial English" (11). The system utilizes word divisions, prefixes, and suffixes, and it is presented in English words. Multisyllablic words often are broken up into unnatural units. For example, the word "butterfly" in SEE-1 would be signed as BUTTER–FLY. This method is no longer widely used in the United States, and few studies exist to document its effectiveness.

In contrast, signing exact English, SEE-2, enjoys great popularity within total communication programs. Developed by a deaf woman and her colleagues, SEE-2 bases its lexicon on ASL signs, but it provides a complete replication of English grammar and morphology through the use of suffixes, prefixes, and tenses (12). Thus, SEE-2 users are able to sign exactly what they say. "Butterfly" in SEE-2 would be signed as a single sign because, if the word were broken down into smaller units, those units would not mean anything in relation to the whole word (*butter* has nothing to do with *butterfly*). Encouraging findings have been reported on the English achievement skills of students educated using a complete SEE-2 system (13,14).

Pidgin sign English, PSE, is not an invented system but is a contact language resulting from the need of two groups of people who desire to communicate with one another. For example, deaf persons who normally use ASL attempt to make their signs more English in nature when communicating with a hearing person. Similarly, hearing people who normally speak English might attempt to use a few signs, plus gesture and pantomime, to communicate with a deaf person. In each case, the result is a PSE that does not adhere to English grammar and does not encode the meaning of the speech that may accompany it (15). Originally evolved as social language, variations of PSE have been formalized and often are used in educational programs. Students exposed to PSE for instructional purposes have not done as well on tests of English language and reading as have students exposed to oral English, ASL, or the SEE systems (16). This research suggests that for English proficiency to be attained, children need exposure to a complete and complex language in its full form, such as spoken English, ASL, or SEE-2. Thus, parents who visit educational programs must probe deeply into whether a complete system is being utilized in each program, and how the program proposes to assist parents in becoming fluent in the system.

COCHLEAR IMPLANTS: DO THEY COMPLICATE OR SIMPLIFY COMMUNICATION DECISIONS?

In the last 15 years, cochlear implants have become widely available for profoundly deaf children. Design improvements in multichannel implants and implantation at increasingly younger ages have produced excellent results in the majority of children who receive these devices (17–19). Due to the impressive benefit now being documented by pediatric implant users, particularly those implanted at young ages, even children with some residual hearing may now be considered candidates for an implant.

Improved speech production is often the focus of parents and teachers when a child receives a cochlear implant. However, speech production skills do not necessarily ensure language competence. Speech refers to oral production, whereas language is the internalized, abstract knowledge system that is the basis for communication. Language ability is a very strong predictor of reading achievement and, hence, academic success in children. If it could be shown that cochlear implants enhance language development, this would be a compelling argument for selecting these devices for children.

Several recent studies have investigated the effects of multichannel cochlear implants on language development. In one such study (18), the language skills of 23 children who had received the Nucleus 22-channel implant were evaluated using the Reynell Developmental Language Scales-Revised (20). Children were tested at the preimplant interval, and at 6- and 12-month postimplant intervals. A large group of profoundly deaf children without cochlear implants (but who were audiologically candidates for the device) provided comparison data. Reynell data from the unimplanted group suggested that profoundly deaf children without an implant could be expected to make 6 months of receptive and 5 months of expressive language growth in 1 year's time. In contrast, the implanted children made approximately the same amount of language growth as the time that passed (i.e., 12 months of language growth in 12 months' time). The absolute language scores of the implanted subjects remained delayed relative to their normal hearing peers because they started out much farther behind in their language. Nevertheless, that the implanted children demonstrated a rate of language learning that matched that of their peers with normal hearing demonstrates an important consequence of cochlear implantation: the foundation of language development above and beyond that expected as a result of maturation.

Rate of language learning also was used to measure implant benefit across a number of subskills that comprise language competence (21). Aspects of linguistic development found to be enhanced by cochlear implants included receptive and expressive vocabulary and expressive concepts. Implanted children's comprehension of grammatical forms, including syntax and morphology, were not found to improve at the rate seen for other subskills.

How and when the cochlear implant is presented to families as a possible rehabilitation tool is critical.

Because cochlear implants are one of the options on the continuum of service for hearing-impaired children, parents should be informed about them as part of the education process that occurs following a diagnosis of hearing loss. However, we contend that the primary focus of professional guidance by the otologist or audiologist in the first few visits after a diagnosis is made should not be on cochlear implants, which may be misinterpreted as a "cure all" for deafness. Rather, our focus is typically on determining how much residual hearing the child has, with the hope of maximizing this residual hearing using traditional amplification. It has been our experience that pushing the notion of cochlear implants too early in the education process may delay the process in some families. This occurs when families fixate on the cochlear implant as a cure for deafness that they believe will eliminate the need for special schooling or other services. When this happens, the parents' commitment to full-time hearing aid use may be jeopardized, making it difficult or impossible for the audiologist to estimate hearing loss accurately.

If adequate progress in communication development is not achieved using hearing aids and appropriate rehabilitation techniques, cochlear implantation should occur as soon as possible. This allows us to maximize the young child's ability to learn a new linguistic code and to teach skills during critical periods of development. Age at implantation has consistently emerged as one of the strongest predictors of implant success in children (22).

The cochlear implant is best presented to families, as suggested by the team at Johns Hopkins University, as "an *opportunity,* not a *cure*." Educational and communication choices may certainly be affected by the decision to implant a child. Successful children with implants may be found in both the oral and the total communication settings. However, it is clear that an environment that emphasizes listening and speaking development is mandatory if children are to receive maximum benefit from the device. Cochlear implants have the potential to dramatically improve a deaf child's ability to perceive spoken language and to speak intelligibly. If those two skills are not essential goals within an educational program, it is considered an inappropriate placement for an implanted child.

IMPORTANCE OF EARLY INTERVENTION

It is our position that every child diagnosed with a hearing loss should undergo a hearing aid evaluation and fitting of loaner hearing aid(s). As maximal use of residual hearing is an important factor in the success of every communication method, other than ASL, consistent, full-time use of optimal amplification is set as a goal from the earliest point of interaction with the fam-

ily. Only by wearing the best-fitted aids on a full-time basis will we be able to judge how much residual hearing the child has (something that is not adequately revealed by auditory brainstem response). This information is also imperative if we are to determine which children cannot be helped with traditional hearing aids and, thus, may be appropriate candidates for cochlear implantation.

In addition to early identification of hearing loss and early fitting of amplification, best practices mandate that young hearing-impaired children be enrolled in a parent–child intervention program. Such early intervention has been shown to enhance language development, academic achievement, and social and emotional development (23). In addition, research in psycholinguistics indicates the existence of a critical period for language acquisition, which peaks at 2 to 4 years and declines steadily after that. Any effort to take advantage of a deaf child's capacity for language acquisition must therefore be an early effort.

EDUCATIONAL PLACEMENT ISSUES FOR DEAF CHILDREN

Least Restrictive Environment

The legal guidelines for determining appropriate educational placement for hearing-impaired children, as dictated by Public Laws 94-142 and 101-476, are the same as for other handicapped children. Central to these guidelines is the notion of placing the child in the least restrictive environment in which he or she may succeed educationally. The law also stipulates that each child's unique needs and educational goals must be outlined in an individual educational plan (IEP), which serves as a contract between the school and family and which is rewritten each academic year. The importance of the least restrictive environment is balanced by "most appropriate placement." A child should be in an environment where he or she has "full access to curricular information." The benefits of educational inclusion for the implanted child cannot be overemphasized. These benefits include a higher standard of educational performance in regular classrooms, better communication models provided by normal hearing peers, and improved speech intelligibility, to name but a few (24).

Although these benefits are powerful and persuasive, they are only enjoyed by those who can achieve in the mainstream environment. In other words, the goal is not to place children with hearing impairment in regular classrooms at all costs, but to choose that environment because the child has the skills to succeed there. Hearing-impaired children have a unique linguistic problem that can severely restrict their ability to profit from an unplanned language presentation in the regular classroom. Unless the language levels of deaf children are within a year or two of the levels of those in the regular class in which they are placed, they will be virtually cut off from the entire verbal input process that is basic to educational experiences.

A deaf child who is ill prepared for the regular classroom, due to language and academic deficits, may fall even further behind his or her peers in that environment if he or she cannot keep up with the accelerated rate of learning. In addition, the sense of failure and loss of confidence that comes from performing poorly are not risks to be taken lightly. The key to successfully mainstreaming any child with hearing loss, including the implanted child, is to ensure that the child is adequately prepared for placement in the mainstream through early intervention, use of audition, and through a concentrated rehabilitation program of language and communication development.

ASSISTING FAMILIES IN MAKING CHOICES

As we guide families of newly identified hearing-impaired children, our goal is not just to talk to them about all the information they need to know, but also to listen to what they can tell us. By establishing this type of dialogue, we make it clear that hearing what a family has to tell us about their lifestyle, the goals for their child, and the support systems available within the larger family (among other factors) is as important as what we have to tell them. This is a fundamentally different approach than one that views the professional as possessing a vast body of knowledge that the family must absorb and implement as quickly as possible. We have learned that we guide families best when we help them select a communication mode that is the right fit for their child, within the larger context of the family. This includes a sensitivity to the unique situation of culturally deaf parents who view deafness as a difference, not a handicap, and who may have strong negative opinions about cochlear implants.

The decision to select a communication methodology is an ongoing process, not a single act, and, as noted earlier, it begins with educating the parents about the various options that are available. Once the family is familiar with the options and has hopefully had the opportunity to actually visit centers that utilize these options, our role is to guide the family in their decision. This guidance varies greatly across families, depending on their unique characteristics. As we guide families in this way, we continue to reiterate three notions to them:

1. *Make a decision that is appropriate for the here and now.* This decision does not have to be made for a lifetime. Any decision is temporary and can be changed if necessary.

2. *Use one approach at a time.* Once you choose a method, commit to it fully and carry it out to the best of your ability. We cannot judge the effectiveness of a communication method unless it is implemented correctly and completely. Do not mix methods at this early stage of learning.

3. *Keep a watchful eye on how well the chosen methodology works for your child.* Be a diagnostician and note whether your child is responding well to the chosen method. Noticeable progress should be seen after 3 months of therapy. Your child's teacher should provide other criteria for measuring ongoing improvement. If progress is not occurring, meet with the teacher and express concern.

How easily a family moves through this process depends on the individual characteristics of that family. Luterman and Ross (25) have identified five characteristics of well-functioning families. These include open communication, flexible roles with shared responsibilities, affirmation, resolution of conflict, and flexibility in times of crisis and change.

As Matkin (2) noted, how well a family deals with hearing loss is largely related to how well the family copes with life in general.

ROLE OF THE OTOLOGIST

The management and education of deaf and hard-of-hearing individuals is an exceedingly complex process that involves a wide range of professionals in partnership with families. Otologists, in combination with audiologic colleagues, have several crucial roles at critical junctures:

1. Early identification of hearing loss falls within the medical and audiologic domains.

2. Initial recommendations and implementation of appropriate technology, whether it be hearing aids, assistive listening devices, cochlear implants, or tactile devices, must be made.

3. Affirmation of the need for a multidisciplinary approach must be provided and the introduction to the broad range of educational options given.

SUMMARY

The educational and communication decisions that families of newly identified hearing-impaired children must make are difficult and important ones. In this chapter, we reviewed the options available to families and presented suggestions for guiding parents through the decision-making process. Our goal is to find the program and philosophy that best meets the needs of the child and parents, recognizing the extraordinary uniqueness of each family we serve.

ACKNOWLEDGMENT

Supported by NIH-NIDCD RO1 DC 00064 and RO1 DC 00423.

SUMMARY POINTS

- Three premises should form the basis of dealing with families of newly identified deaf children. These are:
  1. Families deserve to learn about all available methodologies.
  2. Families will choose the communication methodology that most closely fits their child's and family's need.
  3. No communication method is right for all deaf children.
- Communication approaches for hearing-impaired children may be grouped under three broad headings: auditory-oral, bilingual/bicultural, and total communication approaches.
- Research results with multichannel cochlear implants have revealed impressive results for speech perception and speech production skills, particularly for those children implanted at early ages (by 5 years of age).

- Recent investigations suggest that multichannel cochlear implants enhance language to a greater extent than would be expected from maturation. The rate of language learning matched or exceeded that of peers with normal hearing.
- Placing a child with hearing loss into a regular educational environment is the long-term goal. However, such mainstreaming is ill advised until such time as the child is linguistically and academically prepared to meet the challenges of the regular classroom environment.
- Early intervention is critically important for all children with hearing loss.
- As parents make communication and educational choices for their child, they should watch carefully to ensure that the child is making adequate progress. If not, changes in the program are warranted.

EDUCATIONAL RESOURCES FOR FAMILIES OF CHILDREN WITH HEARING LOSS

- Alexander Graham Bell Association for the Deaf
  (202) 337-5220
  www.aagbell.com
- American Speech-Language-Hearing Association (ASHA)
  (800) 638-8255
  www.asha.org
- Auditory-Verbal International
  (215) 253-6616
  www.auditory-verbal.org
- Cochlear Implant Club International
  (716) 838-4662
  www.cici.org
- John Tracy Clinic
  (213) 748-4481
  www.johntracyclinic.org
- Self Help for Hard of Hearing (SHHH)
  (301) 657-2248
  www.shhh.org

REFERENCES

1. Northcott W. *Curriculum guide: hearing-impaired children and their parents.* Washington, DC: AG Bell, 1978.
2. Matkin N. The challenge of providing family-centered services. In: Bess FH, ed. *Children with hearing impairment: contemporary trends.* Nashville, TN: Vanderbilt Bill Wilkerson Press, 1998:299–304.
3. Geers A, Kuehn G, Moog JS. Evaluation and results. In: Calvert D, ed. EPIC: experimental project in instructional concentration. *Am Ann Deaf* 1981;126:929–964.
4. Geers A, Moog JS, Schick B. Acquisition of spoken and signed English by profoundly deaf children. *J Speech Hear Dis* 1984;49:378–388.
5. Yoshinaga-Itano C, Pollack D. *A retrospective study of the acoupedic method.* Denver: The Listen Foundation, 1988.
6. Goldberg DM, Flexer C. Outcome survey of auditory-verbal graduates: study of clinical efficacy. *J Am Acad Audiol* 1993;4:189–200.
7. Cummins J. A theoretical framework of bilingual special education. *Except Child* 1989;56:111–119.
8. Cummins J. Language development and academic learning. In: Malave LM, Duquette G, eds. *Language, culture, and cognition.* Philadelphia: Multilingual Matters, 1991:203–221.
9. Mayer C, Wells G. Can the linguistic interdependence theory support a bilingual-bicultural model of literacy education for deaf students? *J Deaf Stud Deaf Educ* 1996;1:93–107.
10. Strong M, Prinz P. A study of the relationship between American Sign Language and English literacy. *J Deaf Stud Deaf Educ* 1997;2:37–46.
11. Anthony D. *Seeing essential English manual.* Anaheim, CA: Sign Press, 1971:21.
12. Gustason G, Pfetzing D, Zawolkow E. *Signing exact English.* Rossmoor, CA: Modern Signs Press, 1973;21.
13. Schick B, Moeller MP. What is learnable in manually-coded English sign systems? *Appl Psycholing* 1992;13:313–340.
14. Luetke-Stahlman B, Moeller MP. Enhancing parents' use of SEE-2: progress and retention. *Am Ann Deaf* 1990;135:371–378.
15. Luetke-Stahlman B, Luckner J. *Effectively educating students with hearing impairments.* White Plains, NY: Longman Publishing, 1991.
16. Luetke-Stahlman B. The benefit of oral English-only as compared with signed input to hearing-impaired students. *Volta Rev* 1988;90:349–361.
17. Miyamoto RT, Osberger MJ, Todd SL, Robbins AM. Speech perception skills of children with multichannel cochlear implants. In: Hochmair-Desoyer I, Hochmair E, eds. *Advances in cochlear implants.* Vienna: Manz, 1994:503–507.
18. Robbins AM, Svirsky MA, Kirk KI. Children with implants can speak, but can they communicate? *Otolaryngol Head Neck Surg* 1997;117:155–160.
19. Waltzman S, Cohen N, Shapiro W. Use of a multichannel cochlear implant in the congenitally and prelingually deaf population. *Laryngoscope* 1992;102:395–399.
20. Reynell JK, Huntley M. *Reynell developmental language scales, revised,* 2nd ed. Windsor, England: NFER Publishing, 1985.
21. Robbins AM, Svirsky MA, Miyamoto RT. Language development. In:

Waltzman S, Cohen N, eds. *Cochlear implants.* New York: Thieme Medical Publishers, (in press).

22. Fryauf-Bertschy H, Tyler RS, Kelsay D, Gantz BJ, Woodworth GG. Cochlear implant use by prelingually deafened children: the influences of age at implant and length of device use. *J Speech Hear Res* 1997;40: 183–199.

23. Carney AE, Moeller MP. Treatment efficacy: hearing loss in children. *J Speech Hear Res* 1998;41:S61–S84.

24. Ross M. *Hard of hearing children in regular schools.* Englewood Cliffs, NJ: Prentice Hall, 1982.

25. Luterman D, Ross M. *When your child is deaf.* Parkton, MD: York Press, 1991.

The Ear: Comprehensive Otology,
edited by R. F. Canalis and P. R. Lambert.
Lippincott Williams & Wilkins, Philadelphia © 2000.

CHAPTER 39

Cochlear Implants

Bruce J. Gantz, Brian P. Perry, and Jay T. Rubinstein

Approximately 1 in 1,000 persons have hearing loss that imposes an obstacle to effective communication. If the loss occurs before the acquisition of speech (prelingual deafness), additional difficulties in reading and language result. Djourno and Eyres in 1957 performed the first studies using electric current to stimulate the auditory nerve in a deaf person. After considerable research, the first portable implant system, complete with a speech processor, was implanted in adults in 1972 at the House Ear Clinic. Twelve years later the U.S. Food and Drug Administration approved clinical use of a single-channel cochlear implant (CI) by adults with postlingual deafness. Rapid advances in implant technology and speech processor design have changed these once experimental devices to a standard form of treatment for profound hearing loss. This tremendous advance toward the elimination of deafness is the treatment of choice of children and adults with postlingual deafness and of children older than 18 months of age with prelingual deafness. Because of their safety and efficacy, CIs are an accepted form of aural rehabilitation for deaf children and adults by the American Medical Association, American Academy of Otolaryngology–Head and Neck Surgery, Medicare and Medicaid, and medical insurers.

    B. J. Gantz, B.P. Perry, and J.T. Rubinstein: Department of Otolaryngology–Head and Neck Surgery, The University of Iowa Hospitals and Clinics, Iowa City, Iowa 52242-1078

COCHLEAR IMPLANT DEVICES

Whereas a hearing aid functions to amplify and filter acoustic energy and deliver it to the external ear, a CI processes sound energy by changing it into electric energy for delivery to the auditory nerve. Most causes of neurosensory deafness are related to hair cell loss, thus the implant replaces the transducer function of the damaged cochlear inner hair cells. Although they continually undergo upgrades and modifications, all currently available CIs have the same basic components, which change an acoustic signal into an electric signal, process it, and deliver the signal to the surviving elements of the auditory nerve (Fig. 1). A microphone receives analog sound and sends it to the speech processor, which converts the sound into a digital electric signal. Processing of the electric signal involves band-pass filtering, amplification (gain control), and compression. Filters are used to separate the information into discrete frequency bands that are delivered to the appropriate regions of the cochlea to provide spectral information about the speech signal. After the gain (level) of the signal is increased, the information must be compressed to fit the narrow dynamic range of electric stimulation. The electric signal is sent by radio frequency from a transmitter coil or through a percutaneous connection through the skin to an internal, implanted receiver-stimulator. The signal is decoded and sent to an electrode array within the scala tympani of the

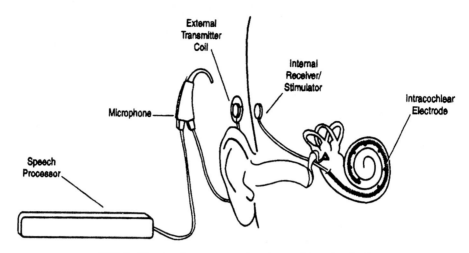

FIG. 1. The basic components of a cochlear implant.

cochlea, which distributes the information to the auditory nerve.

At least two electrodes are needed to complete an electric circuit—an active electrode and a ground electrode. The debate over the superiority of multichannel implants over single-channel implants has been definitively resolved (1–4). Current multichannel devices have 4 to 24 electrodes. Because of its proximity to the osseous spiral lamina and spiral ganglion cells, the electrode array is placed within the scala tympani through a cochleostomy near the round window. Extracochlear electrode placement (positioning on the promontory,

round window, and medial wall of the middle ear) has been shown to be less efficient (5). Electrode placement within the scala vestibuli has been performed and also has been abandoned for being inefficient (6).

Some multichannel CIs can be programmed to function in either a monopolar or bipolar stimulation pattern. In a monopolar paradigm the active electrode is close to the nerve, and the ground electrode is placed farther away to stimulate a larger population of neurons at a lower current level (Fig. 2). The advantages are reduced energy requirements from the speech processor–transmitter and lower current levels within the cochlea. In a bipolar para-

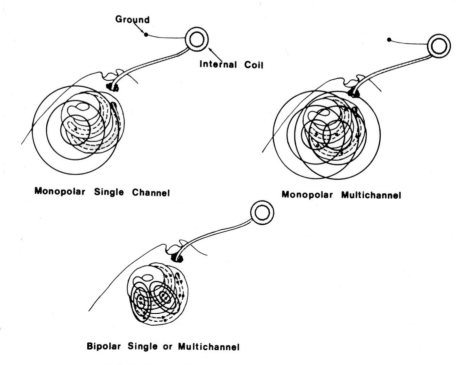

FIG. 2. Monopolar versus bipolar electrode arrays.

digm electrodes are equidistant from the auditory nerve. Theoretically this would stimulate discrete populations of spiral ganglion cells, improve spectral detail, and, one would think, improve word recognition. Clinical evidence for this is lacking however. The electrode pairs may be placed either longitudinally or radially within the cochlea (see Fig. 2). CI-22 and Clarion devices often work with a bipolar strategy, and CI-24 and Med-El devices work on the monopolar paradigm. The energy needed to stimulate small, closely spaced electrodes in a bipolar array is considerably greater than with a monopolar device, requiring patients to change batteries as often as every day.

Three multichannel CI systems are currently being implanted in the United States: the Nucleus, Clarion, and Med-El devices. Whereas the Nucleus (Cochlear Corporation) and Clarion (Advanced Bionics Corporation) devices have been approved for general use by the FDA, the Med-El device is undergoing FDA clinical trials. Still used by some patients but no longer being implanted are the House-3M single-channel system, and the Ineraid percutaneous multichannel system (Smith and Nephew, Richards). For the multichannel systems, the exact number of electrodes may not be as important as the speech-processing strategy. The Nucleus, Clarion, and Med-El systems have multiple electrodes within the scala tympani that deliver temporal and intensity cues by means of varying the rate and pattern of stimulation and the amount of stimulating current. These systems work with a nonsimultaneous stimulation paradigm, which prevents stimulation of more than one channel at a time and reduces channel interaction.

The Nucleus devices (CI-22 and CI-24) are the devices most commonly implanted in the United States. The CI-22 device consists of 22 banded electrodes, which can be programmed into 21 separate bipolar channels. With 24 electrodes, the Nucleus CI-24 device offers both monopolar and bipolar capability with a maximum rate of stimulation of 2400 pulses per second per channel. The Nucleus CI-24 device can work with a variety of speech-processing algorithms, such as spectral peak processing (SPEAK), advanced combination encoding, or continuous interleaved sampling (CIS).

The Advanced Bionics Clarion device was introduced in 1991. The electrode array has eight staggered pairs of electrodes arranged in a radial bipolar configuration. The external processor can be programmed with either the CIS or compressed analog (CA) processing strategies. Both strategies can function in either the monopolar paradigm (the eight medial electrodes are active and referenced to the case of the internal receiver) or the bipolar paradigm (the lateral and medial electrodes make up to eight pairs).

The Med-El device has 16 electrodes in a monopolar array and works by means of the CIS speech-processing strategy. It is used in Europe and is undergoing FDA trials in the United States. Other devices used in Europe are

the Digisonic MXM (France) and the Phillips Laura (Belgium).

SPEECH-PROCESSING STRATEGIES

The development of speech-processing strategies for CIs includes both proprietary and public domain algorithms. The latter were created in university laboratories and ported to commercial devices. The former were created by manufacturers specifically for their products. Early in their history, the proprietary and public domain approaches represented greatly contrasting philosophies and technologies and had little in common. Today they have evolved into highly similar strategies that differ only in details.

The earliest multichannel speech-processing strategy was the CA approach in the Ineraid device developed at the University of Utah. This strategy, based on vocoder technology, is a spectral approach that in the Ineraid involves four band-pass filters that deliver analog signals to each of four monopolar intracochlear electrodes (Fig. 3). Compression is necessary to map the wide dynamic range of the normal acoustic environment onto the limited dynamic range of electric stimulation.

An early competitor of CA was a speech feature extraction approach, the F0F2 strategy of the first device from Cochlear Corporation. This algorithm determined the fundamental frequency or pitch (F0), and second formant of speech (F2). F2 was used to determine which electrode would be activated, and F0 to determine the rate of pulsatile stimulation. F0F2 was subsequently enhanced through the addition of first formant information to F0F1F2 and implemented in the first Cochlear Corporation devices to be widely implanted in the United States. An early study from Iowa demonstrated equivalent speech perception of subjects using the CA strategy on the Ineraid device and F0F1F2 on the Cochlear Corporation CI-22 device (1,7). This was surprising given the radically different speech-processing philosophies represented: analog spectral analysis versus pulsatile feature extraction.

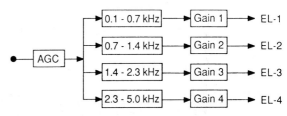

FIG. 3. Block diagram of the main processing steps in the compressed analog speech processing strategy. (From Wilson BS, Finley CC, Lawson DT, Wolford RD, Eddington DK, Rabinowitz WM. Better speech recognition with cochlear implants. *Nature* 1991;352:236–238, with permission from Macmillan Magazines Ltd.)

Subsequent developments at Cochlear Corporation involved a shift toward spectral processing. The MPEAK (multi-PEAK) strategy added spectral information at frequencies above F2. Upgrade studies have failed to prove a significant difference in consonant recognition when changing from F0F1F2 to MPEAK; however, average open-set performance appears modestly better with MPEAK (8–10). The advent of the SPEAK strategy represented the Cochlear Corporation abandonment of feature extraction in favor of spectral analysis. SPEAK is the proprietary version of what is called a *spectral maxima speech processor* (Fig. 4). Six to ten spectral maxima or peaks are identified within the speech signal, and their amplitudes are mapped onto electrodes chosen by the frequency of the maxima. Upgrade studies suggest that SPEAK is superior to MPEAK for most persons (11,12).

While Cochlear Corporation was migrating away from feature extraction to its current spectral processing, CA evolved into its pulsatile offspring, CIS. Work at the Research Triangle Institute in North Carolina and the

Massachusetts Eye and Ear Infirmary sought to solve the problem of current spread and channel interactions through the use of interleaved pulses, whereby pulse amplitude represents the envelope of a band-pass filter output (Fig. 5) (13). Within-subject comparisons suggested that for most subjects with Ineraid devices, CIS was substantially better than CA (14), although it often requires a learning period to demonstrate improved speech reception (15).

The Clarion and Med-El implants both implement a version of the CIS strategy. The Med-El processor supports very high pulse rates, and the Clarion device allows digital emulation of CA, the so-called simultaneous analog strategy. Preliminary studies from the manufacturer suggest that certain patients may prefer and perform better with simultaneous analog strategy. Comparisons of large populations of subjects using the SPEAK strategy on the CI-22 and CI-24 devices versus CIS on the Clarion device are complicated by a number of factors and fail to document a significant difference in speech reception attributable specifically to speech-processing strategy.

Current research suggests that increases in processor rate may yield future performance improvements (14–15). N (filters) of M (electrodes) strategies are being investigated in clinical trials of the CI-24 device. These so-called advanced combination encoders combine theoretic advantages of SPEAK and CIS by implementing SPEAK

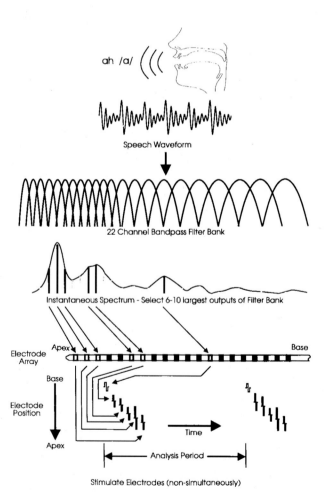

FIG. 4. SPEAK speech-processing strategy. (From Clark GM, Cowan RSC, Dowell RC, eds. *Cochlear implantation for infants and children.* San Diego: Singular Publishing Group, 1997:130, with permission.)

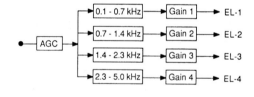

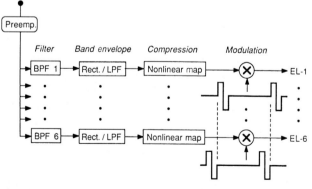

FIG. 5. Comparison between compressed analog and continuous interleaved sampling speech-processing strategies. (From Wilson BS, Finley CC, Lawson DT, Wolford RD, Eddington DK, Rabinowitz WM. Better speech recognition with cochlear implants. *Nature* 1991;352:236–238, with permission from Macmillan Magazines Ltd.)

at higher rates and on more than 6 to 10 channels. The theoretic benefits of higher rates or numbers of channels are being investigated at multiple sites worldwide with transcutaneous devices, proprietary devices, laboratory speech processors, and devices that allow patients percutaneous access to their electrode array. Competition in the implant industry and research funded by the National Institutes of Health are giving patients and clinicians a wider variety of increasingly versatile technologies, which should yield ongoing improvement in auditory perception.

NEURAL RESPONSE TELEMETRY

Newer devices, such as the CI-24, Clarion, and Med-El implants, include an impedance telemetry system. The CI-24 device has the additional capability of recording and transmitting electrically evoked whole-nerve, compound action potentials from the auditory nerve. Measurement of these potentials allows estimation of the recruitment and recovery properties of the residual auditory nerve. Auditory whole-nerve action potentials, as developed by Brown and Abbas (16), can be recorded through the implant. The capability of identifying the functional properties of the residual auditory nerve may allow more precise fitting of the speech-coding algorithm to the individual patient. Auditory nerve action potential measures correlate with speech perception skills with an implant. Good correlations have been observed between the electrically evoked action potential (EAP) threshold and the psychophysical detection threshold and between EAP refractory recovery functions and the psychophysical forward masking functions (17). One interpretation of these findings is that these psychophysical measures are related to the excitability of the auditory nerve to electric stimulation and that these measures are related to CI performance (17). This interpretation is based, presumably, on the number of surviving auditory neurons and the integrity of the fibers. It may be possible to use these techniques to identify different areas within the cochlea that have larger surviving neural populations (18).

Data from studies of the Nucleus CI-24 neural response telemetry system in which EAP threshold was compared with behavioral measures used to program the speech processor are encouraging. It has been shown that EAP thresholds fall within the subject's dynamic range (17). With this device, considerable variations in growth and recovery functions are observed between subjects and between electrodes. This may be indicative of differences in the temporal response capabilities of the stimulated neural population (17). These differences may be evidence of heterogeneity of the neural population caused by variable myelination, dendritic population, and axon integrity of the residual auditory nerve. Ongoing studies of residual auditory nerve function may demonstrate an important method of enhancing perfor-

mance in individual patients and fitting the speech processor.

COCHLEAR IMPLANT SURGERY

Skin flap design is of paramount importance in both children and adults who undergo implant operations. Incisions are placed to provide adequate access and preserve blood supply. Several different skin incisions have been used with success. Proper flap design and delicate handling of soft tissues is critical because flap breakdown is the most common serious complication of CI surgery (19,20). The incision used at The University of Iowa is shown in Figure 6. It provides excellent exposure of the pars squamosa and temporalis muscle insertion and ensures that no incision line overlies the hardware or interferes with an ear-level speech processor. A large Palva flap is made with exposure of the entire mastoid cortex. A posterior extension of the Palva incision is made along the linea temporalis and angled superiorly 3 to 4 cm. This provides a two-layer closure over the receiver-stimulator and mastoid process.

Complete mastoidectomy is performed with preservation of an overhanging ledge of bone in the tegmen mastoideum. The facial recess is opened without preservation of the incus buttress. The round window is located 1.5 cm inferior to the oval window; both windows should be well visualized before cochleostomy (Fig. 7; see color plate 27 following page 484). An appropriately sized well is drilled in the mastoid cortex just posterior to the sinodural angle for the implant to sit securely. Drill holes are made on either side of the well, and 4-0 nylon stay sutures are placed to further secure the implant. Two additional drill holes are made in the tegmen mastoideum overhang for sutures to support the electrode and prevent migration (Fig. 8).

A cochleostomy anteroinferior to the round window membrane is made for placement of the electrode in the

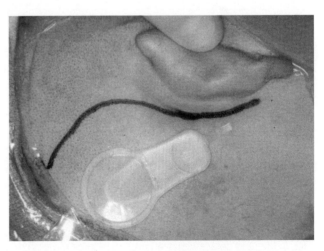

FIG. 6. Scalp incision for cochlear implant operation.

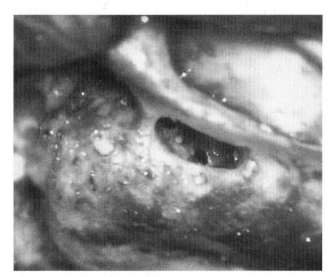

FIG. 7. Round window exposure through a facial recess approach, right ear.

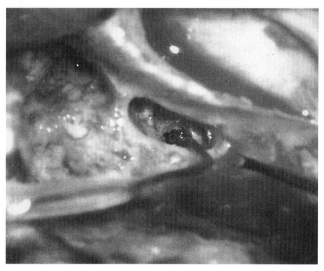

FIG. 9. Placement of a cochlear implant electrode through round window into scala tympani.

scala tympani. Bony or fibrous cochlear obstruction may be encountered in patients who have had meningitis, labyrinthitis, otosclerosis, or trauma. Surgical techniques to overcome this problem have been described in great detail (6,21,22). The electrode array is passed into the cochleostomy (Fig. 9; see color plate 28 following page 484). The Clarion electrode is precoiled and has a larger diameter than does the Nucleus device. A special insertion tool has been designed to allow easy insertion of the electrode into the scala tympani. The Clarion device does require a larger facial recess and cochleostomy to allow the inserter tube access to the scala tympani. This has not resulted in complications or decreased performance. The goal should always be complete insertion of all active and stiffening electrodes. A fascia or muscle plug is used to close the cochleostomy.

Sutures are placed to secure both the electrode and the receiver to the mastoid. The ground electrode of the

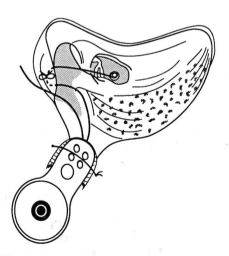

FIG. 8. Mastoid defect with overhanging tegmen mastoideum for support suture placement. Securing suture is placed over receiver.

Nucleus CI-24 system is placed under the temporalis muscle toward the zygoma. The extended Palva flap is used to cover the receiver and the mastoid defect. The wound is closed in two layers over a Penrose drain, and a mastoid dressing is applied. The patient receives perioperative antibiotics for 7 days.

CIs have been placed in children and adults with inner ear abnormalities. The only absolute contraindications are agenesis of the inner ear (Michel syndrome) and absence of the cochlear nerve (23). Cochlear implantation has been successful in management of both Mondini deformity (24) and common cavities (25). Careful attention to the facial nerve is required in these congenital disorders because of the high rate of dehiscence and possible aberrancy; facial nerve monitoring is essential in these situations.

Successful implantation has been performed in children younger than 18 months. Special attention must be given to skull thickness and the position of the facial nerve. By 1 year of age the anatomy of the mastoid process, facial recess, and inner ear of children is similar to that of adults in terms of size and location. Careful removal of bone with a diamond bur is critical in operations on young children, because dural exposure is necessary for secure seating of the receiver-stimulator in most instances.

Insertion of a CI into an obstructed and obliterated cochlea necessitates a different technique (21). Radical mastoidectomy is performed with removal of the posterior canal wall, tympanic membrane, malleus, and incus. The external auditory canal is oversewn, the middle ear mucosa removed, and the eustachian tube obliterated. To reduce pain on stimulation, Jacobson's nerve is eliminated. The round window niche is removed for complete visualization of the window and annulus. The bone within the obliterated scala tympani is white compared with the yellow bone of the otic capsule. With care not to disturb the modiolus, a trough is made in the cochlea with a diamond bur. A 22 to 24 mm trough is drilled after the first and part of the second cochlear turns. The multichannel electrode is coiled around the stump of the modiolus while small chips of bone are used to secure the implant, and a large piece of temporalis fascia is draped over the area. The electrode is anchored and the internal receiver-stimulator secured as in routine implant procedures.

COMPLICATIONS OF COCHLEAR IMPLANTATION

The complications associated with cochlear implantation fortunately are few, and those that do occur tend to be related to aspects of the operation that are least frequently performed by the surgeon. Cohen et al. (19,26) reviewed the complications associated with the Nucleus device. The complications associated with the other devices are similar (Table 1).

Serious complications of CI surgery are rare and often are related to the experience of the surgeon (27). Implant extrusion and infection should be rare, but when either occurs, it can be devastating for a patient who has regained useful hearing (20). Several flap designs are used for cochlear implantation. We use an inverted J incision with a very low rate of flap complications. Before use of this flap, the original C-shaped incision was used in more than 250 operations without skin breakdown. Soft-tissue technique must be meticulous to preserve blood supply to the flap. Other complications, such as facial nerve injuries, are uncommon. In a review by Cohen and Hoffman (18), all complications were temporary with the exception of one nerve transection in an ear with a congenital anomaly that required nerve grafting. Lack of reliability of implant hardware is one of the most common complications; manufacturers continue to eliminate design flaws and improve hardware construction materials. Although new bone growth around the cochleostomy and fibrous tissue growth in the facial recess and basal turn of the cochlea have been found during reimplantation operations, the audiologic results are equal or better with the second device (28,29). Definitive technologic improvements often justify revision surgery to upgrade the device (3).

Minor complications of cochlear implantation are as uncommon as serious complications. They include electrode migration, facial nerve stimulation, perilymphatic gusher, dizziness, and tinnitus (19). The rate of these

complications combined is less than 5%. Facial nerve stimulation is not a surgical complication but is a result of current flow. It usually is associated with instances of otosclerosis in which the otic capsule is less dense. Perilymphatic gusher is uncommon in implant operations; with firm packing of the cochleostomy site the leak is sealed permanently. Postoperative dizziness is uncommon and generally abates within several days.

That trauma to the inner ear can be caused by insertion of a CI has been well established (30–33). Placement of an electrode array within the scala tympani injures the spiral ligament, Reissner's membrane, stria vascularis, basilar membrane, and the organ of Corti. No damage to the modiolus housing the spiral ganglion is typically observed. Because the membranous cochlea is severely dysfunctional before implantation, the degree of damage may not be clinically significant (28). Concern remains that damage to the basilar membrane in animals causes degeneration of the spiral ganglion (34).

AUDIOLOGIC CRITERIA

Adults

Cochlear implantation is limited to persons with bilateral profound deafness, although the selection criteria continue to evolve as hardware and software become more reliable in improving speech understanding. The average hearing thresholds for pure tones at 500 Hz, 1 kHz, and 2 kHz should be 90 dB or poorer. If speech is detected at 65 dB sound pressure level (SPL) or better, a series of comprehensive speech perception tests are performed bilaterally (best-aided condition) in a sound field at 65 dB SPL. A comprehensive hearing aid evaluation is performed. If speech is not detected in a sound field with the assistance of an appropriately fit hearing aid, the patient is considered an audiologic candidate. Persons who can understand some speech in the test conditions are still considered candidates if they score less than 40% on the Iowa (35), Central Institute for the Deaf (CID) (36), or Banford-Kowal-Bench sentence tests (37) or less than 10% on monosyllabic word tests. Each of the sentence tests is a representation of everyday spoken English. Patients must recognize key words in each sentence. The results are reported as percentage of key words correctly identified (e.g., Where are you going?). Monosyllabic word tests are phonemically balanced words that occur frequently in spoken English (e.g., *cat*).

Successful restoration of speech reception in adults has been limited to persons with postlingual deafness (acquired after having learned spoken language). CIs placed in adults with prelingual deafness have provided sound awareness and enhanced speech-reading ability; however, open-set word understanding has not been achieved in this group (38). Apparently if the central auditory pathways are not stimulated (electrically or acoustically) before puberty, central neural processing of auditory information is not possible with available technology.

TABLE 1. *Complications of cochlear implantation*

Complication	Adults (%) (n = 3,064)	Children (%) (n = 1,905)
Flap related	3.46	1.6
Device failure	2.5	3.6
Implant extrusion	1.2	0.2
Electrode migration	1.2	1.3
Facial nerve injury	0.6	0.6
Meningitis	0.03	0.05

Children

In children, contributing factors such as age at onset and identification of the hearing loss, amount of residual hearing, communication mode, and family involvement affect the development of verbal communication with an implant. Consistent use of amplification and early identification of hearing loss are essential in the development of auditory skills. Teenagers with congenital deafness who have never used amplification find sound not useful and possibly even distracting while communicating. If given early amplification, these children may develop the advanced auditory skills necessary for speech comprehension. The amount of residual hearing possessed by a child with profound deafness also affects auditory potential. Some children retain hearing within the speech frequencies, whereas others may not have any speech detection at any frequency with amplification. Children with some residual hearing may detect segmental (vowel and consonant) cues and suprasegmental (duration and intensity) cues of speech.

Three basic educational environments have been developed for children with profound hearing loss: auditory-oral, bilingual-bicultural, and total communication. The *auditory-oral* approach emphasizes spoken language only. With early amplification, this strategy usually is selected for children with severe hearing losses. The *bilingual-bicultural* strategy teaches the child American Sign Language as the primary method of communication, and reading and writing English are secondary. Proponents of this system align themselves with the deaf community. A reduced English-reading comprehension level is the norm for those educated in this system. *Total communication* is the most common educational system in the United States for deaf children. Total communication involves all communication modalities, including speech, signs, gestures, finger spelling, speech reading, reading, and writing. This strategy maximizes the residual auditory information the child can receive. Total communication incorporates signed English with simultaneous speech; this cannot be done with American Sign Language because it has no verbal correlate. Proponents of total communication believe that it leads to better competence with the English language. If cochlear implantation is to be considered, auditory-oral and total communication education with a strong emphasis on oral communication and early amplification are thought to be essential. A strong family commitment to oral rehabilitation is important to successful outcome with a CI.

Auditory criteria for cochlear implantation in children continue to evolve and may vary from center to center depending on participation in FDA trials of expanded criteria. Similar to adult candidates, profound hearing loss among children is defined by a pure tone average greater than 90 dB hearing level (HL) at 500, 1,000, and 2,000 Hz (39). In general children must be 18 months of age and have undergone extensive hearing aid evaluation and

a trial with an aid. The hearing aid trial ensures that speech recognition test results are accurate and allows for evaluation of improvement with an aid. Use of tactile devices is no longer encouraged, the results having been proved inferior to results with a CI (40–42).

The focus of the audiologic assessment is to evaluate the child's aided speech recognition ability with either open-set or closed-set tests, depending on the child's age and language skills, presented by means of audiotape (43). A child unable to detect speech at 60 dB HL or greater with an appropriately fitted hearing aid should be considered a candidate for an implant. If some speech detection at 60 dB HL is present, further testing is needed. Open-set speech recognition tests, such as Phonetically Balanced Kindergarten Words (PBK) or the Lexical Neighbor Test, should be used to assess candidates for CIs. The limited language and cognitive skills of some children often preclude the use of these measures and necessitate closed-set tests such as the Word Intelligibility by Picture Identification (44) or Early Speech Perception Test four choice spondees (45). The discrimination after training test without training (46) or the CID low verbal test battery are used for children with less sophisticated language skills. Children who score less than 20% on an open-set measure of word recognition and less than 40% on an open-set measure of sentence recognition (e.g., CID everyday sentences) with appropriate hearing aids are candidates for CIs. Children who do not score above chance on two closed-set tests appropriate for the child's language skills and cognitive abilities should also be considered candidates for implants.

ADDITIONAL SELECTION CONSIDERATIONS

A history of chronic otitis media or recurrent acute otitis media should be sought from the patient during the implant evaluation; however, neither is a contraindication to surgical treatment. If chronic ear disease is quiescent, the mastoid process and middle ear can be obliterated during the implant procedure. The presence of active ear disease necessitates medical or surgical attention before implantation. In children, pressure equalization tubes have been placed postoperatively without complications. Some surgeons believe, however, that obliteration of the ear is a better solution to the problem (47). Existing, draining mastoid cavities must be obliterated before placement of an implant.

There is no significant relation between the cause of deafness and audiologic success with a CI. The exception can be meningitis with resultant cochlear ossification and near-total loss of auditory nerve ganglion cells. Nadol and Hsu (48) showed that a higher percentage of auditory neural depletion is associated with labyrinthitis ossificans. This is one of the few indications for promontory stimulation testing to determine whether a patient perceives sound. Lack of response still is not a contraindication to surgical treatment. Other indications for promontory stimulation are deafness due to temporal bone fracture, intracranial operation, or head trauma to determine whether the auditory nerve is intact.

A history of otosclerosis or previous stapedectomy should alert the surgeon that the cochlear anatomy might be distorted with obliteration of the round window niche. These conditions cause a loss of anatomic landmarks needed to locate a cochleostomy. Stimulation of the facial nerve by the electrode array might also be caused by demineralization of the otic capsule. Hearing loss after stapedectomy might result in intracochlear fibrosis, which might be encountered during implantation. Intracochlear bony or fibrous growth is not a contraindication to implantation; if present in the basal turn only, it can be removed through the routine surgical approach (22). Extensive ossification might necessitate a circumodiolar drill-out procedure (21).

All candidates for cochlear implantation should undergo high-resolution computed tomography of the temporal bones to identify any inner ear abnormalities (49). The only absolute radiologic contraindications to implantation are Michel syndrome (absence of the cochlea) and absence of the auditory nerve (seen as a narrow internal auditory canal containing only the facial nerve). Congenital malformations such as Mondini dysplasia and common cavity deformity are not contraindications to implantation. These abnormalities should alert the surgeon to the possibility of a perilymph gusher during the procedure, and the parents should be cautioned about the chance of a limited hearing outcome (24,25). Imaging studies might help to detect intracochlear ossification and fibrosis; however, the amount of obstruction usually cannot be ascertained (50). Magnetic resonance imaging can provide additional information about cochlear patency, reduced cochlear fluid content, and the presence of fibrosis but cannot ensure cochlear patency.

The patient interview should determine any medical conditions that might result in a poor outcome with a CI. General medical health should be assessed with regard to the ability to undergo general anesthesia. A detailed account of the history of hearing loss is important to determine which ear heard sound most recently; this ear should receive the implant if all other factors are equal. A congenitally deaf ear in an adult with postlingual deafness should not receive an implant. Evidence suggests that these ears perform similarly to those of adults with prelingual deafness (38,51). The physical examination should focus on any active or inactive chronic ear disease that might have to be addressed either before or during the operation.

RESULTS OF COCHLEAR IMPLANTATION

Evaluating of users of CIs has been modified from traditional audiologic assessment because existing test materials often were too difficult. In some instances, tests were used so frequently that patients soon learned the appropriate responses. Tyler (43) demonstrated that testing requires special age- and language-dependent test materials for children. A battery of tests of varying difficulty should be administered to assess the temporal and intonation patterns of speech and to evaluate speechreading enhancement. Speech perception material should be presented from standardized audio- or videotapes.

Adults with Postlingual Deafness

Considerable data have proved the efficacy of CIs in adults with postlingual deafness (1,10,52). Multichannel implant strategies have been shown to provide these patients with more auditory information than single-channel devices in comparative studies (1) and a prospective randomized trial (2). As speech coding strategies have advanced, results on open-set sentence and monosyllabic word tests have improved among users of multichannel implants. Initial prospective, randomized clinical trials of the four-channel Ineraid device (CA coding) and the Nucleus CI-22 implant (feature extraction, F0F1F2 coding) demonstrated an average open-set sentence score of 30% to 38% after 9 months of device experience (53). The same study demonstrated monosyllabic Northwestern University Test 6 (NU-6) word score averages between 9% and 12%. Performance was evaluated at 3.5 years of use for the same patients. Individual performance varied greatly for both implant groups, from approximately 10% to 85%; mean scores were 49% for the Ineraid patients and 44.4% for the Nucleus patients (7). Results of sentence tests ranged from 0 to 100%, and NU-6 performance ranged from 10% to 60%. Although average scores of 14% to 20% word recognition and 43% to 49% word recognition in sentences are a real change in communication ability, considerable disability remained (7).

Speech scores improved among adults with postlingual deafness with implementation of the CIS speech-coding strategy of the Clarion device and the SPEAK strategy of the Nucleus CI-22 device. After only 9 months of experience with the Clarion device, patients had an average performance comparable with or superior to that of users of Ineraid and Nucleus CI-22 (F0F1F2 coding) devices with more than 36 months of experience (54). The average sentence score for the Clarion CIS implant were shown to be approximately 65% and for NU-6 word scores to be 30% to 38% (55,56). Similar results were obtained with the Nucleus CI-22 implant with the SPEAK speech-coding strategy (57). The average monosyllabic word score with 3 to 6 months of experience with SPEAK on the Nucleus CI-22 and CI-24 devices currently is 48% among the last 46 persons who received implants (4).

Two preoperative variables have been identified as predictive of outcome with a CI: duration of deafness and preoperative sentence recognition (4,53). Duration of deafness has long been the best individual predictor of postoperative speech reception (53) and spiral ganglion survival (58). Each additional year of profound deafness results in a nearly 1% decrease in expected postoperative Consonant-Nucleus-Consonant (CNC) word recognition (4). Although much of the improvement in speech perception scores that has occurred in the past 15 years is attributable to advances in speech-processing strategy, it must be remembered that the implant inclusion criteria have been broadened to include persons with residual hearing. Persons who have received implants within the last 5 years have had much more residual hearing than those who received implants in the 1980s.

Preoperative sentence recognition is predictive of postoperative CI results. For each additional 2% of preoperative CID sentence recognition, an increase of 1% CNC word recognition is expected postoperatively (4). The ability to understand speech presumably necessitates a larger proportion of surviving spiral ganglion cells, or a more intact central auditory pathway. The residual inner hair cells may protect the spiral ganglion from the deleterious effects of a long duration of deafness (4). The improved performance of these patients with new implants may be directly related to the greater number of surviving auditory neurons. To a lesser degree, cognitive ability and speech-reading ability have an effect on implant performance (53). A likely source for these variations is the amount of residual auditory nerve function; ongoing studies at our institution are seeking to test this hypothesis.

Adults with Prelingual Deafness

A small number of adult implant recipients have either congenital or very early onset of hearing loss. These patients have a very long period of auditory deprivation. Outcomes of implantation reveal consistent effects of deprivation evidenced by significant negative correlations between accuracy of speech perception and duration of profound deafness before implantation (51). At The University of Iowa, adults with prelingual deafness rarely receive implants. Implantation among this group is for awareness of environmental sounds.

Children with Postlingual Deafness

Children who have lost hearing after the acquisition of spoken language (usually after 3 years of age) are categorized as having postlingual deafness. These children have been shown to derive considerable improvement in speech perception scores within the first year of implant use (59). In most instances, their speech perception skills are at the upper end of adult performance curves for sentence and monosyllabic word understanding. Average score on the monosyllable trochee spondee word understanding test was 85% for this group after 1 year and 100% after 3 years of implant experience (59). By 3 years after implantation, results of the word recognition tests also were 100% among these children. This study also demonstrated that children attain rapid improvement dur-

ing the first 6 months of implant use and continue to improve their speech perception skills beyond 2 years of experience, which is in contrast to the situation for adult users, whose scores plateau during the second year (59). It is likely that the short duration of deafness and a young, adaptive central nervous system are responsible for the outstanding results. Other variables that affect a child's performance with an implant include the child's rehabilitation, personality, level of parental and educational support, and motivation to use oral language (60).

Children with Prelingual Deafness

Cochlear implantation in children with congenital prelingual deafness has raised the greatest controversy with the deaf community. Proponents of implantation for this group claim that the device has a dramatic effect on improving the acquisition and use of spoken language by deaf children and has subsequent social and psychological benefits (61). Opponents in the deaf community suggest that the CI deprives the deaf child of his or her deaf culture and does not provide enough sound information to make the child accepted by the hearing world (62). Although children with prelingual deafness respond differently to CIs, many studies have found very high levels of speech perception performance after 2 years of implantation (59,63–66). Progress might be slow and often not evident for a year or more. Parents must be aware of this possibility before implantation. Parental involvement in rehabilitation is an important variable that contributes to the successful use of CIs. Other variables that affect performance include the child's age at onset of deafness, length of auditory deprivation, age at implantation, mode of communication, and method of rehabilitation (67).

All children at The University of Iowa undergo rehabilitation by means of total communication. A wide range of performance has been demonstrated among children with prelingual deafness who use CIs. Vowel, consonant, and phoneme recognition usually is poor during the first year of use, but with increased experience, substantial improvement occurs. Unlike adults, children may continue to improve for as long as 8 years after implantation. Open-set word recognition is unlikely during the first 1 to 2 years of use. After 4 years, 85% of these children can understand some speech in a sound-only condition (59). Five years after implantation some children correctly identify 86% of phonemes (67). Improvements in expressive and receptive language skills after cochlear implantation have been well documented (68).

Electrophysiologic data obtained during implantation from children with deafness due to meningitis and congenital causes are quite different. Cochlear nerve recovery functions are slower and growth of amplitude input-output functions is more shallow among patients with meningitis (59). These measures suggest poorer auditory nerve survival and function among children with deafness caused by meningitis. Preliminary results demonstrate that children with congenital prelingual deafness perform on speech perception tests at the same level as or a higher level than children with acquired prelingual deafness due to meningitis (69).

It has been shown that children with prelingual deafness up to the age of 14 years have benefited from CIs (69). Children before the age of 8 years perform at a higher level than those who receive implants at a later age (70). Children who receive implants before the age of 4 years have demonstrated the greatest improvement (71). Results of PBK word tests demonstrate that children who receive implants before 5 years of age ultimately are able to use audition only to repeat words, whereas children who receive implants after 5 years of age rarely score better than 20% on this task (67). Long-term follow-up study with these children indicates that most children derive benefit from their implant for speech perception tasks. Those who do not achieve high test scores might still benefit from recognition of their name, awareness of communication, and awareness of environmental sounds (67). As has been demonstrated with adults, children with hearing loss in the severe to profound range receive considerable benefit from an implant. Thirteen children with substantial residual hearing (mean 17% PBK) had considerable enhancement in speech perception (mean 75% PBK open-set test) after implantation (72).

PROFESSIONAL RESPONSIBILITY

Physicians and audiologists interested in CIs must be trained in each implant device they wish to provide to their patients. Different equipment is required for each implant, including hardware, software, and surgical instruments. Appropriate space for programming, testing, and rehabilitation is critical. At least one dedicated audiologist is essential for any CI program to effectively treat patients. In-depth knowledge of the rehabilitation of persons with severe to profound deafness is required because most patients undergoing implant evaluation are not appropriate candidates because of residual hearing ability. These patients need extensive hearing aid evaluation and fitting and procurement of assistive listening devices. Surgeons who perform cochlear implantation are responsible for the total rehabilitation of their patients.

CONCLUSION

The reliability and performance of CIs and the indications for the use of these devices have broadened substantially over the past 15 years. Cochlear implantation is the treatment of choice of profoundly deaf children and of adults with postlingual deafness. Improvements in speech processing and device programming are continuing to expand the use of this technology. In the future, electronic speech processing may become a management strategy for less severe hearing loss; it is the only way to improve speech discrimination.

SUMMARY POINTS

- A CI replaces the transducer function of the cochlear inner hair cells by changing sound energy into electric energy for delivery to the auditory nerve.
- The devices currently used in the United States (Nucleus, Clarion, Med-El) have multiple electrodes that are placed within the scala tympani to deliver temporal and intensity cues by varying the rate and pattern of stimulation and the amount of stimulating current.
- Comparisons of large populations of subjects using the SPEAK speech-processing strategy of Nucleus devices and the CIS strategy of Clarion and Med-El devices do not document a significant difference in speech reception specifically attributable to speech-processing strategy.
- The capability of identifying the functional properties of the residual auditory nerve by means of neural response telemetry devices may allow more precise fitting of the speech-coding strategy to the individual patient.
- The only absolute contraindications to cochlear implantation are aplasia of the inner ear (Michel syndrome) and absence of the cochlear nerve.
- Serious complications of CI surgery are rare, and those that occur often are related to the experience of the surgeon.
- Adults with postlingual deafness are eligible for cochlear implantation if they score less than 40% on sentence tests or less than 10% on monosyllabic word tests.
- Children who score less than 20% on an open-set measure of word recognition and less than 40% on an open-set measure of sentence recognition with appropriate hearing aids are candidates for a CI.
- The average monosyllabic word score among adults with postlingual deafness with 3 to 6 months of experience using SPEAK is 48%.
- Average monosyllabic trochee spondee word understanding is 85% after 1 year and 100% after 3 years of experience among children with postlingual deafness.
- Children with prelingual deafness correctly identify 86% of phonemes after 5 years of experience with a CI.

REFERENCES

1. Gantz BJ, Tyler RS, Knutson JF, et al. Evaluation of 5 different cochlear implant designs. *Laryngoscope* 1988;98:1100–1106.
2. Cohen NL, Rosenberg R, Goldstein S. A prospective, randomized study of cochlear implants. *N Engl J Med* 1993:328:233–237.

3. Rubinstein JT, Parkinson WS, Lowder MW, Gantz BJ, Nadol JB, Tyler RS. Single-channel to multichannel conversions in adult cochlear implant subjects. *Am J Otol* 1998;19:461–466.

4. Rubinstein JT, Parkinson WS, Tyler RS, Gantz BJ. Residual speech recognition and cochlear implant performance: effects of implantation criteria. *Am J Otol* 1999;20:445–452.

5. Gantz BJ. Cochlear implants: an overview. *Adv Otolaryngol Head Neck Surg* 1987;1:171–200.

6. Steenerson RL, Gary LB, Wynens MS. Scala vestibuli cochlear implantation for labyrinthine ossification. *Am J Otol* 1990;11:360–363.

7. Tyler RS, Lowder MW, Parkinson AJ, Woodworth GG, Gantz BJ. Performance of adult Ineraid and Nucleus cochlear implant patients after 3.5 years of use. *Audiology* 1995;34:135–144.

8. Skinner MW, Holden LK, Holden TA, et al. Performance of postlinguistically deaf adults with the wearable speech processor (WSP III) and the mini speech processor (MSP) of the nucleus multi-electrode cochlear implant. *Ear Hear* 1991;12:3–22.

9. Parkinson AJ, Tyler RS, Woodworth GG, Lowder MW, Gantz BJ. A within-subject comparison of adult patients using the Nucleus F0F1F2 and F0F1F2B3B4B5 speech processing strategies. *J Speech Hear Res* 1996;39:261–277.

10. Waltzman SB, Cohen NL, Fisher S. An experimental comparison of cochlear implant systems. *Semin Hear* 1992;13:195–207.

11. Skinner MW, Clark GM, Seligman PM, et al. Evaluation of a new spectral peak coding strategy for the Nucleus 22 cochlear implant system. *Am J Otol* 1994;15:15–27.

12. Holden LK, Skinner MW, Holden TA. Speech recognition with the MPEAK and SPEAK speech coding strategies of the Nucleus cochlear implant. *Otolaryngol Head Neck Surg* 1997;116:163–167.

13. White MW, Merzenich MM, Gardi JN. Multichannel cochlear implants: channel interactions and processor design. *Arch Otolaryngol* 1984;110:493–501.

14. Wilson BS, Finley CC, Lawson DT, Wolford RD, Eddington DK, Rabinowitz WM. Better speech recognition with cochlear implants. *Nature* 1991;352:236–238.

15. Eddington DK. Third quarterly progress report: NIH contract N01-DC-6-2100—speech processors for auditory prostheses, neural prosthesis program. Bethesda, Md: National Institutes of Health, 1996.

16. Brown CJ, Abbas PJ, Gantz BJ. Electrically evoked whole nerve action potentials: data from human cochlear implant users. *J Acoust Soc Am* 1990;88:1385–1391.

17. Brown CJ, Abbas PJ, Gantz BJ. Auditory nerve potentials recorded using the neural response telemetry system of the Nucleus CI-24 cochlear implant: preliminary data. *Am J Otol* 1998;19:320–327.

18. Gantz BJ, Brown CJ, Abbas PJ. Intraoperative measures of electrically evoked auditory nerve compound action potential. *Am J Otol* 1994;15:137–144.

19. Cohen NL, Hoffman RA. Complications in cochlear implant surgery in adults and children. *Ann Otol Rhinol Laryngol* 1991;100:708–711.

20. Rubinstein JT, Gantz BJ, Parkinson WS. Management of cochlear implant infections. *Am J Otol* 1999;20:46–49.

21. Gantz BJ, McCabe BF, Tyler RS. Use of multichannel cochlear implants in obstructed and obliterated cochleas. *Otolaryngol Head Neck Surg* 1988;98:72–81.

22. Balkany T, Gantz B, Nadol J. Multichannel cochlear implants in partially ossified cochleas. *Ann Otol Rhinol Laryngol* 1988;97[Suppl 135]:3–7.

23. Shelton C, Luxford WM, Tonokawa LL, Lo WW, House WF. The narrow internal auditory canal in children: a contraindication to cochlear implants. *Otolaryngol Head Neck Surg* 1989;100:227–231.

24. Miyamoto RT, Robbins AJ, Myres WA, Pope ML. Cochlear implantation in the Mondini inner ear malformation. *Am J Otol* 1986;7:258–261.

25. Jackler RK, Luxford WM, House WF. Sound detection with the cochlear implant in five ears of four children with congenital malformations of the cochlea. *Laryngoscope* 1987;97[Suppl 40]:15–17.

26. Cohen NL, Hoffman RA, Stroschein M. Medical and surgical complications related to the Nucleus multichannel cochlear implant. *Ann Otol Rhinol Laryngol* 1988;97:8–13.

27. Hoffman RA, Cohen NL. Complications of cochlear implant surgery. *Ann Otol Rhinol Laryngol* 1995;104[Suppl]:420–422.

28. Gantz BJ, Lowder MW, McCabe BF. Audiological results following reimplantation of cochlear implants. *Ann Otol Rhinol Laryngol* 1989;98[Suppl 142]:12–16.

29. Woolford TJ, Saeed SR, Boyd P, Hartley C, Ramsden RT. Cochlear reimplantation. *Ann Otol Rhinol Laryngol* 1995;104[Suppl 166]:449–453.

30. Linthicum FH, Fayad J, Otto SR, et al. Cochlear implant histopathology. *Am J Otol* 1991;12:245–311.

31. Shepherd RK, Clark G, Pyman BC, et al. Banded intracochlear electrode array: evaluation of insertional trauma in human temporal bones. *Ann Otol Rhinol Laryngol* 1985;94:55–59.

32. Kennedy DW. Multichannel intracochlear electrodes: mechanisms of insertional trauma. *Laryngoscope* 1987;97:42–49.

33. Welling DB, Hinojosa R, Gantz BJ, Lee JT. Insertional trauma of multichannel cochlear implants. *Laryngoscope* 1993;103:995–1001.

34. Leake PA, Snyder RL, Hradek GT. Spatial organization of the inner hair cells synapses and cochlear spiral ganglion neurons. *J Comp Neurol* 1993;333:257–270.

35. Tyler RS, Preece JH, Tye-Murray N. The laser video disc sentence test, laser videodisc. Iowa City, Ia: The University of Iowa Department of Otolaryngology–Head and Neck Surgery, 1986.

36. Silverman SR, Hirsh IJ. Problems related to the use of speech in clinical audiometry. *Ann Otol Rhinol Laryngol* 1955;64:1234–1244.

37. Bench J, Bamford J. *Speech-hearing tests and the spoken language of hearing-impaired children.* London: Academic Press, 1979.

38. Zwolan TA, Kileny P, Telian SA. Self report of cochlear implant use and satisfaction by prelingually deafened adults. *Ear Hear* 1996;17:198–210.

39. Boothroyd A. Profound deafness. In: Tyler RS, ed. *Cochlear implants: audiological foundations.* San Diego: Singular Publishing Group, 1993:1–34.

40. Hesketh LJ, Fryauf-Bertschy H, Osberger MJ. Evaluation of a tactile aid and a cochlear implant in one child. *Am J Otol* 1991;12:182–186.

41. Geers AE, Moog JS. Evaluating the benefits of cochlear implants in an educational setting. *Am J Otol* 1991;12[Suppl]:116–125.

42. Osberger MJ, Robbins AM, Miyamoto RT, et al. Speech perception abilities of children with cochlear implants, tactile aids, or hearing aids. *Am J Otolaryngol* 1991;12:105–115.

43. Tyler RS. Speech perception in children. In: Tyler RS, ed. *Cochlear implants: audiological foundations.* San Diego: Singular Publishing Group, 1993:191–256.

44. Ross M, Lerman J. *Word intelligibility by picture identification.* Pittsburgh: Stanwix House, 1971.

45. Moog JS, Geers AE. *Early speech perception test.* St. Louis: Central Institute for the Deaf, 1990.

46. Thielemeir MA. *Discrimination after training test.* Los Angeles: House Ear Institute, 1982.

47. Donnelly MJ, Pyman BC, Clark GM. Chronic middle ear disease and cochlear implantation. *Ann Otol Rhinol Laryngol* 1995;104[Suppl 166]:406–408.

48. Nadol JB, Hsu W. Histopathologic correlation of spiral ganglion cell count and new bone formation in the cochlea following meningogenic labyrinthitis and deafness. *Ann Otol Rhinol Laryngol* 1991;100:712–716.

49. Yune HY, Miyamoto RT, Yune ME. Medical imaging in cochlear implant candidates. *Am J Otol* 1991;12:11–17.

50. Jackler RK, et al. Cochlear patency problems in cochlear implantation. *Laryngoscope* 1987;97:801–805.

51. Tyler RS, Summerfield AQ. Cochlear implantation: relationships with research on auditory deprivation and acclimation. *Ear Hear* 1996;17:38–50.

52. Tyler RS, Lowder MW. Audiological management and performance of adult cochlear implant patients. *Ear Nose Throat J* 1992;71:117–128.

53. Gantz BJ, Woodworth GG, Abbas PJ, Knutson JF, Tyler RS. Multivariate predictors of audiological success with multichannel cochlear implants. *Ann Otol Rhinol Laryngol* 1993;102:909–916.

54. Gantz BJ, Tyler RS, Woodworth GG. Preliminary results with the Clarion cochlear implant in postlingually deafened adults. *Ann Otol Rhinol Laryngol* 1995;104:268–269.

55. Tyler RS, Gantz RS, Woodworth GG, Parkinson AJ, Lowder MW, Schum LK. Initial independent results with the Clarion cochlear implant. *Ear Hear* 1996;17:528–536.

56. Schindler RA, Kessler DK. Clarion cochlear implant: phase 1 investigational results. *Am J Otol* 1993;14:263–272.

57. Hollow RD, Dowell RC, Cowan RSC, Skok MC, Pyman BC, Clark GM. Continuing improvements in speech processing for cochlear implant patients. *Ann Otol Rhinol Laryngol* 1995;104[Suppl 166]:292–294.

58. Nadol JB Jr, Young YS, Glynn RJ. Survival of spiral ganglion cells in profound sensorineural hearing loss: implications for cochlear implantation. *Ann Otol Rhinol Laryngol* 1989;98:411–416.

59. Gantz BJ, Tyler RS, Woodworth GG, Tye-Murray N, Fryauf-Bertschy H. Results of multichannel cochlear implants in congenital and acquired prelingual deafness in children: five year follow-up. *Am J Otol* 1994;15[Suppl 2]:1–7.

60. Fryauf-Bertschy H. Pediatric cochlear implantation: an update. *Am J Audiol* 1993;2(3):13–16.

61. Osberger MJ, Maso M, Sam L. Speech intelligibility of children with cochlear implants, tactile aids, or hearing aids. *J Speech Hear Res* 1993;36:186–202.

62. Lane, H. Cochlear implants: boon for some—bane for others. *Hear Health* 1993;9(2):19–23.

63. Waltzman SB, Cohen NL, Gomolin RH, Shapiro WH, Ozdamar SR, Hoffman RA. Long term results of early cochlear implantation in congenitally and prelingually deafened children. *Am J Otol* 1994; 15[Suppl]:9–13.

64. Miyamoto RT, Osberger MJ, Robbins AM, Myres WA, Kessler K. Prelingually deafened children's performance with the Nucleus multichannel cochlear implant. *Am J Otol* 1993;14:437–445.

65. Shea JJ, Domico EH, Lupfer M. Speech perception after multichannel cochlear implantation in the pediatric patient. *Am J Otol* 1993;15:66–70.

66. Staller SJ, Beiter AL, Brimacombe JA, Mecklenburg DJ, Arndt P. Pediatric performance with the Nucleus 22 channel cochlear implant system. *Am J Otol* 1991;12:126–136.

67. Fryauf-Bertschy H, Tyler RS, Kelsay DMR, Gantz BJ, Woodworth GG. Cochlear implant use by prelingually deafened children: the influences of age at implant and length of device use. *J Speech Lang Hear Res* 1997;40:183–199.

68. Robbins AM, Osberger MJ, Miyamoto RT, Kessler KS. Language development in young children with cochlear implants. Paper presented at the Second European Symposium on Pediatric Cochlear Implantation; May 26–28, 1994; Montpellier, France.

69. Gantz BJ. Long term results of cochlear implants in children: a case for implanting children with residual hearing. Paper presented at the annual meeting of the Canadian Society of Otolaryngology–Head and Neck Surgery; June 16–19, 1996; London, Ontario, Canada.

70. Tyler RS, Fryauf-Bertschy H, Gantz BJ, Kelsay DM, Woodworth GG. Speech perception in prelingually implanted children after four years. *Adv Otorhinolaryngol* 1997;52:187–192.

71. Tyler RS, Gantz BJ, Woodworth GG, Fryauf-Bertschy H, Kelsay DMR. Performance of two and three year old children and predicting four-year and one-year performance. *Am J Otol* 1997;18:S157–S159.

72. Gantz BJ, Rubinstein JT, Tyler RS, et al. Long term results of cochlear implants in children with residual hearing. *Ann Otol Rhinol Laryngol* (in press).

The Ear: Comprehensive Otology,
edited by R. F. Canalis and P. R. Lambert.
Lippincott Williams & Wilkins, Philadelphia © 2000.

CHAPTER 40

Vertigo of Peripheral Origin

Robert W. Baloh

DIFFERENTIATING TYPES OF DIZZINESS

Dizziness is a nonspecific term that describes a sensation of altered orientation in space. Because visual, vestibular, and somatosensory signals provide the main

R. W. Baloh: Departments of Neurology and Surgery (Head and Neck), University of California, Los Angeles, School of Medicine, Los Angeles, California 90095-1769

source of information about the position of the head and body in space, damage to any of these afferent signals can lead to the symptom of dizziness. The initial task of the examining physician is to determine what the patient means by dizziness. Less than half of patients who report dizziness actually have vertigo. Because diagnostic evaluation and management vary markedly depending on the cause of the dizziness, it is critical to obtain a detailed

TABLE 1. *Common types of dizziness*

Type	Mechanism	Common causes
Vertigo	Imbalance of tonic vestibular signals	Benign positional vertigo, Meniere's syndrome, neurolabyrinthitis
Disequilibrium	Loss of vestibulospinal, proprioceptive, cerebellar function	Ototoxicity, peripheral neuropathy, stroke, cerebellar atrophy
Presyncopal light-headedness	Diffuse cerebral ischemia	Orthostatic hypotension, vasovagal episode, cardiac arrhythmia, hyperventilation
Ocular dizziness	Visual vestibular mismatch caused by impaired vision	Change in magnification, oculomotor paresis
Multisensory dizziness	Partial loss of multiple sensory systems	Diabetes mellitus, aging
Physiologic dizziness	Sensory conflict caused by unusual combination of sensory signals	Motion sickness, height vertigo, *mal de debarquement*
Psychophysiologic dizziness	Impaired central integration of sensory signals	Anxiety, panic attacks, phobias

Adapted from Baloh RW, Honrubia V. *Clinical neurophysiology of the vestibular systems,* 2nd ed. Philadelphia: FA Davis, 1990, with permission.

history regarding the type of dizziness before proceeding with a diagnostic evaluation (Table 1) (1).

MECHANISM OF VERTIGO

The afferent nerves from the otoliths and semicircular canals of each labyrinth maintain a balanced tonic rate of firing into the vestibular nuclei. Asymmetric involvement of this baseline activity leads to an illusion of movement, that is, vertigo. Damage to a semicircular canal or its afferent nerve produces a sensation of angular rotation in the plane of that canal similar to the sensation experienced during physiologic stimulation. More commonly, lesions involve all the canals and otoliths of one labyrinth or the entire vestibular nerve, producing a sensation of rotation in the plane determined by the balance of afferent signals from the opposite intact labyrinth. The illusion of rotation is near the horizontal plane because the vertical canals and otolith signals largely cancel out. If a patient with a unilateral peripheral vestibular lesion attempts to fixate on an object, the object appears blurred and seems to move in the direction opposite that of the slow phase of the patient's spontaneous nystagmus (i.e., away from the side of the lesion). This illusion of movement occurs because the brain interprets the target displacement on the retina as object movement rather than eye movement. An illusion of linear movement or tilting suggests isolated involvement of an otolith or its afferent nerve.

FEATURES OF PERIPHERAL VERTIGO

Time Course

The nervous system has a remarkable capability to compensate for an imbalance within the vestibular system, and thus vertigo caused by peripheral vestibular lesions usually occurs in episodes. Of the commonly encountered peripheral vestibular syndromes, brief episodes of vertigo lasting only seconds are typical of so-called benign positional vertigo. During the acute phase such patients may report a nonspecific feeling of disorientation and imbalance along with nausea and vomiting that lasts for hours to days. With careful questioning the examiner can identify recurrent brief attacks of positional vertigo interspersed with more persistent nonspecific dizziness. Vertigo during a typical bout of Meniere's disease lasts 3 to 6 hours, although the patient often describes a vague sense of dizziness for a day or so thereafter. Viral neurolabyrinthitis is characterized by the subacute onset of severe vertigo over hours followed by a gradual decrease in intensity over several days. The rapidity of compensation depends on the patient's age and the functional status of the other body-orienting systems. A young, healthy patient who sustains an acute peripheral vestibular insult usually is able to return to work in 2 to 4 weeks. By comparison, older patients may take months to recover from a similar insult. Continuous dizziness without fluctuations for a long time is not typical of peripheral vestibular disorders.

Precipitating Factors

Vertigo caused by peripheral vestibular lesions usually is worsened by rapid head movements, inasmuch as the new stimulus is sensed differently by the intact and abnormal labyrinths, and existing asymmetries are accentuated. Episodes may be precipitated by turning over in bed, sitting up from a lying position, extending the neck to look up, or bending over and straightening up. Patients with a perilymph fistula have brief episodes of vertigo precipitated by coughing or sneezing. Loud noises sometimes induce transient vertigo among patients with Meniere's syndrome (Tullio phenomenon).

Associated Symptoms

Autonomic symptoms such as sweating, pallor, nausea, and vomiting commonly accompany vertigo caused by peripheral vestibular lesions. Vegetative symptoms sometimes are the only manifestation of such a lesion. Numerous interconnecting pathways between vestibular and autonomic brainstem centers account for this close association between vestibular and autonomic symptoms.

The site of a peripheral vestibular lesion determines the symptoms that accompany vertigo. Besides vertigo, lesions of the labyrinth commonly produce auditory symptoms such as hearing loss, tinnitus, a sensation of pressure or fullness in the ear, or pain in the ear. Lesions involving the eighth cranial nerve also produce hearing loss and tinnitus and may be associated with ipsilateral facial weakness caused by involvement of the closely approximated seventh cranial nerve. As with vertigo, the time course of associated hearing loss can help determine the cause. Fluctuating hearing loss and tinnitus are characteristic of Meniere's disease. Patients with this disorder usually notice a buildup of pressure in the ear just before the onset of hearing loss, tinnitus, and vertigo. Abrupt complete unilateral deafness and vertigo occur with viral involvement of the labyrinth or eighth nerve. Slow progressive unilateral hearing loss suggests the existence of an acoustic neuroma.

Compensation

The severity of symptoms that follow a peripheral vestibular lesion depends on the extent of the lesion, whether the lesion is unilateral or bilateral, and the rapidity with which the functional loss occurs. Patients who slowly lose vestibular function bilaterally (e.g., after exposure to ototoxic drugs) often do not report vertigo but do report oscillopsia with head movement and instability when walking (caused by loss of the vestibuloocular and vestibulospinal reflexes, respectively). If a patient slowly loses vestibular function on one side over a period of months to years (e.g., with an acoustic neuroma), vertigo may not occur. A sudden unilateral loss of vestibular function, however, is a dramatic event. The patient describes severe vertigo and nausea, is pale and perspiring, and usually vomits repeatedly. He or she prefers to lie quietly in a dark room but can walk if forced to (falling toward the side of the lesion). Brisk, spontaneous nystagmus interferes with vision. These symptoms and signs are transient, however, and the process of compensation begins almost immediately. Within 1 week of appearance of the lesion, a young patient can walk without difficulty and with fixation can inhibit the spontaneous nystagmus. Within 1 month, most patients return to work with few if any residual symptoms. It is very important that patients begin compensation exercises as soon as possible after sustaining a unilateral peripheral vestibular lesion.

Predisposing Factors

Although uncommon in the antibiotic era, chronic middle ear infections may lead to bacterial labyrinthitis or serous labyrinthitis. Patients with bacterial meningitis can contract bacterial labyrinthitis through the direct spinal fluid–perilymph connections. Patients with viral neurolabyrinthitis frequently report an upper respiratory tract illness either within 2 or 3 weeks before or at the time of onset of vertigo. Head injury often causes labyrinthine trauma and produces a single, prolonged episode of vertigo or more commonly recurrent episodes of positional vertigo. Vertigo can be caused by surgical intervention in or about the ear. The medical history should focus on chronic medical illnesses that might predispose the patient to damage to the peripheral vestibular system, such as diabetes mellitus, atherosclerotic vascular disease, syphilis (congenital or acquired), and systemic autoimmune illness. Important disorders with genetic predisposition include otosclerosis and neurofibromatosis. Congenital malformations of the inner ear often are associated with other congenital malformations. Ototoxic drugs, such as aminoglycosides, sometimes cause vertigo but more often produce imbalance from bilateral symmetric damage to the vestibular end organs.

BENIGN POSITIONAL VERTIGO

Clinical Features

Benign positional vertigo is a syndrome that can be the sequela of several different inner ear diseases; in about half of cases no cause can be found (2). Patients with benign positional vertigo have brief episodes of vertigo (usually lasting less than 30 seconds) with position change. The most common precipitating movements are turning over in bed, getting in and out of bed, bending over and straightening up, and extending the neck to look up and back. So-called top-shelf vertigo, in which a person experiences an episode of vertigo while reaching for an object on a high shelf, is nearly always caused by benign positional vertigo.

In about half of cases of benign positional vertigo a likely cause can be determined (Table 2) (2). When a

TABLE 2. *Diagnoses for 240 patients with benign positional vertigo*

Diagnosis	No. of patients
Idiopathic	118
Posttraumatic	43
Viral neurolabyrinthitis	37
Miscellaneous	42
Labyrinthine infarction	11
Meniere's syndrome	5
Ear surgery	5
Ototoxicity	4
Luetic labyrinthopathy	2
Chronic otomastoiditis	2
Other	13

Adapted from Baloh RW, Honrubia V, Jacobson K. Benign positional vertigo: clinical and oculographic features in 240 cases. *Neurology* 1987;37:371–378, with permission.

cause can be identified, the two most common diagnostic categories are posttraumatic and postviral. With the former, patients have typical benign positional vertigo after a blow to the head, in many cases a blow that does not lead to loss of consciousness. Patients with an antecedent episode of viral neurolabyrinthitis experience typical benign positional vertigo months to years after resolution of the viral syndrome. Among persons with idiopathic vertigo, women outnumber men at least two to one (2,3). Age at onset peaks in the sixth decade among persons with idiopathic vertigo and in the fourth and fifth decades for those with postviral vertigo. It is evenly distributed over the second to sixth decades among persons with posttraumatic vertigo.

Mechanism of Benign Positional Vertigo

Although originally attributed to a lesion of the otolith organs (4), there is now convincing evidence that benign positional vertigo usually originates from the posterior semicircular canal of the ear on the bottom when positional vertigo and nystagmus are induced. Torsional vertical positional nystagmus is in the plane of the posterior semicircular canal and is identical to that induced in animals when the afferent nerve from the posterior semicircular canal is electrically stimulated (2,5). Surgical sectioning of the ampullary nerve from the posterior semicircular canal (6) or blocking the posterior semicircular canal with a bone plug (7) immediately stops the positional vertigo and nystagmus for nearly all patients who have undergone such procedures.

Schuknecht and Ruby (8,9) introduced the concept of cupulolithiasis when they found basophilic deposits on the cupula of the posterior semicircular canal in patients who manifested benign positional vertigo before death of unrelated disease. The deposits were greatest on the side that was on the bottom when benign positional vertigo was induced. Schuknecht proposed that otoconia from a degenerating utricular macula settled on the cupula of the posterior canal and caused it to become heavier than the surrounding endolymph. The typical features of benign positional vertigo are better explained, however, by the presence of otoconial debris freely floating within the posterior semicircular canal under the influence of gravity (so-called canalithiasis) (10–12). With the patient sitting upright, a clot of calcium carbonate crystals forms at the most dependent portion of the posterior semicircular canal (Fig. 1). Movement back and to the side in the plane of the posterior canal (as with the Dix-Hallpike positioning test) causes the clot to move in an ampullofugal direction and produces ampullofugal displacement of the cupula as the clot moves within the narrow canal (see Fig. 1). Fatigability with repeated positioning is explained by dispersion of single particles from the clot that makes the plunger less effective. Reactivation of positional vertigo after pro-

longed bed rest is explained as the particles reform into a clot. The induced vertigo and nystagmus are brief because once the clot reaches its lowest position within the canal with respect to the earth's surface, the cupula returns to the primary position because of cupular elasticity. Latency before onset of nystagmus is explained by the delay in setting the clot into motion.

Support for the canalithiasis mechanism of benign positional vertigo was provided in surgical procedures designed to block the posterior semicircular canal with a bony plug. In the process of exposing the membranous labyrinth of the posterior semicircular canal for the plugging operation, a chalky white substance was observed in the endolymph of the posterior semicircular canal (7). This finding indicated that the debris was calcium carbonate crystals floating freely within the endolymph. Probably the most convincing argument for the canalithiasis theory is the dramatic response of the posterior canal variant of benign positional vertigo to the positional maneuver designed to relocate the clot from the posterior canal into the utricle (see Fig. 1).

Diagnosis

The diagnosis of benign positional vertigo rests on observing the characteristic fatigable paroxysmal positional nystagmus of a patient with a typical history of positional vertigo. The nystagmus is induced by rapidly moving the patient from the sitting to the head-hanging position, the so-called Dix-Hallpike test. The direction of nystagmus is consistent with the known anatomic connections between the posterior semicircular canal of the bottom ear and the eye muscles. It is torsional and vertical, the upper pole of the eye beating toward the ground. It is readily seen at visual inspection, and the diagnosis can be made at the bedside. Nystagmus fatigues (decreases with repeated positioning) among more than 90% of patients, but some patients with otherwise typical positional vertigo and nystagmus have minimal fatigue. The presence of positional nystagmus correlates with the clinical symptoms. Unless the patient takes the test during a period of acute episodes of vertigo, positional nystagmus is not observed.

In rare instances, benign positional vertigo can result from dysfunction of the horizontal semicircular canal (13). The history is similar to that associated with the posterior canal variety, but the positional nystagmus is different. This variety is induced by rapidly turning the patient's head to either side while he or she is lying in the supine position. A burst of horizontal nystagmus is induced, beating toward the ground. The positional nystagmus is greatest when the abnormal ear is on the bottom, although a lesser horizontal positional nystagmus occurs when the abnormal ear is on the top. The mechanism of horizontal positional nystagmus is presumably similar to that of the posterior canal variety (i.e., debris

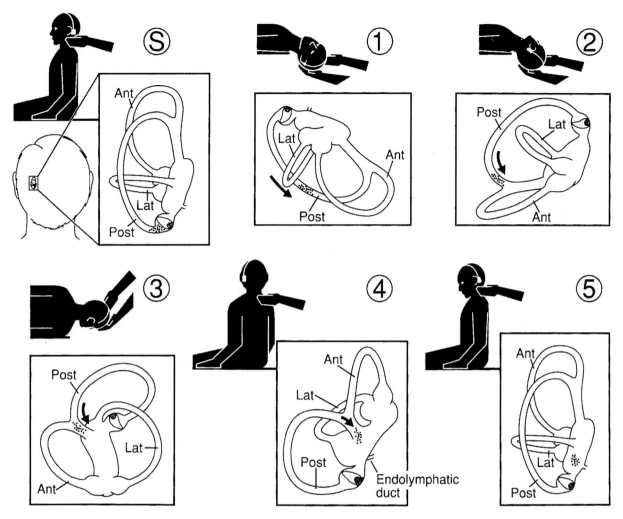

FIG. 1. Positional maneuver designed to remove debris from the posterior semicircular canal. *Dark figure* shows side view; *boxes* show operator's exposed view of left labyrinth and gravitational canaliths. *S*, Start. In the sitting position, the clot of calcium carbonate crystals lies at the lowest position within the posterior canal. *1,* Movement to the head-hanging position causes the clot to move away from the cupula and produces an excitatory burst of activity in the ampullary nerve from the posterior canal (ampullofugal displacement of the cupula). *2,* Movement across to the other head-hanging position causes the clot to move further around the canal. *3,* The patient rolls onto the side, facing the floor, and the movement causes the clot to enter the common crus of the posterior and anterior semicircular canals. *4* and *5,* Finally the patient sits up and the clot disperses into the utricle. The maneuver is repeated until no nystagmus is induced. The patient is instructed not to lie flat for 48 hours after the procedure to prevent the debris from reentering the canal. (From Epley JM. The canalith repositioning procedure for treatment of benign paroxysmal positional vertigo. *Otolaryngol Head Neck Surg* 1992;107:399–404, with permission.)

enters the endolymph of the horizontal semicircular canal).

Treatment

The positioning maneuver designed to liberate the clot of material from the posterior semicircular canal is performed after the diagnosis is established with the Dix-Hallpike positioning test. A modified Epley maneuver for removing the particles from the posterior semicircular canal is illustrated in Figure 1. With the maneuver, the patient is rotated in the plane of the posterior semicircular canal so that the clot rotates around the canal and enters the utricle. The positioning maneuver should be repeated until the patient has no symptoms. Sometimes a vibrator pressed against the mastoid can loosen particles that are stuck in the canal, but for most patients, the maneuver alone performed at the bedside is curative. The patient is instructed to avoid lying flat for at least 2 days after the maneuver to prevent the clot from reentering the posterior semicircular canal. Ten to twenty percent of patients have an exacerbation within the 2 weeks after the maneuver is performed, and about 50% eventually have an exacerbation. It is presumed that some patients are unable to clear the calcium carbonate material from the utricle. Patients can be taught to perform the maneuver on their own at home should they have a recurrence.

The positional maneuver for managing the horizontal canal variant of benign positional vertigo rotates the patient's head in the plane of the horizontal semicircular canal (12). The patient starts in the supine position, is rapidly rolled 90 degrees to the normal side (the side with lesser nystagmus), and then in 90-degree steps to prone, to the abnormal side, and back to supine. The patient is kept in each position for about 60 seconds and is instructed to avoid lying flat for the next 48 hours. Having the patient lie for a prolonged period on the side with the abnormal ear on the bottom also can cure the horizontal canal variant of benign positional vertigo (14).

For rare patients with prolonged intractable benign positional vertigo unresponsive to conventional therapy, surgical procedures have been developed either to cut the ampullary nerve from the posterior semicircular canal crista (6) or to block the posterior semicircular canal with a plug (7). With ampullary nerve section the main complication is sensorineural hearing loss, which occurs among about 8% of patients. Hearing loss may occur with canal blockage but usually is reversible and not as severe as after nerve section. Transection of the vestibular nerve through either a middle cranial fossa or retrolabyrinthine approach is another procedure that can relieve the positional vertigo while preserving hearing, but it is associated with greater potential risks than the other two surgical procedures and rarely is indicated (see Chapter 43).

INFECTIONS OF THE INNER EAR

Labyrinthitis is an inflammatory process of the labyrinth. The inflammation may involve primarily the bony or membranous labyrinth, but for symptoms to occur the membranous labyrinth and its contents must be involved. Bacterial infections and syphilis initially affect the bony labyrinth. Viral infections, however, initially affect the membranous labyrinth, presumably through hematogenous spread.

Bacterial Infections

Two types of labyrinthitis are associated with acute and chronic bacterial infections of the temporal bone: (a) serous or toxic labyrinthitis, in which bacterial toxins or chemical products invade the inner ear, and (b) suppurative labyrinthitis, in which bacteria invade the inner ear. The former usually produces mild symptoms such as an insidious high-frequency sensorineural hearing loss. The latter typically leads to profound combined auditory and vestibular loss with little or no recovery.

Serous labyrinthitis can occur after acute or chronic middle ear infections. With acute otitis media, bacterial toxins and enzymes diffuse through the round window into the scala tympani. Acute and chronic inflammatory cells also infiltrate the round window, and a fine, serofibrinous precipitate forms just medial to the round window membrane. The toxins or inflammatory cells may penetrate the basilar membrane and invade the endolymph at the basal turn of the cochlea. This probably explains the high incidence of high-frequency sensorineural hearing loss among patients with chronic otitis media (15). Vestibular symptoms, including episodic vertigo and unsteadiness, can occur, although they are less common than hearing loss.

Acute suppurative labyrinthitis has become relatively rare because of the introduction of antibiotics, but it produces a clinical syndrome that is easily recognized. Symptoms include a sudden onset of severe vertigo, nausea, vomiting, and unilateral hearing loss. The infection can originate either in the middle ear in association with chronic otitis media or in the cerebrospinal fluid with meningitis. In the latter case bacteria enter the perilymphatic space through the cochlear aqueduct or internal auditory canal. Meningogenic bacterial labyrinthitis often is bilateral, whereas direct invasion from chronic otitis is unilateral. The most common route for direct bacterial invasion of the labyrinth is a horizontal semicircular canal fistula associated with cholesteatoma. Meniere's disease can be a sequela of both serous and suppurative labyrinthitis (16).

Viral Neurolabyrinthitis

Viral infection of the inner ear can cause sudden deafness, acute vertigo, or a combination of auditory and vestibular symptoms. It usually is not possible to differentiate primary end organ and eighth-nerve involvement. Various terms have been used to describe this disease, including viral labyrinthitis, viral neuritis, cochleitis, vestibular neuronitis, and vestibular neuritis. The phrase *viral neurolabyrinthitis* is sufficiently general to encompass all possible sites of involvement and is used in this chapter.

Virus-induced hearing loss often is called *sudden deafness,* although the onset usually occurs over several hours and may even extend over several days. Hearing loss often is profound and may be permanent, although it reverses at least partially in many cases. Tinnitus and fullness in the involved ear are common.

Virus-induced vestibular dysfunction typically is manifested by the gradual onset of vertigo, nausea, and vomiting over several hours. The symptoms usually reach a peak within 24 hours and then gradually resolve over several weeks. During the first day there is severe truncal unsteadiness and imbalance, and the patient has difficulty focusing because of spontaneous nystagmus. Most patients have a benign course with complete recovery within a month or two. There are important exceptions to this rule, however. Some patients, particularly older persons, have intractable dizziness that persists for many months to years. Twenty to thirty percent of patients have at least one recurrent bout of vertigo (usually less severe than the initial episode) (17). This may represent reactivation of a latent virus, inasmuch as it often is associated with a systemic viral illness. A small percentage of these patients have several recurrent episodes of vertigo, which lead to profound bilateral vestibulopathy (so-called bilateral sequential vestibular neuritis) (18). The episodic vertigo is replaced by persistent disequilibrium and oscillopsia.

A clear example of a viral syndrome involving the eighth cranial nerve is herpes zoster oticus (19). It is presumed that the zoster virus remains dormant in the ganglia associated with the seventh and eighth nerves and is reactivated during a period of lowered immunity. The patient initially has deep, burning pain in the ear followed a few days later by a vesicular eruption in the external auditory canal and concha. At some time after the onset of pain, either before or after the vesicular eruption, the patient may have hearing loss, vertigo, and facial weakness. These symptoms may occur singly or collectively. A small percentage of patients with idiopathic facial palsy (Bell's palsy) have a rise in complement fixation antibodies to zoster antigen (20).

Probably the most convincing evidence for a viral cause of the aforedescribed auditory and vestibular syndromes comes from studies of the temporal bones of patients with typical clinical histories (21,22). The atrophy of the nerves and end organs is identical to that associated with well-documented viral disorders, such as mumps or measles (Fig. 2). These pathologic findings are supported by experimental studies with animals in which

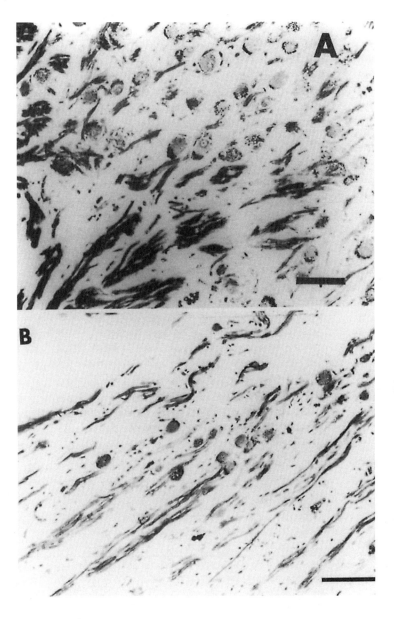

FIG. 2. Sections through comparable areas of the inferior division of Scarpa's ganglion on the normal side **(A)** and on the side with absent caloric response **(B)** stained with toluidine blue. Only a few small neurons remain in **B**. *Bar,* 100 μm. (From Baloh RW, Lopez I, Ishiyama A, Wackym P, Honrubia V. Vestibular neuritis: clinical-pathological correlation. *Otolaryngol Head Neck Surg* 1996;114:586–592, with permission.)

it was shown that several viruses selectively infect the labyrinth and eighth cranial nerve (23,24).

Syphilitic Infections of the Inner Ear

Syphilitic infections produce auditory and vestibular symptoms through two different pathophysiologic mechanisms: (a) meningitis with involvement of the eighth nerve and (b) osteitis of the temporal bone with associated labyrinthitis. The former typically occurs as an early manifestation of acquired syphilis; the latter occurs as a late manifestation of both congenital and acquired syphilis. With early congenital syphilis lymphocytic infiltration of both the membranous labyrinth and eighth nerve may lead to profound bilateral deafness. Spirochetes have been found in temporal bones obtained at autopsies of such patients. With early acquired syphilis the predominant pathologic finding is basilar meningitis that affects the eighth nerve, particularly the auditory branch.

Both congenital and acquired forms of syphilis produce temporal bone osteitis and labyrinthitis as a late manifestation. The congenital variety is approximately three times as common as the acquired variety (25). The time of onset of congenital syphilitic labyrinthitis is anywhere from the first to the seventh decades; the peak incidence is in the fourth and fifth decades. The congenital variety often is associated with other stigmata of congenital syphilis, such as interstitial keratitis, Hutchinson's teeth, saddle nose, frontal bossing, and rhagades. Of these associated signs, interstitial keratitis is by far the most common, occurring among approximately 90% of patients (25).

The natural history of syphilitic labyrinthitis is slow, relentless progression to profound or total bilateral loss of vestibular and auditory function (26). This progression is marked by episodes of sudden deafness and vertigo and fluctuation in the magnitude of hearing loss and tinnitus.

Differential Diagnosis of Labyrinthitis

The features in the history, examination, and laboratory evaluation that help differentiate the types of labyrinthitis are summarized in Table 3. Suppurative labyrinthitis invariably results in fulminant, profound loss of both auditory and vestibular function, usually with only minimal recovery. Serous labyrinthitis may produce only high-frequency sensorineural hearing loss if toxic products remain confined to the basilar region of the cochlea. The diagnosis of viral neurolabyrinthitis is based on finding the characteristic clinical profile and

TABLE 3. *Differential diagnosis and therapy for labyrinthitis*

Type	History	Examination	Laboratory	Treatment
Bacterial	Abrupt onset of vertigo, associated with hearing loss, prior ear infections	May be signs of chronic otitis or acute meningitis	ENG: unilateral absent caloric response Audio: profound unilateral hearing loss CSF: pleocytosis CT: possible cholesteatoma	Local management of infection, parenteral antibiotics, vestibular suppressants, vestibular exercises ASAP
Viral	Vertigo develops over hours, resolves over days, prior flu-like episode, may or may not have associated hearing loss	Spontaneous nystagmus and imbalance for first few days; ears appear normal	ENG: Unilateral caloric hypoexcitability, usually returns to normal Audio: usually normal	High-dose steroids during acute phase, vestibular suppressants, vestibular exercises ASAP
Serous	Mild dizziness and disequilibrium, mild hearing loss	Signs of acute or chronic otitis	ENG: usually normal Audio: high-frequency loss CT: acute or chronic infection of middle ear	Parenteral antibiotics, vestibular suppressants if needed
Syphilitic	Recurrent episodes of vertigo lasting hours, associated tinnitus and hearing loss, prior congenital or acquired syphilis	May be stigmata of congenital syphilis, rarely associated signs of neurosyphilis	ENG: unilateral or bilateral decreased caloric response Audio: low-frequency hearing loss Serology: positive FTA-ABS CSF: usually normal	Penicillin IV or IM, steroids, vestibular suppressants for acute attacks

ENG, Electronystagmography; *Audio,* audiogram; *CSF,* cerebrospinal fluid; *CT,* computed tomography; *ASAP,* as soon as possible; *FTA-ABS,* fluorescent treponemal antibody absorption test.

laboratory evidence of peripheral auditory or vestibular dysfunction in the absence of neurologic symptoms and signs. Syphilitic labyrinthitis might initially be confused with rapidly progressive Meniere's disease. The key to the diagnosis of syphilitic labyrinthitis is the finding of a positive serum fluorescent treponemal antibody absorption test result for a patient with the typical clinical history of fluctuating hearing loss and vertigo (27). A serum Venereal Disease Research Laboratory (VDRL) test result is positive in only about 75% of cases, making it an unreliable test for syphilitic labyrinthitis (25). Cerebrospinal fluid examination, however, may show a positive VDRL test or the presence of lymphocytes.

Treatment

Treatment of patients with bacterial labyrinthitis is directed at the associated infection of the middle ear, mastoid process, or meninges. Any patient with acute or chronic bacterial ear disease associated with sudden or rapidly progressive inner ear symptoms should be admitted to the hospital and treated with local cleansing and topical antibiotic solutions in the affected ear and parental antibiotics capable of penetrating the blood-brain barrier. Surgical intervention to eradicate the middle ear and mastoid infection usually is performed after a few days of antibiotic treatment. Labyrinthitis caused by primary meningitis is best managed by means of addressing the underlying meningitis.

The treatment of patients with isolated episodes of auditory or vestibular loss caused by presumed viral syndromes is controversial because the pathophysiologic features often are uncertain. Unless there is convincing evidence of a vascular or nonviral infectious cause, the patient should be treated as having presumed viral neurolabyrinthitis. Symptomatic treatment with vestibular suppressants is helpful during the acute stage, and vestibular exercises should be started immediately after the acute nausea and vomiting subside. These exercises are continued until dizziness and imbalance are minimal. Results of preliminary studies suggest that steroids may be helpful for aborting the acute vertigo syndrome, presumably because of their antiinflammatory effects (28). A methylprednisolone dose pack should be started as soon as possible after the onset of symptoms. Antiviral agents such as cytosine arabinase and acyclovir have been used for treating children with systemic viral illnesses. Results of several studies suggest that acyclovir given within the first 2 to 6 days after the onset of herpes zoster oticus improves the outcome, at least with regard to residual facial nerve paralysis (29). Some physicians recommend combining steroids and acyclovir (30). Further controlled studies are needed to assess the use of steroids and antiviral agents to manage viral neurolabyrinthitis syndromes.

Penicillin is the therapy of choice for the otologic manifestations of syphilis, although the optimal regimen for each variety remains uncertain. For labyrinthitis that is a late manifestation of both congenital and acquired syphilis, a combination of steroids and penicillin appears to be superior to penicillin alone (25,26). Numerous penicillin regimens have been used, the most popular being benzathine penicillin (2.4 million units weekly for 6 weeks to 3 months). Along with penicillin, prednisone, beginning at a dose of 60 mg per day on an alternate-day regimen, is given for 3 months followed by tapering. If symptoms recur during the tapering, a more long-term maintenance dose of prednisone may be needed. Most patients can be expected to stabilize or improve with this therapeutic regimen (26).

MENIERE'S DISEASE

Clinical Features

Meniere's disease is characterized by fluctuating hearing loss, tinnitus, episodic vertigo, and a sensation of fullness or pressure in the ear. In typical instances the patient feels fullness and pressure along with decreased hearing in one ear. Vertigo rapidly follows, reaching a maximum intensity within minutes and then slowly subsiding over the next several hours. In the early stages the hearing loss is frequently reversible, but in later stages there is residual hearing loss. Tinnitus may persist between episodes but usually increases in intensity immediately before or during the acute episode. It is typically described as a roaring sound (the sound of the ocean or a hollow sea shell). Such episodes occur at irregular intervals for years with periods of remission unpredictably intermixed (31). At least 50% of patients, however, have marked remission within 2 years of onset. The typical natural history of the disease is development of severe permanent hearing loss and diminution in the severity and frequency of the episodic vertigo. Bilateral involvement eventually occurs among about one third of patients.

Some patients with well-documented Meniere's disease experience abrupt episodes of falling to the ground without loss of consciousness or associated neurologic symptoms. These episodes were called *otolithic catastrophes* by Tumarkin (32) because of his suspicion that they represent acute stimulation of the otoliths from endolymphatic hydrops (33). Patients often report feeling as if they were pushed to the ground by an external force. These episodes are particularly dangerous because often the patient sustains blows to the head or fractures a bone. So-called delayed endolymphatic hydrops develops in an ear that has been damaged years before, usually by a viral or bacterial infection (34,35). With this disorder the patient reports a history of hearing loss since early child-hood followed many years later by typical symptoms and signs of Meniere's disease. If the hearing loss is profound, as it often is, the episodic vertigo is not accompanied by fluctuating hearing levels and tinnitus. Delayed Meniere's disease can be unilateral or bilateral, depending on the extent of damage at the time of the original insult.

Mechanism of Endolymphatic Hydrops

With Meniere's disease the membranous labyrinth progressively dilates until the saccular wall makes contact with the stapes footplate and the cochlear duct occupies the entire vestibular scala (36). The cochlear and vestibular end organs and nerves show minimal pathologic changes. Herniation and rupture of the membranous labyrinth are common, the latter frequently involving Reissner's membrane and the walls of the sacculus, utriculus, and ampullae. Sometimes rupture is followed by complete collapse of the membranous labyrinth.

Several diseases are known to produce endolymphatic hydrops, but in most instances the cause is unknown. The basic underlying mechanism is thought to be damage to the fluid resorptive mechanism caused by dysfunction of the endolymphatic duct and sac. Multiple etiologic possibilities have been proposed for Meniere's disease, including immunologic dysfunction, endocrine disturbance, and infection. Developmental hypoplasia of the endolymphatic duct and sac may be an important predisposing factor. The similarity in pathologic findings between so-called delayed Meniere's disease and idiopathic Meniere's disease has suggested a possible common viral cause. Subclinical viral infection might damage the resorptive mechanism of the inner ear and eventually cause decompensation in the balance between secretion and absorption of endolymph (21).

Endolymphatic hydrops can be reliably produced in animals by means of blocking the endolymphatic duct or destroying the endolymphatic sac (37,38). Although the extent of hydrops in the cochlea and vestibular labyrinth is similar to that with Meniere's disease, the characteristic ruptures in the membranous wall that allow mixing of endolymph and perilymph are rarely seen in the animal model.

Diagnosis

The key to the diagnosis of Meniere's disease is to document fluctuating hearing levels in a patient with a characteristic clinical history (39). A shift of more than 10 dB at two different frequencies is significant. In the early stages, sensorineural hearing loss usually is greater in the lower frequencies. Speech discrimination is relatively preserved, and recruitment often is consistent with a cochlear site of dysfunction. Brainstem auditory evoked responses and stapedius reflex measurements are normal. Electronystagmographic examination may reveal peripheral spontaneous nystagmus and either vestibular paresis or directional preponderance at caloric testing. Electrocochleography shows an enlarged summating potential to action potential ratio among 50% to 70% of patients with Meniere's disease. The test appears to have the greatest sensitivity if performed when the patient is having active symptoms, such as aural fullness, tinnitus, or vertigo.

Treatment

Treatment of patients with Meniere's disease consists of vestibular suppression (Table 4) for the acute spells of vertigo and long-term prophylaxis with salt restriction and diuretics (40,41). The mechanism by which a low-salt diet decreases the frequency and severity of attacks in Meniere's disease is unclear, but there is strong empirical evidence for its efficacy. We recommend beginning with salt restriction of 1 g sodium per day, with a minimum therapeutic trial of 2 to 3 months. If a good response is obtained, the level of salt intake can be gradually increased while symptoms and signs are carefully monitored. Fluid and food intake should be regularly distributed throughout the day, and binges, particularly with foods with high sugar or salt content, should be avoided. Some patients find that certain foods (e.g., alcohol, coffee, chocolate) precipitate attacks. Diuretics (50 mg diazide once a day, 250 mg acetazolamide once or twice

TABLE 4. *Drugs commonly used for vestibular suppression*

Class	Drug	Dosage	Comments
Anticholinergic	Scopolamine	0.6 mg orally q 4–6 h or 0.5 mg transdermally q 3 d	Minimal sedation, dry mouth common; may cause pupillary dilatation; avoid use in older patients
Antihistamine	Dimenhydrinate (Dramamine)	50 mg orally q 4–6 h or 100 mg suppository q 8 h	Available without prescription, mild sedation, minimal side effects
	Meclizine (Antivert)	25–50 mg orally q 4–6 h	Mild sedation, minimal side effects
	Promethazine (Phenergan)	25–50 mg orally, IM, or suppository q 4–6 h	Good for nausea and vertigo, more sedating, rare extrapyramidal side effects
Benzodiazepine	Diazepam (Valium)	5 or 10 mg orally q 6–8 h	Prominent sedation, little effect on nausea; avoid chronic use

a day) provide additional benefit to some patients, although these drugs cannot replace the salt-restriction diet. In 1977 Torok (42) wrote a 25-year review of more than 800 articles pertaining to medical therapy for Meniere's disease and concluded that a 60% to 80% success rate can be expected with a variety of approaches. In a more recent review of approximately 75 articles published between 1977 and 1990, Ruchenstein et al. (43) concluded that no specific oral medical therapy has been shown conclusively to ameliorate the symptoms of Meniere's disease. Surgical management of Meniere's disease is discussed in Chapter 43.

VASCULAR DISEASES OF THE INNER EAR

Labyrinthine Ischemia

Occlusion of the internal auditory artery leads to sudden, profound loss of both auditory and vestibular function. Hearing loss usually is permanent, and vestibular imbalance remains, although symptoms gradually improve with central compensation. Pathologic studies involving such patients reveal widespread necrosis of inner ear tissues with subsequent proliferation of fibrous tissue and new bone formation (16). Most documented cases have been seen in association with ischemia in the distribution of the anterior inferior cerebellar artery accompanied by infarction of the dorsolateral pontomedullary region. Infarction of the labyrinth sometimes is preceded by episodes of vertebrobasilar insufficiency and in some cases isolated episodes of vertigo (44).

Intralabyrinthine Hemorrhage

Spontaneous hemorrhage into the inner ear typically occurs in patients with an underlying bleeding diathesis (16). Leukemia is the most common cause. Such patients experience a sudden onset of unilateral deafness and severe vertigo. Pathologic examination of the inner ear reveals hemorrhage into the perilymphatic space with smaller focal hemorrhages in the endolymphatic space. A similar condition may follow from a blow to the head without bony fracture (so-called labyrinthine concussion).

Diagnosis

The diagnosis of ischemia or infarction of the labyrinth rests on finding the characteristic clinical features of the sudden onset of hearing loss or vertigo in a patient with known cerebral vascular disease or a patient with risk factors for vascular occlusion, such as vasculitis, hypercoagulation, or hyperviscosity. With infarction of the labyrinth, hearing loss is profound, and auditory evoked potentials and caloric responses are absent. Diagnosis of intralabyrinthine hemorrhage is based on finding a sud-den auditory and vestibular loss in a patient with an underlying bleeding diathesis or a patient who has received a blow to the head. As with infarction, hearing loss and vestibular loss are profound and usually permanent.

Treatment

Treatment of patients with labyrinthine infarction or hemorrhage is primarily symptomatic. Vestibular suppression can help relieve acute vertigo and nausea (see Table 4). Vestibular exercises should be started as soon as the patient is able to cooperate. Management of underlying blood dyscrasia is indicated whenever possible.

TUMORS OF THE EAR AND TEMPORAL BONE

A wide variety of benign and malignant tumors involve the ear and temporal bone. Tumors involving the middle ear produce symptoms of fullness or conductive hearing loss early, whereas tumors in the temporal bone or outside the middle ear can become quite large without producing symptoms. The tumor may not become apparent until it erodes into the external auditory canal and produces conductive hearing loss or through the mastoid cortex into the skin. Because of the resistance of the enchondral layers, neoplasms rarely invade the inner ear. When they do, hearing loss and vertigo typical of peripheral auditory and vestibular loss occur.

Malignant Tumors

Squamous cell carcinoma is the most frequent histologic type of malignant tumor involving the middle ear and mastoid process. Prognosis is good for tumors confined to the auricle and external canal but not for those invading the middle ear and mastoid process (45). The latter frequently are associated with prominent ear symptoms, which include vertigo, hearing loss, pain, otorrhea, mastoid swelling, and facial paralysis. In general, carcinoma occurs among an older age group, whereas sarcoma occurs among the young. Rhabdomyosarcoma is the most common malignant tumor of the middle ear among young persons. It typically occurs among children younger than 5 years. The initial symptom often is facial paralysis, which may be misdiagnosed as idiopathic (Bell's) palsy. Metastatic involvement of the temporal bone also is common. The most common sites of origin, in order of frequency, are breast, kidney, lung, stomach, larynx, prostate, and thyroid.

Benign Tumors

Glomus tumor is the most common tumor of the middle ear and after schwannoma is the most common tumor of the temporal bone (46). Glomus tumors arise in the glomera of the chemoreceptor system, which are located along the vagus nerve, glossopharyngeal nerve, tympanic branch of the ninth cranial nerve, and the postauricular branch of the tenth cranial nerve. Glomus jugulare tumors may involve the labyrinth and cranial nerves; glomus tympanicum tumors usually produce only local symptoms, such as conductive hearing loss and pulsatile tinnitus. Invasion of the labyrinth is an uncommon but serious prognostic sign and often is associated with extension to the petrous apex and into the middle and posterior fossae.

TRAUMA

Temporal Bone Fractures

Fractures of the temporal bone most commonly result from direct lateral blunt trauma to the skull in the parietal region of the head (47). Because the otic capsule surrounding the inner ear is very dense bone, the fracture usually courses around it to involve the major foramina in the skull base, usually those of the carotid artery and the jugular bulb. Longitudinal fractures account for 70% to 90% of temporal bone fractures. They pass parallel to the anterior margin of the petrous pyramid and usually extend medially from the region of the gasserian ganglion to the middle ear and laterally to the mastoid air cells.

Transverse fractures of the temporal bone are much less common, but the neurologic symptoms are more pronounced. They run orthogonally to the long axis of the petrous pyramid. Unlike longitudinal fractures, transverse fractures usually pass through the vestibule of the inner ear, tear the membranous labyrinth, lacerate the vestibular and cochlear nerve, and produce complete loss of vestibular and cochlear function. Vertigo, nausea, and vomiting are prominent for several days after the fracture, typical of unilateral peripheral vestibular loss. Facial paralysis is present in about 50% of cases, and loss of function may be permanent unless surgical intervention is instituted (see Chapter 46).

Labyrinthine Concussion

Auditory and vestibular symptoms, isolated or in combination, frequently follow blows to the head that do not result in temporal bone fracture (48). The absence of associated brainstem symptoms and signs and the usual rapid improvement in symptoms following injury support peripheral localization in most instances. Although protected by a bony capsule, the delicate labyrinthine membranes are susceptible to blunt trauma. Sudden deafness following a blow to the head without associated vestibular symptoms often is partially or completely reversible. It is probably caused by intense acoustic stimulation from pressure waves produced by the blow that are transmitted through the bone to the cochlea, just as pressure waves are transmitted from air through the conduction mechanism (49).

Posttraumatic Positional Vertigo

The most common neurologic sequela of head injury is benign positional vertigo. It is presumed that the trauma dislodges calcium carbonate crystals from the macula of the utriculus. The crystals then interfere with function of the posterior semicircular canal (see Benign Positional Vertigo). The prognosis for patients with posttraumatic benign positional vertigo is good (50). They respond to the particle repositioning maneuver (see Fig. 1) similar to patients with other causes of benign positional vertigo (12). Recurrences are common, however.

Perilymph Fistula

Perilymph fistula results from disruption of the limiting membranes of the labyrinth, usually at the oval or round window. The cause of the fistula is obvious when there is disruption of the otic capsule or a tear in the membranous labyrinth associated with trauma. Spontaneous fistulas are more difficult to explain. Rupture of the round or oval window can occur with sudden negative or positive pressure change in the middle ear from violent nose blowing, sneezing, or barotrauma (51). A second mechanism involves a sudden increase in cerebrospinal fluid pressure with transmission of this pressure wave to the perilymph associated with lifting, straining, coughing, or vigorous activity. Perilymph fistulas may also be associated with developmental abnormalities of the middle ear and otic capsule.

Differential Diagnosis of Posttraumatic Inner Ear Disorders

High-resolution computed tomography (CT) with bone windows is the radiologic procedure of choice for evaluating trauma to the temporal bone and skull base. With CT one often is able to identify multiple fracture lines spreading throughout the base of the skull. Magnetic resonance imaging can be of some use for identifying soft tissue lesions but is of little use for identifying fractures. Once the patient's condition is stabilized, systematic evaluation of the auditory, vestibular, and facial nerves should be undertaken.

The classic presentation of acute perilymph fistula is a sudden, audible pop in the ear immediately followed by hearing loss, vertigo, and tinnitus. The key to the diagnosis is to identify the characteristic precipitating factors mentioned earlier. There is no pathognomonic test for perilymph fistula (52). A positive fistula test (see Chapter 8) is suggestive but not specific. False-negative test results are common, and false-positive results occur with Meniere's disease and after stapedectomy. Dizziness and

TABLE 5. *Differential diagnosis of dizziness after trauma to the ear*

Diagnosis	Dizziness	Examination	Laboratory
Temporal bone fracture	Immediate onset, severe, gradual improvement	Blood in external or middle ear, step deformity in external canal, spontaneous nystagmus	CT shows fracture lines ENG: caloric paralysis
Labyrinthine concussion	Immediate onset, moderately severe, gradual improvement	External ear and drum normal, spontaneous nystagmus	ENG: caloric paresis
Benign positional vertigo	Delayed onset, brief episodes, position induced	Fatigable positional nystagmus	Normal
Perilymph fistula	Fluctuating, induced by . coughing, sneezing, straining, etc.	Positive fistula test	ENG: caloric paresis

CT, Computed tomography; *ENG,* electronystagmography.

imbalance also are sometimes reported by healthy persons when air pressure in the external auditory canal changes during routine pneumatoscopy (Table 5).

Treatment

There is no specific therapy for vertigo or sensorineural hearing loss caused by temporal bone trauma unless there is evidence of perilymph fistula. Initial management consists of vestibular suppression to control vertigo and nausea followed by vestibular exercises as soon as the patient is able to perform them. Posttraumatic positional vertigo responds to positional maneuvers similar to other varieties of benign positional vertigo (see Fig. 1). Persistent fluctuating vestibular symptoms may indicate the presence of a perilymphatic fistula and necessitate exploration of the middle ear. It is important, however, to recognize that most perilymphatic fistulas heal spontaneously without surgical intervention. For this reason, most authors advocate conservative management with an initial period of bed rest, sedation, head elevation, and measures to decrease straining (53). One exception to this conservative approach might be acute barotrauma, in which immediate exploration has been advocated (54). Persistent auditory and vestibular symptoms are indications for exploration of the middle ear after an initial trial of conservative management. Even in these cases, however, only about one half to two thirds of ears are found to have fistulas.

METABOLIC DISORDERS

Diabetes Mellitus

Vestibular symptoms and signs are common among patients with diabetes mellitus, but convincing evidence does not exist for a specific vestibular lesion. Among patients with diabetes and vestibular dysfunction whose temporal bones and nervous systems have been studied at necropsy, pathologic changes can be explained on the basis of associated vascular disease (16,55). The most common finding in the labyrinth at necropsy among patients with diabetes mellitus is periodic acid–Schiff–positive thickening of the capillary walls, most prominent in the vascular stria of the cochlea, where it probably accounts for the progressive high-frequency hearing loss characteristic of the disease (56). Similar changes are found in the vestibular end organs, which with degeneration of the vestibular nerve and ganglion might explain the frequent reports of chronic disequilibrium and dizziness among persons with diabetes.

Uremia

Multiple causes of auditory and vestibular symptoms can be identified among patients with chronic renal disease (57). The same pathologic process can affect both the kidneys and the labyrinth, as in patients with Alport's syndrome (hereditary nephritis and deafness), diabetes mellitus, and Fabry's disease. Immunosuppressant therapy for the primary renal disorder or to avoid transplant rejection predisposes the patient to otic infections, often with saprophytic organisms. Patients with renal disease are particularly vulnerable to the ototoxic effects of aminoglycoside antibiotics and loop diuretics because of their inability to clear these substances from the blood. Ototoxicity is probably the most common cause of auditory and vestibular symptoms among patients with uremia. Reversible hearing loss and dizziness can occur among patients undergoing long-term hemodialysis. In some cases the cause is hyponatremia (58), but most often symptoms occur without any obvious metabolic correlate.

Hypothyroidism

Symmetric, mild to moderate sensorineural hearing loss is commonly associated with sporadic, nonendemic hypothyroidism. Vertigo may occur among patients with hypothyroidism, although no vertiginous syndrome is characteristic of this disorder. Some investigators have found a high incidence of hypothyroidism among patients with idiopathic Meniere's disease, but most have not.

Otosclerosis

Although otosclerosis is primarily a disorder of the auditory system, vestibular symptoms and signs are more common than generally appreciated (59). Abnormalities at electronystagmographic testing have been found among as many as 50% of patients tested; the most common abnormality is unilateral hypoexcitability to caloric stimulation (60). The mechanism of production of vestibular symptoms and signs among patients with otosclerosis is poorly understood. Direct mechanical deformation of the labyrinth or chemical abnormalities of inner ear fluids are likely possibilities. Endolymphatic hydrops has been identified in a few temporal bones with multiple foci of otosclerosis. Sando et al. (61) studied four temporal bones of two patients with otosclerosis who reported prominent vestibular symptoms and found otosclerotic foci in opposition to the superior vestibular nerve in each. Vestibular nerve degeneration distal to these foci also was present, and three of the four temporal bones exhibited marked degeneration of the sensory epithelium of the cristae of the lateral semicircular canals.

Paget's Disease

Hearing loss is a common symptom of Paget's disease, initially described by Paget himself and subsequently studied in detail by numerous investigators (62,63). Progressive, combined sensorineural and conductive hearing loss usually is found. The vestibular labyrinth may be progressively destroyed, resulting in unsteadiness of gait and in rare cases episodic vertigo. In the late stages complete destruction of the bony labyrinth may occur with invasion of the inner ears, fractures, and degeneration of the membranous labyrinth.

Management of Inner Ear Metabolic Disorders

There is no specific therapy for the neurotologic manifestations of diabetes mellitus. It is presumed that the likelihood of inner ear complications decreases with good control of blood glucose level. Although it has been suggested that auditory and vestibular dysfunction occurs in the prediabetic state, similar to the retinal and renal changes, no controlled studies have supported this premise. The single most important aspect of preventing auditory and vestibular dysfunction among patients with uremia is to avoid the use of potentially ototoxic drugs. Careful management of the electrolytes of patients undergoing long-term renal dialysis may prevent fluctuating auditory and vestibular symptoms. Bilateral sen-

sorineural hearing loss associated with acquired hypothyroidism improves in a small percentage of patients after thyroid hormone replacement.

There is convincing evidence that sodium fluoride is effective in retarding the progression of otosclerosis (64). The usual dosage is 40 to 50 mg sodium fluoride per day given most conveniently as Florical (8.5 mg sodium fluoride and 364 mg calcium carbonate per capsule) plus 500 mg vitamin D daily. Side effects occur among as many as 20% of patients, the most common being gastrointestinal upset and musculoskeletal pain. Whether sodium fluoride can reverse the vestibular abnormalities associated with otosclerosis is unproved. The two main drugs used for the management of Paget's disease are calcitonin, a peptide that inhibits calcium release from bone, and disodium etidronate, an agent that selectively inhibits bone resorption by osteoclasts with minimal effect on formation by osteoblasts. Calcitonin is typically given in twice-weekly injections of 50 units. The usual dose of disodium etidronate is 400 mg per day (two 200-mg tablets). Therapy with both of these agents usually is continued for 6 months, and remissions may be protracted, sometimes for several years.

ACUTE ALCOHOL INTOXICATION

Alcohol intoxication is typically associated with unsteadiness of gait, slurring of speech and, occasionally, vertigo. The gait ataxia and slurring of speech suggest cerebellar dysfunction, but an additional vestibular component may be involved. Patients with acute alcohol intoxication typically display positional vertigo. This is associated with direction-changing positional nystagmus initially beating toward the ground during the acute intoxication phase and later beating away from the ground as the alcohol is cleared from the blood (65). This so-called alcohol positional nystagmus probably results from a differential effect of alcohol on the specific gravity of the crista and the surrounding endolymph (66). Alcohol first rapidly diffuses into the crista because of the proximity of this structure to blood capillaries and slowly diffuses into the surrounding endolymph. The cupula then has a lower specific gravity than that of the endolymph and acts as a gravity-sensing organ, maintaining a slight deflection as long as the lateral position is held. After approximately 3 hours, the endolymph and cupula have approximately the same alcohol concentration, and the positional nystagmus disappears. As blood alcohol level falls, the reverse situation occurs, the cupula being heavier than the surrounding endolymph, and the secondary phase of positional nystagmus occurs.

OTOTOXINS

Patients who take ototoxic drugs often are bedridden and have multiple symptoms of systemic illness, so additional symptoms of auditory and vestibular dysfunction may be overlooked. Vestibular symptoms of imbalance and oscillopsia are particularly difficult to identify in this setting. Only after the patient begins to recover and tries to walk do the devastating effects of vestibular loss become apparent. By this time the damage is probably irreversible.

Aminoglycosides

Although each of the aminoglycosides can produce both auditory and vestibular damage, streptomycin and gentamicin are relatively specific for the vestibular system, whereas kanamycin, tobramycin, and amikacin produce more selective damage to the auditory system (67,68). The newer aminoglycosides such as dibekacin and netilmicin are overall less ototoxic than the older aminoglycosides (69).

The aminoglycosides are excreted almost exclusively through glomerular filtration; they are not metabolized. Patients with renal impairment cannot excrete the drugs, so these agents accumulate in the blood and inner ear tissues. The ototoxicity of the aminoglycosides has been shown convincingly to be caused by hair cell damage in the inner ear. The earliest effect of the vestibulotoxic compounds such as streptomycin and gentamicin is selective destruction of type 1 hair cells in the crista. With the cochleotoxic agents such as kanamycin and amikacin, there first is selective destruction of the outer hair cells in the basal turn of the cochlea. This is followed by total hair cell loss throughout the cochlea as the dose and duration of treatment are increased. Because of the highly selective effect on the vestibular end organ, streptomycin and gentamicin have been used to produce chemical vestibulectomy among patients with episodic vertigo or Meniere's disease.

Salicylates

Treatment with high-dose salicylates commonly causes hearing loss, tinnitus, dizziness, loss of balance, and sometimes vertigo. All symptoms and signs are rapidly reversible after cessation of salicylate ingestion (usually within 24 hours). As are the aminoglycosides, salicylates are highly concentrated in the perilymph. Preliminary evidence suggests they interfere with enzymatic activity of the hair cells and cochlear neurons.

Cis-platinum

Cis-platinum is commonly associated with both auditory and vestibular toxicity. The incidence of aminoglycoside ototoxicity is about 10%, whereas the incidence of cis-platinum ototoxicity is approximately 50% (69). Tinnitus and hearing loss are extremely common. Vestibular loss identified with caloric or rotational testing parallels the hearing loss. The critical cumulative ototoxic dose of cis-platinum has been reported to be in the range of 3 to 4 mg per kg of body weight (70). The ototoxic effects may be decreased with use of slow infusions and dividing the doses over several months. As with aminoglycosides, vestibular toxicity may be overlooked because the patient has multiple symptoms of the underlying malignant disease. Cis-platinum ototoxicity may be caused by inhibition of the activity of adenylate cyclase in the inner ear tissues.

Diagnosis of Ototoxicity

The key to the diagnosis and prevention of ototoxic drug damage is a keen awareness by the examining physician of the potential auditory and vestibular toxicity. The patient should be asked about auditory and vestibular symptoms daily, and if possible, the drug should be discontinued at the first indication of ototoxicity. Because hearing loss due to ototoxic drugs usually begins in the high-frequency range, a screen of the high frequencies usually identifies early loss. Bedside vestibular testing is not satisfactory, but spontaneous and positional nystagmus often can be identified when fixation is inhibited with Frenzel glasses. For patients who can cooperate, a dynamic visual acuity test can help to identify early functional impairment of the vestibuloocular reflex. Patients are asked to read a Snellen visual acuity chart while holding the head still and then rapidly shaking the head, either in the horizontal or vertical planes. A decrease in visual acuity during head shaking of more than two lines suggests the possibility of impairment of the vestibuloocular reflex.

Treatment

The key to management of ototoxicity is prevention. Kidney function should be measured before a patient starts taking any potentially ototoxic drug. Patients in high-risk groups, particularly those with known impaired renal function or existing sensorineural hearing loss, should be monitored with periodic auditory and vestibular testing. As with other causes of bilateral vestibular loss, treatment of patients with permanent bilateral vestibular loss caused by ototoxins should be directed at retraining the nervous system to use other sensory signals to replace the lost vestibular signals. Practical suggestions on how to avoid head-movement–induced oscillopsia (stopping and holding the head still when attempting to read a sign) and gait unsteadiness (having a light on throughout the night) are useful accompanied by an active exercise program to force central compensation. Younger patients often return to nearly normal activity over a period of years, but elderly patients are rarely able to compensate fully for the vestibular loss.

AUTOIMMUNE INNER EAR DISEASE

Clinical Features

Autoimmune inner ear disease is an uncommon but important cause of progressive bilateral loss of auditory and vestibular function (71). It can be confined to the inner ears, but more often it is part of a general systemic autoimmune disorder that involves the inner ears and other target organs. Clinical symptoms often begin with fluctuating hearing loss, ear pressure and tinnitus, along with vertigo, suggesting the diagnosis of Meniere's disease. Unlike Meniere's disease, however, these symptoms rapidly progress to involve the opposite side over weeks to months. Sometimes there is slowly progressive bilateral sensorineural hearing loss accompanied by progressive bilateral loss of vestibular function (loss of response to caloric and rotational stimulation).

Pathophysiology

The blood-labyrinth barrier is analogous to the blood-brain barrier with respect to immunoglobulin equilibrium, and the inner ear is capable of responding to an antigen challenge just as the brain is. A few pathologic studies have been performed on temporal bones from patients with autoimmune inner ear disease (16). Surprising was that the studies did not show localized vasculitis, even among patients with prominent vasculitis in other organs. The most consistent finding was diffuse degeneration of all neural elements in the inner ear. Endolymphatic hydrops was found in one case.

Diagnosis

The diagnosis of autoimmune inner ear disease is based on finding the characteristic clinical course and laboratory evidence of altered immune function. Cogan's syndrome is defined as autoimmune inner ear disease accompanied by interstitial keratitis (72). Patients may begin with isolated inner ear involvement or Cogan's syndrome and later have a more generalized systemic autoimmune disorder such as polyarteritis or rheumatoid arthritis. Blood tests for an elevated erythrocyte sedimentation rate, cryoglobulins, or serum complement are helpful but not diagnostic. Although there have been several specific antibody tests suggested for the diagnosis of autoimmune inner ear disease, at present there is no completely reliable test for the disorder (71). Most patients with sensorineural hearing loss have serum antibodies to inner ear proteins, particularly heat shock protein 70 (73).

Treatment

Many different therapeutic regimens have been tried for autoimmune inner ear disease, and the reported results have varied from report to report. There is general agreement, however, that the initial treatment should be with high doses of steroids (60 to 100 mg prednisone or 12 to 16 mg dexamethasone per day in divided doses for a minimum of 10 days), followed by tapering to a maintenance dose (10 mg of prednisone or 2 to 4 mg of dexamethasone every other day for 3 to 6 months). Response to treatment seems to be more effective if the steroids are begun early in the course, although there have been reports of recovery among patients with near-total deafness (72). The disease process can be reactivated after a period of stability without steroid administration. Cytotoxic drugs such as methotrexate and cyclophosphamide have been used successfully with or without steroids to treat patients who did not respond to steroids (74,75).

SUMMARY POINTS

- Benign positional vertigo is caused by freely floating otoconial debris, usually within the posterior semicircular canal (canalithiasis).
- Benign positional vertigo can be diagnosed at the bedside with the Dix-Hallpike positioning test and cured with a particle repositioning maneuver designed to move the otoconial debris from the posterior semicircular canal into the utricle.
- Viral neurolabyrinthitis can present itself as sudden deafness, acute vertigo gradually resolving over several days, or with combined hearing loss and vertigo.
- Meniere's disease is characterized by fluctuating hearing loss, tinnitus, episodic vertigo, and a sensation of fullness or pressure in the ear.
- Autoimmune inner ear disease and syphilitic labyrinthitis can present themselves as rapidly progressive Meniere's disease.
- Infarction of the labyrinth often is associated with other symptoms and signs of vertebrobasilar insufficiency.
- Benign positional vertigo is the most common neurotologic sequela of head trauma.
- Perilymphatic fistula can be induced by violent nose bleeds, sneezing, barotrauma, or a sudden increase in cerebrospinal fluid pressure associated with lifting, straining, coughing, or vigorous exercise.
- The aminoglycosides streptomycin and gentamicin selectively damage the vestibular system, so monitoring auditory function is of little use in preventing ototoxicity with these drugs.
- The hearing loss associated with autoimmune inner ear disease typically responds dramatically to immunosuppression with high doses of steroids.

ACKNOWLEDGMENTS

This work was supported by NIH grants AG09063 and PO1 DC02952.

REFERENCES

1. Baloh RW, Honrubia V. *Clinical neurophysiology of the vestibular system*, 2nd ed. Philadelphia: FA Davis, 1990.
2. Baloh RW, Honrubia V, Jacobson K. Benign positional vertigo: clinical and oculographic features in 240 cases. *Neurology* 1987;37:371–378.
3. Katsarkas A, Kirkham TH. Paroxysmal positional vertigo: a study of 255 cases. *J Otolaryngol* 1978;7:320–330.
4. Dix M, Hallpike C. The pathology, symptomatology and diagnosis of certain common disorders of the vestibular system. *Ann Otol Rhinol Laryngol* 1952;61:987–1016.
5. Harbert F. Benign paroxysmal positional nystagmus. *Arch Ophthalmol* 1970;84:298–302.
6. Gacek RR. Singular neurectomy update, II: review of 102 cases. *Laryngoscope* 1991;101:855–862.
7. Parnes LS, McClure JA. Free floating endolymphatic particles: a new operative finding during posterior semicircular canal occlusion. *Laryngoscope* 1992;102:988–992.
8. Schuknecht H. Cupulolithiasis. *Arch Otolaryngol* 1985;14:1.
9. Schuknecht H, Ruby R. Cupulolithiasis. *Adv Otorhinolaryngol* 1973; 20:434–43.
10. Epley JM. The canalith repositioning procedure: for treatment of benign paroxysmal positional vertigo. *Otolaryngol Head Neck Surg* 1992;107:399–404.
11. Brandt T, Steddin S. Current view of the mechanism of benign paroxysmal positional vertigo: cupulolithiasis or canalithiasis? *J Vestib Res* 1993;3:373–382.
12. Baloh RW. Benign positional vertigo. In: Baloh RW, Halmagyi GM, eds. *Disorders of the vestibular system*. New York: Oxford University Press, 1996:328–339.
13. Baloh RW, Jacobson K, Honrubia V. Horizontal canal variant of benign positional vertigo. *Neurology* 1993;43:2542–2549.
14. Vannuchi P, Giannoni B, Pagnini P. Treatment of horizontal semicircular canal benign paroxysmal positional vertigo. *J Vestib Res* 1997;7: 1–6.
15. Paparella MM, Goycoolea MV, Meyerhoff WL. Inner ear pathology and otitis media: a review. *Ann Otol Rhinol Laryngol* 1980;89:249–253.
16. Schuknecht HF. *Pathology of the ear*, 2nd ed. Philadelphia: Lea & Febiger, 1993.
17. Coats AC. Vestibular neuronitis. *Acta Otolaryngol* 1969;251:1–32.
18. Schuknecht HF, Witt RL. Acute bilateral sequential vestibular neuritis. *Am J Otolaryngol* 1985;6:255–257.
19. Robillard RB, Hilsinger RL, Adour KK. Ramsay Hunt facial paralysis: clinical analysis of 185 patients. *Otolaryngol Head Neck Surg* 1986;95: 292–297.
20. Peitersen E, Anderson P. Spontaneous course of 220 peripheral non-traumatic facial palsies. *Acta Otolaryngol (Stockh)* 1966;[Suppl 224]: 296–300.
21. Schuknecht HF. Neurolabyrinthitis: viral infections of the peripheral auditory and vestibular systems. In: Nomura Y, ed. *Hearing loss and dizziness*. Tokyo: Igaku–Shoin, 1985:1.
22. Baloh RW, Lopez I, Ishiyama A, Wackym PA, Honrubia V. Vestibular neuritis: clinical-pathological correlation. *Otolaryngol Head Neck Surg* 1996;114:586–592.
23. Davis LE, Johnsson LG. Viral infections of the inner ear: clinical, virologic and pathologic studies in humans and animals. *Am J Otolaryngol* 1983;4:347–362.
24. Nomura Y, Kurata T, Saito K. Sudden deafness: human temporal bone studies and an animal model. In: Nomura Y, ed. *Hearing loss and dizziness*. Tokyo: Igaku–Shoin, 1985:58.
25. Morrison AW. Late syphilis. In: Morrison AW, ed. *Management of sensorineural deafness*. Boston: Butterworth, 1975:109.
26. Steckelberg JM, McDonald TJ. Otologic involvement in late syphilis. *Laryngoscope* 1984;94:753–757.
27. Hughes GB, Rutherford I. Predictive value of serologic tests for syphilis in otology. *Ann Otol Rhinol Laryngol* 1986:95:250–259.
28. Areyasu L, Byl FM, Sprague MS, Adour KK. The beneficial effect of

29. Uri N, Meyer W, Greenberg E, Kitzes-Cohen R. Herpes zoster oticus: treatment with acyclovir. *Ann Otol Rhinol Laryngol* 1992;101:161–162.
30. Murakami S, Hato N, Horiuchi J, Honda N, Gyo K, Yanagihara N. Treatment of Ramsay Hunt syndrome with acyclovir-prednisone: significance of early diagnosis and treatment. *Ann Neurol* 1997;41: 353–357.
31. Eggermont JJ, Schmidt PH. Meniere's disease: a long-term follow–up study of hearing loss. *Ann Otol Rhinol Laryngol* 1985;94:1–9.
32. Tumarkin I. Otolithic catastrophe: a new syndrome. *Br Med J* 1936;2: 175–177.
33. Baloh RW, Jacobson K, Winder AT. Drop attacks with Meniere's syndrome. *Ann Neurol* 1990;28:384–387.
34. Nadol JB, Weiss AD, Parker SW. Vertigo of delayed onset after sudden deafness. *Ann Otol* 1975;84:841–846.
35. Schuknecht HF. Delayed endolymphatic hydrops. *Ann Otol* 1978;87: 743–748.
36. Paparella MM. Pathology of Meniere's disease. *Ann Otol Rhinol Laryngol* 1984;93[Suppl 112]:31–35.
37. Beal D. Effect of endolymphatic sac ablation in the rabbit and cat. *Acta Otolaryngol (Stockh)* 1968;66:333–346.
38. Kimura RS. Experimental blockage of the endolymphatic duct and sac and its effect on the inner ear of the guinea pig: a study on endolymphatic hydrops. *Ann Otol Rhinol Laryngol* 1967;76:664–687.
39. Santos PM, Hall RA, Snyder JM, Hughes LF, Dobie RA. Diuretic and diet effect on Meniere's disease evaluated by the 1989 Committee on Hearing and Equilibrium guidelines. *Otolaryngol Head Neck Surg* 1993;109:680–689.
40. Boles R, Rice DH, Hybels R, Work WP. Conservative management of Meniere's disease: Furstenberg regimen revisited. *Ann Otol Rhinol Laryngol* 1975;84:513–517.
41. Jackson CG, Glasscock ME 3d, Davis WE, Hughes GB, Sismanis A. Medical management of Meniere's disease. *Ann Otol* 1981;90:142–147.
42. Torok N. Old and new in Meniere's disease. *Laryngoscope* 1977;87: 1870–1877.
43. Ruchenstein MJ, Rutka JA, Hawke M. The treatment of Meniere's disease: Torok revisited. *Laryngoscope* 1991;101:211–218.
44. Grad A, Baloh RW. Vertigo of vascular origin: clinical and ENG features in 84 cases. *Arch Neurol* 1989;46:281–285.
45. Stell PM, McCormick MS. Carcinoma of the external auditory meatus and middle ear: prognostic factors and a suggested staging system. *J Laryngol Otol* 1985;99:847–850.
46. Brown JS. Glomus jugulare tumors revisited: a ten-year statistical follow-up of 231 cases. *Laryngoscope* 1985;95:284–288.
47. Cannon CR, Jahrsdoerfer RA. Temporal bone fractures: review of 90 cases. *Arch Otolaryngol* 1983;109:285–288.
48. Davies RA, Luxon LM. Dizziness following head injury: a neuro-otological study. *J Neurol* 1995;242:222–230.
49. Schuknecht H, Neff W, Perlman H. An experimental study of auditory damage following blows to the head. *Ann Otol Rhinol Laryngol* 1951; 60:273–289.
50. Barber HO. Positional nystagmus especially after head injury. *Laryngoscope* 1964;74:891–944.
51. Goodhill V. Leaking labyrinth lesions, deafness, tinnitus, and dizziness. *Ann Otol Rhinol Laryngol* 1981;90:99–106.
52. Simmons FB. Perilymph fistula: some diagnostic problems. *Adv Otorhinolaryngol* 1982;28:68–72.
53. Wall C III, Rauch SD. Perilymphatic fistula. In: Baloh RW, Halmagyi GM, eds. Disorders of the vestibular system. New York: Oxford University Press, 1996:396–406.
54. Pullen FW, Rosenberg GH, Cabeza CH. Sudden hearing loss in divers and fliers. *Laryngoscope* 1979;84:1373–1377.
55. Makishima K, Tanaka K. Pathological changes of the inner ear and central auditory pathways in diabetics. *Ann Otol Rhinol Laryngol* 1971;80: 218–228.
56. Jorgensen M. The inner ear in diabetes mellitus. *Arch Otolaryngol* 1961;74:373.
57. Bergstrom L, Jenkins P, Sando I, English GM. Hearing loss in renal disease: clinical and pathological studies. *Ann Otol Rhinol Laryngol* 1973; 82:555–576.
58. Yassin A, Badry A, Fatt-Hi A. The relationship between electrolyte balance and cochlear disturbances in cases of renal failure. *J Laryngol* 1970;84:429–435.

59. Cody DTR, Baker HL: Otosclerosis: vestibular symptoms and sensorineural hearing loss. *Ann Otol Rhinol Laryngol* 1978;87:788–796.
60. Virolainen E. Vestibular disturbances in clinical otosclerosis. *Acta Otolaryngol (Stockh)* 1972;[Suppl 306]:1–34.
61. Sando I, Hemenway WG, Miller DR. Vestibular pathology in otosclerosis temporal bone histopathological report. *Laryngoscope* 1974;84:593–605.
62. Clemis J, Boyles J, Harford ER, Petasnick JP. The clinical diagnosis of Paget's disease of the temporal bone. *Ann Otol Rhinol Laryngol* 1967;76:611–623.
63. Davies D. Paget's disease of the temporal bone: a clinical and histopathological survey. *Acta Otolaryngol (Stockh)* 1968;[Suppl 242]:3–7.
64. Snow JB Jr. Current status of fluoride therapy for otosclerosis. Am J Otol 1985;6:56–58.
65. Aschan G, Bergstedt M. Positional alcoholic nystagmus (PAN) in man following repeated alcohol doses. *Acta Otolaryngol (Stockh)* 1975;330:15–29.
66. Money KE, Myles WS. Heavy water nystagmus and effects of alcohol. *Nature* 1974;247:404–406.
67. Fee WE. Aminoglycoside ototoxicity in the human. *Laryngoscope* 1980;90:1–19.
68. Smith CR, Lipsky JJ, Laskin OL, et al. Double blind comparison of the nephrotoxicity and auditory toxicity of gentamicin and tobramycin. *N Engl J Med* 1980;302:1106–1109.
69. Roland JT Jr, Cohen NL. Vestibular and auditory ototoxicity. In: Cummings CW, et al., eds. *Otolaryngology head and neck surgery.* St Louis: Mosby, 1998:3186–3197.
70. Hayes DM, Cvitkovic E, Golbey RB, Scheiner E, Helson L, Krakoff IH. High dose cis-platinum diamine dichloride: amelioration by mannitol diuresis. *Cancer* 1977;39:1372–1381.
71. Harris JP, O'Driscoll K. Autoimmune inner ear disease. In: Baloh RW, Halmagyi GM, eds. *Disorders of the vestibular system.* New York: Oxford University Press, 1996:374–380.
72. McDonald TJ, Vollersten RS, Younger BR. Cogan's syndrome: audio-vestibular involvement and prognosis in 18 patients. *Laryngoscope* 1985;95:650–654.
73. Bloch DB, San Martin JE, Rauch SD, et al. Serum antibodies to heat shock protein 70 in sensorineural hearing loss. *Arch Otolaryngol Head Neck Surg* 1995;121:1167–1171.
74. McCabe BF. Autoimmune sensorineural hearing loss. *Ann Otol Rhinol Laryngol* 1979;88:585–589.
75. Sismanis A, Wise CM, Johnson GD. Methotrexate management of immune-mediated cochleovestibular disorders. *Otolaryngol Head Neck Surg* 1997;116:146–152.

The Ear: Comprehensive Otology,
edited by R. F. Canalis and P. R. Lambert.
Lippincott Williams & Wilkins, Philadelphia © 2000.

CHAPTER 41

Vertigo of Central Origin

Robert W. Baloh

DIFFERENTIATING CENTRAL AND PERIPHERAL CAUSES OF VERTIGO

Vertigo, defined as an illusion of movement, indicates an imbalance within the vestibular system, but the same sensation can result from both peripheral and central lesions. Several features in the history can help the clinician differentiate peripheral and central causes of vertigo

R.W. Baloh: Departments of Neurology and Surgery (Head and Neck), University of California, Los Angeles, School of Medicine, Los Angeles, California 90095-1769

(Table 1) (1). Autonomic symptoms such as nausea and vomiting typically are relatively less severe with central than with peripheral vestibular lesions. Patients with central lesions can have prominent vertigo and nystagmus without associated autonomic symptoms. Accompanying symptoms are most helpful in differentiating peripheral from central causes of vertigo. Although common with peripheral lesions, hearing loss is rare with central lesions. Because of the proximity of other neuronal centers and fiber tracts in the brainstem and cerebellum, it is unusual to find lesions in these areas that produce iso-

TABLE 1. *Differentiation between peripheral (end organ and nerve) and central causes of vertigo*

Cause	Nausea and vomiting	Ataxia	Hearing loss	Oscillopsia	Neurologic symptoms	Compensation
Peripheral	Severe	Rare	Common	Mild	Rare	Rapid
Central	Moderate	Common	Rare	Severe	Common	Slow

Adapted from Baloh RW, Honrubia V. *Clinical Neurophysiology of the vestibular system*, 2nd ed. Philadelphia: FA Davis, 1990.

lated vestibular symptoms. Lesions of the brainstem invariably are associated with other cranial nerve and long-tract symptoms. For example, vertigo caused by transient vertebrobasilar insufficiency usually is associated with other brainstem and occipital lobe symptoms such as diplopia, hemianoptic field defects, drop attacks, weakness, numbness, dysarthria, and ataxia. Lesions of the cerebellum may be relatively silent but are always associated with extremity and truncal ataxia in addition to vertigo. Although patients with acute peripheral vestibular lesions do have imbalance, they are able to walk with only slight veering to the side of the lesion, even during the acute stage. By contrast, patients with cerebellar lesions exhibit profound ataxia and often cannot stand with their feet together, even with their eyes open.

Despite severe initial symptoms, patients with peripheral vestibular lesions rapidly compensate for their deficits over a few days to a few weeks. In contrast, patients with central vestibular lesions (e.g., Wallenberg's syndrome or cerebellar infarction) often show only minimal compensation for vestibular imbalance after months or years. The central pathways necessary for vestibular compensation often are damaged with these central lesions.

NEUROLOGIC COMPLICATIONS OF EAR INFECTIONS

Intracranial complications of temporal bone infection can produce severe clinical symptoms and signs and cause pronounced balance disturbances. Among these space-occupying lesions are epidural and brain abscesses.

Epidural Abscess

Probably the most common intracranial complication of chronic otic infections is extradural abscess, a collection of purulent fluid between the dura mater and the bone of the middle or posterior fossa. The dura mater usually is an effective barrier, and the infection remains localized outside the nervous system. Extradural abscesses are frequently asymptomatic and are incidental findings during mastoidectomy for acute or chronic disease (2). Extradural abscesses in the middle fossa may become large and compress the temporal lobe, whereas abscesses in the posterior fossa remain small because of the tight attachment of the dura. Initial symptoms of fever, severe headache, and vomiting without focal neurologic signs can create a diagnostic and therapeutic quandary.

Brain Abscess

Brain abscesses associated with ear infections originate predominantly from venous thrombophlebitis rather than direct extension through the dura mater (3). The temporal lobe is most commonly involved, followed by the cerebellum. Both aerobic and anaerobic organisms are found in pure and mixed cultures within brain abscesses. Multiple organisms are found in more than half of cases (4). Neurologic signs associated with temporal lobe abscesses often are subtle, particularly if the patient has received inadequate antibiotic therapy. The signs of cerebellar abscesses usually are more prominent. The patient reports severe neck stiffness and holds the head rigid in a tilted position. Neurologic examination reveals ataxia, dysrhythmia, and dysmetria of the ipsilateral extremities, and gait is markedly ataxic if the patient can walk at all. Asymmetric gaze-evoked nystagmus usually is present with larger amplitude directed toward the side of the abscess.

Diagnosis

Intracranial complications of otic infection should be considered when a patient with a known ear infection continues to have severe pain and headache despite appropriate antibiotic therapy (Fig. 1). The presence of fever, neck rigidity, and a positive Kernig's or Brudzinski's sign supports the initial impression. Focal neurologic signs may develop late in the course, even with localized brain abscesses, so one must have a high degree of suspicion based on the clinical presentation. After a detailed history and a careful physical examination, computed tomography (CT) with contrast infusion is the initial diagnostic test. CT depicts bone erosion, collections of pus within the intracranial cavity, and thrombosis of the venous sinuses. However, small collections of extradural or subdural pus and early stages of brain abscess formation can be missed, but the signs might be identified with magnetic resonance (MR) imaging. If a mass lesion has been ruled out, lumbar puncture is performed for analysis of the cerebrospinal fluid (CSF).

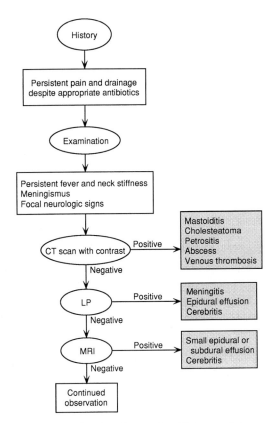

FIG. 1. Algorithm for the diagnosis of intracranial complications of ear infection. *CT,* Computed tomography; *MRI,* magnetic resonance imaging; *LP,* lumbar puncture. (From Baloh RW, Honrubia V: *Clinical neurophysiology of the vestibular system,* 2nd ed. Philadelphia: FA Davis, 1990, with permission.)

TABLE 2. *Frequency of associated symptoms among 42 patients with vertebrobasilar insufficiency*

Symptom	No. of patients
Visual dysfunction	29
Drop attacks	14
Unsteadiness, lack of coordination	9
Extremity weakness	9
Confusion	7
Headache	6
Hearing loss	6
Loss of consciousness	4
Extremity numbness	4
Dysarthria	4
Tinnitus	4
Perioral numbness	2

From Grad A, Baloh RW. Vertigo of vascular origin: clinical and ENG features in 84 cases. *Arch Neur* 1989;46;281–285.

Treatment

Management of intracranial complications of ear infections is directed along two lines: (a) eradication of the infection with appropriate antibiotics and (b) establishment of adequate drainage and excision of infected tissue when necessary (5).

VASCULAR DISEASE

Vertebrobasilar Insufficiency

Vertebrobasilar insufficiency is a common cause of vertigo among older patients (6,7). Whether the vertigo originates from ischemia of the labyrinth, brainstem, or both structures is not always clear inasmuch as the blood supply from both structures arrives from the vertebrobasilar system. Vertebrobasilar insufficiency is abrupt in onset, usually lasts several minutes, and is frequently associated with nausea and vomiting. Invariably the vertigo is associated with other symptoms resulting from ischemia in the remaining territory supplied by the posterior circulation (Table 2) (8). These symptoms occur in episodes either in combination with the vertigo or in isolation. Vertigo may be an isolated initial symptom of vertebrobasilar insufficiency or may be mixed with more typical episodes of vertebrobasilar insufficiency, but long-standing, recurrent episodes of vertigo without other symptoms should suggest another diagnosis (6,8–10). The cause of vertebrobasilar insufficiency usually is atherosclerosis of the subclavian, vertebral, or basilar arteries (11). Other less common causes of arterial occlusion include dissection, arteritis, emboli, polycythemia, thromboangiitis obliterans and hypercoagulation syndromes.

Infarction of the Brainstem and Cerebellum

Lateral Medullary Infarction

The zone of infarction that produces the lateral medullary syndrome consists of a wedge of the dorsolateral medulla just posterior to the olive. Although the syndrome is commonly known as that of the posterior inferior cerebellar artery, it usually results from occlusion of the ipsilateral vertebral artery and only rarely from occlusion of the posterior inferior cerebellar artery. Major symptoms include vertigo, nausea, vomiting, intractable hiccuping, ipsilateral facial pain, diplopia, dysphagia, and dysphonia. At neurologic examination the following abnormalities may be found: ipsilateral Horner's syndrome, ipsilateral loss of pain and temperature sensation on the face, ipsilateral paralysis of the palate, ipsilateral facial and lateral rectus weakness, ipsilateral dysmetria, dysrhythmia and dysdiadochokinesia, and contralateral loss of pain and temperature sensation on the body. Hearing loss does not occur because the lesion is caudal to the cochlear nerve entry zone and cochlear nuclei.

Lateral Pontomedullary Infarction

Ischemia in the distribution of the anterior inferior cerebellar artery usually results in infarction of the dorsolateral pontomedullary region and, less frequently, the inferior lateral cerebellum (10). Because the labyrinthine artery arises from the anterior inferior cerebellar artery in about 85% of cases, infarction of the membranous labyrinth is a common accompaniment. Severe vertigo, nausea, and vomiting may be the initial and most prominent symptoms. Other symptoms include unilateral hearing loss, tinnitus, facial paralysis, and cerebellar asynergy. In addition to the signs of ipsilateral hearing loss, facial weakness and cerebellar dysfunction, the examination discloses ipsilateral loss of pain and temperature sensation on the face and contralateral decreased pain and temperature sensation on the body.

Cerebellar Infarction

Cerebellar infarction can occur in isolation from brainstem involvement, particularly with embolic occlusive disease (11). The initial symptoms are typically severe vertigo, vomiting, and ataxia; because the brainstem is not involved, a mistaken diagnosis of acute peripheral labyrinthine disorder might be made (12). The key differential point is the finding at examination of prominent cerebellar signs including asymmetric gaze-evoked nystagmus and severe truncal ataxia. After a latent interval of 24 to 96 hours, some patients have progressive brainstem dysfunction due to compression by a swollen cerebellum. A relentless progression to quadriplegia, coma, and death follows unless the compression is surgically relieved (13).

Hemorrhage into the Brainstem and Cerebellum

Spontaneous intraparenchymal hemorrhage into the brainstem or cerebellum produces a dramatic clinical syndrome that frequently progresses to loss of consciousness and death (14). The cause of hemorrhage in most cases is hypertensive vascular disease, although anticoagulation therapy, cryptic arteriovenous malformations, and bleeding diathesis are important etiologic factors, whether alone or in combination with hypertension. Because of its potential for reversibility, cerebellar hemorrhage deserves particular emphasis. The initial symptoms of acute cerebellar hemorrhage are vertigo, nausea, vomiting, headache, and inability to stand or walk. As with cerebellar infarction, these symptoms may be confused with an acute peripheral vestibular lesion. Unlike the latter, however, examination in the initial period usually reveals nuchal rigidity, prominent cerebellar signs, ipsilateral facial paralysis, and ipsilateral gaze paralysis. The pupils often are small bilaterally but reactive. Approximately 50% of patients lose consciousness within 24 hours of the initial symptoms, and 75% become comatose within 1 week of onset (15). The condition often is fatal unless surgical decompression is performed.

Diagnosis of Vascular Causes of Vertigo

The diagnosis of vertebrobasilar transient ischemic attacks rests on finding the characteristic combination of symptoms in Table 2. The symptoms typically occur in episodes that last minutes. One often can find multiple risk factors for atherosclerotic vascular disease, and usually there is a history of myocardial infarction or occlusive peripheral vascular disease. Between episodes a neurologic examination usually has normal findings, although there may be residual signs of prior brainstem or cerebellar infarction. CT and MR images of the brain are normal unless there was prior infarction. MR angiography is a rapidly evolving technology that is now replacing conventional angiography for evaluation of the posterior circulation.

The diagnosis of lateral medullary and lateral pontomedullary infarction when complete is readily apparent when based on the characteristic combination of symptoms and signs listed earlier. Isolated cerebellar infarction is the most difficult to identify, although careful neurologic examination should demonstrate ataxia beyond that which would occur with peripheral vestibular lesions. Modern neuroimaging techniques are most useful for differentiating cerebellar infarction from benign peripheral causes of vertigo. CT scans usually are normal in the acute phase, but cerebellar infarction becomes apparent within a few days. With MR imaging, both brainstem and cerebellar infarctions can be identified easily (Fig. 2A) (16).

CT usually is superior to MR imaging in identifying intraparenchymal blood. Any patient with vertigo of acute onset and prominent ataxia of the torso or extremities should undergo CT of the brain. If CT shows normal findings, MR imaging might show evidence of cerebellar infarction.

Treatment

Treatment of patients with vertebrobasilar insufficiency consists of controlling risk factors (diabetes, hypertension, hyperlipidemia) and using antiplatelet drugs (330 mg aspirin a day or 250 mg ticlopidine twice a day) (17). Anticoagulation is reserved for patients with frequent incapacitating episodes or patients with symptoms and signs of a stroke in evolution, particularly basilar artery thrombosis. In these instances heparin is used in an intravenous bolus of 5,000 units followed by continuous infusion of 1,000 units per hour. The dose is titrated to keep partial thromboplastin time at approximately 2.5 times control. After 3 or 4 days, warfarin is begun in an oral dose of 15 mg. The daily dose is adjusted (5 to 15 mg) until the international normalization ratio (INR) is 2 to 3 times normal. Heparin is then discontinued. Among some patients symptoms and signs recur as heparin is discontinued, and the heparin must be restarted and tapered more gradually.

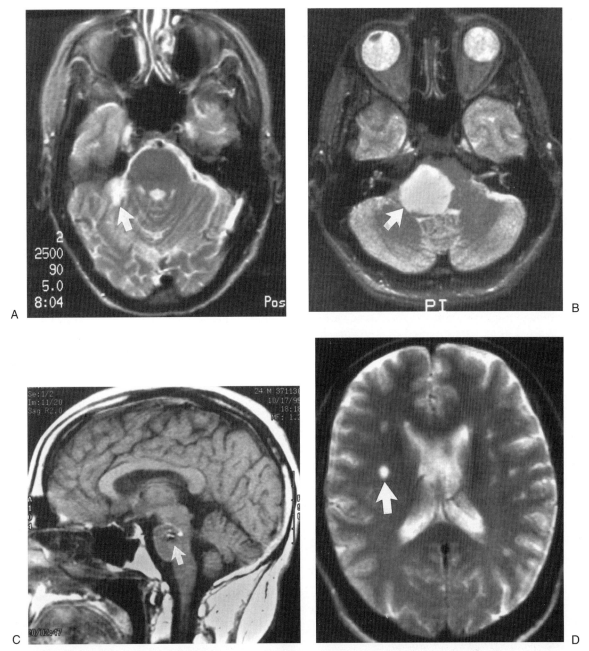

FIG. 2. Magnetic resonance images. **A:** T2-weighted image shows infarction in the distribution of the right anterior inferior cerebellar artery. **B:** T2-weighted image shows brainstem glioma involving the root entry zone of the right eighth cranial nerve. **C:** T1-weighted image shows cavernous hemangioma of the pons. **D:** T2-weighted image shows subcortical white matter lesions of multiple sclerosis.

Management of brainstem or cerebellar infarction is primarily symptomatic. The clinical course is typically that of acute onset followed by gradual, incomplete recovery. Vertigo may persist for months because of damage to central structures needed for compensation (18). Antivertigo medications generally are less effective for controlling vertigo of central origin than controlling vertigo of peripheral origin.

Hemorrhage into the cerebellum can be fatal unless surgical decompression is performed. The earlier the syn-

drome is recognized, the more likely it is that surgical treatment will be successful. Once the patient is comatose, survival is rare. Small hemorrhages into the brainstem and cerebellum may resolve spontaneously.

MIGRAINE

Clinical Profile

Migraine is a syndrome characterized by periodic headaches along with many other symptoms, including dizziness and vertigo. The classic migraine headache begins with an aura and continues with a severe, throbbing, usually unilateral headache. The aura slowly progresses over several minutes, lasts 15 to 60 minutes, and gradually abates. For about 25% of patients, however, the onset is abrupt. The headache begins as the aura diminishes, usually reaching its peak in about an hour and gradually subsiding over the next 4 to 8 hours. Nausea and vomiting typically accompany the onset of head pain. Common migraine can best be described as a sick headache. Vague prodromal symptoms precede it, but aural phenomena are absent. The headache can be unilateral or bilateral, build slowly in intensity, and continue for several days. Nausea, vomiting, diarrhea, chills, and prostration often accompany the headache.

Vertigo is a common symptom with both classic and common migraine (19,20). It can occur with the headaches or in separate, isolated episodes, and it can predate the onset of headache. Bickerstaff (21) first described a type of migraine similar to the classic variety in that it consisted of an aura followed by headache but was different in that the aura consisted of posterior fossa symptoms such as vertigo, ataxia, dysarthria, and tinnitus along with visual phenomena consistent with ischemia in the distribution of the posterior cerebral arteries. The headache following the aura usually is unilateral, occipital, or frontal, but it can occur anywhere. So-called posterior fossa or basilar migraine is estimated to affect 10% to 24% of patients with migraine (22,23) One must be alert for the possibility of posterior fossa migraine in any patient with transient vertigo and other posterior fossa symptoms. Some patients are unaware that migraine is the cause of their headaches and are much more concerned with the aura. If vertigo is prominent, the patient may not mention the headache, believing it is unimportant. Such patients may receive an incorrect diagnosis of peripheral labyrinthine disease.

Migraine Equivalents

Benign Paroxysmal Vertigo of Childhood

Basser (24) described an episodic disorder among children younger than 4 years that he called *benign paroxysmal vertigo*. A completely healthy child suddenly becomes frightened, cries out, clings to the parent, staggers as though drunk, and exhibits pallor, diaphoresis, and often vomiting. Symptoms are accentuated by head movement, and sometimes nystagmus or torticollis is observed. Some children report a spinning sensation, but most have difficulty describing what they are experiencing. The spells typically last for several minutes. Afterward the child feels normal immediately and can resume playing as though nothing had happened.

These spells typically begin before 4 years of age and can occur several times a month. After a 1 to 3 year period the spells decrease in number and gradually disap-

pear. Most children have no further spells after the age of 7 or 8 years. The cause of benign paroxysmal vertigo of childhood is not known, but most authors have concluded that this is probably a migraine equivalent. Follow-up studies of patients with typical benign paroxysmal vertigo during childhood indicate that more than 50% subsequently had migraine (25,26).

Other migraine equivalents among children may appear as cyclic vomiting, attacks of abdominal pain or even ophthalmoplegia. As the child matures, these nonspecific and often puzzling symptoms either cease or are supplanted by more typical migraine headaches.

Benign Recurrent Vertigo

Slater (27) and Moretti et al. (28) described patients who between the ages of 7 and 55 years began to experience repeated episodes of vertigo, nausea, vomiting, and diaphoresis. The attacks often occurred on awakening in the morning and were particularly common around menstrual period among women. Duration varied from a few minutes to as long as 3 or 4 days, with the vertigo becoming primarily positional toward the end of the spell. Nearly all patients had no symptoms between spells. There were no auditory symptoms with the episodes, and most patients had either migraine headaches themselves or a strong family history of migraine. The episodes of vertigo had several features in common with migraine, including precipitation by alcohol, loss of sleep, emotional stress, and a female preponderance.

Transient Migrainous Accompaniments

Symptoms of migraine equivalents can begin in adulthood. Isolated episodes of scintillating scotoma are common after 40 years of age. Fisher described 60 patients who exhibited attacks of paresthesia, aphasia, dysarthria, paresis, and diplopia with or without the visual manifestations of migraine (29). None of these patients had associated headache. Normal angiographic findings, long-term follow-up evaluation, and in a few cases necropsy suggested a migrainous syndrome despite the absence of associated headaches.

Mechanism of Vertigo with Migraine

The mechanism of vertigo associated with migraine is poorly understood (30). Constriction of the internal auditory artery might explain some symptoms, although one might expect a higher incidence of hearing loss accompanying vertigo. Although hearing loss does occur with migraine, it is infrequent compared with the incidence of vertigo. Phonophobia and tinnitus are much more common than hearing loss, the former being particularly prominent during the period of severe headache (19). Brief attacks of vertigo lasting minutes are probably caused by the same mechanism as other migraine aura phenomena, either constriction of intracranial arteries or possibly the so-called spreading wave of depression of Lao. More prolonged attacks of vertigo lasting hours to several days that are commonly associated with severe nausea and recurrent vomiting may be caused by the same mechanism as the headache phase of migraine, that is, release of neuroactive peptides such as substance P and calcitonin gene-related peptide into the inner ear and brainstem vestibular structures (20).

The possible association between migraine and Meniere's disease, initially mentioned by Meniere himself, complicates the situation further. Numerous case reports show migraine and Meniere's attacks occurring in the same patients (30). The patient has classic migraine episodes for many years before experiencing symptoms and signs of Meniere's disease. There is correspondence in the laterality of the hearing loss and migrainous headache and in the occurrence of headache and attacks of vertigo. Genetic defects in ion channels shared by the brain and inner ear might explain the combined symptoms (30).

Diagnosis

The diagnosis of migraine is relatively easy when the headaches are the main feature and there is a strong family history. Among patients in whom headache is less prominent or among patients with migraine equivalents, the diagnosis can be missed if one is unaware of the diversity of this syndrome. The following diagnostic criteria have been suggested for the diagnosis of migraine headaches (31,32): (a) recurrent headaches separated by symptom-free intervals and (b) any three of the following six symptoms: abdominal pain, nausea or vomiting during the headache, hemicrania (a throbbing, pulsatile quality of pain), complete relief after a brief period of rest, an aura (visual, sensory, or motor), and a history of migraine headaches in one or more members of the immediate family. Motion sickness (particularly car sickness) has been reported by more than half of adults (30) and 45% of children (33) with migraine and has been recommended for inclusion as a minor criterion for diagnosis.

Treatment

A complete review of the many possible therapies for migraine is beyond the scope of this chapter. In overview, however, treatment can be divided into two general categories—symptomatic and prophylactic. Antivertigo and antiemetic medications are useful for treating patients for whom vertigo and nausea are prominent features. Promethazine (25 or 50 mg orally or by suppository) is particularly effective for relief of both vertigo and nausea. These drugs also have a sedative effect, which usually is acceptable to a patient who is eager to sleep.

Prophylactic treatment is necessary when migraine attacks are frequent or the severity cannot be ameliorated with symptomatic medicines. It is the only effective therapy for migraine equivalents, particularly episodic vertigo. Propranolol is the most commonly used drug for the prevention of migraine symptoms. It is contraindicated for patients with asthma, congestive heart failure, peripheral vascular disease, diabetes, or hypothyroidism. Propranolol is the only β-adrenergic blocking agent approved by the USDA for use in migraine. As many as 70% of treated patients respond to the drug (34,35). The mechanism of action in migraine is not known, but it may be related to interference with serotonin or ion channel metabolism rather than with β-adrenergic blockade. The principle side effects are fatigue and lethargy, but weakness, hypotension, nonspecific dizziness, insomnia, depression, gastrointestinal symptoms, and weight gain have occurred. Side effects can be minimized by means of slowly increasing the dosage from a low starting level. Adults usually need 120 to 360 mg per day for maximum effect (average 180 mg per day). Usually the first sign of effectiveness is a decrease in severity of individual attacks or improved response to symptomatic medication during an acute attack rather than an actual decrease in the frequency of episodes.

Other medications that may be useful in the prophylaxis of migraine symptoms include tricyclic amines such as amitriptyline, calcium channel blockers such as verapamil, carbonic anhydrase inhibitors such as acetazolamide, and the serotonin antagonist methysergide. No controlled studies have been performed on the effectiveness of any of these migraine prophylactic medications for migraine-associated vertigo. On the basis of my professional experience, I recommend a trial of migraine prophylaxis to any patient with episodic vertigo of unknown causation who has a history or strong family history of migraine (20).

TUMORS

Tumors of the Cerebellopontine Angle

Tumors within the cerebellopontine (CP) angle typically produce slowly progressive compression of the seventh and eighth cranial nerves, resulting in sensorineural hearing loss, tinnitus, and in rare instances facial paresis, that evolves insidiously over months to years. Vertigo is uncommon with such lesions because the nervous system adapts to the gradual loss of vestibular function. Most often tumors begin in the internal auditory canal and grow outward into the CP angle, inasmuch as it is the path of least resistance. After the eighth nerve, the fifth cranial nerve is most commonly involved with tumors of the CP angle, causing ipsilateral facial numbness. In later stages of progression, involvement of the sixth, ninth, and tenth nerves may give rise to diplopia, dysphonia, and dysphagia. Compression of the brainstem and cerebellum causes ipsilateral gaze dysfunction and dysmetria of the extremities. In a series of 2,000 tumors of the CP angle reported by Brackman and Bartels (36), 92% were vestibular schwannoma (acoustic neuroma), 3% meningioma, 2.5% epidermoid cyst, and 1% facial nerve schwannoma.

Schwannoma

Tumors arising from the sheaths of the cranial and peripheral nerves have been called neuroma, neurilemoma, and neurofibroma, but convincing evidence that they represent a proliferation of sheath-producing Schwann cells makes *schwannoma* a more appropriate term. These tumors compose about 5% of intracranial neoplasms and are by far the most common tumor found in the temporal bone (36). They arise from the vestibular nerve in more than 90% of cases and much less frequently from the facial, acoustic, or trigeminal nerve. The general term *acoustic neuroma* therefore is inappropriate on two accounts.

By far the most common symptom associated with the vestibular schwannoma is slowly progressive unilateral hearing loss (37). Some patients experience fluctuating or sudden hearing loss, apparently from compression of the labyrinthine vasculature. Many patients describe inability to understand speech when using the telephone, even before they are aware of a loss of hearing. Unilateral tinnitus is the next most common symptom. Vertigo occurs among less than 20% of patients, although about half report mild impairment of balance.

Meningioma

Meningioma composes about 14% of intracranial tumors, and after schwannoma is the most common primary tumor of the CP angle (38). Meningioma arises from arachnoid fibroblasts, usually in the posterior aspect of the petrous pyramid near the sigmoid and petrosal sinuses. It displaces cranial nerves and compresses the brainstem and cerebellum but does not invade brain tissue. Because they arise outside the internal auditory canal, these tumors often become very large before producing symptoms and signs. As with schwannoma, the most common symptoms are hearing loss and tinnitus. Large tumors compress the brainstem and cerebellum and stretch the fifth and seventh cranial nerves, producing facial numbness and weakness.

Epidermoid Cysts

Epidermoid cysts arise from congenital epithelial inclusion rests in the area of the petrous apex. They slowly enlarge to fill the CP angle, stretching nearby cranial nerves and eventually compressing the brainstem and cerebellum. Because these cysts are slow-growing, the symptoms do not become manifest until the second to fourth decades of life. As with other CP angle tumors, involvement of the eighth nerve is a common early feature, but unlike the situation with other tumors in this area, hemifacial spasm is a frequent early distinguishing feature.

Cholesterol Granuloma

Cholesterol granuloma arises in the pneumatized spaces of the temporal bone when a small hemorrhage into the air cells causes a foreign-body reaction and progressive granuloma formation (39). A lesion within the temporal bone expands and can compress the structures in the CP angle. As with other CP angle lesions, eighth-nerve involvement is most common, and hearing loss is the most frequent presenting symptom. This is an important lesion to recognize because the surgical management is quite different from that of other tumors of the CP angle.

Diagnosis of Tumors of the Cerebellopontine Angle

The logic for differentiating the common types of tumors of the CP angle is outlined in Figure 3. By far the most common presentation of CP angle tumor is slowly progressive unilateral sensorineural hearing loss. Unilateral tinnitus is the next most common symptom, and vertigo is an infrequent symptom. Sudden onset of vertigo and unilateral hearing loss occurs occasionally with benign tumors but should suggest the possibility of a malignant tumor. After an audiogram, brainstem auditory evoked response is the most sensitive special audiometric test for documenting eighth-nerve involvement. The brainstem auditory evoked response is abnormal among 95% to 98% of patients with vestibular schwannoma (40). MR imaging is superior to CT for identifying vestibular schwannoma (41). MR imaging is even more sensitive when accompanied by contrast (gadolinium) infusion. CT is most useful for identifying bony erosion or calcification within tumors.

Management of Tumors of the Cerebellopontine Angle

Surgical management of tumors of the CP angle is discussed in Chapter 53.

Tumors of the Brainstem and Cerebellum

Glioma of the brainstem typically presents itself with relentless, progressive involvement of one brainstem center after another, often ending with destruction of the vital cardiorespiratory centers of the medulla (42). Vestibular and cochlear symptoms and signs are common, occurring in approximately 50% of cases, and the brainstem origin

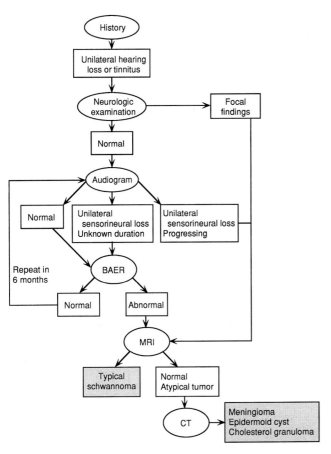

FIG. 3 Algorithm for diagnosis of tumors of the cerebellopontine angle. *ABR,* Auditory brainstem response; *MRI,* magnetic resonance imaging; *CT,* computed tomography. (From Baloh RW, Honrubia V: *Clinical neurophysiology of the vestibular system,* 2nd ed. Philadelphia: FA Davis, 1990, with permission.)

usually is obvious because of the multiple associated findings (see Fig. 2B). Although these tumors are five to ten times more common among children than adults, they still constitute approximately 1% of adult intracranial tumors (43). Tumors originating in the pons or midbrain usually cause long-tract signs, cranial nerve deficits, and ataxia. Although less common, glioma originating in the medulla may present itself with recurrent vertigo and vomiting.

Medulloblastoma is a rapidly growing tumor that occurs primarily among children and adolescents. The highly cellular tumors typically arise in the posterior midline or vermis of the cerebellum and invade the fourth ventricle and adjacent cerebellar hemispheres (44). Vertigo and disequilibrium are common initial symptoms. Positional vertigo and nystagmus are very common with medulloblastoma and may be the initial presenting symptom and sign (45). Headaches and vomiting also occur early from an obstructive hydrocephalus and associated increased intracranial pressure. Other fourth ventricle tumors that produce similar clinical features include

ependymoma, papilloma, teratoma, epidermoid cyst, and in endemic areas cysticercosis.

Glioma of the cerebellum may be relatively silent until it becomes large enough to obstruct CSF circulation or compress the brainstem. The most common symptoms are headache, vomiting, and gait imbalance. As with medulloblastoma, positional vertigo sometimes is the initial symptom of cerebellar glioma (46). The associated paroxysmal positional nystagmus is central in type because it is induced in several positions and is nonfatigable. Other tumors that present identical symptoms and signs include teratoma, hemangioma, and hemangioblastoma (see Fig. 2C).

Diagnosis of Brain Tumors

MR imaging is the diagnostic procedure of choice for identifying brainstem and cerebellar tumors (see Fig. 2B, 2C) (47). CT is not very useful for identifying soft-tissue lesions of the posterior fossa. Glioma of the posterior fossa is particularly difficult to identify with CT because it often is isodense; the only evidence of a lesion is enlargement of the brainstem or compression of the fourth ventricle. MR imaging can reliably depict both brainstem and cerebellar glioma and other tumors mentioned earlier. In some cases, CT can complement MR imaging by helping to differentiate tumor and associated edema.

Treatment of Brain Tumors

When possible, biopsy and surgical resection of the tumor is the treatment of choice. For nonresectable tumors, radiation therapy often is beneficial. Survival for more than 5 years is not uncommon with more benign astrocytoma. Medulloblastoma also is sensitive to radiation therapy.

BRAIN TRAUMA

Mechanism of Brain Injury

The most common mechanism of brain injury with blunt head trauma is movement and deformation of the brain within the skull. When the rapidly moving head is suddenly stopped, the viscoelastic brain continues to move and may rotate in the skull around the axis of the brainstem. The internal shearing and stress forces traumatize neurons and disrupt axons and blood vessels. The latter may cause multifocal petechial hemorrhage or even massive intracerebral hemorrhage. The term *concussion* refers to a brief loss of consciousness after head trauma unassociated with focal neurologic signs or radiologic evidence of structural brain damage. Loss of consciousness usually lasts for only a few minutes, although residual symptoms may last for months to years. The mechanism of such a brief loss of consciousness and rapid recovery is unknown, but diffuse release of neurotransmitters has been postulated (48).

Brainstem Contusion

Brainstem injury from blunt head trauma is not a common cause of isolated auditory and vestibular symptoms. Severe head blows may produce hemorrhage or infarction in the brainstem, but the patient loses consciousness and has multiple neurologic signs. As a rule, isolated episodes of vertigo occurring after brain trauma should not be attributed to brainstem injury.

Postconcussion Syndrome

Postconcussion syndrome has long been the center of medicolegal controversy (49,50). Symptoms include dizziness, headache, increased irritability, insomnia, forgetfulness, mental obtuseness, and loss of initiative, all of which occur after a concussion. Because of the ill-defined nature of these symptoms it is difficult to localize the site of the lesion, and patients frequently receive the diagnosis of psychoneurosis (51). The dizziness associated with postconcussion syndrome is nearly always nonspecific; patients use terms such as "swimming," "lightheaded," "floating," "rocking," and "disoriented" to describe the sensation. If vertigo is present, an additional labyrinthine lesion should be suspected.

Diagnosis of Persistent Dizziness after Head Trauma

Persistent dizziness after a blunt head injury often poses a difficult diagnostic problem (see Chapter 40, Table 5). A careful neurotologic examination should reveal most syndromes that necessitate specific treatment. The history is most helpful for separating peripheral and central causes. Examination of the ear may reveal evidence of a temporal bone fracture or perilymph fistula. Positional testing may reveal benign paroxysmal positional nystagmus, and neurologic examination may reveal signs of brainstem damage. Standard audiometric, brainstem auditory evoked response, and electronystagmographic testing are useful to assess the functional status of the auditory and vestibular systems. Neuroimaging usually is helpful only when there are focal findings at the neurologic examination.

Treatment

Treatment of brainstem contusion usually is directed at controlling the underlying symptoms. Physical rehabilitation programs can be helpful, but overall expectations should be modest because the structures important in compensation often are part of the damaged tissue. Therapy for postconcussion syndrome begins with reassuring

the patient that there is no evidence of structural damage, that symptoms are not unusual after head injury, and that the symptoms nearly always disappear with time. The patient should be encouraged to return to a normal exercise level gradually, even though dizziness and other symptoms may be aggravated at first. Although there is a positive correlation between the severity of head injury and the length of postconcussion symptoms, one cannot reliably base the prognosis for recovery on the nature of the head injury.

CEREBELLAR DEGENERATION SYNDROMES

Alcohol Cerebellar Degeneration

In addition to the peripheral labyrinthine dysfunction (positional vertigo) of acute alcohol intoxication (52,53), cerebellar dysfunction can result from chronic alcohol consumption. Cerebellar involvement causes a dramatic clinical syndrome manifested by severe truncal ataxia with relative sparing of the upper extremities (54). At examination, such patients exhibit severe ataxia of stance and gait with instability of the torso while standing and severe incoordination on heel-to-shin testing. At neuropathologic examination, atrophy is remarkably localized to the anterior cerebellar vermis, which can readily be identified with MR imaging. The cerebellar atrophy is probably caused by both malnutrition and direct alcohol toxicity, because some symptoms and signs associated with this acute cerebellar degeneration can be reversed with large doses of thiamine (55).

Familial Ataxia Syndromes

Auditory and vestibular symptoms and signs occur with several of the common hereditary ataxia syndromes (54). In addition, isolated families with atypical ataxia syndromes associated with hearing loss and abnormal vestibular function have been reported. Clinical cerebellar findings, however, usually overshadow the loss of vestibular function, and patients experience ataxia and incoordination. For most patients the symptoms are slowly progressive, although for some they are episodic. In some instances only after performing caloric or rotational testing can the physician recognize impaired vestibular function. Vertigo usually is not present because the vestibular loss occurs gradually in a bilateral, symmetric manner. The combination of clinical symptoms and signs is the key to differentiating the ataxia syndromes.

Diagnosis

MR imaging is the most useful laboratory test for differentiating cerebellar degeneration syndromes. With alcohol cerebellar degeneration the atrophy is remarkably localized to the anterior cerebellar vermis. With olivo-pontocerebellar atrophy, both the pons and cerebellum are atrophic, producing characteristic flattening of the belly of the pons. With late-onset cerebellar cortical atrophy the entire cerebellum is involved, although the posterior vermis is involved earliest and shows the most pronounced degree of atrophy. Minimal or no cerebellar atrophy is seen among patients with Friedreich's ataxia or patients with familial periodic vertigo and ataxia. Several of the inherited spinocerebellar ataxia syndromes can be diagnosed with blood tests to identify the abnormal gene (54).

Treatment

Alcoholic cerebellar degeneration may respond, at least partially, to thiamine replacement (55). Diener et al. (56) demonstrated that patients with alcoholic cerebellar degeneration who stopped drinking exhibited a marked and sometimes dramatic decrease in body sway measured with posturography compared with patients who continued drinking. This improvement after abstinence from alcohol may have resulted from central plastic changes or recovery of function when structural damage was not complete. Ron et al. (57) reported that the cortical shrinkage and ventricular dilatation seen at CT of the cerebellum were partially reversible with abstinence from alcohol.

Because the genetic defects are not reversible in most of the familial cerebellar degeneration syndromes, treatment is symptomatic. Patients are encouraged to use a cane or walker to improve sensory input and to avoid falls. Regular physical therapy to maintain range of motion about all joints is critical to avoid painful contractions. Acetazolamide is remarkably effective for relieving the episodic symptoms in patients with familial periodic vertigo and ataxia (58). These patients manifest long-standing recurrent episodes of vertigo and ataxia, sometimes associated with other brainstem symptoms such as diplopia, weakness, and dysarthria. The disorder results from a mutation in a gene that codes for a calcium channel subunit primarily expressed in the cerebellum (59). The usual dosage of acetazolamide is 250 mg twice a day. A therapeutic trial should be considered for any patient with early-onset episodic vertigo or ataxia who has a family history of similar episodes.

DISORDERS OF THE CRANIAL-VERTEBRAL JUNCTION

Mechanism of Brain Damage

Disorders of the cranial-vertebral junction can cause a range of brainstem and lower cranial nerve symptoms, including vertigo, hearing loss, and tinnitus (60). The basic mechanism for these symptoms is compression of the nervous system at the upper spinal cord and medulla. The rostrocaudal extent of compression is variable, and the impingement can be ventral, dorsal, or both. A less common but important cause of symptoms is vascular insufficiency due to angulation, stretching, or extrinsic compression of the anterior spinal or vertebral arteries.

Basilar Impression

In basilar impression the cervical spine moves upward into the normally convex skull base (61). The odontoid process projects intracranially to compress the ventral aspect of the medulla, and the cerebellum is compressed posteriorly by the first and second cervical vertebrae. Basilar impression often is associated with Paget's disease, rheumatoid arthritis, osteomalacia, osteogenesis imperfecta, cretinism, and rickets (62).

Atlantoaxial Dislocation

During flexion and extension of the neck, congenital fusion of the occiput to the atlas increases strain on the structures that normally restrict the motion of the atlas on the axis, especially if there is fusion of other cervical vertebrae as well. The transverse ligament that normally secures the odontoid process against the anterior aspect of the arch of the atlas may weaken because of this repeated strain, and the resultant laxity allows the odontoid to move posteriorly into the lumen of the foramen magnum. Flexion or extension of the neck may then produce symptoms depending on whether the predominant neural compression is anterior to the odontoid or posterior to the posterior arch of C1. Atlantoaxial instability is associated with a number of congenital and acquired disease processes. It is common with Down syndrome, Hurler's syndrome, Morquio syndrome, and achondroplastic dwarfism. Twenty-five percent of patients with rheumatoid arthritis have atlantoaxial instability due to destruction of normal stabilizing mechanisms by inflammatory rheumatoid tissue in the synovial membrane (63,64).

Arnold-Chiari Malformation

In Arnold-Chiari malformation, which is congenital, the brainstem and cerebellum are elongated downward into the cervical canal. The deformity most frequently manifests itself in the first few months of life and is associated with hydrocephalus and other nervous system malformations (Arnold-Chiari malformation type 2). Less frequent but more important to neurotologists are instances in which the onset of symptoms and signs is delayed until adult life (Arnold-Chiari malformation type 1). These cases often become evident with subtle neurologic symptoms and signs that usually are unassociated with other developmental defects (65). The most common neurologic symptom is slowly progressive unsteadiness of gait, which the patient frequently describes as dizziness. Vertigo and hearing loss occur among about 10% of patients (66). Dysphagia, hoarseness, and dysarthria can result from stretching of the lower cranial nerves, and obstructive hydrocephalus can result from occlusion of the basilar cisterns.

Diagnosis

In general, congenital abnormalities of the cranial-vertebral junction are associated with morphologic abnormalities of the neck, such as low hairline, short neck, abnormal head position, limitation of motion, and painful torticollis. Accentuation of symptoms with coughing, straining, or change in head position is common. Clinical manifestations of cervical medullary compression usually are relentless and severe, progressing over months to years. Occipital pain with radiation toward the vertex is a common presenting symptom. Other symptoms can be related to brainstem and cranial nerve dysfunction from compression. The diagnosis of basilar impression is confirmed when lateral radiographs of the skull demonstrate that the tip of the odontoid process extends above Chamberlain's line (a line drawn from the posterior edge of the hard palate to the posterior lip of the foramen magnum). With atlantoaxial dislocation, the critical assessment is whether the abnormality is reducible and the direction of encroachment on the cervical medullary region. CT is performed in the frontal and lateral projections; the lateral scans are obtained with the patient's head in both neutral and extended positions (67). MR imaging is now the procedure of choice for assessing the degree of soft-tissue compression associated with Arnold-Chiari malformations. Midline sagittal sections are ideal for identifying the level of the cerebellar tonsils.

Treatment

A series of operations have been developed to correct bony deformities of the cranial-vertebral junction, to eliminate cervical medullary compression, and to prevent recurrence. They are designed to reduce the odontoid process from its cranial position, to remove any bony ligamentous or inflammatory soft-tissue compression on the cervical-medullary junction, and to fix the skull to the cervical-vertebral column in the reduced position when necessary. Among patients with Arnold-Chiari malformations type 1, suboccipital decompression of the foramen magnum region can stop the progression and occasionally improve neurologic symptoms and signs (68,69).

MULTIPLE SCLEROSIS

Clinical Profile

Multiple sclerosis is a demyelinating disorder of the central nervous system of unknown causation that typi-cally runs a course of alternating remissions and exacerbations (65). Demyelination is confined to the central nervous system myelin, which is produced by oligodendrogliocytes. Peripheral nerve myelin produced by Schwann cells is minimally affected. However, because both peripheral and central cranial nerves contain central nervous system myelin at their root entry zones, demyelinated plaques involving the root entry zone may produce signs of peripheral nerve dysfunction. Plaques involving the vestibular and auditory nerve root entry zones can explain the frequent findings of unilateral caloric hypoexcitability and hearing loss among patients with multiple sclerosis. Whether the remissions and exacerbations typical of multiple sclerosis are related to repair of demyelinated regions or physiologic changes in nerve conduction unrelated to demyelination is debated. It has been repeatedly shown, however, that there often is poor correlation between clinical symptoms and findings on MR images of the brain or pathologic findings at necropsy.

Although many symptoms occur with multiple sclerosis, certain ones deserve emphasis because of their consistent appearance. Blurring or loss of vision caused by demyelination of the optic nerve (retrobulbar neuritis) is an initial symptom of multiple sclerosis among approximately 20% of patients. Diplopia, weakness, numbness, and ataxia also occur early in the disease. Vertigo is the initial symptom among about 5% of patients and is reported some time during the disease by as many as 50% (70). Hearing loss occurs among about 10% of patients.

Diagnosis

The key to the diagnosis of multiple sclerosis is to find disseminated signs of central nervous system involvement manifested in an alternating remitting and exacerbating course. In most long-standing cases, there are signs of involvement of the pyramidal tracks, cerebellum, sensory tracks, and visual pathways. No specific laboratory tests exist for multiple sclerosis, but abnormalities in CSF can be identified among about 80% to 90% of patients at some time in the disease course. Findings include elevated gamma globulin level, increased gamma globulin synthesis, oligoclonal banding of gamma globulin, and elevated levels of myelin basic protein (71). T2-weighted MR images of the brain depict white-matter lesions among about 95% of patients with multiple sclerosis, although similar lesions sometimes occur among patients without the clinical criteria for the diagnosis of multiple sclerosis (see Fig. 2D) (72).

Treatment

There is no curative therapy for multiple sclerosis. Steroids and corticotropin (ACTH) may hasten the remission of symptoms and signs after an acute exacerbation, but no evidence indicates that these drugs alter the natural history of multiple sclerosis. Interferon beta lessens the number and severity of exacerbations and also reduces the progression of MR-detected lesions (73).

VERTIGO AND FOCAL SEIZURE DISORDERS

Clinical Profile

Vertigo and other sensations of altered orientation occur with focal epileptic discharges from several different areas of the cortex. In Penfield and Kristiansen's series of 222 patients with focal seizures in which the irritable focus was identified at operation, 9 patients reported an ictal sensory experience of vertigo (74). In 8 of these patients the causal lesion was found in the posterior half of the superior temporal gyrus or at the parietotemporal junction. Electrostimulation of these areas produced episodes of vertigo similar to those experienced during a spontaneous seizure. Other investigators have found vertiginous auras with lesions in other parts of the temporal and parietal lobes, suggesting that the cortical-vestibular projections are somewhat diffuse.

As in the evaluation of most patients with dizziness, the history is critical for determining whether the dizziness can be caused by a focal seizure disorder. One must obtain an accurate description of the typical ictal event. An eyewitness often can provide the key information. Was the patient unresponsive? Were there associated stereotyped motor phenomena? Episodic vertigo as an isolated manifestation of a focal seizure disorder is a rarity if it occurs at all.

Diagnosis and Treatment

An electroencephalogram is the most useful diagnostic test for evaluating patients with suspected seizures. Patients with temporal lobe seizures often show unilateral or bilateral independent anterior temporal lobe spikes. Complex partial seizures often are difficult to control with anticonvulsant medications, even when patients are maintained on high therapeutic blood levels.

SUMMARY POINTS

- Intracranial complications of otic infection should be considered when a patient with a known ear infection continues to have severe pain and headaches despite appropriate antibiotic therapy.
- Episodes of vertigo typically lasting minutes suggest a vascular cause, particularly if the patient has known vascular risk factors.
- Vertigo can be an initial isolated symptom of vertebrobasilar insufficiency, but long-standing recurrent episodes of vertigo without other neurologic symptoms should suggest another diagnosis.
- Although isolated cerebellar infarction can become evident with symptoms similar to an acute peripheral labyrinthine disorder, the key differential point at examination is the finding of prominent cerebellar signs, including asymmetric gaze-evoked nystagmus and severe truncal ataxia.
- Infarction or hemorrhage in the cerebellum can cause delayed, progressive brainstem dysfunction due to compression by a swollen cerebellum.

- Isolated repeat episodes of vertigo among children and young adults are nearly always caused by migraine. About 25% of patients with migraine have episodes of vertigo at some time during their life.
- Acoustic neuroma rarely becomes evident with episodic vertigo because gradual compression of the vestibular nerve is compensated for at the level of the vestibular nuclei.
- By far the most common presenting symptom of a tumor of the CP angle is slowly progressive unilateral hearing loss with or without tinnitus.
- Alcohol ingestion can cause a cerebellar degeneration syndrome with atrophy localized to the anterior vermis of the cerebellum.
- Plaques involving the vestibular and auditory nerve root entry zones explain the frequent finding of unilateral caloric hypoexcitability and hearing loss among patients with multiple sclerosis.

ACKNOWLEDGMENTS

This work was supported by NIH grants AG09063 and PO1 DC02952.

REFERENCES

1. Baloh RW, Honrubia V. *Clinical neurophysiology of the vestibular system,* 2nd ed. Philadelphia: FA Davis, 1990.

2. Holt GR, Gates GA. Masked mastoiditis. *Laryngoscope* 1983;93: 1034–1037.
3. Hirsch JF, Roux FX, Sainte-Rose C, Renier D, Pierre-Kahn A. Brain abscess in childhood: a study of 34 cases treated by puncture and antibiotics. *Childs Brain* 1983;10:251–265.
4. Harrison MJ. The clinical presentation of intracranial abscesses. *Q J Med* 1982;204:461–468.
5. Neely JG. Complications of temporal bone infection. In: Cummings CW, et al, eds. *Otolaryngology–head and neck surgery.* St Louis: Mosby, 1993:2840–2864.

6. Fisher CM. Vertigo in cerebrovascular disease. *Arch Otolaryngol* 1967; 85:529–534.

7. Fife TD, Baloh RW, Duckwiler GR. Isolated dizziness in vertebrobasilar insufficiency: clinical features, angiography, and follow-up. *J Stroke Cerebrovasc Dis* 1994;4:4–12.

8. Grad A, Baloh RW. Vertigo of vascular origin: clinical and ENG features in 84 cases. *Arch Neurol* 1989;46:281–285.

9. Caplan LR. Treatment of patients with vertebrobasilar occlusive disease. *Compr Ther* 1986;12:23–28.

10. Oas J, Baloh RW. Vertigo and the anterior inferior cerebellar artery syndrome. *Neurology* 1992;42:2274–2279.

11. Caplan LR. Brain embolism, revisited. *Neurology* 1993;43:1281–1287.

12. Huang CY, Yu YL. Small cerebellar strokes may mimic labyrinthine lesions. *J Neurol Neurosurg Psychiatry* 1985;48:263–265.

13. Barth A, Bougousslavsky J, Regli F. The clinical and topographic spectrum of cerebellar infarcts: a clinical–magnetic resonance imaging correlational study. *Ann Neurol* 1993;33:451– 456.

14. Dinsdale HB. Spontaneous hemorrhage in the posterior fossa: a study of primary cerebellar and pontine hemorrhage with observations on the pathogenesis. *Arch Neurol* 1964;10:200–217.

15. Brennan RW, Bergland RM. Acute cerebellar hemorrhage: analysis of clinical findings and outcome in 12 cases. *Neurology* 1977;27:527–523.

16. Baloh RW. Vestibular disorders due to cerebrovascular disease. In: Baloh RW, Halmagyi GM, eds. *Disorders of the vestibular system.* New York: Oxford University Press, 1996:418–429.

17. Kistler JP, Ropper AH, Heros RC. Therapy of ischemic cerebral vascular disease due to atherothrombosis. *N Engl J Med* 1984;311:27–34.

18. Igarashi M, Ishikawa K. Post-labyrinthectomy balance compensation with preplacement of cerebellar vermis lesion. *Acta Otolaryngol* 1985; 99:452–428.

19. Kayan A, Hood JD. Neuro-otological manifestations of migraine. *Brain* 1984;107:1123–1142.

20. Cutrer FM, Baloh RW. Migraine-associated dizziness. *Headache* 1992; 32:300–304.

21. Bickerstaff ER. Basilar artery migraine. *Lancet* 1961;1:15–17.

22. Harker LA. Migraine-associated vertigo. In: Baloh RW, Halmagyi GM, eds. *Disorders of the vestibular system.* New York: Oxford University Press, 1996;407–417.

23. Harker LA, Rassek HC. Episodic vertigo in basilar migraine. *Otolaryngol Head Neck Surg* 1987;96:239–249.

24. Basser LS. Benign paroxysmal vertigo of childhood. *Brain* 1964;87: 141–152.

25. Lanzi G, Ballotin U, Fazzi E, Mira E, Piacentino G. Benign paroxysmal vertigo in childhood: a longitudinal study. *Headache* 1986;26:494–497.

26. Watson P, Steele JC. Paroxysmal disequilibrium in the migraine syndrome of childhood. *Arch Otolaryngol* 1974;99:177–179.

27. Slater R. Benign recurrent vertigo. *J Neurol Neurosurg Psychiatry* 1979;42:363–367.

28. Moretti G, Mannzoni GC, Caffarro P, Parma M. Benign recurrent vertigo and its connection with migraine. *Headache* 1980;20:344–346.

29. Fisher CM. Late-life migraine accompaniments as a cause of unexplained transient ischemic attacks. *J Can Sci Neurol* 1980;7:9–17.

30. Baloh RW. Neurotology of migraine. *Headache* 1997;37:615–621.

31. Prensky AL, Sommer D. Diagnosis and treatment of migraine in children. *Neurology* 1979;29:506–510.

32. Olesen J. Headache classification Committee of the International Headache Society: classification and diagnostic criteria for headache disorders, cranial neuralgias and facial pain. *Cephalgia* 1988;8(Suppl 7):1–96.

33. Barabas G, Matthews WS, Ferrari M. Childhood migraine and motion sickness. *Pediatrics* 1983;72:188–190.

34. Diamond S, Kudrow L, Stevens J, Shapiro DB. Long-term study of propranolol in the treatment of migraine. *Headache* 1982;22:268–271.

35. Ziegler DK, Hurwitz A, Hassanein RS, Kodanaz HA, Preskorn SH, Mason J. Migraine prophylaxis: a comparison of propranolol and amitryptiline. *Arch Neurol* 1987;44:486–489.

36. Brackman DE, Bartels LJ. Rare tumors of the cerebellopontine angle. *Otolaryngol Head Neck Surg* 1980;88:555–559.

37. Kim HN, Jenkins HA. Vestibular schwannomas and other cerebellopontine angle tumors. In: Baloh RW, Halmagyi GM, eds. *Disorders of the vestibular system.* New York: Oxford University Press, 1996: 461–475.

38. Granick MS, Martuza RL, Parker SW, Ojemann RG, Montgomery WW. Cerebellopontine angle meningiomas: clinical manifestations and diagnosis. *Ann Otol Rhinol Laryngol* 1985;94:34–38.

39. Gherini SG, Brackmann DE, Lo WW, Solti-Bohman LG. Cholesterol granuloma of the petrous apex. *Laryngoscope* 1985;95:659–664.

40. Musiek FE, Josey AF, Glasscock ME. Auditory brain stem response in patients with acoustic neuromas: wave presence and absence. *Arch Otolaryngol Head Neck Surg* 1986;112:186–189.

41. Valvassori GE. Diagnosis of retrocochlear and central vestibular disease by magnetic resonance imaging. *Ann Otol Rhinol Laryngol* 1988; 97:19–22.

42. Hirose G, Halmagyi GM. Brain tumors and balance disorders. In: Baloh RW, Halmagyi GM, eds. *Disorders of the vestibular system.* New York: Oxford University Press, 1996:446–460.

43. White HH. Brain stem tumors occurring in adults. *Neurology* 1963;13: 292–300.

44. Pobereskin L, Treip C. Adult medulloblastoma. *J Neurol Neurosurg Psychiatry* 1986;49:39–42.

45. Grand W. Positional nystagmus: an early sign of medulloblastoma. *Neurology* 1971;21:1157–1159.

46. Gregorius FK, Crandall PH, Baloh RW. Positional vertigo in cerebellar astrocytoma: report of two cases. *Surg Neurol* 1976;6:283–286.

47. Bradac GB, Schorner W, Bevder A, Felix R. MRI (NMR) in the diagnosis of brain stem tumors. *Neuroradiology* 1985;27:208–213.

48. Cooper P, ed. *Head injury,* 2nd ed. Baltimore: Williams & Wilkins, 1987.

49. Binder LM. Persisting symptoms after mild head injury: a review of the post concussive syndrome. *J Clin Exp Neuropsychol* 1986;8: 323–346.

50. Stuss DT. A sensible approach to mild traumatic brain injury. *Neurology* 1995;45:1251–1252.

51. Miller H. Mental after-effects of head injury. *Proc R Soc Med* 1966;59: 257–261.

52. Aschan G, Bergstedt M. Positional alcoholic nystagmus (PAN) in man following repeated alcohol doses. *Acta Otolaryngol Suppl (Stockh)* 1975;330:15–29.

53. Money KE, Myles WS. Heavy water nystagmus and effects of alcohol. *Nature* 1974;247:404–406.

54. Fife TD, Baloh RW. Cerebellar ataxia syndromes. In: Baloh RW, Halmagyi GM, eds. *Disorders of the vestibular system.* New York: Oxford University Press, 1996:430–445.

55. Graham JR, Woodhouse D. Massive thiamine dosage in an alcoholic with cerebellar cortical degeneration. *Lancet* 1971;2:107.

56. Diener HC, Dichgans J, Bacher M, Hulser J, Liebich H. Improvement of ataxia in alcoholic cerebellar atrophy through alcohol abstinence. *J Neurol* 1984;231:258–262.

57. Ron MA, Acker W, Shaw GK, Lishman WA. Computerized tomography of the brain in chronic alcoholism: a survey and follow-up study. *Brain* 1982;105:497–514.

58. Baloh RW, Winder AT. Acetazolamide responsive vestibulo-cerebellar syndrome: clinical and oculographic features. *Neurology* 1991;41: 429–433.

59. Ophoff RA, Terwindt GM, Vergouwe MN, et al. Familial hemiplegic migraine and episodic ataxia type-2 are caused by mutations in the Ca2-channel gene CACNL1A4. *Cell* 1996;87:543–552.

60. Bertrand G. Anomalies of the craniovertebral junction. In: Youmans JR, ed. *Neurological surgery,* 2nd ed., vol. 3. Philadelphia: WB Saunders, 1982.

61. Elies W, Plester D. Basilar impression: a differential diagnosis of Meniere's disease. *Arch Otolaryngol* 1980;106:232–233.

62. Menezes AH, Van Gilder JC, Graf CJ, McDonnell DE. Craniocervical abnormalities: a comprehensive surgical approach. *J Neurosurg* 1980; 53:444–455.

63. Bland JH. Rheumatoid arthritis of the cervical spine. *J Rheumatol* 1974;1:319–326.

64. Nakano KK, Schoene WC, Baker RA, Dawson DM. The cervical myelopathy associated with rheumatoid arthritis: analysis of 32 patients, with 2 post mortem cases. *Ann Neurol* 1978;3:144–151.

65. Bronstein AM, Rudge P. Vestibular disorders due to multiple sclerosis, Arnold-Chiari malformations, and basal ganglia disorders. In: Baloh RW, Halmagyi GM, eds. *Disorders of the vestibular system.* New York: Oxford University Press, 1996:476–495.

66. Saez RJ, Onofrio BM, Yanagihara T. Experience with Arnold-Chiari malformation: 1960 to 1970. *J Neurosurg* 1976;45:416–422.

67. Kumar A, Jafar J, Mafu M, Glick R. Diagnosis and management of anomalies of the craniovertebral junction. *Ann Otol Rhinol Laryngol* 1986;95:487–497.

68. Levy WJ, Mason L, Hahn JF. Chiari malformation presenting in adults: a surgical experience in 127 cases. *Neurosurgery* 1983;12: 377–390.

69. Spooner JW, Baloh RW. Arnold-Chiari malformation: improvement in eye movements after surgical treatment. *Brain* 1981;104:51–60.

70. Grenman R. Involvement of the audiovestibular system in multiple sclerosis: an otoneurologic and audiologic study. *Acta Otolaryngol Suppl (Stockh)* 1985;420:1–95.

71. Waxman SG. The demyelinating diseases. In: Rosenburg RN, ed. *The clinical neurosciences,* vol. 1. Philadelphia: Harper & Row, 1983.

72. Stone LA, Albert PS, Smith ME, et al. Changes in the amount of diseased white matter over time in patients with relapsing-remitting multiple sclerosis. *Neurology* 1995;45:1808–1814.

73. The IFNB Multiple Sclerosis Study Group and the University of British Columbia MS/MR Analysis Group. Interferon beta-1b in the treatment of multiple sclerosis: final outcome of the randomized controlled trial. *Neurology* 1995;45:1277–1285.

74. Penfield W, Kristiansen K. *Epileptic seizure patterns: a study of the localizing value of initial phenomena in focal cortical seizures.* Springfield, IL: Charles C Thomas, 1951.

The Ear: Comprehensive Otology,
edited by R. F. Canalis and P. R. Lambert.
Lippincott Williams & Wilkins, Philadelphia © 2000.

CHAPTER 42

Vestibular Rehabilitation

Steven A. Telian and Neil T. Shepard

Vertigo or disequilibrium may persist because of poor central nervous system compensation after any acute injury to the vestibular system, even if there is no ongoing labyrinthine dysfunction. Some patients develop maladaptive postural control strategies that are destabilizing in certain settings. These patients often benefit from a program of vestibular rehabilitation therapy. Although the concept of using exercises as part of the treatment of patients with persistent vertigo was introduced several decades ago, structured vestibular rehabilitation therapy programs have only recently been introduced. These programs are customized to the needs of the individual patient and generally include habituation exercises designed to extinguish pathologic responses to head motion, postural control exercises, and general conditioning activities. This chapter

  S. A. Telian: Division of Otology/Neurotology, Department of Otolaryngology–Head and Neck Surgery, University of Michigan Health System, Ann Arbor, Michigan 48109-0312
  N. T. Shepard: Department of Otorhinolaryngology, University of Pennsylvania; Speech Pathology and Balance Center, Department of Otorhinolaryngology, Hospital of the University of Pennsylvania, Philadelphia, Pennsylvania 19104

reviews the concept of central nervous system compensation for vestibular disturbances, the current status of vestibular rehabilitation therapy, and patient selection criteria for rehabilitative techniques.

PHYSIOLOGIC RATIONALE FOR VESTIBULAR REHABILITATION

A unique feature of the central nervous system is its capability of adaptive plasticity in the setting of vestibular system lesions. This property allows remarkably reliable adaptation to asymmetries in peripheral vestibular afferent activity and sometimes rectifies sensory errors due to central nervous system lesions. The process of adaptation is called *vestibular compensation* and results from active neuronal and neurochemical processes in the cerebellum and brainstem nuclei in response to sensory conflicts produced by vestibular abnormalities. In most instances, this process reliably relieves vestibular symptoms, provided that the lesion is either stable or producing only gradually progressive deterioration.

The stimulus for recovery from an acute vestibular lesion seems to be repeated exposure to the sensory conflicts produced by movement. Once the severe symptoms are resolved, vestibular suppressant medications are discontinued and an informal program of increased activities is encouraged. For most patients, recovery is rapid and nearly complete. For some, the symptoms of vestibular dysfunction may persist. These patients with chronic balance disorders are candidates for formal programs of vestibular rehabilitation. Such programs are most effective when customized to the needs of the individual patient and supervised by an appropriately trained physical therapist (1,2).

Four features of the nervous system underlie the physiologic basis behind vestibular rehabilitation. These qualities collectively enhance the therapeutic effect of customized exercise programs. They are as follows:

1. *Adaptive plasticity* of the central nervous system. It is possible to modify the mechanisms of postural control, the vestibuloocular reflex, and the ocular control mechanisms for saccades. These activities take advantage of short-term central nervous system adaptation to produce a change in the automatic mapped response to a familiar stimulus. To accomplish this, repeated exposure to particular environmental conditions or specific stimuli are needed. This factor is exploited primarily for managing disorders of postural control and gait difficulties.
2. *Central sensory substitution.* This feature involves the limited ability of the nervous system to substitute one sensory input (vision, vestibular, or somatosensory-proprioception) for another one that is virtually absent. For example, vision may substitute for loss of cutaneous proprioceptive input on the plantar surface of the foot, or it may help control eye movements among patients with bilateral paresis of the peripheral vestibular system. Although many patients naturally use substitution, some need specific targeted activities in a vestibular rehabilitation program to optimize this effect.
3. *Tonic rebalancing* of neural activity at the level of the vestibular nuclei in response to persistent asymmetry of input from the two sides of the peripheral vestibular system. This usually results from an acute insult to the peripheral system or an ablative surgical procedure. The acute (static compensation) phase of recovery should take place without active head movement exercises. However, some patients do not progress through the chronic (dynamic compensation) phase and need a formalized program of head movement exercises to promote this process.
4. *Habituation.* This is long-term reduction in a neurologic response to a particular noxious stimulus facilitated by repeated exposure to the stimulus. In the vestibular system, the unpleasant response usually is a vertiginous sensation, often associated with nausea, in response to certain head movements. Even with

the first three mechanisms firmly in place and functioning properly, deficiencies in the overall compensation process may persist. If so, certain specific head movements, position changes, or motion in the visual environment may predictably provoke brief spells of vertigo or disequilibrium. To reduce or eliminate these undesirable responses to daily activity, habituation exercises are prescribed that repeatedly expose the patient to the stimuli that provoke the abnormal responses. When this process is complete, the changes appear to be long lasting.

Acute Compensation for Vestibular Lesions

Vertigo of acute onset usually results from a pathologic condition associated with the vestibular nerve or the labyrinth. The vertigo is accompanied by nystagmus and a variety of undesirable vegetative symptoms, such as nausea and vomiting. As acute compensation for the peripheral vestibular insult proceeds, the subjective symptoms are greatly reduced, and nystagmus typically occurs only when visual fixation is eliminated (3). This acute compensation occurs initially through the influence of the cerebellum and probable neurochemical changes at the level of the vestibular nuclei (4). The changes are designed to minimize side to side discrepancies between tonic firing rates in the second-order neurons originating in the nuclei. This provides relief from the most intense symptoms within 24 to 72 hours. Nevertheless, the patient continues to have considerable disequilibrium because the inhibited system is unable to respond appropriately to the labyrinthine input produced by head movements involved in normal daily activities. Even after intense vertigo has been controlled, it is common to have continued motion-provoked vertigo until chronic (dynamic) compensation is achieved.

Chronic Compensation

To eliminate disequilibrium and residual motion-provoked vertigo, the system must reestablish symmetric tonic firing rates in the vestibular nuclei and accurate responses to head movement (5). If the peripheral lesion is extensive, the ipsilateral vestibular nucleus becomes responsive to changes in the contralateral eighth-nerve firing rate through activation of commissural pathways. This feature of the compensation process is critical to recovery after ablative vestibular operations, such as labyrinthectomy or vestibular nerve section. If the peripheral lesion is incomplete, the injured labyrinth produces disordered responses to movement that necessitate adjustment to the central system for proper reinterpretation of the input from the damaged side. If the lesion is unstable, as in Meniere's disease or perilymphatic fistula, compensation is nearly impossible unless the lesion can be stabilized. When the sensory input from the two ears is asymmetric, error signals are produced in the nervous system. These provide the stimulus for the compensation process and are necessary for recovery from acute peripheral lesions. The process of habituation should extinguish the pathologic responses to these error signals and is a critical element of chronic compensation. Although these adjustments usually are made quickly and are reasonably accurate, the central system requires consistency in the inputs to properly use them for habituation. It is not surprising that central compensation is enhanced by head movement but delayed by inactivity (6).

Neuropharmacology of Vestibular Compensation

Although they may provide satisfactory relief during an acute labyrinthine crisis, sedating medications are potentially counterproductive with respect to central vestibular compensation, especially if used for extended periods (7). Drugs that are typically used to manage acute symptoms of vertigo, such as meclizine, scopolamine, and benzodiazepines, all cause sedation and may prevent or delay compensation (8). The role of the cholinergic system in vestibular compensation has been studied most extensively. Multiple studies have confirmed that neurons in the vestibular nuclei have acetylcholine (ACh) receptors (9). ACh also is believed to be the neurotransmitter most likely involved in eighth nerve terminals. Some investigators, however, have demonstrated resistance to both muscarinic and nicotinic antagonists at synapses between the eighth nerve and the medial vestibular nucleus (10). Behavioral studies offer considerable evidence that pharmacologic agents that affect ACh activity affect vestibular compensation. These studies suggest that ACh agonists (e.g., carbachol, arecoline) and acetylcholinesterase inhibitors (e.g., physostigmine) cause decompensation in animals that have recovered from a vestibular insult, whereas ACh antagonists (e.g., atropine, scopolamine) reduce acute spontaneous nystagmus and may ultimately improve compensation (11).

There is evidence that inhibitory amino acids, including glycine and γ-aminobutyric acid (GABA) play a role in vestibular compensation. These compounds mediate commissural input between the vestibular nuclei; GABA alone mediates inhibitory input from the cerebellar Purkinje cells (12). Studies of administration of inhibitory amino acid agonists suggest that these substances play a role in potentiating the inhibitory effects of the commissural pathways on the deafferented vestibular nucleus. Glycine antagonists, however, seem to accelerate compensation and may even cause overcompensation of static postural measures such as head tilt in previously compensated animals (13). These findings are consistent with disinhibition of the deafferented vestibular nucleus by means of reduction of the commissural inhibitory input. There need not be any significant plasticity involved in these changes; rather the deafferented vestibular nucleus may simply be more susceptible to changes in the neurotransmitter levels because it receives less excitatory input from the periphery than the vestibular nucleus on the normal side.

Administration of benzodiazepines such as diazepam potentiates the action of GABA at GABA type A binding sites (14). Administration of diazepam has been shown to decrease the response of type I and II neurons in the medial vestibular nucleus to rotational stimuli in cats (15). Some authors have suggested that administration of diazepam should retard compensation. Animal data have not always supported this concept. An early study with cats showed no delay in return of medial vestibular nucleus activity with use of diazepam after labyrinthectomy (16). The authors also found behavioral benefits in the treated group and suggested that this may have resulted from elimination of the symptoms of acute vestibular loss, led to earlier locomotion and head motion, and promoted compensation. Peppard (7) found in experiments with cats that although the antihistamine dimenhydrinate delayed compensation of the vestibuloocular reflex, diazepam had little effect. A study with squirrel monkeys documented an increase in early disequilibrium along with the expected reduction of intensity of nystagmus in response to diazepam (17). However, the study found no apparent differences in physiologic measurements 3 weeks after labyrinthectomy and documented a fairly dramatic benefit among the diazepam-treated group as measured by time required for return to baseline performance on a locomotor balance task.

Decompensation

A relapse of vestibular symptoms after apparently successful compensation does not necessarily imply ongoing or progressive labyrinthine dysfunction (18). Although remarkably reliable, central vestibular compensation appears to be a somewhat fragile, energy-dependent process. Even after it is apparently complete, there may be occasional periods of symptomatic relapse due to decompensation. This may be triggered by a period of inactivity, extreme fatigue, change in medications, general anesthesia, or an intercurrent illness.

CLINICAL ASSESSMENT OF VESTIBULAR COMPENSATION

Role of the Clinical History

A complete neurotologic history is probably the single most important component in the diagnostic evaluation of a patient with a balance disorder. This also is true in the assessment of compensation status. The history should include a detailed description of the first episode of vertigo and emphasize the intensity and duration of that attack. The clinician should seek information about the nature and duration of typical spells and the progression of symptoms over time. Certain clues in the history suggest that the patient has incomplete compensation even though the vestibular lesion is stable. If the patient describes a severe vestibular crisis at onset without equally intense symptoms on any occasion since that time, an uncompensated lesion is the likely diagnosis. This is particularly true if the current symptoms are characterized as continuous unsteadiness following recovery from the severe crisis. In this setting there may still be intermittent vertigo, but it is exclusively provoked by rapid head motions or certain head positions. Intensity and duration of current spells equal to or greater than the initial insult suggest an unstable or progressive vestibular lesion. The utility and importance of this distinction might be illustrated by considering two relatively common clinical examples.

First, consider a patient with vertigo who is deaf in the right ear. The clinical history suggests severe viral labyrinthitis 2 years previously with sudden sensorineural hearing loss and severe vertigo lasting 2 days. Imaging findings were normal. The patient now seeks medical attention for disabling vertigo. Two very different situations might cause this symptom. The patient may find that although the intense vertigo resolved within 2 days, any rapid head motion since then has been associated with a brief but intense burst of vertigo that lasts as long as 10 seconds, preventing work with heavy manufacturing equipment. This suggests uncompensated labyrinthitis, and the patient is best treated with vestibular rehabilitation and weaning from long-term use of vestibular suppressants. On the other hand, the patient might report satisfactory recovery from the initial vertigo, resulting in a symptom-free interval of several months. If the patient begins to experience recurrent spontaneous spells of intense vertigo that last as long as 2 hours, delayed endolymphatic hydrops after labyrinthitis is suspected. Of course, this is managed quite differently. If medical therapy with salt restriction and diuretics is ineffective, labyrinthectomy will almost certainly relieve the symptoms. In the first scenario, a labyrinthectomy is both unnecessary and unlikely to be successful.

Secondly, consider a patient who seeks care regarding motion-provoked vertigo that seems to be worst when the patient lies on the right side. Audiographic and imaging findings are normal. The Hallpike maneuver produces subjective symptoms, and rapid positioning nystagmus is recorded at electronystagmography (ENG). The history is critical in determining proper treatment. If the patient reports that the initial spell of vertigo occurred when rolling onto the right ear in bed, lasted 10 to 15 seconds, and was identical to subsequent spells, the correct clinical diagnosis is benign paroxysmal positional vertigo (BPPV). Specific therapies for BPPV, such as particle-repositioning maneuvers, singular neurectomy, or posterior semicircular canal occlusion, might be undertaken

with success. If, however, the patient reports a severe vestibular crisis at onset with intense persistent vertigo and vomiting for 24 hours followed by slow resolution to the current symptoms, the diagnosis and treatment are very different. Although the current symptoms mimic classic BPPV, the patient most likely has uncompensated vestibular neuritis with secondary BPPV. Specific treatments directed at classic BPPV caused by canalithiasis would most likely be ineffective, and the patient would be best treated with a customized program of vestibular habituation exercises.

Role of Vestibular Testing

The purpose of balance function studies encompasses three major goals (19). The most traditional is site-of-lesion testing to determine whether the lesion is likely to be of central or peripheral origin. Second, the patient's functional ability to use the sensory input systems in an integrated manner is assessed. The third assessment goal is to evaluate the current degree of physiologic and functional vestibular compensation, factors critical in determining whether the patient is a candidate for rehabilitation therapy. Clinically significant spontaneous nystagmus, positional nystagmus, or a directional preponderance during the traditional ENG battery provides evidence for failure of physiologic compensation in the vestibuloocular reflex. Rotational chair testing provides information about the vestibuloocular system that is not obtained with traditional ENG (19,20). In general, although abnormalities in the timing (phase lead) or amplitude (gain) of the eye movements produced by the vestibuloocular reflex provide evidence for peripheral vestibular dysfunction, they do not address the issue of compensation within the central system. Persistent asymmetry (bias) in the slow-phase eye velocity responses produced by rightward versus leftward rotation, however, strongly suggests that the peripheral lesion is physiologically uncompensated.

Dynamic posturography can provide helpful adjunctive information about balance system function that is not available through the other vestibular testing modalities (19,21). The sensory organization portion of dynamic posturography is primarily a test of functional capabilities. By measuring the degree of postural sway under several test conditions, this test determines whether the patient is able to make proper use of sensory inputs from the visual, vestibular, and somatosensory systems for maintaining stable stance. It can document pathologic conditions in the vestibular system, but does not differentiate peripheral and central lesions. It may also demonstrate sensory preference abnormalities, in which the incorrect choice among conflicting sensory cues is selected inappropriately. This information is helpful in patient counseling and design of the rehabilitation program. The movement coordination battery of dynamic posturography may be used to assess automatic motor output from the central nervous system in response to perturbations of stance. Abnormalities detected may help to explain findings in the sensory organization test, especially the somatosensory and vestibular dysfunction pattern. It also may provide indications of previously undiagnosed but clinically important problems such as peripheral neuropathy or biomechanical deficits.

EFFICACY OF AND PATIENT SELECTION CRITERIA FOR VESTIBULAR REHABILITATION

The utility and success of vestibular rehabilitation therapy appear to be population specific. Patients with uncompensated or decompensated unilateral peripheral lesions have the best prognosis. The percentage of patients who dramatically or completely improve with therapy increases from 30% among those with symptoms due to head injury to more than 90% for those without head injury whose symptoms occur only with rapid head movement. Among patients with substantial loss of function in one or more of the sensory systems responsible for balance function (vestibular, visual, or somatosensory), prognosis for success in therapy is reduced. This does not imply that treatment should be withheld from these groups. The effect of oscillopsia and other deficits caused by bilateral vestibular paresis may be reduced with practice of rehabilitation exercises and the extensive educational benefit of the therapy program.

Controlled Studies of Efficacy

Norre (22) demonstrated in a controlled study that patients with BPPV seem to benefit from habituation exercises. The active treatment group demonstrated results dramatically superior to those of a sham-exercise group and an untreated control group. He also studied the use of traditional vestibular suppressant therapy during habituation training and found that those taking medications were approximately half as likely to achieve complete resolution of symptoms. Horak et al. (23) performed a controlled study comparing the benefits of a customized program of vestibular rehabilitation with results for two control groups. One group received medical therapy with meclizine or diazepam, and the other group performed a program of sham exercises, involving aerobic exercise and strength training. All three groups reported subjective decreases in dizziness; the benefit was dramatic for the vestibular rehabilitation group. Posturography and other measures of balance ability showed a beneficial effect only among the vestibular exercise group.

Shepard and Telian (24) conducted a randomized trial comparing the efficacy of customized rehabilitation programs with that of a generic program of vestibular exercises. The customized-therapy group showed statistically significant resolution of spontaneous nystagmus and rotational chair asymmetries by the end of therapy and significant reduction in motion sensitivity. They also had improved performance on clinical measures of static and dynamic balance ability. The only statistically significant change in performance measures for the generic program was in static balance ability, probably reflecting that one of the generic exercises was identical to one of the outcome measures in this category. The results of this study suggested that the level of vestibular compensation achieved in a customized program of rehabilitation is far superior to the level anticipated from a generic program and justifies the expense required to involve a trained physical therapist in the treatment of patients with chronic vestibular symptoms.

Uncompensated Unilateral Peripheral Lesions

Vestibular rehabilitation therapy is appropriate in any condition characterized by a stable unilateral vestibular deficit when the patient's natural compensation process appears to be incomplete. If medical evaluation reveals no evidence of a progressive process, it is likely that therapy will produce a satisfactory resolution of symptoms. This intervention is certainly preferable to long-term use of vestibular suppressants and may contribute meaningfully to the patient's future well-being and productivity. Regarding the patient's suitability for vestibular rehabilitation, the nature of the symptom complex is more important than the underlying diagnosis. Even chronic lightheadedness or disequilibrium may be treatable, provided that there is evidence of poor vestibular compensation. If any intense vertigo is experienced, it should be primarily provoked by rapid head motion. There should be no evidence of progressive or fluctuating labyrinthine dysfunction that leads to spontaneous vertigo spells such as those resulting from endolymphatic hydrops. Patients with stable central nervous system lesions or mixed central and peripheral lesions need not be excluded from treatment, although their prognosis may be more limited than that of the average patient with a stable peripheral injury. Although the therapeutic activities are best customized to the needs of the patient, Appendix 1 is an example of a program prescribed for a patient with an uncompensated peripheral lesion.

Positional Vertigo

One important group of patients with vestibular disorders treated with exercises are those with BPPV. In the studies cited earlier, the authors included patients with BPPV who were treated with conventional rehabilitation protocols. This approach is almost universally effective and is recommended as an appropriate treatment modality for patients with this diagnosis. The use of noncustomized programs such as Cawthorne exercises has a long and fairly successful history for the management of this problem (25). For some patients, the Cawthorne program is too intense and provokes disturbing vestibular symptoms, often associated with nausea or vomiting. These undesirable side effects may discourage the patient from continuing. A preferred generic (noncustomized) program for BPPV that addresses the needs of most patients with this diagnosis is provided in Appendix 2. When this program does not bring relief, it is appropriate to provide a customized habituation program or consider a treatment protocol uniquely designed for BPPV.

Specific treatment programs for BPPV have been designed that attempt to reposition particulate material, perhaps displaced otoconia, that are pathologically located in the ampulla (cupulolithiasis) or floating freely in the endolymphatic compartment (canalithiasis) of the posterior semicircular canal. These treatments are uniquely appropriate for patients with classic BPPV and are unlikely to be helpful to patients with other types of positional vertigo. Brandt and Daroff (26) advocated that patients lie down quickly from the sitting position onto the side that provoked the vertigo. After waiting for the vertigo to abate, the patients were to sit up quickly, wait again for symptoms to clear, and lie quickly onto the other ear. The patients were instructed to perform the maneuver repeatedly at each session until no vertigo was noticed and to repeat the exercises every 3 hours until they could no longer induce vertigo. Many of those who benefited from this approach may have been habituating centrally, although sudden cures did sometimes occur, possibly from repositioning of the offending particles.

The liberatory maneuver of Semont involves planes of motion similar to Brandt and Daroff's maneuver, yet is an attempt to dislodge and reposition the otoconia in a single session (27). Usually a physician or therapist has the patient quickly assume the offending position, waits for 2 to 3 minutes, then rapidly turns the patient through the original sitting position and onto the other ear. The patient is returned to the sitting position and advised to remain upright for the next 48 hours. Semont et al. (27) reported a greater than 90% rate of complete symptomatic relief among more than 700 patients after one or two treatments with this technique. Epley (28) and Parnes and Price-Jones (29) reported similarly high rates of success with particle-repositioning maneuvers. These techniques feature deliberately slow, passive manipulation of the head through planes of rotation specifically designed to allow the particles in the posterior canal to filter back into the vestibule. Variations on these particle-repositioning techniques have gained widespread acceptance and clinical application in recent years. Similar techniques with different planes of rotation can be used to manage the less common superior or horizontal canal variants of BPPV.

The clinician should attempt to differentiate pure BPPV and positional vertigo resulting from poor compensation

after a labyrinthine injury. The key feature is lack of a vestibular crisis at the onset of symptoms in BPPV. Although the first attack of BPPV usually is quite memorable because of its novelty to the patient, it is rarely any more intense than the subsequent attacks. In cases of positional vertigo due to poor compensation, even when positive Hallpike maneuvers are observed, particle repositioning maneuvers are much less likely to be successful. This point was illustrated to us when we used the particle-repositioning maneuver described by Parnes and Price-Jones (29). After one attempt at the particle-repositioning maneuver, we initiate a customized program of vestibular rehabilitation if the symptoms are not completely resolved. Only 28% of patients believed to have pure BPPV needed habituation programs because of failure of the particle-repositioning maneuver. Seventy percent of those believed to have positional vertigo from uncompensated vestibular lesions needed additional rehabilitation. It was interesting, however, that 63% of the patients with secondary positional vertigo reported substantial reduction of symptoms after the particle-repositioning maneuver.

Disequilibrium of Aging

Another indication for vestibular rehabilitation as a primary treatment modality is in the setting of multifactorial balance difficulties, such as those that occur among the elderly (30). This becomes especially important when other treatment options are unavailable or have been exhausted. These patients may benefit greatly from postural control exercises and individualized conditioning programs. The relationship with the therapist frequently assumes a strong counseling function, and the use of assistive devices for safety in walking can be introduced as needed. Given the public health effect of complications of falls among the elderly, any therapeutic program that can decrease functional disabilities due to disequilibrium and balance and gait problems is highly desirable. Prospective observational results from our laboratory suggest that both objective and subjective therapy outcome measures are not significantly poorer for those older than 65 years compared with younger persons. The only significant difference found among the older population was a longer time needed to maximize the benefit from therapy. Anecdotally we also find that the percentage of patients who need repeated contact with a therapist who supervises the exercise program, as opposed to an independent home-based program, is higher among the elderly population. A representative customized program for an elderly patient with imbalance and dizziness is presented in Appendix 3.

Use after Vestibular Surgery

When a surgeon treats a fluctuating vestibular disorder such as Meniere's disease by performing labyrinthectomy or vestibular nerve section, the goal is to stabilize the vestibular system by producing a complete unilateral lesion. Many of the unsatisfactory outcomes after such surgical treatment of properly selected patients can be attributed to incomplete or delayed postoperative compensation (31). All surgical patients should be instructed regarding the importance of central compensation in the success of vestibular surgery, and vestibular rehabilitation can be helpful in optimizing the outcome achieved. It is appropriate for the therapist to offer counseling and general instructions to any patient who undergoes a procedure that causes unilateral loss of vestibular function. Patients who demonstrate particularly slow recovery should be referred for customized vestibular rehabilitation. Patients at particular risk for poor recovery because of complicating central nervous system conditions, use of sedating medications, or poor motivation for recovery should be encouraged to pursue a customized program of vestibular rehabilitation early in the postoperative course.

Head Injury

Patients who have sustained head injuries often have substantial disability from vestibular symptoms. Because the deficits often include headaches and cognitive and central vestibular disturbances, vestibular rehabilitation techniques are best used as a supplement to a comprehensive, multidisciplinary head injury program. An important subgroup within this population is patients who may have perilymphatic fistula. Use of vestibular rehabilitation may seem counterintuitive for such patients, because rapid head movements should make the symptoms worse. However, because the diagnostic criteria for this condition are uncertain, a trial of vestibular exercises may be appropriate for patients whose hearing is stable. If there is clear improvement within the first 4 to 6 weeks of treatment, perilymphatic fistula is quite unlikely. Subjective improvement in symptoms, ranging from mild improvement to complete resolution of dizziness, occurred among 63% of patients in our series with evidence of fistula. There was no change in symptoms among 25% and worsening of symptoms among 12%. Surgical exploration is recommended to patients who become worse during the course of therapy, because failure of rehabilitation therapy provides strong evidence of an unstable labyrinth in this setting.

Malingering

When a patient may be malingering or embellishing the degree of disability associated with vestibular symptoms, it may be helpful to refer him or her for vestibular testing and a vestibular therapy evaluation. Dynamic posturography often can help identify malingering, because the patients typically demonstrates inconsistent or nonphysiologic results. They may perform poorly on the easier conditions of posturography even though they perform

the eyes-closed Romberg test without difficulty at clinical examination. Their performance often is within the normal range on the more difficult trials despite poor performance on the simpler trials. Experience suggests that persons seeking or receiving disability compensation and those involved with pending litigation are unlikely to experience substantial functional gains in vestibular rehabilitation therapy. Nevertheless, a therapist experienced in treating patients with vestibular disorders can be helpful in discriminating true physiologic disability from psychological or socioeconomic issues. This information might be helpful to a physician called on to provide written documentation or legal testimony in such cases. If the patient seems to have legitimate dysfunction and demonstrates a good-faith effort to cooperate with the therapy program, the physician is much more likely to support a disability claim or testify confidently on the patient's behalf.

Panic Disorder and Other Anxiety Disorders

Patients with panic disorder and other anxiety disorders often seek management of ill-defined vestibular symptoms. After an evaluation is performed, vestibular rehabilitation may be recommended as an adjunctive measure for their condition. If the anxiety is mild, vestibular rehabilitation activities function as a behavioral intervention similar to exposure therapy for phobias. If the anxiety component is substantial, particularly if panic attacks are frequent, psychiatric intervention is needed.

Meniere's Disease

In rare instances patients with Meniere's disease report positional vertigo or other chronic vestibular symptoms between their definitive attacks. Although such patients are candidates for vestibular rehabilitation, they must proceed with the understanding that the likelihood of lasting relief of chronic symptoms is reduced if the spontaneous attacks of Meniere's disease occur more than once a month. If the attacks are rare, or the acute phase of Meniere's disease has resolved, the prognosis improves considerably.

Diagnostic Trial

It is not always possible for a physician to determine whether the patient's symptoms are caused by stable vestibular disease with inadequate compensation or unstable labyrinthine function. In the setting of diagnostic uncertainty, a trial of vestibular rehabilitation is appropriate. It clarifies this important distinction and prevents premature surgical treatment when a course of rehabilitation will suffice. Failure to improve with vestibular rehabilitation lends further credibility to the diagnostic impression that the lesion is unstable or progressive. It is then suitable to proceed with appropriate surgical management.

Inappropriate Candidates

Patients whose symptoms occur only in spontaneous episodes, as with Meniere's disease, are unlikely to benefit from vestibular rehabilitation. If there are no provocative movements or changes in body position that reliably produce spells and no postural control abnormalities are found during the evaluation, the patient is best treated with alternative medical or surgical strategies. Nonetheless, such patients should be encouraged to remain active and optimize their general health through physical activities appropriate for their age and general health.

COMMON TECHNIQUES OF VESTIBULAR REHABILITATION

Habituation of Pathologic Responses

For most patients with positional or motion-provoked symptoms, the primary goal is to extinguish the pathologic responses that remain because of incomplete or disordered compensation. The therapist identifies the typical movements that produce the most intense symptoms and provides the patient with a list of exercises that reproduce these movements (32). These exercises are performed twice a day unless limited by severe nausea or dizziness. Patients should be counseled that symptoms are typically aggravated by the exercises at first but that gradual improvement will follow. Patients often are encouraged by experiencing short-term habituation at the end of an exercise session. If they can persevere with the program, most patients begin to notice dramatic relief of positional vertigo within 4 to 6 weeks.

Postural Control Exercises

When chronic imbalance is noticed by the patient and abnormalities of postural control are detected in the assessment, postural control exercises are a critical component of the vestibular rehabilitation program prescribed. Programs can be designed to correct weight-bearing asymmetries, limited mobility about the center of gravity, and problems with sensory input selection. For example, if the patient is found to depend on somatosensory input despite the availability of accurate visual cues, the program may involve exercises that require balancing on thick foam. This exercise would be performed initially with eyes open and eventually with eyes closed.

Visual-Vestibular Interaction

For patients with bilateral vestibular paresis or disorders of visual-vestibular interaction, exercises may be needed that optimize the use of visual system input for maintaining equilibrium and gaze stability (33). These may be incorporated with hand-eye coordination exercises when needed. Such exercises may be helpful in vestibular rehabilitation programs designed for patients with a high degree of sensitivity to movement within the visual environment.

Conditioning Activities

Most patients with vertigo and balance disorders adopt a sedentary lifestyle to avoid their symptoms. Although it may be understandable, this behavior contributes to ongoing perceived and actual disability and prevents recovery. All patients who receive customized vestibular rehabilitation programs are provided with suggestions for a general exercise program suited to their age, health, and interests. For most patients, this involve at least a graduated walking program. For some, a more strenuous program is suggested that may include jogging, treadmill walking, aerobics, or bicycling. Activities that involve coordinated eye, head, and body movements such as golf and racquet sports may be appropriate. Swimming is approached cautiously because of the disorientation experienced by many patients with vestibular disorders in the relative weightlessness of the aquatic environment.

Maintenance of Initial Results

Once the patient has completed the initial period of treatment, progress is assessed and adjustments are made in the program. Exercises that no longer produce symptoms are eliminated and replaced with others that were not originally included because of lower priority. This process is continued until the improvements begin to plateau. When this point is reached, it is important to provide the patient with counseling and a program of maintenance exercises to ensure stability of the initial improvements. The maintenance program typically includes continuing the prescribed conditioning exercises and any unique postural control activities that were required. The patient is instructed to resume the habituation exercises if a relapse of positional symptoms occurs.

Role of the Therapist in Patient Education

A key role of the therapist in the care of patients with balance disorders is to educate patients about the illness. Considerable misinformation often must be addressed. The supportive function of the therapist is particularly essential in the care of patients with a less favorable prognosis. Patients who are well educated regarding the nature of vestibular dysfunction understand the rationale for vestibular rehabilitation. They recognize that these measures are primarily a management technique rather than a cure. Because the patients take a great deal of responsibility for the outcome of therapy, it is critical that they understand and embrace the theoretic framework on which the treatment is founded. This focus takes patients from a passive to an active role in recovery from dizziness and disequilibrium. Although relapses can be anticipated during periods of illness or fatigue, experienced patients reinstitute their exercise programs and regain a well-compensated state. A patient who is not successful should be reevaluated by the physician and the therapist.

Role of the Physician

Otologists increasingly recognize the need to develop a successful program of vestibular rehabilitation to serve patients with balance disorders. This program is best pursued by a qualified team of professionals that includes an otologist, vestibular testing staff, and a physical therapist specifically trained in vestibular assessment and treatment. A working relationship with insightful neurologic and psychiatric consultants also is helpful. In optimal settings the physical therapist understands something of the diagnostic aspects of neurotology and the strengths and limitations of conventional medical and surgical modalities. The otologist likewise must appreciate the role of the therapist in the treatment of this challenging patient population. A mutually supportive and interactive environment is ideal for responding to the diverse needs encountered in a busy vestibular treatment program. The otologist finds that the time investment required for education and team development pays considerable dividends in terms of treatment outcome and patient satisfaction.

SUMMARY POINTS

- After injury to the vestibular system, the central nervous system undergoes a stereotyped process of recovery, including both an acute (static compensation) stage and a longer and less reliable chronic (dynamic compensation) stage.
- Vestibular rehabilitation therapy is designed to optimize compensation after vestibular system injuries by a variety of mechanisms including adaptive plasticity of the central nervous system, central sensory substitution, and habituation of pathologic responses.
- A clinical history of a vestibular crisis followed by gradual but incomplete recovery of vestibular function is helpful in identifying the patient with an uncompensated vestibular lesion.

- Vestibular testing may help to identify the uncompensated patient by detecting spontaneous or positional nystagmus, asymmetrical responses on rotational chair studies, and persistent postural control abnormalities.
- Vestibular rehabilitation may be appropriate treatment for patients with uncompensated peripheral or central lesions, benign paroxysmal positional vertigo, or disequilibrium of aging, or after vestibular system surgery is undertaken to treat an unstable labyrinthine lesion.
- Although generic vestibular rehabilitation programs may offer meaningful benefits, customized programs that are designed by a physical therapist to address the specific deficits of the individual patient have proven to be more effective.

APPENDIX 1

SAMPLE PROGRAM FOR A PATIENT WITH A UNILATERAL UNCOMPENSATED LESION

HISTORY

A 41-year-old man with the diagnosis of uncompensated vestibular neuritis reports sudden onset of motion-provoked spells of vertigo without a marked peripheral vestibular crisis at onset. Symptoms improve over a 6-month period and suddenly return. Vertigo spells occur several times a day and last for less than 1 minute. Multiple head movements and visual scanning tasks such as shopping in store aisles cause the symptoms. Aural fullness is present in the left ear without hearing loss. Balance testing shows persistent, low-amplitude left-beating nystagmus throughout the study. All other test results are normal. The initial evaluation for therapy shows a motion sensitivity quotient (MSQ) of 21% and moderate to severe disability. There are no balance or gait difficulties unless the head is moving while the patient is walking.

TREATMENT

On the basis of the therapist's findings the following customized program of exercises was prescribed for twice daily use:

1. Sit upright with your legs in front of you. Rapidly lie down straight on your back with your eyes

APPENDIX 1 (CONT.)

open, wait 10 seconds or until symptoms return to baseline, and rapidly roll to the right side. Again wait 10 seconds or until symptoms return to baseline, and roll to your back. Wait 10 seconds or until symptoms return to baseline, and quickly sit back upright. Do this 3 more times.

2. While sitting rapidly bend down and bring your nose to your right knee. Wait 10 seconds or until symptoms return to baseline, and rapidly sit back upright. Do this 3 more times.

3. While sitting turn your head to the right and then to the left leading with your eyes as if you were watching a tennis match. Go back and forth 5 times, then wait for 10 seconds or until symptoms return to baseline. Repeat the entire process 3 times.

4. While sitting bend your head down while looking at the floor, then look up at the ceiling moving both your head and eyes. Do this 5 times. Wait 10 seconds or until symptoms return to baseline. Do the entire exercise 3 more times.

5. While standing make a rapid left about-face pivot with eyes open. Wait until symptoms return to baseline and repeat. Wait 20 seconds or until symptoms return to baseline and repeat the entire process to the right. Do this entire maneuver 3 more times.

OUTCOME

The patient was 100% compliant with the program for 6 weeks. At the follow-up visit, MSQ was reduced to 7%, and the patient reported considerable subjective improvement with occasional symptoms. There was no residual disability. He was advised to continue the exercise program for several weeks and change to a maintenance program.

APPENDIX 2

UNIVERSITY OF MICHIGAN VESTIBULAR REHABILITATION PROGRAM FOR BENIGN PAROXYSMAL POSITIONAL VERTIGO

INSTRUCTIONS

Perform the following exercises *twice a day,* once in the morning and again in the evening. Perform them in an *open area,* where you cannot injure yourself if you fall. If any of the exercises causes *pain,* stop and notify your physician or therapist so the program can be modified. You will probably become dizzy while performing these exercises. This dizziness may become worse over the first week. If the dizziness continues to worsen after 7 days, discontinue the program and contact your physician or therapist.

Perform these exercises faithfully until they no longer cause dizziness. From that point, continue to perform them twice a day for at least 2 more weeks to ensure complete relief of symptoms. You may want to continue them once a day indefinitely. If your dizziness returns, start the program again. If you do not notice an improvement in your symptoms within 6 weeks, you might need an exercise program customized to your needs. In this event, contact your physician or therapist for more information.

EXERCISES

1. Sit upright on the edge of the bed with your feet flat on the floor or dangling straight down. Quickly lie down onto your *left/right* side and swing your feet up onto the bed. Stay in this position for 30 seconds, even if dizziness occurs. Then swing your feet back over the edge of the bed and sit up quickly into the original position. Wait 30 seconds, and do this exercise 3 more times.

2. Sit upright in a comfortable chair and bend your head quickly up and down 5 times looking alternately at the floor and the ceiling (as if nodding your head "yes"). Wait 10 seconds or longer until the dizziness passes, and do the whole exercise 3 more times.

3. Still sitting in a chair, tilt your head up and to the *left/right* looking up at the ceiling. Hold the position for 30 seconds, then return your head to the original neutral position. Wait 30 seconds again. Do the exercise three more times.

APPENDIX 3

SAMPLE PROGRAM FOR
AN ELDERLY PERSON

HISTORY

An 84-year-old woman reports a gradual onset of unsteadiness while standing and walking without a history of falls. She denies any vertigo and reports unsteadiness as being provoked whenever she is up and moving and no symptoms if she is sitting or lying down. She has a history of arthritis, osteoporosis, and hypertension that are controlled medically. Mild bilateral loss of hearing necessitates use of hearing aids. Balance testing shows evidence of an abnormally low time constant during rotational chair testing, which suggests peripheral involvement, normal findings of all oculomotor tests, and sporadic left-beating positional nystagmus. Caloric irrigations produced normal responses. Posturography shows abnormal results on condition 6 only, suggesting sensitivity to visual motion stimuli when foot support surface cues are not accurate.

The initial evaluation for therapy shows no motion sensitivity. The patient cannot stand on thin or thick foam with eyes closed for 10 seconds without a fall or step. She can do an unsteady tandem walk, stepping off the line 3 times in 20 steps. Regular walking shows drift to the right that increases with head movements. The patient can rise from a chair without use of hands. The functional problems appear to result from possible peripheral vestibular involvement and marked fear of falling.

TREATMENT

The patient is treated in a supervised outpatient setting twice a week for 3 weeks with the following supplementary customized home program.

Find a straight path in your house. Place a chair at each end of the path with their backs toward each other. Now set a timer for 5 to 10 minutes and perform the following activities:

1. Walk from one chair to the other turning your head slowly from side to side.
2. When you get to the other chair practice standing on one leg while you lightly touch the chair. Shift your weight onto the right leg. Slowly lift and lower the left leg 5 times. Shift your weight onto the left leg. Slowly lift and lower the right leg 5 times.
3. Turn and walk back to the other chair slowly tilting your head up and down.
4. When you get to the chair practice standing on one leg again.

OUTCOME

At the final therapy visit the patient could stand with eyes open or closed on a firm surface and thin foam without fall reactions and on thick foam with minimal fall reactions, even with eyes closed. Walking with head movements still caused some drift, but the patient was able to correct this without stumbles or fall reactions. She could step up and down a 6- to 8-inch curb without assistance for the first time in several years. She remained fearful of falling but noticed marked subjective improvement in balance. She was given a maintenance program to be continued indefinitely.

REFERENCES

1. Shepard NT, Telian SA, Smith-Wheelock M, Raj A. Vestibular and balance rehabilitation therapy. *Ann Otol Rhinol Laryngol* 1993;102: 198–205.
2. Shumway-Cook A, Horak FB. Rehabilitation strategies for patients with vestibular deficits. *Neurol Clin* 1990;8:441–457.
3. Igarashi M. Vestibular compensation: an overview. *Acta Otolaryngol (Stockh)* 1984;406[Suppl]:78–82.
4. Smith PF, Darlington CL. Neurochemical mechanisms of recovery from peripheral vestibular lesions. *Brain Res Brain Res Rev* 1991;16: 117–133.
5. Smith PF, Curthoys IS. Mechanisms of recovery following unilateral labyrinthectomy. *Brain Res Brain Res Rev* 1989;14:155–180.
6. Mathog RH, Peppard SB. Exercise and recovery from vestibular injury. *Am J Otolaryngol* 1982;3:397–407.
7. Peppard SB. Effect of drug therapy on compensation from vestibular injury. *Laryngoscope* 1986;96:878–898.
8. Zee DS. Perspectives on the pharmacologic therapy of vertigo. *Arch Otolaryngol* 1985;111:609–612.
9. Matsuoka I, Itol J, Takahashi H, Sasa M, Takaori S. Experimental vestibular pharmacology: a minireview with special reference to neuroactive substances and antivertigo drugs. *Acta Otolaryngol (Stockh)* 1985;419:62–70.
10. Cochran SL, Kasik P, Precht W. Pharmacological aspects of excitatory synaptic transmission to second order vestibular neurons in the frog. *Synapse* 1987;1:102–123.
11. Sekitani T, McCabe BF, Ryu JH. Drug effects on the medial vestibular nucleus. *Arch Otolaryngol* 1971;93:581–589.
12. Obata K, Takeda K, Shinozaki H. Further study on pharmacological properties of the cerebellar-induced inhibition of Deiter's neurons. *Exp Brain Res* 1970;11:327–342.
13. Flohr H, Lüneburg U. Neurotransmitter and neuromodulator systems involved in vestibular compensation. In: *Gaze control: facts and theories*. Amsterdam: Elsevier, 1985:269–277.
14. Pettorossi VE, Troiani D, Pterosini L. Diazepam enhances cerebellar inhibition on vestibular neurons. *Acta Otolaryngol (Stockh)* 1982;93: 363–373.
15. Sekitani T, Ryu JH, McCabe BF. Drug effects on the medial vestibular nucleus: perrotatory responses. *Arch Otolaryngol* 1971;94:401–405.
16. Bernstein P, McCabe BF, Ryu JM. The effect of diazepam on vestibular compensation. *Laryngoscope* 1974;84:267–272.

17. Ishikawa K, Igarashi M. Effect of diazepam on vestibular compensation in squirrel monkeys. *Arch Otorhinolaryngol* 1984;240:49–54.
18. Katsarkas A, Segal B. Unilateral loss of peripheral and vestibular function in patients: degree of compensation and factors causing decompensation. *Otolaryngol Head Neck Surg* 1988;98:45–47.
19. Shepard NT, Telian SA. Evaluation of balance system function. In: Katz J, ed. *Handbook of clinical audiology*, 4th ed. Baltimore: Williams & Wilkins, 1994:424–447.
20. Wall C. The sinusoidal harmonic acceleration rotary chair test: theoretical and clinical basis. *Neurol Clin* 1990;8:269–286.
21. Voorhees RL. The role of dynamic posturography in neurotologic diagnosis. *Laryngoscope* 1989;99:940–957.
22. Norre ME. Rationale of rehabilitation treatment for vertigo. *Am J Otolaryngol* 1987;8:31–35.
23. Horak F, Jones-Rycewicz C, Black FO, Shumway-Cook A. Effects of vestibular rehabilitation on dizziness and imbalance. *Otolaryngol Head Neck Surg* 1992;106:175–180.
24. Shepard NT, Telian SA. Programmatic vestibular rehabilitation. *Otolaryngol Head Neck Surg* 1995;112:173–182.
25. Cawthorne T. The physiological basis for head exercises. *J Chart Soc Physiother* 1944:106–107.
26. Brandt T, Daroff RB. Physical therapy for benign paroxysmal positional vertigo. *Arch Otol Rhinol Laryngol* 1980;106:484–485.
27. Semont A, Freyss G, Vitte E. Curing the BPPV with a liberatory maneuver. *Adv Otorhinolaryngol* 1988;42:290–293.
28. Epley JM. The canalith repositioning procedure for treatment of benign paroxysmal positional vertigo. *Otolaryngol Head Neck Surg* 1992;107: 399–404.
29. Parnes LS, Price-Jones RG. Particle repositioning maneuver for treatment of benign paroxysmal positional vertigo. *Ann Otol Rhinol Laryngol* 1993;102:325–331.
30. Smith-Wheelock M, Shepard NT, Telian SA, Boismier T. Balance retraining therapy in the elderly. In: Kashima H, Goldstein J, Lucente F, eds. *Clinical geriatric otolaryngology*. Philadelphia: BC Decker, 1992:71–80.
31. Monsell EM, Brackmann DE, Linthicum FH. Why do vestibular destructive procedures sometimes fail? *Otolaryngol Head Neck Surg* 1988;99:472–479.
32. Smith-Wheelock M, Shepard NT, Telian SA. Physical therapy program for vestibular rehabilitation. *Am J Otol* 1991;12:218–225.
33. Telian SA, Shepard NT, Smith-Wheelock M, Hoberg M. Bilateral vestibular paresis: diagnosis and treatment. *Otolaryngol Head Neck Surg* 1991;104:67–71.

The Ear: Comprehensive Otology,
edited by R. F. Canalis and P. R. Lambert.
Lippincott Williams & Wilkins, Philadelphia © 2000.

CHAPTER 43

Surgical Treatment of Vertigo

Joel A. Sercarz and Rinaldo F. Canalis

Surgery for Meniere's Disease	Destructive Procedures
Conservative Procedures	**Procedures for Benign Positional Paroxysmal Vertigo**
Vestibular Nerve Section	**Vascular Decompression**

Most patients with vertigo undergo effective medical therapy and do not need an operation. Surgery plays a primary role in the management of vestibular nerve neoplasia, labyrinthine fistula, and some cases of temporal bone trauma. Controversy exists over the surgical management of some of the common causes of intractable vertigo, including labyrinthine hydrops and benign paroxysmal positional vertigo (BPPV). Management of acoustic neuroma and labyrinthine fistula is addressed in Chapters 25 and 53. This discussion focuses on the surgical management of Meniere's disease and BPPV. The two strategies for treatment of patients with Meniere's disease are (a) ablation of vestibular function and (b) enhancement of endolymphatic drainage. The mode of treatment may be divided into conservative and destructive on the basis of effect on residual hearing. Conservative approaches include endolymphatic sac operations and vestibular nerve section. Destructive operations are based on various types of labyrinthectomy. The approaches to BPPV are ablative, addressing the singular nerve or the posterior semicircular canal.

SURGERY FOR MENIERE'S DISEASE

Conservative Procedures

Endolymphatic Sac Surgery

A detailed discussion of the pathophysiology and medical management of Meniere's disease is presented in Chapter 40. The endolymphatic sac is believed to be instrumental in absorption of endolymph. Endolymphatic sac

procedures are based on the hypothesis that hydrops is caused by a faulty reabsorption mechanism and that surgical intervention will drain the excess fluid. This theoretic basis for endolymphatic sac surgery, although predicated on current understanding of inner ear pathophysiology, has never been conclusively proved.

The history of endolymphatic sac surgery dates to 1927, when on the basis of research experience with animal models and anatomic studies, Portmann (1) performed the first shunt operation in humans. His procedure involved simple mastoidectomy followed by opening and decompression of the endolymphatic sac. Although Portmann had some success with this technique, it did not gain widespread popularity and was performed rarely until 1962, when House (2) described the endolymphatic to subarachnoid shunt.

For many otologists, an endolymphatic sac operation is the preferred initial surgical management of Meniere's disease for patients whose medical therapy has failed and who have serviceable hearing. This preference is based on the rarity of serious complications of sac surgery and the good results that these surgeons have reported. However, the procedures have remained controversial because most studies evaluating their effectiveness have been retrospective and may be profoundly influenced by patient selection. This issue was discussed in detail by Kerr et al. (3). Those authors stated that given a hypothetically harmless operation, more aggressive surgeons can expect a higher percentage of successes because they will be operating on more patients who would, regardless of therapy, have spontaneous remission (60% to 80%) (4,5). The controversy has been further complicated by a Danish trial of sham surgery versus endolymphatic shunt (6). The authors found no significant difference in outcome between two small groups of patients, even 9 years after the procedures

J. A. Sercarz and R.F. Canalis: Department of Surgery, University of California, Los Angeles, School of Medicine, Los Angeles, California 90095-1624

(6,7). This study has been criticized for its methods and interpretation of results and has failed to clarify the controversy (8). Although a variety of techniques have been described, two endolymphatic sac procedures are most commonly reported—endolymphatic to mastoid and endolymphatic to subarachnoid shunts.

Endolymphatic Subarachnoid Shunt

The introduction of the endolymphatic-subarachnoid shunt by House (2) in 1962 began the modern era of endolymphatic sac surgery. The goal of the procedure is to provide drainage of endolymph from the high-pressure endolymphatic space into the low-pressure subarachnoid space. The procedure begins with simple mastoidectomy, including removal of mastoid air cells from the area of the lateral and posterior semicircular canals. Exposure is extended to the posterior fossa plate posterior and inferior to the labyrinth and jugular bulb. The endolymphatic sac is identified. The outer wall is entered with a scalpel, and the lumen is exposed. The medial wall of the sac is opened, and a blunt instrument is passed to the cerebellopontine angle. The shunt tube is inserted with the bevel directed toward the cerebellum. It is not entirely clear how the subarachnoid shunt functions, but it is believed that it drains excess endolymph when the patient is upright and cerebrospinal fluid (CSF) pressure is lower in the cerebellopontine cistern, producing a gradient.

The most comprehensive report of endolymphatic subarachnoid shunt was by Brackmann and Anderson (4), who described 125 cases in 1980. Vertigo was cured in 61% of patients, hearing was improved in 25%, and 29% ultimately underwent other procedures, the most common of which was vestibular nerve section. Complications of the procedure included hearing loss, which occurred in 7% of the patients; none of the hearing loss was pro-

found. There was one CSF leak and one case of meningitis. These authors recommended revision subarachnoid shunts for patients who had recurrences after an initially successful procedure and retained serviceable hearing. Eleven of 18 revision shunts performed in their series were judged successful. Complications were infrequent; 7% of patients had some loss of hearing. One patient had CSF leak, meningitis, and superficial wound infection. There were no cases of facial paralysis. Glasscock et al. (9) described results of 112 consecutive subarachnoid shunts. Sixty-six percent of patients had complete relief of vertigo. Thirty-five percent of patients, however, had a decrease in hearing of 15 dB or 15% in discrimination. Three patients had total hearing loss.

Endolymphatic-Mastoid Shunt

The endolymphatic sac to mastoid shunt is based on Portmann's original decompression operation. The procedure is similar to the subarachnoid shunt, except an incision is made into the lateral-posterior wall of the sac and is connected to the mastoid process with a tube or polymeric silicone splint (Fig. 1).

Several variations in shunt material have been proposed. Shea (9a) described a polytetrafluoroethylene (Teflon)–containing shunt, and Paparella and Hanson (10) proposed placing a T tube within the endolymphatic sac to serve as the shunt. Arenberg et al. (11) reported use of a unidirectional valve implant. Their results were better than those reported for endolymphatic-subarachnoid shunts and as effective as with other types of shunts. In their series 87.3% of 205 patients experienced complete elimination of vertigo after the procedure; 60% to 75% had improvement or hearing stabilization, depending on whether the best or worst audiogram was used for comparison. These results have not yet been duplicated in other centers.

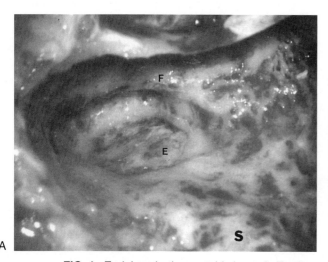 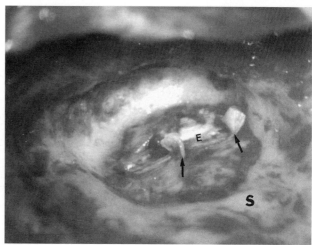

FIG. 1. Endolymphatic-mastoid shunt. **A:** Total canal-wall-up mastoidectomy has been completed. The facial nerve (*F*) and sigmoid sinus (*S*) have been outlined. The endolymphatic sac has been exposed (*E*). **B:** The leaves of the endolymphatic sac have been opened (*arrows*).

The incidence of hearing loss following sac surgery has been low, generally less than 1%. Citing this low risk, Morrison (12) advocated operating on the better- or only-hearing ear. In 129 cases of sac operations on the only- or better-hearing ear, there was one case of total hearing loss. Morrison's view is controversial; we believe that surgery is generally contraindicated in an only-hearing ear.

It appears that endolymphatic sac surgery is not effective in advanced Meniere's disease. Maddox (13) reported that among patients who sought treatment late in the course of disease, only 55% obtained long-term relief of vertigo after surgery. Brackmann and Anderson (4), however, found no difference in results on the basis of duration of symptoms or degree of hearing loss. They nonetheless recommended that the operation be performed early, before marked hearing loss has occurred. Maddox (14) reported better results among patients treated with endolymphatic-mastoid shunts for early hydrops. There was control of vertigo among 70% of patients with early hydrops, whereas only 55% of patients treated after 5 years of clinical symptoms were improved. The decrease in shunt effectiveness among patients treated late in the course of disease suggests that the better results obtained through operating earlier in the course of disease may be, at least in part, due to inclusion of patients who had a high possibility of spontaneous remission.

Sacculotomy and Cochleosacculotomy

Sacculotomy and cochleosacculotomy have as a common goal decompression of the endolymphatic space through a conveniently located structure accessible through the external auditory canal under local anesthesia. Like transcanal labyrinthectomy, these procedures can be performed on elderly patients who are at high anesthetic risk.

Fick (15) described sacculotomy in 1964. The procedure depends on the presence of a dilated saccule and begins with an endaural incision to expose the oval window. A pick is introduced through the stapes footplate, and the dilated saccule is punctured to produce a permanent fistula and allow endolymph to escape into the perilymphatic space. The goal is equalization of pressure between the endolymph and perilymph maintained by a membrane formed across the saccular wall. This membrane has greater permeability than the normal saccular wall and allows endolymph filtration. Although Fick reported success rates as high as 92%, other surgeons were unable to duplicate his results and reported a higher degree of hearing loss (16).

The tack procedure of Cody et al. (17) is a modification of sacculotomy in which a stainless steel tack is placed through the stapes footplate. This approach was designed to maintain decompression of the endolymphatic space by means of periodic repuncturing of the saccular wall. Vertigo control with this operation is similar to that reported for the Fick sacculotomy. Wielinga and Smyth (18) compared methods of sacculotomy and found that vertigo was relieved in 82% of Fick cases and in 89% of tack procedures. They suggested that sacculotomy may be an option in the treatment of elderly patients with Meniere's disease. In their series, hearing was preserved in only 36% of patients undergoing the Fick procedure and 77% undergoing the tack procedure. The tack procedure is not often performed today.

Cochleosacculotomy, another form of otic-periotic shunt, was introduced by Schuknecht (19) in 1982. The procedure was designed to produce a lasting fistula in the cochlear duct. Like sacculotomy, the procedure is an attempt to decompress the endolymphatic system by releasing distention and elevated pressure. The operation is performed through a posterior tympanomeatal flap. Bone is removed, if necessary, from the canal wall to expose the entire round window membrane. A 3-mm right-angled pick is advanced through the round window membrane in the direction of the oval window. According to Schuknecht, this causes fracture-disruption of the osseous spiral lamina and cochlear duct. It is important for the surgeon to adhere to the lateral wall of the inner ear to ensure penetration of the cochlear duct.

Schuknecht (19) described 51 cases and found that 70% of patients experienced no vertigo after the procedure and that an additional 18% experienced only mild vertigo. Twelve percent had recurrence of vertigo, equal to preoperative level. Sixty-five percent of patients had hearing loss greater than 20 dB at 4,000 Hz. Two patients in the series had profound sensorineural hearing loss after the operation.

Other otologists have had lesser success. Silverstein (20) found that cochleosacculotomy was successful in curing vertigo in 70% of patients at short-term follow-up evaluations, but 8 of 14 patients had sensorineural loss greater than 15 dB. Morrison (21) criticized cochleosacculotomy because the procedure is relatively blind, and the surgeon may not penetrate the cochlear duct as intended.

Many practitioners have abandoned use of sacculotomy and cochleosacculotomy. There has been general concern that the fistula made in these procedures will heal with time, a fact supported in animal experiments (20). It is also unclear which patients should be considered for this procedure. Elderly patients with poor hearing who might not fully compensate for the effects of labyrinthectomy may be the best candidates. Most surgeons would exclude patients with early Meniere's disease and serviceable hearing in the involved ear because of the high incidence of hearing loss.

Vestibular Nerve Section

Selected patients with Meniere's disease refractory to medical therapy with serviceable hearing are candidates for vestibular nerve section. Unlike destructive procedures, nerve section has the advantage of preservation of cochlear function, so the patient has the option of cochlear implantation. Nerve section is accepted as the most effective therapy for vertigo with hearing preservation.

The approaches most commonly used are retrolabyrinthine (RL), retrosigmoid, and middle fossa vestibular neurectomy (MFVN). The results have been excellent, success rates ranging from 90% to 95% regardless of approach. Nerve section is indicated for patients with incapacitating peripheral vestibulopathy who can tolerate general anesthesia. Some neurotologists prefer nerve section as a first surgical therapy for their patients. Vestibular neurectomy can be complicated by hearing loss and is therefore contraindicated in an only hearing ear.

The history of vestibular neurectomy dates to the early twentieth century, when Dandy (22) and other neurosurgeons first performed it through a suboccipital approach. The procedure was frequently successful in vertigo control, but enthusiasm was limited by a high incidence of hearing loss and facial paralysis, even when the procedure was performed by experienced surgeons. Vestibular nerve section was abandoned until House described the middle fossa technique in the 1960s.

For successful vestibular nerve section, the patient should have a unilateral vestibular lesion and a normal central vestibular system to allow normal compensation postoperatively. Compensation may be a problem for some patients, particularly the elderly and those with vestibular neuritis. With improvement in approaches to the internal auditory canal (IAC) and cerebellopontine angle, vestibular nerve section has been performed more frequently in recent years. One advantage of nerve section is that if bilateral disease develops and progresses to total deafness, the patient remains a candidate for cochlear implantation. Another advantage over labyrinthectomy is avoidance of traumatic neuroma, which is a possible complication of labyrinthectomy (23).

Retrolabyrinthine and Retrosigmoid Approaches to the Internal Auditory Canal

In the RL approach the nerve is accessed at the cerebellopontine angle. Silverstein and Norrell (24) first outlined the RL approach to nerve section. As with other techniques for vestibular nerve section, the procedure is performed with facial and cochlear nerve monitoring. Complete mastoidectomy is performed; exposure of the facial nerve is not necessary. Bone is removed over the sigmoid sinus and approximately 2 cm posterior to the sinus. The mastoid air cells adjacent to the posterior semicircular canal must be systematically removed to provide maximal exposure of the posterior fossa dura. The dura is incised anterior to the sigmoid sinus and raised anteriorly.

The vestibular division of the eighth cranial nerve is superior to the cochlear nerve. In some persons a small vessel separates the two nerves because actual separation of these structures is absent (Fig. 2). The facial nerve be identified by means of gentle retraction of the eighth cranial nerve.

House et al. (25) reported on a series of 42 patients who underwent RL vestibular nerve section. Twenty-five had Meniere's disease and previous shunt surgery had failed. Twenty-seven patients experienced complete relief of vertigo, and two had improvement. The results were poorer for patients with diagnoses other than Meniere's disease. The authors reported no cases of hearing loss or facial weakness. One patient had CSF rhinorrhea and one had meningitis. Kemink et al. (26) described their experience with RL nerve section in 42 consecutive patients with disorders other than Meniere's disease. Uncompensated vestibular neuritis was the most common diagnosis. Only 9 patients were cured, and 7 improved. The authors attributed the disappointing results to poor central compensation among patients with vestibular neuritis.

The retrosigmoid approach involves suboccipital craniectomy and exposure of the VII–VIII nerve complex at the IAC (Fig. 3). Separation between the cochlear and

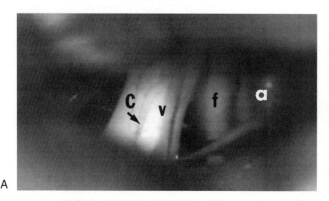
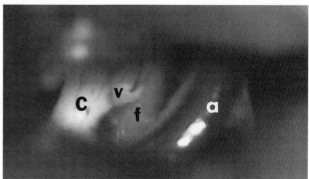

A   B

FIG. 2. Retrolabyrinthine vestibular nerve section. **A:** Initial exposure. **B:** Vestibular nerve section completed. *C,* Cochlear nerve; *V,* vestibular nerve; *f,* facial nerve; *a,* anterior inferior cerebellar artery.

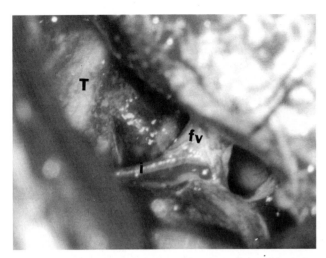

FIG. 3. Retrosigmoid approach to the cerebellopontine angle. *T,* Trigeminal nerve; *fv,* cochleovestibular nerve complex with labyrinthine artery (*i*) overriding it.

vestibular nerves may be found by pressing along their fibers. A difference in color between the two structures may be noted. With a sharp pick the fibers are separated and the vestibular branch divided. Throughout the procedure the facial nerve is repeatedly identified anatomically and by means of electrical stimulation.

A more extensive dissection called the *retrosigmoid IAC* (RSG-IAC) approach was described by Silverstein et al. (27). An incision is made 4 cm from the postauricular crease and extended into the neck. A 3-cm circular craniotomy is made behind the sigmoid sinus. The dura is opened along the sigmoid sinus to create a posteriorly based dural flap. The seventh and eight cranial nerves are exposed in the cerebellopontine angle. The IAC dura is opened, the superior and inferior vestibular nerves are identified (Fig. 4), and the vestibulofacial fibers are care-

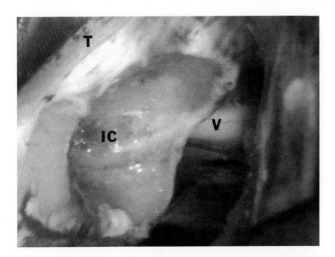

FIG. 4. Retrosigmoid exposure of the cerebellopontine angle and dissection of the internal auditory canal (*IC*) before opening of the dural lining. *T,* Tentorium; *V,* vestibular nerve.

fully separated. Vaporization of the superior vestibular nerve is performed with a laser while the facial nerve is protected with wet gelatin foam sponge. Finally, the posterior ampullary nerve and saccular nerves are avulsed with preservation of the cochlear nerve. All 10 patients treated with this technique were cured of vertigo and had no response to ice water caloric stimulation. One patient had 25 dB sensorineural hearing loss, and another had a 28% loss in speech discrimination. There were no other complications in this initial series.

Silverstein et al. cited the advantages of the RSG-IAC approach. The procedure is shorter than the RL approach and is easier and safer to perform than the middle fossa procedure. The RSG-IAC approach results in a more complete section of the vestibular nerve fibers than the RL. It is not yet clear whether the findings in this study will be replicated when the procedure is performed more widely.

Middle Fossa Approach

Use of MFVN approach for the treatment of intractable vertigo dates to House's work during the early 1960s. The middle fossa approach also is used for resection of acoustic neuroma, decompression of the IAC, and eustachian tuboplasty. The main disadvantage of this approach is that it is technically difficult.

House initially advocated superior vestibular nerve section, but he abandoned the procedure because of poor control of vertigo. Glasscock et al. (28) and Fisch (29) modified the procedure to resect the superior and inferior vestibular nerves and Scarpa's ganglion with improved results.

The operation is performed under general anesthesia, with the patient in the supine position. An incision is made at the level of the zygomatic arch 1.5 cm anterior to the tragus and carried posteriorly toward the vertex. The temporalis muscle is incised to expose the outer table of the skull. Craniectomy is performed to elevate a 3 cm by 3 cm bone flap. The middle fossa dura is exposed and bluntly dissected off the overlying cranium. A House-Urban middle fossa retractor is used to gently lift the temporal lobe. The greater superficial petrosal nerve and the superior semicircular canal are used as landmarks for identification of the IAC.

The bone overlying the IAC is removed to its lateral extent. The dura of the IAC is opened, and the bony crista separating the superior vestibular nerve from the facial nerve is identified (Fig. 5). The superior vestibular nerve, located posteriorly, is dissected, and any vestibulofacial anastomoses are divided. This nerve is avulsed with a right-angled hook and sectioned proximal to Scarpa's ganglion. With retraction of the superior vestibular nerve, the inferior vestibular nerve including the singular branch is identified and cut. Serious complications are rare. Fisch (29) reported a 3% incidence of transitory facial paralysis and a 2.8% rate of deafness.

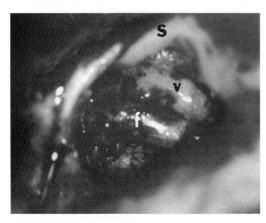

FIG. 5. Exposure of the internal auditory canal through the middle fossa approach. *S,* Superior canal; *V,* vestibular nerve; *f,* facial nerve.

The results of MFVN are generally favorable. Among 80 consecutively treated patient reported by Glasscock et al. (28), 94% of patients were relieved of vertigo when total vestibular nerve section was performed, compared with 71% when superior nerve section alone was used. Glasscock's group (28) reported that stabilization or improvement of hearing was observed among 68% of their patients. Fisch (29) had a similar experience, 78% of patients reporting hearing improvement or stabilization.

Bohmer and Fisch (30) reported use of bilateral MFVN to treat two patients with bilateral Meniere's disease. After the second procedure, symptoms of disequilibrium were absent or mild, and some preservation of vestibuloocular reflexes was found. The deficit, according to these authors, was less than that produced by ototoxic vestibular ablation and probably was caused by incomplete sectioning of vestibular fibers (30).

Green et al. (31) described use of the middle fossa approach when RL neurectomy had failed. The authors' hypothesis was that in revision surgery the MFVN results in a higher incidence of cure because it allows more complete nerve section. Of the 11 patients treated in the series, 6 had successful vertigo control.

In comparing the RL neurectomy and MFVN, not all neurotologists agree. Glasscock et al. (28) contend that the RL approach is riskier because of brainstem exposure and proximity to the anterior inferior cerebellar artery. They also believe that identification of the vestibular nerve is more difficult with the RL approach because the surgeon is relying on an indistinct cleavage plane rather than a bony landmark, as in MFVN.

Although both RL neurectomy and MFVN preserve hearing in most instances, de la Cruz et al (32) reported a statistically significant advantage to the RL approach from the standpoints of both hearing preservation and control of vertigo. Silverstein et al. (27), however, reported that MFVN resulted in a higher rate of vertigo control.

The possibility of transitory facial nerve paralysis is greater with MFVN because the nerve has to be retracted to expose the vestibular nerves before section. The nerve also is more likely to be traumatized by the drill during dissection. RL neurectomy may be preferable in the care of elderly patients because of adherence of the dura and the need to retract the temporal lobe (25).

Destructive Procedures

Patients with disabling vertigo caused by unilateral vestibular dysfunction and without serviceable hearing are candidates for destructive operations. The two procedures used most commonly are transcanal and transmastoid labyrinthectomy. Some surgeons advocate chemical vestibulectomy, performed through simple mastoidectomy and vestibulotomy into the lateral semicircular canal. The aim of labyrinthectomy is to cure patients with peripheral vertigo through surgical ablation of the end organ. In our experience and that of others the procedure has a success rate of approximately 90% (33). Failures may be caused by persistence of a central component to the vertigo or incomplete ablation of the labyrinth. Progressive disease in the contralateral ear must be excluded before labyrinthectomy.

Transcanal Labyrinthectomy

Transcanal labyrinthectomy is particularly suited for a patient with intractable vertigo, a nonhearing ear, and high anesthetic risk. Transcanal approaches to treat vertigo date to early in the twentieth century. In 1903, Crockett (34) reported results of stapedectomy for the management of vertigo. Lempert (34a) reported aspiration of the contents of the vestibule through a transcanal incision in 1948. The modern technique of transcanal labyrinthectomy was described by Schuknecht (35) and Cawthorne (36) in 1957.

Under local anesthesia, the middle ear is exposed through a tympanomeatal flap (Fig. 6A). The incudostapedial joint is divided, and the stapes is removed to expose the vestibule (Fig. 6B). A cutting bur is used to remove bone from the promontory until the round and oval windows are connected (Fig. 6C). A right-angled hook is used to avulse the neuroepithelium from the vestibule. The macula of the saccule and utricle are bluntly removed through the oval window with a right-angled hook. Neuroepithelium is removed systematically from the semicircular canals, utricle, and saccule (Fig. 6C). The labyrinth is packed with gentamicin-impregnated gelatin film (Fig. 6D).

Hammerschlag and Schuknecht (37) reported 124 cases of transcanal labyrinthectomy. Most of the patients had Meniere's disease and were selected because of disabling symptoms and pure-tone thresholds of 50 dB or greater and speech discrimination of 50% or less. The

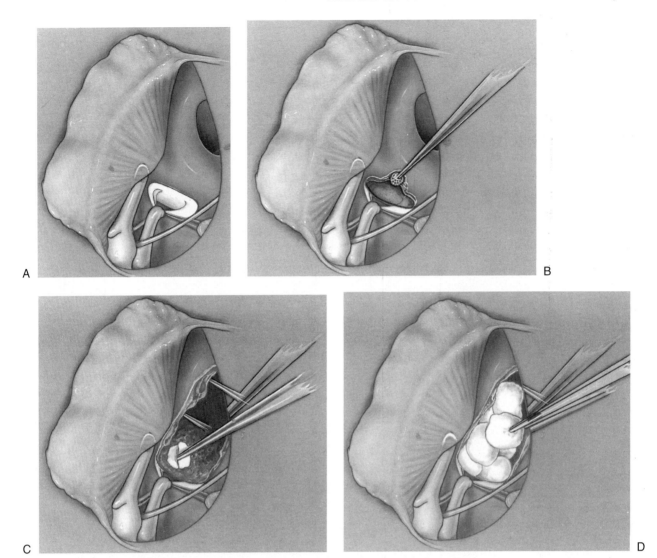

FIG. 6. Transcanal labyrinthectomy. **A:** Exposure of the middle ear through a tympanomeatal flap. **B:** Initial exposure of the vestibule after stapes removal. **C:** Round and oval windows have been joined by means of removal of the intervening promontory. The sensory epithelium is removed with a small pick. **D:** The defect is filled with gentamicin-impregnated gelatin film.

authors reported cessation of severe episodic vertigo in all cases. Four patients had persistence of moderate disequilibrium. Three of these subsequently underwent successful revision labyrinthectomy. Pulec (38) reported 28 cases of transcanal labyrinthectomy. Twenty-five of 28 patients were free of vertigo, and only one patient was not improved.

Transmastoid Labyrinthectomy and Translabyrinthine Nerve Section

The widest exposure for destruction of the labyrinthine neuroepithelium is through the mastoid cavity. Before the labyrinth is addressed, the facial nerve, semicircular canals and sigmoid sinus are skeletonized (Fig. 7A). The horizontal canal is opened first and them the posterior and superior canals (Fig. 7B, 7C). The vestibule is opened last (Fig. 7D), and all remaining neuroepithelium is avulsed under direct vision. The facial nerve is at risk at the ampullated ends of the posterior and horizontal canals; the surgeon must stay within the otic capsule to avoid the nerve.

The results of transmastoid labyrinthectomy (TML) appear to be slightly better than those of transcanal labyrinthectomy and are consistent with the more precise destruction of the neuroepithelium by this route. Kemink et al. (33) reported on 110 patients 88% of whom achieved complete relief and 9% partial relief of vertigo. Nine percent of patients continued to have troublesome but only 3% disabling disequilibrium after TML.

The translabyrinthine approach to vestibular nerve section allows removal of all vestibular neuroepithelium and

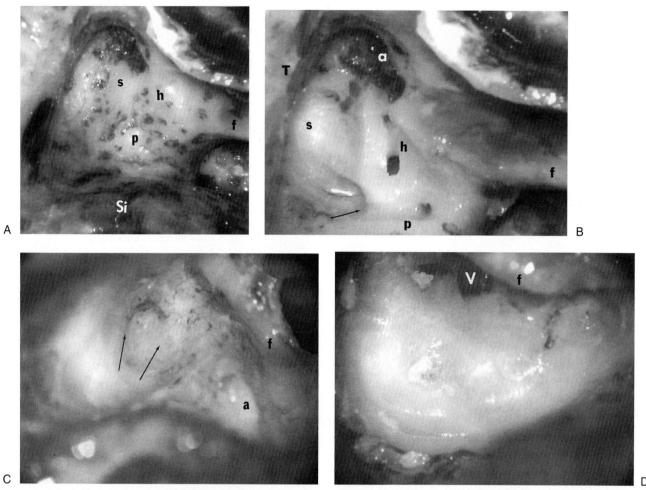

FIG. 7. Transmastoid labyrinthectomy. **A:** Initial exposure of the semicircular canals. *Si,* Sigmoid sinus; *f,* facial nerve canal; *h,* horizontal semicircular canal; *p,* posterior semicircular canal; *S,* superior vestibular canal. **B:** Triple canal labyrinthectomy. *f,* Facial nerve; *a,* attic; *T,* mastoid tegmen; *h,* opened horizontal canal; *p,* opened posterior canal; *S,* opened superior canal; *arrow,* crus commune. **C:** Labyrinthectomy completed. *Arrows* indicate position of the internal auditory canal. *f,* Facial nerve; *a,* posterior fossa plate. **D:** Initial opening of the vestibule through the transcanal labyrinthectomy approach. *f,* Facial nerve; *v,* vestibule.

preganglionic section of the nerve. This procedure is reserved for patients who have a low anesthetic risk and a nonserviceable ear. Although this approach would apparently result in more complete ablation of all afferent stimulation from the labyrinth, it is unclear whether this improves the results considerably. The patient is no longer a candidate for cochlear implantation after either type of labyrinthectomy.

Some surgeons have advocated adding nerve section to labyrinthectomy because of concern about the development of traumatic neuroma. Linthicum et al. (23) in 1979 reported two cases of traumatic neuroma after transcanal labyrinthectomy. Some surgeons believe residual stimulation from Scarpa's ganglion is possible after labyrinthectomy. Brackmann (39) and Pulec (38) prefer translabyrinthine nerve section to TML because it is the most certain method of ablating all labyrinthine function.

Kemink et al. (33) counter that they observed no additional benefit from nerve section compared with TML and recommended this operation for patients without serviceable hearing. The two procedures have never been compared prospectively.

Chemical Vestibulectomy

Chemical vestibulectomy with streptomycin represents an attempt to selectively destroy the vestibular neuroepithelium in patients with Meniere's disease. Although this technique involves toxic ablation of the labyrinth, preservation of hearing usually is possible (40). The use of streptomycin with hearing preservation in the management of Meniere's disease was first reported by Schuknecht in 1956; he delivered the drug intramuscularly (41).

Shea (42) first described perfusion of the inner ear with streptomycin. The technique involves transmastoid exposure of the ampulla of the horizontal semicircular canal. A small area of the membranous duct is exposed approximately 2 mm from the ampulla. A flake containing 125 μg streptomycin is placed on gelatin foam between the bony canal and the membranous duct.

Results of streptomycin infusion have been variable. Monsell and Shelton (43) reported the preliminary findings of a multicenter trial of labyrinthotomy and streptomycin infusion. Four of 13 surgeons in the study found the incidence of hearing loss (68%) to be unacceptable and abandoned the approach. In an accompanying editorial, Shea and Orchik (44) criticized the study as poorly designed and defended the use of the procedure when properly performed.

Gentamicin Infusion

The simplest method of toxic vestibular ablation is through the middle ear. In 1957, Schuknecht described a technique of perfusion of streptomycin into the middle ear through a transtympanic catheter (35). Gentamicin now is preferred because it is less ototoxic than streptomycin. The gentamicin solution presumably diffuses into the labyrinth through the round window membrane, although other routes are possible.

The goal of gentamicin ablation is to damage the labyrinth without producing severe hearing loss. The optimal dose of gentamicin has been determined empirically. If less than complete vestibular destruction is achieved, control of vertigo is possible without causing unacceptable ototoxicity. Murofushi et al. (45) treated 18 patients with Meniere's with intratympanic gentamicin using a long 22-gauge needle to instill the antibiotic into the middle ear. Fourteen patients had no further vertigo attacks. There was greater than 30 dB hearing loss in only 6 of the patients. Hirsch and Kamerer (46) reported on 28 patients with Meniere's disease treated with intratympanic gentamicin given by means of serial titration to allow monitoring of vertigo and hearing loss between treatments. An average of 3.4 injections were used, and substantial control of vertigo was achieved by 92% of patients (46). The pure tone average hearing level was reduced among 31% of the patients. The authors suggested that titration reduces the risk for hearing loss (46).

In a study from the Karolinska institute, the overall success among 14 of 17 patients (82%) was achieved with one or two infusions (47). The authors found that control of vertigo was more effective among patients with residual hearing in the involved ear.

Gentamicin infusion is well tolerated with the exception of the risk for hearing loss. Few patients experience severe postprocedural vertigo. The advantages of toxic ablation compared with labyrinthectomy are its low cost and lack of surgical morbidity. Among healthy patients with normal hearing, vestibular nerve section is preferable because of hearing preservation. The ideal patient for gentamicin ablation has vertigo and poor residual hearing in the involved ear. The procedure also is appropriate for a patient who wants to avoid surgery or is a poor surgical candidate on the basis of anesthetic risk.

PROCEDURES FOR BENIGN POSITIONAL VERTIGO

BPPV is a common entity. The natural history of this disorder generally includes spontaneous resolution within 1 year. However, a small group of patients have persistent debilitating vertigo that does not respond to vestibular exercises and medical management (see Chapter 42). These patients can be considered for one of several forms of surgical therapy.

The site of the disturbance in BPPV is the crista of the posterior semicircular canal, which is innervated by the singular nerve. The pathologic correlate is cupulolithiasis of the crista. Singular neurectomy has been advocated as a method of selective treatment of patients with BPPV and serviceable hearing in the involved ear. The procedure is performed through a tympanomeatal flap. The bony overhang of the round window niche is removed. The intermediate segment of the singular nerve is accessed at the posterior portion of the round window membrane, and the nerve is cut with a sharp pick. Spontaneous nystagmus is noticed immediately when complete neurectomy is achieved.

Gacek (48) first described the technique in 1974 and updated his experience in 1991 (49). He reported relief of symptoms in 97% of 102 consecutive cases of singular neurectomy. Four patients experienced sensorineural hearing loss which was believed to be caused by a diffuse labyrinthine insult. Five patients (7%) had an inaccessible singular canal. Silverstein and White (49a) reported a variation on singular neurectomy that included a wide postauricular exposure in an attempt to lessen the risk for damage to the cochlea. Nonetheless, an incidence of sensorineural hearing loss of 6% followed surgical intervention.

Although it is effective therapy for BPPV, singular neurectomy is difficult to perform. Other approaches have been devised to avoid the technical problems of singular neurectomy. Posterior semicircular canal (PSCC) partition involves blue lining the canal and applying an argon laser to the exposed area. This procedure has been performed successfully on two patients (50). Transmastoid PSCC occlusion has been proposed (51). During this procedure, a small puncture is made into the PSCC with a diamond bur. The canal is plugged with bone chips.

Pulec (52) described a series of 17 patients who underwent PSCC ablation for BPPV designed to prevent movement of endolymph in the canal. The procedure involves making a 4-mm fenestra in the PSCC and packing fibrous tissue into each end of the opening in the canal. None of the patients in Pulec's report had hearing loss after the procedure, and each experienced resolution of BPPV symptoms (52). Thus far, there is no adequate experience to recommend these newer forms of alternative surgery for BPPV.

VASCULAR DECOMPRESSION

In 1984, Jannetta et al. (53) proposed a new balance disorder that did not conform to entities such as Meniere's disease and BPPV. The syndrome was called *disabling positional vertigo* and is characterized by constant positional vertigo and severe nausea. The disorder tends to worsen with time. According to Jannetta et al., the patients do not have loss of either hearing or vestibular function. The authors found that these symptoms are associated with vascular compression of the intracranial eighth nerve.

In 1990, Møller (54) reported on 41 patients treated for disabling peripheral vertigo with vascular decompression. Thirty patients had total relief of vertigo or experienced considerable improvement. Two patients had minimal improvement, and 9 had no change. Two of the patients had total hearing loss after the procedure; there were no other serious complications.

Although other otologists have described vascular loops as a cause of vertigo, including 8 cases reported by McCabe and Harker (55), there has been a lack of documentation to support the concept of microvascular decompression. Verification of this entity will require further research and correlation of intraoperative findings with objective tests of vestibular function.

SUMMARY POINTS

- The central problem in surgical treatment of patients with Meniere's disease is that peripherally caused vertigo can be successfully controlled only with procedures accompanied by hearing loss (labyrinthectomy) or with procedures with a small risk for serious complications (vestibular nerve section). More conservative therapies generally have a lower rate of success, sometimes only slightly higher than the spontaneous rate of remission of untreated Meniere's disease.

- Because of the wide variety of surgical procedures available to manage intractable vertigo, the practitioner must frequently rely on personal experience and clinical judgment when devising therapy for individual patients. Several factors affect management, including the status of hearing, the willingness of the patient to undergo an intracranial procedure, the health of the patient, and the training of the surgeon.

REFERENCES

1. Portmann G. Surgical treatment by opening saccus endolymphaticus. *Arch Otolaryngol* 1927;6:309–319.
2. House W. Subarachnoid shunt for drainage of endolymphatic hydrops. *Laryngoscope* 1962;72:713–728.
3. Kerr AG, Toner JG, McKee GJ, Smyth DL. Role and results of cortical mastoidectomy and endolymphatic sac surgery in Meniere's disease. *J Laryngol Otol* 1989;103:1161–1166.
4. Brackmann DE, Anderson RG. Meniere's disease: treatment with the endolymphatic subarachnoid shunt—a review of 125 cases. *Otolaryngol Head Neck Surg* 1980;88:174–182.
5. Thomsen J, Kerr A, Bretlau P, Olsson J, Tos M. Endolymphatic sac surgery: why we do not do it—the non-specific effect of sac surgery. *Clin Otolaryngol* 1996;21:208–211.
6. Thomsen A, Bretlau P, Tos M, Johnsen NJ. Placebo effect in surgery for Meniere's disease. *Arch Otolaryngol* 1981;107:271–277.
7. Bretlau P, Thomsen J, Tos M, Johnsen NJ. Placebo effect in surgery of Meniere's disease: nine-year follow-up. *Arch Otolaryngol* 1981;107:271–277.
8. Pillsbury HC, Arenberg KI, Ferraro J, Ackley RS. Endolymphatic sac surgery: the Danish sham surgery study—an alternative analysis. *Otolaryngol Clin North Am* 1983;16:123–127.
9. Glasscock ME, Miller GW, Drake FD, Kanok MM. Surgical management of Meniere's disease with the endolymphatic subarachnoid shunt: a five-year study. *Laryngoscope* 1977;87:1668–1675.
9a. Shea JJ. Teflon film drainage of the endolymphatic sac. *Arch Otolaryngol* 1966;83:316–319.
10. Paparella MM, Hanson DG. Endolymphatic sac drainage for intractable vertigo. *Laryngoscope* 1976;86:697–702.
11. Arenberg EK, Zoller SA, Van de Water SM. The results of the first 300 consecutive endolymphatic system-mastoid shunts with valve implants for hydrops. *Otolaryngol Clin North Am* 1983;16:153–175.
12. Morrison AW. Sac surgery on the only or better hearing ear. *Otolaryngol Clin North Am* 1983;16:143–151.
13. Maddox HE. Endolymphatic sac surgery. *Laryngoscope* 1977;87:1676–1679.
14. Maddox HE. Medical treatment of Meniere's disease compared to early sac surgery. *Otolaryngol Clin North Am* 1983;16:129–133.
15. Fick I. Decompression of the labyrinth: a new surgical procedure for Meniere's disease. *Arch Otolaryngol* 1964;79:447–456.
16. Cody DTR. Meniere's disease. *Adv Otorhinolaryngol* 1973;19:342–384.
17. Cody DTR, Simonton KM, Hallberg OE. Automatic repetitive decompression of the saccule in endolymphatic hydrops (tack operation). *Laryngoscope* 1967;77:1480–1501.
18. Wielinga EW, Smyth GD. Long-term results of sacculotomy in older patients. *Ann Otol Rhinol Laryngol* 1989;98:803–806.
19. Schuknecht HF. Cochleosacculotomy for Meniere's disease: theory, technique, and results. *Laryngoscope* 1982;92:853–858.
20. Silverstein H, Hyman S, Silverstein D. Cochleosacculotomy. *Otolaryngol Head Neck Surg* 1984;92:63–66.
21. Morrison AW. Cochleostomy or endolymphatic sac surgery for advanced Meniere's disease. *Otolaryngol Clin North Am* 1983;16:135–141.
22. Dandy WE. Meniere's disease: its diagnosis and a method of treatment. *Arch Surg* 1928;16:1127–1152.
23. Linthicum FH, Alonso A, Denia A. Traumatic neuroma. *Arch Otolaryngol* 1979;105:654–655.
24. Silverstein H, Norrell H. Retrolabyrinthine surgery: a direct approach to the cerebellopontine angle. *Otolaryngol Head Neck Surg* 1980;88:462–469.
25. House JW, Hitselberger WE, McElveen J, Brackmann DE. Retrolabyrinthine section of the vestibular nerve. *Otolaryngol Head Neck Surg* 1984;92:212–215.
26. Kemink JL, Telian SA, El-Kashlan H, Langman AW. Retrolabyrinthine vestibular nerve section: efficacy in disorders other than Meniere's disease. *Laryngoscope* 1991;101:523–528.
27. Silverstein H, Norrell H, Haaberkamp T. A comparison of retrosigmoid IAC, retrolabyrinthine, and middle fossa vestibular neurectomy for treatment of vertigo. *Laryngoscope* 1987;97:165–173.
28. Glasscock ME, Kveton JF, Christiansen SG. Middle fossa vestibular neurectomy: an update. *Otolaryngol Head Neck Surg* 1984;92:216–220.
29. Fisch U. Vestibular and cochlear neurectomy. *Trans Am Acad Ophthalmol Otolaryngol* 1974;78:252–257.

30. Bohmer A, Fisch U. Bilateral vestibular neurectomy for treatment of vertigo. *Otolaryngol Head Neck Surg* 1993;109:101–107.

31. Green JD, Shelton C, Brackmann DE. Middle fossa vestibular neurectomy in retrolabyrinthine neurectomy failures. *Arch Otolaryngol Head Neck Surg* 1992;118:1058–1060.

32. de la Cruz A, McElveen JT. Hearing preservation in vestibular neurectomy. *Laryngoscope* 1984;94:874–877.

33. Kemink JL, Telian SA, Graham MD, Joynt L. Transmastoid labyrinthectomy: reliable surgical management of vertigo. *Otolaryngol Head Neck Surg* 1989;101:5–9.

34. Crockett EA. The removal of the stapes for the relief of auditory vertigo. *Ann Otol Rhinol Laryngol* 1903;12:67–72.

34a. Lempert J. Lempert decompression operation for hydrops of the endolymphatic labyrinth in Meniere's disease. *Arch Otolaryngol* 1948;47:551–570.

35. Schuknecht H. Ablation therapy in Meniere's disease. *Acta Otolaryngol (Stockh)* 1957;61[Suppl 132]:1–42.

36. Cawthorne T. Meniere's disease. *Ann Otol Rhinol Laryngol* 1957;56:18–38.

37. Hammerschlag PE, Schuknecht HF. Transcanal labyrinthectomy for intractable vertigo. *Arch Otolaryngol* 1981;107:152–156.

38. Pulec JL. Labyrinthectomy: indications, technique, and results. *Laryngoscope* 1974:1552–1573.

39. Brackmann DE. Surgical treatment of vertigo. *J Laryngol Otol* 1990;104:849–859.

40. Norris CH, Amedee RG, Risley JA, Shea JJ. Selective chemical vestibulectomy. *Am J Otol* 1990;11:395–400.

41. Schuknecht HF. Ablation therapy for relief of Meniere's disease. *Laryngoscope* 1956;66:859–870.

42. Shea JJ. Perfusion of the inner ear with streptomycin. *Trans Am Otol Soc* 1988;75:89–91.

43. Monsell EM, Shelton C. Labyrinthotomy with streptomycin infusion: early results of a multicenter study. *Am J Otol* 1992;13:416–422.

44. Shea JJ, Orchik DJ. Special commentary. *Am J Otol* 1992;13:422–425.

45. Murofushi T, Halmagyi GM, Yavor RA. Intratympanic gentamicin in Menieréis disease: results of therapy. *Am J Otol* 1997;18:52–57.

46. Hirsch BE, Kamerer DB. Intratympanic gentamicin therapy for Meniere's disease. *Am J Otol* 1997;18:44–51.

47. Hessen Soderman CA, Ahlner K, Bagger-Sjoback D, Bergenius J. Surgical treatment of vertigo: the Karolinska Hospital policy. *Am J Otol* 1996;17:93–98.

48. Gacek RR. Transection of the posterior ampullary nerve for relief of benign paroxysmal positional vertigo. *Ann Otol Rhinol Laryngol* 1974;83:596–605.

49. Gacek RR. Singular neurectomy update, II: review of 102 cases. *Laryngoscope* 1991;101:855–862.

49a. Silverstein H, White DW. Wide Surgical exposure for singular neurectomy in the treatment of benign positional vertigo. *Laryngoscope* 1990;100:701–706.

50. Anthony PF. Partitioning of the labyrinth: application in benign paroxysmal positional vertigo. *Am J Otol* 1991;12:388–393.

51. Parnes LS, McClure JA. Posterior semicircular canal occlusion for intractable benign paroxysmal positional vertigo. *Ann Otol Rhinol Laryngol* 1990;99:330–334.

52. Pulec JL. Ablation of posterior semicircular canal for benign paroxysmal positional vertigo. *Ear Nose Throat J* 1997;76:17–22,24.

53. Jannetta PJ, Møller MB, Møller AR. Disabling positional vertigo. *N Engl J Med* 1984;310:1700–1705.

54. Møller MB. Results of microvascular decompression of the eighth nerve as a treatment for disabling positional vertigo. *Ann Otol Rhinol Laryngol* 1990;99:724–729.

55. McCabe BF, Harker LA. Vascular loop as a cause of vertigo. *Ann Otol Rhinol Laryngol* 1983;92:542–543.

The Ear: Comprehensive Otology,
edited by R. F. Canalis and P. R. Lambert.
Lippincott Williams & Wilkins, Philadelphia © 2000.

CHAPTER 44

Examination and Diagnostic Techniques in Facial Nerve Disorders

James C. Andrews and Eduardo H. Rubinstein

The results of a facial nerve disorder are blatantly obvious yet the cause can be subtle and difficult to diagnose. Although most facial nerve disorders result in paresis or paralysis, a few produce hyperkinetic or spasmodic responses. For the most part, this chapter addresses the evaluation of facial nerve disorders that are paretic or paralytic in nature. Techniques of examination and diagnosis of the facial nerve are primarily directed at (a) measuring the severity of a facial nerve disorder, (b) determining an anatomic site of the lesion affecting the facial nerve, and (c) finding a cause of the disorder.

FACIAL NERVE ANATOMY

The tortuous course of the facial nerve through the temporal bone, although intimidating anatomy for the student, provides a key landmark or road map and orientation to the temporal bone for the experienced surgeon (1). For the purpose of anatomic discussion, the facial nerve can be separated by its course through the intracranial, intratemporal and extratemporal segments of the head (Fig. 1).

J. C. Andrews: Division of Head and Neck Surgery, UCLA Medical Center, Los Angeles, Los Angeles, California 90095

E. H. Rubinstein: Department of Anesthesiology, University of California, Los Angeles, School of Medicine, Center for the Health Sciences, Los Angeles, California 90095

COMPONENTS OF THE FACIAL NERVE

The facial nerve derives from multiple sources and as a result is composed of motor, sensory, and parasympathetic fibers (2). Special visceral efferent fibers supplying the facial muscles form the motor root and constitute the bulk of the facial nerve. The intermediate nerve of Wrisberg accompanying the special visceral efferent fibers carries afferent and general visceral efferent fibers. General visceral efferent fibers innervate the submandibular, sublingual, minor salivary, and lacrimal glands. Special visceral afferent fibers provide taste to the anterior two thirds of the tongue. Somatic afferent fibers supply innervation to the skin of the external auditory canal and postauricular region.

CENTRAL NERVOUS SYSTEM ANATOMY OF THE FACIAL NERVE

The special visceral efferent fibers to the musculature of the face originate from the facial motor nucleus. This nucleus consists of a gray mass approximately 4 mm long in the lateral aspect of the pons lying just dorsal to the superior olivary complex (Fig. 2). The facial motor nucleus can be divided into four subgroups that are specific in regional innervation. The dorsomedial subgroup innervates the auricular and occipital muscles, the ven-

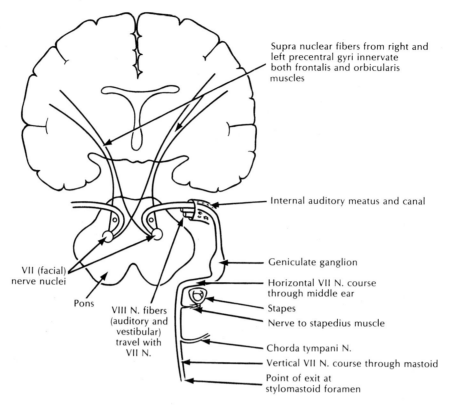

FIG. 1. Schematic shows seventh (facial) nerve pathway from origins in precentral gyri, to pontine nuclei, through internal auditory canal, middle ear, and mastoid, to exit at stylomastoid foramen. (From Goodhill V. Seventh nerve diagnostic techniques. In: Goodhill V, ed. *The ear: diseases, deafness, and dizziness.* Hagerstown, MD: Harper & Row, 1979, with permission.)

tromedial subgroup innervates the platysma muscle, the intermediate subgroup supplies the frontal, ocular, and zygomatic muscle groups, and the lateral group innervates the buccal muscle groups. The facial nucleus derives afferent input from various sources, including the following:

1. Fibers from the spinal trigeminal nucleus that provide trigeminofacial reflexes, such as the corneal blink reflex.
2. Direct and indirect corticobulbar fibers from the pre- and postcentral gyri of the temporal lobe through the reticular formation that provide voluntary facial

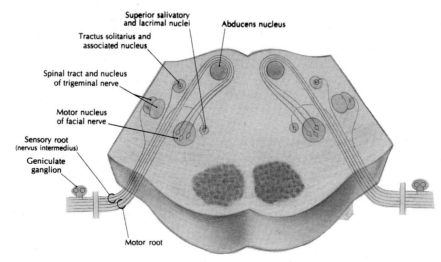

FIG. 2. Facial nerve projections within the pons. (From LaRouere MJ, Lundy LB. Anatomy and physiology of the facial nerve. In: Jackler RJ, Brackmann DE, eds. *Neurotology.* St. Louis: Mosby–Year Book, 1994, with permission.)

movement. Fiber tracts to the middle and lower face are crossed only while those to the upper face are bilaterally represented.

3. Secondary auditory fibers that relay facial motor reflex responses such as stapedial contraction in response to loud sounds.

4. Crossed rubrobulbar fibers that project only to the upper facial muscles.

After emerging from the dorsal aspect of the facial nucleus, the efferent fibers take a sinuous course, passing dorsomedially along the floor of the fourth ventricle, and ascend medially to the abducens nucleus. As the fibers reach the superior aspect of the abducens nucleus, they turn laterally to exit the brainstem between the olivary and restiform bodies near the caudal border of the pons.

General visceral efferent fibers that provide preganglionic parasympathetic innervation to the submandibular, sublingual, and minor salivary glands and the lacrimal gland originate from the superior salivatory nucleus in the dorsolateral region of the reticular formation. In the distal aspect of the pons, these neurons join the motor fibers of the facial nerve. They are carried transiently by way of the facial nerve to secretory tissue. Some of these fibers branch through the greater superficial petrosal nerve and pass through the sphenopalatine ganglion eventually to reach the lacrimal and palatine glands. Other fibers leave the facial nerve through the lesser superficial petrosal nerve, pass through the otic ganglion, and supply the parotid gland along with glossopharyngeal fibers. The remaining preganglionic parasympathetic fibers exit through the chorda tympani nerve, where they traverse the submandibular ganglion and eventually supply the submandibular and sublingual glands.

Visceral afferent fibers that provide taste have their cell bodies in the geniculate ganglion. These fibers pass from the facial nerve through the chorda tympani and then by way of the lingual nerve to taste buds in the anterior two thirds of the tongue. The central projections of these neurons are with the facial nerve and then through the intermediate nerve of Wrisberg at the level of the internal auditory canal and then to the solitarius tract within the brainstem to eventually end in the nucleus solitarius.

INTRATEMPORAL FACIAL NERVE

The fallopian canal is the bony canal within the temporal bone through which the facial nerve courses from the fundus of the internal auditory canal to its exit through the stylomastoid foramen. As it leaves the brainstem, the facial nerve with the intermediate nerve of Wrisberg immediately posterior to it travels a short direct course to the anterosuperior quadrant of the internal auditory canal, where it comes to lie anterior to the vestibular

nerves and superior to the cochlear nerve (Fig. 3). The meatal segment refers to the facial nerve within the internal auditory canal. A thin bony plate at the fundus, the crista falciformis, divides the canal into superior and inferior compartments. A vertical crest of bone from the superior aspect of the internal auditory canal (also called Bill's bar) divides the canal into anterior and posterior halves. Just before being channeled into bony canals, the vestibulofacial anastomosis interconnects the facial nerve and the superior branch of the vestibular nerve.

The labyrinthine part of the facial nerve is the 2.5-mm segment of the fallopian canal that travels from the internal auditory canal to the geniculate ganglion by making an anterior oblique bend of 130 degrees over the ampullae of the superior semicircular canal and vestibule of the inner ear. The entrance to the labyrinthine segment is the most constricted site of passage for the facial nerve as the fallopian canal becomes narrow and a dense ring of epineurium encases the nerve.

The geniculate ganglion contains the cell bodies for the special visceral and somatic afferent fibers of the facial nerve. Here the nerve and and its bony canal form a bulbous widening while they bend 75 degrees posteriorly. This is referred to as the first or medial genu, which is the beginning of the course of the nerve through the middle ear. The intermediate nerve of Wrisberg joins the distal aspect of the geniculate ganglion and fuses with the facial nerve. The greater superficial petrosal nerve, which car-

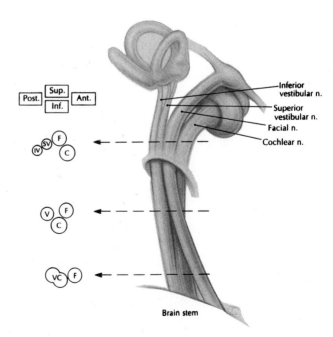

FIG. 3. Relation of the facial nerve to the cochlear and vestibular nerves from the cerebellopontine angle through the external auditory canal. (From LaRouere MJ, Lundy LB. Anatomy and physiology of the facial nerve. In: Jackler RJ, Brackmann DE, eds. *Neurotology.* St. Louis: Mosby–Year Book, 1994, with permission.)

ries preganglionic parasympathetic fibers, branches from the facial nerve at the geniculate ganglion and takes an anterior course as a continuation of the labyrinthine segment of the facial nerve. The greater superficial petrosal nerve passes through the greater superficial petrosal canaliculus to the sphenopalatine ganglion, where the fibers synapse with those relayed to the lacrimal and palatine glands. The lesser superficial petrosal nerve branches from the geniculum anterior to the greater superficial petrosal and continues in this course through its own bony canaliculus to the otic ganglion, where it synapses with postganglionic fibers along with fibers from the glossopharyngeal nerve that provide secretory innervation to the parotid gland.

The continuation of the facial nerve distal to the geniculate ganglion is referred to as the *horizontal segment* (Fig. 4). Its course through the middle ear is straight as it passes posteriorly and at an angle of 10 degrees laterally. The nerve courses medial to the cochleariform process and above the level of the oval window as it heads for the lateral prominence of the horizontal semicircular canal to form a conspicuous bulge over the region of the vestibule. The bone covering the nerve in this region is thin and often dehiscent.

As the nerve passes just anterior to the lateral prominence of the horizontal semicircular canal, it forms the second or lateral genu as it makes a gentle right angle turn from the horizontal segment in the middle ear to the vertical segment that will pass inferiorly through the mastoid. The lateral semicircular canal lies at an approximately 30-degree angle off the horizontal. The facial nerve follows the anterior aspect of the lateral semicircular canal and initially passes deep to come close to the ampullae of the posterior semicircular canal. As the nerve passes inferiorly, it deviates approximately 10 degrees laterally to reach the stylomastoid foramen and exit from the skull.

While coursing through the mastoid process, the facial nerve gives off two branches. In the region of the pyramidal eminence, the nerve to the stapedius muscle diverges. Farther inferiorly the chorda tympani nerve separates from the midvertical segment of the facial nerve at an angle of 150 degrees such that it appears to take a redundant course superiorly through the temporal bone. At approximately the level of the round window the chorda tympani enters the middle ear just medial to the annulus of the tympanic membrane. The chorda tympani courses superiorly and then passes anteriorly through the middle ear lateral to the long process of the incus and medial to the long process of the malleus, eventually exiting the tympanic cavity in its own canal, the iter chorda anterius, in the petrotympanic fissure. The chorda tympani carries preganglionic parasympathetic fibers to the

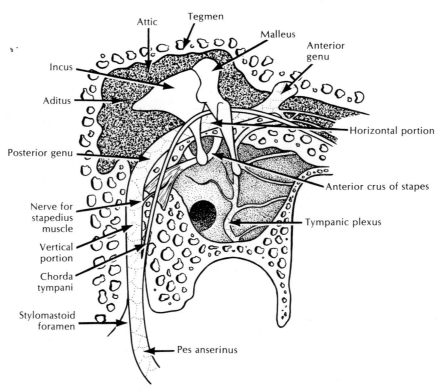

FIG. 4. Intratympanic course of the seventh cranial nerve. (From Goodhill V. Seventh nerve diagnostic techniques. In: Goodhill V, ed. *The ear: diseases, deafness, and dizziness.* Hagerstown, MD: Harper & Row, 1979, with permission.)

submandibular ganglion, which pass to the submandibular and sublingual glands and sensory fibers to the distal lingual nerve, which supplies taste to the anterior two thirds of the tongue (Fig. 5).

The blood supply to the intracranial segment of the facial nerve derives initially from the anterior inferior cerebellar artery (3). In the internal auditory canal, the facial nerve is supplied by the labyrinthine artery. The geniculate ganglion derives arterial blood from the superficial petrosal branch of the middle meningeal artery. At the stylomastoid foramen, the stylomastoid artery (a branch of the posterior auricular or occipital artery) enters to supply the distal temporal segment of the nerve (3a).

EXTRACRANIAL COURSE OF THE FACIAL NERVE

The facial nerve exits the skull through the stylomastoid foramen, just lateral and posterior to the styloid process and at the same level as the site of insertion of the digastric ridge in the temporal bone. Almost immediately after its exit, the posterior auricular nerve branches from the facial nerve and courses superiorly and posteriorly to

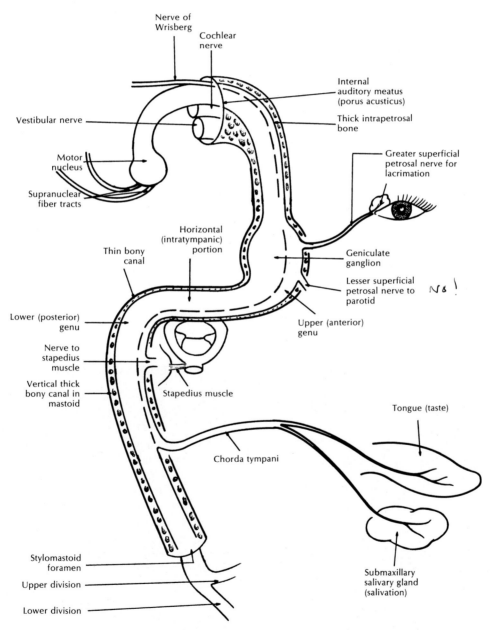

FIG. 5. Intratemporal course of the seventh cranial nerve. (From Goodhill V. Seventh nerve diagnostic techniques. In: Goodhill V, ed. *The ear: diseases, deafness, and dizziness.* Hagerstown, MD: Harper & Row, 1979, with permission.)

supply the occipitalis and the posterior, superior, and intrinsic auricular muscles. The facial nerve takes an anterior bend and enters the substance of the parotid gland to separate the gland into superficial and deep lobes. After passing 1 to 2 cm anteriorly into the parotid gland, the nerve divides at the pes anserinus into superior and inferior branches. Branching of the facial nerve can be quite variable, and numerous branches interconnect the distal facial nerve fibers to form a network plexus of fibers. The following five main divisions are theoretically described: the frontal, zygomatic, buccal, marginal mandibular, and cervical branches. In practicality, these divisions are regions of distribution, and there is overlap between them and the muscles they supply.

STRUCTURAL ANATOMY OF THE FACIAL NERVE

The basic unit of the facial nerve is a highly differentiated axon derived from the neuronal cell body in the pontine facial nucleus of the brainstem (Fig. 6). The axonal

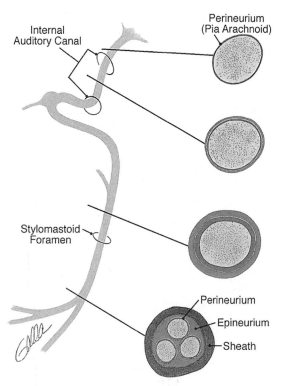

FIG. 6. Topographic arrangement of the cornerstone tissue components of the facial nerve. In the cerebellopontine angle the nerve is monofascicular and bound by only the perineurium that arises from pia and arachnoid tissue. Within the internal auditory canal the nerve gains epineurium. As the nerve enters the middle ear and mastoid segments, the perineurium and epineurium thicken. Where it exits the stylomastoid foramen, the nerve becomes polyfascicular and enclosed within a dense nerve sheath. (From Nadol JB, Schuknecht HF, eds. *Surgery of the ear and temporal bone.* Philadelphia: Raven Press, 1993, with permission.)

processes of the facial nerve are surrounded by a concentric myelin sheath that begins a short distance from the cell body. Within the central nervous system the myelin sheath is derived from the oligodendrocyte. In the peripheral system Schwann cells are responsible for this encasing structure. At regular intervals there are small constrictions in the myelin sheath, the nodes of Ranvier, which consist of the axon surrounded by only a basement membrane and a thin, finger-like process of myelin. The nodes of Ranvier allow for rapid propagation of the action potential along the nerve (3b).

Each axon with its myelin covering is individually ensheathed with endoneurium, a delicate connective tissue layer. The perineurium, a more dense connective tissue, surrounds the endoneurium and groups the nerve fibers into larger nerve trunks. The perineurium is composed of longitudinal strands of collagen and fibroblasts, which provide structural support for the nerve and a barrier to metabolism and diffusion. Epineurium provides another dense collagenous layer that ensheathes the nerve and is contiguous with the dura mater. The facial nerve has no epineurium as it passes from the brainstem to the internal auditory canal, and even within the meatal segment of the nerve, the epineurium is quite thin. Within the labyrinthine segment and distal to this region, the epineurium is well developed. The vascular supply to the nerve runs within this layer.

The facial nerve is composed of a single fascicle until it reaches the distal aspect of the mastoid segment, where it divides into three to four distinct fascicles (4). At the level of the stylomastoid foramen, the nerve has branched into six to ten fascicles. Compartmental topography within the facial nerve that differentiates the axons dispersed to innervate specific muscle groups occurs approximately within the midvertical mastoid segment (5).

PHYSICAL EXAMINATION

Examination of the symmetry of movements of the face are most important in making a diagnosis of unilateral facial paresis or paralysis and the severity of such a problem. Although bilateral facial paresis or paralysis can occur, this condition is rare. All branches of the facial nerve should be evaluated and the two sides compared.

The length of time a facial nerve condition exists can play a role in the degree of symmetry present at the time of examination. With chronic complete paralysis, gross asymmetry even at rest is obvious. With acute paralysis, asymmetry at rest may be subtle; this is even more problematic when the paralysis is incomplete. To express paresis or paralysis, it is beneficial to have the patient maximize facial movement in all branches, including raising the brow, tightly closing the eyes, wrinkling the nose, smiling widely, and grimacing.

As with many subjective diagnostic modalities, the experience of the examiner is important. A number of

TABLE 1. *House-Brackmann classification of facial nerve dysfunction*

Classification	Description	Gross	At rest	Motion
I	Normal	Normal	Normal	Normal
II	Mild dysfunction	Slight weakness, very mild synkinesis	Normal symmetry and tone	Forehead: moderate to good Eye: complete closure with minimal effort Mouth: slight asymmetry
III	Moderate dysfunction	Obvious but not disfiguring difference between two sides; noticeable but not severe synkinesis, contracture, or hemifacial spasm	Normal symmetry and tone	Forehead: slight to moderate movement Eye: complete closure with effort Mouth: slight asymmetry with maximal effort
IV	Moderately severe dysfunction	—	Normal symmetry and tone	Forehead: none Eye: incomplete closure Mouth: asymmetry with maximal effort
V	Severe dysfunction	Barely perceptible movement	Asymmetry	Forehead: none Eye: incomplete closure Mouth: slight movement
VI	Total paralysis	No movement	—	—

From House JW, Brackmann D. Facial nerve grading system. *Otolaryngol Head Neck Surg* 1985;93: 146–147.

scales have been designed to aid in determining the severity of facial paresis. The scale most used and accepted by the American Academy of Otolaryngology–Head and Neck Surgery is the House-Brackmann Classification (Table 1) (6). In addition to providing a guide to diagnosing the severity of a facial paresis, this scale is useful as a means to following the course of a facial disorder and maintaining a standard for reporting in the literature. Other scales have been proposed with definite benefits, but their level of acceptance makes them less useful (7,8,8a).

CENTRAL VERSUS PERIPHERAL FACIAL PARALYSIS

One of the initial considerations in evaluating a patient with facial paresis or paralysis is where along the course of the facial nerve the lesion lies. Although radiographic imaging is commonly used for anatomic isolation of a lesion, one also must understand the physiologic mechanisms and test results used to localize the problem. Within this pathophysiologic regard of facial nerve anatomy and function, the first step is to identify the lesion as central or peripheral. A central problem usually can be discerned with a neurologic examination because most brain lesions are not so specific as to be isolated only to the facial nerve. At the cortical level, tracts near the facial nerve include the ipsilateral upper extremity and tongue. At the brainstem level, nearby tracts include the vestibular and abducens. Because the facial nerve tracts from the brain cortex to the upper face are innervated bilaterally and to the lower face only unilaterally, a cortical lesion resulting in facial paralysis involves only the lower face. There is, however, topographic represen-

tation of facial function within the facial nerve well distal to the geniculate ganglion, making it possible to have a lesion that causes paresis or paralysis of the lower division of one facial nerve. Therefore isolated lower facial paralysis is not pathognomonic of a central lesion.

TOPOGRAPHIC FACIAL NERVE TESTING

Most lesions that cause facial paresis or paralysis are peripheral in nature. After it is discerned that a facial nerve lesion is peripheral, the precise anatomic site of the lesion comes into question. The history, physical examination, and specific physiologic test results can be useful in locating the lesion by means of determining which branches of the facial nerve are affected.

A lesion that affects only specific facial muscle groups is likely to involve only the very distal facial nerve beyond the pes anserinus. Again, there is a topographic spatial organization to the various muscle groups represented in the facial nerve distal to the geniculate ganglion. Therefore an incomplete lesion of the facial nerve might affect only certain muscle groups. A facial nerve lesion usually affects all branches at the level of and distal to the lesion.

A lesion at the level of or proximal to the chorda tympani affects taste in the anterior two thirds of the tongue, secretory function in the submaxillary and sublingual glands, and sensation in the posterior wall of the external auditory canal. The most common symptom of a nonfunctioning chorda tympani is abnormal taste, sometimes described as metallic. Atrophy of the taste papillae on the tongue can occur within 5 to 10 days after interruption of the chorda tympani. Taste can be qualitatively compared from different sites of the tongue with various local applications of common taste stimuli with a cotton swab (e.g. salt, coffee, sugar, lemon juice). Although not commonly used, quantitative measurements of taste can be recorded by specialized laboratories.

Decreased salivary flow from the submaxillary and sublingual glands is almost never noticed by the patient because of the abundance of oral salivary tissue. Submaxillary gland flow can be quantified and compared by means of cannulation of Wharton's ducts and collection of saliva over a set period of time, usually in response to a sialogogue. A differential between the affected and the normal side can then be established. This testing is not commonly used today.

The stapedial nerve is a motor branch of the facial nerve to the stapedius muscle of the middle ear. The stapedial reflex is routinely measured at impedance audiometry in response to acoustic stimulation, usually a pure tone or white noise of 65 dB or greater. The reflex is bilateral, that is, acoustic stimulation of either ear should elicit a reflex contraction response in both stapedial muscles, which move the stapes and other ossicles. Measurement of the response is through alteration in acoustic immitance.

At the geniculate ganglion, the greater superficial petrosal nerve leaves the facial nerve to supply secretory motor fibers to the lacrimal gland. A lesion at the level of or proximal to the geniculate ganglion interferes with secretions of these glands. The lacrimal gland is accessible and can be evaluated for secretory ability by questioning and examining the patient for a dry eye. Lacrimal gland function can be quantified with the Schirmer test. Schirmer paper or filter paper strips are inserted between the lower lid and the conjunctiva of each eye. The length of paper moistened over a determined period of time is compared between the normal and affected sides. A difference of 25% or less compared with the normal side is considered abnormal.

In the clinical assessment of facial nerve paresis or paralysis, measurement of the stapedial reflex has the greatest utility because it is easy to obtain. The Schirmer test sometimes is used if a lesion between the geniculate ganglion and the stapedial branch of the nerve is suspected. The Schirmer, submandibular salivary flow, and taste tests are less commonly performed because of difficulty in obtaining accurate results and the concept that these test results rarely influence the care of the patient. Refinements in radiographic imaging often allow direct visualization of the lesion.

CLASSIFICATION OF NERVE INJURY

Determining the severity of a peripheral nerve injury is important in predicting the potential for spontaneous recovery of function. A classification scheme has been described by Sunderland (9) that is an amplification of the description by Seddon. This system is based on the histologic changes and physiologic implications of the injury (Table 2).

First-degree injury, or neurapraxia, is neural block as a result of increased intraneural pressure. Such an injury does not allow conduction of an action potential across the site of compression. Electrical stimulation of the nerve is possible distal to the site of injury. With relief of compression, complete recovery is expected.

Second-degree injury, or axonetmesis, occurs when pressure is great enough to obstruct vascular flow. Axoplasm flow is interrupted such that there is no exchange of nutrients or waste products, which eventually results in breakdown of the axons. If the compression is relieved, recovery requires axon regeneration. Because the endoneural tubes are intact, axon regeneration with no crossover to other axons is expected.

Third-degree injury, or neurotmesis, occurs when pressure is great enough or long enough to cause breakdown of the endoneural tube. Because of the loss of continuity of the endoneural tube, spontaneous recovery often is incomplete because of the potential of axons to migrate out of the endoneural tube or to other endoneural tubes during regeneration. This causes a mixture of axons and results in poor to moderate recovery with synkinesis.

Fourth-degree injury results from partial disruption of the nerve. In addition to breakdown of the endoneurium, there is discontinuity of the perineurium. All that holds the nerve together is the epineurium. Spontaneous recovery results in minimal mass movement of the face if there is any movement.

Fifth-degree injury occurs with complete disruption of the nerve. No spontaneous recovery is expected.

TABLE 2. *Classification of peripheral nerve injuries and potential for spontaneous recovery*

Injury	Histologic findings	Physiologic injury	Recovery potential
First degree	Neurapraxia	Increased intraneural pressure	Complete recovery
Second degree	Axonotmesis	Increased intraneural pressure with vascular compromise	Good to complete recovery
Third degree	Neurotmesis	Loss of endoneural tubes	Incomplete recovery, synkinesis
Fourth degree	Partial transection	Disruption of endoneural tubes and perineurium	Poor recovery, synkinesis
Fifth degree	Complete transection	Disruption of entire nerve	No recovery

ELECTROMYOGRAPHY

Electromyography (EMG) amplifies and records the spontaneous, evoked, and voluntary electrical responses of the muscle motor endplate (10). Needle electrodes are inserted into the facial muscle, which normally causes a brief burst of electrical activity characteristically measured as a sharp, high-amplitude peak and narrow waveform response at EMG. Among patients with decreased facial muscle function or fibrosis as a result of chronic facial neuropathy, this needle insertion activity is reduced.

After electrode placement, muscle activity at rest can be studied and normally consists of spontaneous discharge activity, which appears as biphasic or triphasic discharge potentials of 50 to 1,500 mV occurring every 30 to 50 ms. In a denervated muscle, there are spontaneous involuntary contractions which appear on EMG as fibrillation potentials consisting of frequent, small-amplitude (20- to 100-mV) waveforms. Fibrillation potentials require 14 to 21 days to develop after facial nerve injury which is dependent on the distance from the site of injury to the facial musculature (11,12).

Voluntary contractions cause a motor discharge which is biphasic or triphasic with an amplitude of 0.3 to 5 mV and a duration of 3 to 16 ms. Diminished or no response to voluntary contraction can occur after facial nerve injury. With recovery or regeneration after facial nerve injury, return of function can be predicted by the presence of polyphasic potentials (a complex waveform with more than three phases). This can occur even before there is clinically evident facial nerve function or excitability of the facial nerve trunk by other means of electrical stimulation.

Overall EMG has limited utility in the evaluation of facial nerve disorders. Because 21 days after a facial nerve injury are needed for any useful information to be recorded, decisions based on this information are too delayed to be clinically useful. This testing is valuable in determining facial nerve regeneration, because polyphasic action potentials can be detected before any visible facial activity is present or any other available test results can be obtained. EMG should be performed before any facial reinnervation procedure is declared a failure (13).

ELECTRICAL TESTING OF THE FACIAL NERVE

The purposes of electrical testing are to determine the degree of injury to the facial nerve and to assess the potential for spontaneous recovery (11). In some third- and all fourth- and fifth-degree injuries, facial nerve recovery may be better with surgical intervention. Electrical testing is useful as a means to follow the clinical course of a patient with facial paresis or paralysis to determine improvement or deterioration (14).

Electrical testing is an attempt to analyze the segment of the facial nerve distal to the site of the lesion by determining the degree of distal axonal degeneration. The distal nerve segment is stimulated to produce an action potential that is conducted orthodromically (in the direction that action potentials normally propagate) to the facial musculature. By means of assessing the facial muscle response to stimulation, an analysis of axonal degeneration is made that is predicted to correlate with the degree of facial nerve injury. Immediately after injury, a normal distal stimulation response is expected. Three days elapse before axonal degeneration of the facial nerve distal to the site of injury fully develops and nerve function and the degree of injury can be accurately analyzed with electrical testing. Thus electrical testing lags the clinical course by 3 days.

The most widely available technique is stimulation of the nerve with pulsed, constant-current stimulation, as produced with a Hilger nerve stimulator (Fig. 7) (15). This device delivers stimulation with a bipolar probe that consists of two steel-ball electrodes placed 2 to 4 cm apart on the skin overlying the facial nerve. As the amperage of the stimulus is increased, the examiner looks for facial muscle twitching at a frequency that corresponds to the output of the stimulator. The most sensitive site for stimulation is the upper branch of the facial nerve with observation of the lower eyelid for a muscle-twitch response. Other stimulation sites include the middle and lower branches of the facial nerve while observing movement of the nasal ala and the lateral commissure of the mouth.

The minimal nerve excitability test is used to determine the current threshold for a barely perceptible facial muscle response (16). The paretic side is compared with the normal side, and the difference correlates with the extent of degeneration. A minimal difference should show complete recovery. A significant difference is considered a current difference of 2 to 3.5 mA or greater. Such a result is considered to be associated with nerve-fiber degeneration and may be expected to show incomplete recovery.

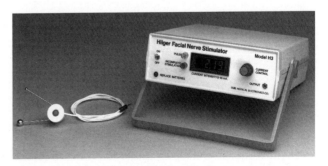

FIG. 7. Hilger nerve stimulator used for electrical testing of the facial nerve. (Courtesy of WR Medical Electronics.)

In the maximal stimulation test facial muscle contraction is elicited with the highest current the patient can tolerate (e.g., 8 to 9 mA) (13). The test results are expressed as the difference in facial response between the normal and affected sides of the face. The degree of difference is ranked as minimal, moderate, severe, or no response. The extent of denervation is considered to correlate with the degree of observed difference, including complete denervation, which correlates with no notable response.

ELECTRONEURONOGRAPHY

Electroneuronography (ENoG) is the recording of compound action potentials from the facial musculature in response to transcutaneous electrical stimulation of the facial nerve trunk at the stylomastoid foramen (17,18). A bipolar stimulating electrode is used, and the response to a maximal stimulation is recorded with a bipolar electrode pair placed peripherally on the face (usually in the nasolabial groove) and measured as the amplitude of the response in millivolts (Fig. 8). Responses between the two sides of the face are then compared and should average within 3% among healthy persons (19,20). The percentage response relative to the normal side is considered proportional to the percentage of degenerated fibers or axonal units within the paretic nerve (21). As in other electrical facial nerve tests, the clinical course precedes ENoG changes by 3 days. Although dedicated instrumentation exists for performing ENoG, most auditory brainstem response recording units can be used for this test with the addition of stimulating and recording electrodes and software.

ENoG is useful in determining when surgical intervention should be considered (22). In Bell's palsy, patients reaching 90% degeneration are considered candidates for

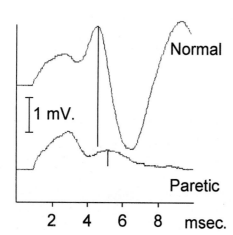

FIG. 8. Electroneuronogram of a patient with unilateral Bell's palsy. The response of the paretic side of the face is approximately 13% of that of the normal side of the face. There is a delay in waveform response on the paretic side of the face compared with normal.

surgical decompression because there is a high chance of a poor result with medical management alone (10,23). Some physicians use ENoG as a means for determining the need for surgical intervention in traumatic injuries to the facial nerve (24). In evaluating patients with tumors of the cerebellopontine angle, some surgeons find ENoG can help predict difficulty in dissecting the facial nerve from the tumor (25). ENoG is also helpful in following facial paresis and determining improvement or deterioration on the basis of the number of active neurons (26).

ENoG can be used to measure nerve conduction velocity (27). The distance between the stimulating and recording electrodes is divided by the time for an electrical stimulus to reach the recording electrodes. As might be expected, a paretic nerve has increased conduction velocity relative to a normal nerve. This measurement has found limited clinical application.

MAGNETIC STIMULATION OF THE FACIAL NERVE

Tests in which a strong magnetic field, such as that generated by an electrical coil directed at the facial motor cortex, have been used successfully to generate a facial nerve response (28). Magnetic stimulation has the potential benefit of stimulating the facial nerve intracranially and therefore proximal to the site of injury (29). The response can be measured as an action potential within the facial musculature and produce waveforms similar to those generated with ENoG (30). One benefit of this form of testing is that the technique is not as painful as electrical testing.

RADIOGRAPHY

Continued imaging improvements have allowed understanding of the structural nature of the facial nerve. To a large extent magnetic resonance imaging and computed tomography have replaced many topographic tests. Rather than inference about a suspected site as in some of the physiologic tests, direct imaging of a lesion provides more clinically useful information.

TRIGEMINAL-FACIAL REFLEX TESTING

Electrodiagnostic testing of facial nerve function as described earlier relies on techniques that directly stimulate or depolarize the nerve and elicit contraction of the facial muscles measured either by means of observing a response or measuring EMG function. The rationale for the use of this kind of testing is based on the expected decrease and cessation of nerve conduction distal to the site of a lesion. However, there is a considerable time lag (3 days) in providing clinical information after a peripheral facial nerve lesion. This discrepancy in testing may be obviated with use of a technique that activates the nerve through reflex excitation of the facial motor neurons at the brainstem level. The advantage of reflex testing is that the motor neuronal discharge is conducted proximal to the site of the lesion and therefore should be more sensitive and especially useful during the initial period after a lesion is inflicted on the nerve.

The trigeminal-facial (T-F; eye blink) reflex consists of recording the EMG activity of the orbicularis oculi muscle in response to stimulation of the supraorbital division of the ophthalmic branch of the trigeminal nerve (Fig. 9) (31). In recording of nerve-conduction velocities, two components are typically recognized: R1, an early response with a latency of 10 to 12 ms, and R2, a late response with a latency of 30 to 40 ms. Both components of the reflex are integrated in the mesencephalon. The R1 response represents oligosynaptic processing within the pons, whereas the R2 response represents polysynaptic activity between the pons and lateral medulla (32). The R2 component can be recorded bilaterally; the R1 response is always unilateral to the side of trigeminal stimulation. This reflex response has been evaluated in various disorders affecting the facial nerve. The advantage is objective measurement of the latency and voltage of the reflex evoked EMG response (7,33–41). The disadvantage of T-F reflex testing is that only the superior division of the facial nerve is assessed.

Recognition of a subclinical problem might find usefulness in management of disorders, especially tumors, involving the facial nerve (35,42,43). This would require

an extremely sensitive test that could detect subtle changes in nerve function, such as latency or morphologic changes in the EMG response. Reflex testing provides greater sensitivity because the entire response is reflex evoked; a large suprathreshold current is not used to induce depolarization of the nerve.

Intraoperative monitoring has shown that the T-F reflex is completely inhibited by general anesthesia. The transition between wakefulness and profound sedation can be monitored through progressive disappearance of first the R2 component and later the R1 component. The T-F reflex response is blocked well before the onset of unconsciousness and up to 30 minutes after emergence from general anesthesia (44). These are important considerations in attempts to evaluate facial nerve reflex function before and during the induction of general anesthesia or in the postanesthetic state.

In a few clinical conditions, the T-F reflex response is exaggerated, and facial muscles other than the orbicularis oculi are activated during supraorbital nerve stimulation. Hemifacial spasm is a condition in which the T-F reflex may be simultaneously recorded in the orbicularis oculi, oris, and mentalis muscles. This finding constitutes objective evidence of synkinetic contractions during volitional contraction of a single muscle group, such as voluntary eye closure (40).

ANTIDROMIC TESTING

Antidromic testing of the facial nerve involves a response *opposite* to the direction that action potentials normally propagate in that the facial nerve is stimulated peripherally and the response is measured centrally. Such evoked facial nerve potentials can produce polyphasic waves similar to an auditory brainstem response (45). The waveforms, however, are variable and dependent on the site of stimulation and whether the nerve is directly stimulated or stimulated through the skin (12).

Antidromic potential refers to the EMG response that follows within a relatively short latency that triggered with direct stimulation of the motor fibers that innervate a specific muscle group (46–48). It is assumed that this indirect response is not a reflex but is the result of the pulse generated during electrical stimulation of the peripheral nerve (Fig. 10). During nerve stimulation, the axons are depolarized, and action potentials travel in the direction of the muscle (orthodromic), triggering a direct response (M wave). Antidromic action potentials simultaneously travel along the nerve and reach the facial nucleus at the brainstem level, resulting in depolarization of the motor neurons and generating a new secondary orthodromic action potential that activates the muscle (F wave). The likelihood of observing this indirect muscular response is a function of (a) the integrity of the nerve fibers in the motor nerve, (b) the excitability of the motor neuron pool, and (c) the relation between the duration of

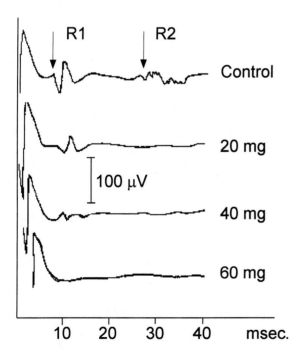

FIG. 9. Trigeminal-facial reflex demonstrated for various incremental doses of propofol in milligrams. The *R2* and then the *R1* waves disappear progressively with increasing levels of anesthetic agent.

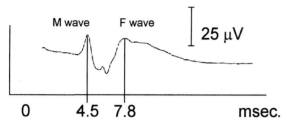

FIG. 10. Antidromic facial nerve potential from stimulation of the facial nerve at the stylomastoid foramen. One stimulation has resulted in the *M wave* from direct orthodromic stimulation and the *F wave* from antidromic stimulation that occurs back to the brainstem with a subsequent second impulse carried peripherally.

the M wave and the latency of the F wave. Such testing is especially useful in the assessment of hemifacial spasm (49).

Although more complicated, it is possible to use the T-F reflex to generate and assess the F and M waves. Because the F wave is maintained during general anesthesia, this form of testing may have utility in intraoperative facial nerve monitoring (50). For a few patients with pathologic processes involving the facial nerve (e.g., acoustic neuroma, cholesteatoma, and various parotid tumors), we have identified an enhanced T-F reflex–generated F wave with patients awake and during general anesthesia.

SUMMARY POINTS

- The facial nerve contains motor, sensory (to skin of external auditory canal and postauricular region), and parasympathetic fibers.
- The parasympathetic fibers innervate the submandibular, sublingual, minor salivary, and lacrimal glands. Special visceral afferent fibers carry taste from the anterior two thirds of the tongue.
- Motor input to the lower two thirds of the face originates from the contralateral motor cortex only. There is bilateral cortical input to each facial nerve nucleus for motor fibers to the forehead.
- The fallopian canal encloses the intratympanic portion of the facial nerve. It extends from the fundus of the internal auditory canal to the stylomastoid foramen and includes the labyrinthine, tympanic, and mastoid segments of the facial nerve.
- The geniculate ganglion contains the cell bodies for the special visceral sensory (taste) fibers and the somatic sensory fibers.
- The facial nerve consists of a single fascicle until the mastoid segment. At the stylomastoid segment it consists of six to ten fascicles.
- Lesions of the peripheral facial nerve often can be localized by means of examining function of the var-

ious branches, such as tearing (greater superficial petrosal branch), the acoustic reflex (stapedial branch), and taste (chorda tympani branch). Of these topographic tests, the acoustic reflex is the easiest to obtain and the most reliable.
- Nerve injury can be classified as neurapraxia (conduction block), axonetmesis (loss of axon), neurotmesis (loss of endoneural tubes), and nerve disruption (loss of perineurium and epineurium).
- Neurapraxia can be differentiated from more severe degrees of facial nerve injury by means of electrical stimulation tests (minimal and maximal nerve excitability tests, ENoG).
- EMG is used to measure spontaneous facial muscle activity and can be used to identify denervation (fibrillation potentials) and early reinnervation (polyphasic potentials).
- The T-F reflex consists of recording the EMG activity of the orbicularis oculi muscle in response to stimulation of the supraorbital division of the trigeminal nerve. The advantage is objective measurement of the latency and voltage of the reflex evoked response.

REFERENCES

1. Wetmore SJ. Surgical landmarks for the facial nerve. *Otolaryngol Clin North Am* 1991;24:505–530.
2. Proctor B. The anatomy of the facial nerve. *Otolaryngol Clin North Am* 1991;24:479–504.
3. Guerrier Y. Surgical anatomy, particularly vascular supply of the facial nerve. In Fisch U, ed. *Facial nerve surgery.* Birmingham, AL: Aesculapius, 1977:13–23.
3a. Miehlke A. *Surgery of the facial nerve.* Philadelphia: WB Saunders, 1973.
3b. Parnes SM. The facial nerve. In: Jahn AF, Santos-Sacchi J, eds. *Physiology of the ear.* New York: Raven Press, 1988:125–142.
4. Radpour S, Gacek R. Anatomic organization of the cat facial nerve. *Otolaryngol Head Neck Surg* 1985;93:591–596.
5. Gacek R, Radpour S. Fiber orientation of the facial nerve: an experimental study in the cat. *Laryngoscope* 1982;92:547–556.

6. House JW, Brackmann D. Facial nerve grading system. *Otolaryngol Head Neck Surg* 1985;93:146–147.
7. Taylor N, Jebsen RH, Tenckoff HA. Facial nerve conduction latency in chronic renal insufficiency. *Arch Phys Med Rehabil* 1970;51:259–267.
8. Wood DA, Hughes GB, Secic M, Good TL. Objective measurement of normal facial movement with video microscaling. *Am J Otol* 1994;15: 61–65.
8a. Rickenmann J, Jaquenod C, Cerenko D, Fisch U. Comparative value of facial nerve grading systems. *Otolaryngol Head Neck Surg* 1997;117: 322–325.
9. Sunderland S. *Nerves and nerve injuries,* 2nd ed. Edinburgh: Churchill Livingstone, 1978.
10. Esslen E. Electro neuronography and electromyography. In Fisch U, ed. *Facial nerve surgery.* Birmingham, AL: Aesculapius, 1977:93–100.
11. Alford BR. Electrodiagnostic studies in facial paralysis. *Arch Otolaryngol* 1967;85:259–264.

12. Cramer HB, Kartush JM. Testing facial nerve function. *Otolaryngol Clin North Am* 1991;24:555–570.

13. May M, Blumenthal F, Klein SR. Acute Bell's palsy: prognostic value of evoked electromyography, maximal stimulation and other electrical tests. *Am J Otol* 1983;5:1–7.

14. Yangihara N, Kishimoto M. Electrodiagnosis in facial palsy. *Arch Otolaryngol* 1972;95:376–382.

15. Lewis BI, Adour KK, Kahn JM, Lewis AJ. Hilger facial nerve stimulator: a 25-year update. *Laryngoscope* 1991;101:71–74.

16. Gates G. Nerve excitability testing: technical pitfalls and threshold norms using absolute values. *Laryngoscope* 1993;103:379–385.

17. Bauer CA, Coker NJ. Update on facial nerve disorders. *Otolaryngol North Am* 1996;29:445–454.

18. Dennis JM, Coker NJ. Electroneuronography. *Adv Otorhinolaryngol* 1997;53:112–131.

19. Gantz BJ, Gmuer AA, Holiday M, Fisch U. Electroneurographic evaluation of the facial nerve. *An Otol Rhinol Laryngol* 1984;93:394–398.

20. Hughes G, Nodar R, Williams G. Analysis of test-retest variability in facial electroneuronography. *Otolaryngol Head Neck Surg* 1983;91:290–293.

21. Halvorson DJ, Coker NJ, Wang-Bennett LT. Histologic correlation of the degenerating facial nerve with electroneurography. *Laryngoscope* 1993;103:178–184.

22. Fisch U. Surgery for Bell's palsy. *Arch Otolaryngol* 1981;107:1–11.

23. Fisch U. Prognostic value of electrical tests in acute facial paralysis. *Am J Otol* 1984;5:494–498.

24. Coker NJ, Jenkins HA, Psifidis A. Electrophysiological prognostication of acute facial nerve trauma. In Fisch U, Valavanis A, Yasargil MG, eds. *Neurological surgery of the ear and skull base.* Amsterdam: Kugler & Ghedini, 1989: 355–362.

25. Syms CA, House JR, Luxford WM, Brackmann DE. Preoperative ENoG and facial nerve outcome in acoustic neuroma surgery. *Am J Otol* 1997;18:401–403.

26. Danielides V, Skevas A, Van Conevenberge P. A comparison of ENoG with facial nerve latency testing for prognostic accuracy in patients with Bell's palsy. *Eur Arch Otolaryngol* 1996;253:35–38.

27. Ruboyaianes JM, Adour KK, Santos DQ, von Doersten PG. The maximal stimulation and facial nerve conduction latency tests: predicting the outcome of Bell's palsy. *Laryngoscope* 1994;104:1–6.

28. Lavanne J, Rimpilainen I, Karma P, Eshola H, Hakkinen V, Laipalla P. A comparison of transcranial magnetic stimulation with ENoG as a predictive test in patients with Bell's palsy. *Eur Arch Otorhinolaryngol* 1995;252:344–347.

29. Mills K, Mrura N, Hess C. Magnetic and electrical transcranial brain stimulation: physiologic mechanisms and clinical applications. *Neurosurgery* 1987;20:164–168.

30. Seki Y, Krain L, Yamada T, Kimura J. Transcranial magnetic stimulation of the facial nerve: recording technique and estimation of the stimulated site. *Neurosurgery* 1990;26:286–290.

31. Kimura J. Clinical uses of the electrically elicited blink reflex. In Desmedt JE, ed. *Motor control mechanisms in health and disease,* vol. 39. New York: Raven Press, 1983:773–786.

32. Hiraoka M, Shimamura M. Neural mechanisms of the corneal blinking reflex in cats. *Brain Res* 1977;125:265–272.

33. Kimura J, Giron LT, Young SM. Electrophysiological study of Bell's palsy: electrically elicited blink reflex in assessment of prognosis. *Arch Otorhinolaryngol* 1976;102:140–149.

34. Kimura J, Lyon LW. Orbicularis oculi reflex in the Wallenberg syndrome. *J Neurol Neurosurg Psychiatry* 1972;35:228–235.

35. Kimura J, Lyon LW. Alteration of orbicularis oculi reflex by posterior fossa tumors. *J Neurosurg* 1973;38:10–22.

36. Kimura J, Powers JM, Van Allen MW. Reflex response of the orbicularis oculi muscle to supraorbital nerve stimulation: study in normal subjects and in peripheral facial paresis. *Arch Neurol* 1969;21:193–201.

37. Kimura J, Rodnitzky RL, Okawara S. Electrophysiologic analysis of aberrant regeneration after facial nerve paralysis. *Neurology* 1975;25:989–913.

38. Kimura J, Wilkinson JT, Damasio H. Blink reflex in patients with hemispheric cerebrovascular accident (CVA). *J Neurol Sci* 1985;67:15–21.

39. Kimura J. Disorder of interneurons in Parkinsonism: the orbicularis oculi reflex to paired stimuli. *Brain* 1973;98:87–96.

40. Moller AR, Janetta PJ. Blink reflex in patients with hemifacial spasm. *J Neurol Sci* 1986;72:171–182.

41. Nielsen VK. Pathophysiology of hemifacial spasm, II: lateral spread of the supraorbital nerve reflex. *Neurology* 1984;34:427–431.

42. Eisen A, Danon J. The orbicularis oculi reflex in acoustic neuromas: a clinical and electrodiagnostic evaluation. *Neurology* 1974;24:306–317.

43. Lyon LW, Van Allen MW. Alteration of the orbicularis oculi reflex by acoustic neuroma. *Arch Otorhinolaryngol* 1972;95:100–108.

44. Mahajan A, Rubinstein EH. Changes in the eye blink (trigeminal-facial) reflex during sedation and after induction and emergence from general anesthesia. Presented at the annual meeting of the California Society of Anesthesiology; 1997; Monterey, Calif.

45. Niparko JK, Kartush JM, Bledsoe SC, Graham MD. Antidromically evoked facial nerve response. *Am J Otolaryngol* 1985;6:353–357.

46. Magladery JW, McDougal DB. Electrophysiological studies of nerve and reflex activity in normal man, I: identification of certain reflexes in the electromyogram and the conduction velocity of peripheral nerve fibers. *Bull Johns Hopkins Hosp* 1950;86:265–290.

47. Mayer RF, Feldman FG. Observations in the nature of the F-wave in man. *Neurology* 1967;17:147–156.

48. Trontelj JV, Trontelj M. F-responses of human facial muscles. *J Neurol Sci* 1973;20:211–222.

49. Ishikawa M, Ohira T, Namiki J, Gotoh K, Takase M, Toya S. Electrophysiological investigation of hemifacial spasm: F-waves of the facial muscles. *Acta Neurochir (Wien)* 1996;138:24–32.

50. Moller AR, Janetta PJ. Microvascular decompression in hemifacial spasm: intraoperative electrophysiological observations. *Neurosurgery* 1985;16:612–618.

The Ear: Comprehensive Otology,
edited by R. F. Canalis and P. R. Lambert.
Lippincott Williams & Wilkins, Philadelphia © 2000.

CHAPTER 45

Inflammatory Disorders of the Facial Nerve: Bell's Palsy, Ramsay Hunt Syndrome, Otitis Media, and Lyme Disease

Kedar K. Adour

The two most common forms of facial paralysis are Bell's palsy, for which the incidence is 20 cases per 100,000 persons annually (1), and herpes zoster oticus (Ramsay Hunt syndrome), for which the incidence is 5 cases per 100,000 persons annually (2,3).

FACIAL NERVE DISORDERS

Causes

Bell's palsy is a demyelinating, virally induced immune response that is caused by herpes simplex virus type 1 (HSV-1) reactivation in the ganglia of the head and neck. Herpes zoster virus (HZV, varicella-zoster virus) was identified as the causative agent in Ramsay Hunt syndrome in 1907 (4), but the cause of Bell's palsy remained elusive. In 1919, using only physical diagnostic methods, Antoni (5) correctly labeled Bell's palsy "acute infectious polyneuritis cerebralis acusticofacialis." The signs and symptoms are similar to those in herpes zoster oticus. Forty years later, Dalton (6) correctly postulated that herpes zoster facial paralysis rep-

resented a more florid form of Bell's palsy. Another 10 years later, herpes simplex virus (HSV) was suggested to cause Bell's palsy (7,8). This hypothesis was not confirmed until 1996, when Murakami and colleagues (9) explored the link between HSV-1 and Bell's palsy and established that Bell's palsy is a viral disease. Their study included 23 patients (14 with Bell's palsy and 9 with Ramsay Hunt syndrome) in whom surgical decompression was performed. Endoneurial fluid was collected from the facial nerve, and a polymerase chain reaction was used to analyze samples for the presence of HSV-1, HZV, and Epstein-Barr virus genomes. The researchers concluded, "HSV-1 infection in the facial nerve is directly related to the pathogenesis of Bell palsy just as the varicella-zoster virus is directly related to the pathogenesis of the Ramsay Hunt syndrome" (p. 30). An editorial published in the same issue of *Annals of Internal Medicine* (10) stated, "One might now question whether we should continue using the term 'Bell palsy' to mean 'idiopathic facial paralysis' or whether we should now recognize Bell palsy as 'herpetic facial paralysis'" (p. 64).

Although the disease is herpetic, the term "Bell's palsy" is used here because it is most commonly used and to prevent confusion with HZV facial paralysis. In some instances, the term "Bell's palsy (HSV)" appears.

K. K. Adour: Cranial Nerve Research Clinic, Department of Head and Neck Surgery, Kaiser Permanente Medical Center, Oakland, California 94611-5693

BELL'S PALSY VERSUS RAMSAY HUNT SYNDROME

As herpetic diseases, Bell's palsy and Ramsay Hunt syndrome can be described as "mononeuritis multiplex": they can exist in mononeuritic or polyneuritic form. Both affect the cranial nerves equally (Table 1); the difference is one of severity. HZV is more likely than Bell's palsy to cause complete clinical paralysis, complete electrical denervation, and incomplete recovery with contracture and synkinesis as late complications (1,2).

Major damage to the facial nerve occurs within 10 days in patients with Bell's palsy but does not occur until 2 to 3 weeks after onset of paralysis in patients with HZV, as electrical tests have shown (11). This is consistent with HZV nerve destruction seen in animal models. Therefore, prognosis for recovering facial function can be predicted within 10 to 14 days in patients with Bell's palsy but not until 3 weeks after onset in patients with HZV (12,13).

Pathophysiology of Herpetic Facial Paralysis

The mechanism by which HZV is activated remains obscure, but certain steps in the human pathophysiology of herpes simplex activity are well understood. During recovery from primary HSV infection, the virus becomes latent in the trigeminal and other cranial and spinal sen-

TABLE 1. *Percentage of other cranial nerves affected in patients with Bell's palsy and herpes zoster virus facial palsy*

Cranial nerve	Bell's palsy (%; n = 48)	Herpes zoster virus (%; n = 47)
V (sensory)	5	6
V (motor)	4	11
VIII (vestibular)	42	36
VIII (cochlear)	29	26
IX (sensory)	35	23
X (superior laryngeal)	19	19

sory ganglia (14–16). Through a method not yet elucidated, the virus is reactivated and replicates within the sensory ganglion cells, where it is protected from the circulating antibodies. During replication, local damage to the ganglia causes hypofunction of these nerves, appearing clinically as hypesthesia of the face, pharynx, head, and neck. Replication of HZV within special sensory cells controlling taste in the geniculate or glossopharyngeal ganglion causes dysgeusia. The virus then passes down the axons to induce radiculitis and passes upward along the nerve to the brainstem to induce local meningoencephalitis as evidenced by increased protein in the cerebrospinal fluid and lymphocytic pleocytosis. This inflammatory response has been shown by gadolinium-enhanced magnetic resonance imaging (MRI).

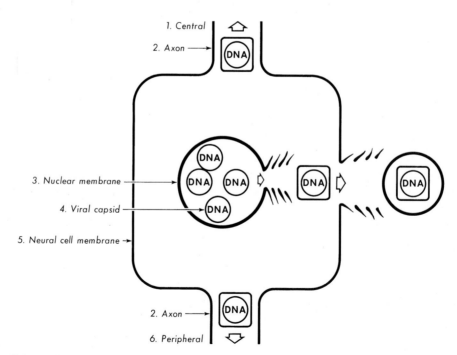

FIG. 1. Schematic representation of herpes simplex virus (HSV) replication within sensory ganglion cells shows centripetal and centrifugal migration and envelopment of portions of neural cell protein. (From Adour KK, Hilsinger RL Jr, Byl FM. Herpes simplex polyganglionitis. *Otolaryngol Head Neck Surg* 1980;88:273, with permission.)

At this point, two events occur: (a) the virus infects Schwann cells in the affected nerve, causing inflammation; and (b) because the virus accumulates a protein coat from the nerve cells as it extrudes through their membranes (Fig. 1), a damaging, virally induced immune response to nerve cell membrane ensues (17).

Lymphocytic infiltration of the peripheral nerve fiber follows, leading to fragmentation of myelin, demyelinization, and chromatolysis of the facial nucleus cells. These cells thus are impaired but may be retrieved if the distal disease process resolves. Motor nerves traversing the ganglion are affected as "innocent bystanders" (18). The paralysis is caused by segmental demyelinization and not by compression. Suprasystolic pressure is needed to cause sufficient compression to stop the nerve action potential (19,20). Inflammatory edema greater than intraarteriolar pressure is physiologically impossible; inflammatory edema is only possible when the intraarteriolar pressure is greater than the pressure in the surrounding tissue.

When the inflammation and virally induced immune reaction resolve, remyelinization ensues and functional muscle enervation is reestablished. The degree and rate of recovery depend directly on the degree and rate of damage.

Diagnosis

Medical History and Physical Examination

Bell's palsy and Ramsay Hunt syndrome can be diagnosed by medical history and by observing the patient's initial signs and symptoms; they are not diagnoses of exclusion. The more knowledge clinicians have about these diseases, the more confidently the diseases can be diagnosed and treated and the more reassurance clinicians can offer patients. Obtaining an accurate medical history and performing a complete physical examination often can yield sufficient information for diagnosis or to suggest which diagnostic tests are needed.

A positive family history of Bell's palsy is noted in about 10% of all patients. The annual incidence of Bell's palsy is about 20 cases per 100,000 population; however, age-corrected figures indicate increasing incidence in each decade of life, with the incidence reaching 30 to 35 cases per 100,000 in patients older than 60 years (Fig. 2) (1).

The ratio of male to female patients affected with Bell's palsy is about equal. However, the condition is twice as common in women aged 10 to 19 years, whereas it is 1.5 times more common in men after age 40 years (Fig. 3) (1). This distribution suggests a relation to menarche and menopause (21). The rate of occurrence in menstruating women is highest during the first menstrual day; secondary peaks of incidence are seen on the eleventh through seventeenth day of the menstrual cycle

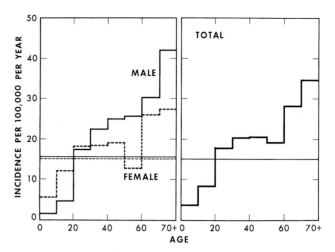

FIG. 2. Graphic representation of age-corrected incidence figures for patients with Bell's palsy seen in a defined geographic area. (From Adour KK, Byl FM, Hilsinger RL Jr, Kahn ZM, Sheldon MI. The true nature of Bell's palsy: analysis of 1,000 consecutive patients. *Laryngoscope* 1978;88:789, with permission.)

and are probably related to ovulation (21). The frequency of Bell's palsy in pregnant women is 45 cases per 100,000 births; per year of exposure, these women have 3.3 times the risk as nonpregnant women in the same age group. Bell's palsy is statistically more likely to occur during the third trimester or immediate postpartum period (21).

Bell's palsy recurs at a rate of about 10%, and recurrence can be ipsilateral or contralateral. Persons who have one recurrence are more likely to have a second recurrence; and 50% of those who have three recurrences will

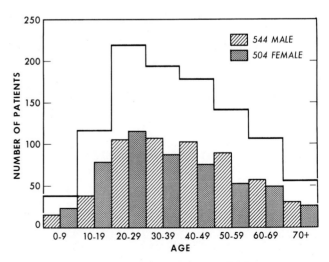

FIG. 3. Graphic representation of age distribution among 1,048 patients with Bell's palsy. (From Adour KK, Byl FM, Hilsinger RL Jr, Kahn ZM, Sheldon MI. The true nature of Bell's palsy: analysis of 1,000 consecutive patients. *Laryngoscope* 1978;88:789, with permission.)

RANDOM DATA IN 684 BELL'S AND 131 ZOSTER PALSY CASES

	BELL'S PALSY		HERPES ZOSTER	
	Number	Percent	Number	Percent
Right	326	48	75	57
Left	355	52	55	42
Bilateral	3	0.4	1	0.8
Previous paralysis	64	9.4	9	6.9
Family history of paralysis	54	8	16	12.2
Hypertension	91	13.3	10	7.6
Diabetes	78	11.4	9	6.9

FIG. 4. Random data tabulated for 684 patients with Bell's palsy and 131 patients with herpes zoster oticus.

probably have a fourth (22). Of patients who have recurrences, one third are likely to have abnormal glucose tolerance test results without necessarily having clinical diabetes. Nonetheless, Bell's palsy is 4.5 times more likely to occur in diabetic patients than in nondiabetic patients (23).

Otologic complications of Bell's palsy and Ramsay Hunt syndrome include facial paralysis, hearing loss, hyperacusis (dysacusis), vertigo, and dysgeusia. In HZV mononeuritis multiplex, balance problems are severe and in the elderly are often incapacitating.

At physical examination, the clinician should exclude lesions that can mimic Bell's palsy. This is done by documenting four points: (a) all facial nerve branches are involved diffusely; (b) findings from otoscopic examination are normal; (c) no ipsilateral parotid masses are present; and (d) presence or absence of skin blebs or blisters around the ear (herpes zoster). These points distinguish Bell's palsy and Ramsay Hunt syndrome from infection, tumor, trauma, and stroke. In Bell's palsy, the left and right sides of the face are equally affected; less than 1% of occurrences are bilateral (Fig. 4).

The definition of central versus peripheral lesions causing Bell's palsy is not clear. Sparing of forehead function, inequality of voluntary and emotional facial muscle motion, ipsilateral motor weakness of the arm or leg, dysarthria, or confusion all indicate presence of a "central" lesion. Herpetic facial paralysis accounts for 90% to 95% of all cases (1) and is considered "periph-

eral," although inflammation is often seen from the brainstem to the stylomastoid foramen.

Onset of paralysis is best defined as acute or progressive. In acute cases, patients have paralysis that reaches maximum severity within 2 weeks after onset. Cases of Bell's palsy are similar in history, natural course, and outcome. Onset of paralysis is often preceded by a viral syndrome. Symptoms and signs during the early phase of facial paralysis include facial numbness, epiphora, dysgeusia (aberrant taste), hyperacusis (dysacusis), and decreased tearing (Table 2). Facial numbness is diagnostic for trigeminal nerve involvement; no somatic sensory fibers have been found in the facial nerve. The pain usually is retroauricular, indicating inflammation of the second or third cervical nerve: however, the pain can and does radiate into the face (cranial nerve V) or into the neck (cervical C2, C3, or both) and arm (cervical C4, C5, and C6). Dysgeusia suggests dysfunction of the geniculate ganglion, which contains the cell bodies of the chorda tympani nerve and is probably the site of HSV reactivation. These symptoms usually are unilateral, but they can

TABLE 2. *Presenting signs and symptoms in patients with Ramsay Hunt syndrome and Bell's palsy*

Symptom	Ramsay Hunt syndrome (%; n = 102)	Bell's palsy (%; n = 772)
Pain	100	55
Dysgeusia	67	57
Hyperacusis	52	30
Decreased tears	42	24
Facial hypesthesia	34	52
Vertigo	11	1
Hearing loss and tinnitus	21	0

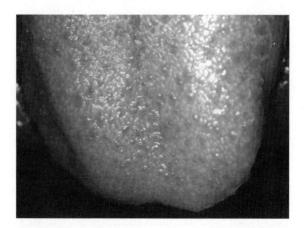

FIG. 5. Bilateral inflammation (more on the left than right) of fungiform papillae of tongue in a patient with Bell's palsy, indicating neural inflammatory disease in chorda tympani nerve. (From Adour KK, Byl FM, Hilsinger RL Jr, Kahn ZM, Sheldon MI. The true nature of Bell's palsy: analysis of 1,000 consecutive patients. *Laryngoscope* 1978;88:798, with permission.)

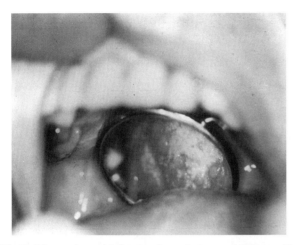

FIG. 6. Mirror view of inflammation of circumvallate papillae of the tongue in a patient with Bell's palsy, with left glossopharyngeal hypesthesia, dysgeusia, and paresis of the left superior laryngeal nerve. (From Adour KK, Byl FM, Hilsinger RL Jr, Kahn ZM, Sheldon MI. The true nature of Bell's palsy: analysis of 1,000 consecutive patients. *Laryngoscope* 1978; 88:799, with permission.)

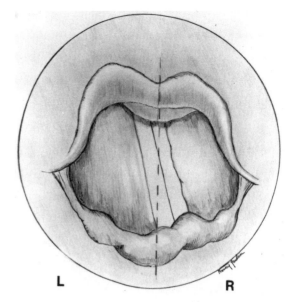

FIG. 8. Shortening of right true vocal cord with rotation of posterior larynx caused by palsy of the right superior laryngeal nerve in a patient with Bell's palsy. (From Adour KK, Schneider GD, Hilsinger RL Jr. Acute superior laryngeal nerve palsy: analysis of 78 cases. *Otolaryngol Head Neck Surg* 1980;88:419, with permission.)

be contralateral (24). The hyperacusis is more accurately labeled as dysacusis because it represents intolerance to noise and not more acute hearing. Dysacusis is not related to stapedial muscle paralysis but probably represents loss of inhibition to the cochlea (25). After evaluating more than 4,000 patients affected with all forms of facial paralysis, we have accumulated statistical evidence indicating that dysgeusia or dysacusis in a patient with acute facial paralysis leads to definitive diagnosis of HSV or HZV mononeuritis multiplex.

Physical findings include inflammation of the fungiform (always) and the circumvallate (occasionally) papillae of the tongue (Figs. 5 and 6) and hypesthesia of cranial nerves V and IX and of cervical C2 (1). Motor paralysis of branches of the vagus nerve manifests as unilateral shift of the palate (Fig. 7) (26) or as shortening of one vocal cord with rotation of the posterior larynx to the affected side (Fig. 8) (27). Bell's palsy thus can be diagnosed when facial paralysis is peripheral in origin, when systemic disease is not evident, when onset is acute, and when concomitant sensory cranial polyneuritis is evident (Fig. 9) (28). No further diagnostic tests are needed.

HZV facial paralysis is differentiated from the HSV form by increased severity of symptoms, presence of auricular vesicles (Ramsay Hunt syndrome), and rising titer of antibody to varicella-zoster virus (Fig. 10; see color plate 29 following page 484) (2,29). HSV may produce segmental focal lesions resembling zoster (30), and HZV reactivation is known to occur without pathognomonic vesicles (zoster sine herpete). In one study using HZV-complement fixation titers for 892 patients with "Bell's palsy," 73 (8.2%) were diagnosed as having zoster sine herpete (31). A "zosterlike" form of Bell's palsy exists without vesicles or antibodies diagnostic for HZV (32). Patients with this syndrome have a higher risk of both nerve degeneration and subsequent poor outcome. Classic vesicular eruption of the pinna (Fig. 11) is not always present. If vesicles appear, they can appear before, during, or after the facial paralysis (28).

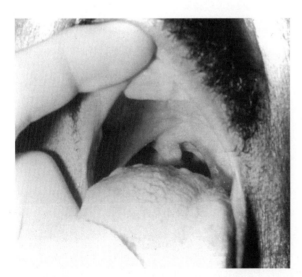

FIG. 7. Patient with Bell's palsy in whom unilateral palatal weakness is apparent when the tongue is used to stretch palatal folds (Byl sign). (From Adour KK, Hilsinger RL Jr, Byl FM. Herpes simplex polyganglionitis. *Otolaryngol Head Neck Surg* 1980;88:272, with permission.)

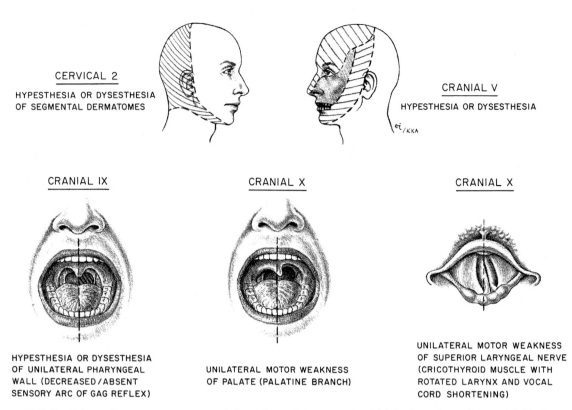

CERVICAL 2

HYPESTHESIA OR DYSESTHESIA
OF SEGMENTAL DERMATOMES

CRANIAL V

HYPESTHESIA OR DYSESTHESIA

CRANIAL IX

HYPESTHESIA OR DYSESTHESIA
OF UNILATERAL PHARYNGEAL
WALL (DECREASED/ABSENT
SENSORY ARC OF GAG REFLEX)

CRANIAL X

UNILATERAL MOTOR WEAKNESS
OF PALATE (PALATINE BRANCH)

CRANIAL X

UNILATERAL MOTOR WEAKNESS
OF SUPERIOR LARYNGEAL NERVE
(CRICOTHYROID MUSCLE WITH
ROTATED LARYNX AND VOCAL
CORD SHORTENING)

FIG. 9. Schematic summary representation of cranial nerve physical findings in patients with Bell's palsy (HSV) and with Ramsay Hunt syndrome (HZV). (From Adour KK. Facial nerve testing and evaluation. In: House JW, O'Connor AF, eds. *Handbook of neurotological diagnosis.* New York: Dekker, 1987:209, with permission.)

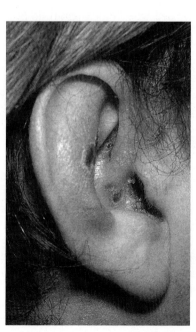

FIG. 10. Healing vesicles on the auricle of a patient with a facial paralysis secondary to Ramsay Hunt syndrome.

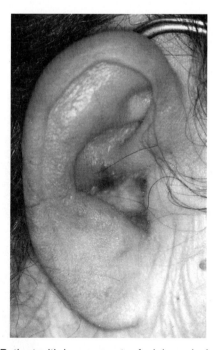

FIG. 11. Patient with herpes zoster facial paralysis (Ramsay Hunt syndrome) shows classic auricular vesicles seen in this condition. (From Adour KK. Facial nerve testing and evaluation. In: House JW, O'Connor AF, eds. *Handbook of neurotological diagnosis.* New York: Dekker, 1987:202, with permission.)

Topographic Testing

Many researchers and clinicians have shown use of topographic tests in facial paralysis to be completely unreliable (11,33–37). Topographic diagnosis is founded on the physiologic anatomy of the facial nerve, i.e., that it includes three types of nerve fibers: branchial motor, visceral motor, and visceral sensory (Fig. 12) (28). This diagnostic technique thus purports to relate particular motor, sensory, and secretory deficits resulting from facial paralysis to extent and site of the lesion. However, many patients have decreased tearing and intact stapedial reflex (25), which are findings that would defy topographic localization. Gadolinium-enhanced MRI shows that multiple sites of demyelination can occur at any point from the brainstem to the periphery. Inflammation and demyelination occur longitudinally and not perpendicularly to the facial canal. Topographic diagnostic tests are only useful to supplement other diagnostic information. They are partial indicators of severity and therefore are only relative indicators of prognosis (13).

Stapedial Reflex Testing

We refer to the stapedial reflex test as "the otologists' electromyography" because the stapedial muscle is the first muscle to be innervated by the facial nerve and is the first muscle to demonstrate reinnervation. The stapedial reflex test is therefore the most objective and reproducible of all the topographic tests (25). Although the accuracy of stapedial reflex testing in determining site of lesion is not absolute, its prognostic value is unquestioned. An intact stapedial reflex indicates incomplete paralysis with excellent prognosis. An intact reflex also should redirect the clinician's attention to the possibility of an intraparotid or mastoid lesion involving the facial nerve. If the stapedial reflex is absent but returns before day 21, prognosis is again excellent.

Audiometry

A pure tone audiogram should be recorded for all patients affected with facial paralysis. If hearing is normal or if sensorineural hearing loss is symmetric, speech discrimination and brainstem evoked auditory response tests are not indicated for assessing paralysis. For some patients who have acute facial paralysis with normal hearing, evoked auditory response testing in a research setting can yield information confirming that the brainstem is affected, but this finding has no therapeutic or prognostic significance.

Auditory testing can suggest cochlear and retrocochlear pathology (38–40), which is consistent with pathologic findings at autopsy (41) or with MRI. Bell's

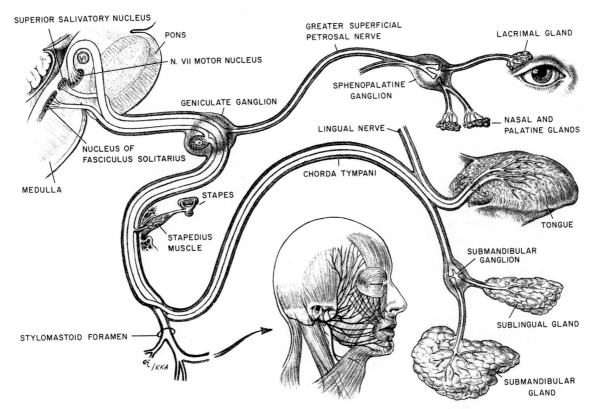

FIG. 12. Anatomic diagram of facial nerve function typically used to discuss topographic diagnosis and "site of lesion testing." (From Adour KK. Facial nerve testing and evaluation. In: House JW, O'Connor AF, eds. *Handbook of neurotological diagnosis.* New York: Dekker, 1987:181, with permission.)

palsy facial paralysis with sensorineural hearing loss statistically portends a final diagnosis of HZV and probably is pathognomonic for this condition (9). Recovery of hearing is problematic, and recovery is incomplete in those who regain hearing.

Radiography and MRI

Neither radiography nor MRI is needed to assess herpetic disease. When a soft-tissue or other inflammatory mass is suspected, MRI is a far superior choice in enabling accurate diagnosis (42,43). MRI produces unique high-resolution images that provide exquisite anatomic definition and can distinguish subtle biochemical changes. Except in patients whose facial paralysis is associated with skull fracture, MRI has replaced computed tomographic scanning.

When using gadolinium-enhanced MRI, clinically significant enhancement of the geniculate ganglion was observed in 37 (88.1%) of 46 patients with Bell's palsy and in 6 (100%) of 6 patients with Ramsay Hunt syndrome (44). Paradoxically, however, these diseases show no difference in either the intensity or the pattern of facial nerve enhancement. In patients who have internal auditory symptoms such as vertigo or tinnitus, enhancement can be seen not only in the facial nerve but also in the vestibular and cochlear nerves (45).

Evoked Electromyography

Evoked electromyography, often called electroneurography (ENoG), not only permits study of muscle excitability and state of muscle fibers, but it also provides useful information regarding conduction properties of nerve fibers. Evoked electromyography is the basis for determining conduction time (also known as *latency* and expressed as milliseconds) and motor nerve conduction (also known as *velocity* and expressed as meters per second). When testing the facial nerve, the distance between the stimulation and recording electrodes is only 10 to 12 cm, and facial nerve latency is traditionally preferable to conduction velocity as a measure of nerve function.

The stimulating electrode is placed over the nerve trunk at the stylomastoid foramen; the surface recording electrode is placed over the muscle group to be tested. The nerve then is given a supramaximal stimulus. The functional status of the nerve is assessed by comparing amplitudes of the compound muscle action potentials on both sides of the face. The interval between nerve stimulation and start of the muscle potential—the facial nerve latency—can be accurately measured and is an acceptable indication of nerve function.

Maximal Stimulation Testing

To obtain greater reliability than provided by minimal nerve excitability testing, a modification called the max-

TABLE 3. *Averaged results of maximal stimulation test in a hypothetical patient*

Branch tested	Visual muscle response	Numeric score
Forehead	Minimally decreased	3
Eye	Moderately decreased	2
Mouth	Severely decreased	1
Averaged score (3 + 2 + 1 ÷ 3)		2

imal stimulation test (MST) was developed (46,47). In this diagnostic technique, in which the observer's location allows both sides of the patient's face to be seen simultaneously, the stimulating probe is applied to the nerve branch at the intensity that produces a barely visible muscle twitch. When the first contraction is observed, the area is explored to find the most sensitive point (i.e., the point that shows the most muscle motion). Current then is increased 1 to 2 mA above this threshold to stimulate maximal nerve excitement. Test results are expressed as the difference between facial muscle movement of the affected and normal sides of the face; results are recorded as equal (numeric score of 4) or decreased movement (numeric score of 3, 2, or 1). In addition, the observer notes whether any decreased response of the affected side is minimally (score = 3), moderately (score = 2), or severely (score = 1) decreased compared with the unaffected side. Findings equate well with degree of denervation. No response indicates complete denervation of the nerve branch being tested. A hypothetical example of this computation is shown in Table 3.

In this example, the facial nerve is "moderately" degenerated, and recovery would be delayed and followed by sequelae. A score of ≤2.7 has 94% accuracy in predicting incomplete final recovery with midface contracture and synkinesis (Table 4) (48).

Although facial nerve excitability testing is a simple procedure, determining the location of the peripheral branches requires experience (Fig. 13) (49). The branch to the frontal muscle usually is located about 1 cm lateral to the eye; the branch to the orbicular muscle of the eye

TABLE 4. *Prediction of recovery based on averaged maximal stimulation test scores*

Maximal stimulation test score	Percent recovery	Time (wk)	Sequelae[a] (severity)
4	100	3–6	None
3–3.9	75–100	4–8	Minimal
2–2.9	75	6–12	Moderate
1–1.9	50–75	8–12	Moderate/severe
0–0.9	<50	12+	Severe

[a]Contracture with synkinesis.

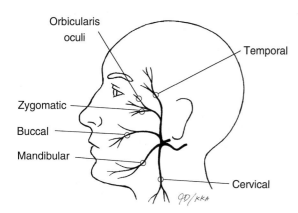

FIG. 13. Schematic drawing depicting the location of facial nerve branches to be stimulated when performing maximal stimulation tests (MST). (Courtesy of Juan Domingo. From Adour KK. Who's afraid of the facial nerve? In: Lucente FE, ed. *American Academy of Otolaryngology—Head and Neck Surgery. Highlights of the instructional courses, volume 8.* St. Louis: Mosby–Year Book, 1995:258, with permission.)

is stimulated at the lateral border of the orbit. Location of the branch to the orbicular muscle of the mouth varies the most of all three peripheral branches, but this branch usually is located just anterior to the notch where the facial artery traverses the mandible. The stimulating probe may need to be moved to determine the point of maximal response because the facial nerve can branch in many directions beyond the stylomastoid foramen.

Comparison of Electrical Tests

In a prospective study, we compared results of ENoG, facial nerve latency testing, and MST in 150 patients affected with facial paralysis (48). To facilitate statistical analysis, we modified the method of reporting MST response to resemble reporting of electromyographic findings and thus to show more comprehensively the status of the peripheral branches. The degree of denervation is not always equal in every branch. Electromyography technicians estimate the degree of muscle action potentials (known as the interference pattern) on a scale of 0 to 4, with a score of 0 indicating no muscle action pattern and a score of 4 indicating a normal response. By assigning a score of 4 to equal response, a score of 3 to minimally decreased response, a score of 2 to moderately decreased response, a score of 1 to severely decreased response, and a score of 0 to no response, we could now compute mean MST score for the entire face (49).

MST has the disadvantage of relying on a visual end point, whereas ENoG has the advantage of recording an often reproducible end point (i.e., the muscle's action potential). However, ENoG has the disadvantage of relying on stimulation of the nerve trunk. A stronger stimulus is required because the facial nerve trunk is deep in the stylomastoid foramen, and this stronger stimulus often trig-

gers a reaction in the masseter muscle—the "trigeminal nerve artifact." Moreover, ENoG results are interpreted on the basis of muscle reaction in only one portion of the face; if the upper part of the facial nerve is cut, ENoG records muscle response equal to that of the other side. MST, which records activity in the peripheral branches, can accurately show this abnormal muscle response (26,50). The electrical impulse can stimulate only neurapraxic fibers. Because no tests distinguish between axonotmesis and neurotmesis, tests do not distinguish between injuries of second and third degree. The compound action potential recorded for a nerve in which 25% of fibers are neurapraxic remains the same, regardless of whether the other fibers are in a state of axonotmesis or neurotmesis.

The ostensible goal of facial nerve decompression is to prevent neural degeneration; therefore, the after-the-fact nature of ENoG makes it an insufficiently sensitive indicator of the need for decompression surgery in patients with herpetic facial palsy (HSV or HZV). Nonetheless, because ENoG offers a recorded and often reproducible end point, ENoG has become the preferred tool for determining which patients with Bell's palsy will benefit from surgical facial nerve decompression.

However, universal lack of understanding, lack of normative experimental data, and lack of control variables for ENoG still have not led to standardization in ENoG testing (4,51–53). Hughes (54) suggested standardized lead placement (Fig. 14) (49) of the recording electrode, but despite careful controls, test-retest variability can significantly influence ENoG measurements; and test-retest variability between both sides of the face and between test results on different days ranges as high as 50% with a mean difference of 20%, which is in agreement with our early research findings (27). Fisch (55) advocated changing the positions

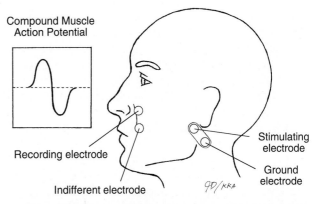

FIG. 14. Schematic drawing showing suggested standardized lead placement of stimulating and recording electrodes for electroneurography (ENoG) and a compound muscle action potential. (Courtesy of Juan Domingo. From Adour KK. Who's afraid of the facial nerve? In: Lucente FE, ed. *American Academy of Otolaryngology—Head and Neck Surgery. Highlights of the instructional courses, volume 8.* St. Louis: Mosby–Year Book, 1995:260, with permission.)

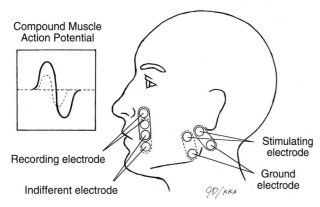

FIG. 15. Schematic drawing showing the optimized lead placement of stimulating and recording electrodes for electroneurography (ENoG) and the possible variation in the size of compound muscle action potentials. (Courtesy of Juan Domingo. From Adour KK. Who's afraid of the facial nerve? In: Lucente FE, ed. *American Academy of Otolaryngology—Head and Neck Surgery. Highlights of the instructional courses, volume 8.* St. Louis: Mosby–Year Book, 1995:260, with permission.)

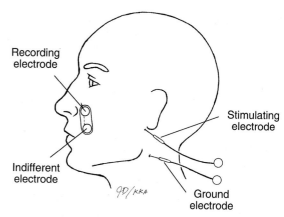

FIG. 16. Schematic drawing showing placement of the recording electrode for electroneurography (ENoG) and insertion of stimulating needle electrodes as suggested by Kobayashi. (Courtesy of Juan Domingo. From Adour KK. Who's afraid of the facial nerve? In: Lucente FE, ed. *American Academy of Otolaryngology—Head and Neck Surgery. Highlights of the instructional courses, volume 8.* St. Louis: Mosby–Year Book, 1995:260, with permission.)

of the stimulating and recording electrodes (optimized lead placement) (Fig. 15) to obtain maximum compound summation muscle action potential as the end point for comparison between both sides of the face but also suggested that repeated and averaged measures for a given patient can increase the precision of ENoG.

Kartush et al. (56) conducted a clinical and experimental study to determine the reasons for inaccuracy of ENoG in some patients. The authors advised optimized lead placement and still found intertest result variance of 18%. The authors further commented that a supramaximal level of stimulation was achieved less often using standardized lead placement because pain or masseter muscle artifact prevented this level of stimulation.

Kobayashi et al. (26) reemphasized three disadvantages of using surface-stimulating electrodes: inconsistent and possibly suboptimal placement of electrodes; variability of electrical characteristics of the skin owing to inconsistent temperature, moisture, and thickness of the soft tissue covering the nerve; and variations in patient's tolerance to pain. The authors devised a method whereby a stimulating needle electrode is inserted subcutaneously to a depth of about 1 cm (Fig. 16) (49) and in which the threshold for nerve excitability ranged from 2 to 70 mV; in contrast, the excitability threshold for surface electrodes ranged from 30 to 160 mV. Some patients who had not responded to nerve excitability testing using conventional surface electrodes made a complete recovery when the needle electrodes were used because the needle method more effectively stimulated the nerve in these patients. Kobayashi et al. stated that by using the needle stimulation electrode, "We believe that unnecessary risk of early decom-

pression surgery for Bell's palsy or Hunt's syndrome can be avoided" (26).

The diagnosis of HSV (Bell's palsy) or HZV facial paralysis should be in question when any of the following occur:

1. *Partial* facial paralysis that either does not resolve within 3 to 6 weeks or is accompanied by electrical evidence of nerve degeneration;
2. Any facial paralysis accompanied by evidence of chronic otitis media or previous ear surgery;
3. Total facial paralysis with no return of facial motion within 4 months. Even after total loss of nerve excitability, 99% of all patients with Bell's palsy or Ramsay Hunt syndrome have nerve regeneration with midface contracture and synkinesis. Return of stapedial reflex is the earliest sign of regeneration; the next sign is evidence of mouth motion with voluntary forced closure of the eyes (synkinesis);
4. Any facial paralysis accompanied by electrical evidence of nerve degeneration that resolves without midface contracture or synkinesis. HSV or HZV paralysis with facial nerve degeneration followed by regeneration will show some midface contracture and/or synkinesis;
5. Facial paralysis that progresses for weeks or months. Damage to the nerve is complete by day 14 in patients with Bell's palsy and by day 21 in patients with Ramsay Hunt syndrome (49).

Treatment

No reliable, widely available test for early identification of HZV infection currently exists. Because HZV carries a considerably poorer prognosis than does HSV, patients infected with HZV require longer follow-up, longer treatment, and greater emotional support (2). As in the past, medical history and results of physical examination are crucial for identifying patients who will benefit from aggressive treatment. If a patient complains of concomitant severe pain or has sensorineural hearing loss, consider the diagnosis to be HZV (and not Bell's palsy, HSV) and administer aggressive treatment.

Pharmacologic Agents

Corticosteroid agents remain the best treatment for inflammatory, virally induced, immune-mediated disease. Because Bell's palsy can progress from mild, incomplete paresis to severe, complete paralysis, all patients should be given corticosteroid agents; progression to the severe form of the disease cannot be predicted. If treatment is delayed until severity is determined, irreversible nerve damage may occur. Patients should receive both prednisone and acyclovir (57), and treatment should be tailored to the degree of disease severity. Prednisone treats the inflammatory, immune response; acyclovir treats the causative agent, HSV.

For adults, a daily total of 1 mg prednisone per kilogram of body weight should be taken in divided doses in the morning and evening. From a practical viewpoint, 30 to 40 mg prednisone given twice daily is therapeutic, and we suggest it be taken with food at breakfast and dinner (Table 5) (58). Acyclovir has been replaced by newer antiviral agents (Table 6). Famciclovir is a prodrug of penciclovir, which is chemically similar to acyclovir. Valacyclovir is the prodrug of acyclovir. Both famciclovir and valacyclovir are absorbed more rapidly and extensively than acyclovir.

TABLE 5. *Prednisone treatment schedule*

Day	Breakfast	Dinner
1	30 (40) mg	30 (40) mg
2	30 (40) mg	30 (40) mg
3	30 (40) mg	30 (40) mg
4	30 (40) mg	30 (40) mg
5	30 (40) mg	30 (40) mg
6	25 (35) mg	25 (35) mg
7	20 (30) mg	20 (30) mg
8	15 (25) mg	15 (25) mg
9	10 (20) mg	10 (20) mg
10	5 (15) mg	5 (15) mg
11	(10) mg	(10) mg

The cost of generic prednisone is negligible. There is no advantage to giving dexamethasone (Decadron) or methylprednisolone (Medrol).
Adapted from Adour KK. Idiopathic facial paralysis. In: Gates GA, ed. *Current therapy in otolaryngology–head and neck surgery*, 6th ed. St. Louis: Mosby, 1998:97, with permission.

TABLE 6. *Acyclovir recommendations*

Drug used	Dosage
Acyclovir	200 (400) mg five times daily
Famciclovir	500 mg three times daily
Valacyclovir	500 mg three times daily

The newer forms of acyclovir—famciclovir and valacyclovir—are given three times daily.
Adapted from Adour KK. Idiopathic facial paralysis. In: Gates GA, ed. *Current therapy in otolaryngology–head and neck surgery*, 6th ed. St. Louis: Mosby, 1998:97, with permission.

Patients should be seen on the fifth or sixth day after onset of paralysis. If paralysis is incomplete, prednisone dosage can be tapered to zero during the next 5 days, and acyclovir can be discontinued. If severity or progression is questionable, the full dose of prednisone and acyclovir should be continued for another 7 to 10 days, and the prednisone then should be tapered to zero beginning at day 10.

Surgical Intervention

In the past, when facial paralysis was considered to be idiopathic and surgical decompression of the facial nerve was a viable treatment option, patients were referred to the otolaryngologist to rule out other causes of the paralysis. In the present system of managed health care, patients may not be seen by an otolaryngologist, or, more probably, patients may be referred to an otolaryngologist days, weeks, or months after onset of paralysis. Moreover, selection of patients, timing of surgery, and extent of surgical decompression may become moot issues. The admonition by Jongkees (59,60) in the 1960s that surgery cannot benefit a viral disease gained further validity in the 1990s. Today, the primary role of the otologist treating Bell's palsy is again as it was in the 1930s: to rule out other diseases as the cause of paralysis.

Prognosis

In the early stages of facial paralysis, a reliable prognosis is difficult to make. Electrodiagnostic testing attempts to predict prognosis by determining the physiologic extent of nerve damage (48,61,62). However, the results of available electrical tests (nerve excitability, facial nerve latency, evoked and volitional electromyography, and strength duration determination) do not show abnormality until several days or weeks after onset of degeneration. In the case of a severed nerve, nerve excitability, facial nerve latency, and ENoG results are normal for 72 hours (63–65). All stimulatory nerve tests reflect events that occurred 3 days earlier, and volitional electromyography results do not become abnormal for 2 to 3 weeks (66–68). Moreover, once stimulatory electrical tests become abnormal, they remain abnormal and cannot be used to monitor regeneration and reinnervation. For patients in whom nerve regeneration is expected, electrical tests are good prognostic indicators but yield different interpretations depending on the bias of the individual author.

To establish prognosis in cases of facial paralysis, findings from all electrical testing must be correlated with the clinical and pathologic process causing the paralysis (69,70). In general, the tests are useful only during the first weeks of the disease. Because the degree of regeneration is related to the degree and rate of denervation, tests of electrical response are done serially. If denervation has progressed from minimal to severe degeneration within 7 to 10 days, a greater and earlier return of volitional muscle motion can be expected than in patients whose denervation progresses from minimal to severe within 3 to 4 days (37,50,71).

If testing indicates equal muscle response on both sides of the face, the patient can be expected to have complete return of facial function within 3 to 6 weeks without complications of faulty nerve regeneration. The most common complications of faulty nerve regeneration are contracture, synkinesis (associated facial motion), and facial spasms (tics). An uncommon complication is gustatory tearing ("crocodile tears") (1).

OTITIS MEDIA

Facial paralysis may occur in either acute or chronic otitis media; however, in acute otitis media, facial paralysis is a relatively unimportant sign, whereas in chronic otitis media it has serious practical bearing on diagnosis, prognosis, and treatment.

In an epidemiologic study in Denmark, researchers calculated an annual incidence of 2.3 cases of otitis media facial paralysis per million inhabitants (72). In the preantibiotic era, facial palsy was estimated to develop in 0.5% of patients who had acute otitis media. These figures indicate a decrease of this complication by a factor of 100, to 0.005%. Although 14 (61%) of the 23 patients in the study were children, the risk of acute otitis media being complicated by facial palsy seems highest in adults (who have low incidence of acute otitis media). Complete remission was seen in all but one patient.

Pathophysiology

Facial paralysis in chronic otitis media indicates that a pathologic process, such as cholesteatoma, is eroding bone and that a defect exists in the fallopian canal. In acute otitis media, infection is confined to the mucosa or mucoperiosteum of the middle ear cleft (73). The mucosal infection can affect the facial nerve only if its protective canal has a preexisting defect; in practice, this defect indicates congenital dehiscence, which most frequently occurs in the nerve's tympanic segment. An intact facial canal protects the facial nerve from middle ear infection.

The pathogenesis of facial paralysis in otitis media remains open to conjecture because of limitations imposed on biopsy and controlled study. The pathophysiology by which acute suppuration results in early facial paralysis also remains open to speculation. Vascular congestion and edema in the loose fibrous tissue of the nerve commonly are perceived as important factors. More controversial is the proposal that the paralysis results from toxins released by bacteria. The suggestion that the pathophysiology is a compressive phenomenon associated with purulent fluid under increased pressure is not valid; physiologically purulent fluid can never be greater than systolic blood pressure. If paralysis is to occur by compression, the pressure must be suprasystolic (19,20).

Facial paralysis occasionally may develop from acute suppurative otitis media early in the course of infection and may progress for 2 to 3 days. In adults affected with acute suppurative otitis media, onset of paralysis is equally gradual but often is delayed (72).

Diagnosis

Diagnostic evaluation for otitis media facial paralysis includes otologic and neurologic examination and awareness of other possible causes of facial paralysis. For this reason, diagnostic testing in children should probably include computed axial tomographic scans.

Treatment

Our practice is to treat children with acute otitis media using antibiotics, prednisone, decongestants, and observation. Myringotomy often is advised, but no studies have documented its benefit or lack of benefit for facial nerve recovery. In the rare case in which surgical exploration is done, we advise against cutting the nerve sheath; doing so would expose the nerve trunk to active bacterial inflammation. Prednisone shortens the clinical course of the otitis media, but the effect of this drug on facial nerve recovery is not known.

LYME DISEASE

Another cause of facial nerve dysfunction is Lyme disease, a multisystem inflammatory illness caused by infection with the spirochete *Borrelia burgdorferi*. The disease is widespread but tends to occur in geographically defined areas. In the United States it is most prevalent in the northeastern states and on the west coast, although cases have been reported in at least 46 states. The principal vectors for Lyme disease in the United States are the deer ticks *Ixodes dammini* and *I. pacificus*. Transmission of the spirochete is mostly by the ixodid nymphs, given that the larvae are rarely infected. Adult ticks are less likely to transmit *B. burgdorferi* to humans because there are fewer of them, they are more easily seen and removed, and they appear in colder months, which is a time when fewer people venture into tick habitats and, if they do, are protected by layers of clothing (74).

Although clinicians seem to disagree about timing of clinical symptoms, they unanimously categorize clinical symptoms as *early localized*, *early disseminated*, or *late*.

Erythema migrans is the only pathognomonic sign of early localized Lyme disease. It manifests as a spreading rash at the site of the tick bite 3 to 32 days after the person is bitten. The skin lesion is painless, does not burn or itch, and within a few days spreads in a pattern of concentric circles with a white zone in the center. Many patients have no symptoms or have only nonspecific respiratory "flulike" symptoms (75).

Early disseminated Lyme disease is caused by hematogenous spread of the spirochete and occurs within the first few months after the person is bitten. Neurologic symptoms are caused by cranial neuropathy and include unilateral or bilateral facial paralysis as well as lymphocytic and painful radiculopathies. The facial nerve is the most frequently affected cranial nerve.

Late Lyme disease occurs months to years after the patient is bitten. The condition manifests as polyarthralgia, arthritis, tendinitis, fibromyalgia, and progressive neurologic symptoms, such as polyneuritis or mental disorder.

Diagnosis

Lyme disease is a clinical diagnosis confirmed by serologic testing that uses enzyme-linked immunosorbent assay and Western blot techniques. However, results of antibody detection tests must be interpreted carefully (76). A negative serologic result most often means the patient has not been infected with *B. burgdorferi*. In early disease, when immunoglobulin M has not had a chance to develop, results of serologic testing may be negative; therefore, negative serologic test results do not contraindicate treatment when clinical evaluation suggests the presence of Lyme disease. Antibiotic treatment very early in the course of Lyme disease may abrogate the antibody response; thus, in some patients who have negative serologic test results and are given antibiotics for other conditions (but in dosages inadequate to treat Lyme disease), illness may progress.

Positive serologic test results are useful in confirming the diagnosis of Lyme disease. However, positive results of antibody testing may be misleading when results of clinical evaluation are nonspecific, reflecting either a false-positive result (from cross-reacting antibodies) or a true-positive result related to prior exposure to the organism but *unrelated* to the patient's current complaints (77).

The Western blot technique is useful to distinguish false-positive from true-positive results, but it cannot substitute for clinical judgment in the latter situation (78). In Göttingen, Germany, Lyme borreliosis proved to be the most frequently verifiable cause of acute peripheral facial palsy in children, causing half the incidence of this disorder in summer and autumn. Similar findings were reported from Japan (79). In contrast, a French multicenter study indicated that unless clinical signs suggest borreliosis, patients with facial palsy need not be tested for Lyme disease. However, the study suggested that in areas where Lyme disease is endemic, this condition should always be suspected, especially in children who have acute facial paralysis (76).

Although immunoglobulin M (80) and enzyme-linked immunosorbent assay (79) are adequate methods of diagnosis, the most specific laboratory test probably is measurement of antibody concentration in cerebrospinal fluid. Therefore, when Lyme disease is suspected in a patient affected with facial paralysis, analysis of cerebrospinal fluid may be indicated. Polymerase chain reaction, antigen detection assays, and borreliacidal assays are now being studied (and may be more specific) for application in confirming the diagnosis of Lyme disease (81).

The pathophysiology of facial paralysis in Lyme disease is unknown but because this condition is caused by a spirochete, neural invasion is suspected.

Treatment

A great deal of controversy concerns treatment protocols because so few data are available. Early treatment may reasonably be offered when results of clinical evaluation suggest the diagnosis. The effect of any treatment on outcome of facial paralysis is unknown and thus is anecdotal at best. For early, localized Lyme disease or isolated facial palsy when cerebrospinal fluid is normal, a reasonable treatment approach has been suggested (75).

For early, localized Lyme disease or isolated facial palsy when cerebrospinal fluid is normal:

1. 100 mg doxycycline taken orally twice daily; or
2. 500 mg amoxicillin taken orally three times daily; or
3. 500 mg cefuroxime axetil (Ceftin) taken orally twice daily.

For all other manifestations (including facial palsy):

1. 2 gm ceftriaxone (Rocephin) taken intravenously once daily; or
2. 3 gm cefotaxime (Claforan) taken intravenously twice daily; or
3. 4 million U penicillin G taken intravenously every 4 hours.

All regimens should be administered for 21 to 28 days (75).

SUMMARY POINTS

- The two most common forms of facial paralysis are Bell's palsy and herpes zoster oticus (Ramsay Hunt syndrome).
- Bell's palsy is a demyelinating, virally induced immune response that is caused by HSV-1 reactivation in the ganglia of the head and neck.
- Bell's palsy and Ramsay Hunt syndrome can be diagnosed by medical history and by observing the patient's initial signs and symptoms. They are not diagnoses of exclusion.
- Selection of patients, timing of surgery, and extent of surgical decompression may become moot issues because surgery cannot benefit a viral disease.
- To establish prognosis in cases of facial paralysis, findings from all electrical testing may be correlated with the clinical and pathologic process causing the paralysis.
- Facial paralysis may occur in either acute or chronic otitis media; however, in acute otitis media, facial paralysis is a relatively unimportant sign, whereas in chronic otitis media it has serious practical bearing on diagnosis, prognosis, and treatment.
- Facial paralysis in chronic otitis media indicates that a pathologic process is eroding bone and that a defect exists in the fallopian canal. Unchecked erosion may permit spread of infection to the inner ear and to the cranial cavity.
- Another cause of facial nerve dysfunction is Lyme disease, a multisystem inflammatory illness caused by infection with the spirochete *B. burgdorferi*.

ADDENDUM

Since acceptance of this chapter for publication, an additional study has confirmed the beneficial effects of acyclovir and prednisone in the treatment of Bell's palsy. Early treatment started within 3 days was highly effective in preventing nerve degeneration (Hato N, Murakami S, Honda N, Aono H, Yanagihara N. Treatment of Bell's palsy with oral acyclovir and prednisolone. *Facial Nerve Res Jpn* 1998;18:145).

Sunderland's classification of nerve injuries is based on trauma perpendicular to a specific section of the nerve and is not applicable to viral demyelinating disease. Virally induced demyelinization causes multiple patches of damage in a horizontal pattern. Therefore, a new classification of nerve injury is needed to accurately describe the pathophysiology of viral demyelinization.

Questions arise concerning use of electrical physiotherapy treatment for delayed return of facial muscle function after any form of facial paralysis, even though Mosforth and Taverner concluded no significant advantage could be demonstrated from use of galvanic stimulation for Bell's palsy (Mosforth J, Taverner D. Physiotherapy for Bell's palsy. *Br Med J* 1958;2:675–677). Further, animal research by Hisashe Aono, et al. demonstrated that electrical stimulation given to paralyzed muscles suppresses nerve regeneration (Aono H, Murakami S, Honda N, Hato N, Yanagihara N. Therapeutic effects of electrical stimulation of the reinnervated orbicularis oculi muscle in guinea pigs: a preliminary report. *Facial Nerve Res Jpn* 1997;17:39).

ACKNOWLEDGMENT

The Medical Editing Department, Kaiser Foundation Research Institute, provided editorial assistance.

REFERENCES

1. Adour KK, Byl FM, Hilsinger RL Jr, Kahn ZM, Sheldon MI. The true nature of Bell's palsy: analysis of 1,000 consecutive patients. *Laryngoscope* 1978;88:787–801.
2. Robillard RB, Hilsinger RL Jr, Adour KK. Ramsay Hunt facial paralysis: clinical analyses of 185 patients. *Otolaryngol Head Neck Surg* 1986;95:292–297.
3. Adour KK. Otological complications of herpes zoster. *Ann Neurol* 1994;35:S62–S64.
4. Hunt JR. On herpetic inflammations of the geniculate ganglion: a new syndrome and its complications. *J Nerv Ment Dis* 1907;34:73–96.
5. Antoni N. Herpes zoster med Forlamning. *Hygiea* 1919;81:340–353. (Cited by Moller F. Critical viewpoints on the pathogenesis in Bell's palsy. *Acta Neurol Scand* 1967;43:228–238.)
6. Dalton GA. Bell's palsy: some problems of prognosis and treatment. *Br Med J* 1960;1:1765–1770.
7. Adour KK, Bell DN, Hilsinger RL Jr. Herpes simplex virus in idiopathic facial paralysis (Bell palsy). *JAMA* 1975;233:527–530.
8. McCormick DP. Herpes-simplex virus as cause of Bell's palsy. *Lancet* 1972;1:937–939.
9. Murakami S, Mizobuchi M, Nakashiro Y, Doi T, Hato N, Yanagihara N. Bell palsy and herpes simplex virus: identification of viral DNA in endoneurial fluid and muscle. *Ann Intern Med* 1996;124:27–30.
10. Baringer JR. Herpes simplex virus and Bell palsy [Editorial]. *Ann Intern Med* 1996;124:63–65.
11. Wayman DM, Pham HN, Byl FM, Adour KK. Audiological manifestations of Ramsay Hunt syndrome. *J Laryngol Otol* 1990;104:104–108.
12. Adour KK, Hetzler DG. Current medical treatment for facial palsy. *Am J Otol* 1984;5:499–502.
13. Kerbavaz RJ, Hilsinger RL Jr, Adour KK. The facial paralysis prognostic index. *Otolaryngol Head Neck Surg* 1983;91:284–289.
14. Baringer JR, Swoveland P. Persistent herpes simplex virus infection in rabbit trigeminal ganglia. *Lab Invest* 1974;30:230–240.
15. Nahmias AJ, Roizman B. Infection with herpes-simplex viruses 1 and 2. *N Engl J Med* 1973;289:781–789.
16. Warren KG, Brown SM, Wroblewska Z, Gilden D, Koprowski H, Subak-Sharpe J. Isolation of latent herpes simplex virus from the superior cervical and vagus ganglions of human beings. *N Engl J Med* 1978; 298:1068–1069.
17. Adour KK, Hilsinger RL Jr, Byl FM. Herpes simplex polyganglionitis. *Otolaryngol Head Neck Surg* 1980;88:270–274.
18. Adour KK. Cranial polyneuritis and Bell palsy. *Arch Otolaryngol* 1976; 102:262–264.
19. Tzadik A, Babin RW, Ryu JH. Hypotension-induced neurapraxis in the cat facial nerve. *Otolaryngol Head Neck Surg* 1982;90:163–167.

20. Devriese PP. Experimental facial nerve decompression in the cat. *Arch Otolaryngol* 1972;95:350–355.
21. Hilsinger RL Jr, Adour KK, Doty HE. Idiopathic facial paralysis, pregnancy, and the menstrual cycle. *Ann Otol Rhinol Laryngol* 1975;84: 433–442.
22. Pitts DB, Adour KK, Hilsinger RL Jr. Recurrent Bell's palsy: analysis of 140 patients. *Laryngoscope* 1988;98:535–540.
23. Adour KK, Wingerd J, Doty HE. Prevalence of concurrent diabetes mellitus and idiopathic facial paralysis (Bell's palsy). *Diabetes* 1975; 24:449–451.
24. Safman BL. Bilateral pathology in Bell's palsy. *Arch Otolaryngol* 1971; 93:55–57.
25. Citron D III, Adour KK. Acoustic reflex and loudness discomfort in acute facial paralysis. *Arch Otolaryngol* 1978;104:303–306.
26. Kobayashi T, Kudo Y, Chow M-J. Nerve excitability test using fine needle electrodes. *Acta Otolaryngol Suppl (Stockh)* 1988;446:64–69.
27. Adour KK, Schneider GD, Hilsinger RL Jr. Acute superior laryngeal nerve palsy: analysis of 78 cases. *Otolaryngol Head Neck Surg* 1980; 88:418–424.
28. Adour KK. Facial nerve testing and evaluation. In: House JW, O'Connor AF, eds. *Handbook of neurotological diagnosis*. New York: Dekker, 1987:175–219.
29. Selmanowitz VJ. Neurocutaneous herpes simplex. *Int J Dermatol* 1971; 10:227–232.
30. Slavin HB, Ferguson JJ Jr. Zoster-like eruptions caused by the virus of herpes simplex. *Am J Med* 1950;8:456–467.
31. Shiotani M, Yuda Y, Wakasugi B. Comparison of prognosis in Bell's palsy, Ramsay Hunt syndrome and zoster sine herpete. *Facial Nerve Res Jpn* 1991;11:207–210.
32. Djupesland G, Berdal P, Johannessen TA, Degré M, Stien MI, Skrede S. Viral infection as a cause of acute peripheral facial palsy. *Arch Otolaryngol* 1976;102:403–406.
33. Adour KK, Wingerd J. Idiopathic facial paralysis (Bell's palsy): factors affecting severity and outcome in 446 patients. *Neurology* 1974;24: 1112–1116.
34. Hughes GB. Prognostic tests in acute facial palsy. *Am J Otol* 1989;10: 304–311.
35. Tonning FM. The reliability of level-diagnostic examinations in acute, peripheral facial palsy. *Acta Otolaryngol (Stockh)* 1977;84:414–415.
36. Adour KK, Hilsinger RL Jr, Callan EJ. Facial paralysis and Bell's palsy: a protocol for differential diagnosis. *Am J Otol* 1985;6[Suppl]:68–73.
37. Adour KK. Medical management of Antoni's palsy (acute infectious polyneuritis cerebralis acusticofacialis). In: Shambaugh GE, Shea JJ, eds. *Proceedings of the Sixth Shambaugh International Workshop on Otomicrosurgery and Third Shea Fluctuant Hearing Loss Symposium, March 2–7, 1980, Chicago, Illinois*. Huntsville, AL: Strode, 1981: 64–172.
38. Byl FM, Adour KK. Auditory symptoms associated with herpes zoster or idiopathic facial paralysis. *Laryngoscope* 1977;87:372–379.
39. Blackley B, Friedman I, Wright I. Herpes zoster auris associated with facial nerve palsy and auditory nerve symptoms: a case report with histopathological findings. *Acta Otolaryngol (Stockh)* 1967;63: 533–550.
40. Harbert F, Young IM. Audiologic findings in Ramsay Hunt syndrome. *Arch Otolaryngol* 1967;85:632–639.
41. Hope-Simpson RE. The nature of herpes zoster: a long-term study and a new hypothesis. *Proc R Soc Med* 1965;58:9–20.
42. Tien R, Dillon WP, Jackler RK. Contrast-enhanced MR imaging of the facial nerve in 11 patients with Bell's palsy. *AJNR Am J Neuroradiol* 1990;11:735–741.
43. Jonsson L, Engström M, Thuomas K-Å, Stålberg E. Correlation between gadolinium-enhanced MRI and neurophysiology in Bell's palsy: a preliminary study. In: Proceedings of the VIIth International Symposium on the Facial Nerve, Cologne, June 9–14, 1992. *Eur Arch Otorhinolaryngol Suppl* 1994:S330–S331.
44. Matsumoto Y, Yanagihara N, Sadamoto M. Gd-DTPA-enhanced MR imaging in peripheral facial palsy. *Facial Nerve Res Jpn* 1991;11: 93–95.
45. Ushiro K, Yanagida M, Iwano T, Hosoda Y. Gd-DTPA enhanced MRI in patients with Ramsay Hunt syndrome. *Facial Nerve Res Jpn* 1991; 11:133–138.
46. May M, Harvey JE, Marovitz WF, Stroud M. The prognostic accuracy of the maximum stimulation test compared with that of the nerve excitability test in Bell's palsy. *Laryngoscope* 1971;81:931–938.
47. May M, Blumenthal F, Klein SR. Acute Bell's palsy: prognostic value of evoked electromyography, maximal stimulation, and other electrical tests. *Am J Otol* 1983;5:1–7.
48. Ruboyianes JM, Adour KK, Santos DQ, Von Doersten PG. The maximal stimulation and facial nerve conduction latency tests: predicting the outcome of Bell's palsy. *Laryngoscope* 1994;104[Suppl 61]:1–6.
49. Adour KK. Who's afraid of the facial nerve? In: Lucente FE, ed. *American Academy of Otolaryngology—Head and Neck Surgery. Highlights of the instructional courses, volume 8*. St. Louis: Mosby–Year Book, 1995:249–264.
50. Lewis BI, Adour KK, Kahn JM, Lewis AJ. Hilger facial nerve stimulator: a 25-year update. *Laryngoscope* 1991;101:71–74.
51. Gavilan J, Gavilan C, Sarria MJ. Facial electroneurography: results on normal humans. *J Laryngol Otol* 1983;5:1–7.
52. Raslan WF, Wiet R, Zealear DL. A statistical study of ENoG test error. *Laryngoscope* 1988;98:891–893.
53. Smith IM, Murray JAM, Prescott RJ, Barr-Hamilton R. Facial electroneurography: standardization of electrode position. *Arch Otolaryngol Head Neck Surg* 1988;114:322–325.
54. Hughes GB, Nodar RH, Williams GW. Analysis of test-retest variability in facial electroneurography. *Otolaryngol Head Neck Surg* 1983;91: 290–293.
55. Fisch U. Maximal nerve excitability testing vs. electroneurography. *Arch Otolaryngol* 1980;106:352–357.
56. Kartush JM, Lilly DJ, Kemink JL. Facial electroneurography: clinical and experimental investigations. *Otolaryngol Head Neck Surg* 1985;93: 516–523.
57. Adour KK, Ruboyianes JM, Von Doersten PG, et al. Bell's palsy treatment with acyclovir and prednisone compared with prednisone alone: a double-blind, randomized, controlled trial. *Ann Otol Rhinol Laryngol* 1996;105:371–378.
58. Adour KK. Idiopathic facial paralysis. In: Gates GA, ed. *Current therapy in otolaryngology—head and neck surgery*, 6th ed. St. Louis: Mosby–Year Book, 1998:96–98.
59. Jongkees LBW. Bell's palsy: a surgical emergency? *Arch Otolaryngol* 1965;81:497–501.
60. Jongkees LBW. The timing of surgery in intratemporal facial paralysis. *Laryngoscope* 1969;79:1557–1561.
61. Olsen PZ. Prediction of recovery in Bell's palsy. *Acta Neurol Scand Suppl* 1975;61:1–121.
62. Thomander L, Stålberg E. Electroneurography in the prognostication of Bell's palsy. *Acta Otolaryngol (Stockh)* 1981;92:221–237.
63. Coker NJ, Fordice JO, Moore S. Correlation of the nerve excitability test and electroneurography in acute facial paralysis. *Am J Otol* 1992; 13:127–133.
64. Richardson AT, Wynn Parry CB. The theory and practice of electrodiagnosis. *Ann Phys Med* 1957;4:3–16.
65. Taverner D. Electrodiagnosis in facial palsy. *Arch Otolaryngol* 1965; 81:470–477.
66. Denny-Brown D, Brenner C. Paralysis of nerve induced by direct pressure and by tourniquet. *Arch Neurol Psychiatry* 1944;51:1–26.
67. Taverner D. Bell's palsy: a clinical and electromyographic study. *Brain* 1955;78:209–228.
68. Denny-Brown D, Brenner C. Lesion in peripheral nerves resulting from compression by spring clip. *Arch Neurol Psychiatry* 1944;52: 1–19.
69. Gilliat RW, Taylor JC. Electrical changes following section of the facial nerve. *Proc R Soc Med* 1959;52:1080–1083.
70. Seddon HJ. Three types of nerve injury. *Brain* 1943;66:237–288.
71. Sunderland S. *Nerves and nerve injuries*, 2nd ed. Edinburgh: Churchill Livingstone, 1978.
72. Ellefsen B, Bonding P. Facial palsy in acute otitis media. *Clin Otolaryngol* 1996;21:393–395.
73. Diamond C, Frew I. *The facial nerve*. Oxford: Oxford University Press, 1979:80–81.
74. Frank E. Lyme disease and ehrlichiosis. In: Rakel RE, ed. *Conn's current therapy*. Philadelphia: WB Saunders, 1996:136–138.
75. Steere AC. Lyme disease. *N Engl J Med* 1989;321:586–596.
76. Smouha EE, Coyle PK, Shukri S. Facial nerve palsy in Lyme disease: evaluation of clinical diagnostic criteria. *Am J Otol* 1997;18:257–261.
77. Halperin JJ, Golightly M. Lyme borreliosis in Bell's palsy. Long Island Neuroborreliosis Collaborative Study Group. *Neurology* 1992;42: 1268–1270.
78. Christen HJ, Hanefeld F, Eiffert H, Thomssen R. Epidemiology and

clinical manifestations of Lyme borreliosis in childhood: a prospective multicentre study with special regard to neuroborreliosis. *Acta Paediatr Suppl* 1993;386:1–75.

79. Ikeda M, Kawabata M, Kuga M, Nakazato H. Anti-Borrelia burgdorferi antibodies in patients with facial paralysis. *Eur Arch Otorhinolaryngol* 1993;249:488–491.

80. Jain VK, Hilton E, Maytal J, Dorante G, Ilowite NT, Sood SK. Immunoglobulin M immunoblot for diagnosis of Borrelia burgdorferi infection in patients with acute facial palsy. *J Clin Microbiol* 1996;34:2033–2035.

81. Mouritsen CL, Wittwer CT, Litwin CM, et al. Polymerase chain reaction detection of Lyme disease: correlation with clinical manifestations and serologic responses. *Am J Clin Pathol* 1996;105:647–654.

The Ear: Comprehensive Otology,
edited by R. F. Canalis and P. R. Lambert.
Lippincott Williams & Wilkins, Philadelphia © 2000.

CHAPTER 46

Traumatic and Neoplastic Disorders of the Facial Nerve

Jennifer L. Maw and Jack M. Kartush

Managing a patient with traumatic or neoplastic facial paralysis is a challenging endeavor. For traumatic etiologies, determining the need for surgical intervention is hindered by current limitations in accurately assessing the site and severity of nerve injury. For tumors with little facial weakness, the decision to sacrifice the facial nerve is an extremely difficult one for both the patient and surgeon. This chapter reviews traumatic and neoplastic disorders of the facial nerve, with an analysis of current diagnostic and treatment options.

TRAUMATIC DISORDERS OF THE FACIAL NERVE

The facial nerve may sustain penetrating or blunt injuries due to temporal bone trauma or iatrogenic injury. There is extensive dispute in the literature concerning the role of surgery in the management of traumatic facial nerve paralysis. Strong viewpoints are backed only by uncontrolled retrospective reviews. The lack of evidenced-based treatment, be it aggressive or conservative, is striking. Among the proponents of surgical treatment, there is controversy with regard to timing, approach, and technique of facial nerve decompression and repair. This section focuses on facial nerve trauma classified by mechanism and site of injury, reviews pertinent literature,

and rationalizes our approach to traumatic facial nerve paralysis.

Penetrating Trauma

Extracranial Nerve Injury

Penetrating trauma to the extracranial facial nerve and its branches may be caused by facial and neck stab wounds or lacerations, mandibular fractures, gunshot wounds, and a variety of surgical procedures. Crush injuries may occur following maxillofacial, gunshot, or iatrogenic trauma from instruments or ligatures and may coincide with area(s) of transection.

Transections of the main trunk and the temporozygomatic and the cervicofacial primary branches should be repaired, although assessing the exact site and severity of injury without surgical exploration can be difficult or impossible. Injuries of branches distal to the lateral canthus and nasolabial crease are too small for reanastomosis and do not require repair. Extensive arborization of the buccal and zygomatic branches results in minimal disfigurement and excellent recovery of local weakness. Repair of these branches therefore is unnecessary, as is repair of the platysmal branch.

Primary repair should be performed at the time of wound closure but may be precluded if the patient's general medical condition is unstable or if there is gross wound contamination, inadequate equipment, or insuffi-

J. L. Maw and J.M. Kartush: Michigan Ear Institute, Farmington Hills, Michigan 43334

cient surgical experience. In these situations, the nerve endings should be identified and tagged and the wound closed. Tagging is important as identifying the ends of the nerve during the repair procedure can be difficult even in the early posttraumatic period. When gross contamination is present, the wound should be debrided, irrigated with antibiotic solution, and closed. If severe contamination is present, wound closure should be delayed and intravenous antibiotics given. To optimize results, facial nerve repair is performed in a clean, well-vascularized bed.

The optimal timing for facial nerve repair following transection has been debated for decades. Previous historical papers demonstrated maximal proteosynthetic ability of the nerve cell body at 21 days (1). Repair during this period was hypothesized to allow regrowth of the nerve cells across the anastomosis site while minimizing the amount of fibrosis. More modern approaches favor the earliest possible repair (2); however, other factors such as age, blood supply, and surgical technique probably impact outcome more significantly than the timing of repair. May (3) demonstrated superior results when facial nerve grafting is performed within 30 days. If the ends of the transected nerve were not identified and tagged, then repair should preferably be undertaken within 3 days, as this is the time period during which the distal nerve can still be stimulated electrically.

Primary end-to-end anastomosis should be performed whenever possible, but tension across the anastomosis site must be avoided. The proximal stump may be lengthened by mastoidectomy and rerouting of the vertical segment, and the distal stump by parotidectomy. An interposition graft should be used if tension will exist. The greater auricular nerve is the graft of choice for defects less than 10 cm and the sural nerve for larger ones. In selective branch injury, a less important branch can be sacrificed and used to repair the more important temporal or ramus mandibularis branch.

Intratemporal Nerve Injury

Gunshot Wounds

The majority of penetrating trauma causing intratemporal facial nerve injuries are caused by gunshot wounds. Temporal bone involvement occurs in approximately 20% of gunshot wounds to the head. Approximately one third of patients will have associated central nervous system or vascular injury (4).

The ipsilateral infraorbital region is the most common entrance site and occurs three times more commonly than other trajectory paths (5). The bullet, its fragments, or secondary fracture (usually mixed or comminuted) of the temporal bone all may cause facial nerve injury. Extensive nerve injury and multiple sites of injury are the rule, and combined intratemporal and extracranial injury may

occur. Immediate, total facial nerve paralysis usually results.

The first steps of management are within the domain of the trauma specialist: airway, breathing, circulation, assessment of neurologic deficits and cervical spine injuries, and management of increased intracranial pressure are the priorities. Computed tomographic (CT) scan of the head is performed to assess the intracranial injury, ballistic pathway, and location of bullet fragments. Carotid angiography with venous phase should be considered even in the absence of clinical or CT evidence of vascular injury, as occult injury is common (4).

After stabilization and care of critical neurologic and vascular injuries, further radiologic assessment of the temporal bone can be performed using bone windows in 1-mm cuts in the axial and coronal planes. The external canal, middle ear, mastoid, and inner ear frequently are injured in combination. Audiometric evaluation is performed.

Patients with immediate paralysis or those with delayed palsy who progress to complete paralysis with evidence of degeneration on electrophysiologic testing are candidates for facial nerve exploration once the patient is medically and neurologically stable. When serviceable hearing is present, a middle fossa craniotomy is combined with transmastoid exploration for injuries involving the perigeniculate area and proximal. Concomitant canaloplasty, tympanoplasty, and ossicular repair can be performed when indicated. When serviceable hearing is absent, the labyrinthine and geniculate areas of the facial nerve are exposed by a translabyrinthine approach. Impacted skin elements should be debrided from the middle ear and mastoid, and a dehiscent posterior bony canal should be repaired or taken down. Persistent cerebrospinal fluid (CSF) leaks that have not stopped at the time of exploration should be repaired.

Blunt Trauma

Extracranial Injury

Facial nerve paresis or paralysis has been described following an impact or compression injury to the preauricular face or stylomastoid foramen (6). Prognosis in the few case reports of this injury has generally been good without surgical intervention.

Intracranial Injury

Facial nerve paralysis occurs in 10% to 25% of temporal bone injuries, and its treatment is the most controversial among facial nerve injuries. Management remains variable from center to center, and evidence-based treatment is sparse. Reported series suffer from lack of follow-up due to poor compliance in this population of patients and, until recently, inconsistent reporting of facial function. Although all facial nerve grading scales are subjective and have inherent weaknesses, the House-Brackmann facial nerve grading scale (Table 1) (7) is an easy to use and well-accepted scale, although it is poorly discriminating with only six categories (see Chapter 44).

Classification of Fractures

Temporal bone fractures can be classified into longitudinal and transverse types according to the plane of their fracture lines. Seventy to eighty percent of fractures are longitudinal and cause facial nerve injury in 10% to 20% of cases. The paresis or paralysis often is delayed, and the majority of longitudinal fractures injure the perigeniculate segment of the facial nerve with occasional injury at the second genu. Mechanisms of injury include impingement of bony spicules, edema, intraneural hematoma, and disruption (4,5,8,9). Transverse fractures comprise 10% to 30% and cause facial weakness in 40% to 50%, which is frequently immediate. The most frequent mechanisms of injury have been said to include avulsion or laceration (5); however, bony compression and edema of the labyrinthine segment also has been reported (9). Trans-verse fractures most commonly are associated with injury at the geniculate and tympanic areas.

This classification system is somewhat artificial, and high-resolution CT scanning will demonstrate a mixed fracture in 10% of injuries. The clinical separation of these fractures into longitudinal and transverse types based on the absence or presence of sensorineural hearing loss (SNHL) and vertigo probably is more useful. The identification on CT scan of severe comminution, displacement of fragments, and evidence of fracture lines passing through the facial canal is of much more clinical significance than attempting to classify the fracture type.

Clinical Assessment

A careful history of the trauma, site of blow to the head, loss of consciousness, and onset of facial paralysis is obtained. Associated symptoms of hearing loss, tinnitus, vertigo, and disequilibrium are documented. The inquiry should include questions relevant to the status of the eye, function of the other cranial nerves, as well as symptoms of CSF leakage. On physical examination, the grade of facial function should be documented. Raccoon eyes or Battle's sign (postauricular ecchymosis) may be present as

TABLE 1. *House-Brackmann facial nerve grading system*

Grade	Characteristics
I. Normal	Normal facial function in all areas
II. Mild dysfunction	Gross 　Slight weakness noticeable on close inspection. 　May have very slight synkinesis. 　At rest, normal symmetry and tone. Motion 　Forehead: moderate-to-good function 　Eye: complete closure with minimal effort 　Mouth: slight asymmetry
III. Moderate dysfunction	Gross 　Obvious, but not disfiguring difference between the two sides. 　Noticeable but not severe synkinesis, contracture, or hemifacial spasm. 　At rest, normal symmetry and tone. Motion 　Forehead: slight-to-moderate movement 　Eye: complete closure with effort 　Mouth: slightly weak with maximum effort
IV. Moderately severe dysfunction	Gross 　Obvious weakness and/or disfiguring asymmetry. 　At rest, normal symmetry and tone. Motion 　Forehead: none 　Eye: incomplete closure 　Mouth: asymmetric with maximum effort
V. Severe dysfunction	Gross 　Only barely perceptible motion. 　At rest, asymmetry. Motion 　Forehead: none 　Eye: incomplete closure 　Mouth: slight movement
VI. Total paralysis	No movement

evidence of basal skull fracture. Longitudinal fractures may demonstrate a lacerated posterior superior canal wall or drum with or without leakage of CSF. Results of tuning fork tests typically are consistent with a conductive hearing loss. The ear canal usually is normal in transverse fractures, but hemotympanum is common. A hearing loss, primarily SNHL, usually is present. The examination may demonstrate spontaneous nystagmus and other evidence of labyrinthine dysfunction on neurotologic exam.

There have been reports of finding complete facial nerve transection in patients who were stated to have delayed or partial facial weakness (3). This is secondary to an incomplete or erroneous assessment of facial movement. Incomplete assessment sometimes is unavoidable, because the patient is comatose or uncooperative after head injury. A grimace in response to painful stimulation occasionally can be the only assessment possible. Erroneous assessment may occur for various reasons. In a young patient, facial symmetry may be markedly preserved despite the presence of total facial paralysis because of excellent muscle tone. If active facial contraction is not examined for, the extent of the injury may be underestimated and patients with immediate paralysis may be erroneously classified as delayed. Error also may be made in the assessment of eye closure. Passive closure of the eye occurs via relaxation of the levator palpebra muscle innervated by the third cranial nerve. It is active contraction of the orbicularis oculi muscles that must be assessed. In some patients, near-complete eye closure may still be present in the upright position despite total facial paralysis and may mislead an inexperienced examiner into believing some function is intact. Conversely, complete facial paralysis may be overcalled if the minute contractions of the face with grade V paralysis are not sought or noted. The necessity for assessment of active facial movement and documentation of such in the immediate posttrauma period is important.

Investigations

Many patients with temporal bone fractures have suffered multiple trauma. The workup for facial paralysis should be deferred until the patients are medically and neurologically stable. Investigations should include audiometry and high-resolution CT scanning with bone windows in the axial and coronal planes. Electronystagmography is considered when inner ear symptoms are present. The value of topognostic testing is controversial and rarely is used at our institution. More than 80% of fractures involve the geniculate ganglion, as it is the transition site between pneumatized and compact bone (10). It is therefore almost always included in surgical exploration at our institution regardless of lacrimation status (Schirmer's test).

Because the distal segment of a transected nerve will still conduct an electrical stimulus for 2 to 3 days after the injury, electrical testing is not performed until 72 hours after the onset of complete paralysis to allow for wallerian degeneration. During the first week, testing is repeated on several occasions. Although they have limitations, electrodiagnostics are the best clinical tools available for distinguishing neurapraxia (conduction block) from more severe forms of nerve injury (axon loss).

Management

Management of facial paralysis from closed head injuries previously depended on the timing of paralysis. Exploration was reserved for those who demonstrated paralysis immediately after head trauma, whereas delayed paralysis was treated with expectant observation. Several studies have argued against surgery in delayed-onset paralysis. The largest of these reported a 94% complete recovery rate in 34 cases of delayed paralysis (11). Other studies demonstrated complete recovery rates of 76% (12) to 84% (13), the latter stating that surgery is "rarely, if ever, warranted, since the natural recovery is very good." The prognosis for recovery is very good. Most patients with delayed facial paralysis do not require surgery; however, a small percentage will. Therefore, all patients with paralysis, immediate or delayed, are followed clinically and electrically so that early treatment can be offered to those patients who fall in the poor prognostic group. Steroids are used if there are no contraindications. Patients with paresis have a very good prognosis for recovery and are treated with steroids and followed clinically. Electrical testing is begun only if there is progression to paralysis.

There are many who believe that all cases of immediate facial nerve paralysis after trauma should be explored, because the likelihood of transection or severe crush injury is high. Again, poor outcome is not universal, as some patients in this category recover completely. Although imperfect, electrophysiologic testing is the single best prognostic tool available today. A complete discussion of these tests is found in Chapter 44. Patients are considered for facial nerve exploration when a complete facial paralysis is present and electroneurography (ENoG) demonstrates 90% or more degeneration within 2 to 3 weeks of onset of paralysis.

Pathologic Considerations. The majority of injured nerves demonstrate impingement, contusion, stretching, intraneural hematoma, or partial crush injury rather than complete transection. The final common pathway of these mechanisms of injury is inflammation and edema. It is likely that compression of the nerve in the restricted bony confines of the canal and secondary ischemia cause an intact nerve to degenerate.

Goals of Exploration. The goals of exploration are (a) decompression to prevent prolonged ischemic injury and to allow the return of normal microvascular circulation, (b) removal of bony fragments impinging on the nerve and potentially interfering with reinnervation, and (c) reestablishment of the nerve's continuity when it has been partially or completely interrupted.

Timing of Exploration. Controversy exists as to the appropriate timing of exploration. An immediate "don't let the sun set" approach is not necessary; however, the extensive experience of May (3) demonstrated that when grafting is required, results are superior when performed within 30 days of injury. Most surgeons would agree that if surgery is indicated, it should be performed as soon as possible. In reality, medical and neurologic status and the time lapse before referral to a neurotologist usually dictate the timing of the surgical treatment. We counsel patients according to the amount of benefit that can be gained from decompression at the various time intervals during which the patients present.

Early presentation. Maximal benefit is likely achieved if decompression is performed within the first week of injury. One practical consideration and argument for decompression within the first week is that it is much easier at this stage to wash away blood around the nerve to properly visualize and assess its integrity. Congealed blood and the presence of granulation tissue make assessment difficult at a later date.

Delayed presentation. For patients presenting between 2 to 4 weeks after trauma, some benefit may still be gained from surgical exploration. Although the window of opportunity for release of pressure and ischemia is likely past, removal of an impinging bone spicule or relief of compression in a fracture line may still be beneficial within the first few weeks after injury. Careful review of the CT scan may demonstrate marked bony displacement and fragmentation near the nerve, which strongly suggest that benefit may be obtained.

Late presentation. Patients commonly present between 2 to 6 months after injury and are the most challenging to assess and advise. These patients are usually one of two types: patients with multiple trauma who were in a poor prognostic category for recovery but were too ill to undergo earlier surgical intervention, or patients who were thought to be in a good prognostic category but who have not shown signs of recovery after nonsurgical treatment. A patient whose paralysis is secondary to neurapraxia should show signs of improvement within 4 weeks. ENoG is not helpful in predicting prognosis at the late presentations, because it cannot reliably assess wallerian degeneration beyond 3 weeks after paralysis. Asynchronous depolarization, differing conduction velocities, poor summation of the action potentials, and poor muscular contraction are all factors limiting late ENoG testing (14). Some nerves that are recovering will demonstrate "100% degeneration" on ENoG. Decisions must be made based on history, physical examination, CT findings, and electromyographic results. Some believe that only those who demonstrated immediate paralysis should be candidates for late exploration. May (3) states that facial nerve disruption is more likely in patients with complete onset

facial paralysis, loss of consciousness, CSF otorrhea, and those in whom marked disruption of the temporal bone fragments is noted radiologically. The absence of voluntary motor units or denervation potentials is the electromyographic criterion for considering exploration in the later stages.

Arguments for late exploration include the need for removal of bony fragments and fibrosis that may impede the spontaneous regeneration of motor neurons across the injury site. As only minimum benefit likely can be obtained from surgical decompression at this stage, some adopt a conservative approach and observe the patient for another 3 to 4 months. If no return of facial function is noted 6 to 12 months after trauma and electromyographic testing shows no evidence of reinnervation potentials, exploration is indicated and a nerve graft most likely will be necessary (10). After 12 months, transpositional nerve grafting (e.g., hypoglossal to facial nerve) or reanimation procedures such as temporalis muscle transposition are recommended.

Surgical Approach. The majority of nerves are injured at the geniculate ganglion, although some have additional areas of injury, especially in the region of the second genu (15). A total nerve exploration/decompression usually is indicated. When serviceable hearing is present, a middle fossa craniotomy combined with transmastoid exploration is used (Fig. 1). Tympanoplasty and ossicular chain reconstruction can be performed at the same time. Transmastoid-extralabyrinthine techniques have been described (16,17); however, they do not provide sufficient exposure for decompression of the labyrinthine segment or grafting. When serviceable hearing is absent, a translabyrinthine approach is used (Fig. 2). Decompression usually is sufficient, although a severely crushed nerve is best resected and grafted or rerouted and primarily anastomosed.

Traumatic Facial Paralysis in the Neonate

The incidence of newborn facial paralysis reported in the literature has ranged from 0.05% to 0.23% (18,19). The majority of cases are presumed secondary to trauma; however, proof of traumatic etiology often is lacking, and a careful search for congenital and other causes of acquired facial paralysis must be undertaken.

As facial paralysis occurs with similar frequencies in normal vaginal deliveries, forceps deliveries, and cesarean sections, trauma from forceps likely is not the etiology. The superficial position of the facial nerve at the stylomastoid foramen and the softness of the temporal bone make it vulnerable to injury by other presumed mechanisms, including compression against the infant's shoulder or maternal sacral prominence in cephalopelvic disproportion. Fracture of the temporal bone is rare, as its softness makes it more likely to indent and compress the nerve rather than to fracture and lacerate it.

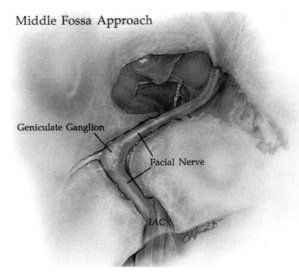

Facial Recess Approach

EAC

Chorda
Tympani N.

Facial Recess

Facial Nerve in Canal

A

Middle Fossa Approach

Geniculate Ganglion

Facial Nerve

IAC

B

FIG. 1. Total facial nerve decompression for patients with serviceable hearing is accomplished by combining the transmastoid-facial recess approach **(A)** with the middle fossa approach **(B)**. (From Huang MY, Lambert PR. Temporal bone trauma. In: Hughes G, Pensak ML, eds. *Clinical otology.* New York: Thieme Medical Publishers, 1997:262, with permission.)

Differentiating traumatic facial paralysis from other causes can be difficult. The history may reveal a long and/or difficult delivery or cephalopelvic disproportion leading to forceps delivery or cesarean section, but their absence does not exclude a traumatic cause. On physical examination, a traumatic process usually presents as a unilateral paralysis or palsy of all divisions of the facial nerve. Bruising of the face and/or skull, palpable indentation of the squama, and hemotympanum also may be present.

Möbius' syndrome is the most common of the congenital causes of facial paralysis; they are reviewed else-

where (18). Congenital causes of paralysis are associated with partial facial nerve deficits or the presence of other cranial nerve paralyses, dysmorphic features of the skull, face, or ear, and other abnormalities of the chest, limbs, and cardiovascular and genitourinary systems.

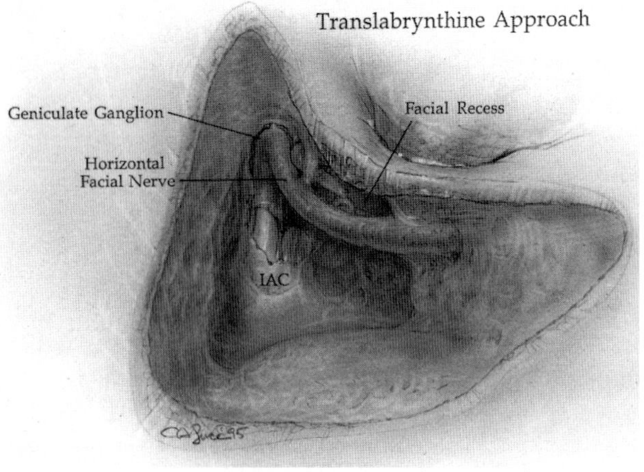

CT scan rarely may show bony injury or congenital anomalies. Auditory brainstem response testing can be used to document hearing. Topographic testing in neonates has been of limited use. Electrophysiologic testing can have both diagnostic and prognostic value. Developmental causes of facial paralysis usually are abnormal immediately at birth, whereas traumatic causes of facial paralysis initially are normal and become abnormal at 3 to 7 days of age as wallerian degeneration proceeds (18).

The prognosis of facial paralysis from birth trauma is excellent; more than 90% of infants recover spontaneously (20,21). Complete facial nerve transection from birth trauma has never been reported. For these reasons, a conservative approach nearly always is indicated. Facial palsy and delayed paralysis usually are treated with expectant observation. Only neonates with immediate, total facial paralysis need to be followed with electrical testing. Facial nerve exploration or reanimation procedures rarely will be necessary.

Translabrynthine Approach

Geniculate Ganglion

Facial Recess

Horizontal
Facial Nerve

IAC

FIG. 2. Translabyrinthine approach used for total facial nerve decompression in patients without serviceable hearing. (From Huang MY, Lambert PR. Temporal bone trauma. In: Hughes G, Pensak ML, eds. *Clinical otology.* New York: Thieme Medical Publishers, 1997:263, with permission.)

Iatrogenic Facial Nerve Injury

Iatrogenic facial nerve injury may be penetrating or blunt, and it may be expected (intentional or mandatory) or unexpected (accidental). Deliberate section of the facial nerve may be necessary during the removal of parotid and skull base malignancies, facial nerve tumors, and large acoustic neuromas. Modern surgical techniques and the advent of intraoperative facial nerve electromyographic monitoring have decreased the incidence of facial nerve injury during tumor resection (22–24). Routine intraoperative monitoring relies on the mechanically evoked responses that blunt manipulation and traction may create during tumor dissection; however, sharp dissection may evoke little or no response even with complete transection of the nerve. Stimulating dissection instruments are a set of insulated instruments that have been designed to circumvent this problem (Fig. 3). They allow simultaneous monopolar mapping with sharp dissection and alert the surgeon to the proximity of the nerve before a cutting maneuver is performed (25).

Accidental surgical injury to the facial nerve is a recognized complication of facial plastic, head, neck, and otologic surgery. The frequency of facial nerve injury has been reported to be between 0.6% and 3.6% of all otologic cases and is the second most common reason for malpractice lawsuits in otology (26). Intraoperative facial nerve monitoring is gaining acceptance as a means to decrease this risk in nontumor surgery. Monitoring technology must be well understood by the surgeon to be effective. Its use is not a substitute for experience and knowledge of temporal bone anatomy.

Most otologic facial nerve injuries occur when the anatomy has been distorted by congenital malformations, cholesteatoma, infection, previous surgery, or trauma. However, even the most routine case is never free of risk. Bony dehiscence of the tympanic facial canal can be visualized or palpated in 5% to 30% of cases (27), but the inferior surface may be dehiscent in 40% to 50% (28). Variations in the course of the facial nerve may occur without other heralding congenital anomalies; however, one should be alert for subtle anomalies of the auricle.

Prevention of Injury

The prevention of facial nerve injury begins with otologic training and temporal bone dissection to cultivate a solid understanding of temporal bone anatomy. It is also essential to understand when the facial nerve is at greatest risk during specific procedures.

Stapedectomy

The risk of injury is low during stapedectomy, but injury can occur from mechanical or thermal means. Heat from a laser, or mechanical or thermal injury from a bur may injure the nerve. If a markedly prolapsed facial nerve is discovered, the case can be terminated and referred to an experienced otologist.

Mastoid Surgery

The majority of injuries following mastoid surgery occur at the second genu and vertical segment and are caused by a cutting bur. Revision surgery for iatrogenic facial paralysis frequently reveals a small antrotomy and insufficient exposure of the tegmen because of fear of injury to the middle fossa dura. As a result, the "antrotomy" is made too inferiorly, and the genu is traumatized. Adequate soft tissue exposure and wide beveling of the cavity to optimize visibility are essential.

Labyrinthectomy

During labyrinthectomy, the nerve is at greatest risk while drilling near the amputated ends of the semicircular canals. The posterior canal courses medial to the genu of the facial nerve. Aggressive removal of this canal's ampullated end can traumatize the medial surface of the facial nerve. The tympanic portion is 0.5 mm from the lateral canal ampulla and is at highest risk in the right ear when the clockwise rotating bur may skip inferiorly (Fig. 4A). One technique to avoid injury is to reverse the drill and use a diamond bur when near the ampullae. The use of a "cup" technique also prevents the bur from skipping over the facial nerve. This involves drilling a cuplike depression in the subarcuate fossa and proceeding with the labyrinthectomy by gradual enlargement of the cup (Figs. 4B and 4C). Its rim then prevents skipping of the bur out of the cup. The ampullated ends of the superior and horizontal canals are deferred to the last step, as they are closest to the nerve.

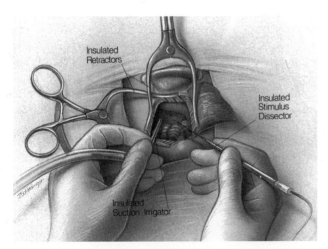

FIG. 3. Kartush stimulus dissectors are a set of insulated instruments that allow simultaneous monopolar mapping during sharp surgical dissection. (From Kartush JM, LaRouere MJ, Graham MD, et al. Intraoperative cranial nerve monitoring during posterior skull base surgery. *Skull Base Surg* 1991;1:85–92, with permission.)

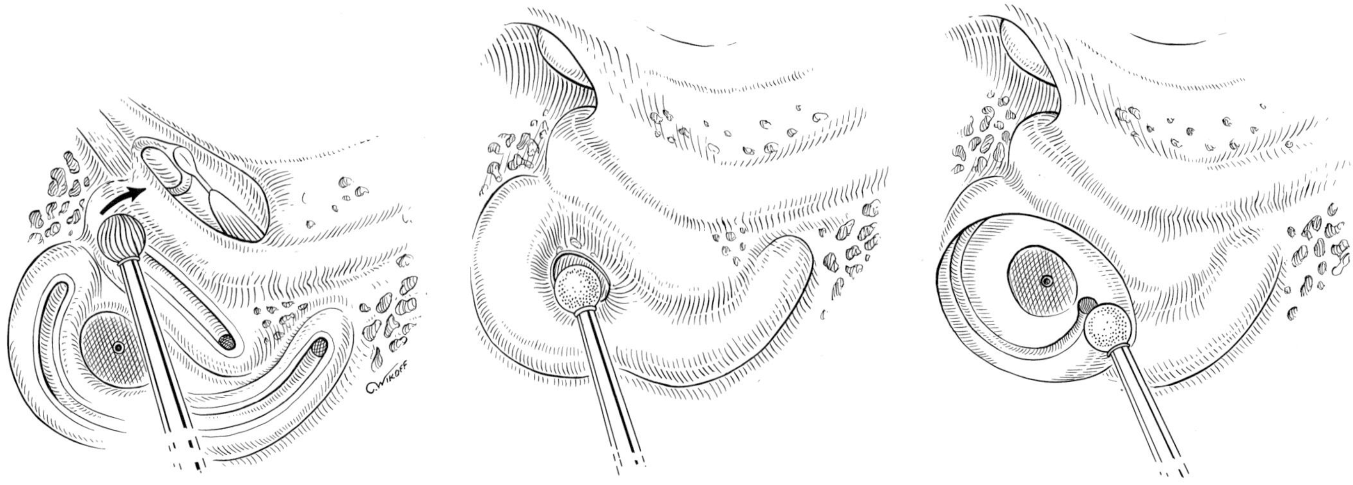

FIG. 4. A: Conventional labyrinthectomy. The incus has been removed and the facial recess opened. A cutting bur is used. The canals are fenestrated on their edges. In the right ear, the facial nerve is at risk while fenestrating the horizontal canal, as the bur is rotating clockwise and may skip onto the facial nerve. (Illustration by Christopher Wikoff.) **B:** "Cup" technique labyrinthectomy. The incus has not been removed and the facial recess remains closed. The labyrinthectomy is begun with the creation of a cup in the subarcuate fossa, which is gradually enlarged. A diamond bur is used. (Illustration by Christopher Wikoff.) **C:** The cup has been widened and deepened. The canals are fenestrated within the cup and the cup maintains the drill within it and prevents the bur from skipping onto the facial nerve. The ampullated ends of the superior and horizontal canals are deferred for the last step. (Illustration by Christopher Wikoff.)

Tumor Surgery

Facial nerve injury during neurotologic approaches can be reduced by intraoperative monitoring, stimulating dissection instruments, Brackmann fenestrated suction tips, and the use of lasers. During translabyrinthine and middle fossa resections of a tumor, prophylactic decompression of the facial nerve at the meatal foramen has been used at our institution, as this is the likely site of edematous entrapment of the facial nerve in delayed postoperative facial paralysis (29). At the completion of dissection of the tumor, the lowest level at which the nerve can be stimulated is documented. Nerves that have thresholds higher than 0.2 mA typically demonstrate some degree of facial weakness postoperatively (25). If considerable facial nerve stretching occurs during the case, steroids are administered and continued postoperatively if there is facial weakness. Acyclovir also has been used in an attempt to prevent activation of a dormant virus that has been hypothesized to be one cause of delayed postoperative paralysis (30).

When there is marked attenuation of the facial nerve by the tumor, preservation of facial nerve integrity may be impossible. In this situation, as for brainstem involvement, staged surgery has been used at our institution to allow decompression of the structures of the cerebellopontine angle (CPA). During the second procedure, the facial nerve commonly is observed to have regained mass and become less adherent to the tumor remnant. If a second stage is required, a piece of 0.04-inch-thick Silastic is implanted at the brainstem and along the cerebellum to maintain dissection planes and protect the underlying structures at reentry (Fig. 5) (31).

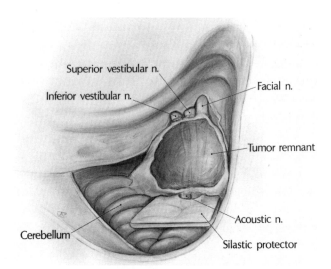

FIG. 5. Subtotal tumor resection via the translabyrinthine approach. Silastic is placed to improve safety at reentry in revision surgery. (From Kartush JM, Brackmann DE. Acoustic neuroma update. *Otolaryngol Clin North Am* 1996; 29:373–392, with permission.)

Management

Injury Recognized Intraoperatively

When facial nerve injury is suspected intraoperatively, the site of the possible injury should be explored and electrically stimulated to verify integrity of the nerve. Decompression of the immediate proximal and distal areas should be performed. In mild injuries such as tearing of the epineurium, decompression is adequate surgical treatment and facial function usually is not compromised. Steroids may be started if there are no significant contraindications. If nerve fibers are found to be herniating through an epineural tear, the epineural sheath should be opened more widely with an arachnoid knife to reduce the herniation. Prognosis is favorable.

The management of more severe injuries is controversial and challenging, as it is difficult to assess the severity of injury. If the nerve is found to be partially disrupted, the surgeon should discuss the complication with the patient's family and document the injury and discussion. If the surgeon is inadequately trained to proceed, then further treatment can be delayed and/or intraoperative consultation with an otologist sought.

Judgment must be used on whether to decompress the disrupted segment and realign the fibers or to proceed to segmental resection. If more than 50% of the circumference of the nerve has been disrupted, it should be repaired (9,32). The extent of the facial nerve injury usually is underestimated, and other authors have advocated repair if a 35% disruption is visualized (5). There are multiple methods of repair reported in the literature. An inlay nerve graft may be used to fill the site of the partially transected nerve. Alternatively, the entire segment of the nerve may be resected and a primary anastomosis or interposition graft repair performed, depending on the length of the defect. The reader is referred to the third section of this chapter for details of facial nerve repair.

Injury Recognized Postoperatively

When facial nerve dysfunction is recognized postoperatively, the ear packing should be loosened if a canal-wall-down procedure was performed. Facial function should be reassessed over a few hours to allow local anesthesia to wear off. If facial function does not recover with the passage of time, further investigation is indicated. Previous approaches to iatrogenic facial nerve injury were based on the dogma of "Never let the sun set on a facial nerve injury." In time, the dictum that all immediate paralyses required surgical exploration and all delayed paralyses required conservative treatment was adopted. Although the onset of paralysis is an important consideration in determining the need for reexploration, other critical factors include completeness of the palsy, the experience and assessment of the surgeon, and the results of radiographic and electrical testing.

Incomplete and delayed paralysis indicate that the nerve has not been completely transected, and both carry favorable prognoses. Steroids can be considered for a postoperative palsy, and facial function should be observed and documented regularly. If it progresses to complete paralysis, electrical testing is started on the second or third day of paralysis. Greater than 90% degeneration on ENoG within the first 3 weeks indicates a poor prognosis for rapid or complete restoration of facial function, and surgical exploration is considered.

Immediate postoperative facial paralysis carries a much worse prognosis. Although exploration within 24 hours has been proposed by some (26,28), other studies have not demonstrated a difference in facial outcome between patients explored early versus those delayed more than 7 days after injury (33). The experience and findings of the primary surgeon is of importance. If the injury occurred in the hands of an experienced surgeon who identified the nerve's course and believes it was not directly injured, then a more conservative approach may be taken. Steroids, antibiotics, corneal protection, and observation are indicated for the first 2 to 3 days. Electrophysiologic testing can be used as an adjunct in the decision to reexplore. Evidence of 90% nerve degeneration within the first week suggests severe injury and indicates the need for reexploration. Although degeneration will occur in most immediate, complete paralyses (19 of 22 cases in a modern series) (33), the delay of a few days may allow appropriate time for consultation among colleagues, education of patient and family, administration of steroids and antibiotics, and documentation of nerve function and hearing. A high-resolution CT scan may help to indicate the likely site of injury.

Some series have reported complete facial nerve transection in patients who were stated to have delayed or partial facial nerve function postoperatively. This emphasizes the necessity for proper assessment of active facial function in the immediate postoperative period. Furthermore, it demonstrates that history should be only one of a number of factors considered in determining the need for surgical exploration.

NEOPLASMS OF THE FACIAL NERVE

The facial nerve can be compressed or invaded by neoplasms along its course from the pons to the parotid gland. Involvement of the facial nerve by cholesteatoma, paraganglioma, and other temporal bone neoplasms are discussed in other chapters. This section will discuss primary tumors of the intratemporal facial nerve.

Facial nerve tumors cause approximately 5% of peripheral facial nerve palsies (4–7). Their rarity, the subtle progression of variable symptoms, and the shortcomings of radiologic tests often result in delayed or misdiagnosis for even the most experienced clinicians.

Pathology of Facial Nerve Neoplasms

Facial Neuromas

The various nomenclatures used in the past and present to describe this category of tumor are confusing. The terms neuroma, neurinoma, schwannoma, neurilemoma, and neurofibroma have been used interchangeably. "Neuroma" is not a pathologic entity; it simply refers to any benign swelling of a nerve. Within this category, facial schwannomas, neurofibromas, and perineuromas are benign neoplasms that arise from the nerve sheath. Traumatic neuromas are not neoplasms per se, but they fall within this category of benign swellings of the facial nerve.

Immunopathologic stains are now available to aid in defining these closely related tumors, but these stains are tedious and their distinction can remain uncertain. Many pathologists therefore refer to these as "benign nerve sheath tumors." The term "facial neuroma," although inexact, is still the favored name for facial schwannomas, as is "acoustic neuromas" for vestibular schwannomas.

Schwannomas

Facial schwannomas were first described by Schmidt (34) in 1930. The exact incidence of these tumors is unknown, as many are likely missed or misdiagnosed. One cadaver study found their incidence to be 0.8% (35); however, this is now believed to be an overestimation of the true incidence. Another study estimates the incidence to be 0.15% (36). Facial schwannomas may occur at any age and have been found to be more common in females. They may arise from any segment of the facial nerve, but purely intracranial schwannomas are rare. They may arise from the nerve's branches, and schwannomas of the greater superficial petrosal, stapedius, and chorda tympani nerves have been reported (37). They have been found to arise (in descending order) from the tympanic, vertical, geniculate and labyrinthine, meatal, and cerebellopontine segments (37). They frequently extend intracranially and thus can be difficult to diagnose preoperatively. Facial schwannomas are solitary encapsulated tumors that arise from the Schwann cell. They appear as gray or tan, lobulated, firm swellings. Their lobulated nature may mimic multicentricity. In tumors that appear truly multicentric, studies have demonstrated intraneural connections between the apparently discrete lesions (38,39). Microscopically, they are composed of areas of compact spindle cells (Antoni A areas) and those of loose, hypocellular zones (Antoni B areas). The relative proportions of these areas varies from tumor to tumor. Areas of nuclear palisading may be present and are called Verocay bodies. Axons, if present, are located at the periphery beneath the capsule.

Neurofibromas

Neurofibromas may be sporadic solitary lesions, or they may occur in neurofibromatosis type 1 or 2. The origin of these benign tumors is controversial; however, they currently are believed to arise from, and be principally composed of, Schwann cells (40). They are circumscribed but unencapsulated tumors. Neurofibromas have ill-defined borders and expand the nerve in a fusiform manner. Axons may be seen diffusely throughout the lesion. For this reason, they are clinically more difficult or impossible to dissect off the nerve and require transection for removal. They are composed of interlacing bundles of spindle cells separated by a myxomatous stroma, and they lack Antoni areas and Verocay bodies.

Traumatic Neuromas

Traumatic neuromas are nonneoplastic proliferations of traumatized nerves that develop secondary to a proliferative-reparative process. They occur most frequently from the proximal end of a severed nerve, but they can occur after a crush injury (41). They have been reported to occur from an exposed facial nerve after relatively minor trauma or secondary to contact with chronic inflammatory disease (42). They likely arise secondary to inadequate proximal axonal regenerative growth into distal endoneurial tubes. They are common after severe facial nerve injury, but they usually remain inconspicuous. Why some lesions continue to proliferate to extensive sizes remains unknown; however, a growth factor produced at the site of injury has been postulated as the causative agent (43). Radiographic signs include a progressively enlarging fallopian canal on successive scans after facial nerve trauma. They are white or gray, firm, and well-circumscribed lesions. Histologically they are unencapsulated and are composed of disrupted axons, proliferating Schwann cells, and endoneurial and perineurial fibroblastic cells. The axons are myelinated proximally but unmyelinated distally to the site of injury. The cells are surrounded by a dense collagenous matrix. They lack the organized features of the neoplasms discussed previously.

Vascular Tumors

There is controversy as to the origin and classification of vascular tumors of the head and neck, and no less so of those that arise from the facial nerve. Modern thinking is that they are vascular hamartomas rather than true neoplastic growths. Some believe they are congenital lesions that are manifested in adulthood. Hemangiomas of the facial nerve are now being reported more frequently than in the past, but this is likely secondary to improved imaging and diagnosis rather than a true increase in incidence.

Some authorities describe hemangiomas as being composed of thin-walled vascular spaces (which can be classified into capillary and cavernous types based on their lumen size) and describe vascular malformations as thick-walled vascular spaces lined by a single layer of endothelium surrounded by fibroblasts and collagen (38). Others describe cavernous hemangiomas as being composed of thin-walled sinusoidal spaces without any elastic membrane or intervascular neural tissue, and consider them a vascular malformation rather than a true neoplasm (44). Batsakis (45) classifies vascular tumors according to their stage of development. Tumors with characteristics of both hemangioma and vascular malformation have been described. An absolute histologic definition, it seems, cannot always be made. Osseous hemangiomas are a subset that grow among bone trabeculae and may form bone (46).

These vascular tumors are benign, nonencapsulated lesions that grow slowly and usually are less than 1 cm in diameter at diagnosis. They are thought to arise from the rich vascular plexus around the facial nerve and originate (in descending order of frequency) from the geniculate ganglion, internal auditory canal (IAC), and tympanic and mastoid segments of the facial nerve (47). Cavernous hemangiomas rarely arise in the IAC. As hemangiomas arise eccentrically from the nerve, sometimes they can be removed in the early stages with preservation of the facial nerve (47).

Other Tumors of the Facial Nerve

Other benign tumors of the facial nerve have been reported. They are rare and include perineuroma, angiofibroma, and paraganglioma. Malignant counterparts of these tumors are extremely rare. Neurogenic sarcomas are found in association with neurofibromas or as a separate neoplasm in 5% to 15% of patients with neurofibromatosis (45). Only three malignant schwannomas of the facial nerve have been recorded (48), all of which presented with facial pain.

Management of Facial Nerve Neoplasms

Diagnosis

The presenting symptoms of primary facial nerve tumors are extremely variable. Although disturbance in facial nerve function is the most common presenting complaint, a review of the world literature of intracranial and intratemporal facial neuromas demonstrated that some degree of facial weakness was reported in only 73% (37). Nearly one fourth of these patients therefore do not manifest facial weakness. Facial weakness usually is gradual, with paresis of a part of the face progressing (sometimes to full paralysis) over a variable period of time. In patients with paralysis, a sudden loss occurs in 16% (37). Patients who present with sudden paralysis may be diagnosed initially with Bell's palsy. One should be suspicious of any patient who does not show signs of recovery from Bell's palsy after 6 months. Fluctuation of paresis is common and although fluctuation from complete paralysis to full recovery is rare, it may occur. These patients may be labeled as having recurring episodes of Bell's palsy. The more common pattern is recurrent paralysis with incomplete recovery after attacks. It has been said that a patient with fluctuating facial nerve function should be considered to have a neoplasm unless proven otherwise. Facial spasm or fasciculation is reported to occur in 17% of patients with facial weakness and is highly suggestive of a tumor (37).

Facial nerve weakness is also the most common symptom of vascular tumors. However, in one series of seven cavernous hemangiomas of the IAC, only two patients had facial weakness (49). A common characteristic of vascular tumors is their ability to cause facial paresis out of proportion to that expected from other primary tumors of the same size. They may cause facial weakness by extrinsic nerve compression or by a vascular steal phenomenon, which is more plausible given that most are small lesions.

Hearing loss is the second most common symptom caused by primary tumors of the facial nerve, occurring in approximately half of patients. The loss may be conductive, cochlear, or retrocochlear, depending on the site of the lesion and its extent. If conductive hearing loss is the sole symptom, the lesion may be discovered during exploratory tympanotomy or found serendipitously during an intended stapedectomy. Biopsy, although tempting, should be resisted in most cases. as postoperative facial paralysis usually ensues. A dehiscent, prolapsed facial nerve may be mistaken for a facial nerve tumor. Tinnitus may occur secondary to the presence of a conductive loss or to cochlear or retrocochlear involvement. It may be pulsatile in the case of a vascular tumor. Vertigo and dizziness may occur and occasionally may be the presenting problem. Some of these tumors lie mainly in the CPA, simulating acoustic neuromas, and their true identification as facial schwannomas is made intraoperatively.

Other less common presentations include a visible mass behind the tympanic membrane or in the ear canal, otorrhea secondary to infection, and loss of taste. Pain is a rare symptom, usually associated with a secondary complication such as otitis media or externa or direct intracranial extension. Extracranial neuromas may present as palpable masses within the parotid gland. Finally, facial nerve tumors may remain totally asymptomatic and be found at autopsy (35). Facial neoplasms occasionally may remain clinically silent for extended periods of time and be very large lesions when finally diagnosed.

Patients should undergo a complete neurotologic history and examination with documentation of facial and auditory function. Video or photographic documentation is valuable. Auditory brainstem response testing may suggest retrocochlear pathology when it is not previously suspected. The usefulness of electrical testing of the facial nerve has been questioned. When tumor growth causes paralysis of slow onset, both degeneration and regeneration may be present and invalidate electrical testing (25,50,51). These tests are most useful when paralysis is sudden. Electronystagmography should be performed when symptoms suggest vestibular involvement. Topognostic tests are rarely useful tests of site of lesion, as the presence of the tumor may not completely interrupt electrical transmission along the facial nerve (52).

Radiographic assessment is the most definitive of the diagnostic tools. Complete assessment may require both high-resolution CT scan and gadolinium-enhanced magnetic resonance imaging (MRI) of the temporal bone and CPA. Signs of facial nerve tumor on CT scan include widening of the fallopian canal or IAC, bone destruction, soft tissue mass, or erosion of the ossicular chain. Labyrinthine fistulas may be detected, but these usually are occult. CT scan findings of vascular tumors may include irregular or indistinct bone margins, honeycomb bone, and intratumoral bone spicules (47). In general, CT lacks the soft tissue definition to accurately assess the smallest of neurogenic tumors (53). The diagnosis of facial nerve neoplasms has been greatly aided by advancements in gadolinium-enhanced MRI scanning. It is now considered to be the most sensitive diagnostic tool in the search for a facial nerve tumor, localizing the site of lesion and assessing extension (53). Facial schwannomas enhance brightly after administration of gadolinium. On MRI, vascular tumors demonstrate increased signal intensity on both T1- and T2-weighted sequences, which distinguishes them from schwannomas (49). It should be remembered, however, that MRI is relatively nonspecific, demonstrating facial nerve enhancement in Bell's palsy, trauma, and meatal arachnoiditis (53). It may give a false appearance of a facial nerve lesion or overestimate its extent. Although preoperative evaluation has improved greatly, perfect accuracy still is not possible.

Angiographic assessment of hemangiomas and vascular malformations are disappointing, as tumor blush is not seen. Angiography is only useful in differentiating these from other vascular tumors such as the paragangliomas.

The need for careful assessment of every patient with Bell's palsy cannot be overemphasized. A high index of suspicion of neoplasm is required in patients without signs of recovery by 6 months and those with recurring facial weakness. Despite vast improvements in diagnosis, the most extensive of searches for a tumor may be unfruitful in the case of small neoplasms. A high index of suspicion must sometimes be the sole basis for recommending a total facial nerve exploration (54).

Treatment

Surgical Timing and Procedure

It has been said that the ideal goals of treatment of facial nerve neoplasms are complete removal of the tumor, preservation or restoration of facial function, and conservation of hearing (50). Only rarely can these ideal goals be fully realized. In young patients with poor or absent facial movement (grades IV through VI), there is little difficulty in advising complete resection of tumor as early as possible. Controversy arises in deciding the appropriate surgical timing when there is mild or no facial weakness.

The potential for facial nerve preservation is higher for vascular tumors than for neuromas. The eccentric origin of the vascular tumors from the facial nerve often allows for development of a tissue plane and facial nerve conservation without compromising the oncologic resection. Increased weakness often occurs postoperatively secondary to stretch or manipulation, but it is usually temporary and improvement beyond preoperative status is possible (47). Early resection of vascular tumors offers the best chance for good facial recovery, because, with time, a perineural reaction to the tumor may occur and preclude complete removal without facial nerve disruption. When perineural reaction is present, resection with facial nerve sacrifice even in the presence of normal preoperative facial function has been recommended in the past (46).

There have been a few reports of neuroma removal with preservation of the continuity of the facial nerve (39,55–58), but this is rarely feasible with schwannomas and impossible for neurofibromas. In general, total removal of the neurogenic facial tumors requires sacrifice of the nerve.

Some authors have advocated aggressive, early removal of facial neuromas with transection of the facial nerve even in the presence of normal or near-normal facial function (50,53,59,60). Others have advocated the need for surgery at the earliest sign of facial weakness (61). The possibility of delaying surgery in patients with normal facial nerve function has been proposed (51), and decompression of facial schwannomas has been recommended for older patients with good nerve function (60). Partial resection also has been advocated (55).

The main argument for an aggressive approach is that the ultimate facial nerve function will be poorer if the nerve is allowed to degenerate prior to sacrifice and grafting (3). Tumor growth can cause progressive degeneration and regeneration of facial nerve fibers that lead to collagenization of the distal portion of the nerve. A sixth category of Sunderland's classification of degeneration has been proposed for schwannomas (62). The hypothesis that early resection in the presence of mild or absent facial weakness will lead to improved ultimate function is reasonable but has never been tested in a prospective manner. The majority of studies proposing early resection are based on retrospective analyses that showed the poorest outcome occurred in patients with prolonged paralysis. The extrapolation that all neuromas should be removed as soon as possible has not been validated.

Many primary tumors of the facial nerve are indolent, slow-growing lesions (63). Cases have been reported where patients maintained good facial function for years following the onset of paresis (64,65); one patient maintained a "20 percent" left facial weakness for 25 years (66). The best expected outcome after resection and grafting is grade III, and synkinesis is always present. It has been our experience that young patients prefer to maintain excellent to good facial function as long as is safely feasible. Grade III dysfunction has been considered by one author to be a prerequisite for excision of neuroma (37). We agree that the results of grafting will likely be poor if total paralysis has been allowed to develop, but we believe that allowing degeneration to grade II or III function does not significantly impact the ultimate result.

A second argument for early resection is prevention of intracranial extension. Older studies focused on the uncertainty of judging tumor extension on the polytomograms or CT images of their times. Modern-day imaging techniques are more reliable and often can identify cases in which intracranial extension is imminent.

A final argument for early aggressive resection is prevention of hearing loss. Early tumor extirpation may prevent destruction of the ossicular chain, posterior canal wall, and labyrinthine fistulization. The exact incidence of fistula formation is unknown, but it has been reported (66). Erosion of the otic capsule occurred in 29% in one series (59), but the average length of facial paralysis was 4 years.

Our experience with young patients has been that they often value continued excellent or good facial function over the possibility of hearing loss and that this preference should be respected as long as contralateral hearing is normal. We believe that with close clinical and radiographic follow-up, patients with small extracranial tumors and some with small intracranial tumors and normal facial nerve function can be treated conservatively for a period of time with either expectant observation or decompression. Subtotal removal of an intracranial tumor with a second stage planned after degeneration to grade II to III function has been performed with success at our institution.

In short, we believe that the rarity of these tumors and the previously reported retrospective series do not provide convincing evidence for "the earlier the better" surgical approach. The decision of when to remove facial neuromas in the presence of normal facial function is difficult. Extensive patient counseling is essential. We consider tumor size and location, personal wishes, symptoms, age, and health in the formation of each individual's treatment plan.

Approach

Careful preoperative assessment of the location and extension of these lesions is essential, but the surgeon must be prepared to expose the entire intratemporal and even the extratemporal course of the facial nerve. Lesions involving the vertical segment may require extratemporal exposure if there is extension through the stylomastoid foramen or if exposure is required for grafting. Lesions of the proximal extratemporal nerve may require mastoidectomy for the same reasons.

Tumors involving the tympanic and mastoid segments of the facial nerve are removed via a transmastoid approach. A middle fossa mass is approached through a temporal craniotomy. Labyrinthine and intracanalicular lesions are exposed via a middle fossa or translabyrinthine approach. The decision as to which of these will be used depends on age, health, and hearing. For example, tumors involving the CPA in patients with severe SNHL are best removed via the translabyrinthine approach, whereas the middle fossa is used for tumors of the geniculate ganglion and proximal.

Technique

Intraoperative facial nerve monitoring and the use of stimulating instruments can assist in removal of the tumor from the nerve's surface and help confirm nerve integrity and function at the completion of resection. As noted previously, removal of facial neuromas generally requires transection of the nerve. Previous authors have advocated the need for resection of a length of the normal-appearing nerve for frozen section exclusion of intraneural diffusion of the tumor (37,50). Fisch (53) discussed the difficulties of the pathologist in defining the limits of neurogenic tumors on frozen section and their tendency to cautiously err in favor of tumor presence. The use of intraoperative frozen sections, therefore, can be a misleading guide to tumor extension, and the extent of resection must ultimately depend on the clinical judgment of the surgeon. Immunohistochemical markers may allow "Mohs' surgery" of the facial nerve in the future, but presently they are cumbersome techniques and are not available for frozen section determination of tumor boundaries.

After removal of most facial nerve tumors, the size of the resultant defect usually does not permit rerouting of the nerve and end-to-end anastomosis. Cable grafting is the preferred technique of repair. A XII–VII anastomosis may be required if there is an insufficient proximal nerve stump.

TECHNIQUES OF FACIAL NERVE REPAIR

Partial Injury/Transection

If the facial nerve is partially transected, an onlay nerve graft may be used to fill the site of the partially transected nerve. Alternatively, the entire segment of the nerve may be resected.

Complete Transection

A primary anastomosis or interposition graft can be performed depending on the length of the defect. In the extratemporal or perigeniculate segments, if the defect is less than 1 cm, mobilization of proximal and distal segments for primary anastomosis may be performed. In the mastoid, the mobilization procedure is of little benefit because further injury and nutrient vessel disruption may occur. Grafting is the favored repair technique for the horizontal and vertical segments.

Direct Anastomosis

The type of neurorrhaphy is determined by the extent and site of injury. The connective tissue and fascicular characteristics change along the course of the facial nerve. A precise end-to-end anastomosis that is tension-free is essential. The nerve ends should be handled atraumatically with microinstruments. Beveling the nerve endings can increase the surface area and help compensate for two nerve ends of unequal diameter (Fig. 6). For the distal intratemporal nerve, several perineural sutures are preferred to epineural, and a few millimeters of the latter can be trimmed away from the nerve endings when present (Fig. 6). An anastomosis in the extratemporal or perigeniculate regions should be performed with interrupted perineural sutures of 9 or 10-0 monofilament. Due to limited exposure within the CPA, intermittent pooling of CSF, and the delicate nature of the nerve, repair usually is performed using one or two sutures. Materials such as oxidized cellulose, Avitene, collagen splints, and fibrin glue have been used if suture placement was not possible (67).

Grafting

Interpositional grafts are used when a defect larger than 1 cm is present, when end-to-end anastomosis would be under tension, or when decompression and primary anastomosis would be unfavorable because of compromised microcirculation. The greater auricular nerve is most commonly used because of its appropriate diameter and accessibility. A sural nerve graft is used for defects larger than 10 cm. The graft should be reversed to avoid loss of regenerating axons through small transected nerve branches. In the tympanic and mastoid segments, the remaining trough of the fallopian canal helps to support the sites of anastomosis (Fig. 6). Although some surgeons prefer to avoid sutures and use blood, fibrin glue, and other tissue adhesives to stabilize the graft, we prefer perineural sutures. Sutures should always be used distal to the stylomastoid foramen.

Reroutement

Reroutement is used sparingly to avoid devascularization, except when tumor removal obligates transposition for exposure. Grafting is preferred for most defects of the tympanic and mastoid segments. Before reroutement, the facial nerve should be well decompressed to reduce trauma during displacement. Once adequate length is assured, repair is performed as described previously. Anterior transposition for exposure of the infratemporal fossa provides additional length to achieve a primary anastomosis if the nerve must be sectioned near the stylomastoid foramen. Posterior transposition is useful for repair at the CPA and the perigeniculate area (Fig. 7).

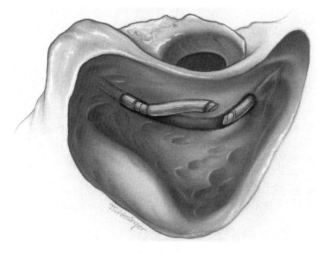

FIG. 6. Interposition grafting of a mastoid defect. The epineurium has been trimmed and the ends beveled. The facial canal helps to support the repair.

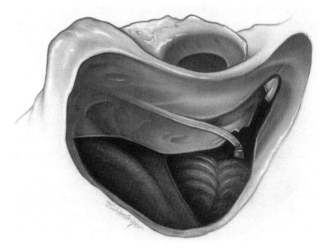

FIG. 7. Translabyrinthine repair of the facial nerve in the cerebellopontine angle (CPA) by posterior transposition of the nerve. A graft is used if a tension-free primary anastomosis is not possible.

SUMMARY POINTS

- Traumatic facial paresis and delayed paralysis both carry good prognosis for spontaneous recovery.
- Patients with traumatic facial paralysis require careful clinical and electrodiagnostic assessment to determine those with poor prognosis so that surgery can be considered.
- The perigeniculate facial nerve is the most common area injured following temporal bone fracture. When surgery is indicated, a total facial nerve decompression is required via a transmastoid-middle fossa or translabyrinthine approach, depending on hearing status.
- The amount of benefit possible from facial nerve decompression following blunt head trauma depends to a large extent on the time interval from injury. Ideally, surgery is performed within the first 2 weeks after injury.
- Preventing iatrogenic injury to the facial nerve begins with understanding when the nerve is at greatest risk during otologic and neurotologic procedures.
- Facial nerve neoplasms cause 5% of acute "idiopathic" facial paralysis. A high index of suspicion is required in patients who show no recovery within 6 months or who have recurrent paralysis.
- Patients with facial neoplasms may present with normal facial function. Tumor resection with preservation of facial function is achieved only occasionally. Decompression or "watchful waiting" are two controversial alternatives.

REFERENCES

1. McCabe BF. Injuries to the facial nerve. *Laryngoscope* 1973;82:1891–1896.
2. Barrs DM. Facial nerve trauma: optimal timing for repair. *Laryngoscope* 1991;101:835–848.
3. May M. Trauma to the facial nerve. *Otolaryngol Clin North Am* 1983;16:661–670.
4. Duncan NO, Coker NJ, Jenkins HA, Canalis RF. Gunshot injuries of the temporal bone. *Otolaryngol Head Neck Surg* 1986;94:47–55.
5. Adkins WY, Osguthorpe JD. Management of trauma of the facial nerve. *Otolaryngol Clin North Am* 1991;24:587–611.
6. Simo R, Jones NS. Extratemporal facial nerve paralysis after blunt trauma. *J Trauma* 1996;40:306–307.
7. House JW, Brackmann DE. Facial nerve grading system. *Otolaryngol Head Neck Surg* 1985;93:146–147.
8. Eby T, Pollak A, Fisch U. Histopathology of the facial nerve after longitudinal temporal bone fracture. *Laryngoscope* 1988;98:717–720.
9. Coker NJ, Kendall KA, Jenkins HA, Alford BR. Traumatic intratemporal facial nerve injury: management rationale for preservation of function. *Otolaryngol Head Neck Surg* 1987;97:262–269.
10. Lambert PL, Brackmann DE. Facial paralysis in longitudinal temporal bone fractures: a review of 26 cases. *Laryngoscope* 1984;94:1022–1026.
11. Turner JW. Facial palsy in closed head injuries—the prognosis. *Lancet* 1944;vol 1:756–757.
12. Adour KK, Boyajian JA, Kahn ZM, Schneider GS. Surgical and non-surgical management of facial paralysis following closed head injury. *Laryngoscope* 1977;87:389–390.
13. McKennan KX, Chole RA. Facial paralysis in temporal bone trauma. *Am J Otol* 1992;13:167–172.
14. Coker NJ. Acute paralysis of the facial nerve. In: Byron J, Bailey JB, eds. *Head and neck surgery—otolaryngology.* Philadelphia: JB Lippincott Co., 1993:1711–1728.
15. Hasso A, Ledington J. Traumatic injuries of the temporal bone. *Otolaryngol Clin North Am* 1988;21:295–316.
16. Yanagihara N. Transmastoid decompression of the facial nerve in temporal bone fracture. *Otolaryngol Head Neck Surg* 1982;90:616–621.
17. May M. Total facial nerve exploration: indications and results. *Laryngoscope* 1979;89:906–917.
18. Bergman I, May M, Wessel HB, Stool SE. Management of facial palsy caused by birth trauma. *Laryngoscope* 1986;94:381–384.
19. McHugh HE, Sowden KA, Levitt MN. Facial paralysis and muscle agenesis in the newborn. *Arch Otolaryngol* 1969;89:131–143.
20. Smith JD, Crumley RL, Harker LA. Facial paralysis in the newborn. *Otolaryngol Head Neck Surg* 1981;89:1021–1024.

21. Manning JJ, Adour KK. Facial paralysis in children. *Pediatrics* 1972;49:102–109.
22. Acoustic neuroma. *NIH Consens Dev Conf Consens Statement* 1991;9:1–24.
23. Kartush J, Niparko J, Graham M. Intraoperative facial nerve monitoring: a comparison of stimulating electrodes. *Laryngoscope* 1985;95:1536–1540.
24. Moller A, Janetta P. Preservation of facial function during removal of acoustic neuromas: use of monopolar constant voltage stimulation and EMG. *J Neurosurg* 1984;61:757–760.
25. Kartush JM. Electroneurography and intraoperative facial monitoring in contemporary neurotology. *Otolaryngol Head Neck Surg* 1989;101:496–503.
26. Wiet RJ. Iatrogenic facial paralysis. *Otolaryngol Clin North Am* 1982;15:773–780.
27. Althaus SR, House HP. The facial nerve in middle ear surgery. *Otolaryngol Clin North Am* 1974;2:461–465.
28. Althaus SR. Postoperative facial paralysis: the otologist's dilemma. *Laryngoscope* 1978;88:243–253.
29. Kartush JM, Graham MD, LaRouere MJ. Meatal decompression following acoustic neuroma resection: minimizing delayed facial palsy. *Laryngoscope* 1991;101:674–675.
30. Gianoli G, Kartush JM. Delayed facial palsy after acoustic tumor resection: the role of viral activation. *Laryngoscope* 1996;vol 17, no 4:1–5
31. Kartush JM, Brackmann DE. Acoustic neuroma update. *Otolaryngol Clin North Am* 1996;29:377–392.
32. Kamerer DB. Intratemporal facial nerve injuries. *Otolaryngol Head Neck Surg* 1982;90:612–615.
33. Green JD, Shelton C, Brackmann DE. Surgical management of iatrogenic facial nerve injuries. *Otolaryngol Head Neck Surg* 1994;111:606–610.
34. Schmidt C. Neurimon des nervus facialis. *Zentrabl Hals Nas-Ohren-heilk* 1930;16:329.
35. Saito H, Baxter A. Undiagnosed intratemporal facial nerve neurilemmomas. *Arch Otolaryngol* 1972;95:415–419.
36. Jung TT, Jun B, Paparella MM. Primary and secondary tumours of the facial nerve: a temporal bone study. In: Portmann M, ed. *Proceedings of the 5th international symposium on the facial nerve.* New York: Masson Publishing, 1985;426–432.
37. Lipkin AF, Coker NJ, Jenkins HA, Alford BR. Intracranial and intratemporal facial neuroma. *Otolaryngol Head Neck Surg* 1987;96:71–79.
38. Fisch U, Ruttner J. Pathology of intratemporal tumors involving the facial nerve. In: Fisch U, ed. *Facial nerve surgery.* Birmingham, AL: Aesculapius, 1977:448–456.
39. Horn KL, Crumley RL, Schindler RA. Facial neurilemmomas. *Laryngoscope* 1981;91:1326–1331.

40. Wenig BM. *Atlas of head and neck pathology.* Philadelphia: WB Saunders, 1993.

41. Snyderman C, May M, Berman MA, Curtin HD. Facial paralysis: traumatic neuromas vs. facial nerve neoplasms. *Otolaryngol Head Neck Surg* 1988;98:53–59.

42. Babin RW, Fratkin J, Harker LA. Traumatic neuromas of the facial nerve. *Arch Otolaryngol Head Neck Surg* 1981;107:55–58.

43. Weller RO, Cervos-Navarro J. Tumors of the peripheral nervous system. In: Weller RO, Cervos-Navarro J, eds. *Pathology of peripheral nerves,* 1st ed. Boston: Butterworth Publishers, 1977:90–143.

44. Russel DA, Rubinstein LJ. *Pathology of tumors of the nervous system,* 4th ed. Baltimore: Williams & Wilkins, 1977:127–141.

45. Batsakis JG. Tumors of the peripheral nervous system. In: Batsakis JG, ed. *Tumors of the head and neck. Clinical and pathological considerations,* 2nd ed. Baltimore: Williams & Wilkins, 1979:313–333.

46. Glasscock M, Smith PG, Schwaber MK, Nissen AJ. Clinical aspects of osseous hemangiomas of the skull base. *Laryngoscope* 1984;94:869–873.

47. Lo WW, Brackmann DE, Shelton C. Facial nerve hemangioma. *Ann Otol Rhinol Laryngol* 1989;98:160–161.

48. Kavanagh KT, Panje WR. Neurogenic neoplasms of the seventh cranial nerve presenting as a parotid mass. *Am J Otolaryngol* 1982;3:53–56.

49. Pappas DG, Schneiderman TS, Brackmann DE, et al. Cavernous hemangiomas of the internal auditory canal. *Otolaryngol Head Neck Surg* 1989;101:27–32.

50. Sanna M, Zini C, Gamoletti R, Pasanisi E. Primary intratemporal tumours of the facial nerve: diagnosis and treatment. *J Laryngol Otol* 1990;104:765–771.

51. Pulec JL. Management of intratemporal tumours. In: Fisch U, ed. *Panel discussion no. 15 in facial nerve surgery.* Birmingham, AL: Kugler Amstelveen/Aesculapius, 1977:423–469.

52. Pillsbury HC, Price HC, Gardiner LJ. Primary tumors of the facial nerve: diagnosis and management. *Laryngoscope* 1983;93:1045–1048.

53. Chen JM, Moll C, Wichmann W, Kurrer MO, Fisch U. Magnetic-resonance imaging and intraoperative frozen sections in intratemporal facial schwannomas. *Am J Otology* 1995;16:69–74.

54. Jackson CG, Glasscock ME, Hughes G, Sismanis A. Facial paralysis of neoplastic origin: diagnosis and management. *Laryngoscope* 1980;90:1581–1595.

55. Lundgren N. Neurinoma n. facialis. *Acta Otolaryngol* 1947;35:535–537.

56. Andrieu-Guitaincourt JB. Un cas de schwanno-gliome du nerf facial au neveau de la portion tympanique. *Ann Otolaryngol* 1964;81:384.

57. Shambaugh GE, Arenberg IK, Barney PL, Valvassori GE. Facial neurilemmomas: a study of four diverse cases. *Arch Otolaryngol* 1969;90:90–103.

58. Carachon R, Roux O, Dumas G. Tumeurs du nerf facial. Ann Otolaryngol 1978;95:777–784.

59. O'Donoghue GM, Brackmann DE, House JW, Jackler RK. Neuromas of the facial nerve. *Am J Otol* 1989;10:49–54.

60. Bailey CM, Graham MD. Intratemporal facial nerve neuroma: a discussion of five cases. *J Laryngol Otol* 1983;97:65–72.

61. King TT, Morrison AW. Primary facial nerve tumors within the skull. *J Neurosurg* 1990;72:1–8.

62. Mackinnon SE, Dellon AL. *Surgery of the peripheral nerve.* New York: Thieme Medical Publishers, 1988:39.

63. O'Donoghue GE. Tumors of the facial nerve. In: Jackler RK, Brackmann DE, ed. *Neurotology.* St. Louis: Mosby–Year Book, 1994:1321–1331.

64. Liliequist B. Neurinomas of the labyrinthine portion of the facial nerve canal. *Adv Otorhinolaryngol* 1978;24:58–67.

65. Pulec JL. Facial nerve tumors. *Ann Otol Rhinol Laryngol* 1969;78:962–982.

66. Pulec JL. Facial nerve neuroma. *Laryngoscope* 1972;82:1160–1176.

67. Fisch U, Dobie RA, Gmur A, Felix H. Intracranial facial nerve anastomosis. *Am J Otol* 1987;8:23–29.

The Ear: Comprehensive Otology,
edited by R. F. Canalis and P. R. Lambert.
Lippincott Williams & Wilkins, Philadelphia © 2000.

CHAPTER 47

Facial Reanimation

Mack L. Cheney and Cliff A. Megerian

The surgical management of facial nerve disorders requires an in-depth knowledge of the anatomy and physiology of this structure under normal and pathologic conditions. In addition, an understanding of how the dynamic parts of the face function in an integrated manner and of how disease and trauma result in a variety of complex clinical situations is critical to maximize the chances of optimal rehabilitation. Patients who are candidates for reparative surgery are primarily those with a nerve transection injury or long-standing facial paralysis (over 1 year's duration), and no physical or electrical evidence of recovery (1). Conservative therapy with the expectation of spontaneous recovery usually is indicated in less severe injuries. A limited number of patients with congenital abnormalities of facial function and those suffering from hyperkinetic syndromes, including hemifacial spasm and blepharospasm, are candidates for surgical intervention.

The surgical management of the paralyzed face varies and in many ways depends on the individual needs and desires of the patient. Other factors that must be considered prior to the formulation of a surgical plan are the causes and duration of the dysfunction, the patient's age, and the presumed condition of the facial nerve and muscles. The most important goals to be achieved are corneal protection, bilateral symmetry of the face at rest, and restoration of a symmetric smile. The surgeon must be certain that the patient is clear about the surgical objectives and be able to balance the importance of functional versus aesthetic objectives.

This chapter is organized around specific surgical procedures aimed at the rehabilitation of facial function, including decompression, primary nerve repair, interposition nerve grafting, reinnervation techniques, dynamic and static reanimation, and neurotization. In addition, the surgical management of hyperkinetic disorders is discussed.

ANATOMY OF FACIAL EXPRESSION

A detailed description of the central and peripheral anatomy of the facial nerve can be found in Chapter 44.

  M.L. Cheney: Department of Otolaryngology, Harvard Medical School; and Division of Facial Plastic and Reconstructive Surgery, Massachusetts Eye and Ear Infirmary, Boston, Massachusetts 02114

  C.A. Megerian: Department of Otolaryngology, University of Massachusetts Medical School; and Department of Otolaryngology UMass Memorial Medical Center, Worcester, Massachusetts 01655

The information provided here is limited to those structural elements fundamental to the treatment of facial nerve disorders. Human communication depends in large part on emotions conveyed through different facial expressions, resulting from the action of various muscle groups. Although there are 18 paired muscles involved with facial expression, clinical assessment of facial dysfunction primarily depends on the evaluation of the frontalis, orbicularis oculi, zygomaticus major, orbicularis oris, and lip depressors muscles (Fig. 1) (1). Two functional elements are especially important in assessing facial dysfunction prior to treatment: the status of the nasolabial fold and the dynamics of smile formation.

The nasolabial fold consists of dense fibrous tissue, the levator muscles of the upper lip, and striated muscle bundles originating in the fold's fascia. The shape and depth of the nasolabial fold can vary greatly. Superiorly, the nasolabial fold begins where the alar nasi, cheek, and upper lip meet. From this point, the curve of the fold descends with a lateral orientation and terminates in the corner of the mouth. The fold can assume a straight, convex, or concave course (2).

A smile is formed mainly by the levator muscles of the upper lip that pass through the orbicularis oris, inserting into the dermis and the vermilion line. A smile is divided into two stages. In the first stage, all the levator and fold muscles contract, elevating the upper lip to the nasolabial fold against the resistance given by the cheek fat, which limits the superior excursion of the upper lip. In the second stage, the levator superior, zygomaticus major, and caninus muscles raise the lip and the fold upward (2). The levator muscles of the upper lip pass through the orbicu-

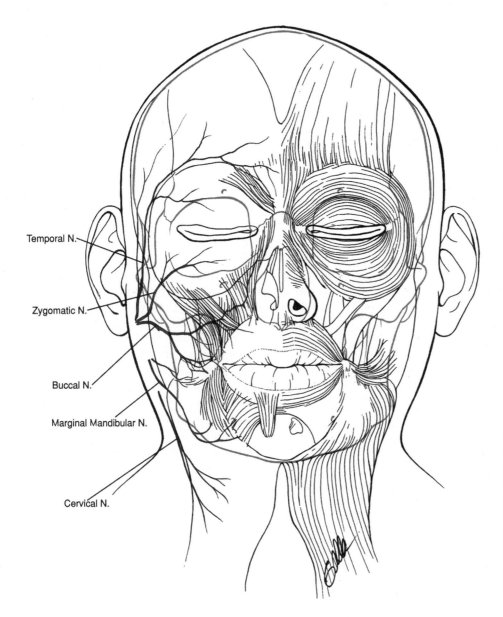

Temporal N.

Zygomatic N.

Buccal N.

Marginal Mandibular N.

Cervical N.

FIG. 1. Peripheral distribution of the facial nerve. Distal to the stylomastoid foramen, the facial nerve branches into five major divisions at the pes anserinus. The nerve first bifurcates into upper and lower divisions. The upper division gives rise to the temporal and zygomatic branches and the lower to the buccal, mandibular, and cervical branches. The temporal branch serves the forehead musculature (frontalis, corrugator), and the zygomatic branch serves the orbicularis oculi. The buccal branch elevates the corner of the mouth, and the marginal mandibular serves the orbicularis oris and depressor labii oris. The cervical branch supplies the platysma. (From Megerian CA, McKenna MJ, Cheney ML. Facial paralysis: etiology, physiology, and principles of repair. In: Cheney ML, ed. *Facial surgery: plastic and reconstructive.* Baltimore: Williams & Wilkins, 1997;629–654, with permission.)

laris oris, inserting into the dermis of the upper lip and the cutaneous vermilion line.

Smiles differ in their line of contracture, point of insertion, and the varying strengths of each muscle group. The interaction of these components results in one of three basic patterns: the zygomaticus major smile, the canine smile, and the full-denture smile. The zygomaticus major is the most common type, occurring 67% of the time; it is dominated by the zygomaticus major muscle (Fig. 2A).

The second most common is the canine smile, mainly due to the action of the levator labii superioris; it occurs approximately 31% of the time (Fig. 2B). The least common is the full-denture smile, occurring in 2% of the population; it results from contraction of elevator and depressor muscles of the lips and the angles of the mouth (Fig. 2C). In this chapter the House-Brackmann classification is used throughout when referring to facial dysfunction and degrees of rehabilitation.

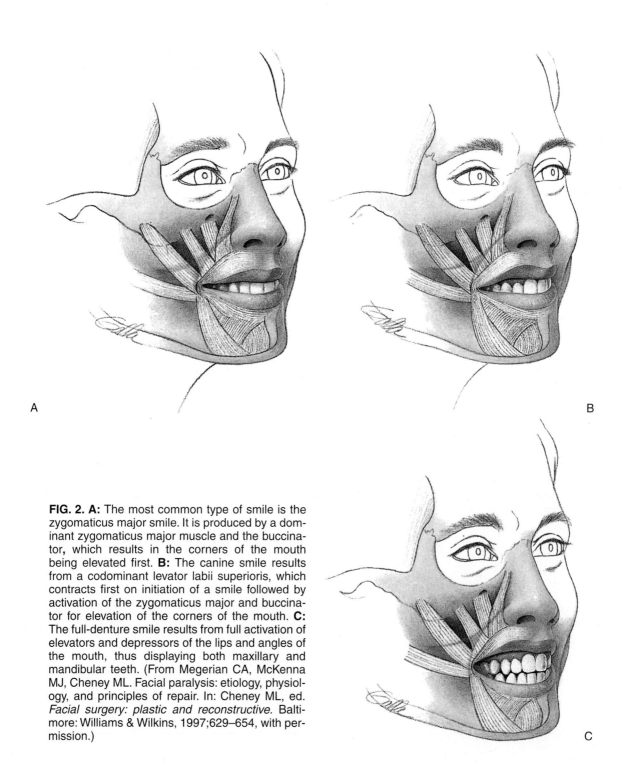

A

B

C

FIG. 2. A: The most common type of smile is the zygomaticus major smile. It is produced by a dominant zygomaticus major muscle and the buccinator, which results in the corners of the mouth being elevated first. **B:** The canine smile results from a codominant levator labii superioris, which contracts first on initiation of a smile followed by activation of the zygomaticus major and buccinator for elevation of the corners of the mouth. **C:** The full-denture smile results from full activation of elevators and depressors of the lips and angles of the mouth, thus displaying both maxillary and mandibular teeth. (From Megerian CA, McKenna MJ, Cheney ML. Facial paralysis: etiology, physiology, and principles of repair. In: Cheney ML, ed. *Facial surgery: plastic and reconstructive.* Baltimore: Williams & Wilkins, 1997;629–654, with permission.)

TABLE 1. *Classification of nerve injuries*

Seddon	Sunderland (degree)	MacKinnon and Dellon
Neurapraxia	I	
Axonotmesis	II	VI
	III	(combination of any Sunderland I–V) (5)
	IV	
Neurotmesis	V	

CLASSIFICATION OF NERVE INJURIES

Study of injuries sustained during World War II provided the basis for a systematic classification of nerve injuries. In 1943, Seddon (3) introduced the first comprehensive classification system, identifying three types of nerve injuries: neurapraxia, axonotmesis, and neurotmesis. Sunderland, using histopathologic criteria, expanded it into five categories (Tables 1 and 2). Mac-Kinnon and Dellon added a sixth degree, which combines various degrees of nerve injury occurring in a single nerve.

First-degree Injury

This type consists of interruption of nerve conduction at the injury site and corresponds with Seddon's category of neurapraxia. It usually is caused by compression or ischemia. The continuity of the axon is preserved and there is no Wallerian degeneration. There are minor, if any, local changes. Motor nerves are more susceptible to this type of injury than sensory nerves, and thick nerves are more susceptible than thin ones. Sympathetic nerves show the greatest resistance to first-degree nerve injury and are the first to recover when affected. Failure of nerve fiber function occurs in the following order: motor, proprioreceptive, touch, temperature, pain, and autonomic (sympathetic). The recovery sequence occurs in the reverse order. The period of dysfunction is short, and recovery is rapid and complete, usually without muscle wasting.

Clinically there is painless loss of function. There may be paresis instead of complete paralysis, and there are no signs of muscular fibrillation or degeneration.

First-degree injuries may present in two forms: (a) delayed conduction block and (b) conduction block superimposed on a recovered second-degree injury. The former can be described as an injury sustained for a prolonged period of time, which begins to improve following exploration and simple neurolysis, and then follows the pattern of a first-degree injury. The latter refers to a second-degree injury that fails to achieve the desired sensory and motor recovery following axon regeneration, and proceeds to display characteristics of a delayed conduction block.

Second-degree Injury

This category formulated by Sunderland corresponds to the axonotmesis classification described by Seddon. Pathologically, the changes encountered include fiber degeneration distal to the site of injury resulting from a severed axon or extreme disorganization of axonal function. Continuity of the endoneurial sheath and basal lamina of the Schwann cell is preserved. Regenerating axons will be directed toward the original targets because these are retained within the confines of the endoneurial tube.

The clinical characteristics of a second-degree nerve injury are loss of motor, sensory, and sympathetic function at the site of injury. Axon degeneration occurs between 24 and 72 hours after injury, at which time nerve conduction is lost distal to the lesion. Denervated muscle often displays fibrillation, electrical indications of denervation, and finally atrophy. Recovery rate is dictated by the severity and level of the injury and occurs in a proximal to distal fashion. Functional restoration is complete. Time of recovery is measured in months as opposed to weeks, as is the norm in first-degree injuries.

Third-degree Injury

There are two common causes for this type of injury: (a) traction, when it is of sufficient intensity to rupture the nerve fibers and endoneurium, but not so severe that the fasciculi are disrupted; and (b) compression, occurring either directly or indirectly by ischemia.

TABLE 2. *Classification of nerve injuries*

Degree of injury	Histopathologic changes					Tinel's sign	
	Myelin	Axon	Endoneurium	Perineurium	Epineurium	Present	Progresses daily
I Neurapraxia	+/–					–	–
II Axonotmesis	+	+				+	+
III	+	+	+			+	+
IV	+	+	+	+		+	–
V Neurotmesis	+	+	+	+	+	+	–
VI	Various fibers and fascicles demonstrate various pathologic changes					+	+/–

This type of injury is intrafascicular and may range from an isolated segment to sizable nerve lengths. It is associated with Wallerian degeneration and axonal decomposition, and there is loss of continuity in the endoneurial tube. However, the fasciculi remain in continuity, and their arrangement within the nerve is preserved. Intrafascicular damage may be complicated by hemorrhage, edema, vascular stasis, and ischemia. The resulting intrafascicular fibrosis markedly hinders the regeneration process. In addition, when compared to first- and second-degree insults, the number of viable neurons and axons available for regeneration is reduced. Axon regeneration is often delayed, as the time needed for cell recovery is greater, and complete recovery of function may not occur. With the loss of confinement to its endoneurial tube, a regenerating axon may follow other incomplete conduits, producing a loss of continuity. As a result of one or a combination of these factors, functional recovery tends to be incomplete.

Motor and sensory functions are lost in the field of the injured nerve, and the recovery period is longer than in first- and second-degree injuries. The recovery sequence may be irregular, as axons encountering fewer obstacles recover at a more rapid rate than those impeded by scar and edema. Muscles that are reinnervated following prolonged denervation may recover incompletely or not at all.

Fourth-degree Injury

In this type of injury, the nerve trunk is undisturbed, but the injured site is a distorted mass of ruptured fasciculi, scarred Schwann cells, and regenerating axons. Wallerian degeneration follows the usual pattern and neuroma formation is possible. Factors altering the reinnervation process are similar to those of the third-degree level, but they are more serious and debilitating. There is complete loss of motor, sensory, and sympathetic functions in the field of injury. Occasionally there may be some spontaneous recovery, but never to an acceptable degree. Aberrant interfascicular regeneration commonly results in synkinesis producing mass movement of the face on recovery of any function.

Fifth-degree Injury

This category, as formulated by Sunderland, corresponds to the neurotmesis classification of the Seddon system. It consists of loss of continuity of the nerve and a generalized disruption of all structures in the immediate area of injury. Retrograde neuronal function is severely disturbed, and few neurons survive. Regenerating axons often fail to reach fasciculi, and although surgical repair is useful, return of function usually is incomplete and synkinesis is the rule (4,5).

TECHNIQUES OF FACIAL NERVE REPAIR

The most common situation in which facial nerve exploration is considered is following trauma, especially in the context of temporal bone fractures. Patients with immediate facial paralysis following temporal bone fracture proven by computed tomography (CT) and electroneurography showing 90% or greater nerve fiber degeneration are candidates for surgical exploration. Occipital or frontal head injuries are the most common causes of transverse temporal bone fractures, which carry a 50% incidence of facial nerve paralysis (see Chapter 49). Patients with delayed-onset paralysis have an intact nerve; the dysfunction is likely due to neuropraxia that tends to resolve spontaneously. Steroids (prednisone 60 mg per day initially, over a 10- to 12-day taper) often are used, but their benefit has yet to be proven conclusively in trauma. Routine supportive measures are included, especially eye protection with lubrication and taping, and in some cases tarsorrhaphy and gold weight implantation. Patients with immediate facial paralysis following temporal bone fracture are evaluated by fine section (1.0 to 1.5 mm) CT scanning. Those in whom discontinuity of the facial canal is demonstrated are surgical candidates. There are no current controlled, prospective, randomized studies to support surgical decompression of all traumatic facial paralyses. We have found that it is best utilized in patients who have immediate paralysis with radiographic evidence of discontinuity of the fallopian canal and in patients with either delayed or immediate paralysis, with no evidence of nerve discontinuity, who fail to show signs of recovery (6,7).

Once a surgical decision is made and the patient is cleared of related injuries such as subdural hematoma, cervical spine fracture, and concussion, the appropriate route of access to the nerve is selected. When hearing is present in the involved ear, the middle fossa or transmastoid route is chosen depending on the site of injury. When audiometric and clinical examinations indicate anacusis, the translabyrinthine approach should by considered. Sites of facial nerve injury in both transverse and longitudinal temporal bone fractures most frequently involve the geniculate ganglion and labyrinthine segment. At exploration the nerve often is found to be compressed or partially lacerated. In these cases, the nerve is to be decompressed and the epineurium opened. If the nerve is completely transected or clearly devitalized, excision of the involved segment is performed, followed by primary repair or interposition (cable) nerve grafting. Suture reapproximation of nerve ends often is not necessary, or possible, for intratemporal defects. The graft should be interposed between two clean ends of the native nerve and stabilized with Surgicel and temporalis fascia. Signs of reinnervation begin to appear over the course of 6 months, continuing for 12 to 18 months thereafter. A House-Brackmann grade III level of recovery may be expected in the majority of cases (7).

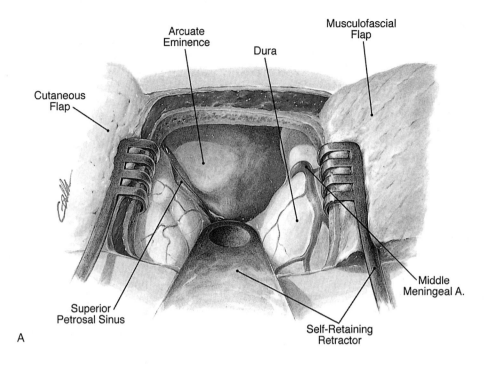

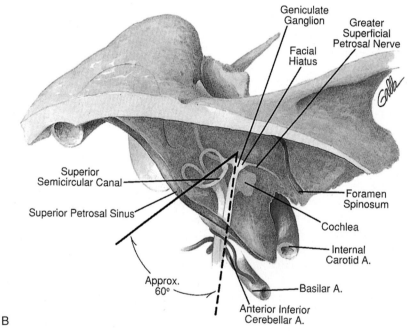

FIG. 3. A: Middle fossa approach to geniculate ganglion and labyrinthine segment of the facial nerve. Elevation of the middle cranial fossa dura reveals the arcuate eminence. The geniculate ganglion lies anteromedially. To access the geniculate ganglion and labyrinthine segment, the greater superficial petrosal nerve is identified anteriorly and followed proximally to the ganglion. Alternatively, the internal auditory canal is exposed and the nerve is identified as it enters the labyrinth segment anterolaterally. **B:** Anatomic relationships of the intratemporal facial nerve as viewed from above the left middle cranial fossa. (From Megerian CA, McKenna MJ, Cheney ML. Facial paralysis: etiology, physiology, and principles of repair. In: Cheney ML, ed. *Facial surgery: plastic and reconstructive.* Baltimore: Williams & Wilkins, 1997;629–654, with permission.)

SURGICAL APPROACHES TO THE FACIAL NERVE

Middle Cranial Fossa

The middle cranial fossa approach is used to expose the internal auditory canal (IAC) and labyrinthine segment of the facial nerve when preservation of hearing is desired. A middle fossa craniotomy is performed after administration of 100 g of mannitol and 20 mg of furosemide intravenously. Once the dura is slack, it is elevated from the floor of the middle cranial fossa and a self-retaining retractor is placed (Fig. 3). After the intervening branch of the middle meningeal artery is cauterized, elevation proceeds with care to prevent injury to the exposed geniculate ganglion (5% of cases). The greater superficial petrosal nerve is identified and transected. The tip of the middle fossa dural retractor is placed at the petrous ridge medially and the arcuate eminence identified. The superior semicircular canal may be blue-lined with a diamond bur and the IAC is located by removing bone 60 degrees anterior to the superior semicircular canal. The IAC is exposed 180 degrees, with care taken not to enter the basal turn of the cochlea in its lateral end. The dura of the IAC and labyrinthine segment of the facial nerve are skeletonized to the geniculate ganglion and the tympanic segment is exposed as it courses posteriorly from it. Thinned bone and bony spicules are removed from the nerve. Compression injury is relieved with epineurolysis of the labyrinthine segment using a microscalpel.

Transmastoid Approach

For cases in which the mastoid or tympanic segment of the facial nerve is compromised, a transmastoid approach is preferred. A postauricular incision is used to perform a complete mastoidectomy. Both the vertical and horizontal portions of the nerve can be exposed and decompression is done following the directives outlined earlier. When the tympanic segment is affected, incus removal facilitates exposure of the nerve, but it does not allow adequate visualization of the geniculate ganglion or labyrinthine segment without sacrifice of the ampulla of the lateral semicircular canal. Removal of the facial ridge often improves exposure to the nerve.

Translabyrinthine Approach

For cases of temporal bone fractures with deafness, the translabyrinthine approach allows total facial nerve exposure (Fig. 4). Following mastoidectomy, a labyrinthectomy is performed and the IAC is skeletonized. Bone is removed 180 to 270 degrees around the IAC, and the

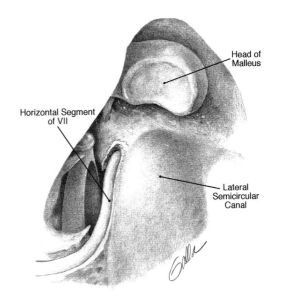

A

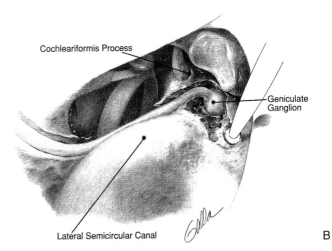

B

FIG. 4. A: Translabyrinthine facial nerve decompression. Following canal-wall-down mastoidectomy, the horizontal segment of the facial nerve is decompressed after removal of the incus. **B:** Translabyrinthine facial nerve decompression. The geniculate ganglion is decompressed. To completely expose the ganglion, labyrinthine segment, and internal auditory canal, a labyrinthectomy is commonly performed. (From Megerian CA, McKenna MJ, Cheney ML. Facial paralysis: etiology, physiology, and principles of repair. In: Cheney ML, ed. *Facial surgery: plastic and reconstructive.* Baltimore: Williams & Wilkins; 1997;629–654, with permission.)

labyrinthine segment of the facial nerve is identified medial and superior to the superior vestibular nerve. Thinned bone is removed along the course of the nerve from geniculate ganglion to stylomastoid foramen. The epineurium can be incised using a microscalpel over areas of edema. Dura over the IAC is opened to expose the intracanalicular portion of the facial nerve. Opening of the posterior fossa dura allows visualization of the cerebellopontine cistern. In lesions that require excision of the nerve, an interposition graft can be sutured into the stump of the proximal nerve in the cerebellopontine angle (CPA) or IAC and approximated to the distal end of the bony fallopian canal. At the end of the procedure, the eustachian tube and mastoid are obliterated with abdominal fat. Rerouting of the facial nerve may be necessary when large sections of nerve have been lost. In such cases, the labyrinthine and transverse segments can be mobilized via the translabyrinthine or middle fossa approach and the freed nerve coapted to the vertical segment. If excessive tension exists across the suture line, a greater auricular nerve interposition graft is indicated.

Illustrative Case

A 25-year-old man suffered a blow to the right temporoparietal region resulting in a complete right facial paralysis (Fig. 5A), cerebrospinal fluid otorrhea, and anacusis. A CT scan demonstrated a transverse temporal bone fracture with discontinuity of the geniculate ganglion (Fig. 5B). Otoscopy revealed a fracture line through the floor of the external auditory canal and a ruptured tympanic membrane. Electroneurography was consistent with complete denervation. The patient underwent translabyrinthine decompression of the facial nerve from the labyrinthine segment to the stylomastoid foramen. A transected geniculate ganglion and a markedly contused tympanic segment were identified. The labyrinthine segment was excised and repaired with a greater auricular nerve graft secured to the proximal and distal nerve stumps (Fig. 5C) using a single 9-0 nylon epineural suture. Facial nerve recovery was noted to be House-Brackmann grade III after 6 months (Fig. 5D).

Technique of Primary Nerve Repair

A neuron consists of a cell body with dendritic and axonal extensions. The axon is surrounded by a Schwann

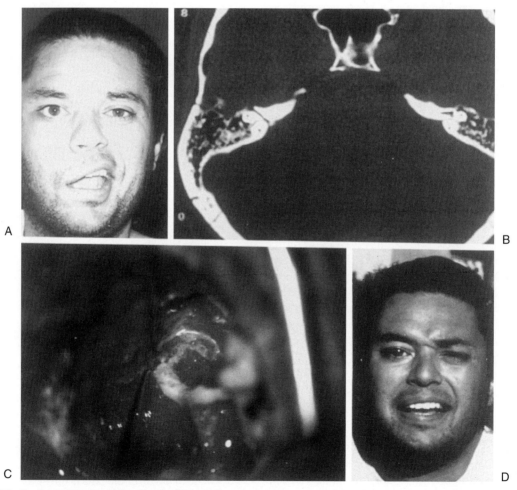

FIG. 5. A: A 25-year-old patient with a right transverse temporal bone fracture and complete facial paralysis. **B:** Computed tomogram showing a comminuted transverse temporal bone fracture. **C:** Translabyrinthine exploration showing a devitalized and necrotic labyrinthine segment of facial nerve. A greater auricular cable nerve graft is used for repair. **D:** Early postoperative photograph (4 months) shows onset of recovery to House-Brackmann grade III.

cell sheath. The communication between the axon of one nerve and the dendrite of another is termed a synapse. Individual axons are enclosed by a microscopic endoneurium and arranged in groups of fascicles, each of which is surrounded by a distinct perineurium. The fascicles and surrounding perineurium are enclosed by an inner loose areolar epineurium containing multiple vascular channels. The outer circumferential epineurium encloses bundles of fascicles and encases the entire peripheral nerve. Of these anatomic elements, three are

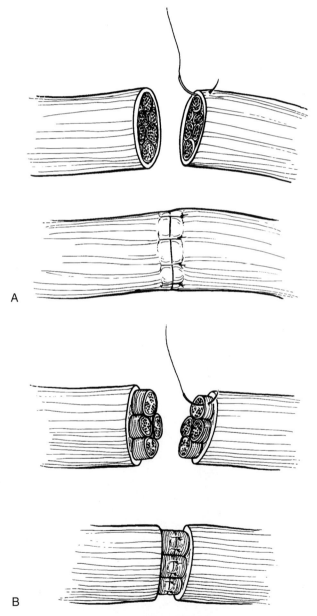

FIG. 6. A: Schematic diagram of the epineural repair technique. **B:** Schematic diagram of group fascicular repair technique. (From Megerian CA, McKenna MJ, Cheney ML. Facial paralysis: etiology, physiology, and principles of repair. In: Cheney ML, ed. *Facial surgery: plastic and reconstructive.* Baltimore: Williams & Wilkins, 1997;629–654, with permission.)

crucial for the surgical correction of severed nerves: the outer epineurium, which is sutured in neural repair; the inner epineurium, which is sutured in fascicular bundle and perineurium repair; and the perineurium, which is sutured in fascicular repair. Peripheral nerve sheaths are well vascularized and include two intracommunicative systems: (a) the perifascicular system, located in the epineurium; and (b) the intrafascicular system, located in the endoneurium. Proximal to the stylomastoid foramen, the facial nerve usually is monofascicular (8,9).

A transected facial nerve is best repaired by primary end-to-end anastomosis. The nerve ends should be reapproximated without tension to prevent fibrous tissue growth into the anastomosis. In cases where the pathology requires resection of 17 mm or less of the nerve's trunk, primary neurorrhaphy can still be accomplished by rerouting it. Given a stable patient, extratemporal facial nerve transection repair should be performed within the first 72 hours after injury to ensure distal segment excitability, thus facilitating its identification. After exposure of the severed ends, all devitalized tissue is removed with a fine scalpel. The epineural sheath then is approximated with 9-0 nonabsorbable sutures. Defects longer than 17 mm require placement of an interposition graft. Epineural sutures should be used for repair of nerves divided within the temporal bone and proximal to the pes anserinus. Although fascicular sutures would appear to be ideal to maintain the precise anatomic direction of the fibers, they are difficult to place and most surgeons do not use them. Furthermore, the extratemporal nerve lacks sufficient identifiable topographic orientation to be useful in fascicular repair, and the nerve is monofascicular proximal to the stylomastoid foramen. During repair, the surgeon should take small bites of the epineurium so that the underlying nerve substance is not distorted or injured (Fig. 6). This is best accomplished by careful preparation of the nerve prior to suturing by removing all fibrous tissue and debris from the epineurium. In intratemporal repair the horizontal segment rarely is accessible to suture repair; therefore, the nerve ends should be carefully approximated and held in place with Surgicel (10–12).

Interposition Grafting

Cable grafts are used when the nerve cannot be reapproximated or the repair is under tension (13). The most common donor grafts are the ipsilateral greater auricular nerve and sensory nerves of the superficial cervical plexus. Other graft sources are the sural and the the medial antebrachial cutaneous nerves. The greater auricular nerve is ideal for defects less than 6 cm in length. The only contraindication to its use is the presence of malignancy in the surgical field. The graft must be carefully harvested, cleaned with normal saline solution, and set at the repair site following removal of extraneous tissue and complete hemostasis. The results of cable grafting generally are favorable. The quality and quantity of axonal regrowth are best when repair is done as soon as possible after disruption of the nerve. Negative factors are poor technique, infection, anastomotic tension, and poor graft match. Radiotherapy delays reinnervation but does not impede it. In most cases, return of movement is first noted 6 months after surgery. Usually improved muscle tone precedes voluntary movement. Recovery often is heralded by a tingling sensation in the facial skin (Tinel's sign) and improved tone. Movement usually is first noted in the middle third of the face and over time extends superiorly toward the eye. Improvement may be expected over the course of 12 to 18 months. Movement tends to lack coordination, resulting in a variable degree of synkinesis. A House-Brackmann grade III recovery level is expected in the majority of cases (7).

Nerve Graft Harvesting

Greater Auricular Nerve

Several features make the greater auricular nerve particularly useful in facial nerve reconstruction. These include proximity to the facial nerve, cross-sectional diameter, and limited functional morbidity following its harvest. Its usefulness is limited in the reconstruction of long defects and of branching nerve gaps because it rarely yields more than two divisions, which are of small caliber and often short.

The greater auricular nerve runs over the sternocleidomastoid muscle at a point midway between the mastoid tip and the angle of the mandible. The nerve will bisect a line drawn between these two points at the anterior aspect of the sternocleidomastoid muscle, posterior to the external jugular vein (Fig. 7). It may be harvested through an extension of a postauricular incision or by a separate neck incision.

Sural Nerve

The sural nerve is commonly used in peripheral nerve repair. The factors that contribute to its utility are its length (40 cm), accessibility, and relatively low morbidity deriving from its sacrifice. Two teams may work simultaneously at the donor and recipient sites, thereby reducing surgical time (Fig. 8) (14–17). On the negative side, the caliber of this nerve is variable (often too large), making graft approximation difficult, and the scar resulting from its harvest may be unsightly.

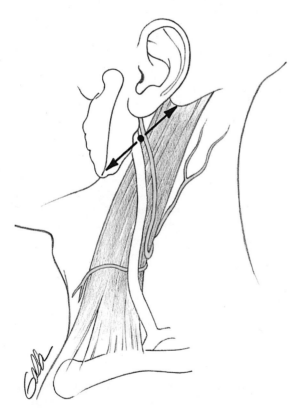

FIG. 7. The greater auricular nerve can be located on the lateral surface of the sternocleidomastoid muscle at the midpoint of a line drawn between the mastoid tip and the angle of the mandible. (From Nadol JB Jr. Schwannomas of the facial nerve. In: Nadol JB, Schuknecht HF, eds. *Surgery of the ear and temporal bone.* Philadelphia: Raven Press, 1993;418, with permission).

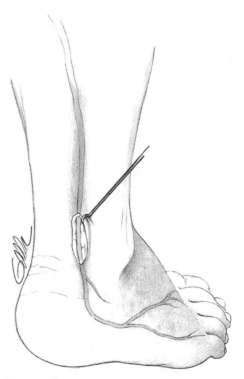

FIG. 8. The sural nerve can be located in a subcutaneous plane posterior to the lateral fibular malleolus. It runs in parallel with the small saphenous vein. (From Nadol JB Jr. Schwannomas of the facial nerve. In: Nadol JB, Schuknecht HF, eds. *Surgery of the ear and temporal bone.* Philadelphia: Raven Press, 1993;419, with permission).

The sural nerve is formed by the union of the medial sural cutaneous nerve and a single communicating branch of the lateral sural cutaneous branch of the peroneal nerve. The dominant contributor, the medial sural cutaneous nerve, arises from the tibial nerve in the popliteal fossa between the superior heads of the gastrocnemius muscle. The nerve runs deep to the muscular fascia for a variable distance down the posterior calf and then pierces the fascia to lie in close association with, but deep to, the short saphenous vein at the lateral malleolus. The nerve and vein run in a lateral compartment between the lateral malleolus and the tendon of the calcaneus. At this point, the nerve divides into several branches that pass around the malleolus distally and supply the skin of the foot. The nerve is devoid of major branches until it divides into two dependable branches on the lateral aspect of the foot. As the nerve courses proximally over the lateral head of the gastrocnemius muscle, it can be traced in a superficial plane over the muscular fascia if additional nerve graft length is required (15,18).

The nerve may be harvested through multiple transverse incisions or a longitudinal incision. Nerve and tendon strippers may be used to isolate and harvest the nerve from the lower leg. The sural nerve is identified through a small incision posterior to the lateral malleolus and then dissected proximally with the stripping instrument. Proximal division can be accomplished by placing gentle longitudinal traction on the nerve and then utilizing the cutting edge of the instrument to sever it. This technique is only appropriate when a simple nonbranching nerve graft is required. Peripheral branches of the nerve cannot be preserved when using this instrument. A direct approach to the nerve is achieved through a longitudinal incision starting behind the lateral malleolus and then extending it up the leg until adequate nerve length is obtained. Neuroma formation at the distal end of the transected nerve is a potential complication. It may be prevented by suturing the distal end of the nerve within the body of the gastrocnemius muscle (18–21).

Medial Antebrachial Cutaneous Nerve

The medial antebrachial cutaneous nerve (MACN) is a sensory nerve of the arm that has been used extensively for the repair of peripheral nerve defects in the extremities and recently has been reported as a useful choice for facial nerve repair (22–25).

The MACN arises from the medial cord of the brachial plexus, adjacent to the ulnar nerve. It carries fibers from the eighth cervical and first thoracic nerves. It lies medial to the axillary artery and more distally, anterior and medial to the brachial artery. At the junction of the middle and lower thirds of the arm, it pierces the brachial fascia medially and becomes closely associated with the basilic vein. At this point, it divides into anterior and posterior (ulnar) branches (Fig. 9). The branches travel parallel to the basilic vein until the posterior branch turns

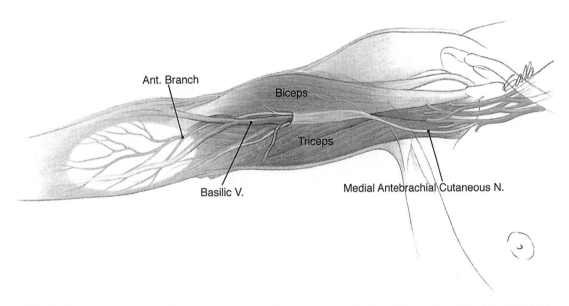

FIG. 9. The medial antebrachial cutaneous nerve arises primarily from the medial cord of the brachial plexus with contributions from the ventral rami of eighth cervical and the first thoracic nerve. As it enters the arm, it lies superficial to the brachial artery and lies in close proximity to the basilic vein. At the elbow, it divides into posterior and anterior branches that supply sensation to the ulnar aspect of both the flexor and extensor surfaces of the forearm. (From Cheney ML, Megerian CA, McKenna MJ. Rehabilitation of the paralyzed face. In: Cheney ML, ed. *Facial surgery: plastic and reconstructive.* Baltimore: Williams & Wilkins, 1997;655–684, with permission.)

toward the ulna. The anterior branch divides into three to five branches between 6 cm proximal and 5 cm distal to the elbow (26–29).

The anterior branch of the MACN may pass superficial or deep to the medial cubital vein, and divide into several branches that are distributed to the anterior and medial surfaces of the forearm as far as the wrist. The posterior branch passes posteriorly, anterior to the medial condyle of the humerus, and divides into branches to supply the skin on the posteromedial aspect of the forearm.

Important topographic landmarks for harvesting this nerve are the medial epicondyle of the humerus, the biceps tendon, and the basilic and medial cubital veins. The fascial plane separating the biceps brachii muscle and the triceps brachii muscle should be palpated and outlined. The use of a proximal sterile tourniquet allows for easy identification of the basilic vein. The upper extremity is prepped and draped from the axilla to the wrist. The donor site can be continuous with the head and neck ablative field. The donor area can be accessed by a second surgical team at the time of surgical ablation, thus expediting reconstruction.

A longitudinal lazy (S) incision is made from the mid arm to the mid forearm, just medial of the midsagittal plane of the extremity. Dissection is begun superiorly through the subcutaneous tissue. The basilic vein is always identified where it pierces the brachial fascia to become superficial. The vein is always the best landmark for identifying the MACN, as the nerve runs in close association with this vessel. In approximately 50% of specimens, the nerve will travel superficial to the medial cubital vein at the elbow.

Once the nerve is identified, its anterior branches are traced distally until an adequate length of nerve and branching pattern is obtained. The anterior branch of the nerve divides distally into three to five large branches. In patients with a thick adipose layer in the upper arm, the dissection of the nerve and vein may be more difficult. It is important not to dissect deep to the muscular fascia, as this may risk injury to the median nerve that lies directly deep to the MACN.

The wound is closed in two layers. No drain is necessary and the upper extremity is dressed with a compressive wrap. Dissection of this nerve results in an average nerve graft of 18.7 cm (if the dissection is taken proximally to the origin from the medial cord) with a potential length of 24 to 26 cm. Proximally the nerve graft diameter averages 3 to 4 mm.

The donor site has the advantage that the incision is well concealed on the medial aspect of the arm. The cutaneous sensory innervation distribution includes that distal arm anteromedially, the antecubital fossa, the posterior olecranon, and the area from the midline of the forearm ventrally to the midline dorsally. Leaving the posterior branch intact ensures that sensation over the elbow and medial border of the forearm remains intact.

The sensory deficit over the forearm is normally limited to a 6 × 6 cm area of the forearm, which decreases over a 6- to 12-month period and usually recovers fully by 3 years.

The truncal and divisional diameters of this graft are similar to that of the facial nerve and its branches, thereby providing an excellent size match for both the proximal and distal neurorrhaphy. The distal branching pattern provides four to six branches for facial nerve repair, thereby eliminating the need for multiple grafts. In addition, MACN grafts may be used when the greater auricular nerve is the field of tumor. They have the advantage, over the sural nerve, of rapid postoperative rehabilitation because ambulation is unimpaired and the risk of cellulitis is avoided in patients with peripheral vascular disease.

Reinnervation Techniques

In cases of known facial discontinuity in which primary repair or cable grafting is impossible, reinnervation of the facial nerve should be considered. Because muscle atrophy and structural degeneration of the nerve proceed rapidly, early reinnervation produces more favorable results. In patients with intracranial injury or idiopathic or traumatic facial paralysis in which neural continuity is preserved but function has not returned spontaneously, it is best to wait at least 1 year before considering surgical reinnervation. In the paralyzed face with potential recovery of function, electromyography often demonstrates evidence of polyphasic reinnervation potentials. The lack of reinnervation potentials and normal action potentials and the presence of fibrillation potentials 1 year after injury provide evidence of permanent denervation and are prerequisites to reinnervation surgery. In patients who present long after the injury (more than 2 years) and in whom electromyography shows no reinnervation potentials, a muscle biopsy should be performed. This is important because evidence of atrophy and neurofibrosis in the muscle are predictive of a poor functional result following reinnervation surgery and are indications for rehabilitation with muscle transfer techniques (30–32).

Facial reinnervation has been performed with the hypoglossal, contralateral facial, trigeminal (motor), and spinal accessory nerves. The accessory and trigeminal nerves are seldom used. Sacrifice of the spinal accessory nerve results in trapezius muscle paralysis and significant shoulder morbidity. The motor branch of the trigeminal is very difficult to access, except during infratemporal approaches, and experience with it as a reinnervation source is limited. Cross-facial transfers may be successful in experienced hands, but their use requires multiple procedures and may produce some dysfunction in the donor side. Hypoglossal-facial reinnervation remains the most practical and frequently used method of facial nerve reinnervation (33).

Hypoglossal-facial Anastomosis

The technique is contraindicated when there is ipsilateral vagal paralysis because it may result in severe swallowing dysfunction. A modified Blair parotidectomy incision is made in the preauricular crease and extended inferiorly to the cervical crease, approximately 2 to 3 cm below the mandible. The facial nerve is identified between the styloid process and the mastoid tip and then dissected distal to the pes anserinus. To identify the hypoglossal nerve the sternocleidomastoid muscle is retracted posteriorly and followed superiorly to identify the posterior belly of the digastric muscle. Once this muscle is retracted superiorly, the hypoglossal nerve is found coursing inferiorly. The hypoglossal nerve is within 2 to 3 cm of the main trunk of the facial nerve (Fig. 10) and can be identified as it gives rise to the ansa hypoglossis. It may be electrically stimulated to document tongue motion. The nerve is followed anteriorly and medially into the tongue musculature and freed of fascial attachments. The hypoglossal nerve is transected distal to the ansa hypoglossis and the facial at the stylomastoid foramen.

Anastomosis of the nerve is performed as described for primary anastomosis. The two stumps should be free of tension and cut sharply to allow for precise coaptation. The ends should be approximated with 9-0 epineural sutures in each quadrant. A modification of this technique is the par-

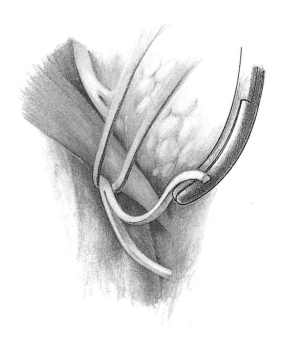

FIG. 11. The hypoglossal nerve is split distal to the ansa hypoglossi. A 30% section is taken from the superior aspect of the nerve trunk. (From Cheney ML, Megerian CA, McKenna MJ. Rehabilitation of the paralyzed face. In: Cheney ML, ed. *Facial surgery: plastic and reconstructive.* Baltimore: Williams & Wilkins, 1997;655–684, with permission.)

tial XII–VII transfer, which limits tongue atrophy and dysfunction. A donor nerve, usually the greater auricular, is harvested. One end of the graft is sutured to the proximal segment of a partially severed twelfth nerve and the other to the trunk of the severed seventh nerve (Figs. 11 and 12).

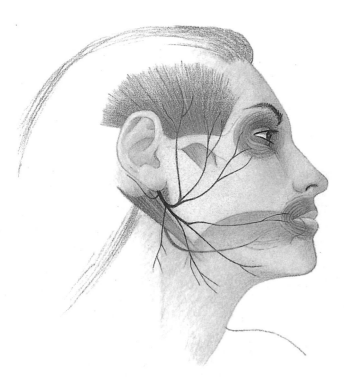

FIG. 10. At the location of the posterior belly of the digastric muscle, the hypoglossal nerve lies within 2 to 3 cm of the main trunk of the facial nerve. (From Cheney ML, Megerian CA, McKenna MJ. Rehabilitation of the paralyzed face. In: Cheney ML, ed. *Facial surgery: plastic and reconstructive.* Baltimore: Williams & Wilkins, 1997;655–684, with permission.)

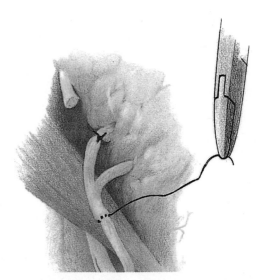

FIG. 12. The main trunk of the facial nerve is divided and the split segment of hypoglossal nerve is reflected superiorly and anastomosed to it. (From Cheney ML, Megerian CA, McKenna MJ. Rehabilitation of the paralyzed face. In: Cheney ML, ed. *Facial surgery: plastic and reconstructive.* Baltimore: Williams & Wilkins, 1997;655–684, with permission.)

In approximately 6 months, the patient can be expected to show improved facial tone and symmetry. Rehabilitation then focuses on teaching the patient to smile by moving the tongue. The goal is to achieve as close a symmetric smile pattern as possible. Mass movement can be decreased with exercise and biofeedback training (Fig. 13). A blink reflex cannot be reproduced, and corneal exposure and xerophthalmia may require adjunctive lid procedures (33,34).

Cross-facial Nerve Grafting

The goal of this procedure is to reinnervate the paralyzed side using a crossover graft from the contralateral facial nerve. This is accomplished most commonly with a sural nerve graft, which connects the distal segments of the paralyzed side to a corresponding branch of the contralateral healthy facial nerve. Approximately 25 to 30 cm of sural nerve is necessary for this procedure. When successful, the technique results in restitution of the emotional smile and synchronous eye blinking. The disadvantages are that the sural nerve has to be secured from a second surgical site, and, most importantly, there is surgical violation of the normal facial nerve. Four techniques for cross-facial nerve grafting have been described. Scaramella transects the buccal division of the normal side and routes the sural nerve graft subcutaneously under the lip into the stump of the facial nerve on the paralyzed side. Fisch (7) uses dual grafts, in which a branch of the zygomaticus of the normal side is transected and attached to the zygomaticus portion of the paralyzed side while the buccal division of the normal side is cable grafted to the marginal mandibular division of the paralyzed side. Anderl advocates four separate grafts from the temporal, zygomatic, buccal, and marginal mandibular divisions of the normal nerve grafted to the corresponding individual divisions on the paralyzed side. Baker and Conley transect the entire lower division, including the marginal mandibular and cervical branches on the normal side and graft them to the main trunk of the nerve on the paralyzed side. A separate jump graft is used to reinnervate the lower branches of the facial nerve on the normal side (34,35).

Reanimation Techniques

In cases where mimetic muscles are atrophic, as demonstrated by biopsy and histologic study, or when early facial reanimation is desired, innervated regional muscle transfers should be considered. The temporalis and masseter are the most frequently used muscles because they are regional and can be transferred with their nerve supply. Most surgeons prefer to use them for oral reanimation and rehabilitate the eye separately with upper lid gold weight implantation and lower lid suspension (31,36).

The temporalis muscle transfer provides movement and improves symmetry to the paralyzed side of the mouth. It is short, thin, and has contractile capabilities ranging from 1 to 1.5 cm. The middle 2 to 2.5 cm of the muscle is best

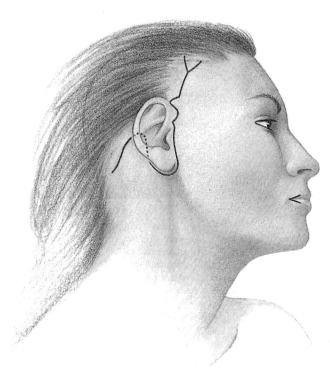

FIG. 14. The incisions used for access to the temporalis muscle include preauricular incision, which can be extended into the postauricular sulcus and posterior hairline, if necessary. In addition, there is a tangential incision made over the midsection of the temporalis muscle to allow access to the temporoparietal fascia and the temporalis muscle. (From Cheney ML, Megerian CA, McKenna MJ. Rehabilitation of the paralyzed face. In: Cheney ML, ed. *Facial surgery: plastic and reconstructive.* Baltimore: Williams & Wilkins, 1997;655–684, with permission.)

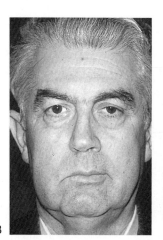 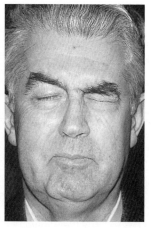

A,B

FIG. 13. A: Patient at rest after hypoglossal facial nerve transfer. **B:** Mass movement is noted with the tongue used to trigger a facial movement. This illustrates well the problem with mass movement and synkinesis associated with hypoglossal facial nerve transfer.

suited for transfer, as the length is adequate and resists the forces of soft tissue fibrosis. The internal maxillary artery provides vascular supply to the undersurface of the muscle and the trigeminal nerve (V2) innervation to the muscle in an arcadian pattern. Exposure of the temporalis muscle is gained through an incision running from the mid portion of the superior auricular helix to the superior temporal line (Fig. 14). Superiorly the incision extends 5 to 6 cm above the hair line and inferiorly to the pretragal area to allow soft tissue dissection in the midface. A temporoparietal fascia flap should be harvested before exposing the temporalis fascia, because this flap is used to recontour the donor site defect (Fig. 15). Thereafter, a 4.5-cm area is undermined, extending from the zygomatic arch to the oral commissure. At the oral commissure, a vermilion incision is made extending 1.5 to 2 cm along the upper and lower lips to expose the lateral aspect of the orbicularis muscle. A subcutaneous tunnel is then developed between the upper incision and the oral commissure. It is considered complete when the surgeon is able to pass the index and medial fingers through it (Fig. 16). In cases where the anatomy is restricted, a rhytidectomy flap may be used to facilitate the transfer. The central temporalis muscle flap is detached from its origin at the temporal line and elevated with at least 2 cm of underlying pericranium (Fig. 17). The vascular and neural supplies to the muscle flap are preserved. A centrally placed incision represents the point of attachment

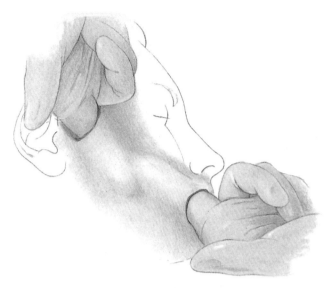

FIG. 16. The cheek flap is elevated for transfer of the temporalis muscle into the midface. This should be wide enough so that two fingers can be introduced from the oral commissure to the zygomatic arch. (From Cheney ML, Megerian CA, McKenna MJ. Rehabilitation of the paralyzed face. In: Cheney ML, ed. *Facial surgery: plastic and reconstructive.* Baltimore: Williams & Wilkins, 1997;655–684, with permission.)

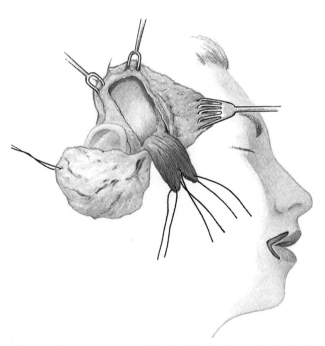

FIG. 15. A temporoparietal fascial flap is harvested prior to elevation of the temporalis muscle. This is based on the superficial temporal artery and vein and is mobilized laterally prior to transfer of the midportion of the temporalis muscle. (From Cheney ML, Megerian CA, McKenna MJ. Rehabilitation of the paralyzed face. In: Cheney ML, ed. *Facial surgery: plastic and reconstructive.* Baltimore: Williams & Wilkins, 1997;655–684, with permission.)

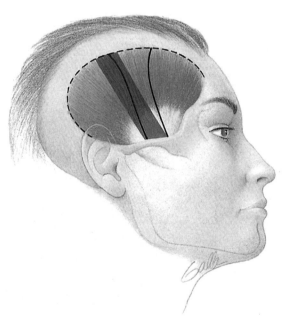

FIG. 17. The temporalis muscle is elevated with muscular fascia and underlying pericranium. The orientation of the muscle can be varied to accommodate individual smile patterns. The dark segment indicates the most common segment used for transfer, which accentuates a horizontal smile pattern. The more vertically oriented pattern is well suited to provide additional midline elevation of the lip, mimicking a type II smile pattern. (From Cheney ML, Megerian CA, McKenna MJ. Rehabilitation of the paralyzed face. In: Cheney ML, ed. *Facial surgery: plastic and reconstructive.* Baltimore: Williams & Wilkins, 1997;655–684, with permission.)

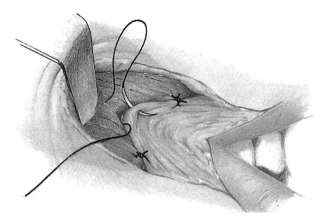

FIG. 18. The distal end of the temporalis muscle flap should be sutured to the lateral aspect of the orbicularis oris muscle with Prolene suture. It is important that muscle-to-muscle contact be achieved, as this is believed to improve the dynamic nature of the procedure. (From Cheney ML, Megerian CA, McKenna MJ. Rehabilitation of the paralyzed face. In: Cheney ML, ed. *Facial surgery: plastic and reconstructive.* Baltimore: Williams & Wilkins, 1997;655–684, with permission.)

of the transferred flap at the commissure. The flap is sutured into the orbicularis muscle using 3-0 Prolene sutures (Fig. 18). Overcorrection of the commissure and nasolabial fold is critical. The second or third molar of the upper dental arch should be exposed at the completion of the procedure (Fig. 19). The wound is closed with 6-0 nylon sutures at the oral commissure. The previously developed temporoparietal fascial flap is used to fill the

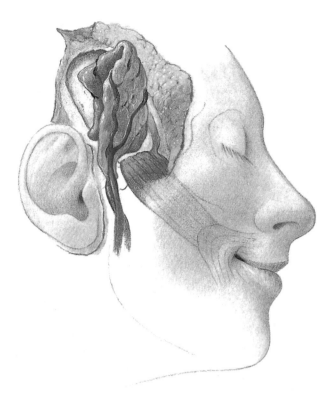

FIG. 20. After completion of the transfer over the zygomatic arch and stabilization of the orbicularis oris muscle, the temporoparietal facial flap is used to recontour the donor site. This is draped into the temporal fossa and stabilized with a 4-0 clear polydioxanone suture (PDS). Special attention is given to creating a proper transitional zone between the muscle at the zygomatic arch and the donor site defect. (From Cheney ML, Megerian CA, McKenna MJ. Rehabilitation of the paralyzed face. In: Cheney ML, ed. *Facial surgery: plastic and reconstructive.* Baltimore: Williams & Wilkins, 1997;655–684, with permission.)

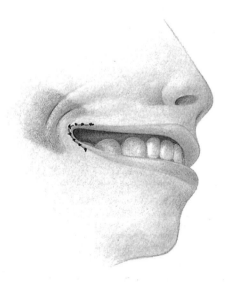

FIG. 19. The resting tension at the completion of muscle transfer should be exaggerated. It is common for the second or third molar of the upper dental arch to be exposed at the completion of the procedure. (From Cheney ML, Megerian CA, McKenna MJ. Rehabilitation of the paralyzed face. In: Cheney ML, ed. *Facial surgery: plastic and reconstructive.* Baltimore: Williams & Wilkins, 1997;655–684, with permission.)

donor site defect (Fig. 20). A Penrose drain and a conforming dressing are placed for 24 to 36 hours. The procedure can provide oral support within 6 weeks. Movement is achieved by clenching the jaws; however, the resulting contraction is not physiologic and rehabilitation requires physical therapy (37,38). Regardless of the degree of preserved innervation some atrophy of the transfer will occur, particularly in elderly and debilitated patients. Additional procedures, such as partial wedge resection of the lower lip and redundant nasolabial fold excision, often are needed for cosmetic and functional reasons.

Free Muscle Grafts and Microvascular Muscle Transfer

Early experience with free muscle transfers relied on myoneurotization and reinnervation of the graft from the orbicularis oris of the nonparalyzed side. However, because most transplanted muscle undergoes atrophy due to its limited vascularization and lack of neurotization, Harii (37) proposed using the gracilis muscle with immediate microvascular anastomosis. This modification allows for survival of the transfer and has been improved further with the addition of microneurovascular anastomosis. The pectoralis minor, latissimus dorsi, and serratus anterior muscles also have been used for this purpose. Cross-facial nerve grafts are utilized to provide for neurotization of the transferred muscle. Harrison (38) described a two-stage procedure. A cross-facial nerve graft is done in the first stage; after confirmation of successful neurotization in 6 months, a microneurovascular pectoralis minor muscle transfer is performed. This approach avoids muscle atrophy secondary to delayed neurotization. Manktelow (39) described a similar technique using the gracilis muscle with excellent results. Microvascular muscle transfers have significant risks and complications, including excessive cheek fullness, distortion of the nasolabial fold, asymmetric smile, and anastomotic failure (40). They are primarily used in the rehabilitation of congenital facial paralysis (Fig. 21) (37–40).

Physical Therapy After Surgical Reanimation

Physical therapy often is necessary after surgical rehabilitation of the paralyzed face, especially after hypoglossal-facial nerve anastomosis, temporalis muscle transposition, and free muscle transfer, and for patients with synkinesis following primary nerve repair.

The primary goals of physical therapy are the achievement of facial symmetry at rest, improved mouth control for a symmetric smile, and reduced synkinesis. Emphasis is on isolation of muscle contraction and in achieving specific facial movements with a reduced effort. Biofeedback helps motor learning and programming with diminished sensory input and aids in the development of cortical impulses involved in voluntary movement. Visual techniques are implemented using a mirror or with electromyographic feedback (41,42).

After hypoglossal-facial nerve anastomosis, patient education is centered on understanding the relationship between tongue action and the resulting facial movement. The ultimate goal is to achieve effective muscle strength and control to produce meaningful facial movement (43).

In temporalis muscle transposition, isometric exercises are initiated 2 to 3 weeks postoperatively. The patient is taught to develop a symmetric smile by biting down, thereby tightening the temporalis muscle segment on the affected side while trying to control movement on the unaffected side. The exercise regimen is gradually advanced to include speaking and smiling, which requires contraction of jaw and cheek muscles on the operated side without biting down. This pattern of muscle contracture is challenging and requires time, a high degree of motivation, and regular sessions to master (44). Patients are recommended to practice frequently at home in front of a mirror. Regular follow-up is indicated to ensure that correct movement patterns are being achieved.

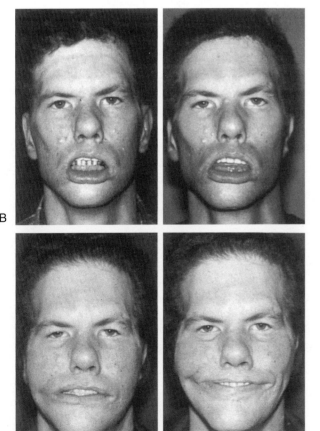

A,B

C,D

FIG. 21. A patient with Möbius' syndrome. **A,B:** Preoperative appearance at rest and an attempt to smile. **C,D:** Result after free tissue transfer of gracilis muscle and neurotization by trigeminal innervation from the masseter muscle. *Continued.*

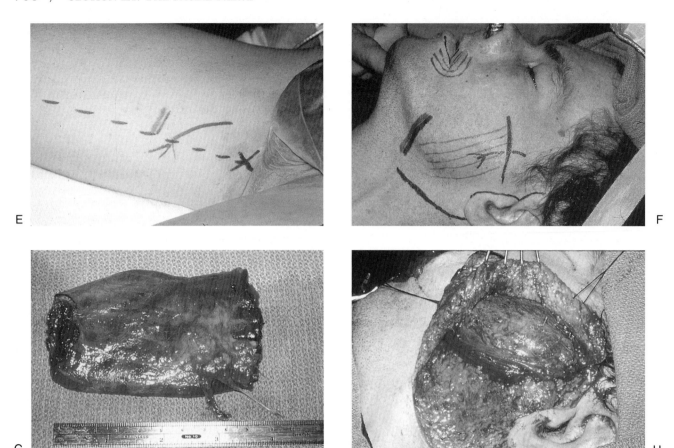

FIG. 21. *Continued.* **E:** Donor site in the leg of the gracilis muscle. **F:** Recipient site with identification of the trigeminal innervation of the masseter muscle and facial artery and vein. **G:** Harvested gracilis muscle with neurovascular pedicle. **H:** Transferred gracilis muscle with attachment at the zygomatic arch and oral commissure. Vascular supply has been reestablished through the facial artery and vein. Neural supply has been reconstituted by trigeminal innervation from the masseter muscle.

Static Facial Reconstruction

Several procedures are available for patients in whom facial reanimation techniques cannot be performed. These include patients who are not candidates for prolonged surgery and reanimation failures. A static procedure offers the patient improved facial symmetry at rest and better control of slurred speech and drooling. Support of the paralyzed face may be obtained with a superficial muscular aponeurotic system plication and a superciliary brow lift and z-plasty of the oral commissure. Limited resections of the lateral lower lip and conservative nasolabial fold resection may further complement these steps. Lower eyelid ectropion may be treated by suspension and lid shortening. Lateral and superior repositioning of the nasal base corrects abnormalities in the nasolabial fold, and shortening of the upper and lower lips prevents drooling and eating and speaking deficits (Fig. 22) (12,44–47).

Neurotization

Spontaneous return of various degrees of facial movement following the deliberate intraoperative sacrifice of the facial nerve without neurorrhaphy has been reported (48–54). A number of hypotheses on the cause of this phenomenon have been proposed, with four currently being considered: aberrant unknown pathways (52), open field regulation, ipsilateral trigeminal innervation, and contralateral facial innervation (53). A case is described that provides clinical and electroneurographic evidence supporting ipsilateral trigeminal neurotization of the facial musculature after facial nerve resection without repair.

Representative Case

A 62-year-old woman who had sustained a left superficial parotidectomy with facial nerve preservation for carcinoma presented 32 years later with left otalgia, facial paralysis, and a 3.8-cm parotid mass (54). CT-guided fine-needle aspiration showed cytologic evidence of mucoepidermoid carcinoma. Excision necessitated radical parotidectomy, partial ablation of the masseter, and sacrifice of the facial nerve, which was sectioned at the stylomastoid foramen. Complete left facial paralysis resulted, but the patient refused reanimation surgery. Approximately 8 months postoperatively, she noted spontaneous left oral

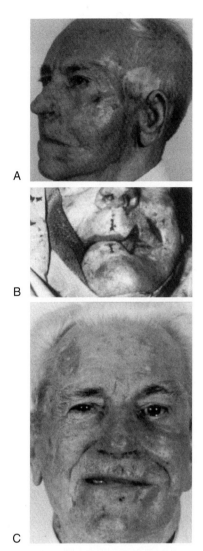

FIG. 22. A: Patient with metastatic squamous cell carcinoma who had a previous resection of the temporalis muscle. **B:** Incisions include upper and lower lip shortening and cheek elevation in preparation for fascial lata transfer for static suspension of the paralyzed face. **C:** Result after 4 weeks.

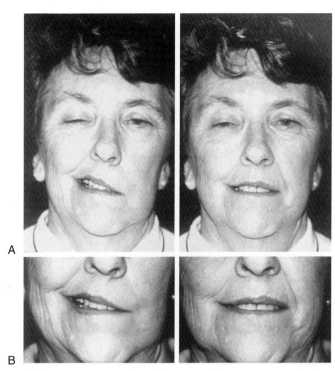

FIG. 23. Facial paralysis 8 months after total parotidectomy. **A:** Facial movement generated by spontaneous smile (**top**) and close-up of spontaneous smile (**bottom**). **B:** Facial movement when biting down on back teeth (**top**) and close-up of smile when biting down (**bottom**).

commissure movement when chewing and facial movement could be demonstrated when she was asked to bite (Fig. 23). Xylocaine injection into the left and right stylomastoid foramina failed to abolish left facial movement.

In some cases, the movement generated by temporalis muscle transfers is more organized and substantial than might be predicted (55–57). It is possible that, as documented in this case, trigeminal myoneurotization of the facial musculature is responsible for such findings.

Management of Specific Deficits

The Eye and Brow

Paresis of the orbicularis oculi muscle results in delayed blinking and lagophthalmos, causing impairment of the nasolacrimal system, a dry eye, and the risk of exposure keratitis, corneal ulceration, and blindness. Surgical correction of paralytic lagophthalmos is aimed at maintaining a normal corneal epithelium. Options include tarsorrhaphy, medial canthoplasty, and procedures designed to increase the range of the blink reflex, including a spring or gold weight implant.

Lateral tarsorrhaphy has proven to be very effective in managing exposure keratitis. A tarsorrhaphy of 5 mm or less generally will not cause eyelid distortion. A tongue-in-groove technique should be incorporated into the procedure to avoid any disturbance of the lash follicles at the anterior lid margin. If a 5-mm lid tarsorrhaphy is not adequate for management, a gold weight should be considered. Some surgeons believe that a gold weight implant is the initial treatment of choice (36).

In some cases, brow ptosis is a significant problem. Open and endoscopic brow lift techniques can be used to raise the forehead pericranium. The elevated brow is stabilized with bone pins and sutures (Fig. 24). A direct brow lift also may be used in some cases.

The Nose

The nasal valve is controlled by the dilator naris muscle, which is responsible for limiting air flow through the nose and provides 70% of nasal inspiratory resistance. In the paralyzed face, collapse of the nasal valve is common.

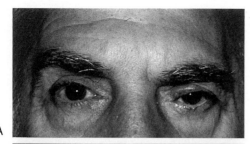

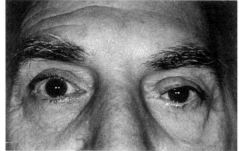

FIG. 24. A: Patient with brow ptosis resulting from facial paralysis. **B:** Result after unilateral endoscopic brow lift.

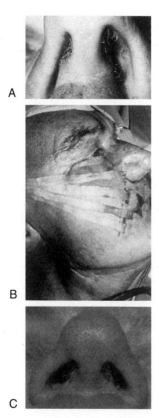

FIG. 25. A: Patient noted to have collapse of the external nasal valve secondary to facial paralysis. **B:** Static suspension is designed to incorporate the base of the nose for lateral displacement. **C:** Result after 2 months of static displacement of the nasal valve and improved nasal function.

Support of the nasal valve laterally helps to maintain a patent airway (Fig. 25).

HYPERKINETIC DISORDERS

Hyperkinetic disorders of the facial nerve are characterized by uncontrolled contractions of the facial muscles, which may persist even when the patient is sleeping. The most common forms of hyperkinesis are hemifacial spasm and blepharospasm.

Hemifacial Spasm

Hemifacial spasm is most common in middle-aged and elderly patients (58). It usually begins periorally with mild and intermittent contractions, which, as the disease progresses, increase in frequency and severity and spread over the entire hemiface. Patients may ultimately develop facial weakness and loss of tone. Some forms of the disorder are believed to be due to aberrant loops of the anterior-inferior cerebellar artery (AICA) impinging on the facial nerve at the brainstem (59). However, other lesions including parotid, temporal bone, and cerebellopontine angle tumors can produce these symptoms; therefore, radiographic imaging of the cerebellopontine angle, temporal bone, and skull base is indicated prior to treatment (60). Medical therapy using anticonvulsant agents such as carbamazepine (Tegretol) usually is not effective. Botulinum toxin injections have been shown to be helpful in alleviating hemifacial spasm (61,62). Botulinum A toxin blocks the myoneural junction by preventing the release of acetylcholine, thus decreasing the tone of the injected muscles. It can eliminate symptoms of blepharospasm from 3 to 6 months. Pretreatment testing is needed to exclude allergy. Injections may be repeated as necessary (63,64). Surgical exploration and vascular decompression of the facial nerve at the brainstem root entry zone is indicated in incapacitating cases and in medical treatment failures. When a compressing vessel loop is found, it can be mobilized away from the nerve by interposing a small Teflon sponge. This technique often is successful.

Blepharospasm

This disorder ranges from mild and infrequent to constant and severe involuntary eyelid spasms. The contraction usually begins unilaterally and eventually becomes bilateral. It predominately affects middle-aged females and is thought to be due to a disorder of the extrapyramidal system. Treatment includes partial destruction of functioning facial nerve axons with phenol injections, neurectomy, and botulinum A toxin injection to the periorbital muscles. All of these measures often produce only transitory control of the problem.

SUMMARY POINTS

- The goals of facial reanimation are corneal protection, symmetry at rest, and smile restoration.
- The status of the nasolabial fold, degree of eye protection, and the dynamic of smile formation are critical in the assessment of facial nerve dysfunction.
- In first-degree nerve injury, the axon is preserved and there is no wallerian degeneration.
- In second-degree nerve injury, there is fiber degeneration distal to the site of injury due to a damaged axon but the endoneurial sheath and basal lamina of the Schwann cell are preserved.
- Third-degree nerve injury may be caused by traction or compression resulting in loss of continuity of the endoneural tube.
- In fourth-degree injury, the nerve trunk is undisturbed but the involved site is a distorted mass of ruptured fasciculi, Schwann cells, and regenerating neurons.
- In fifth-degree injury, there is loss of continuity of the nerve.
- Repair of the facial nerve may be accomplished via the middle cranial fossa, transmastoid, and trans-

labyrinthine approach depending on site of injury and the auditory status of the patient.
- A transected facial nerve is best repaired by primary end-to-end anastomosis. Defects longer than 17 mm require an interposition graft.
- Cable graft sources include the greater auricle, sural, cutaneous cervical, and medial antebrachial nerves. Selection depends on availability, accessibility, and length and diameter of the graft needed.
- When nerve repair or grafting are not possible, a hypoglossal-facial anastomosis provides the best form of repair.
- Reanimation techniques used when reinnervation is not feasible include temporalis and masseter muscle transfers or dynamic options and fascial slings as a static alternative.
- Hyperkinetic facial disorders include hemifacial spasm and blepharospasm. Botulinum toxin injections and vascular decompression are used with variable success in the management of hemifacial spasm.

REFERENCES

1. Anderson RG. Facial nerve disorders. *Select Read Plast Surg* 1991;6:1–34.
2. Rubin LR. Expressions of emotion: the role of the nasolabial fold and the anatomy of the smile. In: Rubin LR, ed. *The paralyzed face.* St. Louis: Mosby-Year Book, 1991:11–15.
3. Seddon HJ. Three types of nerve injury. *Brain* 1943;66:237.
4. Sunderland S. *Nerves and nerve injuries*, 2nd ed. New York: Churchill Livingstone, 1978.
5. MacKinnon SE, Dellon AL. *Surgery of the peripheral nerve.* New York: Thieme Publishers, 1988.
6. Fisch U. Prognostic value of electrical tests in acute facial paralysis. *Am J Otol* 1984;5:494–498.
7. Fisch U. Facial paralysis in fractures of the petrous bone. *Laryngoscope* 1974;184:2141–2154.
8. Orenstein HH, Rohrich RJ: Hand II: peripheral nerve surgery and tendon transfers. *Select Read Plast Surg* 1990;5:1–38.
9. Bremond G, Magnan J. The anatomical and histological features of the facial nerve and their physiopathological consequences. In: Portmann M, ed: *Facial nerve.* New York: Masson, 1985:8–11.
10. Millesi H. Nerve suture and grafting to restore the extratemporal facial nerve. *Clin Plast Surg* 1979;6:333–341.
11. Yarbrough WG, Brownlee RE, Pillsbury HC. Primary anastomosis of extensive facial nerve defects: an anatomic study. *Am J Otol* 1993;14:238–246.
12. Anderson RG. Facial nerve disorders and surgery. *Sel Read Plast Surg* 1994;7:4.
13. Spector JG, Lee P, Petererin J, Roufa D. Facial nerve regeneration through autologous nerve grafts: a clinical and experimental study. *Laryngoscope* 1991;101:537–554.
14. Doi K, Kuwata N, Kawakami F, Tamaru K, Kawai S. The free vascularized sural nerve graft. *Microsurgery* 1984;5:175–184.
15. Doi K, Tamaru K, Sakai K, Kuwata N, Kurafuji Y, Kuwai S. A comparison of vascularized and conventional sural nerve grafts. *J Hand Surg* 1992;17:670–676.
16. May M. *The facial nerve.* New York: Thieme Medical Publishers, 1986.
17. Rubin LR. *The paralyzed face.* St. Louis: Mosby-Year Book, 1991.
18. Hill HL, Vascomez LO, Jurkiewicz MJ. Method for obtaining a sural nerve graft. *Plast Reconstr Surg* 1978;1:177–179.
19. Hankin FM, Jaeger SH, Beddings A. Autogenous sural nerve grafts: a harvesting technique. *Orthopedics* 1955;8:1160.
20. Rindell K, Telaranta T. A new atraumatic and simple method of taking sural nerve grafts. *Ann Chir Gynecol* 1984;73:40–41.
21. MacKinnon SE, Dellon AL. *Surgery of the peripheral nerve.* New York: Thieme Medical Publishers, 1988.
22. McKinnon SE, Dellon AL, Patterson GA, Gruss JS. Medial antebrachial cutaneous–lateral femoral cutaneous neurotization to provide sensation to pressure-bearing areas in paraplegic patients. *Ann Plast Surg* 1985;14:541–544.
23. Masear VR, Meyer RD, Pichora PR. Surgical anatomy of the medial cutaneous nerve. *J Hand Surg* 1987;14A:267–271.
24. Netterville JL, Civantos FJ. Defect reconstruction following neurotologic skull base surgery. *Laryngoscope* 1993;103[Suppl 60]:55–63.
25. Cheney ML, Varvares MA, McKenna MJ, Sizeland AM, Brown MT, MacKinnon SE. The medial antebrachial nerve graft in facial nerve repair. *(submitted).*
26. Millesi H. Technique of peripheral nerve repair. In: Tubiana R, ed. *The hand, volume III.* Philadelphia: WB Saunders, 1988:557–558.
27. Nunley JA, Ugino MR, Golnder RD, Regan N, Ubaniak JR. Use of the anterior branch of the cutaneous nerve as a graft for the repair of defects of the digital nerve. *J Bone Joint Surg* 1989;71:563–567.
28. Race CM, Saldena MJ. Anatomic course of the medial cutaneous nerves of the arm. *J Hand Surg* 1991;16:48–52.
29. Woodburn RT. *Essentials of human anatomy,* 6th ed. New York: Oxford University Press, 1988.
30. Gagnon NB, Molina Negro P. Facial reinnervation after facial paralysis. Is it ever too late? *Arch Otorhinolaryngol* 1989;246:303–307.
31. McKenna MJ, Cheney ML, Borodic G, Ojemann RG. Management of facial paralysis after intracranial surgery. *Contemp Neurosurg* 1991;13:1–8.

32. Hughes GB. Prognostic tests in acute facial palsy. *Am J Otol* 1989;10: 304–311.

33. May M, Sobol SM, Mester SJ. Hypoglossal-facial nerve interpositional jump graft for facial reanimation without tongue atrophy. *Otolaryngol Head Neck Surg* 1991;104:818–825.

34. Conley J, Baker DC. Hypoglossal-facial nerve anastomosis for reinnervation of the paralyzed face. *Plast Reconstr Surg* 1979;63:63–72.

35. Baker DC, Conley J. Facial nerve grafting: a thirty-year retrospective review. *Clin Plast Surg* 1979;6:343–360.

36. Cheney ML, McKenna MJ, Megerian CA, Ojemann RG. Early temporalis muscle transposition for the management of facial paralysis. *Laryngoscope* 1993;9:993-1000.

37. Harii K. Microneurovascular free muscle transplantation for reanimation of facial paralysis. *Clin Plast Surg* 1979;6:361–375.

38. Harrison DH. The pectoralis minor vascularized muscle graft for the treatment of unilateral facial palsy. *Plast Reconstr Surg* 1985;75: 206–216.

39. Manktelow RT. Free muscle transplantation for facial paralysis. *Clin Plast Surg* 1984;11:215–220.

40. Varvares MA, Cheney ML. Free flaps for head and neck reconstruction. In: Cheney ML, ed. *Facial surgery: plastic and reconstructive.* Philadelphia: Williams & Wilkins, 1997:487–507.

41. Schmidt RA. *Motor control and learning: a behavioral emphasis.* Champaign, IL: Human Kinetics Publishing, 1982.

42. Ross B, Nedzelski JM, McLean A. Efficacy of feedback training in long-standing facial nerve paresis. *Laryngoscope* 1991;101:744–750.

43. Brudny J, Hammerschlag PE, Cohen NL, Ransohoff J. Electromyographic rehabilitation of facial function and introduction of a facial paralysis grading scale for hypoglossal-facial nerve anastomosis. *Laryngoscope* 1988;98:405–410.

44. Balch CR. Superficial musculoaponeurotic system suspension and buccinator plication for facial nerve paralysis. *Plast Reconstr Surg* 1980;66:769–771.

45. Martin H, Helsper J. Spontaneous return of facial nerve function following surgical section of the seventh cranial nerve in surgery of parotid tumors. *Ann Surg* 1957;146:715–727.

46. Cerny U, Steidl LJ. Reinnervation after resection of the facial nerve. *Acta Otolaryngol (Stockh)* 1974;77:102–107.

47. Trojaborg W, Siemssen SO. Reinnervation after resection of the facial nerve. *Arch Neurol* 1972;26:17–24.

48. DeLacure MD, Sasaki CT, Petku JG. Spontaneous trigeminal-facial innervation. *Arch Otolaryngol Head Neck Surg* 1990;116:1079–1081.

49. Baumell JJ. Trigeminal-facial nerve communications. *Arch Otolaryngol* 1974;99:34–44.

50. Norris CW, Proud GO. Spontaneous return of facial motion following seventh cranial nerve resection. *Laryngoscope* 1981;91:211–215.

51. Siverstein H, Griffin WL, Balogh K. Teratoma of the middle ear and mastoid processes. *Arch Otolaryngol* 1967;85:243–248.

52. Conley JJ, Papper EM, Kaplan N. Spontaneous return and facial nerve grafting. *Arch Otolaryngol* 1963;77:643–649.

53. Binns PM, Riano A. Facial nerve homographs. *Arch Otolaryngol* 1972; 95:342–347.

54. Cheney ML, McKenna MJ, Megerian CA, West C, Elahi MM. Trigeminal neo-neurotization of the paralyzed face. *Ann Otol Rhinol Laryngol* 1997;106:733-738.

55. Dellon L, MacKinnon SE. Reanimation following facial paralysis by adjacent muscle neurotization: experimental model in the primate. *Microsurgery* 1989;10:251–255.

56. McKenna MJ, Cheney ML, Borodic G, Ojemann RG. Management of facial paralysis after intracranial surgery. *Contemp Neurosurg* 1991;13: 1–8.

57. Cheney ML, McKenna MJ, Megerian CA, Ojemann RG. Early temporalis muscle transposition for the management of complete facial paralysis. *Laryngoscope* 1995;105:993–1000.

58. Fisch U, Esslen E. The surgical treatment of facial hyperkinesis. *Arch Otolaryngol* 1972;95:400–405.

59. Janneta PJ. Observations on the etiology of trigeminal neuralgia, hemifacial spasm, acoustic nerve dysfunction, and glossopharyngeal neuralgia: definitive microsurgical treatment and results in 117 patients. *Neurochirurgia* 1977;20:145–154.

60. Harnsberger HR, Davis RK, Osborn AG, Parkin JL, Smoker W. The tailored CT evaluation of persistent facial nerve paralysis. *Laryngoscope* 1986;96:347–352.

61. Kennedy RH, Bartly GB, Flanagan JC, Waller RR. Treatment of blepharospasm with botulinum toxin. *Mayo Clin Proc* 1989;64: 1085–1090.

62. Borodic GE, Pearce LB, Cheney ML, et al. Botulinum A toxin for treatment of aberrant facial nerve regeneration. *Plast Reconstr Surg* 1992;91:1–4.

63. Borodic GE, Cheney ML, McKenna MJ. Contralateral injections of botulinum toxin for the treatment of hemifacial spasm to achieve increased facial symmetry. *Plast Reconstr Surg* 1990;90:972–977.

64. Borodic GE, Cozzolino D. Blepharospasm and its treatment with emphasis on the use of botulinum toxin. *Plast Reconstr Surg* 1989;83: 546–554.

The Ear: Comprehensive Otology,
edited by R. F. Canalis and P. R. Lambert.
Lippincott Williams & Wilkins, Philadelphia © 2000.

CHAPTER 48

Acoustic Trauma and Noise-induced Hearing Loss

Joel B. Shulman, Paul R. Lambert, and Victor Goodhill

The auditory sensitivity of the normal human cochlea is remarkable. However, this extraordinary auditory capability is vulnerable to the effects of acute acoustic trauma and chronic environmental noise. Noise may be defined as an unpleasant, disagreeable, or unwanted sound, but from the otologic perspective, it is the acoustic energy reaching the ear that is important, not the nature or quality of the sound; beautiful music may inflict as much damage on the ear as a jackhammer if delivered with equal intensity.

Eventually, continued or repeated exposures to high-intensity sound cause inner ear damage and the sequelae of hearing loss, tinnitus, occasional vertigo, and occasional nonauditory systemic effects.

The association between noise exposure and hearing loss has been recognized for centuries. As early as the first century A.D., reference was made to hearing problems in persons living near waterfalls of the Nile. In the 1700s and 1800s, various investigators documented hearing loss in blacksmiths and boilermakers. The term "boilermaker's deafness" became well known, and its high-tone hearing loss characteristics were recognizable with tuning fork tests. During the past half century, increased mechanization and its accompanying noise have caused an inevitable increase in damage to the human ear. Today,

it is estimated that 25% of this nation's industrial work force is exposed to excessive noise levels.

The number of individuals exposed to hazardous noise from other sources such as firearms or power tools exceeds this figure. Annoying environmental sounds such as road traffic noise and construction noise, unrelated to occupation, are increasing as population density grows. Of the 30 million Americans with hearing loss, approximately one third have an impairment at least partially attributable to excessive noise exposure. Noise remains the most common preventable cause of irreversible sensorineural hearing loss.

NOISE CLASSIFICATION

Noise can be classified as transient or continuous. Transient noises are further defined as either impulse or impact. Impulse noises are characterized by a single positive pressure peak followed by rapid return to normal atmospheric pressure; examples include gun fire and explosions. Impact noises are caused by collision of two masses such as occurs with a drop forge or stamping press resulting in a series of positive and negative pressure peaks that slowly dampen.

Continuous noises are defined as sound pressures that remain relatively constant for at least 0.2 second. Continuous noise may fluctuate in intensity or remain steady. In the industrial work place, steady, continuous noise with superimposed impact peaks frequently occurs.

  J. B. Shulman: Otosurgical Group, Los Angeles, California 90067

  P. R. Lambert: Department of Otolaryngology–Head and Neck Surgery, University of Virginia Health Sciences Center, Charlottesville, Virginia 22908-0430

The hearing loss produced by acute noise exposure is referred to as *acoustic trauma*. The hearing loss produced by chronic noise exposure is referred to as *noise-induced hearing loss* (NIHL).

CLINICAL ASPECTS

Acute Acoustic Trauma

History and Physical Findings

The history of the patient with acute acoustic trauma is chronologically definitive. The onset of the sudden hearing loss and tinnitus is related to a single incident or to a brief episode, such as exposure to an intense noise with or without blast or direct trauma to the head or ear. Vertigo may be mentioned as a transient symptom at the time of the acute acoustic trauma.

If the patient with acute acoustic trauma is examined within a few days after onset, there may be otoscopic evidence of vascular congestion in the tympanic membrane. In acute acoustic trauma associated with blast injury, there may be tympanic membrane perforation and possible ossicular damage, as well as cochleovestibular damage with or without a labyrinth window (oval or round window) fistula.

Audiologic Findings

The audiologic sequelae of sudden acoustic trauma may range from a mild sensorineural hearing loss at 4,000 Hz to major losses at all frequencies above 500 Hz. This pure tone loss will be accompanied by concomitant losses in speech reception threshold and speech discrimination scores. In some instances there will be total hearing loss (anacusis). Spontaneous nystagmus may be present, and caloric responses on electronystagmography may be diminished.

Diagnosis and Management

In the differential diagnosis of acute acoustic trauma, the history of sudden hearing loss following exposure to intense noise or blast usually is diagnostic. All of the etiologic factors involved in the sudden hearing loss syndrome (see Chapter 31), however, should be kept in mind.

If the acute acoustic trauma incident is accompanied by obvious damage to the tympanic membrane, appropriate management of that injury is undertaken (see Chapter 49). In total anacusis, immediate surgical exploration may be indicated to locate a possible round window or oval window perilymph fistula (see Chapter 49). If such a fistula is present, early surgical intervention with fistula repair may result in some hearing gain. Even if there is a long delay (4 to 8 weeks) between onset and time of examination in total anacusis resulting from acute acoustic trauma, middle ear exploration may be beneficial. Although hearing

improvement is unlikely, exploration and repair of a fistula, even at a late date, may eliminate a possible route for subsequent intracranial infection.

Following acoustic trauma, the patient should strictly avoid noise exposure while the hearing status is monitored by serial audiograms. Significant improvement is common during the first few days after the insult and the hearing may not stabilize for several weeks. However, fluctuating or decreasing thresholds should raise the suspicion of a perilymph fistula.

Chronic NIHL

History and Physical Findings

The history of a patient with chronic NIHL may be vague. The primary presenting complaint may be tinnitus, usually described as high pitched, with a secondary report of hearing loss. This is especially true in a patient with classic bilateral losses in the 4,000-Hz range but having relatively good hearing in the other frequencies. Vertigo is a rare complaint, and nonauditory symptoms are uncommon. Otoscopic findings usually are normal unless there is another unrelated otologic disease.

In the early phase of chronic NIHL, the patient may not be aware of hearing loss subjectively, with the exception of speech discrimination problems in the presence of background noise. As the degree of hearing loss increases in the major speech frequencies below 4,000 Hz, the hearing capability for ordinary speech, even in quiet areas, decreases. The loss is noticed particularly in consonant identification and in increasing communication difficulties in noisy environments. Frequencies above 1,000 Hz have only approximately 5% of the acoustic power of speech, but contribute more than 50% to speech intelligibility. The lower frequency vowel sounds, from which come most of the power of speech, are affected minimally or not at all by noise. Thus, speech is heard, but it is distorted.

Audiologic Findings

Auditory sequelae of NIHL are (a) specific 4,000-Hz notch, (b) speech reception threshold changes, (c) recruitment of loudness, and (d) diplacusis.

The earliest audiometric finding may be a slight "notch" at 4,000 Hz (Fig. 1A). With further noise-induced hearing damage, the audiologic findings change, with widening and deepening of the 4,000-Hz notch (Fig. 1B). However, there are variations in this susceptibility area, with some patients exhibiting major NIHL notches at 5,000 or 6,000 Hz and occasionally at 3,000 Hz (Fig. 1C). With longer exposure to noise, usually over a period of years, the 4,000-Hz notch not only deepens further but progressively expands to the left to involve 3,000, 2,000, and 1,000 Hz. There is often a lesser expansion to the

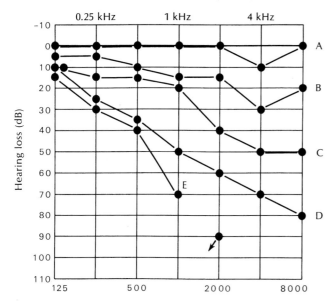

FIG. 1. Five audiometric profiles in noise-induced hearing loss. **A:** Slight notch at 4 kHz (speech discrimination score [SDS], 96%). **B:** Widening and deepening of 4-kHz notch (SDS, 80%). **C:** Major hearing loss at 5 or 6 Hz (SDS, 70%). **D:** Deepening loss over a period of years with shift to the left (SDS, 60%). **E:** Complete loss of high-frequency perception (SDS, 30%).

right with a decrease in thresholds in the 5,000 to 8,000-Hz region (Fig. 1D). As the losses increase, the notch shifts into the shape of a valley and eventually all high-frequency perception may be completely lost (Fig. 1E). Significant threshold changes at 500 Hz and below are unusual, even after chronic noise exposure. It should be noted that some impact and impulse noise can produce atypical audiometric patterns.

Chronic NIHL almost always is bilateral, but some degree of asymmetry is not unusual, especially with lateralized noise sources. For example, firing a rifle tends to injure the ear opposite the side of the trigger finger due to the head shadow effect (e.g., with gun on right shoulder and right trigger finger, left ear exposed to muzzle and right ear protected by head).

Temporary auditory fatigue caused by brief noise exposures is termed a *temporary threshold shift* (TTS), indicating auditory effects that produce no lasting damage. Longer duration exposure to noise produces an irreversible hearing loss described as a *permanent threshold shift* (PTS). The quantitative relationships between TTS measurements and eventual PTS sequelae are unclear. The development of a PTS, however, is almost always due to repetitive episodes of TTS. For a period of time after noise exposure, TTS and PTS may coexist; thus, to determine a stable hearing threshold, it may be necessary to perform serial audiograms while the patient is kept away from noise for at least 48 hours to allow all TTS effects to subside. In general, once the noise exposure ceases the NIHL does not progress significantly (1).

Individual Susceptibility to NIHL

The risk of significant loss of hearing (greater than 25 dB average at 500, 1,000, 2,000, and 3,000 Hz) in individuals chronically exposed to various noise intensities can be estimated from several large studies (*Federal Register* 1981;46:4078–4171) and from the international standard ISO 1999. In general, these data suggest a risk of less than 5% after years of exposure to 80-dBA time-weighted average noise. (The time-weighted average is the sound level that, if constant over an 8-hour day, would result in the same exposure as the noise level in question.) The risk increases to 5% to 15% for an 85-dBA time-weighted average exposure and 15% to 25% for a 90-dBA time-weighted average exposure. For very loud noises, such as those with peak pressure levels greater than 130 to 140 dBA, instantaneous loss of hearing can occur. It should be noted that there is a range of individual susceptibility to NIHL. Although the biologic basis for this difference is unknown, Table 1 lists several factors that might affect the susceptibility to NIHL.

Diagnosis

The diagnosis of NIHL is based primarily on the history of exposure to noise accompanied by a characteristic 4,000-Hz notch or its variants. Such bilateral audiologic findings, unaccompanied by other significant otoscopic or x-ray findings, usually are diagnostic. However, differential diagnostic considerations are extremely important in patients with NIHL. Too frequently the false assumption is made that a history of noise exposure and a high-frequency audiometric notch constitutes clear evidence of NIHL. It is possible for other conditions to coexist and be missed, unless a high index of suspicion regarding differential diagnosis is maintained.

A number of causes other than noise can produce comparable audiometric configurations, e.g., head injuries

TABLE 1. *Factors possibly increasing susceptibility to noise-induced hearing loss*

Factor	Reference
Blue eyes, light skin	Barrenäs and Lindgren (40,41)
	Hood et al. (42)
	Tota and Bocci (43)
Genetic predisposition	Li (44)
Diabetes	Ishii et al. (45)
Cochlear hydrops	Nakai et al. (46)
Iron deficiency	Sun et al. (47)
Vitamin A deficiency	Biesalski et al. (48)
Aminoglycoside therapy	Touma (4)
Cisplastinum therapy	Touma (4)
Older age	Touma (4)
Arteriosclerosis	Touma (4)
Smoking	Touma (4)
Atherogenic diet	Touma (4)
Prematurity	Touma (4)

with or without fractures or concussion, various congenital and postnatal genetic and acquired cochlear lesions (rubella, rubeola, influenza, mumps), and ototoxicity from drugs or industrial chemicals. When some or all of these conditions coexist with a history of noise exposure, quantifying the contributions of the various possible etiologic factors is extremely difficult.

The coexistence of presbycusis poses serious differential diagnostic responsibilities in relative assessment of hearing loss due to noise and hearing loss due to age (see Chapter 33). Both urban and agricultural community environmental noise can produce hearing losses ("socioacusis") and must be reckoned with in all differential diagnostic considerations.

Clinical vigilance must be maintained for proper and complete diagnosis. Even a patient with a typical history and audiometric pattern for NIHL and negative otoscopic findings still deserves a complete otologic evaluation. In cases of significant audiometric asymmetry, with or without complaints of vertigo, an auditory brainstem response test and/or gadolinium-enhanced magnetic resonance imaging are indicated to rule out a concomitant eighth cranial nerve schwannoma.

Management

There is no proven effective treatment for NIHL. Whereas TTS is spontaneously reversible, PTS by definition is irreversible. Remaining in relative silence for a period of time after acoustic trauma may enhance recovery (2). The potential for hearing damage caused by constant noise may be lessened by rest periods between exposures (3). Interestingly, threshold shifts observed after impact noise tend to be less if presented concomitantly with steady noise, presumably because the acoustic reflex, with its attendant sound attenuation, is activated; however, above 100 dB this protective effect disappears (4). In animal studies some protective effects from either the hearing loss or tinnitus have been found from 100% oxygen or hyperbaric oxygen (5,6) or corticosteroids (7). However, the primary management lies in prevention, reduction of the further noise exposure, and measures designed to assist in habilitation. The individual with significant hearing loss may require amplification with a hearing aid(s), but retrieval of normal auditory function cannot be expected.

The problem of tinnitus in NIHL requires careful clinical judgment and management (see Chapter 34). There is no specific treatment for noise-induced tinnitus, although a hearing aid, appropriate for the hearing loss, often helps by amplifying ambient sounds and masking the tinnitus. Alternatively, various masking devices can be tried.

The patient with a diagnosis of NIHL should be counseled regarding avoidance of further noise exposure, not only from the basic etiology (e.g., industrial or military), but also with reference to other causes of such loss unrelated to the patient's occupation, such as loud music, motorcycle noise, firearms, and hobby workshop machinery. The patient should recognize a personal responsibility for prevention of additional cochlear damage.

A recent NIH Consensus Conference (8) offers some practical guidelines to indicate that a particular noise level might be hazardous:

1. The sound is appreciably louder than conversational level.
2. It is difficult to carry on a conversation in the presence of the noise.
3. Tinnitus occurs after exposure to the sound.
4. The ears feel muffled after leaving the noisy environment.

Prevention: Noise Protectors

Exposure to potentially injurious noise levels sometimes is unavoidable. Personal hearing protectors, which include ear plugs, canal caps, and ear muffs, can offer some protection in these settings. Ear plugs can be premolded (or even custom fitted) or formable. Popular types of formable plugs are made from expandable, slow-recovery foam or silicone putty. Canal caps consist of flexible tips on a light-weight, spring-loaded head band. In general, they provide less protection than plugs or muffs. The ease of putting on and taking off canal caps, however, make them ideal for intermittent use. Ear muffs consist of rigid plastic cups filled with sound-absorptive foam that seal around the ear via foam or fluid-filled cushions. Ear plugs can be worn with ear muffs for additional protection. The effectiveness of any protector depends on it being properly fitted and consistently used. For example, failure to use a hearing protector for just 1 hour during an 8-hour day of noise exposure can reduce its overall effectiveness as much as 50%.

In general, hearing protectors provide more attenuation with increasing frequencies (i.e., approximately 10 to 30 dB for frequencies less than 500 Hz and approximately 25 to 45 dB for frequencies from 1,000 to 8,000 Hz). It should be noted that the manufacturer's attenuation data obtained in laboratory testing (noise reduction rating) overestimates by at least 10 dB the protection that these devices provide when used in the field (9). Dry cotton attenuates noise only 5 dB.

PATHOPHYSIOLOGY

Chronic NIHL

In chronic NIHL, the progressive series of traumatic excitations results in an asymmetric amplitude of basilar membrane vibration, which conforms to the basic traveling-wave hypothesis of Von Békésy (10). The 4,000-Hz region in the basal turn of the cochlea is the most vulnerable area. According to Lehnhardt (11), the phenomenon is due to the fact that those regions of the basilar membrane whose characteristic vibration frequencies are higher than the frequency of the stimulating tone are shaken more vigorously than regions having a lower characteristic frequency, namely, those at the cochlear apex. Therefore, all components of a mixed-frequency noise source below the 4,000 Hz will contribute and add their effects to that area. The same may not be true for higher-frequency noise sources. Still, the exact nature of the alteration in hair cell transduction by noise exposure remains uncertain.

Impairment in cochlear blood flow appears to play a major role in the pathogenesis of NIHL. Hawkins (12) clarified the role of vasoconstrictive factors in terms of hair cell damage, dissolution of supporting structures of the organ of Corti, replacement by a flat, undifferentiated epithelium, and subsequent transganglionic degeneration of afferent cochlear nerve fibers. With only 8 hours of noise exposure at 118 to 120 dB, a permanent impairment with hair cell loss was noted. Prolonged hypoxia causes degeneration of capillaries and hair cells (Fig. 2). Axelsson and Vertes (13) demonstrated that noise exposure causes a decrease in cochlear blood flow, specifically to the regions showing the greatest degree of hair cell damage. Using laser Doppler flowmetry in guinea pigs, Okamoto et al. (14) showed further that narrowband noise interferes with blood flow to the specific areas of the cochlea sensitive to those frequencies. The vessels of the spiral ligament and stria vascularis are the most severely affected, with blood stagnation in strial capillaries leading to strial dysfunction (15). Impaired cochlear blood flow leads to progressive damage to increasing

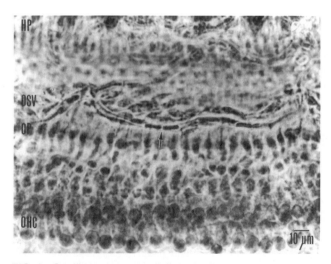

FIG. 2. Capillary vasoconstrictions in the outer spiral vessel, with trapped red cells (*arrow*) directly beneath the hair cells. Noise exposure was 118 to 120 dB for 8 hours. (From Hawkins JE. The role of vasoconstriction in noise induced hearing loss. *Ann Otol Rhinol Laryngol* 1971;80:903–913, with permission.)

numbers of hair cells, the first observed changes often being damage to the stereocilia. However, the vascular changes are not limited to the areas of greatest cell damage, suggesting to Catlin (16) that compensatory vascular shunting may take place within the cochlea.

Acute Acoustic Trauma

One of two things may happen as a result of high-level intensity acute noise exposure. If it is of great magnitude, as exemplified by blast or percussive noise, a tympanic membrane rupture will occur. In such instances, the very rupture may act as a "safety valve" to prevent what otherwise would have been greater damage to the cochlea. In acute acoustic trauma without tympanic membrane rupture, cochlear losses may be total, severe, or moderate.

In acute acoustic trauma resulting from short intense exposures, the basic changes are due, at least in part, to mechanical damage caused by excessive vibration of the basilar membrane by high-amplitude noise levels. Actual tearing of the organ of Corti from the basilar membrane can occur in addition to the structural damage of the hair cells and nerve fibers as described later. In areas of total hair cell loss, adjacent supporting cells form a phalangeal scar.

TEMPORAL BONE HISTOPATHOLOGY

Haberman (17) in 1890 described the findings in the temporal bones of a metal smith with hearing loss of high-pitch tones, who was struck and killed by a train because he was unable to hear it. The microscopic study showed absence of hair cells, nerve fibers, and ganglion cells in the cochleae, especially in the basal turns. These classic observations have since been refined in detail as newer research tools have become available.

Most studies of the effects of noise exposure on the human ear are retrospective. Animal studies have provided the bulk of our current information on this subject. Because the basic mechanisms of acoustic damage seem to be similar in most mammalian auditory systems, cautious extrapolation to humans appears to be justified.

The primary lesion seen on light microscopy is in the 8- to 10-mm region of the cochlea, within which the 4,000-Hz pitch area is located. Loss of outer hair cells and radial nerve fiber damage are noted initially, followed by loss of inner hair cells (Fig. 3).

Lim and Melnick (18) reported a series of guinea pig noise exposure experiments utilizing scanning and transmission electron microscopy. They described the following changes in affected hair cells: (a) an increase in the formation of blebs on the surface of the stereocilia, (b) vesiculation proceeding through vacuolization of the smooth endoplasmic reticulum system, (c) heavy accumulation of lysosomal granules in the subcuticular

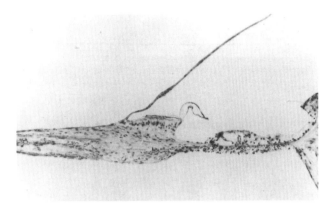

FIG. 3. Acoustic trauma. Note loss of outer hair cells in the organ of Corti from the basal turn.

region, (d) deformation of cuticular plates, and (e) eventual cell rupture and lysis (Fig. 4).

They pointed out further that the space occupied by the destroyed sensory cells was immediately sealed off by processes from neighboring Dieters' cells.

The degeneration patterns in human ears exposed to noise were shown by Johnsson and Hawkins (19) in microdissection studies using phase microscopy. The most common lesion associated with the classic 4,000-Hz audiometric dip was diffuse degeneration in the 9- to 13-mm area of the basal turn of the cochlea (Fig. 5).

It is fair to assume that up to a certain degree of noise exposure, reversible changes occur in and around the hair cells, and with greater noise exposure more permanent changes take place (16). The pathologic changes resulting in TTS are not fully established but may include (a) subtle intracellular changes in hair cells, (b) swelling of auditory

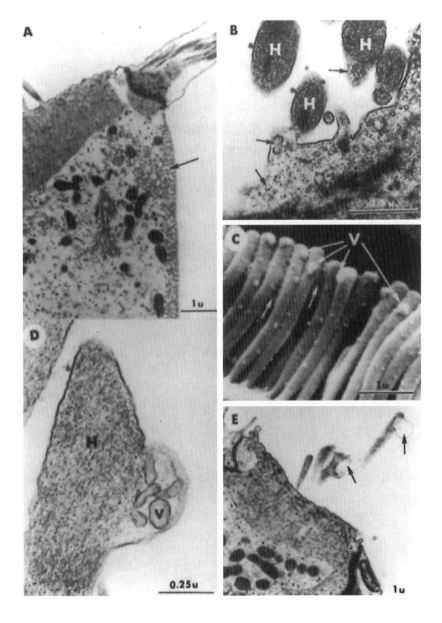

FIG. 4. A: Transmission electron micrograph of upper part of outer hair cell showing early state of vesiculation at basal turn (*arrow*) (300 to 600 Hz, 117 dB SPL, 4-hour exposure). **B:** Trapped vesicles (*arrows*) in the cuticular plate and also inside sensory cells at apical turn (*H*) (300 to 600 Hz, 117 dB SPL, 4-hour exposure). **C:** Scanning electron micrograph showing vesicles (*V*) in sensory hairs of inner hair cells at apex of the cochlea. String-like structures (*arrows*) connect sensory hairs (300 to 600 Hz, 117 dB SPL, 4-hour exposure). **D:** Transmission electron micrograph showing vesicles (*V*) in sensory hairs (*H*) of inner hair cells in the basal turn (300 to 600 Hz, 117 dB SPL, 6-hour exposure). **E:** Ruptured sensory hairs of inner hair cell (*arrows*) in the basal turn (300 to 600 Hz, 117 dB SPL, 24-hour exposure, 17-day recuperation). (From Lim JD, Melnick W. Acoustic damage of the cochlea. *Arch Otolaryngol* 1961;94:294–305, with permission.)

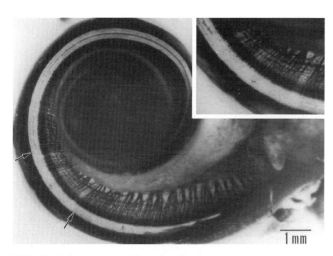

FIG. 5. Left cochlea. Note lesion in the second quadrant between *arrows* **(insert)**, with three small sectors of nerve degeneration corresponding to three areas of complete absence of organ of Corti. (From Johnsson LG, Hawkins JE. Degeneration patterns in human ears exposed to noise. *Trans Am Otolaryngol Soc* 1976;64:52–66, with permission.)

nerve endings, (c) vascular changes, (d) metabolic exhaustion, (e) chemical changes within the hair cells, and (f) a regional decrease in stiffness of the stereocilia (8).

Studies of TTS show profuse vacuolization of the neuropil of the inner hair cells (16). Abnormalities of the stereocilia occur rapidly after high-intensity noise exposure, beginning in the first row of outer hair cells followed by rows two and three and then the inner hair cells. Damage to the inner hair cell stereocilia has a greater effect on auditory function than similar lesions of the outer hair cells (20). Studies suggest that TTS may primarily affect the region around the synaptic pole, whereas PTS is due to damage to the stereocilia at the other end of the hair cell (16).

Once a sufficient number of hair cells is lost, the associated cochlear nerve fibers degenerate, followed by corresponding structural and functional changes in the central auditory system (8,20).

INDUSTRIAL NOISE AND WORKERS' COMPENSATION

Occupational hearing loss can be defined as hearing impairment of one or both ears, partial or complete, arising in or during the course of one's employment. Both acoustic trauma and NIHL may be due to industrial noise.

To assess the potential risk from a noise exposure, it is necessary to know the following parameters of that exposure: intensity of the noise, its frequency spectrum, and the duration of exposure. Noise intensity, or the sound pressure level reaching the ear, is usually expressed in decibels on the *A scale*. Sound levels using the A scale are weighted to approximate the ear's frequency response, thus emphasizing those frequencies most likely to damage the cochlea. The numerical measurements are labeled dBA.

Ambient peak or time-averaged sound levels can be determined using a *sound level meter*. In most cases, these meters use the A-weighted scale. An individual's exposure to noise during a specified time period can best be determined using a *dosimeter*. This instrument is a special sound level meter that integrates a constant or fluctuating sound over time, thus calculating a total noise dose and estimating overall exposure risk.

In the early days of the Industrial Revolution, occupational NIHL was the sole responsibility of the worker. Attitudes have gradually shifted so that today the burden of prevention and compensation is largely on the employer. Since the turn of the century, acute traumatic hearing loss was considered a compensable injury, but not until the 1950s was NIHL covered under the Workers' Compensation statutes in some states. In 1969 the US Department of Labor established noise criteria guidelines in industry under the Walsh-Healy Act. This noise standard covered only workers on projects funded by the federal government. The Occupational Safety and Health Act (OSHA) became effective in April 1971 and applies to most industrial workers in the United States. Noise exposure criteria were modified by Hearing Conservation Amendments in 1981 (21) and 1983 (22).

Current federal law represents a political compromise and can be summarized as follows. If a worker's time-weighted average noise exposure for an 8-hour period is 85 dBA or higher, the employer is required to establish a hearing conservation program, which includes periodic noise surveys and audiometric monitoring of employees, and employee education regarding noise and hearing loss. When the average exposure is higher than 90 dBA, the employer must engineer the workplace to decrease the noise levels, reduce the duration of employee's exposure, and provide hearing protectors. Although a 3-dB increase represents a doubling of sound intensity, in practice a 5-dB exchange rule is used. That is, for each 5-dB increase in intensity, the permissible exposure time is halved (Table 2). The 5-dB rule is based in part on the assumption that noise levels usually fluctuate during an 8-hour exposure, permitting some inner ear reparative processes to occur during the intervals of relative quiet. Workers may not be exposed to steady sound levels greater than 115 dB for any duration without ear protec-

TABLE 2. *Equal risk noise exposures*

Sound level (dBA)	Duration of exposure (h/d)
90	8
95	4
100	2
105	1
110	0.5
115	0.25

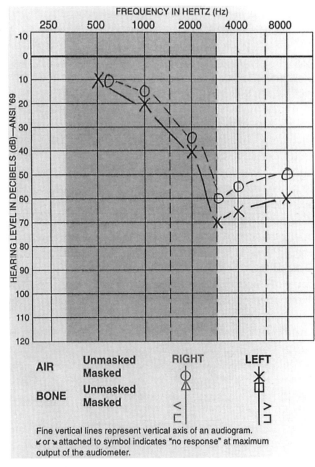

FREQUENCY IN HERTZ (Hz)

AIR	Unmasked	RIGHT	LEFT
	Masked		
BONE	Unmasked		
	Masked		

Fine vertical lines represent vertical axis of an audiogram.
⬐ or ⬎ attached to symbol indicates "no response" at maximum
output of the audiometer.

FIG. 6. Audiogram of a patient with bilateral noise-induced hearing loss.

tion. The upper limit for impact or impulse noise is 140 dB (23).

When compensation is involved, the physician is often called on to validate the auditory status and to apportion the hearing loss rationally among the various potential eti-

ologies. Adequate medical evaluation requires (a) a detailed history, including information about occupational and nonoccupational noise exposure, head injuries, ototoxic drug exposure, other ear diseases, and family history of hearing loss; (b) a complete otolaryngologic physical examination; and (c) a reliable audiogram. If available, prior audiograms, ideally bracketing the nose exposure in question, are invaluable in assessing cause and effect.

Although it is impossible to quantitate the impact of a hearing loss on a particular individual, various methods to calculate hearing handicap have been proposed (24). The most widely accepted formula was developed by the American Academy of Otolaryngology–Head and Neck Surgery in 1979 and adopted by the American Medical Association (25).

The calculations are as follows:

1. The pure tone air conduction thresholds at 500, 1,000, 2,000, and 3,000 Hz are averaged for each ear.
2. Twenty-five decibels is subtracted from this average for each ear, and the remainder is multiplied by 1.5 to calculate the *percent impairment* for the right and left ears (100% impairment is reached at 92 dB).
3. The *binaural hearing handicap* is calculated by multiplying the percent impairment of the better ear by 5, adding the percent impairment of the poorer ear, and dividing the total by 6 (Fig. 6 and Table 3).

Compensation criteria differ from state to state, but all use some variation of this scheme. Adjustments for presbycusis, tinnitus, or speech discrimination loss may or may not be included. Because Workers' Compensation laws are being modified continually, the evaluating physician must keep abreast of the statutes in his or her state.

NONOCCUPATIONAL NOISE

Rosen and coworkers (26), who studied the Mabaans, a primitive African tribe living in an environment of low

TABLE 3. *Calculation of hearing handicap*

	500 Hz	1,000 Hz	2,000 Hz	3,000 Hz
I. Average hearing thresholds				
Right ear	10	15	35	60
Left ear	10	20	40	70
Right ear	$\frac{10 + 15 + 35 + 60}{4}$ = **30** dB			
Left ear	$\frac{10 + 20 + 40 + 70}{4}$ = **35** dB			
II. Monaural impairment				
Right ear	30 dB − 25 dB = 5 dB			
	5 dB × 1.5% = **7.5%**			
Left ear	35 dB − 25 dB = 10 dB			
	10 dB × 1.5% = **15%**			
III. Hearing handicap (binaural)				
Better ear (R)	7.5% × 5 = 37.5%			
Poorer ear (L)	15% × 1 = 15%			
	$\frac{37.5 + 15}{6}$ = **8.75%**			

psychic stress and extremely low sound pressure levels, discovered a singular freedom from presbycusis, even among the very aged. Also significant was the low incidence of coronary arteriosclerotic heart disease in this tribe. Rosen and colleagues hypothesized that the presbycusis seen in civilized countries may well be the cumulative result of a lifetime of exposure to sound pressure levels that, in the ordinary sense, are not considered traumatic.

Noise pollution has become a common concern of all members of society, and noise abatement methods have received a great deal of attention from public health authorities, acoustic physicists, and audiologists. The noise problem is complex and is related to the increase in labor-saving machinery and in transportation. The control of noise at the source (e.g., in building design and community planning) is the primary approach to noise abatement in community life.

In a study of sound power and mechanical power, Shaw (27) compared the relative effects of some transportation vehicles, recreational machines, and power tools. Home power tools (e.g., lawn mowers, gas-powered leaf blowers, chain saws) are capable of producing noise levels in the 100- to 115-dBA range (Table 4). Depending on frequency of use, these devices are potentially damaging to the ear.

Of the common nonoccupational noise sources recently reviewed by Clark (28), hunting and target shooting proved to be the most dangerous. Repeated daily exposure to guns is not necessary, because the impulse noise they generate can cause sudden severe inner ear trauma after a single event. Peak sound pressure levels from rifles and shot guns range from 130 to 170 dB; thus, they are capable of mechanically disrupting the organ of Corti. It has been estimated that 50% of industrial workers are exposed regularly to gun fire from hunting and target practicing. Another more subtle and often overlooked potential cause of hearing loss in already hearing-impaired individuals is overamplification by hearing aids (29).

A change in our music culture during the last few decades has produced a new problem in terms of NIHL.

Flottorp (30) pointed out that the typical feature of modern pop music is its very narrowed dynamic range. The acoustic level of the average rock group is one that far exceeds the normal maximum level of a symphony. Loudspeakers that may be as close as 1 m to the listener result in a sound pressure level at the listener's ear of 120 to 130 dB.

"Audiophiles" often prefer their music loud to better appreciate the high and low extremes of the frequency spectrum to which the ear is less sensitive. The danger of portable radios and tape or compact disk players with earphones often has been cited because of how easily traumatic levels of sound (110 to 120 dB SPL) can be delivered to the ear. If routinely used at the high volume settings for extended periods of time, NIHL could develop.

Both TTS and PTS values have been measured not only in rock musicians but in members of the audience as well. Reddell and Lebo (31) pointed out in a study of the ototraumatic effects of hard rock music that in some instances it is possible to prevent serious cochlear damage by attenuating the amplification to safe levels and by the use of appropriate ear protection devices.

Even classical musicians are at risk for NIHL. Jathko and Hellman (32) studied the problem of acoustic trauma in orchestra musicians and found significant hearing losses, primarily in those professional musicians playing in orchestras utilizing powerful amplifiers and speakers. Such high-frequency losses also may occur in musicians in vulnerable orchestral positions, where they are subjected to acoustic trauma from brass instruments. McBride et al. (33) found trumpet and piccolo players to be at greater risk than string and woodwind players.

A disturbing prevalence of NIHL in children pointed out by Brookhauser (34) highlights the importance of recognizing this public health hazard even in the pediatric age group. Such studies illustrate the enormity of the problem of environmental noise and its effect on society.

CONSTITUTIONAL NONAUDITORY EFFECTS OF NOISE

Tolerance of, and reaction to, noise varies as much with the individual as with the type of noise. Schiff (35) pointed out that noise can alter electroencephalographic patterns during sleep. The rapid eye movement stage of sleep patterns can be interrupted by noise levels as low as 50 dB. Physiologic nonauditory effects of noise include peripheral vasoconstriction and increased depth and diminished rate of respiration. There also may be endocrine and glandular stress responses to environmental noise. Increase in urinary catecholamine levels has been reported in response to loud and long noise exposure, with resultant blood pressure elevation and decreased peripheral circulation. Geber (36,37) reported that gravid women exposed to noise stress experienced an increased incidence of developmental anomalies, apparently related to maternal hor-

TABLE 4. *Noise levels and sources*

dBA	Source
160	
150	Jet take off
140	Shotgun
130	Jackhammer
120	Thunder clap
110	Chain saw, rock concert
100	
90	Power lawn mower
80	Heavy traffic, noisy restaurant
70	
60	Normal conversation
50	
40	
30	Whisper

mone changes producing reduced fetal blood flow and teratogenic biochemical disturbances.

In a summary of multiple aspects of noise exposure, Glorig (38) pointed out that sound pressure levels of 120 to 150 dB or higher may cause undesirable nonauditory effects that cannot be prevented by ear protection. In addition, intense noise with a spectrum primarily in the area below 1,000 Hz can be felt (tactile) as well as heard. The respiratory system is affected in the 40- to 60-Hz range because of resonant characteristics of the chest. Despite these findings, Glorig (38) states: "As far as we can determine from industrial records, we can find no increase in cardiovascular problems or ulcers, or both, and no increase in fatigue or irritability or tendencies to nervousness." Godlee (39) points out that some links have been found between noise exposure and psychiatric illness, cardiovascular disease, hypertension, stroke, and peptic ulcer disease, but the results of these studies are inconclusive.

It appears, therefore, that nonauditory effects of noise exposure are not always clearly defined. The effects of stress, fatigue, and vertigo are difficult to quantify. An enormous spectrum of industrial and nonindustrial noise sources exists in our society today, and the potential for individual exposure is high.

SUMMARY POINTS

- The human ear and its neural pathways are susceptible to damage by noise. Acute acoustic trauma results from high-intensity noise (above 120 to 130 dBA) and can occur even after a brief exposure. NIHL results from long-term (years) exposure (without hearing protectors) to noise above 90 dBA.
- A sensorineural hearing loss around the 4,000-Hz range is usually the initial audiometric finding following noise damage. With continued exposure, the loss will broaden to include the middle and higher frequency ranges.
- Noise damages primarily the hair cells, beginning with the outer row of outer hair cells and progressing to the inner hair cell row. Changes to the stereocilia precede hair cell loss; nerve fiber and ganglion cell loss also can occur.
- Reversible (within hours to few days) sensorineural hearing loss is termed temporary threshold shift (TTS); PTS refers to a permanent threshold shift.
- Formulas exist for calculating hearing impairment and hearing handicap.
- In our increasingly mechanized society, NIHL is a growing health hazard. Noise is the most common preventable cause of irreversible sensorineural hearing loss in the United States.

REFERENCES

1. Segal S, Harell M, Shahar A, Englander M. Acute acoustic trauma: dynamics of hearing loss following cessation of exposure. *Am J Otol* 1988;9:293–298.
2. Flottorp G. Treatment of noise induced hearing loss. *Scand Audiol Suppl* 1991;34:123–130.
3. Clark WW. Recent studies of temporary threshold shift (TTS) and permanent threshold shift (PTS) in animals. *J Acoust Soc Am* 1990;90:155–163.
4. Touma JB. Controversies in noise-induced hearing loss (NIHL). *Ann Occup Hyg* 1992;36:199–209.
5. Hatch M, Tsai M, La Rouere MJ, Nutall AL, Miller JM. The effects of carbogen, carbon dioxide, and oxygen on noise-induced hearing loss. *Hear Res* 1991;56:265–272.
6. Pilgramm M. Clinical and animal experiment studies to optimize the therapy for acute acoustic trauma. *Scand Audiol Suppl* 1991;34:103–122.
7. Henry KR. Noise-induced auditory loss: influence of genotype, naloxone, and methylprednisolone. *Acta Otolaryngol (Stockh)* 1992;112:599–603.
8. Noise and hearing loss—NIH consensus conference. *JAMA* 1990;263:3185–3190.
9. Park MY, Casali JG. A controlled investigation of in-field attenuation performance of selected insert, earmuff, and canal cap hearing protectors. *Hum Factors* 1991;33:693–714.
10. Von Békésy G. *Experiments in hearing.* New York: McGraw-Hill, 1960.
11. Lehnhardt E. The C^5-dip: its interpretation in the light of generally known physiological concepts. *Int Audiol* 1967;6:86–95.
12. Hawkins JE. The role of vasoconstriction in noise induced hearing loss. *Ann Otol Rhinol Laryngol* 1971;80:903–913.
13. Axelsson A, Vertes D. Histologic findings in cochlear vessels after noise. In Hamernik RP, Henderson D, Salvi R, (eds). *New perspectives on noise-induced hearing loss.* New York: Raven Press, 1982:49–68.
14. Okamoto A, Hasegawa M, Tamura T, Komatsuzaki A. Effects of frequency and intensity of sound on cochlear blood flow. *Acta Otolaryngol (Stockh)* 1992;112:59–64.
15. Yamane H, Nakai Y, Kanishi K, Sakamoto H, Matsuda Y, Iguchi H. Strial circulation impairment due to acoustic trauma. *Acta Otolaryngol (Stockh)* 1991;111:85–93.
16. Catlin FI. Noise induced hearing loss. *Am J Otolaryngol* 1986;7:141–149.
17. Haberman J. Ueber die Schwerhorigkeit der Kesselschmiede. *Arch Ohrenheilk* 1890;30:1–25.
18. Lim DJ, Melnick W. Acoustic damage of the cochlea. *Arch Otolaryngol* 1961;94:294–305.
19. Johnsson LG, Hawkins JE. Degeneration patterns in human ears exposed to noise. *Trans Am Otolaryngol Soc* 1976;64:52–66.
20. Saunders JC, Cohen YE, Szymko YM. The structural and functional consequences of acoustic injury in the cochlea and peripheral auditory system: a five year update. *J Acoust Soc Am* 1991;90:136–146.
21. Occupational Safety and Health Administration. Occupational noise exposure: hearing conservation amendment. *Federal Register* 1981;46:4078–4179.
22. Occupational Safety and Health Administration. Occupational noise exposure: hearing conservation amendment. *Federal Register* 1983;48:9738–9785.
23. Osguthorpe JD, Klein AJ. Occupational hearing conservation. *Otolaryngol Clin North Am* 1991;24:403–414.

24. Melnick W, Morgan W. Hearing compensation evaluation. *Otolaryngol Clin North Am* 1991;24:391–402.

25. American Academy of Otolaryngology–Head and Neck Surgery, Committee on Hearing and Equilibrium and the American Council of Otolaryngology, Committee on the Medical Aspects of Noise. Guide for the evaluation of hearing handicap. *Otolaryngol Head Neck Surg* 1979; 87(4):539–551.

26. Rosen S, Bergman M, Plester D, et al. Presbycusis study of a relatively noise-free population in the Sudan. *Ann Otol Rhinol Laryngol* 1962;71: 727–743.

27. Shaw E. Noise pollution—what can be done? *Phys Today* 1975;Jan:46–58.

28. Clark WW. Noise exposure from leisure activities: a review. *J Acoust Soc Am* 1991;90:175–181.

29. Macrae JH. Permanent threshold shift associated with overamplification by hearing aids. *J Speech Hear Res* 1991;34:403–414.

30. Flottorp G. Music—a noise hazard? *Acta Otolaryngol (Stockh)* 1973; 75:345–347.

31. Reddell R, Lebo C. Ototraumatic effects of hard rock music. *Calif Med* 1972;116:1–4.

32. Jathko K, Hellman H. Zur Frage des Larm-und Klangtraumas des Orchestermusikers. *HNO* 1972;20:21–29.

33. McBride D, Gill F, Proops D, Harrington M, Gardiner K, Attwell C. Noise and the classical musician. *Br Med J* 1992;305:1561–1563.

34. Brookhauser PE. Noise-induced hearing loss in children. *Laryngoscope* 1992;102:645–655.

35. Schiff M. Non auditory effects of noise. *Trans Am Acad Ophthalmol Otolaryngol* 1973;77:ORL348–ORL398.

36. Geber WF. Developmental effects of chronic maternal audiovisual stress on the rat fetus. *J Embryol Exp Morphol* 1966;16:1–16.

37. Geber WF. Vascular and teratogenic effects of chronic intermittent noise stress. Presented at the AAAS Symposium on Non-Auditory Effects of Noise, Boston, Massachusetts, December 28–30, 1969.

38. Glorig A. Noise exposure—facts and myths. *Trans Am Acad Ophthalmol Otolaryngol* 1971;75:1254–1262.

39. Godlee F. Noise: breaking the silence. *Br Med J* 1992;304:110–113.

40. Barrenäs ML, Lindgren F. The influence of eye colour on susceptibility to TTS in humans. *Br J Audiol* 1991;25:303–307.

41. Barrenäs ML, Lindgren F. The influence of inner ear melanin on susceptibility to TTS in humans. *Scand Audiol* 1990;19:97–102.

42. Hood JD, Poole JP, Freedman L. The influence of eye color upon temporary threshold shift. *Audiology* 1976;15:449–464.

43. Tota G, Bocci G. The importance of the color of the iris on the evaluation of resistance to auditory fatigue. *Rev Otoneurooftalmol (Bologna)* 1967;42:183–192.

44. Li HS. Influence of genotype and age on acute acoustic trauma and recovery in CBA/Ca and C57BL/6J mice. *Acta Otolaryngol (Stockh)* 1992;112:956–967.

45. Ishii EK, Talbott EO, Findlay RC, D'Antonio JA, Kuller LH. Is NIDDM a risk factor for noise-induced hearing loss in an occupationally noise exposed cohort? *Sci Total Environ* 1992;127: 155–165.

46. Nakai Y, Masutani H, Moriguchi M, Matsunaga K, Sugita M. The influence of noise exposure on endolymph hydrops. An experimental study. *Acta Otolaryngol Suppl (Stockh)* 1991;486:7–12.

47. Sun AH, Wang ZM, Xiao SZ, et al. Noise-induced hearing loss in iron-deficient rats. *Acta Otolaryngol (Stockh)* 1991;111:684–690.

48. Biesalski HK, Wellner U, Weiser H. Vitamin A deficiency increases noise susceptibility in guinea pigs. *J Nutr* 1990;120:726–737.

The Ear: Comprehensive Otology,
edited by R. F. Canalis and P. R. Lambert.
Lippincott Williams & Wilkins, Philadelphia © 2000.

CHAPTER 49

Blunt and Penetrating Injuries to the Ear and Temporal Bone

Rinaldo F. Canalis, Elliot Abemayor, and Joel Shulman

The ear and temporal bone are frequently involved in head and neck trauma, either as isolated sites or in association with other skull and systemic injuries. In this chapter we review the diagnosis and management of injuries that affect all components of the temporal bone and external ear. Because of their clinical importance and increasing frequency, special attention is given to temporal bone fractures and their complications.

AURICULAR TRAUMA

Lacerations

Because of its superficial location, the auricle is highly susceptible to trauma. Lacerations of the cartilaginous framework are repaired with absorbable sutures placed in the perichondrium or through cartilage. Soft tissues are closed meticulously with fine monofilament nylon. Débridement is restricted to nonviable tissue. Because of the exceptionally good blood supply, even tenuous flaps usually survive (Fig. 1). If not managed properly, lacerations may lead to various degrees of perichondritis and its sequelae (Fig. 2; see color plate 30 following page 484).

Avulsion

Partial or complete avulsion of the pinna usually is the result of windshield trauma in motor vehicle accidents or of violent crime, such as slashing knife injuries and human bites. A severed auricle that is preserved and brought with the patient to the emergency department should be placed in sterile, iced saline solution and replanted promptly. In an early report Potsic and Naunton (1) recommended simple reattachment of the pinna, postoperative administration of antibiotics and low-molecu-

  R. F. Canalis: Department of Surgery, University of California, Los Angeles, School of Medicine, Los Angeles, California 90095-1624
  E. Abemayor: Division of Head and Neck Surgery, University of California, Los Angeles, School of Medicine, Los Angeles, California 90095-1624
  J. Shulman: Otosurgical Group, Los Angeles, California 90067

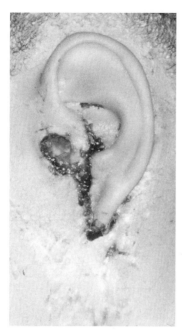

FIG. 1. Appearance 10 days after repair of near-total auricular evulsion.

lar-weight dextran, and heparinization. Although this method has been successful, it is not fully reliable; auricular atrophy and pigmentation changes are to be expected.

When adequate vessels are present, replantation by means of microvascular anastomosis offers the best chance for successful results without substantial atrophy and with good preservation of contour (2,3). However,

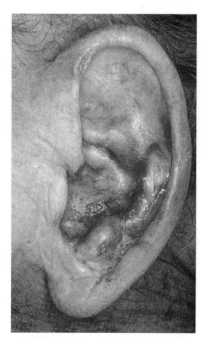

FIG. 2. Perichondritis after trauma to the pinna.

experts in microvascular technique are not always available on an emergency basis, and it often is difficult to find adequate arterial and venous structures in the amputated segment. To overcome these difficulties, other techniques to ensure increased vascular supply to the amputated pinna have been developed. These were pioneered by Mladick et al. (4) and usually require débridement and dermabrasion of the auricle followed by reattachment and implantation under a subcutaneous pocket. After 2 to 4 weeks the ear is removed from the pocket and a skin graft is performed. A one-stage alternative procedure was developed by Bardsley (5) to preserve a large severed ear fragment. He also removed the skin from the amputated pinna and after reattaching the cartilage covered it with a temporoparietal fascial island flap based on the superficial temporal artery. He reported good results with reduction in the degree of atrophy and improved contour. Jenkins and Finucan (6) also used a temporoparietal fascial island flap with good results but emphasized the difficulties encountered in maintaining normal contour.

We have used a modification of a two-stage procedure initially described by Baudet et al. (7) in 1972. In the initial stage, the skin of the medial surface of the auricle excluding the lobe is removed, and a postauricular flap is elevated to develop a large recipient bed (Fig. 3A). Four to six fenestrations are made along the posterior edge of the concha; care is taken to preserve the lateral skin and perichondrium. These fenestrations (Fig. 3B) allow breaking the spring of the chondral cartilage to allow the auricle to flatten against the recipient bed. The auricle is replanted by suturing the edge of the anterior lateral avulsion rim in its normal anatomic position with absorbable interrupted sutures for the cartilage and 5-0 nylon sutures for the skin (Fig. 3C). The edges of the postauricular flap are sutured to the skin edges of the decorticated pinna (Fig. 3D). The patient is given intravenous antibiotics for 5 to 7 days. If replantation is successful, the medial surface of the auricle is freed from the recipient bed 8 weeks after initial repair. A split-thickness skin graft is applied to the decorticated surface (Fig. 3E). Reconstruction of the ear lobe usually necessitates a separate procedure with a folded postauricular flap. Results appear to be comparable with those of other nonmicrosurgical techniques and include a less than perfect contour.

Closed Injury

Blunt trauma to the external ear can cause hematoma. Hematomas are found most often in the subperichondrial plane of the anterior portion of the auricle because the skin is tightly adherent to underlying perichondrium and cartilage. In the posterior aspect the skin is buttressed by a small amount of fat. Such hematomas can stimulate the formation of abundant fibrous tissue and new cartilage, resulting in an auricular deformity commonly called *cauliflower ear*. Prevention of this complication is best

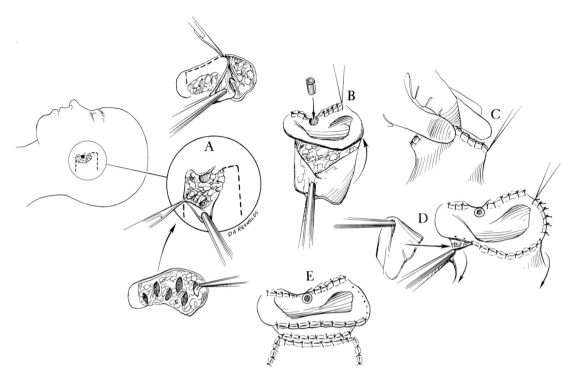

FIG. 3. Auricular replantation. **A:** Decortication of auricular skin and opening of multiple cartilage fenestrations. **B:** Elevation of postauricular flap, anterior reimplantation, and placement of canal stent. **C:** Suturing of auricular rim to elevated flap. **D:** Freeing of postauricular area and resurfacing with a split-thickness skin graft. **E:** Completed reconstruction.

effected with drainage of the hematoma followed by bolstering of the overlying skin. This may be achieved by means of needle aspiration followed by placement of a tight-fitting plastic mold or by means of incision, drainage, and insertion of a small drain (Fig. 4).

Frostbite

Auricular frostbite is rare except in arctic and subarctic climates. It occurs when exposure to freezing temper-

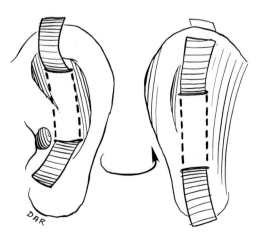

FIG. 4. Management of auricular hematoma with step-ladder incisions and drainage.

atures causes ice crystals to form within the soft tissues of the pinna. Depending on severity, frostbite injuries may be superficial or deep. Pathologic changes (8) are characterized by extreme vasoconstriction followed by subcutaneous edema and as thawing occurs formation of vesicles. Rewarming is associated with reestablishment of circulation, increased capillary permeability, and extravasation of fluid and red blood cells. Twenty to 72 hours after thawing, subcutaneous hemorrhage, edema and areas of devitalization become noticeable. Thereafter tissues revert to normal or progress to diffuse necrosis. Sessions et al. (9) conducted a study of 32 patients with frostbite of the ear. Although the length of time and degree of temperature exposure varied widely (−19°F to −42°F) wind chill factors appeared to play an important role in the severity of the injury. The authors recommended rapid thawing of the auricle by means of application of sterile cotton pledgets maintained at 100°F to 108°F.

Analgesics and sedatives are indicated in the treatment of patients with frostbite of the ear because pain may be associated with rapid rewarming. After emergency treatment the patient is hospitalized with sterile precautions to prevent infection. Intravenous antibiotics are used when deep injuries are diagnosed or suspected. Débridement is contraindicated in the early stage of frostbite. Twenty-four of the patients in the study by Sessions et al. (9) had a superficial injury and recovered without permanent deformity. Eight patients had a deep injury that led to variable degrees of tissue loss, predominantly affecting the helix. Poor prognostic signs are cyanosis, late appearance of dark vesicles, and mummification. A favorable outcome is expected when the auricle retains good color and superficial sensation and when large, clear vesicles occur early in the course of treatment.

Burns

The auricle is involved in 40% to 90% of all facial burns (10,11). These injuries require special attention because the dearth of subcutaneous tissue in the auricle makes it susceptible to severe damage, even when exposed to relatively mild offending agents. Identification of the cause of injury is important. Hot water scalds usually cause second-degree burns; exposure to flame nearly always produces full-thickness loss. Grease and tar burns usually cause second- and third-degree lesions.

Early diagnosis of the degree of injury is critical. First-degree burns, which are characterized by erythema without bleb formation, generally are managed conservatively with antibiotic cream. Patients with second-degree injuries are treated early with conservative débridement and topical antimicrobial agents. Débridement should not continue after initial treatment; eschar that forms should be allowed to separate spontaneously. Dressings and pressure are to be avoided because they may prevent revascularization and cause further cartilage necrosis and infection.

A unique complication of auricular burns is the development of suppurative chondritis, which occurs in as many as one fourth of cases (10–12). Chondritis is suspected in the presence of persistent pain, increased erythema, and swelling. This complication can occur even after the onset of healthy reepithelialization in an apparently sterile field. *Pseudomonas aeruginosa* and *Staphylococcus aureus* are the most frequently cultured infectious agents. Excision of all necrotic cartilage is essential. Appropriate intravenous antibiotic therapy is instituted, but the lack of vascular supply to the affected areas often makes it ineffective. Topical administration of antibiotics after open packing of the defect is continued until healing is complete.

INJURIES TO THE EXTERNAL EAR CANAL

Abrasions, small lacerations, and hematomas generally require no treatment other than topical administration of antiseptics or antibiotics. If flaps of canal skin are elevated, an attempt is made to replace them with absorbable gelatin foam (Gelfoam). An alternative is packing petroleum-impregnated fabric of viscose filament (Adaptic) into the canal for several days to hold the flaps in place. Transection of the ear canal at the osseous-cartilaginous junction frequently is seen in deep lacerations and near

avulsions of the pinna. Splinting with a rubber or silicone tube sutured in place (see Figs. 1 and 3B) for 7 to 10 days prevents canal stenosis in most circumferential injuries. Close follow-up care is important to control the formation of granulation tissue at the line of laceration. When blunt head trauma has produced ear bleeding or external auditory canal tears, middle ear damage and temporal bone fracture are highly likely (see later).

Aggressive cleansing with cotton applicators is a common cause of external canal trauma. The swabs are wielded by persons who harbor the mistaken notion that regular cleaning of the external auditory canal with an applicator is an important part of personal hygiene. One result is that cerumen becomes impacted more deeply in the canal. Because the delicate skin of the canal is easily damaged, infection is promoted. Other injuries such as perforation of the tympanic membrane with ossicular or even facial nerve injury have been caused by these applicators. Consequently the cotton applicator has no use in the ear. The outer ear may be cleaned with a washcloth wrapped over the index finger. For persons with troublesome cerumen accumulation, a trained person can clean the ear periodically under direct vision. If the patient has a history of otorrhea or tympanic membrane perforation, irrigation must be avoided. Debris may be washed into the middle ear through an unseen perforation, or the delicate neomembrane of a healed perforation may be ruptured by the irrigating stream.

TRAUMATIC PERFORATION OF THE TYMPANIC MEMBRANE

Etiology

Perforation of the tympanic membrane is a common injury that can have a variety of causes, including (a) direct trauma by foreign objects, such as cotton applicators, pencils, paper clips, flying objects, or irrigation of the external auditory canal; (b) concussive injury from an explosion or a blow to the ear that suddenly compresses the air within the external auditory canal; (c) barotrauma; and (d) temporal bone fractures. Any of these may produce varying types and sizes of perforations, ranging from minute tears of the pars tensa to massive injuries involving the tympanic membrane, ossicular chain, labyrinthine windows, and facial nerve.

Diagnosis

Accurate and early diagnosis is important in the management of traumatic perforations of the tympanic membrane. The mechanism of injury usually is apparent from the history. Careful examination of the external auditory canal and tympanic membrane with good lighting and magnification (see Chapter 7) helps identify the type and extent of the perforation. Blood and debris may be removed from the canal by means of sterile suction but never by means of irrigation. Particular attention is given to documenting facial nerve and audiovestibular function at initial presentation. This is important before any sedation or intubation of patients with multiple trauma. Hearing status as determined with audiologic studies gives information about possible concomitant injury to the ossicular chain or cochlea. Assessment by means of tuning fork responses can give a good initial impression of the degree and type of hearing loss. Computed tomography (CT) of the temporal bone is essential to evaluate the extent of injury and the possibility of preexisting disease.

Management

A small traumatic perforation that occupies no more than one quadrant of the tympanic membrane, is accompanied by less than 30 dB conductive hearing loss, and has no other sequelae, often can be managed by means of simple paper patching of the perforation as an outpatient procedure. It may be advisable to delay patching for several days after the injury to make sure that there is no foreign body in the middle ear. A sterile piece of cotton is kept in the external auditory canal, and the patient is advised to prevent water from entering the ear.

Very small perforations (less than 2 mm) the edges of which are not curled inward usually close spontaneously without any special treatment. If the perforation remains dry but shows no signs of closing after 4 weeks and if the margins can be easily seen, patching may be performed (Fig. 5). A 3- to 4-mm disk of cigarette paper is moist-

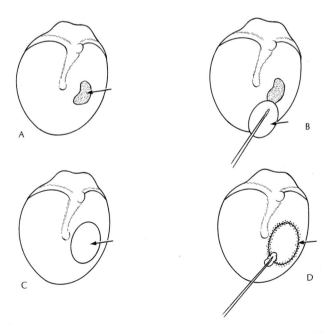

FIG. 5. A–D: Technical steps in paper patching of a small perforation of the tympanic membrane.

ened with 10% silver nitrate and picked up simply by touching it with a fine, cotton-tipped, metal applicator also dampened with silver nitrate. The paper is introduced through a speculum and manipulated into position so that it covers the perforation completely with a margin of at least 1.5 mm. The mildly irritating effect of the silver nitrate stimulates proliferation of the squamous layer of the tympanic membrane. The paper acts as scaffolding under which the epithelium tends to grow. A disk of absorbable gelatin film (Gelfilm) also may be used as a patch. This approach is effective in approximately half of cases. If posttreatment audiometry reveals closure of the air–bone gap, substantial concomitant injury to the ossicular chain is unlikely. A second procedure may be necessary if the patch migrates off the tympanic membrane before healing is complete. A good alternative is adipose tissue myringoplasty, which may be performed as an office procedure under local anesthesia. Careful observation is important to detect secondary infection. If application of a patch is followed by purulent middle ear drainage, the patch is immediately removed and not replaced until the infection is controlled with systemic antibiotic therapy. Large and persistent perforations are managed by means of myringoplasty (see Chapter 27).

Complications

Penetration of the tympanic membrane with a contaminated instrument or from a blast inevitably introduces pathogenic bacteria into the middle ear with or without gross foreign matter. As long as canal irrigation and excessive manipulation are avoided, the incidence of infection is surprisingly low. When otorrhea develops, *S. aureus* or *P. aeruginosa* is the most common organism cultured. Oral antibiotics are initially tried. Otorrhea not controlled with oral antibiotics necessitates parenteral antibiotic therapy and less frequently surgical treatment. In the long-term care of these patients, one must be alert to the possibility of posttraumatic cholesteatoma. This complication may be present even with a dry perforation, minimal hearing loss, and a well-pneumatized mastoid process. Such cholesteatomas are uncommon but have been described as occurring anywhere from the external canal to the middle ear or mastoid process (see later).

SLAG INJURY

Certain occupations, such as welding, involve the hazard of injury from flying beads of hot metal, which produce perforations accompanied by burns of the tympanic membrane and middle ear mucosa (Fig. 6). Because small bits of metal may be hidden within the middle ear, neither patching nor simple myringoplasty suffices. Careful middle ear exploration and in some instances mastoid exploration may be needed before grafting. Repair of slag injuries is less successful than that of uncomplicated per-

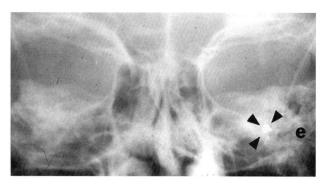

FIG. 6. Plain radiograph shows welding material in the left middle ear space (*arrows*). *e*, External ear canal.

foration, probably because vascular insult to the remaining tympanic membrane prevents ingrowth of viable epithelium. Adequate débridement of the rim of the perforation and mechanical abrasion of the undersurface of the remnant (in medial techniques) are critical for graft take. Burns of the facial nerve may complicate slag injuries.

INJURY TO THE OSSICULAR CHAIN

All the mechanisms described in connection with traumatic perforation of the tympanic membrane may be associated with injuries to the ossicular chain, even without actual rupture of the membrane. Violent, closed-head injuries, especially if the temporal bone is fractured, also can disrupt the ossicular chain. In such instances bleeding from the ear and a period of unconsciousness frequently occur. Considerable damage to the ossicular chain usually produces conductive hearing loss (30 to 60 dB), which does not improve when the tympanic membrane perforation is patched. When the tympanic membrane is intact, impedance audiometry is helpful in detecting ossicular discontinuity (Fig. 7).

The most common traumatic lesion of the ossicular chain is dislocation of the incudostapedial joint with or without fracture of the long process of the incus (see later). The injury is common because of the fragile nature of the joint. However, virtually any imaginable ossicular fracture or dislocation may be found. Surgical exploration for ossicular repair is not urgent and is delayed until hemotympanum, soft-tissue reaction, and posttraumatic effusion have resolved. The various tympanoplasty techniques are discussed in Chapter 27.

TEMPORAL BONE FRACTURES

Fractures involving the temporal bone are the most common fractures of the skull base. Ulrich (13) in 1926 was the first to classify these fractures as longitudinal or transverse according to their relation to the long axis of the petrous pyramid. In 1959 McHugh (14) modified this classification by recognizing mixed fractures as distinct clinical and pathologic entities. The classic distribution of fractures of the temporal bone into longitudinal, transverse, and mixed remains practical for routine clinical use. However, detailed histopathologic studies (15) and the advent of high-resolution CT have greatly improved our understanding of these lesions and challenged the validity of the established classification. Aguilar et al. (16) in a retrospective CT assessment of temporal bone fractures associated with facial nerve dysfunction found that nearly 70% did not fall within traditionally recognized patterns. Ghorayeb and Yeakley (17) proposed that most longitudinal fractures (to date accepted as the most prevalent) actually are oblique. They pointed out that the emphasis on the long axis of the temporal bone as a point of reference does not include the fracture line on the external surface of the skull and restricts it to an artificial vertical plane without tridimensional perspective. In this chapter we adhere to the classic terminology but include these concepts in the discussion of longitudinal fractures.

Longitudinal Fractures

Both longitudinal and oblique fractures run parallel to the long axis of the petrous ridge (Figs. 8–10A) and together account for 75% to 80% of temporal bone fractures. They are usually produced by a blow to the side of the head with the oblique fracture running in a horizontal plane and the longitudinal fracture in a vertical plane. In oblique lesions the fracture extends from the squama through the lateral surface of the mastoid process and divides the external auditory canal into an upper and a lower half. It extends into the glenoid fossa anteriorly and crosses the attic superiorly, breaking the tegmen as it runs parallel to the long axis of the petrous bone. Throughout its course the fracture may involve the facial nerve at the geniculate ganglion, the osseous portion of the eustachian tube, and the carotid canal. Oblique fractures do not involve the inferior surface of the temporal bone. In contrast, true longitudinal fractures extend from the squama

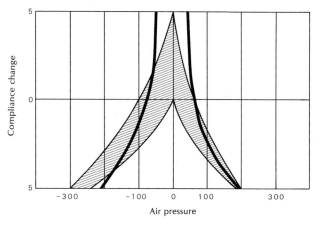

FIG. 7. Open-ended tympanogram in ossicular discontinuity.

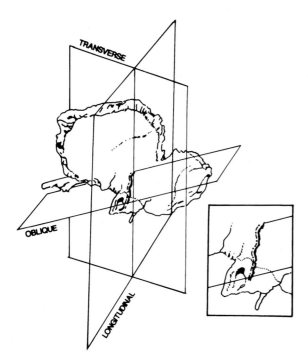

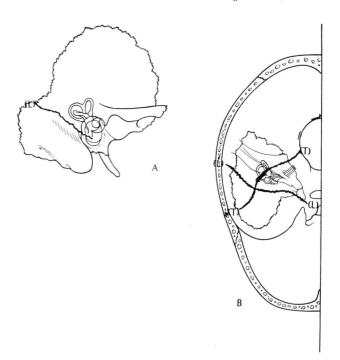

FIG. 8. Oblique, longitudinal, and transverse fracture planes. The right temporal bone is drawn from a medial perspective. The *icon* shows the oblique fracture line (*solid line*), the longitudinal fracture line (*semidotted*), and the transverse fracture line (*dotted line*). The oblique and longitudinal fracture lines are identical in the middle fossa. (From Ghorayeb BY, Yeakley JW. Temporal bone fractures: longitudinal or oblique temporal bone fractures. *Laryngoscope* 1992;102:129–134, with permission.)

FIG. 9. A: Longitudinal fracture running along the squama of the right temporal bone and extending into the posterior-superior wall of the external auditory canal. **B:** Principal lines of rupture in the longitudinal (*L*) and transverse (*T*) types of temporalis fracture.

into the external auditory canal, through the superior portion of the auricular rim into the attic at the level of the incudomalleolar joint, and above the horizontal facial canal into the geniculate ganglion. At the inferior external surface of the temporal bone the fracture follows the petrotympanic fissure and runs anteromedially between the carotid canal and foramen spinosum toward the clivus. In the middle cranial fossa the fracture line is no different from that of an oblique fracture as it courses along the axis of the petrous pyramid.

Fractures that parallel the long axis of the petrous bone usually exhibit a bloody discharge in the external auditory canal that issues from posterosuperior perforation of the tympanic membrane. Battle's sign often is present, and a fracture line may be seen as a stepoff along the posterior-superior aspect of the external auditory canal (Fig. 10B; see color plate 31 following page 484). This defect may extend into the tympanic ring. When the facial nerve is involved (20% to 25% of instances), paralysis often is delayed or is incomplete and rarely progresses to neurotmesis; lacrimation usually is intact. Hearing loss is predominantly conductive and is caused by perforation of the tympanic membrane, hemotympanum, or ossicular damage (Fig. 10C). Mild high-

frequency sensorineural loss may be present and usually is caused by cochlear concussion. Vestibular symptoms seldom are severe, although positional vertigo may persist for many months. Cerebrospinal fluid (CSF) otorrhea is common but usually resolves in a few days or weeks.

Transverse Fractures

Transverse fractures (Figs. 9B, 11) usually are caused by blows to the occipital bone. They represent 15% to 20% of all temporal bone fractures. The fracture line begins in the posterior fossa at or near the foramen magnum, crosses the petrous ridge through the internal auditory canal or the otic capsule, and slants anteriorly to end in the middle cranial fossa near the foramen lacerum. Transverse fractures exhibit a hemotympanum with an intact tympanic membrane. Facial paralysis is present in approximately 50% of patients and appears immediately. There is diminished tearing in the ipsilateral eye as a result of disruption of the facial nerve in the internal auditory canal; recovery often is incomplete. CSF leaks are uncommon. Hearing loss generally is sensorineural and profound because the otic capsule is fractured, but the loss sometimes may be mixed. Vertigo with spontaneous nystagmus is severe until compensation for the destroyed labyrinth occurs.

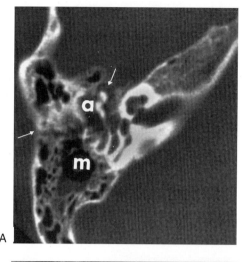

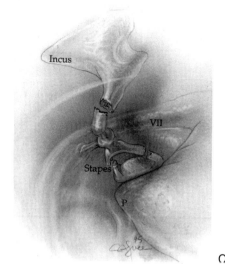

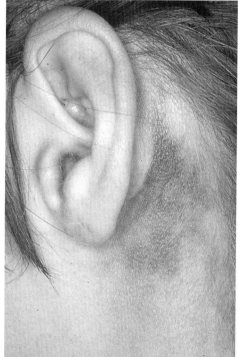

FIG. 10. A: Longitudinal fracture of the temporal bone (*arrows*). Fracture extends into the mastoid process (*m*) and attic (*a*). Ossicular dislocation is present. **B:** Postauricular ecchymosis (Battle's sign) in a longitudinal temporal bone fracture. **C:** Ossicular trauma associated with longitudinal temporal bone fracture.

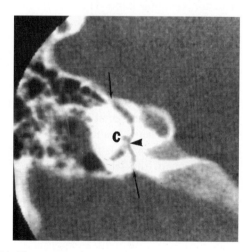

FIG. 11. Transverse fracture (*arrows*) with cochlear disruption (*arrowhead*). *c,* Cochlea.

Mixed Fractures

Pure longitudinal or transverse fractures as described earlier rarely occur but are identified on the basis of their clinical features and predominant lines of rupture. The term *mixed fracture* is used to define lesions in which such predominant lines are not apparent. Complex traumatic lesions of the temporal bone result from severe crushing blows to the head and account for approximately 5% of all fractures of the temporal bone. More than one fourth of these severe injuries are bilateral and are characterized by multiple, irregular breaks involving the middle and inner ear structures in unpredictable combinations. If caused by gunshot injuries, the bony fragments are comminuted and lie anywhere within the temporal bone (see later).

Temporal Bone Fractures in Children

Temporal bone fractures in children are classified the same way as fractures in adults. In 1973 Mitchell and Stone (18) evaluated 1,015 children admitted to a neurosurgical unit because of head trauma. They found that 71 children (7%) had sustained a temporal bone fracture. In 1979 Shapiro (19) evaluated 50 children with temporal bone fractures that occurred in an urban setting. Most patients were 3 to 9 years of age, and there was a distinct male prevalence (68%). Longitudinal fractures were most frequent with an 87.5% incidence; 12.5% of the patients had transverse fractures, and no mixed injuries were described. The most common sources of trauma were motor vehicle accidents (20) and falls (21). Total hearing loss occurred in 6 patients, all with transverse fractures. Partial hearing loss (more frequently sensorineural) occurred in 10 of 42 patients with longitudinal fractures. Facial nerve injury was rare; only one child had total paralysis that necessitated surgical treatment. No permanent perforation of the tympanic membrane occurred, and cerebrospinal otorrhea, which occurred among 45% of the patients, resolved spontaneously in all instances. These findings were corroborated in part by Williams et al. (22) in a study of 27 fractures among 25 children. In this series the prevalent causative agent also was a motor vehicle accident (60% of cases). Williams et al. differentiated longitudinal and oblique fractures and found the most common type was oblique, occurring among 22 patients (88%). One patient had a longitudinal fracture and 2 (8%) had transverse fractures. Conductive hearing loss was present in two thirds of the patients and sensorineural or mixed loss in the rest. The facial nerve was involved in 8 patients (32%), 6 having complete paralysis. Two needed surgical repair.

Analysis of the available information reveals that most temporal bone fractures in children parallel the long axis of the petrous pyramid. These lesions appear to have a better outcome than those in adults; children have a lower incidence of permanent hearing loss and facial nerve dysfunction. Most patients do not need corrective surgical treatment. Complete facial paralysis must be closely evaluated because it is the most common indication for intervention.

Gunshot Injuries

The rise of violent crime has resulted in an increased incidence of temporal bone injuries. Newton et al. (23) analyzed the combined experience of several institutions (including ours) with gunshot wounds of this structure. The charts of 22 patients who survived their injuries were reviewed. Most were young, male crime victims. The most common site of entrance was the infraorbital region with the projectile trajectory running obliquely and laterally into the petrous or mastoid bone.

Most fractures resulting from gunshot wounds are of the mixed variety. Anacusis is frequent, occurring among at least one third of patients. Approximately half of all patients experience facial nerve paralysis that necessitates surgical repair. Vascular damage involving either the carotid artery or the deep venous system occurs in one third of patients and brain injury in 36%.

Management of Temporal Bone Fractures

The basic steps in the management of temporal bone fractures and their complications are presented. The specific management of traumatic perforation of the tympanic membrane, ossicular damage, facial paralysis, and posttraumatic vertigo are discussed in Chapters 27, 42, and 46.

General Principles

Immediate treatment of a patient with head trauma involves a multidisciplinary approach with collaboration on the part of an emergency department physician, general surgeon, neurosurgeon, otolaryngologist, ophthalmologist, and others. Airway maintenance, resuscitation, evaluation, and management of intracranial and vital organ injuries take precedence over otologic problems.

If blood or CSF is draining from the ear, a temporal bone fracture is presumed. A sterile bandage is applied, and further evaluation is deferred until the patient's general condition is stable. Facial nerve function is evaluated as early as possible because the time of onset of traumatic facial paralysis dictates treatment (see Chapter 46). As soon as is practical the affected ear is examined under the microscope and cleaned with sterile instruments. Part of the initial examination includes gross assessment of hearing (whispered voice, fingers rubbed together, and tuning fork tests) and a check for nystagmus. Audiometric, vestibular, and special radiographic studies are performed as soon as the patient's condition allows.

Cerebrospinal Fluid Otorrhea

Management of CSF otorrhea requires close cooperation between otologist and neurosurgeon. Even when mixed with blood, CSF otorrhea can be detected by means of allowing a drop of the discharge to fall on a piece of filter paper, paper towel, or bed linen. CSF migrates faster than blood, leaving a characteristic double ring or halo sign. Strict sterile procedures are followed in examinations of the ear, and a dry, sterile mastoid dressing is placed for protection.

Most cases of posttraumatic CSF otorrhea respond to conservative management consisting of bed rest with head elevation (when possible), drainage of CSF through an indwelling subarachnoid catheter, and dehydrating agents such as acetazolamide. The use of prophylactic antibiotics is controversial.

At least 2 weeks should elapse before surgical intervention. Patients with persistent CSF otorrhea are best examined by means of contrast CT. Fractures of the tegmen tympani or tegmen mastoideum sometimes can be approached through mastoidectomy, and sealing of the leak is achieved with a tissue graft. This procedure may obviate craniotomy. If the fracture is more medial or extensive, a middle fossa approach or formal temporal craniotomy may be necessary to visualize the entire rim and edges of the fracture and achieve adequate closure.

Traumatic Encephalocele and Meningocele

The management of traumatic encephalocele and meningocele depends on its anatomic location (middle or posterior cranial fossa) and whether treatment is immediate or delayed.

Middle Cranial Fossa Defects

The tissue found during the acute phase of trauma usually is composed of traumatized meningeal and cortical brain tissue (Fig. 12). Reduction from the mastoid side is hampered by comminution and instability of the bone fragments surrounding the defect and in general is better accomplished at a later date, after inflammatory changes have subsided. However, the problem may have to be addressed acutely when the injury is associated with facial nerve trauma. In some instances middle fossa craniotomy may be needed to minimize risk for temporal lobe

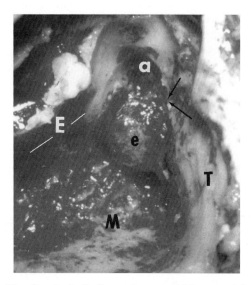

FIG. 12. Surgical findings in a middle cranial fossa encephalocele. *T,* Tegmen; *E,* external ear canal; *a,* attic; *M,* mastoid process; *e,* encephalocele; *arrows,* tegmental fracture line.

injury. Chronic encephaloceles usually are composed of devitalized neural tissue. If the defect is stable, chronic encephaloceles can be debulked by means of low-intensity bipolar cauterization and gently reduced. Bone from the mastoid cortex is shaped so that it can be carefully wedged into the defect to close it.

Posterior Cranial Fossa Defects

Posterior cranial fossa defects are less frequent than middle cranial fossa defects. They tend to occur in complex temporal bone fractures and in those caused by gunshot wounds. Definitive management usually is based on mastoid obliteration. Adipose tissue is most frequently used. These patients are at high risk for posttraumatic cholesteatoma (see later), and close follow-up evaluation over many years is mandatory.

Intracranial Suppuration

Meningitis or intracranial abscesses may occur during the acute phase of injury even when antibiotics are used prophylactically. Late meningitis can occur after temporal bone fractures. The risk is higher in transverse breaks, probably because of inability of the otic capsule to undergo complete osseous regeneration. The fibrous callous thus formed may be insufficient to isolate the intracranial structures from the middle ear–mastoid complex. Tympanomastoiditis, which is not uncommon after traumatic distortion of temporal bone structures, may result in direct extension of infection through this weakened barrier into the brain. Management of these complications is addressed in Chapter 26.

Conductive Hearing Loss

Injuries to the ossicles and tympanic membrane are best managed after resolution of all acute problems, provided there is evidence of serviceable cochlear function. Early middle ear reconstruction often is made difficult by immature scars, incompletely resolved inflammation, and excessive bleeding. Myringoplasty sometimes is performed in a deaf ear to allow an active patient to engage in water sports and prevent chronic infection.

Cholesteatoma

We have found it difficult to estimate the incidence of posttraumatic cholesteatoma because many patients are not available for follow-up studies. We treated 6 patients with this complication, all with severe, complex fractures. Our experience is similar to that of Brookes and Graham (24), who described 3 patients with cholesteatoma of the external auditory canal after skull base fractures. Most cholesteatomas are caused by posttraumatic stenosis, which traps squamous epithelium medial to a ring of fibrous tissue. Gunshot wounds can produce temporal bone cholesteatoma by means of direct implantation of squamous epithelium. These lesions can become symptomatic as early as 2 years after injury. Middle ear epithelial pearls have been found in 2.8% of tympanoplasties for nonhealing traumatic perforations of the tympanic membrane. Invasive cholesteatoma has been reported in as many as 4.8% of posttraumatic perforations among soldiers injured by military blasts (20). Posttraumatic cholesteatoma tends to be large because it occupies a mastoid complex that is not contracted by prior ear infections. Treatment is surgical and frequently involves canal-wall-down mastoidectomy.

BLAST INJURY

Blast trauma is defined as an injury resulting from a sudden explosion. The degree of damage depends on the rate and intensity of pressure-wave buildup and the duration of the pressure wave. Perforation of the tympanic membrane and middle-ear damage are common. Some degree of sensorineural hearing loss with tinnitus is almost universal. The high frequencies are most severely affected, and there is a strong tendency toward rapid spontaneous improvement over the first few hours. The main recovery process is complete within a few days, but some improvement may continue over a period of 6 months or more. After a year any residual loss is considered permanent. Attempts have been made to reduce the amount of permanent hearing loss after blast injury by using steroids, vasodilators, or low-molecular-weight dextran, but compelling evidence for the beneficial effect of these drugs is lacking. Vertigo is unusual after blast exposure and if present suggests perilymphatic fistula.

LABYRINTHINE CONCUSSION

Marked hearing loss with or without vestibular symptoms may be caused by head trauma, even without a demonstrable skull fracture. According to Schuknecht and Davidson (21) labyrinthine concussion occurs most frequently in ears with longitudinal temporal bone fractures. Next in frequency are ears opposite a temporal bone fracture and head trauma without fracture. In the last group of patients auditory damage usually is caused by occipital injury severe enough to produce loss of consciousness.

Characteristic symptoms of labyrinthine concussion are hearing impairment, tinnitus (usually high frequency), aural fullness, and vertigo. Audiometry reveals a variable degree of sensorineural hearing loss maximal in the 4 to 6 kHz range. Special audiometric tests usually indicate a predominantly cochlear loss. Electronystagmography may demonstrate spontaneous nystagmus beating away from the affected ear and ipsilateral vestibular paresis. Hearing loss may be transient or permanent. Some degree of improvement in tinnitus and auditory perception is experienced by most patients with mild to moderate injuries. The duration and degree of vestibular imbalance vary but are distinctly age related. Vartiainen et al. (25) in a study with a group of 61 children 16 years of age or younger showed that only 1.5% of the patients reported dizziness 6 months after injury. Among adults both early and late symptoms are more pronounced and tend to last longer. Some elderly patients may not recover completely. Positional vertigo sometimes is a sequela of labyrinthine concussion (see Chapter 40).

The pathologic changes associated with labyrinthine concussion have been investigated extensively. As early as 1932 Wittmaack (26) demonstrated degenerative changes in the organ of Corti and cochlear neurons in the middle turn of the cochlea of cats receiving skull blows of varying severity. Schuknecht et al. (27) obtained behavioral audiograms on 9 cats subjected to blows to the skull. These animals exhibited hearing losses that were more pronounced in the high frequencies (4 to 8 kHz) and pathologic changes in the middle and basal turns of the cochlea. These ranged from mild alterations of the external hair cells to loss of internal hair cells and flattening or even disappearance of the organ of Corti. In 1964 Igarashi et al. (28) described the temporal bone findings of a patient who had sustained a severe concussion at 53 years of age. Audiometry demonstrated sensorineural loss predominant at 4 kHz and histopathologic loss of external hair cells in the corresponding cochlear turn.

The precise mechanisms of cochlear injury are unclear. The most popular hypothesis is that a blow to the head produces a high-pressure wave that is transmitted to the cochlea by bone conduction. The resulting pathologic process would be analogous to that caused by intense auditory stimuli, a concept predicated on the similarity of changes and site of damage for both types of insult.

The mechanism of injury in vestibular concussion is unclear. Schuknecht and Davidson (21) showed rupture of the utricle and saccule in the ear of a cat that had sustained a blow that produced rapid acceleration of the head. Structural alterations in the cytoarchitecture of the lateral vestibular nuclei (28) and petechial hemorrhages of the brain, brainstem, and cerebellum (29,30) also have been demonstrated in experimental head injuries. According to Schuknecht (31) attacks of positional vertigo, which often occur after concussion, may be caused by disruption of the otolithic membrane of the utricle. Detached otoconia may be trapped in the ampulla of the posterior semicircular canal and produce displacement of the cupula with certain head movements (see Chapter 40).

Immediate management of labyrinthine concussion follows the general principles recommended for severe head trauma. Treatment of the ear itself includes bed rest and symptomatic medication such as meclizine hydrochloride (25 mg by mouth three times a day) or other antivertiginous drugs. Appropriate studies to exclude the presence of temporal bone fracture follows otologic evaluation, including examination under a surgical microscope and basic audiometry.

Middle ear injury and CSF leaks must be excluded. If they are present, appropriate treatment is instituted (see earlier). Isolated concussion is managed expectantly. No study has adequately documented the beneficial use of corticosteroids. However, if no contraindications exist, a short course of prednisone therapy may be considered. In cases of persistent vestibular abnormalities a traumatic perilymphatic fistula may be present and necessitate middle ear exploration (see Chapters 31 and 43). In addition to meclizine hydrochloride, 2 mg to 5 mg diazepam combined with 25 mg promethazine hydrochloride every 8 hours is beneficial symptomatic therapy. In addition to rest and medication Cawthorne's vestibular exercises are valuable after the acute phase of injury (see Chapter 42).

LIGHTNING INJURIES

The devastating force of lightning may cause temporal bone injury through mechanisms that are not yet known. Persons struck by lightning often have burns of the external auditory canal, rupture of the tympanic membrane, ossicular damage, sensorineural hearing loss, vestibular disturbances, and facial nerve injury. In a lightning-damaged temporal bone Bergstrom et al. (32) found hemorrhage and inflammatory exudate in the middle ear and mastoid, perforation of the tympanic membrane, rupture of Reissner's membrane, degenerative changes in the stria vascularis, and facial nerve edema within the internal auditory meatus. These findings represented an extreme degree of an injury that resulted in death. In lesser injuries general initial management includes aural hygiene and prevention of infection. Perforations of the tympanic membrane may be patched with paper or absorbable gelatin film after elevation of infolded edges. However, because of the compromised vascularity caused by burning of local tissues, definitive tympanoplasty is deferred to allow revascularization. There is little experience with facial nerve palsy complicating lightning injury. The possibility of severe thermal injury to the nerve must be taken into account during the initial evaluation of the patient. Such an injury carries a poor prognosis and might necessitate resection of the burned area (if identifiable) and replacement with an interposition graft. The general principles of management of traumatic facial nerve paralysis apply (see Chapter 46).

BAROTRAUMA

A special category of otologic trauma is caused by relatively gradual changes in ambient pressure. Because of the frequency of airplane travel and the increased popularity of deep-sea diving, barotrauma has become an important clinical problem. Damage to the external, middle, and inner ear may occur.

External Ear

Obstruction of the external auditory canal by cerumen or tight-fitting ear plugs during a dive may produce blood-filled vesicles, sometimes with a bloody discharge. These injuries may be painful but are rarely serious and require no treatment.

Middle Ear

When extratympanic pressure decreases in aircraft ascent or after diving, air expands in the middle ear and increases its relative pressure. Equalization occurs passively as air escapes through the eustachian tube to limit buildup of relative positive pressure in the middle ear and effectively prevent injury. During descent, the eustachian tube must actively open by means of muscular contraction or forced inflation (modified Valsalva maneuver or politzerization) to prevent a sustained pressure gradient across the tympanic membrane. When the pressure differential exceeds 90 mm Hg, muscular action can no longer open the eustachian tube, and it is said to become locked. If inflation is not achieved, the tympanic membrane retracts, and otalgia occurs. The process is encouraged by preexisting eustachian tube dysfunction from mucosal congestion (upper respiratory infection, allergy), otitis media, mechanical obstruction (mucosal polyps, surgical scarring), or simply congenital variations in size and patency of the eustachian tubes. Mounting pressure eventually ruptures the tympanic membrane. Keller (33) in a cadaveric study found that pressure differences between 100 to 500 mm Hg were needed to produce a laceration of the tympanic membrane, a ratio that correlates with seawater depths exceeding 4 feet (1.3 m). Farmer (34,35) classifies patients with middle ear barotrauma into three types. Type I patients have mild ear fullness and discomfort and normal otoscopic findings. Type II patients have more severe symptoms, including otalgia and hearing loss; otoscopy reveals tympanic membrane erythema, serous effusion, or hemotympanum. Type III patients have severe middle ear symptoms and perforation of the tympanic membrane.

Therapy for barotitis is based on the use of systemic and intranasal decongestants, antibiotics if infection is present in the ears or nasopharynx, and gentle politzerization as long as the nasopharynx is free of infection.

Myringotomy, with or without intubation, is performed when medical management fails.

Prevention of barotrauma is more desirable than management. Patients are discouraged from flying or diving with upper respiratory infections or during severe nasal episodes of allergies. Airplane passengers should remain awake during descent and actively engage in maneuvers to exercise the eustachian tube (chewing, swallowing, yawning). A gentle Valsalva maneuver (forcible expiration against closed mouth and nose) or the safer but more difficult Frenzel maneuver (contracting muscles of floor of mouth and pharynx with the glottis, mouth, and nose closed) may be added if necessary. Systemic decongestants or topical intranasal vasoconstrictors used 0.5 to 1 hour before descent are helpful. When barotrauma is recurrent, special attention should be paid to correction of obstructive nasal and pharyngeal lesions (polyps, septal deviations), allergies, and chronic sinus infections. The occasional patient who must continue to fly despite recurrent aerotitis resistant to the foregoing measures may need long-term insertion of a transtympanic ventilation tube.

A special type of barotitis media may occur 2 or more hours after breathing high concentrations of oxygen. As the oxygen in the middle ear is absorbed, relative negative pressure develops and causes the typical syndrome of barotitis unless the ears are adequately ventilated. This condition most commonly occurs among fliers who have gone to sleep soon after returning from a flight and awaken with ear pain.

Inner Ear

Compression Problems

When extratympanic pressure increases during descent, the tympanic membrane moves inward, the stapes is depressed into the oval window, and the displaced perilymph bulges the round window membrane outward. Passive opening of the eustachian tube readily equalizes positive intratympanic pressure. However, if this pressure change occurs rapidly or with great force, damage may be inflicted on the membranous structures within the otic capsule, producing sensorineural hearing loss or vertigo (35). A modified Valsalva maneuver performed to clear the ears very rapidly, pulls the stapes outward, reversing the perilymph flow. This is more likely to produce inner ear damage than a more gradual change in ambient pressure. A forceful Valsalva maneuver alone may produce a perilymphatic fistula.

So far all clinical reports of window rupture occurring during diving have involved the round window membrane and have usually resulted in both auditory and vestibular impairment (36,37). However, cases have been reported in which no hearing loss or acute vertigo has occurred or when only one of the two systems has been affected

(38,39). Parell and Becker (40) postulated that in such cases cochleolabyrinthine trauma may occur without oval or round window rupture and may be caused by inner ear bleeding. In patients with predominantly auditory symptoms the prognosis for hearing normalization is excellent. Support for inner ear hemorrhage as a cause of auditory symptoms can be found in several experimental studies. In guinea pigs subjected to ear barotrauma hemorrhage is more frequent in the cochlea than in the semicircular canals; the scala tympani at the basal turn is the prevalent site of damage (41,42).

Management of inner ear barotrauma includes bed rest with 30-degree head elevation. Straining, forceful nose blowing, and vigorous coughing are avoided. Exploratory tympanotomy for fistula identification and repair is controversial. Some authors advocate a period of conservative treatment with close observation, performing exploration only for patients whose condition does not improve or worsens (38,43). Other authors (44,45) believe prompt exploration is indicated when a positive fistula sign is present in association with progressive hearing loss and vestibular symptoms. We believe that prompt exploration is warranted when cochleovestibular symptoms are severe. Divers with permanent inner ear dysfunction should stop diving because further damage is more likely because of scar formation and altered vascularization; there is increased risk for vertigo, nausea, and vomiting; and injury to the undamaged ear may cause additional auditory and vestibular disability (34,35).

Problems at Stable Pressures

Nitrogen narcosis and oxygen poisoning occur as a result of increased partial pressures of nitrogen and oxygen, respectively, in the blood and other body tissues and therefore occur only in superatmospheric pressure situations (diving). Risk for these conditions is directly related to depth and time of exposure. Nitrogen narcosis produces an effect similar to that of alcohol intoxication, with euphoria, giddiness, impaired judgment, confusion, and disequilibrium. To prevent this syndrome, nitrogen is replaced by the less toxic gas helium during deep dives (46). The precise cause of oxygen toxicity is unknown, but it can cause nausea, vertigo, muscle twitching, auditory and visual disturbances, and sudden convulsions. The minimum depth at which oxygen poisoning may occur is about 40 feet (12 m) (47). Some toxic symptoms may develop after one breathes 10% oxygen at a total pressure as low as 380 mm Hg in subatmospheric pressure situations for prolonged periods (e.g., space flight) but data are incomplete (46).

The disturbance in equilibrium that occurs with nitrogen narcosis and oxygen toxicity appears to be related to central nervous system (CNS) effects rather than to any vestibular end-organ dysfunction, but these conditions must be kept in mind by the physician and the diver if dizziness occurs during descent or while the diver is on the bottom. Sudden changes in inspired inert gases at great depths also may lead to vertigo caused by end-organ damage or to CNS disturbance (46).

Problems during Decompression

As a diver or flier ascends, gases in the middle ear (and other body cavities) expand and increase relative to middle ear pressure. If equalization of pressure by the eustachian tube occurs asymmetrically in the two ears, so-called alternobaric vertigo and nystagmus may result. The precise mechanism for this phenomenon is not clear (48).

Cerebral air embolism is a CNS catastrophe in which vestibular symptoms play a minor role. It occurs when a diver does not exhale adequately during ascent. Expanding gases rupture alveoli and air bubbles escape into the arterial circulation. Immediate recompression may prevent permanent CNS damage or death.

Inner ear injuries with hearing loss, tinnitus, or vertigo may be the main or only manifestation of decompression sickness, or the bends, a condition related to the release of nitrogen bubbles into the bloodstream and other body tissues as the solubility of nitrogen is exceeded as pressure decreases (46). The greater the depth, the more nitrogen becomes dissolved and the more slowly the diver must ascend to allow the bubbles to dissipate and be expired in the lungs. Special tables are used to gauge the safe rate of ascent. Other symptoms include itching, paresthesia, joint pain, CNS disturbances (visual problems, paralysis, seizures), and dyspnea. If symptoms occur, prompt recompression is critical if permanent damage is to be avoided. It must be remembered, however, that decompression sickness does not occur in shallow dives (less than 30 feet [9 m]) no matter how long the submersion or how rapid the ascent, and other causes must be sought for symptoms that develop under these conditions. Inner ear injury that may have been sustained during descent brings to mind the possibility of labyrinthine window rupture, and recompression is contraindicated (35).

Decompression sickness may occur during aircraft ascent, but it usually is less severe than a descent during diving and rarely produces long-lasting symptoms. Several factors influence the development of subatmospheric bends. The rate of ascent is less critical than the rate in diving, but the altitude attained and duration of exposure are quite important. For example, decompression symptoms are rare below 20,000 feet (6,000 m). More than 90% of young healthy persons can tolerate 1 hour at 35,000 feet (10,500 m) without symptoms. After 1 hour at 40,000 feet (12,000 m) 20% have symptoms, and 45% cannot tolerate 35,000 feet for 4 hours. Tolerance diminishes with age and with obesity. Exercise increases susceptibility to decompression sickness, as does reexposure within 24 hours. This syndrome is effectively prevented by cabin pressurization

to less than 25,000 feet (7,500 m). Denitrogenization by means of breathing 100% oxygen before flight also is helpful. If the syndrome does occur, recompression by means of simple descent is curative in most instances. In severe cases compression to pressures greater than 1 atmosphere may be necessary.

IRRADIATION

Currently used therapeutic doses of ionizing irradiation to the temporal bone may produce acute and chronic changes. Early acute changes include serous otitis media and transient conductive hearing loss. Chronic changes include fibrosis, osteoradionecrosis, and cochlear damage.

Dias (49) and Schuknecht and Karmody (50) stated that the cochlea tends to be resistant to irradiation at the doses usually given for management of malignant tumors of the head and neck, but this resistance appears to decline when doses greater than 7 Gy are used (51). The effects of ionizing radiation to the inner ear have been under scrutiny since 1905, when Ewald (52) described findings similar to those of labyrinthectomy in pigeons that had radium seeds placed in their middle ears. The structural changes in the organ of Corti after the deliverance of 40 to 70 Gy to the inner ears of guinea pigs were first studied by Winther in 1969 (53). Using surface electron microscope techniques, he found extensive degeneration of the outer hair cells of the two basal turns of the cochlea as early as 6 hours after irradiation. The inner hair cells, the outer hair cells of the apical coils, and the supporting cells remained normal. Borsanyi et al. (54) in 1962 reported on human sensorineural hearing loss after radiation therapy.

In 1965 Leach (55) assessed cochlear damage in 56 patients who had undergone irradiation for head and neck cancer. He documented permanent hearing loss in 3 of 11 patients who were examined before and after treatment. Two of these patients experienced unilateral anacusis 1 and 3 months after treatment, and the other did so gradually over several years. Temporal bone specimens were available for 1 patient with profound hearing loss after high-dose irradiation. They showed diffuse atrophy of the organ of Corti in the treated ear. In 1976 Moretti (56) conducted a study with 137 patients who had received radiation therapy for malignant tumors of the head and neck. He found sensorineural hearing losses in 7 of 13 patients who underwent hearing tests before and after treatment. He concluded that the loss potentially induced by radiation therapy is gradual, sometimes occurring over several years. Moretti also found that all profound hearing losses occurred among patients who received huge doses of radiation (some more than 20,000 rad).

Hoistad et al. (51) compared the temporal bone findings for 5 patients with head and neck cancer who had received radiation with those for 4 patients who had been treated with cisplatinum chemotherapy, 2 who were treated with both modalities, and 4 age-matched healthy control subjects. Decreased numbers of spiral ganglion cells and loss of inner and outer hair cells were found in all treated specimens. Endothelial proliferation, hypertrophy, and fibrosis of vascular walls were found in arterioles around the facial nerve. Fibrotic changes in connective tissue appeared to progress over time. The authors concluded that irradiation and cisplatinum therapy can contribute to considerable temporal bone changes, including sensorineural hearing loss, serous effusion, and progressive fibrosis involving soft tissues and vessels.

Osteoradionecrosis is an infrequent but serious complication of radiation therapy to the temporal bone. Diffuse vascular changes are progressive and widespread, appear to be dose dependent, and likely occur when exposure exceeds 70 Gy (57). Radiation causes obliterative endovasculitis and thrombosis, primarily in small and medium-sized arterioles. These changes may be responsible for obliteration of involved vessels, death of osteocytes, oste-

olysis, a marked decrease in new bone formation, and in the petrous bone loss of marrow (50). Hoistad et al. (51) found some of these changes in all the temporal bones they studied; they also found fibrosis of the ossicular ligaments.

Osteoradionecrosis of the temporal bone tends to be progressive and complicated by fibrosis of the surrounding soft tissues, including the temporomandibular joint capsule, with resulting ankylosis and trismus. Unchecked it may progress along the skull base and is especially serious when the patient has undergone temporal bone resection. In these patients progressive destruction may lead to involvement of the carotid canal, rupture of the artery, and death. Osteoradionecrosis of the temporal bone is difficult to manage. It may be arrested when viable tissue, such as a rotation temporalis muscle flap, is brought in for coverage of exposed bone. Long-term antibiotic therapy and hyperbaric oxygen treatments may slow the process but are not curative.

SUMMARY POINTS

- When adequate vessels are available, complete avulsion of the pinna is best repaired by means of microvascular anastomosis. When vessels are not available, multiple-stage reconstruction with the severed auricle gives good results.
- Failure to drain promptly an auricular hematoma results in a hypertrophic deformity called cauliflower ear.
- Frostbite of the auricle is treated with rapid warming. Débridement is contraindicated in the early stages.
- The auricle is involved in 90% of facial burns. These injuries are frequently complicated by suppurative chondritis due to *P. aeruginosa* and *S. aureus.*
- Perforation of the tympanic membrane may be caused by direct injury, concussive trauma, barotrauma, and temporal bone fractures.
- Traumatic perforation of the tympanic membrane may heal spontaneously; otherwise it is managed with the paper patch technique, adipose tissue myringoplasty when small, or formal tympanoplasty when large.
- The most common traumatic ossicular lesion is incudostapedial dislocation.
- Temporal bone fractures are classified, according to the long axis of the petrous pyramid, as longitudinal, transverse, or complex.
- Longitudinal temporal bone fractures are the most common (75% to 85%) temporal bone fractures. They are frequently associated with conductive hearing loss. The facial nerve is involved in 20% to 25% of cases.
- The facial nerve is involved in 50% of transverse temporal bone fractures. These often are associated with sensorineural hearing loss.

- Other complications of temporal bone fractures include persistent tinnitus, CSF otorrhea, encephalocele, meningocele, intracranial suppuration, and cholesteatoma.
- Labyrinthine concussion may be caused by a high-pressure wave produced by a head blow that is transmitted to the cochlea through bone conduction.
- Barotrauma may cause damage to the external, middle, and inner ear. The inner ear may be injured by compression forces, which if they occur rapidly or with force may produce sensorineural hearing loss and vertigo, which may be caused by oval or round window rupture or bleeding.
- Inner ear injuries may be the main or only manifestation of decompression sickness, which is related to the release of nitrogen bubbles into the bloodstream.
- Ionizing irradiation primarily affects the outer hair cells of the basal turn and causes high-frequency sensorineural hearing loss. As a late result, osteoradionecrosis of the temporal bone may occur.
- The cochlea is relatively resistant to irradiation, but damage is dose related and appears to increase when treatment exceeds 70 Gy.
- Cochlear damage after radiation therapy may progress over months and years. Anacusis may occur but is infrequent.
- Osteoradionecrosis of the temporal bone appears to follow thrombosis and obliteration of small- and medium-caliber arterioles. A decrease in osteogenesis, death of osteocytes, osteolysis, and loss of petrous marrow are characteristic.

REFERENCES

1. Potsic WP, Naunton RF. Reimplantation of an amputated pinna. *Arch Otolaryngol* 1974;100:73–75.
2. Nahai F, Hayhurst JW, Salibian AH. Microvascular surgery in avulsive trauma to the external ear. *Clin Plast Surg* 1978;5:423–429.
3. Pennington DG, Lai MF, Pelly AD. Successful replantation of a completely avulsed ear by microvascular anastomosis. *Plast Reconstr Surg* 1980;65:820–827.
4. Mladick RA, Horton CE, Adamson JE, Cohen BI. The pocket principle: a new technique for the rear attachment of a severed ear. *Plast Reconstr Surg* 1971;48:219–223.
5. Bardsley AF. Primary reconstruction of a severed ear fragment using a flap of temporo-parietal fascia. *Br J Plast Surg* 1986;39:524–525.
6. Jenkins AM, Finucan T. Primary non-microsurgical reconstruction following ear avulsion using the temporoparietal facial island flap. *Plast Reconstr Surg* 1989;83:148–152.
7. Baudet J, Tramond P, Goumain A. A propos d'un procédé original de replantation d'un pavillon de l'oreille totalement separé. *Ann Chir Plast* 1972;17:67–72.
8. Lange K, Boyd CJ, Loewe L. The functional pathology of frostbite and prevention of gangrene in experimental animals and humans. *Science* 1945;102:151–520.
9. Sessions DG, Stallings JO, Mills WJ, Beal DD. Frostbite of the ear. *Laryngoscope* 1971;81:1223–1232.
10. Hammond JS, Ward GC. Burns of the head and neck. *Otolaryngol Clin North Am* 1983;16:679–696.
11. Dowling JA, Foley FD, Moncrief JA. Chondritis in the burned ear. *Plast Reconstr Surg* 1968;42:115–121.
12. Stewart RC, Benson ES. Chondritis of the ear: a method of treatment. *J Trauma* 1979;19:686–690.
13. Ulrich K. Verletzungen des Gehororgans bei schadelbasisfrakturen (eine histologische und klinissche Studie). *Acta Otolaryngol Suppl (Stockh)* 1926;6:1–150.
14. McHugh HE. The surgical treatment of facial paralysis and traumatic conductive deafness in fractures of the temporal bone. *Otolaryngol Head Neck Surg* 1989;101:404–408.
15. Khan AA, Marion M, Hinojosa R. Temporal bone fractures: a histopathologic study. *Otolaryngol Head Neck Surg* 1985;93:177–186.
16. Aguilar EA, Yeakley JW, Ghorayeb BY, et al. High resolution CT scan of temporal bone fractures: association of facial nerve paralysis with temporal bone fractures. *Head Neck Surg* 1987;9:162–166.
17. Ghorayeb BY, Yeakley JW. Longitudinal or oblique: the case for oblique temporal bone fractures. *Laryngoscope* 1992;102:129–134.
18. Mitchell DP, Stone P. Temporal bone fractures in children. *Can J Otolaryngol* 1973;2:156–162.
19. Shapiro RS. Temporal bone fractures in children. *Otolaryngol Head Neck Surg* 1979;87:323–329.
20. McKennan KX, Chole RD. Posttraumatic cholesteatoma. *Laryngoscope* 1989;99:779–783.
21. Schuknecht HF, Davidson RC. Deafness and vertigo from head injury. *Arch Otolaryngol* 1956;63:513–528.
22. Williams WT, Ghorayeb BY, Yeakley JW. Pediatric temporal bone fractures. *Laryngoscope* 1992;102:600–603.
23. Newton OD, Coker N, Jenkins HA, Canalis RF. Gunshot injuries of the temporal bone. *Otolaryngol Head Neck Surg* 1986;94:47–55.
24. Brookes GR, Graham MD. Posttraumatic cholesteatoma of the external ear canal. *Laryngoscope* 1984;94:667–670.
25. Vartiainen E, Karjalainen S, Karja J. Vestibular disorders following head injury in children. *Int J Pediatr Otorhinolaryngol* 1985;9:135–141.
26. Wittmaack K. Uber die traumatische labyrinthdegeneration. *Arch Ohr Nas Kehlkheilk* 1932;131:59–66.
27. Schuknecht H, Neff W, Pearlman H. An experimental study of auditory damage following blows to the head. *Ann Otol Rhinol Laryngol* 1951;60:273–283.
28. Igarashi M, Schuknecht HF, Myers E. Cochlear pathology in human with stimulation deafness. *J Laryngol Otol* 1964;78:115–129.
29. Windle W, Grat R, Fox C. Experimental structural alterations in the brain during and after concussion. *Surg Gynecol Obstet* 1944;79:561–572.
30. Kirikae I, Eguchi K, Okamoto M, Nakamura K. Histopathological changes in the auditory pathway in cases of fatal head injury. *Acta Otolaryngol (Stockh)* 1969;67:341–353.
31. Schuknecht HF. Cupulolithiasis. *Arch Otolaryngol* 1969;90:765–773.
32. Bergstrom L, Neblet L, Sando I, et al. The lightning damaged ear. *Arch Otolaryngol* 1974;100:117–121.
33. Keller AP. A study of relationship of air pressure to myringopuncture. *Laryngoscope* 1958;68:2015–2029.
34. Farmer JC. Ear and sinus problems in diving. In: Bove AA, Davis JC, eds. *Diving medicine,* 2nd ed. Philadelphia: WB Saunders, 1990:200–222.
35. Farmer JC. Otologic barotrauma. In: Britton BH, ed. *Common problems in otology.* St Louis: Mosby–Year Book, 1991:342–353.
36. Goodhill V, Harris I, Brockman S. Sudden deafness in labyrinthine window ruptures. *Ann Otol Rhinol Laryngol* 1973;82:2–12.
37. Seltzer S, McCabe BF. Perilymph fistula: the Iowa experience. *Laryngoscope* 1986;94:37–49.
38. Althans SR. Perilymph fistulas. *Laryngoscope* 1981;91:538–562.
39. Nakashima T, Arao H, Watanabe Y, Yanagita N. Clinical manifestation in labyrinthine window rupture: with reference to so-called "silent fistula." *Pract Otol* 1985;78:1023–1026.
40. Parell GJ, Becker GD. Conservation management of inner ear barotraumas resulting from scuba diving. *Otolaryngol Head Neck Surg* 1985;93:393–397.
41. Lamkin R, Axelsson A, McPharson D, Miller J. Experimental aural barotrauma: electrophysiological and morphological findings. *Acta Otolaryngol Suppl (Stockh)* 1975;335:1–24.
42. Nakashima T, Hob M, Sato M, Watanabe Y, Yanagita N. Auditory and vestibular disorders due to barotrauma. *Ann Otol Rhinol Laryngol* 1988;97:146–152.
43. Love JT, Waguesback RW. Perilymph fistulas. *Laryngoscope* 1981;91:1118–1128.
44. Pullen FW, Rosenberg GJ, Cabera CH. Sudden hearing loss in divers. *Laryngoscope* 1979;89:1372–1377.
45. Caruso VG, Winkelmann PE, Correia MJ, Miltenberger GE, Love JT. Otologic and otoneurologic injuries in divers: clinical studies on nine commercial and two sport divers. *Laryngoscope* 1977;87:508–521.
46. Farmer JC, Thomas WG, Youngblood DG, Bennett DB. Inner ear decompression sickness. *Laryngoscope* 1976;86:1315–1326.
47. Henry RF. Hyperbaric problems as they relate to divers. *Trans Am Acad Ophthalmol Otolaryngol* 1971;75:1322–1332.
48. Ingelsted FS, Ivarsson A, Tjerstrom O. Vertigo due to relative over pressure in the middle ear. *Acta Otolaryngol (Stockh)* 1974;78:1–14.
49. Dias A. Effects on the hearing of patients treated with irradiation of head and neck area. *J Laryngol Otol* 1966;80:276–287.
50. Schuknecht H, Karmody C. Radionecrosis of the temporal bone. *Laryngoscope* 1966;76:1416–1428.
51. Hoistad DL, Ondrey FG, Mutlu C, et al. Histopathology of human temporal bone after cis-platinum, radiation, or both. *Otolaryngol Head Neck Surg* 1998;188:825–832.
52. Ewald I. Die Wirkung des Radiums und das Labyrint. *Zentralbl Physiol* 1905;19:297–298.
53. Winther FO. X-Irradiation of the inner ear of the guinea pig. *Acta Otolaryngol (Stockh)* 1969;68:117.
54. Borsanyi S, Blanchard CL, Thorne B. Effect of ionizing radiation on the ear. *Ann Otol Rhinol Otolarygol* 1962;70:255–262.
55. Leach W. Irradiation of the ear. *J Laryngol Otol* 1965;79:870–880.
56. Moretti JA. Sensorineural hearing loss following radiotherapy to the nasopharynx. *Laryngoscope* 1976;86:598–602.
57. Wang CC, Doppke K. Osteoradionecrosis of the temporal bone: considerations of nominal standard dose. *Int J Radiat Oncol Biol Phys* 1976;1:881–883.

The Ear: Comprehensive Otology,
edited by R. F. Canalis and P. R. Lambert.
Lippincott Williams & Wilkins, Philadelphia © 2000.

CHAPTER 50

Temporal Bone Granulomas and Dystrophies

Edwin M. Monsell and Mark D. Wilson

Osteodystrophies and Dysplasias
    Paget's Disease of Bone
    Fibrous Dysplasia
    Osteogenesis Imperfecta
    Osteopetrosis
    Endosteal Hyperostosis

    Osteitis Fibrosa Cystica
Histiocytic Proliferation
    Langerhans Cell Histiocytosis
Autoimmune Disorders
    Wegener's Granulomatosis
    Sarcoidosis

Granulomatous disease and osteodystrophy are a diverse group of disorders that include osseus dysplasia, histiocytic proliferation, autoimmune disorders, and infectious diseases. Most of these processes are not common, but they are important to otolaryngologists. Local behavior can be aggressive, and audiologic, vestibular, or facial nerve dysfunction can be a result. Many of these disorders are amenable to medical or surgical intervention. Infectious granulomatous disease and osteodystrophy of the temporal bone are discussed in other chapters.

OSTEODYSTROPHIES AND DYSPLASIAS

Osteodystrophy and dysplasia are a group of diseases that vary in causation, manifestations, and treatment, though each is characterized by pathologic bone metabolism. Paget's disease is associated with hearing loss and skeletal deformity. Pain is common when the pelvis, spine, or long bones are involved but is not common with skull involvement. Complete control of the disease is possible through treatment with bisphosphonates. Osteogenesis imperfecta is a group of genetic disorders of collagen synthesis. The associated hearing loss sometimes can be corrected surgically, though results are not as consistent as with stapes surgery for otosclerosis. Osteopetrosis, also of genetic causation, produces intermittent

E. M. Monsell and M.D. Wilson: Department of Otolaryngology–Head and Neck Surgery, Henry Ford Health System and the Henry Ford Health Sciences Center, Detroit, Michigan 48202

facial palsy. The "malignant" form may necessitate bone marrow transplantation.

Paget's Disease of Bone

Osteitis deformans, or Paget's disease of bone, was first described in 1877 by Sir James Paget (1). It is a patchy, focal disorder characterized by a marked increase in the rate of bone remodeling caused by accelerated activity in giant, probably virally transformed, osteoclasts with a secondary osteoblastic response. Paget's disease primarily affects the larger bones, including the skull, pelvis, and axial skeleton. Hearing loss is an important complication of Paget's disease when the temporal bone is affected (Figs. 1, 2). In rare instances pagetic foci undergo sarcomatous change, which has a poor prognosis for survival. Paget's disease can be controlled with antiosteoclastic medical treatment.

Epidemiology

The prevalence of Paget's disease is second only to that of osteoporosis among bone diseases of the elderly. In a population-based study of the prevalence of Paget's disease involving the pelvis the overall prevalence of Paget's disease in the United States was estimated to be 13.4 per 1,000 (confidence interval 8.7 to 19.6) (2). The prevalence of Paget's disease was similar among men and women 45 to 64 years of age but was higher among men than women 65 to 74 years of age (2.1:1) (2). Other investigators (3–5) have estimated that about 3% of the population older than 40 years is affected and that 11% of per-

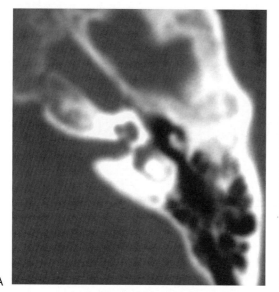
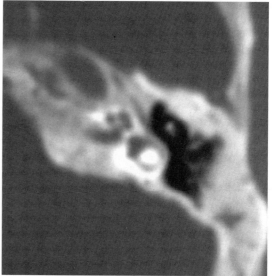

FIG. 1. High-resolution quantitative computed tomograms of normal left temporal bone **(A)** and bone affected by Paget's disease **(B)**. (From Monsell EM, Bone GH, Cody DD, et al. Hearing loss in Paget's disease of bone: evidence of auditory nerve integrity. *Am J Otol* 1995;16:27–33, with permission.)

sons older than 80 years have the disease. The prevalence increases about 0.3% per year after 55 years of age. Paget's disease is rare before 40 years of age. The disease is more prevalent in Europe, North America, and Australia; it is rarely reported in Scandinavia, Spain, Italy, or Asia (6). In the United States Paget's disease is about as common among black persons as white persons. The temporal bone is involved in about 30% of cases (7).

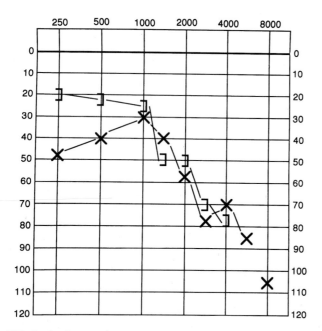

FIG. 2. Audiogram from same ear as in Fig. 1. (From Monsell EM, Bone GH, Cody DD, et al. Hearing loss in Paget's disease of bone: evidence of auditory nerve integrity. *Am J Otol* 1995;16:27–33, with permission.)

Etiology

Although the cause of Paget's disease is unknown, genetic, infectious, endocrine, metabolic, neoplastic, and vascular causes have been proposed. Autosomal dominant transmission has been suggested in familial cases. An association with HLA-D, HLA-A9, and B15 loci has been reported. Risk increases approximately sevenfold among first-degree relatives, but few cases are found among identical twins (8–10). A genetic locus has been identified on chromosome 18q, but its role is uncertain (11). The polyostotic and familial forms of Paget's disease are associated with increased risk for malignant transformation (12). Clinical evidence favoring a slow virus as an etiologic factor includes geographic clustering, a long latency period, a single target organ, and lack of marked inflammatory response. Evidence from electron microscopic, immunohistochemical, and messenger RNA hybridization studies shows involvement of paramyxovirus, including the identification of measles, respiratory syncytial, and canine distemper virus messenger RNA in affected osteoclasts (13–15). No cause and effect relation has been established, however, for these ubiquitous viruses, and virions have not been successfully retrieved or cultured (16).

Interleukin-6 may play an autocrine or paracrine role in osteoclast formation in Paget's disease, and in osteoclastic bone resorption in general (10). An association with bone trauma has been suggested, because weight-bearing bones and those exposed to injury are typical targets of osteoclastic change. Trauma may help determine which bones are affected (17). The pattern of distribution of affected areas suggests that an event occurs in a monocyte stem cell precursor that is disseminated hematogenously throughout bone. Later in life the affected osteoclasts become pagetic wherever they have been distributed.

Pathology

Paget's disease of bone is a result of substantially disordered osteoclastic activity with reactive osteoblastic activity (18). It is focal and is sharply delineated from adjacent normal bone. Three stages are described histologically. First is an osteoclastic or resorptive stage with destruction of the haversian systems; osteoclasts are increased in both size and number and are markedly multinucleated. Second is a mixed phase consisting of resorption tightly coupled with new bone deposition; morphologically normal osteoblasts lay down woven and lamellar bone. Overall bone turnover is increased about 20-fold. Bone is repeatedly resorbed and reformed, and a mosaic pattern of cement lines and reduced structural strength results. The bone mineral density of pagetic cortical bone and otic capsule bone become progressively less than their normal counterparts (19). Marrow is replaced with a cellular fibrovascular material. This leads to the third phase, which occurs when sclerotic bone remains. All three phases can occur simultaneously at different sites (20). Khetarpal and Schuknecht (21) described a fourth phase in the temporal bone that consists of remodeling of pagetic bone and bossing of the porus of the internal auditory canal.

Clinical Features

Paget's disease often is discovered while asymptomatic by means of evaluation because of an elevated serum alkaline phosphatase level. Bowing or asymptomatic enlargement of the long bones is characteristic. The lesions often are warm to the touch, a feature that led early observers to describe the lesion as inflammatory (osteitic). Technetium pyrophosphate or bisphosphonate radionuclide scanning reveals the distribution of lesions. The discovery of new sites of involvement after initial radionuclide scanning is rare. Bone pain occurs in the long bones but not typically in the skull. Severe bone pain at any site of involvement is rare and suggests sarcoma.

The temporal bones usually are involved bilaterally, but the degree of involvement commonly is asymmetric. The frontal bone is the most common facial bone affected. Increased head size or flattening of the occiput with or without frontal bossing occur only in the most advanced cases of skull involvement. Involvement of cranial nerves is rare. Because of the increased vascularity of pagetic bone, prominence of the superficial temporal vessels is common in advanced cases.

The hearing loss associated with Paget's disease typically displays a sloping, high-frequency pure tone pattern (see Fig. 2) (22). An air–bone gap in the low frequencies is characteristic. Both of these effects have been correlated with loss of bone mineral density in the cochlear capsule (19,21). The hearing loss associated with Paget's disease progresses faster than that of presbycusis. The pathophysiologic features of the hearing loss are not well defined; conductive loss is not attributable directly to ossicular fixation, nor is sensorineural loss to cochlear nerve compression (23).

Radiologic Findings

Radiographs (Table 1) reveal the classic cotton wool appearance of Paget's disease of bone (see Fig. 1). This pattern occurs with thickening of the trabecular plates and replacement of marrow and diploic spaces with pagetic bone of low mineral density. The inner and outer tables of the skull may become indistinct. Early changes consist mostly of osteolysis and appear as radiolucent areas called *osteoporosis circumscripta*. Although the diagnosis frequently can be made from plain radiographs, one cannot identify the level of activity of the lesion or identify early lesions. Nuclear imaging with technetium 99 or gallium 67 is highly sensitive (24). These radionuclides are taken up readily by active osteoblasts, and the

TABLE 1. *Radiographic findings in temporal bone osteodystrophy and dysplasia*

Condition	Stenosis of external auditory canal	Middle ear involvement	Otic capsule involvement	Stenosis of internal auditory canal	Radiographic pattern
Paget's disease	Very rare	Rare	Common when temporal bone is involved though not always evident on clinical radiographs (19)	Uncommon	Thickening of cortical bone, obliteration of marrow spaces; lytic and blastic areas; lysis of otic capsular bone
Fibrous dysplasia	Common	Uncommon	Uninvolved	Rare	Pagetoid, ground-glass sclerosis or cystic lucency
Osteopetrosis	Common	Common	Expanded when advanced	Common	Blastic sclerosis
Osteogenesis imperfecta	None	Uncommon	Demineralization in advanced lesions	None	More extensive pericochlear lucency

Adapted from Lustig LR, Jackler RK. Benign tumors of the temporal bone. In: Hughes GB, Pensak ML, eds. *Clinical otology,* 2nd ed. New York: Thieme Medical Publishers, 1997, with permission.

scans are useful in identifying early lesions. Reticuloendothelial technetium uptake decreases in malignant lesions (25). Bone scintigraphy is not specific for Paget's disease, because radionuclide uptake also occurs in processes ranging from osteoarthritis to metastatic disease. Scintigraphic findings must be correlated with the history, examination findings, plain radiographic findings, and laboratory data.

Laboratory Findings

Total serum alkaline phosphatase level is a satisfactory screening test for Paget's disease; however, bone-specific serum alkaline phosphatase level and 24-hour urinary hydroxyproline excretion are better measures of disease activity. Both indices are helpful in assessing disease activity and monitoring response to treatment. Serum and urinary calcium levels remain normal among patients with Paget's disease.

Treatment

Medical treatment is provided to control pain and to prevent the complications of Paget's disease. Pamidronate is the standard therapy for Paget's disease (26). Alendronate also provides excellent control of the disease. These bisphosphonates strongly inhibit the activity of pagetic osteoclasts. Pamidronate must be administered intravenously.

Calcitonin, self-administered by means of subcutaneous injection, has been shown to stabilize hearing (27). The effect of bisphosphonates may persist for as long as a year after cessation of therapy, whereas pagetic activity resumes more quickly after cessation of calcitonin therapy. Etidronate is the original bisphosphonate. It has the advantage of oral administration but may inhibit bone mineralization. As a consequence it typically has been administered for 6 months followed by cessation of treatment and resumption of treatment for 6 months. Etidronate is contraindicated in the treatment of the femoral neck because of risk for a devastating pathologic fracture if demineralization occurs. Early identification and vigorous treatment to normalize serum markers of disease activity are essential in controlling hearing loss due to Paget's disease (27,28).

Fibrous Dysplasia

Fibrous dysplasia is a termed applied in 1938 by Lichtenstein (29) to a localized, proliferative disorder characterized by slow replacement of normal bone with fibrous tissue and abnormal bone. It is classified as monostotic, polyostotic, or McCune-Albright syndrome. McCune-Albright syndrome includes polyostotic fibrous dysplasia with pigmentary and endocrine abnormalities. Conductive hearing loss is common with extensive involvement of the temporal bone caused by replacement of the bony external auditory canal with soft tissue. This tissue collapses, closing the external auditory canal. This condition can be treated surgically when needed. No successful medical intervention is known.

Epidemiology

Fibrous dysplasia is an uncommon disorder, accounting for about 7% of benign bony growths. Temporal bone presentation is rare; fewer than 100 cases have been reported in the world literature. The true prevalence is unknown, because the disorder usually is asymptomatic and often is diagnosed incidentally at plain radiography. Fibrous dysplasia commonly starts in childhood or adolescence. The mean age at presentation is 28 years (30). A slight male preponderance (60%) has been reported, but a review of 10 cases showed an 80% female prevalence (31). There is a clear female majority among patients with McCune-Albright syndrome.

Etiology

Fibrous dysplasia is caused by an activating mutation of the G_s-α protein, which substitutes for Arg 218 (32). Several hypotheses have been proposed, including mesenchymal enzyme derangement, altered calcium and phosphorus metabolism, and osteoblastic hyperplasia (33–35). Evidence suggests that in McCune-Albright syndrome the apparent autonomous hyperfunction of affected tissues is caused by alteration in regulation of cyclic adenosine monophosphate or protein kinase A (36). No hereditary influences are known.

Pathology

The gross appearance of fibrous dysplasia is a red to white focal lesion with a soft, gritty texture. Lesions vary in size from a few centimeters to large lesions that distort normal bony contours. Microscopic examination shows that normal cancellous bone is slowly replaced by nonoriented, immature woven bone and that irregular trabeculae form. This appearance is present in a matrix of fibrovascular tissue, seen as a whorled pattern. The process continues from the inside, expanding the ever-thinning but normal cortical bone around the diseased cancellous bone. Deformity, pathologic fractures, and cranial nerve palsy may result. The squamous, tympanic, mastoid, and petrous temporal bone can be involved. The otic capsule itself is almost always spared.

Clinical Features

Monostotic fibrous dysplasia represents about 70% of cases and is generally milder in its course than polyostotic disease. In order of frequency it affects most commonly the ribs, femur, tibia, maxilla, calvarium, and humerus. The polyostotic form accounts for about 30% of cases, occurs earlier in life than the monostotic form, and tends to be more progressive. Unlike Paget's disease, monostotic fibrous dysplasia of the cranium usually is unilateral (Fig. 3). The monostotic form often arrests during puberty, whereas the polyostotic form progresses. In either case there tends to be decreased activity with increasing age. McCune-Albright syndrome (about 3% of cases) includes polyostotic lesions with skin or mucosal pigmental change and classically precocious puberty among girls. Other endocrine abnormalities may present instead; hyperthyroidism, hyperparathyroidism, Cushing's syndrome, and pituitary modulated skeletal aberration have been described. Short stature caused by early epiphyseal closure can occur.

Monostotic presentations affect the craniofacial bones about 10% of the time. The polyostotic form involves the cranium and facial bones in about 50% of milder cases and nearly all severe cases (37). In order of frequency, the craniofacial bones involved are the frontal (69%), sphenoid (50%), ethmoid (27%), parietal (22%), and temporal (18%) (38). Temporal bone involvement is more likely when the disease is monostotic. It typically presents itself as painless swelling in the mastoid or squamous bone with progression to involve the external auditory canal or temporomandibular joint. Progressive conductive hearing loss is caused by stenosis of the external auditory canal and is the most common otologic finding. Otalgia, otorrhea, and tinnitus are less common.

Sensorineural hearing loss occurs among 14% to 17% of patients. External auditory canal stenosis (about 85% of patients with skull involvement) can lead to cholesteatoma formation. In severe instances the disease may invade the otic capsule or fallopian canal with resultant cochlear hearing loss or facial nerve impairment. The rate of facial nerve involvement has been reported to be as high as 9.4% among persons with advanced temporal bone involvement. Intracranial complications from middle or posterior fossa erosion can occur. Sarcomatous degeneration is rare (39).

Radiologic Findings

On radiographs lesions have a ground glass appearance, which is caused by fibroosseus tissue replacement of normal cancellous bone. Lesions have been categorized as pagetoid (56%, both dense and radiolucent domains), sclerotic (23%, homogenously dense), and cystic (21%, well-delineated lucency). The appearance depends on the relative amounts of fibrous and osseus tissue replacement (40). Computed tomography (CT) can be used to evaluate changes in bone density and loss of trabecular bone; to carefully define the extent of disease, state of the ossicles, patency of the external auditory canal; and suggest the presence of cholesteatoma.

Laboratory Findings

Serum alkaline phosphatase level is elevated in about 30% of patients with fibrous dysplasia with polyostotic disease but otherwise usually is normal. Serum calcium and phosphorus values are within the normal range.

Treatment

Surgical treatment is performed for symptomatic external auditory canal stenosis to correct conductive hearing loss, recurrent infection, or cholesteatoma. Canal-wall-down mastoidectomy with canalplasty and split-thickness skin grafting is indicated, because simple canalplasty results in postoperative recrudescence of stenosis in nearly 90% of cases. Radiation therapy is contraindicated because of the small risk for sarcomatous transformation.

Osteogenesis Imperfecta

Osteogenesis imperfecta (OI) is a group of genetic connective tissue disorders characterized by errors in type-1 collagen synthesis. These errors lead to osteopenia, fracture, and deformity. Otologic lesions include stapedial footplate involvement and conductive hearing loss, which often is amenable to surgical correction. OI in the context of conductive deafness is called *van der Hoeve–de Kleyn syndrome*.

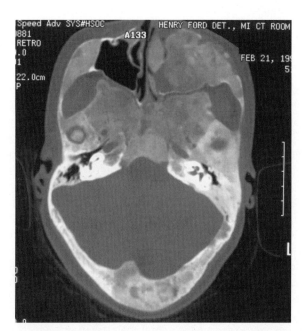

FIG. 3. Axial computed tomogram of the skull of a 9-year-old girl with fibrous dysplasia. Despite extensive involvement of the left temporal bone, hearing was normal. (Courtesy of Edwin M. Monsell.)

Genetics and Epidemiology

Four clinical types of OI are commonly recognized. Type I OI is an autosomal dominant disorder caused by decreased production of type I procollagen. In type II OI glycyl substitutions are fatal in the perinatal period. Type III OI can be autosomal recessive when caused by a frameshift mutation or dominant when caused by a point mutation. Type IV OI is autosomal dominant and is caused by a point mutation. Type I OI is the most common with a prevalence of about 1/30,000. Although this scheme of four types is useful, it is oversimplified. There are many different defects of varying severity, and more probably will be discovered.

Pathology

Bone in OI is weaker than normal bone because of reduced mineralization. Microscopic examination shows absence of normal lamellar bone. In the temporal bone the endochondral and periosteal layers of the otic capsule exhibit finely trabeculated bone and fibrous, vascular replacement. Endosteal bone can be thickened, though the otic capsule usually is not affected. Macroscopic evaluation shows that cortical bone of the temporal squamosa is thinned. Conductive hearing loss may be caused by fracture or fixation of the ossicles. (41,42).

Clinical Features

Sensorineural and mixed losses often are present and progressive. Type I OI is the mildest form. It is characterized by normal stature, nondeforming fractures, blue sclerae, and a normal life span. Hearing loss affects about 50% of patients. In dentinogenesis imperfecta, also an autosomal dominant hereditary disorder, dentin formation is poor. The enamel is discolored and easily fractured. Dentinogenesis imperfecta occurs rarely in association with type I OI. Type II OI usually is lethal in the perinatal period because of respiratory complications. It is characterized by multiple fractures and blue sclerae. Hearing loss is not well documented because of the early lethality. Patients with type III OI have short stature and deformity from recurrent fractures; dentinogenesis imperfecta is common. Scleral hue is variable. Hearing loss is common. Patients with type IV OI have normal sclerae and are of variable stature. Deformity can be mild to moderate. Dentinogenesis imperfecta is common, and hearing loss occurs among some patients. The mechanism of sensorineural hearing loss is unknown.

Radiologic Findings

Plain radiographs of the skull can reveal multiple wormian bones in the skull, which are common in OI but not pathognomonic. CT findings are indistinguishable from those of otosclerosis (43).

Laboratory Findings

Serum laboratory values are generally unremarkable. Some patients have elevated serum alkaline phosphatase and urinary hydroxyproline levels.

Treatment

Supportive care consisting of orthopedic and dental intervention is helpful, but no definitive medical therapy is available. Ossicular repair and stapedotomy are indicated for conductive hearing loss. Because of the fragility of the bone, reparative surgery is best left to experienced stapes surgeons. A platinum ribbon or bucket prosthesis may be preferred over stainless steel wire because it can be attached to the incus with less forceful compression than steel wire (44).

Osteopetrosis

Osteopetrosis, first described by Albers-Schönberg in 1904 and known variously as Albers-Schönberg disease and marble bone disease, is a rare, generalized bone disorder characterized by inability of osteoclasts to resorb cartilage and primitive bone. Bone density increases progressively because of continued osteoblastic function (45,46). The calcified cartilage and bony material accumulate in areas of endochondral bone formation, eventually replacing marrow and causing anemia, infection, and death. Recurrent otitis media, conductive and sensorineural hearing loss, and facial nerve impairment can occur.

Genetics

Osteopetrosis occurs in both autosomal recessive and autosomal dominant forms (47). The former accounts for about 25% of cases and is also called *malignant osteopetrosis* or *osteopetrosis congenita* because of its early presentation in infancy or childhood with rapid progression to death in early adulthood. The autosomal dominant form, *benign osteopetrosis* or *osteopetrosis tarda,* composes the remaining 75% and often presents in adulthood. Half of persons with this disorder have no symptoms and have a normal life expectancy. The others may have pathologic fractures, cranial neuropathy, or osteomyelitis. A less common variant of the autosomal recessive form, *intermediate osteopetrosis,* presents itself in childhood but does appear to alter life expectancy. A second rare autosomal recessive form is osteopetrosis with renal tubular acidosis and cerebral calcification, which is caused by carbonic anhydrase II deficiency. The genetic defect has been localized to chromosome 8. No racial or sex predilection is known.

Pathology

Histologic examination shows poor bone resorption caused by a defect of the osteoclasts. Poor resorption leads to increased net deposition of mineralized osteoid and cartilage, producing islands within mature bony trabeculae. Normal lamellar endochondral bone is replaced with domains of partially calcified cartilage. The squamous temporal bone, which consists of membranous bone, usually is unaffected. In the severe form of the disease the otic capsule is denser with a thickened periosteal layer. Marrow may be absent from the petrous apex. The mastoid is under- or nonpneumatized, the temporal squama is thickened, and the stapes persists in fetal form. The middle ear may have lesions that resemble exostosis. Dehiscence of the tympanic segment of the facial nerve is consistently found, but compression is not. Other neural foramina can be stenotic (48). In the more benign autosomal dominant form, sclerosis of the mastoid, ossicular involvement, and narrowing of the internal and external auditory canals and eustachian tube have been reported (49).

Clinical Features

The autosomal recessive type of osteopetrosis is rapidly progressive and usually apparent in infancy. It is characterized by replacement of functional bone marrow, which causes anemia, thrombocytopenia, hepatosplenomegaly, increased susceptibility to infection and fracture, and stenosis of neural foramina with resulting neuropathy. Nasal congestion and recurrent otitis media are common, as are optic atrophy, facial paresis or paralysis, sensorineural hearing loss, facial hypesthesia caused by trigeminal neuropathy, hydrocephalus, and mental retardation. Conductive hearing loss is more common than sensorineural hearing loss, especially early in the course of the disorder. Facial nerve involvement is characterized by recurrent attacks of facial palsy, which can alternate between sides of the face. This feature is especially characteristic in the sclerosteotic form. Although attacks are intermittent at first, permanent paralysis eventually occurs. Death typically occurs by the second decade of life.

The intermediate form of osteopetrosis causes short stature, cranial neuropathy and macrocephaly in some instances, osteomyelitis of the mandible, anemia, and recurrent fractures. In the benign form recurrent otitis, mastoid obliteration, ossicular involvement, and progressive narrowing of the external auditory canal and eustachian tube contribute to conductive hearing loss, although sensorineural hearing may occur, usually later (50). Bone effects such as macrocephaly, osteomyelitis of the mandible, and susceptibility to fractures are common, but cranial neuropathy does not often occur. Patients with carbonic anhydrase II deficiency are brought for evaluation in infancy or early childhood with fractures, short stature, and failure to thrive and may exhibit developmental delay or mental retardation. Optic nerve compression and malocclusion may be present. Some patients have hypotonia, muscle weakness, and periodic hypokalemia caused by renal tubular acidosis. Life expectancy is not altered (51).

Radiologic Findings

Plain radiographs reveal uniform, sclerotic bone without clear delineation of the two cortical plates. In the skull two types of heritable benign osteopetrosis have been described radiologically: type I with thickening of the cranial vault and type II with selective thickening of the skull base. CT may show sclerosis of the mastoid process, replacement of the petrous marrow, stenosis of the internal and external auditory canals, eustachian tubes, skull base foramina, exostosis-like lesions in the middle ear cleft, and ossicular changes. Patients with carbonic anhydrase II deficiency show findings similar to those of patients with the malignant disease, but slowing or regression over time rather than progression is appreciated.

Laboratory Findings

Serum acid phosphatase level is elevated in some patients. In malignant osteopetrosis, serum calcium levels mirror dietary intake, and hypocalcemia may cause rickets. Laboratory indices are unremarkable in the benign form. Metabolic acidosis occurs among patients with carbonic anhydrase II deficiency.

Treatment

Before considering therapy it is important to establish the nature of the osteopetrosis through careful examination, interviews, and examination of family members and serial radiographic examinations. Management of malignant osteopetrosis consists of supportive therapy for fractures, recurrent infections, and anemia. When the condition is life-threatening, bone marrow transplantation has had some success, possibly because transplanted stem cells may give rise to normal osteoclasts (52). Intervention for the intermediate and benign forms is supportive when needed. Therapy for carbonic anhydrase II deficiency osteopetrosis has been bicarbonate supplementation.

Endosteal Hyperostosis

Endosteal hyperostosis is a rare disorder characterized by progressive sclerosing dysplasia caused by enhanced osteoblastic function (53,54). Autosomal recessive (van Buchem's syndrome) and autosomal dominant (Worth disease) modes of inheritance have been described (55). The term *sclerosteosis* is used when the clinical syndrome includes syndactyly. Microscopic features include thickening of the trabecular plates with osteoid and replacement of marrow bone with lamellar bone. Narrowing of cranial nerve foramina occurs (56). The temporal bone becomes enlarged and sclerotic. Stenosis of the internal auditory canal, fallopian canal, and middle ear cleft may occur. Otologic manifestations include sensorineural, conductive, or mixed hearing loss and facial paralysis. Cranial nerve decompression may be helpful when neuropathy occurs (57).

Osteitis Fibrosa Cystica

Osteitis fibrosa cystica, also known as von Recklinghausen's disease of bone, is a rare temporal bone dystrophy. Overproduction of parathyroid hormone from hyperplasia or adenoma causes increased osteoclastic activity, bone resorption, hypercalcemia, and hypophosphatemia. Generalized osteoporosis, bone cysts, bone pain, marrow fibrosis, and fractures occur. The temporal bone is rarely involved, because this disorder most commonly affects the long bones. The otic capsule can be replaced with fine, loosely arranged trabeculae in marrow that is replaced with fatty, fibrous tissue. Sensorineural hearing loss has been attributed to this condition (58).

HISTIOCYTIC PROLIFERATION

Cells of reticuloendothelial origin called *histiocytes* can undergo transformation of unknown causation that leads to proliferation. Collections of these aberrant histiocytes (Langerhans cells) are responsible for three recognized entities. In order of increasing severity they are eosinophilic granuloma, Hand-Schüller-Christian disease and Letterer-Siwe disease. These are diseases of youth. They may be asymptomatic or associated with otitis media, otitis externa, and hearing loss. They are usually managed by means of observation, curettage, or systemic chemotherapy, depending on the disease.

Langerhans Cell Histiocytosis

Langerhans cell histiocytosis, also known as *histiocytosis X* and *reticuloendotheliosis,* comprises three clinical variants of obscure origin that share a pathogenesis of benign histiocytic proliferation. The three clinical variants are eosinophilic granuloma, Hand-Schüller-Christian disease and Letterer-Siwe disease. Although the first disease is localized and indolent, the latter two are systemic and chronic and have poor prognoses. Disease in the temporal bone may present itself with soft-tissue swelling or hearing loss; facial paralysis is rare.

Epidemiology

Review of the 19 cases of eosinophilic granuloma entered in the Armed Forces Institute of Pathology Tumor Registry from 1940 through 1978 suggests a male predominance and age at presentation of 1 to 33 years. Two thirds of patients are younger than 6 years at the onset of disease (59).

Etiology

The cause of the disorders that constitute histiocytosis X remains unknown. Causes involving metabolic, genetic, infectious, neoplastic, and immunologic factors have been proposed (57). Two cell populations of normal histiocytes have been identified. One line presumably matures in bone marrow, is related to circulating monocytes, and gives rise to tissue phagocytes. The mononuclear phagocyte, or monocyte, and its derivatives, the tissue macrophage, the epithelioid cell, and multinucleated giant cells, form a cellular collection called a *granuloma,* such that which occurs in tuberculosis. The other cell type matures in the thymus and is located in the T zone region of lymph nodes and the spleen. Dermal Langerhans cells are of this type. The two types have different antigenic markers, the former expressing α-1-antitrypsin and α-1-antichymotrypsin and not S-100. T-zone histiocytes lack the first two markers but do express S-100. The T-zone histiocytes appear to have a role in antigen processing. The histiocytes of eosinophilic granuloma, Hand-Schüller-Christian disease and Letterer-Siwe disease are of the T-zone variety and thus are not of the same origin (B cell) as the usual granuloma (60).

Pathology

At gross inspection eosinophilic granuloma is a very localized, soft, gray, yellow, tan, or reddish-brown lesion with a granular consistency. It may have cystic, necrotic, or hemorrhagic foci. Lesions contain histiocytes, eosinophils, lymphocytes, plasma cells, and multinucleated giant cells (Fig. 4). The two systemic presentations have lesions that are mostly histiocytes. Electron microscopic examination reveals Birbeck granules, trilaminar rod-shaped organelles in the histiocyte (Fig. 5) (61). The

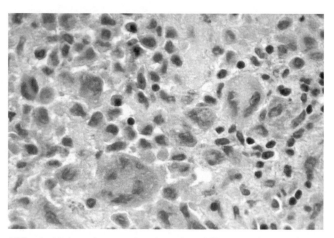

FIG. 4. Light micrograph of eosinophilic granuloma of the temporal bone shows a loose, unorganized array of histiocytes, lymphocytes, and multinucleated giant cells (hematoxylin and eosin, original magnification × 40). (Courtesy of Edwin M. Monsell.)

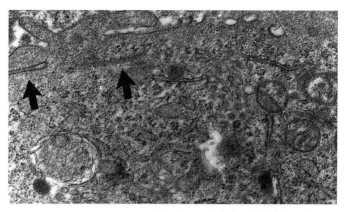

FIG. 5. Electron micrograph of histiocyte nucleus from eosinophilic granuloma exhibits several long, trilaminar bodies, or Birbeck granules *(arrows)*. (Courtesy of Edwin M. Monsell.)

presence of these granules confirms the diagnosis. There is some debate whether the lesions associated with Letterer-Siwe disease represent a version of malignant histiocytosis. In these latter the infiltrates are more monomorphous, mainly consisting of histiocytes with few inflammatory cells, and some atypia may be present. Birbeck granules are rare or absent. Although temporal bone lesions are not uncommon, involvement of the otic capsule or facial nerve is infrequent, and involvement of the jugular fossa and skull base is rare.

Clinical Features

Eosinophilic granuloma typically presents itself during childhood or young adulthood as a solitary skeletal lesion (62,63). The skull, long bones, ribs, pelvis, scapulae, and vertebral bodies are common targets. Pain or swelling are common, although the lesion may be asymptomatic. The prognosis for this benign process is excellent. Spontaneous regression can occur, and treatment usually is effective. Otologic symptoms and temporal bone involvement occur among 15% to 61% of patients. Otitis media, otorrhea with intact tympanic membrane, otitis externa, and aural polyp are the most common otologic problems (64,65). Extension of the process can involve the mastoid process, external auditory canal, or middle ear cleft with resulting conductive or sensorineural hearing loss. The process may mimic cholesteatoma, infectious mastoiditis, or a neoplasm. Vertigo and facial palsy are uncommon. When the temporal bone is involved, the disease is bilateral in about 30% of instances.

Hand-Schüller-Christian disease is the multifocal, chronic form of eosinophilic granuloma. It usually becomes apparent before 5 years of age. There is limited extraskeletal involvement of skin, lymph nodes, and viscera. Systemic signs and symptoms include fever, anorexia, recurrent upper respiratory infections, hepatosplenomegaly, and the otologic problems mentioned ear-

lier. In the classic triad of Hand-Schüller-Christian disease there is skull involvement, exophthalmos from periorbital bony disease, and diabetes insipidus from pituitary-hypothalamic involvement. This triad affects only 10% to 25% of patients. The skull base is more often involved than in isolated eosinophilic granuloma. Chronic debility without death is typical. The most severe presentation is that of systemic Letterer-Siwe disease, which strikes in the first year of life with skeletal and disseminated multiorgan disease. Mortality is high. Presentation includes the systemic and otologic manifestations mentioned earlier and seborrheic or eczematoid rash, oral lesions, blood dyscrasia caused by marrow replacement by multiple lesions, and respiratory failure caused by pulmonary lesions. Facial palsy is rare in eosinophilic granuloma (less than 3% of systemic presentations) (66). A biopsy is appropriate for diagnosis of these disorders and to rule out malignancy.

Radiologic Findings

Skull radiographs reveal a well-defined osteolytic lucency without periosteal reaction. Chest radiography may demonstrate diffuse infiltration in systemic disease, especially in central or perihilar locations. Hilar adenopathy is rare. At magnetic resonance imaging the lesion gives a low signal on both T1 and T2 sequences but becomes well enhanced with gadolinium (67). Because the lesion causes lysis of bone, CT is helpful to delineate its extent.

Treatment

Solitary lesions may initially be followed because they often resolve spontaneously. Lesions may be removed by means of curettage of the margins. Radiation therapy can be used either alone or in combination with surgery. The absence of new lesions within 12 months of therapy for a solitary lesion suggests cure. Intralesional steroids also have been useful in some cases (68). For widely disseminated or visceral involvement, chemotherapy may be considered. Low-dose monotherapy may suffice for Hand-Schüller-Christian disease, whereas combinations of corticosteroids and cytotoxic agents have been used to manage Letterer-Siwe disease (61).

AUTOIMMUNE DISORDERS

Possibly resulting from an interaction between genetic predisposition, infection, and other unidentified factors, autoimmune diseases of otolaryngologic importance include Wegener's granulomatosis, sarcoidosis, and autoimmune inner ear disease. Otitis media and sensorineural hearing loss are the primary otologic manifestations of Wegener's granulomatosis. The most common otologic manifestation of sarcoidosis is facial palsy, which may occur either in isolation or as a component of the uveo-parotid fever of Heerfordt. Sensorineural hearing loss also has been reported. Autoimmune inner ear disease is discussed in Chapter 32.

Wegener's Granulomatosis

Wegener's granulomatosis is a systemic disease of unknown autoimmune origin. It is characterized by necrotizing granulomas of the upper and lower respiratory tracts, focal segmental necrotizing glomerulonephritis, and small-vessel systemic vasculitis. There is a slight male preponderance, and the disease typically presents itself in the fifth decade of life. Head and neck presentation is common; about 90% of patients have involvement of the nose and paranasal sinuses. Common symptoms include headache, cough, pleuritic chest pain, hemoptysis, conjunctivitis, arthralgia, sinusitis, rhinorrhea, and otitis media. Ear involvement occurs among 20% to 40% of patients, most commonly as serous otitis media caused by eustachian tube dysfunction from upper respiratory infection or sinusitis or direct obstruction of the eustachian tube (69,70). Low to moderate sensorineural hearing loss has been reported among as many as 80% of patients (71). Severe or profound hearing loss is not rare. Granulomas may cause single and sometimes multiple perforations of the tympanic membrane. The diagnosis is confirmed with the circulating antineutrophil cytoplasmic antigen test. The disease is managed with steroids, cyclophosphamide, or other chemotherapeutic agents and trimethoprim-sulfamethoxazole (see Chapter 25).

Sarcoidosis

Sarcoidosis is an autoimmune disease of unknown causation characterized by systemic involvement with non-caseating granulomas, especially in the lungs. It is slightly more common among women, ten times more common among black than white Americans, and typically occurs between the ages of 20 and 40 years. Cough, bihilar adenopathy, and skin rash are common; hepatosplenomegaly, keratoconjunctivitis, arthralgia, myalgia, cardiac failure, and central and peripheral neuropathy also may occur. The cranial nerves most commonly involved are the optic and facial nerves. Facial palsy with uveitis and parotitis is called uveoparotid fever of Heerfordt (72). Involvement of the auditory and vestibular systems is known and is hypothesized to be caused by direct granulomatous involvement of the nerves (73). The disease is characterized by bihilar adenopathy, elevated levels of angiotensin I converting enzyme, and sometimes hypercalcemia. The process often is self-limited. Neuropathy and other progressive symptoms may be managed with steroids.

SUMMARY POINTS

- Paget's disease of bone is a treatable cause of hearing loss among the middle-aged and elderly. It presents itself with high-frequency sensorineural hearing loss and a low-frequency air–bone gap. Early identification and vigorous treatment may slow or prevent progressive hearing loss.
- Fibrous dysplasia can lead to cholesteatoma caused by stenosis of the external auditory canal.
- Osteogenesis imperfecta is a group of genetic disorders of collagen synthesis. Mixed hearing loss is common. Langerhans cell histiocytosis includes eosinophilic granuloma, Hand-Schüller-Christian disease and Letterer-Siwe disease.
- Osteopetrosis (marble bone disease) is characterized by the inability of osteoclasts to resorb bone. Cranial nerve deficits (II, VII, VIII) can occur from bony compression of these structures. Recurrent otitis media and conductive hearing loss also occur.
- Eosinophilic granuloma, the most benign subtype, can be managed by means of observation. Expanding lesions can be controlled with curettage.
- Wegener's granulomatosis may present itself with serous otitis media, sensorineural hearing loss, or both.
- Facial paralysis is the most common otologic manifestation of sarcoidosis, an autoimmune disease of unknown causation.

REFERENCES

1. Paget J. On a form of chronic inflammation of bones (osteitis deformans). *Med Chir Trans London* 1877;60:37–63.
2. Altman RD, Hochberg MC, Murphy WA. Paget's disease of bone in the United States [Abstract]. *J Bone Miner Res* 1997;12:S272.
3. Kanis JA. Epidemiology. In: *Pathophysiology and treatment of Paget's disease of bone*. London: Martin Dunitz, 1991;1–12.
4. Davies DG. Paget's disease of the temporal bone: a clinical and histopathological survey. *Acta Otolaryngol (Stockh)* 1968;Suppl 242.
5. Barker DJP. The epidemiology of Paget's disease. In: Barker DJP, ed. *Proceedings of the MRC symposium on Paget's disease*. Scientific Reports No. 5. Medical Research Council, 1983:1–6.
6. Smith R. Disorders of the skeleton: Paget's disease. In: Smith R, ed. *Oxford textbook of medicine*. Oxford, UK: Oxford Medical Publications, 1989:17.19–17.22.
7. Nager GT. Paget's disease of the temporal bone. *Ann Otol Rhinol Laryngol Suppl* 1975;22:1–32.
8. Siris ES, Ottman R, Flaster E, et al. Familial aggregation of Paget's disease of bone. *J Bone Miner Res* 1991;6:495–500.
9. McKusick VA. *Heritable disorders of connective tissue*. St. Louis: CV Mosby, 1972:718.
10. Jones JV, Reed MF. Paget's disease: a family with 6 cases. *Br Med J* 1967;4:90–91.
11. Roodman GD. Paget's disease and osteoclast biology. *Bone* 1996;19:209–212.
12. Wu RK, Trumble TE, Ruwe PA. Familial incidence of Paget's disease

and secondary osteogenic sarcoma: a report of three cases from a single family. *Clin Orthop* 1991;265:306–309.

13. Rebel A, Malkani K, Basle M, Bregeon C. Osteoclast ultrastructure in Paget's disease. *Calcif Tissue Int* 1976;20:187–199.

14. Basle MF, Rebel A, Fournier JG, Russell WC, Malkani K. On the trail of paramyxoviruses in Paget's disease of bone. *Clin Orthop* 1987;217:9–15.

15. Mills BG, Frausto A, Singer FR, et al. Multinucleated cells formed in vitro from Paget's bone marrow express viral antigens. *Bone* 1994;15:443–448.

16. Kahn AJ. The viral etiology of Paget's disease of bone: a new perspective. *Calcif Tissue Int* 1990;47:127–129.

17. Hamdy RC. Trauma and Paget's disease of bone. *Br Med J* 1979;1:1487.

18. Chole RA. Differential osteoclast activation in endochondral and intramembranous bone. *Ann Otol Rhinol Laryngol* 1993;102:616–619.

19. Monsell EM, Cody DD, Bone GH, et al. Hearing loss in Paget's disease of bone: the relationship between pure-tone thresholds and mineral density of the cochlear capsule. *Hear Res* 1995;83:114–120.

20. Siris, ES. Paget's disease of bone. In: Favus MJ, ed. *Primer on metabolic bone diseases and disorders of mineral metabolism.* Richmond, VA: William Byrd Press, 1990:253–259.

21. Khetarpal U, Schuknecht HF. In search of pathologic correlates of hearing loss and vertigo in Paget's disease: a clinical and histopathologic study of 26 temporal bones. *Ann Otol Rhinol Laryngol Suppl* 1990;145:1–16.

22. Harner SG, Rose DE, Facer GW. Paget's disease and hearing loss. *Otolaryngol Head Neck Surg* 1978;86:869–874.

23. Monsell EM, Bone GH, Cody DD, et al. Hearing loss in Paget's disease of bone: evidence of auditory nerve integrity. *Am J Otol* 1995;16:27–33.

24. Fogelman I. Bone scanning in Paget's disease. In: Freeman LM, ed. *Nuclear Medicine Annual.* New York: Raven Press, 1991:99–128.

25. Rudberg U, Ahlback SO, Uden R. Bone marrow scintigraphy in Paget's disease of bone. *Acta Radiol* 1990;31:141–144.

26. Lando M, Hoover LA, Finerman G. Stabilization of hearing loss in Paget's disease with calcitonin and etidronate. *Arch Otolaryngol Head Neck Surg* 1988;114:891–894.

27. Delmas PD, Meunier PJ. The management of Paget's disease of bone. *N Engl J Med* 1997;336:558–566.

28. Hamdy RC. Paget's disease of the bone. *Clin Geriatr Med* 1994;10:719–735.

29. Lichtenstein L. Polyostotic fibrous dysplasia. *Arch Surg* 1938;36:874–898.

30. Nager GT, Kennedy DW, Kopstein E. Fibrous dysplasia: a review of the disease and its manifestation in the temporal bone. *Ann Otol Rhinol Laryngol Suppl* 1982;91(92):1–52.

31. Megerian CA, Sofferman RA, McKenna MJ, et al. Fibrous dysplasia of the temporal bone: ten new cases demonstrating the spectrum of otologic sequelae. *Am J Otol* 1995;16:408–419.

32. Shenker A, Chanson P, Weinstein LS, et al. Osteoblastic cells derived from isolated lesions of fibrous dysplasia contain activating somatic mutations of the Gs alpha gene. *Hum Mol Genet* 1995;4:1675–1676.

33. Lichtenstein L, Jaffe HL. Fibrous dysplasia of bone. *Arch Pathol Lab Med* 1942;33:777–816.

34. Changus GW. Osteoblastic hyperplasia of bone: a histochemical appraisal of fibrous dysplasia of bone. *Cancer* 1957;10:1157–1161.

35. Murray RC, Kirkpatrick HJR, Forrai E. Case of McCune-Albright's syndrome. *Br J Surg* 1946;34:48–57.

36. Lee PA, Van Dop C, Migeon CJ. McCune-Albright syndrome: long-term follow-up. *JAMA* 1986;256:2980–2984.

37. Windolz F. Cranial manifestations of fibrous dysplasia of bone. *AJR Am J Roentgenol* 1947;58:51–63.

38. Van Tilberg W. Fibrous dysplasia. In: Vinken PJ, Bruyn GW, eds. *Handbook of clinical neurology, vol. 14.* Amsterdam: North Holland Publishing, 1972:163–212.

39. Schwartz DT, Alert M. The malignant transformation of fibrous dysplasia. *Am J Med Sci* 1964;247:35–54.

40. Fries JW. The roentgen features of fibrous dysplasia of the skull and facial bones: a critical analysis of thirty-nine pathologically proven cases. *Am J Radiol* 1957;77:71–88.

41. Berger G, Hawke M, Johnson A, Proops D. Histopathology of the temporal bone in osteogenesis imperfecta congenita: a report of 5 cases. *Laryngoscope* 1985;95:193–199.

42. Nager GT. Osteogenesis imperfecta of the temporal bone and its relation to otosclerosis. *Ann Otol Rhinol Laryngol* 1988;97:585–593.

43. Hasso AN, Ledington JA. Imaging modalities for the study of the temporal bone. *Otolaryngol Clin North Am* 1988;22:219–244.

44. Armstrong BW. Stapes surgery in patients with osteogenesis imperfecta. *Ann Otol Rhinol Laryngol* 1984;93:634–635.

45. Albers-Schonberg H. Rontgenbilder einer seltenen, Knochenerkrankung. *MMW* 1904;51:365.

46. Felix R, Hofstetter W, Cecchini MG. Recent developments in the understanding of the pathophysiology of osteopetrosis. *Eur J Endocrinol* 1996;134:143–156.

47. Bollerslev AJ, Mosekilde L. Autosomal dominant osteopetrosis. *Clin Orthop* 1993;294:45–51.

48. Hawke M, Jahn AF, Bailey D. Osteopetrosis of the temporal bone. *Arch Otolaryngol Head Neck Surg* 1981;107:278–282.

49. Milroy CM, Michaels L. Temporal bone pathology of adult-type osteopetrosis. *Arch Otolaryngol Head Neck Surg* 1990;116:79–84.

50. Hamersma H. Total decompression of the facial nerve in osteopetrosis. *ORL J Otorhinolaryngol Relat Spec* 1974;36:21–32.

51. Sly WS. Carbonic anhydrase II deficiency syndrome: osteopetrosis with renal tubular acidosis and cerebral calcification In: Scriver CR, Beaudet AL, Sly WS, Valle D, eds. *The metabolic basis of inherited disease,* 6th ed. New York: McGraw-Hill, 1989:2857–2868.

52. Coccia PF, Krivit W, Cervenka J, et al. Successful bone-marrow transplantation for infantile malignant osteopetrosis. *N Engl J Med* 1980;302:701–708.

53. Beighton P, Barnard A, Hamersma H, et al. The syndromic status of sclerosteosis and van Buchem disease. *Clin Genet* 1984;25:175–181.

54. Stein SA, Witkop C, Hill S, et al. Sclerosteosis: neurogenetic and pathophysiologic analysis of an American kinship. *Neurology* 1983;33:267–277.

55. Whyte MP. Sclerosing bone dysplasias In: Favus MJ, ed. *Primer on metabolic bone diseases and disorders of mineral metabolism.* Richmond, VA: William Byrd Press, 1990:213–219.

56. Nager GT, Stein SA, Dorst JP, et al. Sclerosteosis involving the temporal bone: clinical and radiologic aspects. *Am J Otolaryngol* 1983;4:1–17.

57. Leikin SL. Immunobiology of histiocytosis-X. *Hematol Oncol Clin North Am* 1987;1:49–61.

58. Lindsay JR, Suga F. Sensorineural deafness due to osteitis fibrosa. *Arch Otolaryngol* 1976;102:37.

59. Sweet RM, Kornblut AD, Hyams VJ. Eosinophilic granuloma in the temporal bone. *Laryngoscope* 1979;89:1545–1552.

60. Burns DK, Meyerhoff WL. Granulomatosis disorders and related conditions of the ear and temporal bone. In: Paparella MM, ed. *Otolaryngology.* Philadelphia: WB Saunders, 1991:1549.

61. Starling KA. Chemotherapy of histiocytosis X. *Hematol Oncol Clin North Am* 1987;1:119–122.

62. Alessi DM, Maceri D. Histiocytosis X of the head and neck in a pediatric population. *Arch Otolaryngol Head Neck Surg* 1992;118:945–948.

63. DeNardo LJ, Wetmore RF. Head and neck manifestations of histiocytosis-X in children. *Laryngoscope* 1989;99:721–724.

64. Goldsmith AJ, Myssiorek D, Valderrama E, Patel M. Unifocal Langerhans' cell histiocytosis (eosinophilic granuloma) of the petrous apex. *Arch Otolaryngol Head Neck Surg* 1993;119:113–116.

65. Cunningham MJ, Curtin HD, Jaffe R, Stool SE. Otologic manifestations of Langerhans' cell histiocytosis. *Arch Otolaryngol Head Neck Surg* 1989;115:807–813.

66. Tos M. Facial palsy in Hand-Schüller-Christian disease. *Arch Otolaryngol Head Neck Surg* 1969;90:563–567.

67. Angeli SI, Luxford WM, Lo WW. Magnetic resonance imaging in the evaluation of Langerhans' cell histiocytosis of the temporal bone: case report. *Otolaryngol Head Neck Surg* 1996;114:120–124.

68. Fradis M, Podoshin L, Ben-David J, Grishkan A. Eosinophilic granuloma of the temporal bone. *J Laryngol Otol* 1985;99:475–579.

69. Woolf NK, Harris JP. Cochlear pathophysiology associated with inner ear immune responses. *Acta Otolaryngol* 1986;102:353–364.

70. Kornblut AD, Wolff SM, Fauci AS. Ear disease in patients with Wegener's granulomatosis. *Laryngoscope* 1982;92:713–717.

71. Kempf HG. Ear involvement in Wegener's granulomatosis. *Clin Otolaryngol* 1989;14:451–456.

72. Cohen JP, Lachman LJ, Hammerschlag PE. Reversible facial paralysis in sarcoidosis. *Arch Otolaryngol Head Neck Surg* 1983;109:832–835.

73. Hybels RL, Rice DH. Neuro-otologic manifestations of sarcoidosis. *Laryngoscope* 1976;86:1873–1878.

The Ear: Comprehensive Otology,
edited by R. F. Canalis and P. R. Lambert.
Lippincott Williams & Wilkins, Philadelphia © 2000.

CHAPTER 51

Glomus and Other Benign Tumors of the Temporal Bone

C. Gary Jackson, Samuel Marzo, Akira Ishiyama, and Paul R. Lambert

The evolution of temporal bone surgery has been based on the application of contemporary research and technology to the eradication of inflammatory diseases of the middle ear and mastoid process. As a consequence, advances in antibiotic therapy, microsurgery, and radiology have expanded the limits of otologic surgery and markedly improved the treatment of nonneoplastic lesions of the ear. The management of temporal bone tumors has benefited somewhat less from these advances because of their complex histologic features and anatomic relations, but these challenges have set the stage for the multispecialty efforts that are likely to produce improved results in the near future.

C. G. Jackson: Department of Otolaryngology–Head and Neck Surgery, Otology and Neurotology, Vanderbilt University School of Medicine, Nashville, Tennessee 37203

S. Marzo: Department of Otolaryngology, Loyola University Medical Center, Maywood, Illinois 60153

A. Ishiyama: Division of Head and Neck Surgery, University of California, Los Angeles, School of Medicine, Los Angeles, California 90095

P. R. Lambert: Department of Otolaryngology–Head and Neck Surgery, University of Virginia Health Sciences Center, Charlottesville, Virginia 22908-0430

The temporal bone derives from all germinal layers and contains epithelial, neural, vascular, and cartilaginous structures from which a variety of benign and malignant tumors can develop (1). As part of the skull base the temporal bone is relatively inaccessible, and tumors at this site often become symptomatic only after they reach peripheral structures, such as the middle ear. The spread of temporal bone tumors closely relates to the pneumatized spaces of the temporal bone and the degree of resistance of its contents. For example, the tympanic membrane offers mild resistance to the medial spread of pathologic processes of the external ear, whereas the hard bone of the labyrinth is moderately resistant to tumor spread. The neurovascular and bony foramina may allow tumor extension beyond the confines of the temporal bone into the intracranial space, parotid glands, or infratemporal fossa. Tumor extension by the lymphatic system also must be considered. In addition to the preauricular parotid lymphatic drainage system, which is prominent in diseases of the external auditory canal (EAC), the ear is drained by superior cervical, jugular, postauricular, and posterior cervical lymphatic vessels. Although the inner ear has no known lymphatic drainage, the middle ear, mastoid process, and eustachian tube drain into the deep jugular and retropharyngeal lymph nodes (1).

Most temporal bone lesions are benign. Progression can be so slow that neurologic deficits may undergo simultaneous compensation and remain unnoticed by the patient. These lesions ultimately can cause hearing loss, vestibular dysfunction, and cranial neuropathy, which cause dysphagia, hoarseness, aspiration, facial nerve paresis, and eye problems.

This chapter discusses benign neoplasms of the temporal bone. To provide a general perspective, the most common of these lesions, glomus tumor or nonchromaffin paraganglioma, is examined in detail. The management strategy for this tumor can be broadly applied to most neoplasms of this region. Specific lesions are categorized and discussed in detail.

GLOMUS TUMORS

Glomus tumor is the most frequently diagnosed neurotologic neoplasm after acoustic neuroma. It is most common among white persons (2) and occurs in a female to male ratio of approximately 5:1 (2,3). Glomus tumor has been reported in all age groups from infants to the elderly, but it is most frequent in the fifth and sixth decades of life. It is usually solitary. A hereditary tendency with an autosomal dominant mode of transmission has been identified among some patients (4). For familial tumors, the incidence of other paragangliomas is 25% to 50% (4,5).

The ideal management of glomus tumors is complete surgical resection. Because of technical advances, problems of resectability have given way to issues of functional outcome: the quality of life after surgery. Effective reconstruction of sizable defects and rehabilitation from cranial nerve deficits, now routine, reduce the strength of the most common argument against surgery in the management of these tumors: the *perceived* risk for long-term functional disability. As an alternative, radiation therapy is proposed as a low morbidity, conservation treatment that may arrest growth but does not eradicate the tumor. This section reviews the surgical indications for glomus tumors and gives a radiation therapy management perspective. Intracranial extension, defect reconstruction, and cranial nerve rehabilitation are addressed.

Historical Perspective

Surgery for glomus tumors and acoustic tumors has provided the focal point around which modern neurotologic skull base surgery has evolved over the last 50 years. Surgical adaptation to new challenges has been consistently spurred by diagnostic advances that have allowed surgeons to better define the extent of disease. A brief review of the principal events that led to current treatment outlooks follows.

The Forties and Fifties

In 1945 Rosenwasser (6) resected a middle ear lesion he associated with the characteristics of Guild's (3) original description of a glomus tumor. In 1949, Lundgren (4) attempted jugular bulb resection. However, as late as 1950, operations were limited to exploration of these tumors because of the high morbidity and mortality associated with resection (6). Gastpar (7) advocated total tumor removal and sacrifice of the facial nerve and labyrinth. In 1952 Capps (5) considered facial nerve mobilization and elaborated on basic principles for dealing with the jugular bulb. Suboccipital and other alternative routes were tried without success (8–11). Radiation therapy became the preferred management (12).

The Sixties

Polytomography, retrograde jugulography (13), and conventional and subtraction angiography enhanced tumor delineation and diagnosis and prompted new developments. In 1964, Shapiro and Neues (8) proposed complete glomus tumor resection by means of wide exposure of the neck structures and rerouting of the facial nerve. In 1965 Gejrot (9) stated that jugular bulb resection was a prerequisite for cure. He supported this view with extensive angiographic studies showing that intraluminal tumor was always present. He emphasized proximal and distal isolation of the jugular venous system. In 1969, House (6) first proposed conservation surgery with an extended facial recess approach, which preserved the wall of the EAC and hearing.

The Seventies

Sporadic successful reports of complete tumor resection began to appear in the 1970s (11). Spector et al. (14) presented 46 cases in 1973 and concluded that surgery was the preferred management of glomus tumor. In 1974, Glasscock et al. (15) combined the approaches of Shapiro and Neues and House and reported consistent surgical success among a large group of patients. Gardner et al. (16), however, advocated surgery combined with radiation therapy. Fisch (17) in 1977 proposed infratemporal fossa exposure for disease that extended beyond the confines of the temporal bone. The internal carotid artery (ICA), clivus, and parasellar regions were no longer off limits (18–20).

Current Achievements

Kinney (21) addressed the problem of intracranial extension in 1980 and Fisch did so in 1982 (22). When the tumor was resectable, staging was usually recommended. Jackson et al. (23) described a single-stage approach for lesions extending intracranially. Later they (24) established guidelines for defect reconstruction and prevention of cerebral spinal fluid (CSF) leakage. Emphasis on conservation surgery and functional outcome continues to mount (25–28). Jackson and Netterville (29) further emphasized reconstruction approaches, cranial nerve rehabilitation, and hearing conservation (30).

Classification

Accurate tumor classification is essential for surgical planning and reporting standards. Alford and Guilford (31) in the early 1960s first proposed an anatomic classification of glomus tumors. Current anatomic site classifications are included in Tables 1 and 2. Fisch (17) and Oldring and Fisch (32) in 1979 proposed their A, B, C, and D classification. This system was upgraded first in 1981 (19) and again in 1982 to include intracranial extension (20) as subclasses of type C and D lesions (see Table 1). The Glasscock-Jackson (20,33) classification retained

TABLE 1. *Glomus tumors: Fisch classification*

Type A	Tumors limited to the middle ear cleft
Type B	Tumors limited to the tympanomastoid area with no involvement of the infralabyrinthine compartment
Type C	Tumors involving the infralabyrinthine compartment of the temporal bone and extending into the petrous apex
Type D_1	Tumors with an intracranial extension less than 2 cm in diameter
Type D_2	Tumors with an intracranial extension greater than 2 cm in diameter

TABLE 2. *Glasscock–Jackson glomus tumor classification*

Type	Physical findings
Glomus tympanicum	
Type I	Small mass limited to the promontory
Type II	Tumor completely filling middle ear space
Type III	Tumor filling middle ear and extending into mastoid process
Type IV	Tumor filling middle ear, extending into mastoid or through tympanic membrane to fill external auditory canal; may extend anterior to internal carotid artery
Glomus jugulare	
Type I	Small tumor involving jugular bulb, middle ear, and mastoid process
Type II	Tumor extending under internal auditory canal; may have intracranial extension
Type III	Tumor extending into petrous apex; may have intracranial extension
Type IV	Tumor extending beyond petrous apex into clivus or infratemporal fossa; may have intracranial extension

the basic tympanicum-jugulare divisions and expanded them according to tumor extent. Intracranial extension is expressed as a superscript: for example, glomus tumor type $IV^{2.0}$ is a type IV lesion with 2.0 cm of intracranial extension (see Table 2).

Biology

The term *glomus* is a misnomer because these tumors originate from specific neural crest elements, the paraganglion cells, which with autonomic ganglion cells form the paraganglia (34,35). The paraganglia are part of the neuroendocrine system usually associated with sympathetic ganglia and consist of the adrenal paraganglion (the adrenal medulla) and extraadrenal paraganglia (34,36). Paragangliomas may arise from adrenal and extraadrenal paraganglia and are classified accordingly.

The distribution of craniocervical paraganglia is along the arteries and cranial nerves of the ontogenetic gill arches. They are embryologically derived from the branchiomeric system and may be located along their derivatives as follows:

Jugulotympanic
Intercarotid
Subclavian
Laryngeal
Coronary
Aortic-pulmonary
Orbital
Pulmonary

The vagal paraganglia are considered separate because they are not intimate to arteries (36,37).

Temporal bone–related glomus bodies are ovoid, lobulated structures 0.1 mm to 1.5 mm in diameter (34–37). Vascularized by the inferior tympanic branch of the ascending pharyngeal artery, they average three per side in association with Jacobson's or Arnold's nerve, and more than half are located in the jugular fossa. They are predominantly innervated by the glossopharyngeal nerve, but the vagus nerve may supply some glomus bodies located along Arnold's nerve. Vagal paraganglial cell groups occupy the epineurium of the nerve (34).

The ultrastructural appearance of paragangliomas mimics that of the paraganglia (38). Paraganglia comprise clusters (Zellballen) of epithelial (chief) cells surrounded by sustentacular cells and small blood vessels (35,38). The chief cells are filled with cytoplasmic granules containing catecholamines (35,38–40). These granules have ultrastructural characteristics similar to those of others found in neurosecretory cells (38,41). Two types of chief cells, light and dark, are identified.

Biochemistry

The chief cells of paraganglia are one of 40 types classified within the diffuse neuroendocrine system. These cells are capable of producing neuropeptides and catecholamines that may serve as neurotransmitters, neurohormones, hormones, and parahormones (38–40). The biochemical activity of these tumors is variable and expresses itself in diverse ways as documented in the following findings: intratumoral norepinephrine accumulation (probably because the tumors lack phenylethanolamine-*N*-methyltransferase) (39), dopamine secretion (38,39), serotonin (5-hydroxyindoleacetic acid) production, carcinoid syndrome (40), and paraneoplastic anemia (reported in a malignant glomus tumor) (42). Other neurohormones have been immunohistochemically identified in glomus tumors. These include neuron specific enolase, substance P, cholecystokinin, bombesin, chromogranin, vasoinhibitory peptide, somatostatin, calcitonin, S-100, melanocyte-stimulating hormone, and gastrin (43–46). Symptomatic tumors are known as *functional* or *secretors.* Approximately 1% to 3% of paragangliomas are functional (24,38).

Clinical Correlates

Catecholamines

Catecholamine levels three to five times normal are generally needed to produce symptoms and signs suggestive of catecholamine secretion, such as headaches, excessive perspiration, palpitations, pallor, and nausea. Catecholamine paraneoplasia should be differentiated from pheochromocytoma by means of computed tomography (CT) of the adrenal glands or selective renal vein sampling (46). Perioperative management is essential to safeguard against the potentially life-threatening consequences of catecholamine overload on anesthesia induction or intraoperatively on tumor manipulation. Paraneoplastic syndrome associated with other neurohormones (e.g., anemia, gastrointestinal symptoms) must be sought and identified.

Immunohistochemistry

The presence of immunoreactive peptides can be used to diagnostic advantage. To this effect a somatostatin analogue (47), iodine-labeled type 3 octreotide (octreotide scanning) has been used (48). Histochemical markers also may provide insight into the biologic aggressiveness of a tumor because chief cells and sustentacular cells possess different protein components. Aggressive tumors have been proposed to have scarce sustentacular cell populations and produce fewer neuropeptides than more benign lesions. Tendency toward a malignant character has been implied through immunohistochemical analysis of the ratio of chief cells to sustentacular cells and marker reactivity in the latter (48,49).

Associated Tumors

Pheochromocytoma, thyroid and visceral neoplasms, parathyroid adenoma, and the multiple endocrine neoplasia syndromes have been associated with glomus tumors (43,50,51). In 10% of nonfamilial cases the additional tumor may be ipsi- or contralateral and occurs in one of the branchiomeric paraganglionic stations (50,52). The most common association is between glomus tympanicum or jugulare and ipsilateral carotid body tumor (23, 53,54).

Tumor Growth and Functional Deficit

Multidirectional growth occurs simultaneously as the tumor spreads from the site of origin along tracks of least resistance, predominantly the air-cell tracts of the temporal bone. Vascular lumina, neurovascular foramina, and the eustachian tube allow extratemporal extension. Cochleovestibular destruction is caused by ischemic necrosis (20,24). Intracranial extension is common into the posterior cranial fossa directly through the dura, along cranial nerve roots, or through the internal auditory canal (21). Glomus tumors have a high morbidity because of their location in the skull base adjacent to the posterior cranial fossa and the lower cranial nerves. Cranial nerve paralysis occurs with 35% of glomus jugulare lesions and 57% of vagal paragangliomas (21). Cranial nerves VII through XII and the sympathetic trunk are commonly involved.

Malignancy

Glomus tumors rarely exhibit malignant degeneration. Lattes and Waltner (53) in 1948 first reported a glomus tumor metastatic to the liver. Approximately 30 cases have been reported since then. The incidence of malignant glomus tumor is variously quoted at 1% to 12%, 4% being the most commonly cited figure (55–57). The diagnosis is made only when regional or distant metastasis is confirmed in locations other than those in which paragangliomas may develop (multicentricity). The most common metastatic sites are the regional lymph nodes, skeleton, lung, liver, and occasionally the spleen (58). Glomus vagale tumors have a high malignancy rate, estimated at 19% (55–57). The symptoms tend to be more severe and rapidly progressive in malignant glomus tumor. Cranial nerve deficits are common. Treatment morbidity and mortality are higher than with benign lesions. Prolonged survival periods, however, are possible with evidence of active malignant disease (56,57).

Diagnosis

Clinical Assessment

Complete tumor resection with high levels of functional preservation is possible with early diagnosis. The most common presenting symptom is pulsatile tinnitus (80%) followed by hearing loss (60%) (Table 3). Tumor growth into the mesotympanum causes conductive hearing loss, and cochleolabyrinthine invasion causes sen-

TABLE 3. *Presenting signs and symptoms among patients with glomus tumors*

Presenting symptom	Tumor type	
	Glomus jugulare (n = 106)	Glomus vagale (n = 27)
Pulsatile tinnitus	84	8
Hearing loss	62	4
Otalgia	13	3
Aural fullness	32	3
Hoarseness	12	4
Dysphagia	8	5
Pharyngeal fullness	0	9
Vertigo	15	1
Facial weakness	15	1
Headache	5	0
Dysarthria	0	0
Aural bleeding	2	0

TABLE 5. *Physical findings among patients with glomus tumors*

Physical findings	Tumor type	
	Glomus jugulare (n = 106)	Glomus vagale (n = 27)
Middle ear mass	78	4
External auditory canal mass	7	1
Neck mass	0	11
Pharyngeal fullness	1	7

sorineural loss. Tympanic membrane erosion and bleeding are late symptoms. Cranial nerve dysfunction is common with glomus tumors (Table 4). Lower cranial nerve dysfunction, including dysphagia, loss of airway protection, shoulder drop, tongue paralysis, and voice weakness, suggests an extensive process. Facial paralysis is a sign of advanced disease and is a poor prognostic sign for functional preservation. Symptoms of a "functioning" tumor must be sought and differentiated from those of pheochromocytoma (20,24,31,58).

The most common physical finding in glomus tumor is a middle ear mass (Table 5). A mesotympanic mass is characteristic but may be inapparent on rare occasions. Superior mesotympanic tumors rarely occur and are diagnostically confusing. Unless margins visible 360 degrees around a mesotympanic mass can be seen, differentiating a glomus tympanicum tumor from a glomus jugulare tumor is not possible at otoscopy, and imaging (CT) is necessary (31).

Myringotomy or tympanotomy for biopsy are contraindicated. Biopsy causes brisk bleeding, which necessitates packing and carries risk for structural damage to the ear. If a vascular lesion is suspected and cannot be demonstrated on radiographs, exploration through a postauricular transmastoid approach with all vital anatomic features identified is indicated (23).

TABLE 4. *Preoperative cranial nerve deficits (n = 104)*

Affected nerve	Tumor type	
	Glomus jugulare (n = 7)	Glomus vagale (n = 27)
None	55	8
V	0	0
VI	0	0
VII	7	4
VIII	16	3
IX	13	6
X	16	13
XI	9	4
XII	11	9

Temporal bone involvement by glomus vagale tumors is rare. The lesions present themselves as enlarging parapharyngeal masses that cause high neck fullness. Paralysis of the vagus nerve is a relatively infrequent initial finding. With advanced lesions aspiration and hoarseness, Horner's syndrome, and other cranial neuropathies may be present (58).

Laboratory Tests and Imaging

The following objectives must be met to plan effective treatment for glomus tumors:

- Determination of tumor type, size, and extent
- Exclusion of associated lesions
- Evaluation for neuroendocrine secretion (catecholamine levels)
- Determination of intracranial extension
- Assessment of large-vessel involvement
- Assessment of collateral circulation

Most of these objectives are met with imaging. The extent of the tumor and its relation to the anatomic features of the temporal bone are best identified with CT in both axial and coronal planes (Figs. 1–4). An intact jugu-

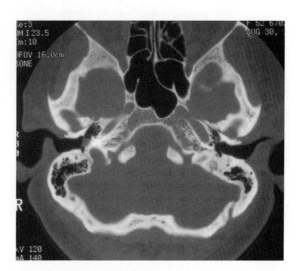

FIG. 1. Axial computed tomographic scan shows right middle ear mass defined as glomus tympanicum tumor by an uninvolved jugular bulb.

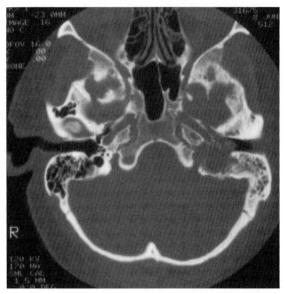

FIG. 2. Axial computed tomographic scan shows left glomus jugulare tumor.

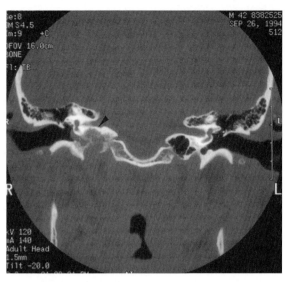

FIG. 4. Computed tomographic scan shows tumor extent within the temporal bone and relation of the tumor to the internal auditory canal *(arrow)*.

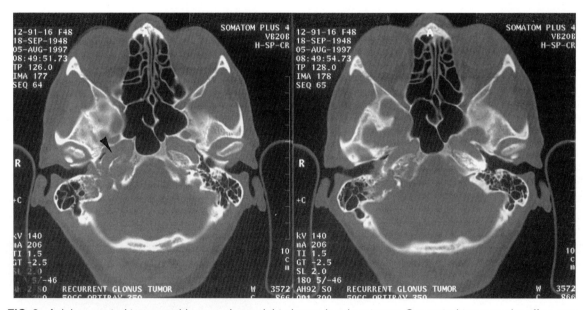

FIG. 3. Axial computed tomographic scan shows right glomus jugulare tumor. Computed tomography offers useful information relative to involvement of the petrous internal carotid artery *(arrow)*.

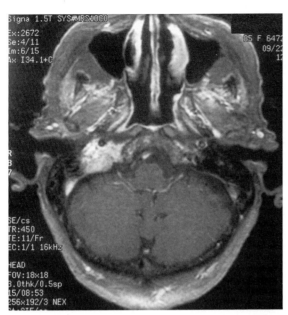

FIG. 5. Magnetic resonance image shows typical appearance of a glomus jugulare tumor *(right)*. Flow voids of vessels are present within the tumor.

lar bulb plate defines a glomus tympanicum tumor. Intracranial extension and the relation between the tumor and regional, neural, and vascular structures are best assessed with magnetic resonance (MR) imaging. MR imaging of the head and neck also helps in assessment of multicentricity (Figs. 5–8).

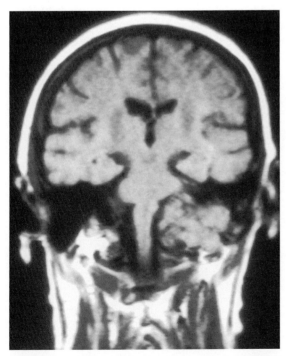

FIG. 6. Magnetic resonance image shows intracranial extension. Image shows proximity of the left glomus jugulare tumor to brainstem.

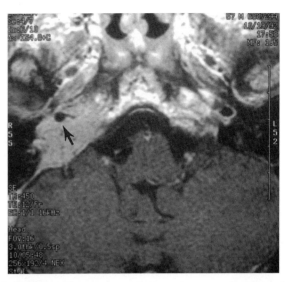

FIG. 7. Magnetic resonance image shows encroachment of right glomus jugulare tumor on the internal carotid artery *(arrow)*.

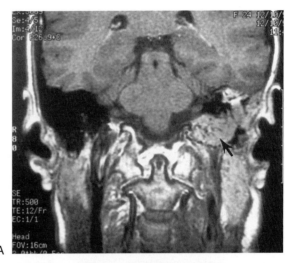

A

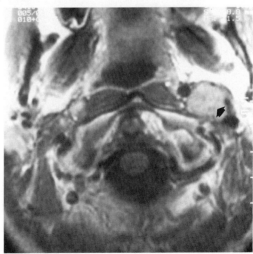

B

FIG. 8. Magnetic resonance (MR) image lesion left skull base *(arrow)* **(A)** and left carotid body tumor *(arrow)* **(B)**. For known glomus tumors of the head and neck, MR imaging should be performed for further evaluation of multicentricity.

Bilateral carotid angiography is performed to evaluate involvement of the ICA by tumor, to assess the blood supply of the lesion, and to identify associated lesions. Preoperative tumor embolization is accomplished in the same session (Figs. 9, 10). Angiography is particularly important in the evaluation of intracranial tumor extension. These lesions can derive blood supply from pial sources, the vertebral artery, the ICA, or the anterior and posterior inferior cerebellar arteries in addition to the external carotid artery branches. The value of embolization in limiting operative blood loss has been well documented (59–61). A diagnostic algorithm is shown in Fig. 11.

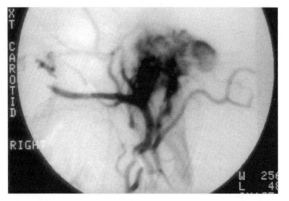

FIG. 9. Angiogram shows glomus tumor blush before embolization.

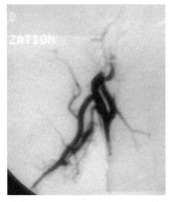

FIG. 10. Successful presurgical embolization of the tumor shown in Fig. 9.

Treatment Planning

Therapy for glomus tumors is palliative or definitive (curative). We consider radiation therapy palliative and surgery curative. Each treatment plan is based on data generated in the diagnostic evaluation and takes into account patient age, tumor type, and general health. The question that always must be addressed is: In the natural course of *this* patient's life expectancy, is the tumor likely to cause death or serious morbidity?

Palliation or simply observation is reserved for elderly persons, persons who are infirm, or those with multicentric lesions for whom definitive treatment is contraindicated. When palliation or observation is chosen, tumor behavior is assessed with yearly imaging studies.

If synchronous lesions are present, the first operation is performed on the most life-threatening lesion. The postoperative neurologic status of the patient determines subsequent recommendations. Bilateral glomus tumors are particularly challenging. If one is resected and the patient emerges neurologically intact, a contralateral operation in 6 months is planned. If considerable cranial nerve loss occurs with the initial operation, such a plan may not be feasible because of risk for devastating laryngeal and pharyngeal denervation that necessitates permanent tracheostomy and gastrostomy. The residual lesions should be followed and palliated when indicated.

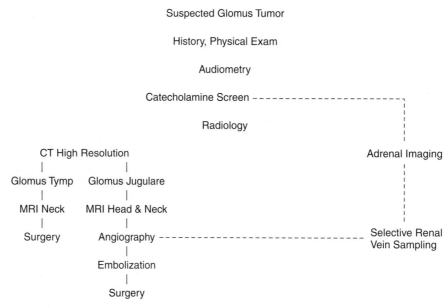

FIG. 11. Algorithm for diagnosis of glomus tumors.

Radiation Therapy

There is a longstanding controversy between surgeons and radiation therapists regarding the treatment modality that provides the best *primary* therapy for glomus tumor. The radiation therapy position was articulated nicely by Cummings et al. (62), who wrote, ". . . the relief of symptoms and the failure of the tumor to grow during the remainder of the patient's lifetime is a practical measure of successful treatment." However, the suggestion that irradiated tumors always consist of benign masses of inert cells is probably inaccurate (63–65). Because of the relative rarity of these tumors and their protracted natural history, it has been difficult to accumulate enough data from which to derive reliable statistical information (66–68). Jackson et al. (24) reviewed 157 studies that addressed irradiation as the therapeutic method for glomus tumors. They found that although growth was arrested in a considerable number of tumors, a high incidence of hearing loss, central nervous system damage, osteoradionecrosis, and radiation-induced malignant growth occurred in these cases. They concluded that the risks of radiation therapy were ongoing, long term and not fully determined.

Surgical Treatment

Basic Principles

Glomus tumors grow along lines of least resistance (Fig. 12). The surgical approach varies depending on tumor extent (Fig. 13). It must allow wide exposure of all tumor margins, including intracranial extension, and exposure and control of vital anatomic structures. Two structures, the facial nerve and the ICA are especially important in glomus tumor surgery.

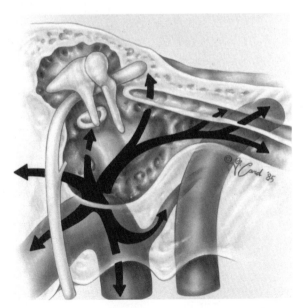

FIG. 12. Potential routes of glomus tumor extension.

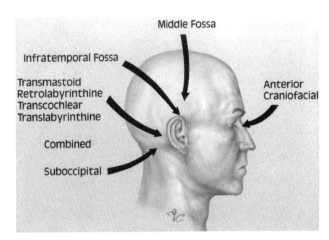

FIG. 13. To individualize an approach, the surgical team must combine a variety of options.

The Facial Nerve

In operations on the lateral skull base, the facial nerve is often an impediment to exposure and frequently must be relocated (23,69). Successful manipulation of the facial nerve is aided by its vascular supply. The facial nerve is fed by branches of the ICA and external carotid artery that form an extrinsic network that courses between the fallopian canal and the epineurium (70). A secondary network of capillaries derived from the same sources courses within the nerve and can support it when relocation interrupts the extrinsic system.

Tumor size and the amount of distal ICA control required determine the degree of nerve mobilization. Options include simple exposure, short or long mobilization, segmental resection, and selective division (71). Short mobilization of the facial nerve limited to the lateral genu usually is attended by normal postoperative facial nerve function. It is indicated in the management of small glomus tumors. Long mobilization is needed for large tumors. It involves nerve detachment from the geniculate ganglion to the pes anserinus. Long-term facial nerve function generally is good (71,72). Selective division with reanastomosis rarely is performed, even in the management of very large lesions. Segmental resection rarely is needed and is undertaken only when the nerve is inextricable from the tumor. When preoperative facial nerve function is normal, microdissection to separate the tumor from the nerve is attempted. Intraoperative monitoring greatly adds to the surgeon's ability to preserve nerve fibers. Preoperative paralysis usually is an indication for nerve resection and interposition graft reconstruction (73).

Internal Carotid Artery

Proximal and distal control of the ICA is fundamental in glomus jugulare surgery (Fig. 14). Control implies circumferential access to an area of normal vessel. In addition to exposing the carotid artery in the neck, the surgeon must be able to access its tympanic, petrous, and intracranial segments.

It is not always possible to ascertain the condition of the ICA before the operation, and guidelines for sacrifice of

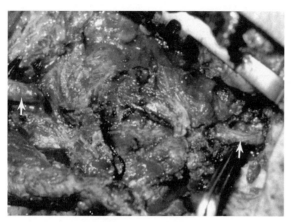

FIG. 14. Intraoperative photograph shows proximal and distal control of the internal carotid artery *(arrows)*.

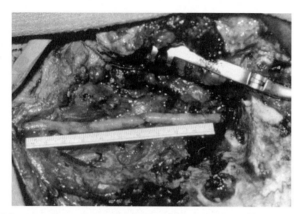

FIG. 15. When the internal carotid artery cannot be salvaged, circulation is reestablished with a venous graft.

the ICA remain uncertain (74). When the tumor invades the walls of the ICA, continuity of the vessel may be restored with an interposition venous graft (Fig. 15). When sacrifice of the ICA is predetermined, the patient does not pass angiographic test occlusion, or reconstruction is not feasible, extracranial bypass is performed before resection (74). Occlusion (sacrifice) of the ICA with detachable intravascular balloons can be performed preoperatively (75,76).

ICA spasm is an extremely serious complication that occurs in response to stretch manipulation of the vessel. When spasm occurs, manipulation should cease and papaverine should be administered immediately, either topically or by means of ICA wall injection. In extreme cases manual dilation or segmental resection of the artery may be needed (69).

Surgical Technique: Glomus Tympanicum Tumors

A type I glomus tympanicum tumor (see Table 2) is characterized by circumferentially visible margins (Figs. 16, 17: see color plates 32 and 33 following page 484). It can be exposed by means of transcanal tympanotomy and avulsed from the promontory. Bleeding is controlled with microbipolar coagulation or light packing (14,24). Resection of type II through IV glomus tympanicum tumors (see Table 2) (margins indistinct at otoscopy) necessitates a

transmastoid approach (14,24). If imaging has been unreliable and exploration reveals a jugulare tumor, resection is aborted and plans are made for a skull base approach in another operation.

The transmastoid approach to glomus tympanicum tumors involves complete mastoidectomy with extended facial recess techniques (25–27). Hypotympanic exposure allows visual assessment of the tumor relative to the jugular bulb, ICA, and remaining anatomic structures of the temporal bone (Fig. 18). Middle ear reconstruction may be needed after tumor resection and usually is performed in the same operation.

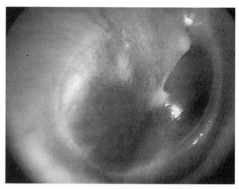

FIG. 16. Glomus tympanicum tumor of right ear involves posterior-inferior mesotympanum.

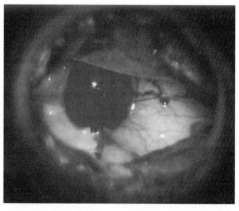

FIG. 17. Glomus tympanicum tumor of left ear attached to inferior promontory.

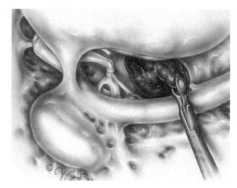

FIG. 18. Extended facial recess provides wide exposure into the hypotympanum for tumor removal.

Surgical Technique: Glomus Jugulare Tumors Types I and II

For tumors confined to the infralabyrinthine chamber and involving only the tympanic segment of the ICA, a hearing-conservation approach can be used (external canal and middle ear structures conserved) (36). The incision should allow access to the temporal bone and neck (Fig. 19). The carotid arteries, internal jugular vein, and cranial nerves X, XI, and XII are isolated and controlled. The extratemporal facial nerve is identified. The ICA is exposed and secured with vascular loops, and the internal jugular vein is ligated. Complete mastoidectomy is performed with removal of the mastoid tip. An extended facial recess exposure is made by means of removal of the inferior tympanic bone and skeletonization of the inferior-anterior EAC. This step allows access to the mesotympanum and exteriorization of the tympanic ICA to the level of the eustachian tube (Fig. 20). The facial nerve undergoes short mobilization (Fig. 21). Proximal control

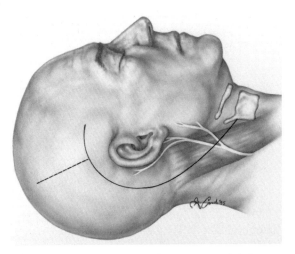

FIG. 19. Incision for glomus jugulare tumors minimizes superior flap necrosis and allows cephalic access as needed.

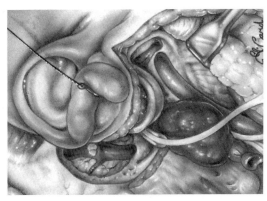

FIG. 20. The extended facial recess approach to small tumors provides ample distal control of the internal carotid artery and allows hearing conservation.

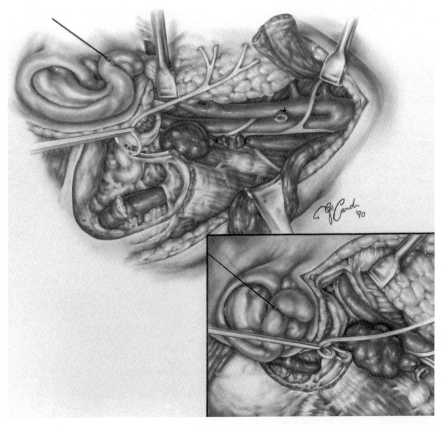

FIG. 21. Tympanic bone removal, skeletonization of the external auditory canal, and facial nerve mobilization.

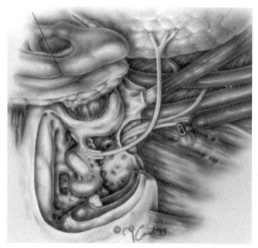

FIG. 22. Tumor removal is complete and all cranial nerves are intact. Sigmoid sinus pack occlusion is visible.

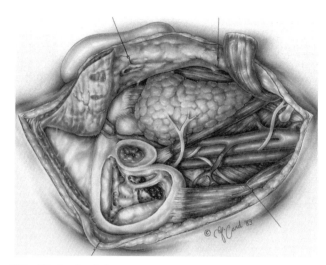

FIG. 23. In the infratemporal fossa approach, the external auditory canal is transected and oversewn.

of the sigmoid sinus is achieved by means of intraluminal packing with oxidized cellulose absorbable hemostat (Surgicel; see Fig. 21). The tumor is dissected from the ICA and mobilized from the infralabyrinthine space. Opening the jugular bulb to remove intraluminal tumor results in bleeding from the inferior petrosal sinus. This bleeding is controlled by means of packing. Delicate dissection of a glomus jugulare tumor from the contents of the pars nervosa and hypoglossal canal is critical to preserve the lower cranial nerve (Fig. 22).

Surgical Technique: Glomus Jugulare Tumors Types III and IV

When the tumor extends beyond the temporal bone into the infratemporal fossa (IFTF) or when control of the petrous ICA is needed, a modified or extended infratemporal fossa approach is necessary. These approaches give access to the deep recesses of the temporal bone, IFTF, clivus, nasopharynx, and cavernous sinus. The posterior, middle, and anterior cranial fossa can be accessed if intracranial extension exists. Complete conductive hearing loss is conceded.

The same incision used for a Type I or II glomus jugulare tumors is executed (see Fig. 19), but the EAC is transected and oversewn (Fig. 23). The EAC, tympanic membrane, and middle ear contents lateral to the stapes are resected (Fig. 24). Access to the petrous ICA and IFTF necessitates anterior and inferior dislocation of the mandible by means of dividing its anteromedial ligaments. The facial nerve undergoes long mobilization (see Fig. 24). Current technical modifications (77–79) preserve the periosteal tissue of the stylomastoid foramen and soft tissues surrounding the facial nerve during translocation (for clarity the illustrations show the facial

nerve alone). Mandibular retraction or segmental resection may be necessary to gain wider exposure.

Access may be extended farther when the anterosuperior extension of the tumor is extreme. When the zygoma and temporomandibular joint are resected as a unit, the temporalis muscle is reflected inferiorly, and the mandible is dislocated anteroinferiorly, the IFTF can be widely accessed (Fig. 25). The eustachian tube is resected, and the contents of the foramen spinosum are preserved as the ICA is exposed and mobilized from the pterygoid region to its precavernous segment (Fig. 26). Access to the middle cranial fossa, nasopharynx, foramen rotundum (maxillary division of cranial nerve V), clivus, posterior cranial fossa, and cavernous sinus is possible. Tumor resection proceeds as described earlier.

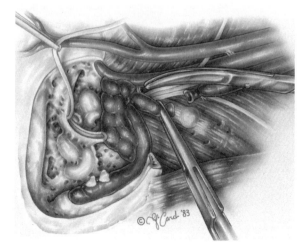

FIG. 24. Tumor dissection from proximal petrous internal carotid artery is facilitated by facial nerve mobilization and mandibular dislocation.

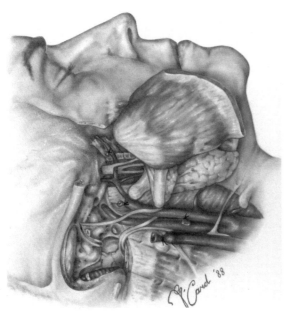

FIG. 25. The mandible, temporalis muscle, and zygoma are reflected as a unit to allow extension into the infratemporal fossa.

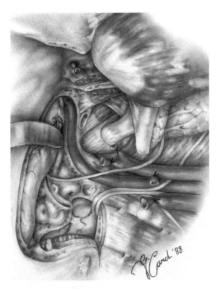

FIG. 26. The internal carotid artery exposure is complete. Middle cranial fossa exposure is excellent. The maxillary division of cranial nerve V in the foramen rotundum is depicted.

Intracranial Extension

Intracranial extension is defined as the spread of tumor through the dura into the subarachnoid space. Until recently it was considered a criterion for unresectability. The temporal bone and intracranial portions of the tumor often were regarded as two separate lesions and were managed as such. The current trend is to excise the entire tumor in a one-stage procedure (21,23).

Posterior fossa extension usually occurs through the dura or along cranial nerves (Fig. 27). Single-stage

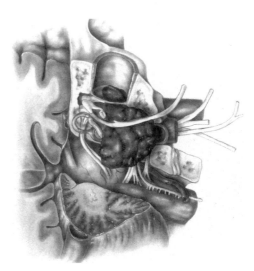

FIG. 27. Transdural extension of tumor occurs along cranial nerve roots or directly.

resection is complicated by reconstruction of dural defects, bone and soft-tissue defects, elevated CSF pressure caused by venous occlusion, regional ischemia from ligation of the external carotid artery, and possibly radiation-induced vascular changes. Resection of intracranial tumors limited to the area of the pars nervosa usually produces a small dural defect. Large intracranial resections are associated with considerable loss of dura and bone.

Defect Reconstruction

Although defect reconstruction is size dependent, the following guidelines apply to every case:

- The dura should be reconstructed with *vascularized* tissue.
- Tissue bulk is added to support the reconstruction and counteract CSF pressure.
- A lumbar drain for CSF decompression is maintained for 5 days.

Successful reconstruction is facilitated by careful preservation and mobilization of regional tissue (80). The skin incision should allow access to the superficial temporal fascia. The skin flap should be elevated deep to the platysma in the neck and in the subcutaneous plane over the mastoid process. A strong sternomastoid musculofascial flap is made by means of cutting along the temporal line up to or beyond the EAC if resection of this structure is contemplated (Fig. 28A). The sternomastoid musculofascial flap is then mobilized posteriorly and inferiorly (Fig. 28B). This facilitates closure through reattachment of this tissue to the deep temporal fascia superiorly and the parotid fascia anteriorly. When the EAC is preserved, this flap is attached to the bone-cartilage junction of the EAC (Fig. 28C).

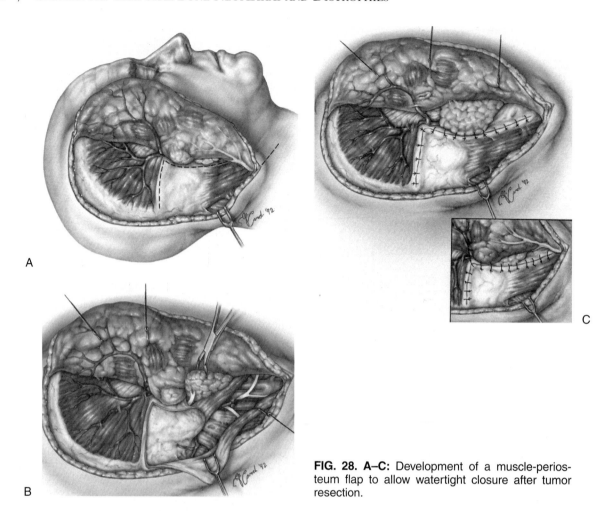

FIG. 28. A–C: Development of a muscle-periosteum flap to allow watertight closure after tumor resection.

Small dural defects are closed with vascularized temporalis (temporal parietal) fascia and free abdominal fat (23,81). The temporalis flap is based on the superficial temporal artery and elevation requires careful dissection in the zygomatic region to maintain the blood supply (Fig. 29A). The superficial temporalis fascia is left attached to the skin flap until need for the fascia is determined. The fascia then is detached and rotated into the dural defect (Fig. 29B). Even when the EAC is left intact and the middle ear is open, this flap is ample enough to wrap around the ear canal, facial recess, and antrum to maintain an aerated middle ear space (23).

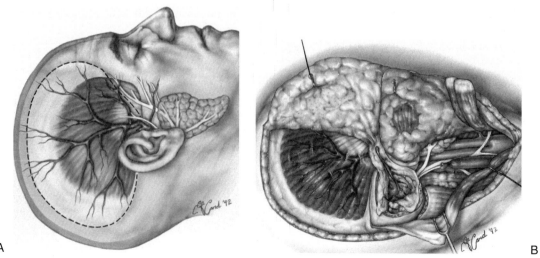

FIG. 29. A, B: Development of a superficial temporalis fascia flap based on the superficial temporal artery. Used for repair after tumor ablation.

For larger defects, revision operations, and operations on irradiated fields, the greater bulk of a musculocutaneous flap is needed. For young women a lower trapezius musculocutaneous flap is preferred (Fig. 30). (82). Free flap reconstruction is an excellent and frequently superior alternative (Fig. 31).

Rehabilitation after Cranial Nerve Loss

In operations on small tumors cranial nerve preservation can be achieved more than 90% of the time (83). In the management of advanced lesions, however, an operation on the lateral skull base exposes cranial nerves VII through XII and the sympathetic trunk to permanent damage. The lower cranial nerves function as a complex unit integrating phonopharyngeal function (Fig. 32). Loss of one nerve rarely interferes with permanent airway protection, swallowing, or speech, but acute loss of multiple lower cranial nerves is poorly tolerated. For elderly patients swallowing rehabilitation may be very difficult and usually leads to a prolonged period of disability. Rehabilitation strategies for each cranial nerve have been described in detail by Netterville et al. (84). The most important steps are vocal cord and arytenoid medialization and cricopharyngeal myotomy, which may obviate tracheostomy, improve speech, facilitate oral intake, and shorten hospital stay.

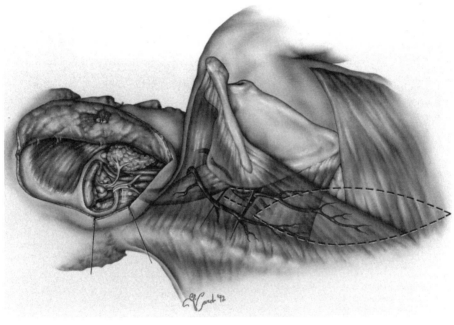

A

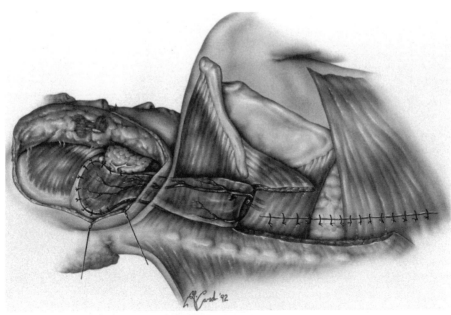

B

FIG. 30. A, B: Development of a lower trapezius flap.

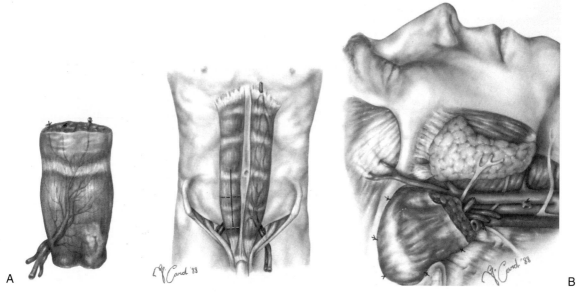

FIG. 31. A, B: Development of a rectus abdominis free flap.

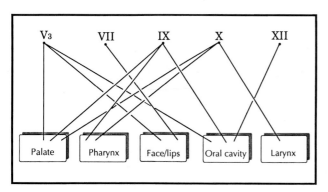

FIG. 32. Interaction of lower cranial nerves in phonopharyngeal function.

Results

Between January 1971 and November 1993, 133 patients underwent surgical treatment by The Otology Group, Nashville, Tenn. Most of the patients (106) had glomus jugulare tumors. Twenty-seven with glomus vagale tumors that required skull base approaches were included in the study. Presenting symptoms (see Table 3), physical findings (see Table 5), sex, age distribution, and multicentricity were analyzed. Seventeen patients had undergone previous operations, and 9 had been treated with radiation; 107 patients had no prior treatment. Previously treated patients were excluded in the analysis of surgical results and preoperative cranial nerve deficits (see Table 4). Five patients were excluded because of inadequate documentation. Tumors were classified with the Fisch and Glasscock-Jackson systems (Table 6).

The male to female ratio was 1:4 for glomus jugulare and 1:2.6 for glomus vagale tumors. Approximately 20%

of glomus jugulare patients had multicentric lesions, as follows: 10 carotid body tumors, 5 glomus jugulare tumors, 3 glomus vagale tumors, 1 bilateral glomus jugulare tumor, and 1 glomus tympanicum tumor. The most common symptom was pulsatile tinnitus followed by hearing loss. Seventy-three percent of patients with a glo-

TABLE 6. *Classification of glomus jugulare tumors*

Classification system	Tumor type	n	Percentage
Fisch	B	25	32
	C	26	33
	D_1	23	30
	D_2	4	5
	Total	78	100
Glasscock–Jackson	1	23	30
	2	13	17
	3	30	38
	4	12	15
	Total	78	100

TABLE 7. *Cranial nerve preservation (n = 102)*

	Tumor type	
Cranial nerve	Glomus jugulare (n = 78)	Glomus vagale (n = 24)
V	78	23
VI	78	24
VII	62	21
VIII	64	22
IX	26	13
X	39	3
XI	41	13
XII	46	9

TABLE 8. *Cranial nerve preservation among patients with glomus jugulare tumors according to tumor size*

Tumor type	n	Cranial nerve VII	Cranial nerve VIII	Cranial nerve IX	Cranial nerve X	Cranial nerve XI	Cranial nerve XII
I	23	19 (83%)	22 (96%)	17 (74%)	21 (91%)	22 (96%)	22 (96%)
II	13	13 (100%)	6 (55%)	6 (46%)	9 (69%)	9 (69%)	10 (78%)
III	30	19 (73%)	7 (30%)	5 (19%)	8 (33%)	7 (30%)	10 (43%)
IV	2	7 (58%)	0	1 (8%)	1 (8%)	1 (8%)	1 (8%)

TABLE 9. *Facial nerve recovery*

Facial class	Intact		Divided		Total
	Fallopian canal	Nerve mobilized	Primary anastomosis	Cable grafted	
I	4	6	0	0	10
II	1	16	0	0	17
III	—	11	5	3	19
IV	—	3	1	5	9
V	—	1	2	0	3
VI	0	0	0	0	0
Total					60

mus jugulare tumor had a red middle ear mass at otoscopy, and 41% of patients with glomus vagale tumors had a palpable neck mass. Six percent of patients had catecholamine-secreting tumors.

The most common deficits produced by glomus jugulare tumors were caused by involvement of cranial nerves X (23%), IX (17%), and XII (15%). The most common preoperative nerve deficit associated with glomus vagale tumors was tenth-nerve paralysis (54%). Nerve deficits were more common among patients with glomus vagale tumors (67%) than among those with glomus jugulare tumors (41%).

Four patients had malignant glomus jugulare tumors (3.8%). Two of these were disease free 3 years after primary resection. One patient was alive with lung metastasis 2 years after resection. One patient who underwent resection of the ICA had a stroke and died in the postoperative period.

Almost half of the patients needed an IFTF approach. Translabyrinthine or transcochlear resection was necessary in 15% of the operations. Data relating to cranial nerve preservation are reported in Table 7. The vagus nerve was preserved in 49% of patients with glomus jugulare tumors and the glossopharyngeal nerve in 32%. The vagus nerve was preserved in only 12% of patients with glomus vagale tumors. The facial nerve was preserved in 80% of patients, and the remaining 20% underwent direct anastomosis, cable grafting, or facial to hypoglossal nerve anastomosis. Table 8 shows cranial nerve preservation in relation to tumor size for glomus jugulare tumors. Facial nerve recovery after surgical treatment is analyzed in Table 9.

Surgical complications are listed in Table 10. The most common perioperative complications were CSF leak (Table 11) and aspiration. There were three perioperative deaths, two as a result of ICA injury during the operation that resulted in a stroke and one of pulmonary embolism.

Long-term follow-up results were reported by Poe et al. (79) on 43 patients with glomus jugulare tumors surgically treated by means of skull-base approaches. Dura-

TABLE 10. *Surgical complications among 102 patients with glomus jugulare or glomus vagale tumors*

Complication	No. of patients	Percentage
Cerebrospinal fluid (CSF) leak	11	11.6
Aspiration	5	5.3
Death	3	2.1
Aural infection	4	4.2
Ileus	2	1.0
Internal carotid artery blowout	1	1.0
Meningitis	2	2.1
Pulmonary embolus	2	1.0
Acute respiratory distress syndrome	1	1.0
Stroke	3	2.1
Respiratory arrest	1	1.0
Bacterial endocarditis	1	1.0
Gastrointestinal bleeding	1	1.0

TABLE 11. *Incidence of postoperative cerebrospinal fluid leak among patients with glomus jugulare tumors according to size (1971–1993)*

Glasscock–Jackson class	No. of patients	No. of leaks
Type I	23	1
Type II	13	0
Type III	30	7
Type IV	11	2
Total	77	10 (13%)

tion of the follow-up period ranged from 2 to 19 years, with a median of 5 years. Four tumors were subtotally resected, and the patients underwent radiation therapy; none has had progression of disease. No tumors recurred after total resection.

GLANDULAR TUMORS OF THE MIDDLE EAR

Primary adenomatous tumors of the middle ear are rare. Their clinical and structural features have been the source of considerable controversy. Although these tumors appear to derive from the glands of the middle ear mucosa as opposed to ectopic salivary tissue, many unclear and even contradictory descriptions of their nature lead to a confusing nomenclature. In 1976, Hyams and Michaels (85) reviewed 20 primary adenomas of the middle ear cleft and found that although the clinical course was benign, the structural pattern varied from clearly glandular to papillary cystadenomatous and occasionally to one lacking a specific structure. These authors further analyzed lesions that adopted aggressive behavior that resulted in destruction of the otic capsule and ossicles. They also found that the tumors lacked the features that typified the adenomas described in their study. This outlook was later supported by Benecke et al. (86) who in a review of their experience with 13 patients found that adenomatous tumors can present themselves as distinctly glandular or adopt a papillary pattern. Papillary tumors exhibited aggressive behavior that eroded bone, grew at a faster rate, and on occasion extended intracranially.

Amble et al. (77) addressed this controversy and reviewed their experience with 16 patients. They proposed a different explanation for the structural origin of these tumors. They believed the lesions arose from middle ear paraganglia and were similar to glomus tumors but had gland formation and positive staining for keratin and chromogranin. They based this hypothesis on the clinical findings for these tumors, which were considered similar to those of paraganglioma, the limited histologic variety of the middle ear lining as a neoplastic source, and the immunohistologic characteristics of the lesions. These findings have not been confirmed by other investigators.

Adenomatous tumors have been described among children and elderly persons but are most common in midlife. There is no sex prevalence. The tumors usually present with hearing loss. Pain and otorrhea develop later. At examination the most common finding is a middle ear mass behind an intact tympanic membrane. When otorrhea is present, the diagnosis often is missed and sometimes is made only at surgical exploration. CT is helpful in outlining the bony limits of the lesion and identifying bone destruction. MR imaging also may be valuable when intracranial involvement is present.

Differentiating benign from malignant adenomatous tumors may be difficult. Bone erosion per se is not an indication of malignancy. There are numerous reports of instances in which this finding was associated with a benign course and surgical cure. Cranial nerve involvement, however, is a poor prognostic sign and usually is associated with persistent disease despite aggressive treatment and eventually death due to tumor (77–79,85,86).

Because of the histologic complexity and rarity of glandular tumors and difficulties predicting their behavior, it is difficult to establish precise guidelines for the management of these tumors. It appears that unless clear signs of malignancy are present, gross surgical resection should be complete but neural function should be preserved. This usually involves radical or modified radical mastoidectomy. Aggressive tumors appear to be radioresistant.

CARCINOID TUMORS

Middle ear carcinoid is a very rare lesion. As with adenomatous and papillary tumors, with which carcinoids often are confused, thorough evaluation of the clinical and especially the histologic findings is critical to reach a correct diagnosis. Among the latter, immunohistochemical and electron microscopic techniques aimed at identifying neurosecretory granules are the most important (80).

Light microscopic study usually shows islands of small, regular cuboidal cells disposed in compact sheets, which often show a tendency to form lumens. The cytoplasm is eosinophilic and contains fine granules. At electron microscopic examination these cells show numerous neurosecretory granules with a diameter of about 200 nm. At immunohistochemical analysis, carcinoid cells are found to contain cytokeratin antibodies and sometimes chromogranin. The most important issue is accurate identification, because the histologic features of carcinoids are similar to those of papillary glandular tumors. The histologic features also resemble those of other neuroendocrine tumors, such as paraganglioma, which contains the same polypeptides as do carcinoids, including serotonin, somatostatin, glucagon, and others (87).

Nyrop et al. (88) reviewed the world literature on carcinoid tumors of the ear and found that only 30 have been reported. There was a slight predominance among men (19:11), and the age at presentation varied between 16 and 59 years. The most common symptom was hearing loss, usually conductive and progressive. At otoscopy the tympanic membrane usually is intact, but it may be erythematous and laterally displaced (mass effect). Most reported tumors have been confined to the middle ear and produce little ossicular destruction.

Complete excision, usually by means of tympanomastoidectomy is the recommended treatment. Radical mastoidectomy may be necessary to manage larger lesions.

The follow-up results reported in the literature are too varied to provide clear information, but recurrences are found to follow incomplete removal.

TUMORS OF THE ENDOLYMPHATIC SAC

Tumors of the endolymphatic sac are low-grade, locally aggressive glandular lesions with frequent intracranial involvement. They have to be differentiated from middle ear adenoma (glandular and papillary), adenocarcinoma, and carcinoid tumor. Tumors of the endolymphatic sac are centered between the sigmoid sinus and the internal auditory canal along the posteromedial petrous bone in the region of the vestibular aqueduct. Posterior fossa involvement is not expected in mastoid and middle ear mucosal tumors. Histologic studies reveal a papillary-cystic architecture with villous formation, typically with a cuboidal or columnar lining epithelium and an underlying spindle or myoepithelial layer. Microscopic examination shows the tumor as a lobular, reddish, highly vascular mass.

Hasserd et al. (89) in 1984 reported the first endolymphatic sac tumor. During an operation on the endolymphatic sac for Meniere's disease, a highly vascular, lobular mass was found centered along the posterior portion of the petrous temporal bone. Both anatomic location and histopathologic findings were highly suggestive of endolymphatic sac origin. Subsequent review of 20 cases by Heffner et al. (90) further supported the hypothesis that this is a distinct entity arising from the endolymphatic sac.

CT commonly shows an osteolytic lesion centered in the area between the internal auditory canal and the sigmoid sinus. Prominent calcification within the mass often is present. MR imaging demonstrates heterogenous foci of low and high signal intensity on both T1- and T2-weighted images and with gadolinium enhancement. Preoperative angiography with embolization to minimize intraoperative blood loss has been suggested (91).

Endolymphatic sac tumor appears to grow slowly and often is not diagnosed or is managed inadequately until extensive local destruction has occurred. Clinical presentation usually is sudden or progressive hearing loss or tinnitus, transient vertigo, and often facial paralysis. Other findings include decreased ipsilateral caloric responses. In a study by Megerian et al. (92), sensorineural hearing loss was diagnosed an average of 10.6 years before the tumor was found. Intracranial involvement is not uncommon because of the delay in diagnosis. Heffner (90) reported tumor extension into the posterior cranial cavity ranging from 4 to 6 cm in 17 of 20 patients in the study. Complete surgical resection of the tumor and long-term surveillance are recommended because these lesions may recur as late as a decade after resection. There is no reported case of metastasis from an endolymphatic sac tumor.

There is a strong association between unilateral and bilateral endolymphatic sac tumors and von Hippel–Lindau disease, an autosomal dominant disorder with retinal and cerebellar angiomatosis. Detection of endolymphatic sac tumors during the patient's annual von Hippel–Lindau radiographic screening might lead to early diagnosis and possibly to a hearing-preservation operation.

CHOLESTEATOMA OF THE PETROUS APEX

Petrous apex cholesteatoma is a rare lesion that can be primary, congenital, or more commonly caused by chronic otitis media. Congenital lesions appear to originate from trapped squamous epithelial rests and usually are insidious with symptoms occurring late in the course (93). Acquired cholesteatoma can gain access to the petrous apex along the supralabyrinthine or subcochlear route (94). CT demonstrates an expansile, nonenhancing mass with scalloped margins. Imaging separates this finding from the more common cholesterol granuloma. On MR images cholesteatoma has a low signal intensity with T1-weighted sequences and a high signal intensity with T2-weighted sequences (94).

Important guidelines for surgical resection include complete matrix removal, facial nerve preservation, and avoidance of CSF leak. Exteriorization usually is needed when the cholesteatoma matrix is extensive and cannot be resected from the ICA and dura. A translyabyrinthine-transcochlear or middle cranial fossa approach is most commonly used. Follow-up evaluation with yearly MR imaging is recommended (93,94).

CHOLESTEROL GRANULOMA

Cholesterol granuloma can occur in any part of the temporal bone and is believed to result from a localized inflammatory reaction to cholesterol crystals (Chapter 25). Improper drainage or locally inadequate aeration of the temporal bone pneumatic system may cause hemorrhage, which gives origin to cholesterol crystals. Cholesterol granuloma typically occurs in a well-pneumatized petrous apex. The natural history of these lesions is not completely understood, but over time they may expand and cause hearing loss, imbalance, and dysfunction of cranial nerves V, VI, and VII.

Diagnosis is made by means of MR imaging (95,96). The lesion exhibits very high signal intensity on both T1- and T2-weighted images, in contradistinction to the pattern of petrous apex cholesteatoma (see earlier). Symptomatic cholesterol granuloma of the petrous apex is managed by means of marsupialization and drainage. The lesion may be approached through the infralabyrinthine, subcochlear, or middle cranial fossa route. Yearly MR imaging is recommended after the operation because recurrences are common.

CHORISTOMA

Choristoma was first described by Taylor and Martin in 1961 (97). It is a rare lesion, approximately 20 cases having been reported to date. Choristoma is not a true neoplasm because it consists of normal, ectopic, usually lobulated salivary tissue in the middle ear. These lesions have been the subjects of reviews by Namdar et al. (98) and Hinni and Beatty (99). They have been described in young children and elderly patients. The most common symptom is hearing loss followed by tinnitus and in rare instances drainage. A middle ear mass usually is evident at otoscopy. Ossicular abnormalities are almost always present. The most important clinical finding in choristoma is an intimate association with the facial nerve. In the review by Namdar et al. (98), a dehiscent nerve was reported in 6 patients, the nerve was obscured by the mass in 4, and the nerve had an abnormal course in 5 patients.

CT shows a middle ear mass, usually posterosuperiorly. Associated ossicular or facial nerve abnormalities, if definable, can aid in the diagnosis. Cholesteatoma (congenital or acquired) and tumor are the principal entities to be considered in the differential diagnosis. When the diagnosis is uncertain, repeated imaging after several months may indicate a stable lesion, which may further substantiate the initial impression. If exploration is undertaken for biopsy, facial nerve monitoring should be performed. Excision is contraindicated in the management of choristoma with a sessile attachment. If the lesion is pedunculated with a fine stalk, excision may be performed, provided the position and course of the facial nerve are clearly outlined and no connections exist between the nerve and the lesion.

Choristomas have *no growth* potential, and there have been no reported instances of tumoral degeneration. Ossicular reconstruction has been attempted but usually unsuccessfully. It would appear from the available experience that a conservative outlook is warranted in the management of these lesions.

CONCLUSION

Although the diagnosis and management of glomus tumors have been reasonably well established, less common neoplastic lesions of the middle ear need further definition. This is especially so for adenomatous and adenoma-like tumors. Differentiation between papillary lesions of the middle ear, carcinoid tumors, and endolymphatic sac tumors, which have locally aggressive behavior, similar histologic features, and immunohistochemical characteristics, is particularly challenging and merits further research to elucidate the nature and origin of these tumors.

SUMMARY POINTS

- Glomus tumors are second only to acoustic neuromas as the most frequently diagnosed temporal bone neoplasm. Less than 5% are malignant.
- Depending on site of origin, glomus tumors are called *tympanicum* (middle ear origin) or *jugulare* (jugular bulb origin). These tumors are further classified according to extent of disease (middle ear, skull base, petrous carotid, and intracranial involvement).
- Glomus tumors originate from the extraadrenal paraganglia, which are groups of neural crest cells located in various sites of the head and neck. These paraganglia are part of the neuroendocrine system, and tumors arising from them may secrete neuropeptides and catecholamines.
- In approximately 10% of cases, multicentric neural crest tumors develop. The most common association is glomus tympanicum or jugulare tumor and ipsilateral carotid body tumor.
- The most common presenting symptom of a glomus tumor is pulsatile tinnitus. Hearing loss may occur early and is caused by ossicular involvement. Bleeding and cranial nerve palsy usually occur late.
- Unless a glomus tympanicum tumor is very small with clear borders apparent circumferentially, it is not possible to differentiate it from a glomus jugulare tumor. Diagnosis of any vascular middle ear mass is made with CT and MR imaging; biopsy is contraindicated.
- For most glomus tumors, especially in otherwise healthy patients, surgical excision is the recommended treatment. Radiation therapy may prevent tumor growth in the long term and should be considered in the care of some elderly patients and those with multicentric lesions.
- Other benign tumors that occur in the middle ear include adenoma (glandular and papillary) and carcinoid tumor. Treatment is complete local excision.
- Endolymphatic sac tumors are low-grade, locally aggressive glandular lesions that present themselves as a vascular mass in the mastoid process, often with extension into the posterior cranial fossa. These tumors are often associated with von Hippel–Lindau disease.
- Choristoma is not a true neoplasm but is an ectopic mass of salivary tissue in the middle ear that does not have growth potential. These tumors often have an intimate connection with the facial nerve.

REFERENCES

1. Anson BJ, Donaldson JA, eds. *Surgical anatomy of the temporal bone.* Philadelphia: WB Saunders, 1981.

2. Jackson CG, Carrasco VN, Glasscock ME. Complications of surgery for glomus jugulare tumors. In: Eisele DW, ed. *Complications in head and neck surgery.* St. Louis: Mosby–Year Book, 1993:628–638.

3. Guild RS. A hitherto unrecognized structure, the glomus jugularis, in man. *Anat Rec* 1941;79[Suppl 2]:28–35.

4. Lundgren M. Tympanic body tumors in the middle ear: tumors of carotid body type. *Acta Otolaryngol (Stockh)* 1949;37:366.

5. Capps FCW. Glomus jugulare tumors of the middle ear. *J Laryngol Otol* 1952;66:302.

6. House W. Management of glomus tumors [Panel discussion]. *Arch Otolaryngol* 1969;89:170.

7. Gatspar H. Die Tumoren des glomus caroticus glomus jugulare–tympanicum und glomus vagale. *Acta Otolaryngol (Stockh)* 1961;54[Suppl 167]:1–45.

8. Shapiro MJ, Neues DK. Technique for removal of glomus jugulare tumors. *Arch Otolaryngol* 1964;79:219.

9. Gejrot T. Surgical treatment of glomus jugulare tumors with special reference to the diagnostic value of retrograde jugulography. *Acta Otolaryngol (Stockh)* 1965;60:150.

10. Kempe L, VanderArk GD, Smith DR. The neurosurgical treatment of glomus jugulare tumors. *Neurosurgery* 1971;35:59.

11. Hilding DA, Greenberg A. Surgery for large glomus jugulare tumor. *Arch Otolaryngol* 1971;93:227.

12. Semmes RE. Discussion: tumor of the glomus jugulare: follow-up study two years after roentgen therapy. *J Neurosurg* 1953;10:672.

13. Gejrot T. Retrograde jugulography in the diagnosis of abnormalities of the superior bulb of the internal jugular vein. *Acta Otolaryngol (Stockh)* 1964;57:177.

14. Spector GJ, Maisel RH, Ogura JH. Glomus tumors in the middle ear, I: an analysis of 46 patients. *Laryngoscope* 1973;93:1652.

15. Glasscock ME, Harris PF, Newsome G. Glomus tumors: diagnosis and treatment. *Laryngoscope* 1974;84:2006.

16. Gardner G, Cocke EW Jr, Robertson JT, et al. Combined approach surgery for removal of glomus jugulare tumors. *Laryngoscope* 1977;87:665.

17. Fisch U. Infratemporal fossa approach for extensive tumors of the temporal bone and base of the skull. In: Silverstein H, Norrel H, eds. *Neurological surgery of the ear,* vol II. Birmingham, AL: Aesculapius Publishers, 1977:34–53.

18. Fisch U. Infratemporal fossa approach for extensive tumors of the temporal bone and base of the skull. *J Laryngol Otol* 1978;92:949.

19. Jenkins HA, Fisch U. Glomus tumors of the temporal regions. *Arch Otolaryngol* 1981;107:209.

20. Glasscock ME, Jackson, CG, Harris PF. Glomus tumors: diagnosis, classification and management of large lesions. *Arch Otolaryngol* 1982;108:401.

21. Kinney SE. Glomus jugulare tumor surgery with intracranial extension. *Otolaryngol Head Neck Surg* 1980;88:531–535.

22. Fisch U. Carotid lesions at the skull base. In: Brackmann DE, ed. *Neurological surgery of the ear and skull base.* New York: Raven Press, 1982:269–281.

23. Jackson CG, Glasscock ME, McKennan KX, et al. The surgical treatment of skull base tumors with intracranial extension. *Otolaryngol Head Neck Surg* 1987;96:175–185.

24. Jackson CG, Johnson GD, Poe DS. Glomus tumors: surgical treatment of glomus tumors. In: Pillsbury H, Goldsmith MM, eds. *Operative challenges in otolaryngology–head and neck surgery.* Chicago: Year Book, 1990:153.

25. Jackson CG, Cueva RA, Thedinger BA, Glasscock ME. Conservation surgery for glomus jugulare tumors: the value of early diagnosis. *Laryngoscope* 1990;100:1031–1036.

26. Jackson CG, Cueva RA, Thedinger BA, Glasscock ME. Cranial nerve preservation in lesions of the jugulare foramen. *Otolaryngol Head Neck Surg* 1991;105:687–693.

27. Jackson CG. Infratympanic extended facial recess approach for anteriorly extensive middle ear disease: a conservation technique. *Laryngoscope* 1993;103:451–454.

28. Jackson CG. Neurotologic skull base surgery for glomus tumors: diag-

29. Jackson CG, Netterville JL. Lateral transtemporal approaches to the skull base, defect reconstruction and cranial nerve rehabilitation. In: AAO–HNS Instructional Courses, volume VI. Alexandria, VA: American Academy of Otolaryngology–Head and Neck Surgery, 1993.

30. Jackson CG. Hearing conservation in surgery for glomus jugulare tumors. *Am J Otol* 1996;17:425–437.

31. Alford BR, Guilford FR. A comprehensive study of tumors of the glomus jugulare. *Laryngoscope* 1962;72:765.

32. Oldring D, Fisch U. Glomus tumors of the temporal region. *Arch Otolaryngol* 1981;107:209.

33. Glasscock ME, Kveton JF. Surgical methods. In: Thawley SE, Panje WR, eds. *Comprehensive management of head and neck tumors.* Philadelphia: WB Saunders, 1987:222–245.

34. Glenner GG, Grimley PM. Tumors of the extra-adrenal paraganglion system (including chemoreceptors). In: *Atlas of tumor pathology,* 2nd series, fasc. 1. Washington, DC: Armed Forces Institute of Pathology, 1974:1–90.

35. Guild SR. The glomus jugulare, a nonchromaffin paraganglioma, in man. *Ann Otol Rhinol Laryngol* 1953;62:1045–1071.

36. Pearse AGE. The diffuse neuroendocrine system: historical review. *Front Horm Res* 1984;12:1–7.

37. Batsakis JG. Paragangliomas of the head and neck. In: *Tumors of the head and neck: clinical and pathological consideration,* 2nd ed. Baltimore: Williams & Wilkins, 1979:269–380.

38. Pearse AGE. The cytochemistry and ultrastructure of polypeptide hormone-producing cells of the APUD series and the embryologic, physiologic and pathologic implications of the concept. *J Histochem Cytochem* 1969;17:303–313.

39. Matsuguchi H, Tsuneyoshi M, Takeshita A, et al. Noradrenalin-secreting glomus jugulare tumor with cyclic change of blood pressure. *Arch Intern Med* 1975;135:1110–1113.

40. Schwaber MK, Glasscock ME, Jackson CG, et al. Diagnosis and management of catecholamine secreting glomus tumors. *Laryngoscope* 1984;94:1008–1015.

41. Schwartz ML, Israel HL. Severe anemia as a manifestation of metastatic jugular paraganglioma. *Arch Otolaryngol* 1983;109:269–272.

42. Spector GJ, Ciralski R, Maisel RH, et al. Multiple glomus tumors in the head and neck. *Laryngoscope* 1975;85:1066–1075.

43. Farrior JB III, Hyams VJ, Benke RH, et al. Carcinoid apudoma arising in a glomus jugulare tumor: review of endocrine activity in glomus jugulare tumors. *Laryngoscope* 1980;90:110–119.

44. Hadley ME. *Endocrinology.* Englewood Cliffs, NJ: Prentice-Hall, 1984:318–343.

45. Belal A Jr, Sanna M. Pathology as it relates to ear surgery, I: surgery of glomus tumors. *J Laryngol Otol* 1982;96:1079–1097.

46. Myers EN, Newman J, Kaseff L, et al. Glomus jugulare tumor: a radiographic-histologic correlation. *Laryngoscope* 1971;81:1838–1851.

47. Spector GJ, Gado M, Ciralsky R, et al. Neurologic implications of glomus tumors in the head and neck. *Laryngoscope* 1975;85:1387–1395.

48. Sternberger LA. *Immunocytochemistry.* New York: John Wiley & Sons, 1979.

49. Smith PG, Schwaber MK, Goebel JA. Clinical evaluation of glomus tumors of the ear and the base of the skull. In: Thawley SE, Panjey WR, eds. *Comprehensive management of head and tumors.* Philadelphia: WB Saunders, 1987:207.

50. Parkin JL. Familial multiple glomus tumors and pheochromocytomas. *Ann Otol Rhinol Laryngol* 1981;90:60–63.

51. Van Barrs F, Van Del Brook P, Cremers C, Veldman J. Familial nonchromatinnic paragangliomas (glomus tumors): clinical aspects. *Laryngoscope* 1981;91:988.

52. Ervin DM, Osguthorpe JD. X-ray study of the month: multicentric paragangliomas. *Ann Otol Rhinol Laryngol* 1984;93:96–97.

53. Lattes R, Waltner JG. Nonchromaffin paraganglioma of the middle ear. *Cancer* 1948;2:447–468.

54. Borsanyi SJ. Glomus jugulare tumors. *Laryngoscope* 1962;72:1336–1345.

55. Zbaren P, Lehmann W. Carotid body paraganglioma with metastases. *Laryngoscope* 1985;95:450–455.

56. Davis JM, Davis KR, Hesselink JR, et al. Malignant glomus jugulare tumor: a case with two unusual radiographic features. *J Comput Assist Tomogr* 1980;4:415–417.

57. Druck NS, Spector GJ, Ciralsky RH, et al. Malignant glomus vagale: report of a case and review of the literature. *Arch Otolaryngol* 1976;102:634–636.

58. Irons GB, Weiland LH, Brown WL. Paragangliomas of the neck: clinical and pathologic analysis of 116 cases. *Surg Clin North Am* 1977;57:575–583.

59. Lasjaunias P, Berenstein A. *Surgical neuroangiography, vol 2: endovascular treatment of craniofacial lesions.* Berlin: Springer-Verlag, 1987.

60. Schick PM, Hieshima GB, White RA, et al. Arterial catheter embolization followed by surgery for large chemodectoma. *Surgery* 1980;87:459–464.

61. Valavanis A. Preoperative embolization of the head and neck: indications, patient selection, goals, and precautions. *AJNR Am J Neuroradiol* 1986;7:943–952.

62. Cummings BJ, Beale FA, Garrett PG, et al. The treatment of glomus tumors in the temporal bone by megavoltage radiation. *Cancer* 1984;52:2635–2640.

63. Cole JM, Beiler D. Long-term results of treatment for glomus jugulare and glomus vagale tumors with radiotherapy. *Laryngoscope* 1994:104:1461–1465.

64. de Jong AL, Coker NJ, Jenkins HA, Goepfert H, Alford BR. Radiation therapy in the management of paragangliomas of the temporal bone. *Am J Otol* 1995;16:283–289.

65. Carrasco V, Rosenman J. Radiation therapy of glomus jugulare tumors. *Laryngoscope* 1993:103:23–26.

66. Brackmann DE, House WF, Terry R, et al. Glomus jugulare tumors: effect of irradiation. *Trans Am Acad Ophthalmol Otolaryngol* 1972;76:1423–1431.

67. Spector GJ, Compaqno J, Perez CA, et al. Gomus jugulare tumors: effects of radio-therapy. *Cancer* 1975;35:1316–1321.

68. Spector GJ, Maisel RH, Ogura JH. Glomus jugulare tumors, II: a clinicopathologic analysis of the effect of radiotherapy. *Ann Otol Rhinol Laryngol* 1974;83:6–32.

69. Smith PG, Killeen TE. Carotid artery vasospasm complicating extensive skull base surgery: cause, prevention and management. *Otolaryngol Head Neck Surg* 1987;97:1–7.

70. Makele M, Franklin DJ, Zhao J, et al. Neural infiltration of glomus temporale tumors. *Am J Otol* 1990;11:1–5.

71. Von Doersten P, Jackson CG, Manolidis S, et al. Facial nerve outcome in skull base surgery for benign lesion. *Laryngoscope* 1998;108:1480–1484.

72. Jackson CG. *Facial nerve paralysis: diagnosis and treatment of lower motor neuron facial nerve lesions and facial paralysis.* Alexandria, VA: American Academy of Otolaryngology–Head and Neck Surgery Foundation, 1986.

73. Brackmann DE. The facial nerve in the infratemporal approach. *Otolaryngol Head Neck Surg* 1987;97:15–17.

74. Sen C, Sekhar LN. Direct vein graft reconstruction of the cavernous, petrous, and upper cervical internal carotid artery: lessons learned from 30 cases. *Neurosurgery* 1992;30:732–742.

75. Awad IA, Spetzler RF. Extracranial-intracranial bypass surgery: a critical analysis in light of the international cooperative study. *Neurosurgery* 1986;19:655–664.

76. Zane RS, Aeschbacher P, Moll C, Fisch U. Carotid occlusion without reconstruction: a safe surgical option in selected patients. *Am J Otol* 1995;16:353–359.

77. Amble FR, Harner SG, Weiland LH, et al. Middle ear adenoma and adenocarcinoma. *Otolaryngol Head Neck Surg* 1993;109:871–874.

78. Pallanch JF, MacDonald TJ, Weiland LH. Adenocarcinoma and adenoma of the middle ear. *Laryngoscope* 1982;92:47–54.

79. Poe DS, Tarlov EC, Thomas CB, Kveton JF. Aggressive papillary tumors of temporal bone. *Otolaryngol Head Neck Surg* 1993;108:80–86.

80. Krouse JH, Nadol JB, Goodman ML. Carcinoid tumors of the middle ear. *Ann Otol Rhinol Laryngol* 1990;99:547–552.

81. Abul-Hassan HS, Ascher GD, Acland RD. Surgical anatomy and blood supply of the fascial layers of the temporal region. *Plast Reconstr Surg* 1986;77:17–23.

82. Maves MD, Panje WR, Shagets F. Extended latissimus dorsi myocutaneous flap reconstruction of major head and neck defects. *Otolaryngol Head Neck Surg* 1984;92:551–558.

83. Leonetti JP, Brackmann DE, Prass RL. Improved preservation of facial nerve function in the infratemporal approach to the skull base. *Otolaryngol Head Neck Surg* 1988:101:74–78.

84. Netterville JL, Jackson CG, Civantos FJ. Thyroplasty in the functional rehabilitation of neurotologic skull base surgery patients. *Am J Otol* 1993;14:460–464.

85. Hyams VJ, Michaels L. Benign adenomatous neoplasm (adenoma of the middle ear). *Clin Otolaryngol* 1976;1:17–26.

86. Benecke TE, Noel FL, Carberry JN, et al. Adenomatous tumors of the middle ear and mastoid. *Am J Otol* 1990;11:20–26.

87. Davies JE, Semeraro D, Knight LC, Griffiths GJ. Middle ear neoplasms slowing adenomatous and neuroendocrine components. *J Laryngol Otol* 1989;103:404–407.

88. Nyrop M, Skov BG, Katholm M, Nielsen HW. Carcinoid tumors of the middle ear. *Ear Nose Throat J* 1994;73:688–693.

89. Hassard AD, Boudreau SF, Cron CC. Adenoma of the endolymphatic sac. *J Otolaryngol* 1984;13:213–216.

90. Heffner DK. Low-grade adenocarcinoma of probable endolymphatic sac origin: a clinicopathologic study of 20 cases. *Cancer* 1989;64:2292–2302.

91. Mukherji SK, Albernaz VS, Lo WW, et al. Papillary endolymphatic sac tumors: CT, MR imaging, and angiographic findings in 20 patients. *Radiology* 1997;202:801–808.

92. Megerian CA, McKenna MJ, Nadol JB. Non-paraganglioma jugular foramen lesions masquerading as glomus jugulare tumors. *Am J Otol* 1995;10:72–77.

93. Levenson MJ, Michaels L, Parisier SC. Congenital cholesteatomas of the middle ear in children: origin and management. *Otolaryngol Clin North Am* 1989;22:941–954.

94. Ishii K, Takahashi S, Matsumoto K, et al. Middle ear cholesteatoma extending into the petrous apex: evaluation by CT and MR imaging. *AJNR Am J Neuroradiol* 1991;12:719–724.

95. Plester D, Steinbach E. Cholesterol granuloma. *Otolaryngol Clin North Am* 1982;15:665–672.

96. Lo WW, Solti-Bohman LG, Brackmann DE, Gruskin P. Cholesterol granuloma of the petrous apex: CT diagnosis. *Radiology* 1984;153:705–711.

97. Taylor GD, Martin HF. Salivary gland tissue in the middle ear. *Arch Otolaryngol* 1961;73:651–653.

98. Namdar I, Smouha EE, Kane P. Salivary gland choristoma of the middle ear: role of intraoperative facial nerve monitoring. *Otolaryngol Head Neck Surg* 1995;112:616–620.

99. Hinni ML, Beatty CW. Salivary gland choristoma of the middle ear: report of a case and review of the literature. *Ear Nose Throat J* 1996;75:422–424.

The Ear: Comprehensive Otology,
edited by R. F. Canalis and P. R. Lambert.
Lippincott Williams & Wilkins, Philadelphia © 2000.

CHAPTER 52

Malignant Tumors of the Temporal Bone

C. Gary Jackson, Samuel Marzo, Akira Ishiyama, and Rinaldo F. Canalis

This chapter addresses the clinical features and current management of malignant tumors of the temporal bone. For the most part it excludes tumors of the external auditory canal (EAC) and pinna, which are covered extensively in Chapter 20. Statistical and clinical information on EAC lesions is included, however, in the section on squamous cell carcinoma (SCCA). This is necessary to clarify the discussion of treatment, because the available literature does not separate EAC lesions from those arising in the middle ear and mastoid process.

Malignant tumors of the temporal bone are encountered infrequently in otologic practice. The National Cancer Institute estimates there are 200 new cases annually, or approximately 6 cases per million population (1). Conley (2) and Rosenwasser (3) estimated that malignant tumors of the temporal bone account for 1 in 5,000 to 20,000 otologic diagnoses, SCCA accounting for most cases. In a study that comprised several series Kuhel et al. (4) determined that approximately 60% to 70% of ear cancers arose in the auricle, 20% to 30% in the external canal, and 10% in the middle ear. In a review Kenyon et al. (5) found 21 documented middle ear carcinomas in 207,000 pathologic reports.

The incidence of mesenchymal and other soft-tissue malignant tumors involving the temporal bone is difficult to assess, because there are no statistically significant series from which to derive this information. This dearth of information is attributed to the rarity of these lesions and difficulties in establishing the site of origin at the time of diagnosis (6,7). Insight into the relative frequency of these lesions may be derived from analysis of two large series of lesions managed by means of infratemporal fossa surgery and reported by Fisch et al. (8). Those authors found 32 malignant salivary tumors (7 adenoid cystic carcinomas) and 7 rhabdomyosarcomas arising from or involving the temporal bone. Table 1 presents an abbreviated classification of malignant tumors of the temporal bone based on cases reported in the U.S. literature.

C. G. Jackson: Department of Otolaryngology–Head and Neck Surgery, Otology and Neurotology, Vanderbilt University School of Medicine, Nashville, Tennessee 37203

S. Marzo: Department of Otolaryngology, Loyola University Medical Center, Maywood, Illinois 60153

A. Ishiyama: Division of Head and Neck Surgery, University of California, Los Angeles, School of Medicine, Los Angeles, California 90095

R. F. Canalis: Department of Surgery, University of California, Los Angeles, School of Medicine, Los Angeles, California 90095-1624

TABLE 1. *Abbreviated classification of malignant temporal bone tumors based on reports from the English language literature*

Primary tumors	
Epithelial	Squamous cell carcinoma, melanoma
Neurogenic	Malignant schwannoma
	Malignant meningioma
Sarcomas	Rhabdomyosarcoma
	Kaposi's sarcoma
	Fibrosarcoma
	Chondrosarcoma
	Osteogenic sarcoma
Glandular	Adenoid cystic carcinoma
	Adenocarcinoma
Reticuloendothelial system	Plasmacytoma
	Histiocytosis
	Primary lymphoma
Vascular	Malignant glomus tumors
	Hemangiopericytoma
Metastatic tumors	
Breast	
Lung	
Kidney	
Melanoma	
Lymphoma	
Leukemia	
Unknown primary	

SQUAMOUS CELL CANCER

Historical Note

Efforts toward successful management of malignant tumors of the temporal bone have been for the most part based on therapy for SCCA. Although findings that suggested temporal bone cancer were described in the late 1700s, these lesions were first identified histologically by Politzer in 1883 (9) and first managed by means of piecemeal removal by Heyer in 1899 (10). No significant progress in treatment followed Heyer's unsuccessful attempt until 1951, when Ward et al. (11) recommended progressive tumor resection to clear margins, and Campbell et al. (12) explored the feasibility of total temporal bone resection. Parson and Lewis (13) first accomplished this even now formidable operation in 1954. Lewis (14) later reported on 100 temporal bone resections with a 5-year survival rate of 27% and a mortality of 5% for SCCA. Conley and Novack (15) in the early 1960s refined the operation, outlined management of recurrent disease, and reported that middle ear involvement is a poor prognostic sign. Conley (16) introduced the hypoglossal-facial transfer operation for simultaneous facial reanimation.

Since these initial efforts several noteworthy contributions have been made. In 1980 Goodwin and Jesse (17) reported on the largest series of malignant tumors of the temporal bone treated surgically. The patients had a 5-year survival rate of 50% overall and of 27% for advanced cancer. Hilding and Selker (18) first recommended distal control of the internal carotid artery (ICA)

to reduce morbidity. Graham et al. (19) in 1982 wrote guidelines for ICA resection. Kinney and Wood (20) reported on 30 patients treated with planned combined surgical and radiation therapy. The patients had a 91% rate of local control of tumors contained within the temporal bone and 45% for advanced lesions. Operative techniques, classification systems, and predictors of outcome have been extensively discussed and revised (21–23).

Etiology

The cause of SCCA of the temporal bone is incompletely understood. During the 1940s and early 1950s radium was used to paint the numerals in clocks and watches to make them visible in the dark. The workers involved in this process would lick the brushes they used to make the tips as fine as possible so that the radioactive substance could be precisely applied. Beal et al. (24) reported a high incidence of mastoid cancer among these workers that appeared to be directly related to their occupation.

The importance of long-standing chronic otitis media as a possible etiologic factor was first described by Whitehead in 1908 (25) and corroborated by several authors thereafter (26–29). Approximately 50% of patients with temporal bone cancer have a history of chronic otitis media, but the mechanisms by which unrelenting ear inflammation induces neoplastic change are unknown. Lodge et al. (29) proposed that middle ear cancer may be induced in a manner similar to the development of malignant lesions of the skin close to actively draining fistulas caused by chronic osteomyelitis. Stell and McCormick

(30) postulated that bacteria liberate toxins that over years produce dysplastic changes and eventually malignant degeneration of the surface epithelium of the middle ear.

There is disagreement regarding the role of cholesteatoma in the causation of SCCA of the temporal bone. Michaels and Wells (31) speculated that long-term middle ear suppuration in the absence of cholesteatoma might represent a factor in the development of SCCA. Previous studies, however, found cholesteatoma predating cancer in a large number of cases of malignant tumors of the temporal bone (17,23). Kenyon et al. (5) addressed this issue in a study involving 21 patients with SCCA of the middle ear. The investigators documented cholesteatoma in 3 patients. Therefore cholesteatoma may sometimes be present in association with temporal bone cancer. Persistent inflammation, however, continues to be the most important element in development of this disease and may not be prevented by adequate mastoid surgery, as shown by Pettigrew (32).

Clinical Features

Most instances of SCCA of the temporal bone are diagnosed in patients in the fifth and sixth decades of life (4,5,26,29). There appears to be no definite sex prevalence, although Kenyon et al. (5) found a slightly higher frequency among women (13:8). Clinical evaluation begins with a thorough neurotologic history and otomicroscopic examination. Kuhel et al. (4) collated the frequency of presenting signs and symptoms among a group of 442 patients with malignant tumors of the temporal bone, including external ear canal cancers, obtained from a review of the literature and summarized them (Table 2). Physical and historical aspects of SCCA often are masked by drainage and inflammation that suggest chronic ear disease. Otorrhea, usually present for 20 years or more, and hearing loss are the most common presenting symptoms followed by pain (22,26,28). As the disease advances, otalgia intensifies and becomes deep seated (26–29).

At examination an isolated middle ear mass and destructive lesions in the EAC or mastoid are not infre-

TABLE 2. *Presenting symptoms of cancer of the external auditory canal and temporal bone*

Symptom	n	Percentage
Otorrhea	396	61
Otalgia	396	51
External auditory canal mass	113	37
Hearing loss	336	29
Periauricular mass	130	19
Facial palsy	441	16
Vertigo	80	15
Tinnitus	156	11

From Kuhel WI, Hume CR, Selesnick SH. Cancer of the external auditory canal and temporal bone. *Otolaryngol Clin North Am* 1996;29:827–852, with permission.

quent. Hearing loss (conductive or mixed) is documented among 50% of patients. Primary involvement of SCCA in the internal auditory canal (IAC) remains, to our knowledge, unreported. Involvement of the IAC sometimes occurs with metastatic lesions or primary mesenchymal tumors (see later), which produce rapidly evolving sensorineural hearing loss (21–29). Direct labyrinthine invasion from SCCA of the middle ear is infrequent because of the resistance of the otic capsule.

Facial paralysis is a sign of advanced disease (17, 21–29). The degree of nerve involvement has been correlated with survival. Patients without facial nerve weakness have a treatment failure rate of 30% and those with only mild paresis 34%. Patients with moderate paresis have a 50% failure rate and those with paralysis 62% (33,34). Involvement of other cranial nerves carries a dismal prognosis for survival (21–29,31,33,34).

The extent of bone involvement is best evaluated with high-resolution, thin-section computed tomography (CT) (35). Regional infiltration into soft-tissue compartments, including the central nervous system, surrounding the temporal bone is best assessed with magnetic resonance imaging. Magnetic resonance angiography may be adequate to determine major vessel involvement; if not, angiography with possible embolization is performed. A metastatic survey, consisting of chest radiography, bone scan, and liver function studies, is performed.

Classification

Because survival is determined in great part by the extent of the tumor, classification of SCCA of the temporal bone might provide a much needed vehicle for accurate representation of clinical data applicable to comparative studies. Arriaga et al. (35) proposed a tumor-nodes-metastasis classification of lesions of the external auditory meatus. For advanced lesions this includes eight areas of extension that can be accurately evaluated by means of CT. These include the middle and inner ears and the principal structures around the temporal bone. Although imaging findings appear to correlate well with tumor extent and may provide the basis for precise distribution of cases, a practical, generally accepted, classification of these tumors is yet to be structured.

Management

Management of malignant tumors of the temporal bone in general and of SCCA in particular poses a formidable challenge. Before the development of current techniques, all patients with these tumors experienced the sequelae of uncontrolled progressive disease: intolerable pain, dysfunction of multiple cranial nerves, intracranial extension, carotid destruction, and death. Management of malignant tumors of the temporal bone is based on en bloc resection of the lesion and its regional pathways of spread. This is rarely possible when the tumor extends beyond the external ear canal. The pneumatic character of the temporal bone and its irregular and rich vascularity often render accurate tumor demarcation virtually impossible, be it by means of imaging or direct examination during a surgical procedure. Nevertheless, histologic mapping of surgical margins at all levels should be attempted as precisely as possible to aid in the establishment of accurate postoperative irradiation fields.

Surgical Treatment

The surgical techniques for the management of malignant tumors of the temporal bone are lateral, subtotal, or total.

Lateral Temporal Bone Resection

Lesions confined to the EAC without middle ear involvement (tympanic membrane intact) can be managed with lateral temporal bone resection (LTBR). EAC cartilage resection or sleeve resection of canal lesions should be avoided because of a high recurrence rate. LTBR (Fig. 1) includes en bloc resection of the EAC, usually with superficial parotidectomy and suprahyoid neck dissection. A wide C-shaped incision from the postauricular region to the anterior part of the neck is used to gain access to the temporal bone, parotid gland, and cervical structures (Fig. 2). An anteriorly based flap is elevated, and the lateral meatus is incised and confirmed to be free of disease by means of histologic frozen section. Complete mastoidectomy is performed with facial recess exposure of the middle ear (Fig. 3). The incus is removed after section of the incudostapedial joint. Tumor extension into the middle ear or mastoid process precludes this operation and mandates subtotal resection (see later). Care is taken not to fenestrate the EAC. The EAC is freed by means of extension of the facial

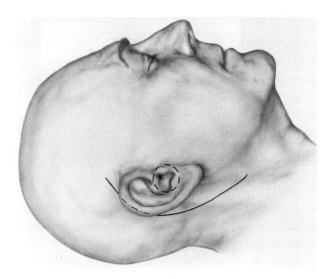

FIG. 2. Design of external auditory canal incision for preservation of the auricle. Postauricular exposure.

recess inferiorly and across the tympanic bone (Fig. 4) (36). This maneuver is done with the trunk of the peripheral facial nerve under direct vision to avoid traumatizing it.

The dissection is carried into the zygomatic root and the posterior-superior wall of the glenoid fossa. At this point the EAC is isolated and can be fractured from the remaining bone with a chisel. The specimen is left attached to the superficial lobe of the parotid gland, which is resected in continuity with the specimen. Total parotidectomy is performed when gross disease involves

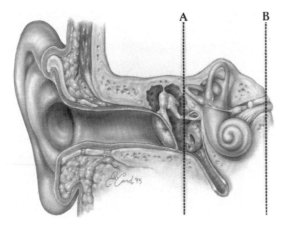

FIG. 1. A: Lesions confined to the external auditory canal that spare the tympanic membrane are suitable for partial lateral temporal bone resection. **B:** When the middle ear is violated, subtotal or total temporal bone resection is required.

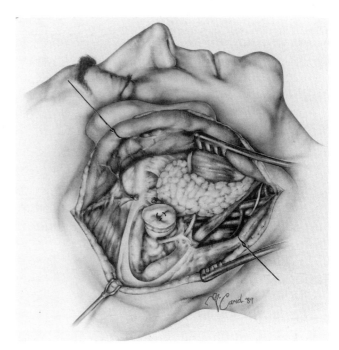

FIG. 3. The external auditory canal is isolated and fractured free of the temporal bone anteriorly.

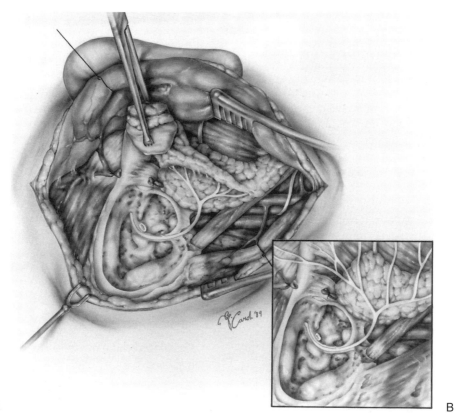

FIG. 4. The specimen is resected en bloc with the superficial parotid gland. **A:** Nodes from the suprahyoid neck are sampled. **B:** The resected field.

the gland. Conventional or modified neck dissection is performed depending on the stage of disease.

Reconstruction of the defect often is difficult. Resurfacing with a split-thickness skin graft, which allows hearing aid placement is often not possible. The loss of EAC support produces a depression behind the angle of the mandible that distorts the position of the auricle. It is an especially vexing problem for men, who find shaving this area difficult. Oversewing the EAC and obliterating the defect with free fat grafts or pedicled flaps is more cosmetically appealing but limits the possibilities for auditory rehabilitation. Five-year survival rates among patients with SCCA bone amenable to LTBR is approximately 50% (34,37).

Subtotal Temporal Bone Resection

Tumors that extend through the tympanic membrane and into the middle ear can be managed with subtotal resection of the temporal bone. Exposure is as for LTBR. The sigmoid sinus and posterior fossa dura are exposed, and a temporal craniotomy is performed to evaluate tumor resectability. Limited involvement of the posterior or middle cranial fossa dura can be resected and grafted. The zygoma and ascending mandibular ramus are sectioned for close inspection of the glenoid fossa and posterior infratemporal space. If these areas are resectable, total

parotidectomy with facial nerve transection and radical neck dissection are performed. The ICA is isolated through the subtemporal craniotomy in its tympanic and petrous portions. The IAC is accessed and its contents divided. Osteotomes can then be used to resect the temporal bone through the ICA canal, lateral IAC, cochlea, and jugular bulb. Cranial nerves IX through XII are not sacrificed. The resulting defect is considerable and best reconstructed with a free flap. Leakage of cerebrospinal fluid and ICA exposure generally preclude use of regional flaps or free adipose tissue grafts. When tumor involves the facial nerve, functional rehabilitation relies on extratemporal measures such as XII–VII anastomosis. The 5-year survival rate is approximately 25% (37–40).

Total Temporal Bone Resection

For extensive disease of the middle ear, total temporal bone resection is required. The procedure begins as for subtotal temporal bone resection to verify resectability. The anterior temporal bone is isolated by means of dissection toward the foramen ovale. The greater superficial petrosal nerve and cartilaginous eustachian tube are divided. The petrous ICA is mobilized or transected. The petroclival suture is isolated and osteotomies are used to free the temporal bone, including the petrous apex. Five-year survival rates are low (33,37–40).

Perspective

The relative rarity of SCCA of the temporal bone has resulted in a large variety of treatment modalities, for the most part based on individual experience. No results of randomized or nonrandomized treatment-control studies have been reported, and the use of surgery, irradiation, or combined techniques has not followed a deliberate philosophy. In an attempt to gain perspective on the role of surgery in the management of malignant tumors of the temporal bone, Prasad and Janecka (36) reviewed the U.S. and U.K. literature to select for an in-depth study 144 patients from 26 publications. Table 3 summarizes their results. The following conclusions may be derived from this study and others: (a) tumors limited to the external ear canal have a 50% overall cure rate after LTBR; (b) postoperative radiation therapy does not appear to improve these results in a statistically significant way; (c) middle ear involvement cuts the 5-year survival rate in half; (d) patients with extensive disease have an extremely poor prognosis.

The morbidity and mortality for subtotal and total temporal bone resection are high, and treatment outcomes are poor. This outlook led Kinney and Wood (21) to propose piecemeal tumor removal and petrosectomy with an otologic drill followed by high-dose irradiation. This approach was used to manage advanced tumors and is different from previously proposed partial resections in that it is aided by modern microsurgical techniques. Preliminary results suggest that it leads to less morbidity; results remain poor but not worse than with other methods.

Radiation Therapy

In general radiation therapy is used as adjunctive therapy for SCCA of the temporal bone. Although survival rates of 23% to 77% have been reported with use of this modality, the consensus is that it is curative in approximately 22% of cases and in selected circumstances (38,41). Tumor electrocoagulation followed by intracavitary radium implantation has yielded disappointing outcomes (17,42,43). Radiation failure probably occurs because low oxygen tensions are present in bone invaded by tumor. Tumor sequestration in this area leads to uncontrollable disease progression. Complications of temporal bone irradiation include central nervous system injury, osteoradionecrosis, delayed wound healing, and in some instances cochlear and vestibular damage.

SARCOMA

Rhabdomyosarcoma

Rhabdomyosarcoma is a rare soft-tissue malignant tumor believed to derive from totipotential mesenchymal cells. They are classified as embryonal, alveolar, or botryoid, and adult pleomorphic tumors. Although all types have a variable architecture, the predominant cell is an elongated element with a hyperchromatic nucleus and occasional cytoplasmic projections. Temporal bone rhabdomyosarcoma occurs almost exclusively among children and almost always is embryonal in type. Despite its rarity it is the most common temporal bone sarcoma. In an extensive

TABLE 3. *Results derived from a literature review by Prasad and Janecka*

Type of disease	Operation	Radiation therapy	Survival rate (%)	Follow-up period
Carcinoma confined to external auditory canal	Lateral TBR	No	44 (4 of 9)	5 y
	Mastoidectomy	Yes	50 (5 of 10)	5 y
	Lateral TBR	Yes	48 (12 of 25)	5 y
	Subtotal TBR	Yes	50 (1 of 2)	5 y
Carcinoma extending into the middle ear space	Mastoidectomy	No	0 (0 of 4)	2 y
	Subtotal TBR	No	100 (3 of 3)	5 y
	Mastoidectomy	Yes	20 (6 of 30)	5 y
	Lateral TBR	Yes	28.7 (2 of 7)	5 y
	Subtotal TBR	Yes	30 (3 of 10)	5 y
	Total TBR	Yes	0 (0 of 4)	1 y
Advanced disease, involvement of				
Petrous apex	Subtotal TBR	Yes	0 (0 of 1)	2 y
	Total TBR	Yes	0 (0 of 4)	2 y
Internal carotid artery	Total TBR and ICA	No	0 (0 of 2)	14 m
	Total TBR	No	0 (0 of 1)	8 m
	Lateral TBR	Yes	0 (0 of 1)	21 d
Temporal lobe	Mastoidectomy	Yes	0 (0 of 2)	14 m
Dura	Dural resection	?	9 (1 of 11)	5 y
	Without dural resection	?	11 (1 of 9)	5 y

TBR, temporal bone resection; *ICA,* internal carotid artery.
From Prasad S, Janecka IP. Efficacy of surgical treatments for squamous cell carcinoma of the temporal bone: a literature review. *Otolaryngol Head Neck Surg* 1994;110:270–280, with permission.

review Naufal (44) found that among 211 sarcomas involving the temporal bone 30% were rhabdomyosarcoma. This tumor accounts for 4% to 7% of all malignant tumors of the temporal bone with 80 to 90 cases so far reported. Rhabdomyosarcoma most commonly arises in the middle ear. Canalis and Gussen (45), however, described the histopathologic findings of a tumor that appeared to be centered in the eustachian tube and predominantly involved the petrous bone. A review revealed that approximately one fourth of previously reported temporal bone rhabdomyosarcomas had a similar site of origin (45).

Rhabdomyosarcoma grows through the temporal bone following paths of least resistance. Three stages of expansion are recognizable in tumors arising in the middle ear (44,45). In the first, the tumor is limited to the middle ear and produces hearing loss and aural discharge; a polypoid, often infected mass may be found at otoscopy. In the second stage infratemporal progression causes increasing pain, further hearing loss, and facial paralysis. Invasion into the skull, brain, neck, and the infratemporal and parapharyngeal spaces typifies the terminal stage. Patients with rhabdomyosarcoma arising in the eustachian tube region and extending intrapetrosally have persistent headaches (often frontal) and diplopia due to abducens nerve paralysis caused by tumor extension into Dorello's canal. The facial, auditory, and vestibular nerves usually are spared in these tumors, which tend to invade the petrosal cells and marrow and bypass the structures protected by the resistant otic capsule. The carotid canal and trigeminal nerve roots become involved where they cross the petrosal ridge or enter Meckel's cave.

At diagnosis 20% of temporal bone rhabdomyosarcomas are metastatic, and the facial nerve is involved in about 50% of patients. The diagnosis is confirmed by means of biopsy. Superficial tissue findings may be inconclusive, and identification may occasionally necessitate mastoidectomy to obtain adequate tissue. Temporal bone staging follows current guidelines for rhabdomyosarcoma of the limbs and is based on surgical findings (46–48), as follows:

Grade I.   Localized disease completely resected
  A. Confined to organ or muscle of origin
  B. Infiltration outside site of origin
Grade II. Compromised or regional resection
  A. Grossly resected tumor with microscopic residual disease; lymph nodes negative
  B. Regional disease, completely resected, with nodes that may be involved or extension of tumor into adjacent organs
  C. Regional disease with involved lymph nodes grossly resected but with evidence of microscopic residual disease
Grade III. Incomplete resection or biopsy with gross residual disease
Grade IV. Distant metastasis present at diagnosis

Complete surgical resection is rarely possible in the management of rhabdomyosarcoma of the temporal bone. Current management involves combined chemotherapy consisting of cyclophosphamide, vincristine, and doxorubicin followed by radiation therapy. Two-year and 5-year survival rates for grade I embryonal types are 79% and 60%, respectively. Skull base extension and recurrence are uniformly fatal within 24 months of diagnosis. The alveolar subtype has a poor prognosis regardless of grade (44–48).

Other Sarcomas

In addition to rhabdomyosarcoma other mesenchymal tumors that occur primarily or as a result of metastatic or regional extension to the temporal bone have been sporadically reported.

Primary Ewing's sarcoma is a very rare lesion. Only 11 cases arising in the skull (3 in the temporal bone) have been reported (49). Unlike the more common lesions of the pelvis and long bones, Ewing's sarcoma of the skull appears less likely to present with systemic metastasis. Excision under the general guidelines of temporal bone resection followed by irradiation and chemotherapy has been proposed as the recommended treatment. Prognosis is uncertain because of the limited available experience.

Osteogenic sarcoma is the most common primary bone cancer, but it is very rare in the skull. Conventry and Dahlin (50) found only three such tumors in a review of 430 cases, none known to be arising from the temporal bone. Schuknecht (51) described the histopathologic findings of an osteoblastic osteosarcoma of the temporal bone in a 21-year-old patient with multiple hereditary osteochondromatosis. The tumor was composed of closely packed spindle and stellate cells. The patient died after receiving a radiation therapy dose of 80 Gy, which failed to produce any appreciable tumor response. Schuknecht (51) also described the pathologic changes of *chondromyxosarcoma* involving the petrous bone in a 27-year-old woman who sought evaluation of serous otitis media and multiple cranial nerve palsies. Hemiparesis followed, probably because of neoplastic obstruction of the petrosal portion of the ICA. Craniotomy and partial tumor removal were performed, but the patient died soon thereafter. The tumor consisted of lobules interspaced by fibrous bands that contained stellate, sometimes multinucleated cells within a myxomatous background.

Chondrosarcoma although uncommon sometimes occurs along the skull base and petroclival region. The differential diagnosis, which for low-grade tumors may be quite difficult, includes chordoma, which may occur in an extraaxial location, and chondroma (52–54). Chondrosarcoma may be amenable to surgical resection. However, recurrences are common, and multiple operations often are needed to control tumor growth. External beam radiation therapy produces uncertain results. The effectiveness of proton radiation therapy and other relatively recent advances, including stereotactic techniques, remains to be elucidated in the management of temporal bone sarcoma.

Kaposi's sarcoma is a multifocal malignant neoplasm of blood vessels that may involve large areas of the skin and later the lungs, spleen, and liver. In the head and neck, it was first described by Naunton and Stoller (55) in 1960 as an isolated lesion of the auricle. Currently Kaposi's sarcoma in the most common malignant expression of acquired immunodeficiency syndrome (AIDS), and auricular involvement occurs almost exclusively among patients with AIDS. This lesion sometimes may involve the EAC and extend into the middle ear (56). Kaposi's sarcoma of the auricle and tympanic membrane is amendable to laser treatment. An argon laser is preferred for lesions that involve the tympanic membrane because the lesion can be eradicated without damage to this structure. Tumors involving the middle ear are best managed with irradiation (56).

MALIGNANT GLANDULAR TUMORS

Adenoid Cystic Carcinoma

Adenoid cystic cancers arising from the external ear canal are discussed in Chapter 20. Those that develop in the middle ear are exceedingly rare. The precise site of origin—salivary (parotid), or apocrine or seromucosinous glands of the external canal—often is impossible to discern when the lesion is advanced. Perzin et al. (57) in a detailed clinicopathologic study of 16 cases of adenoid cystic carcinoma involving the external ear canal reported on two that were likely to have developed in the middle ear. Both patients had a history of chronic otitis media and had undergone previous tympanomastoidectomy. The disease was extensive at diagnosis, and both patients died of disease despite wide resection and radiation therapy.

Adenocarcinoma

Adenocarcinoma is a rare lesion with a controversial histologic origin. Sites of possible development include the middle ear mucosa, eustachian tube, and mastoid air cells. Middle ear adenocarcinoma is further classified into low-grade papillary cystadenocarcinoma and high-grade undifferentiated adenocarcinoma. This lesion usually manifests pain, otorrhea, and hearing loss. Cranial nerve deficits follow. Resection with planned postoperative radiation therapy is the recommended therapy for these tumors (58). The low-grade variety has a 15% mortality rate. No cases of regional or distant metastasis have been reported (59). High-grade tumors usually are metastatic at presentation and have a very poor prognosis. During clinical assessment of these tumors exclusion of metastatic adenocarcinoma from a more common source is mandatory. Low-grade tumors must be differentiated from other glandular tumors, especially from aggressive papillary adenoma. When differentiation is not possible, careful histopathologic and clinical evaluation is critical when considering radical treatment (see Chapter 51).

TUMORS OF THE LYMPHORETICULAR SYSTEM

Plasmacytoma

Plasmacytoma arises from plasma cells, which are derived from the B-lymphocyte lineage and synthesize and secrete the body immunoglobulins. Neoplastic proliferation of plasma cells may produce localized or disseminated disease. The disseminated form, multiple myeloma, is common, whereas localized types are infrequent. There are two varieties of localized plasma cell tumors: solitary plasmacytoma of bone (SPB) and extramedullary plasmacytoma (EMP). SPB tends eventually to become disseminated, and EMP expands locally. AMP accounts for less than 10% of all malignant plasma cell tumors, but when they occur, they most commonly affect the head and neck (60). To date approximately 10 cases of temporal bone plasmacytoma have been reported. Differentiation between SPB and EMP in the temporal bone is particularly difficult because most lesions are fairly advanced when diagnosed, and a mucosal, muscular or bony primary site cannot be established. However, the available information suggests that most reported cases are EMP. Patients with EMP tend to lack elevated serum or urine paraprotein titers, which reflects a limited tumor burden. In most reported cases the tumor was limited to the middle ear and mastoid, suggesting that the tumor is derived from clonal expansion of local lymphocyte deposits. The petrous marrow was involved in only one case, suggesting primarily mucosal involvement in most instances (61).

Patients with EMP have otalgia of rapid onset, otorrhea, and hearing loss. Initial findings resemble those of acute or chronic otomastoiditis. Facial nerve involvement is infrequent even with extensive lesions. CT is fairly nonspecific in revealing a destructive lesion of the mastoid and soft tissues of the middle ear.

Both SPB and EMP are managed with external beam radiation therapy. Although there is no consensus regarding the treatment dose for SPB, EMP is highly radiosensitive with a regional control rate of 80% when doses between 40 and 50 Gy (gray) are used (62).

Histiocytosis X

Histiocytosis X comprises a spectrum of disease processes, including eosinophilic granuloma, Hand-Schüller-Christian disease, and Letterer-Siwe disease. Eosinophilic granuloma, the most common of these processes, occurs among children and usually is limited to a single site. It is characterized by a proliferation of histiocytes, eosinophils, and connective tissue. Refractory otorrhea and otalgia are characteristic symptoms. A lytic lesion of the external ear, middle ear, or mastoid process is seen at CT. Diagnosis is made at histologic examination of the excised tissue. Radiation therapy usually is curative (63,64).

Letterer-Siwe disease is a disorder that affects infants younger than 2 years. Skin, skeletal bone, and extraskclctal tissue lesions occur. This disease is rapidly fatal. Chemotherapy is recommended (64). Hand-Schüller-Christian disease affects children older than 5 years and young adults. Therapy parallels that for Letterer-Siwe disease (64).

VASCULAR MALIGNANT TUMORS

Malignant Glomus Tumors

Approximately 4% of all paragangliomas of the temporal bone are malignant. Glomus tumors are discussed in Chapter 51.

Hemangiopericytoma

Hemangiopericytoma arises from capillary pericytes and may develop anywhere capillaries are found (65). These tumors are most common in the soft tissues of the extremities and have a 15% rate of head and neck involvement. They are rare in the temporal bone; only eight cases have been reported to date. Microscopic examination shows that these tumors are composed of round and spindle-shaped cells around endothelial lined vascular spaces. Mitoses are infrequent. The vascular spaces tend to branch into larger spaces to produce a staghorn appearance (66). These tumors may occur at any age from childhood to senescence. One temporal bone tumor developed in the middle ear and external canal of a 6-year-old boy. Others have presented in the mastoid process, petrous bone, and jugular foramen (diagnosed initially as glomus tumor) (67). Cranial nerve involvement was present in three cases. Patients have been treated with surgical and radiation therapy with good disease control, but the follow-up period has been short. Tumors with intracranial extension are difficult to manage and probably have a high recurrence rate. Hemangiopericytoma has a 15% to 20% rate of metastasis, predominantly to lung and bone. Metastasis to regional lymphatic vessels are rare and may occur several years after initial treatment (65,66).

METASTATIC TUMORS

General Concepts

Metastasis to the temporal bone is uncommon; approximately 200 cases have been reported so far (Fig. 5). In some cases metastasis may be the first evidence of malignant dissemination, but more frequently the diagnosis is unsuspected and made at postmortem examination, possibly because ear symptoms are overshadowed by those deriving from the primary tumor and other metastatic sites (68). Patients with symptoms usually seek treatment late during the course of the disease with hearing loss, otalgia,

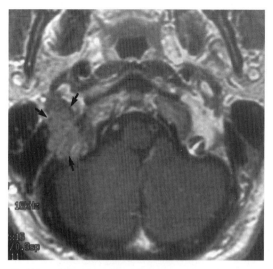

FIG. 5. T1-weighted magnetic resonance image shows petrous bone metastasis from prostate cancer *(arrows)*.

facial nerve paralysis, periauricular swelling, otorrhea, or an aural mass. Tumors of the breast, lung, and kidney are the most common sources of temporal bone metastasis. Cumberworth et al. (69) reviewed 165 cases of temporal bone metastasis and found that 29% were from breast cancer, 11% from the lung, 8% from the prostate, 8% from an unknown primary, and 6% from kidney lesions. Metastasis to the structures of the cerebellopontine angle, including the petrous bone, is discussed in Chapter 53.

Berlinger et al. (70) described five routes of tumor spread to the temporal bone as follows:

- Isolated metastasis from a distinct primary lesion. This situation is the most common, and spread usually is hematogenous.
- Direct extension from a regional primary lesion, such as parotid, auricular, or periauricular cancer
- Meningeal carcinomatosis, which is usually hematogenous
- Leptomeningeal extension from an intracranial primary
- Leukemic or lymphomatous spread

Proctor and Lindsay (71) reported that the petrous marrow may filter and trap circulating tumor cells and give rise to metastatic growth. Viable tumor cells implanted in the temporal bone may proliferate rapidly or remain dormant only to grow later, sometimes even after the primary site is controlled. Nelson and Hinojosa (72) studied 60 temporal bones from 33 patients and found that specific metastatic tumor locations depended on the mode of metastatic spread. The hematogenous route caused petrosal involvement, meningeal pathways involved the IAC, and direct extension more commonly affected the foramen lacerum and the petrous apex. With few exceptions (renal carcinoma), metastatic temporal bone lesions tend to be less differentiated than the primary lesion and to be destructive. Osteoneogenesis sometimes is found in lesions of long standing and in prostate and breast cancer metastasis. The clinical and pathologic findings in various unusual lesions metastatic to the temporal bone, including seminoma, vaginal carcinoma, cardiac myxoma, pilomatrix carcinoma, and others have been described (73–92).

Malignant Lymphoma

Lymphoma is a malignant tumor of the lymphoreticular system that has been reported occasionally to involve the ear. It is classified into Hodgkin's disease and non-Hodgkin's lymphoma. Non-Hodgkin's lymphoma is further classified as nodular or diffuse and, depending on the site of origin, as nodal or extranodal. Temporal bone lymphoma was first studied in detail by Paparella and El-Fiky (93), who reported on 12 lesions metastatic to this site. Other case reports have extended the number of cases available for review to 15 patients with metastatic temporal bone lymphoma (94). Tucci et al. (95) reported on two primary lymphomas of the temporal bone. The patients were a 66-year-old man and a 5-year-old boy. They had otorrhea, hearing loss, and facial paresis. At exploration a fleshly tumor was found to occupy the mastoid process in one patient and the middle ear in the other. For both patients the diagnosis was large-cell, diffuse lymphoma. They were both treated with chemotherapy. The adult patient also received irradiation to the temporal bone, but disseminated disease developed 12 months after treatment. The child had no evidence of recurrence 2 years after treatment. Facial nerve paresis resolved for both patients after therapy. All temporal bone histologic studies showed destructive lesions of the inner ear and middle ear and hemorrhage.

Leukemia

Deafness due to leukemia was first described by Don in 1844 and then by Vidal in 1856 (96). The first histopathologic description was by Politzer in 1894 (97). Since then involvement of the temporal bone by leukemic infiltrates has been studied extensively (98). The incidence of otologic complications of leukemia is approximately 20%. In an early study Druss (99) found that they occurred among 25 of 148 patients. The current incidence may be lower because modern chemotherapy is likely to prevent these complications. Temporal bone leukemia adopts two major forms, one characterized by tumoral infiltration and the other by hemorrhage. A conspicuous site of leukemic involvement is the petrous bone marrow, although the temporal bone air spaces also are frequently involved. Hemorrhage is common and may be limited or diffuse. Involvement of the cochlea and labyrinth sometimes is responsible for sudden losses of auditory and vestibular function. Friedmann (100) described the inner ear findings in a case of chronic lymphocytic leukemia and documented destruction by lymphoid cells of the organ of Corti and infiltration of Reissner's membrane, stria vascularis spiral ligament, and spiral ganglion.

Patients with acute myelogenous leukemia may have focal infiltrates of leukemic cells called *granulocytic sarcoma*. The term *chloroma* also is frequently applied to such deposits because of elaboration of myeloperoxidase by the tumor cells, which at visual examination imparts a greenish hue to the tissue. Chloroma is more common among infants and is more frequently associated with the monocytic cell types of leukemia. This tumor may arise in bones or soft tissue and frequently occurs in the epidural space and around the orbits and skull base, including the temporal bone. Central nervous system involvement consists primarily of meningeal infiltration; parenchymal lesions also are possible. Chloroma may appear before a blast crisis or may herald a relapse (101).

SUMMARY POINTS

- Squamous cell cancer of the temporal bone is a rare malignant lesion. Longstanding chronic otitis media appears to be involved in the pathogenesis of at least half of these tumors.
- Presenting symptoms of temporal bone SCCA include otorrhea, usually present for decades, hearing loss, and pain. Facial paralysis is a sign of advanced disease.
- En bloc resection (LTBR) is possible in the management of SCCA limited to the EAC. The 5-year survival rate is approximately 50%.
- SCCA involvement of the middle ear dramatically lowers the 5-year survival rate to 25% or less. Subtotal or total temporal bone resection is required.
- Although radiation therapy often is used in conjunction with surgical management of SCCA of the temporal bone, its precise role remains to be defined.
- Rhabdomyosarcoma is the most common type of temporal bone sarcoma. It occurs almost exclusively among children.
- Management of temporal bone rhabdomyosarcoma includes surgical intervention, chemotherapy, and radiation therapy.
- Adenocarcinoma rarely occurs in the middle ear. Combined resection and radiation therapy are the recommended treatments.
- Cancer metastatic to the temporal bone is rare. Breast cancer is the most common primary tumor source. Metastatic lesions from lung, prostate, and renal cancer follow in incidence.
- Leukemia and primary and metastatic lymphoma can involve the temporal bone. Otologic complications can occur in approximately 20% of cases of leukemia.

REFERENCES

1. Horn J. Surveillance epidemiology and end results. Rockville, MD: National Cancer Institute, 1987.
2. Conley JJ. Cancer of the middle ear and temporal bone. *NY State J Med* 1974;9:1575–1579.
3. Rosenwasser H. Neoplasms involving the middle ear. *Ann Otol Rhinol Laryngol* 1965;74:555–572.
4. Kuhel WI, Hume CR, Selesnick SH. Cancer of the external auditory canal and temporal bone. *Otolaryngol Clin North Am* 1996;29:827–852.
5. Kenyon GS, Marks PV, Scholtz CL, Dhillon R. Squamous cell carcinoma of the middle ear. *Ann Otol Rhinol Laryngol* 1985;94:273–277.
6. Sekhar L, Pomeranz S, Janecka I, et al. Temporal bone neoplasms: a report on 20 surgically treated cases. *J Neurosurg* 1992;76: 578–587.
7. Ellis M, Pracy R. Carcinoma of the middle ear. *Br Med J* 1954;1: 1413–1415.
8. Fisch U, Fagan P, Valavanis A. The infratemporal fossa approach for the lateral skull base. *Otolaryngol Clin North Am* 1984;17:513–553.
9. Politzer A. *Textbook of diseases of the ear.* Cassels JP, ed and trans. London: Balliere Tindall & Cox, 1883:729–734.
10. Heyer H. Ueber einen fall von Ohrencarcinoma, hehandelt mit Resection des Fesenbeines. *Dtsch Z Chir* 1899;50:552–533.
11. Ward GE, Loch WE, Lawrence W. Radical operation for carcinoma of the external auditory canal and middle ear. *Am J Surg* 1951;134: 397–403.
12. Campbell EH, Volk RM, Burkland CW. Total resection of the temporal bone for malignancy of the middle ear. *Ann Surg* 1951;134:397–403.
13. Parsons H, Lewis JS. Subtotal resection of the temporal bone for cancer of the ear. *Cancer* 1954;7:995–1001.
14. Lewis JS. Temporal bone resection: review of 100 cases. *Arch Otolaryngol* 1974;101:23–25.
15. Conley JJ, Novack AJ. The surgical treatment of malignant tumors of the ear and temporal bone, 1. *Arch Otolaryngol* 1960;71:635–652.
16. Conley J. Cancer of the middle ear. *Ann Otol Rhinol Laryngol* 1965; 74:555–572.
17. Goodwin WJ, Jesse RH. Malignant neoplasms of the external auditory canal and temporal bone. *Arch Otolaryngol* 1980;106:675–679.
18. Hilding DA, Selker R. Total resection of temporal bone for carcinoma. *Arch Otolaryngol* 1965;89:636–645.
19. Graham MD, Staloff RT, Kemink JL. Total en bloc resection of the temporal bone and carotid artery for malignant tumors of the ear and temporal bone. *Laryngoscope* 1984;94:528–533.
20. Kinney SE, Wood BG. Surgical treatment of skull base malignancy. *Otolaryngol Head Neck Surg* 1984;92:158–164.
21. Kinney SE, Wood BG. Malignancies of the external ear canal and temporal bone: surgical techniques and results. *Laryngoscope* 1987; 97:158–164.
22. Kinney SE. Squamous cell carcinoma of the external auditory canal. *Am J Otol* 1989;10:111–116.
23. Arena S, Keen M. Carcinoma of the middle ear and temporal bone. *Am J Otol* 1988;9:351–356.
24. Beal D, Lindsay J, Ward PH. Radiation induced carcinoma of the mastoid. *Arch Otolaryngol* 1965;81:9–16.
25. Whitehead AL. A case of primary epithelioma of the tympanum following chronic suppurative otitis media. *Proc R Soc Med* 1908;1: 34–36.
26. Hahn SS, Kim JA, Goodchild N, Constable WC. Carcinoma of the middle ear and external auditory canal. *Int J Radiat Oncol Biol Phys* 1983;9:1003–1007.
27. Paaske PB, Witten J, Schwer S, et al. Results in treatment of carcinoma of the external auditory canal and middle ear. *Cancer* 1987;59:156–160.
28. Austin JR, Stewart K, Fauzi N. Squamous cell carcinoma of the external auditory canal: therapeutic prognosis based on a proposed staging system. *Arch Otolaryngol Head Neck Surg* 1994;120:1228–1239.
29. Lodge W, Jones HW, Smith MN. Malignant tumors of the temporal bone. *Arch Otolaryngol* 1955;61:535–541.
30. Stell PM, McCormick MS. Carcinoma of the external auditory meatus and middle ear: prognostic factors and suggested staging system. *J Laryngol Otol* 1985;99:847–850.
31. Michaels L, Wells M. Squamous carcinoma of the middle ear. *Clin Otolaryngol* 1986;5:235–248.
32. Pettigrew AM. Histopathology of the temporal bone after open mastoid surgery. *Clin Otolaryngol* 1980;5:227–234.
33. Sataloff RT, Myers DL, Lowry LD, et al. Total temporal bone resection for squamous cell carcinoma. *Otolaryngol Head Neck Surg* 1987; 96:5–14.
34. Medina JE, Park AO, Neely GJ, et al. Lateral temporal bone resections. *Am J Surg* 1990;160:427–433.
35. Arriaga M, Curtin HD, Takahashi H, Kamerer DB. The role of preoperative CT scans in staging external auditory meatus carcinoma: radiologic pathologic correlation study. *Otolaryngol Head Neck Surg* 1991;105:6–11.
36. Neely GJ, Forrester M. Anatomic considerations of the medial cuts in the subtotal temporal bone resection. *Otolaryngol Head Neck Surg* 1982;90:641–645.
37. Prasad S, Janecka IP. Efficacy of surgical treatments for squamous cell carcinoma of the temporal bone: a literature review. *Otolaryngol Head Neck Surg* 1994;110:270–280.
38. Spector JF. Management of temporal bone carcinomas: a therapeutic analysis of two groups of patients and long term follow-up. *Otolaryngol Head Neck Surg* 1991;104:58–66.
39. Go KG, Annyas A, Vermey A, et al. Evaluation of results of temporal bone resection. *Acta Neurochir (Wien)* 1991;110:110–115.
40. Arena S. Treatment of carcinoma of the temporal bone. *Am J Otol* 1983;5:56–61.
41. Gacek R, Goodman M. Management of malignancy of the temporal bone. *Laryngoscope* 1977;87:1672–1634.
42. Tabb HG, Komet H, McLaurin JW. Cancer of the external auditory canal: treatment with radical mastoidectomy and irradiation. *Laryngoscope* 1976;86:405–415.
43. Holmes KS. The treatment of carcinoma of the middle ear by the 4MV linear accelerator. *Proc R Soc Med* 1960;53:242–244.
44. Naufal PM. Primary sarcomas of the temporal bone. *Arch Otolaryngol* 1973;98:44–50.
45. Canalis RF, Gussen R. Temporal bone findings in rhabdomyosarcoma with predominantly petrous involvement. *Arch Otolaryngol* 1980;106: 290–293.
46. Feldman BA. Rhabdomyosarcoma of the head and neck. *Laryngoscope* 1982;92:424–420.
47. Jaffe N, Fuller RM, Farber S. Rhabdomyosarcoma in children: improved outlook with a multidisciplinary approach. *Am J Surg* 1973; 125:482–487.
48. Wiatrak BJ, Pensak ML. Rhabdomyosarcoma of the ear and temporal bone, *Laryngoscope* 1989;99:1188–1192.
49. Watanabe H, Tsubokawa T, Katayama Y, Koyama S, Nakamura S. Primary Ewing's sarcoma of the temporal bone. *Surg Neurol* 1992;37: 54–58.
50. Coventry MB, Dahlin DC. Osteogenic sarcoma: a critical analysis of 430 cases. *J Bone Joint Surg Am* 1957;39:741–758.
51. Schuknecht HF. *Pathology of the ear.* Philadelphia: Lea & Febiger, 1993:452–453.
52. Eriksson B, Guntenberg B, Kindblom LG. Chordoma: a clinicopathologic and prognostic study of a Swedish national series. *Acta Orthop Scand* 1981;52:49–58.
53. Rich T, Schiller A, Suit H, et al. Clinical and pathologic review of 48 cases of chordoma. *Cancer* 1985;56:182–187.
54. Huvos A, Sundaresan N, Bretsky S, et al. Osteogenic sarcoma of the skull: a clinicopathologic study of 19 patients. *Cancer* 1985;56: 1214–1221.
55. Nauton RF, Stoller FM. Kaposi sarcoma of the auricle. *Laryngoscope* 1960;78:1041–1044.
56. Lalwani AK, Sooy CD. Otologic and neurotologic manifestations of the acquired immunodeficiency syndrome. *Otolaryngol Clin North Am* 1992;25:1183–1197.
57. Perzin KH, Gullane P, Conley J. Adenoid cystic carcinoma involving the external auditory canal: a clinicopathologic study of 16 cases. *Cancer* 1982;50:2873–2883.
58. Regine WF, Fontanesi J, Kumar P, et al. Local tumor control in rhabdomyosarcoma following low-dose irradiation: comparison of group II and select group III patients. *Int J Radiat Oncol Biol Phys* 1995;31: 485–491.
59. Raney RB Jr, Lawrence W Jr, Maurer HM, et al. Rhabdomyosarcoma of the ear in childhood: a report from the intragroup rhabdomyosarcoma study-I. *Cancer* 1983;51:2356–2361.
60. Wiltshaw E. The natural history of extramedullary plasmocytoma and its relation to multiple myeloma. *Medicine* 1976;55:217–238.
61. Abemayor E, Canalis RF, Greenberg P, et al. Plasma cell tumors of the head and neck. *J Otolaryngol* 1988;17:376–381.

62. Woodruff RK, Whittle JM, Malpas JS. Solitary plasmocytoma, I: extramedullary soft tissue plasmocytoma. *Cancer* 1979;43:2340–2343.
63. Jones RO, Pillsbury HC. Histiocytosis X of the head and neck. *Laryngoscope* 1984;94:1031–1035.
64. Lahey ME. Histiocytosis X: comparison of three treatment regimens. *J Pediatr Surg* 1975;87:179–183.
65. Cross DL, Nixon C. Temporal bone hemangiopericytoma. *Otolaryngol Head Neck Surg* 1996;114:631–644.
66. Batsakis JG. Tumors of the head and neck: clinical and pathological considerations, Baltimore: Williams & Wilkins, 1979:307–308.
67. Megerian CA, McKenna MJ, Nedol JB. Non paraganglioma jugular foramen lesions masquerading as glomus jugulare tumors. *Am J Otol* 1995;93:477–494.
68. Belal A. Metastatic tumors of the temporal bone. *J Laryngol Otol* 1985;99:839–846.
69. Cumberworth VL, Friedmann I, Glover GW. Late metastasis of breast carcinoma to the external auditory canal. *J Laryngol Otol* 1994;108:808–810.
70. Berlinger NT, Koutropas S, Adams G, Maisel R. Patterns of involvement of the temporal bone in metastatic and systemic malignancy. *Laryngoscope* 1980;11:171–176.
71. Proctor B, Lindsay JR. tumors involving the petrous pyramid of the temporal bone. *Arch Otolaryngol* 1947;46:180–194.
72. Nelson EG, Hinojosa R. Histopathology of metastatic temporal bone tumors. *Arch Otolaryngol Head Neck Surg* 1991;117:189–191.
73. Schuknecht HF, Allam AM, Murakami Y. Pathology of secondary malignant tumors of the temporal bone. *Ann Otol Rhinol Laryngol* 1968;77:5–22.
74. Hill B, Kohut RI. Metastatic adenocarcinoma of the temporal bone. *Arch Otolaryngol* 1976;102:568–571.
75. Worthington P. Secondary malignant tumor of the temporal bone presenting as jaw joint dysfunction. *J Laryngol Otol* 1983;97:1157–1161.
76. Feinmesser R, Lisbon Y, Uziely B, Gay I. Metastatic carcinoma to the temporal bone. *Am J Otol* 1986;7:119–120.
77. Kobayashi K, Igarashi M, Ohashi K, Mcbride RA. Metastatic seminoma of the temporal bone. *Arch Otolaryngol Head Neck Surg* 1986;112:102–105.
78. Morton LA, Butler SA, Khan A, Johnson A, Middleton P. Temporal bone metastasis: pathophysiology and imaging. *Otolaryngol Head Neck Surg* 1987;97:583–587.
79. Johnson A, Hawke M, Berger G. Sudden deafness and vertigo due to inner ear hemorrhage: a temporal bone case report. *J Otolaryngol* 1984;13:201–207.
80. Martin DS, Benecke J, Maas C. Metastatic tumor presenting as chronic otitis and facial paralysis. *Ann Otol Rhinol Laryngol* 1992;101:280–281.
81. Ruah CB, Bohigian RK, Vincent ME, Vaughan CW. Metastatic sigmoid adenocarcinoma to the temporal bone. *Otolaryngol Head Neck Surg* 1987;97:500–503.
82. Hirsch BE, Sehkar L, Kamerer DB. Metastatic atrial myxoma to the temporal bone. *Am J Otol* 1991;12:207–209.
83. Jungreis CA, Sekhar LN, Martinez AJ, Hirsch BE. Cardiac myxoma metastatic to the temporal bone. *Radiology* 1989;170:244.
84. El Fiky FM, Paparella MM. A metastatic glomus jugulare tumor. *Am J Otol* 1984;5:197–200.
85. Saldanha CB, Bennett JD, Evans JN, Pambakian H. Metastasis to the temporal bone, secondary to carcinoma of the bladder. *J Laryngol Otol* 1989;103:599–601.
86. Tan J, Mackenzie I, Duvall E. Metastatic small cell carcinoma of the temporal bone. *J Laryngol Otol* 1984;98:1267–1271.
87. Corey JP, Nelson E, Crawford M, Riester JW, Geiss R. Metastatic vaginal carcinoma to the temporal bone. *Am J Otol* 1991;12:128–131.
88. Vanexan K, Gammel T, Soong VY. Scalp pilomatrix carcinoma as an extra-axial mass. *South Med J* 1991;84:371–373.
89. Yoshihara T, Igarashi M. Poorly differentiated fibrosarcoma (spindle cell carcinoma) involving the temporal bone. *ORL J Otorhinolaryngol Relat Spec* 1986;48:249–255.
90. Cross JP, Ladaga LA. Peripheral synovial sarcoma metastatic to the temporal bone. *Am J Otol* 1986;7:169–171.
91. Jahn AF, Farkashidy J, Berman JM. Metastatic tumors in the temporal bone: a pathophysiologic study. *J Otolaryngol* 1979;8:85–95.
92. Maddox HE. Metastatic tumors of the temporal bone. *Ann Otol Rhinol Laryngol* 1967;76:149–165.
93. Paparella MM, El-Fiky F. Ear involvement in malignant lymphoma. *Ann Otol Rhinol Laryngol* 1972;81:352–363.
94. Nicolaides A, McFerran DJ, Croxson G. Non Hodgkin's lymphoma of the temporal bone. *J Laryngol Otol* 1988;102:928–931.
95. Tucci DL, Lambert PR, Innes DJ. Primary lymphoma of the temporal bone. *Arch Otolaryngol Head Neck Surg* 1992;118:83–85.
96. Vidal JBE. De la leukocytemie splenique, on de l'hypertrophiz de la rate avec alteration du sang consistent dans une augmentation considerable du nombre des globules blancs. *Gaz Hebd Med Paris,*1856;3:53–60.
97. Politzer A. Pathologische Veranderungen in Labyrinthe bei leukamisher Taubheit Cong. *Int Otol Compt Rend* 1894;3:139–150.
98. Schuknecht HF. *Pathology of the ear.* Philadelphia: Lea & Febiger, 1993:489–491.
99. Druss JG. Aural manifestation of leukemia. *Arch Otolaryngol* 1945;42:267–272.
100. Friedmann I. *Pathology of the ear.* Oxford, UK: Blackwell Scientific, 1974:208–210.
101. Batsakis JG. *Tumors of the head and neck: clinical and pathological considerations,* 2nd ed. Baltimore: Williams & Wilkins, 1979:369–380.

The Ear: Comprehensive Otology,
edited by R.F. Canalis and P.R. Lambert.
Lippincott Williams & Wilkins, Philadelphia ©2000.

CHAPTER 53

Acoustic Neuroma and Other Tumors of the Cerebellopontine Angle

Gregory A. Ator, Herman A. Jenkins, Donald P. Becker, and Rinaldo F. Canalis

Neuroma (schwannoma, neurilemoma, neurinoma) of the acoustic (cochleovestibular) nerve is a slow-growing, benign tumor that is the most commonly found mass in the cerebellopontine angle (CPA). In this chapter, we discuss the clinical features and current concepts in the diagnosis and treatment of these tumors and other lesions in this anatomic region.

HISTORICAL NOTE

The first report of a tumor that could be interpreted as an acoustic neuroma was by Sandifort (1), who in 1777 described a hard nodule firmly attached to the inferior portion of the auditory nerve that was encountered during the course of an anatomic dissection. Other sporadic reports of incidental autopsy findings appeared in the literature of the eighteenth century, but none correlated the pathology found with antemortem symptoms. At the beginning of the nineteenth century, Leveque-Lasource (2) described a tumor arising from the left porus acusticus of a 38-year-old woman who had experienced headache, tinnitus, blindness, and later deafness and gait instability. Although the findings were suggestive of an acoustic tumor, Cushing (3), discussing the report, felt that it could have been a meningioma and stated that the first unequivocal description of a vestibular schwannoma was by Charles Bell (4) in 1830. Figure 1 is a photograph of the illustration used by Bell to document his findings. Following Bell's report, several other reports appeared in the literature; those by Cruveilhier (5) and Oppenheim (6) were of special interest because of their detailed clinicopathologic correlations. The first European clinical series was reported by Sternberg (7) in 1900, and the first American series was by Fraenkel and Hunt (8) in 1903.

Although successful surgical treatment of acoustic schwannomas was first achieved by Ballance (9) in 1894,

G. A. Ator: Otologic Center, Inc., Otology/Neurotology, Kansas City, Missouri 64111

H. A. Jenkins: Department of Otolaryngology and Communicative Sciences, Baylor College of Medicine, Houston, Texas 77030

D. P. Becker: Division of Neurosurgery, University of California, Los Angeles, School of Medicine, Los Angeles, California 90095

R. F. Canalis: Department of Surgery, University of California, Los Angeles, School of Medicine, Los Angeles, California 90095-1624

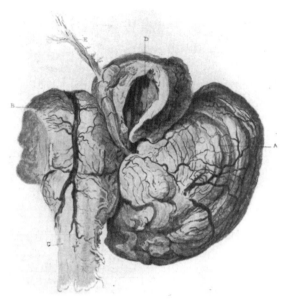

FIG. 1. Bell's 1830 drawing of an acoustic tumor with central degeneration.

problems with asepsis and lack of magnification made these pioneering operations an ordeal for patient and surgeon and carried a mortality rate in excess of 70%. It was not until 1917 when Harvey Cushing (3) introduced the subtotal intracapsular resection technique that the mortality rate was reduced to 30% and the stage was set for the modern era of acoustic neuroma surgery. At the time, reduction of tumor mass was the primary goal of surgery, which was deemed successful when the progression of neurologic symptoms was delayed and the patient's survival was prolonged. Further progress, however, did not take place for almost 50 years, and the incidence of complications such as facial paralysis and other cranial nerve functional impairments remained high.

The next phase in the successful treatment of acoustic schwannomas was determined by technological advances. The introduction of microsurgical techniques to the translabyrinthine and middle fossa approaches by House (10, 11) in the early 1960s and to the suboccipital approach by Rand and Kurze (12) in 1965 resulted in precise control of tumor resection, enhanced preservation of cranial nerve function, and marked reduction in general morbidity and mortality.

Improved radiographic techniques and intraoperative monitoring are responsible for the latest advances in the management of acoustic schwannomas. Among the diagnostic modalities, contrast-enhanced magnetic resonance image (MRI) is especially important because it allows detection of very small tumors before any significant neurologic compromise has occurred. Surgically, ongoing electromyographic monitoring of facial nerve function and tracking of auditory brainstem evoked responses in patients with serviceable hearing are now routinely used with constantly improving functional results.

This brief survey of the history of acoustic tumors reveals three distinct phases, each a reflection of the evolution of modern surgery as an art and science. The first phase occurs toward the end of the enlightenment and is marked by increasing understanding of pathologic changes responsible for clinical symptoms. The second phase takes place during the latter part of the nineteenth century and beginning of the twentieth century, and it is highlighted by the development of successful operative techniques performed in an aseptic field. The third, or current, phase is characterized by the ever increasing availability of sophisticated equipment leading to early diagnosis, total tumor resection, and preservation of function. An exhaustive history of acoustic neuroma surgery was written by House (13) in 1979.

INCIDENCE

Acoustic neuromas account for 10% of all intracranial tumors and are the most common mass presenting in the CPA (14,15). The age of presentation ranges from the second to the ninth decades. The male-to-female ratio is 6:4, with females frequently presenting symptoms at an earlier age. Only 5% of tumors are bilateral, and most of these arise in patients with neurofibromatosis type 2 (NF2) (16,17). The incidence of acoustic tumors in temporal bone collections is 1% to 2% (18), but in the general population the incidence is much lower at about 0.015% (15 of 100,000) (19).

PATHOGENESIS

Acoustic neuromas usually arise from the vestibular portion of the eighth cranial nerve. Tumors of the auditory branch are rare. Vestibular schwannomas typically originate from the internal auditory canal portion of the nerve, anywhere central to the Obersteiner-Redlich zone,

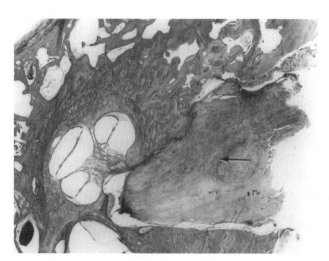

FIG. 2. Histopathologic section of the left temporal bone demonstrating the intracanalicular portion of an acoustic neuroma *(arrow).* (From Tower DB, ed. *The nervous system. Human communication and its disorders, volume 3.* New York: Raven Press, 1975, with permission.)

which is the junction of central myelin produced by glial cells and peripheral myelin produced by Schwann cells (19). Acoustic neuromas probably arise from the inferior and superior divisions of the vestibular nerve in approximately equal frequency. The true ratio is not clear because the nerve of origin sometimes is difficult to identify intraoperatively and the primary histologic evidence is limited to temporal bone studies of asymptomatic cases (20). After the canal is filled with tumor, extension into the CPA ensues (Figs. 2, 3, and 4). Because there is no firm anatomic obstruction to spread, the tumor can grow freely in various directions, extending superiorly to the trigeminal nerve and inferiorly to the vagus and glossopharyngeal nerves. Large tumors can compress the brainstem and produce multiple neurologic deficits.

PATHOLOGY

Cranial nerves arise from the brainstem with a glial support cell covering the neural fibers. At the Obersteiner-Redlich zone within the internal auditory canal the support cells become Schwann cells, which are the cells of origin of acoustic tumors. This differentiates vestibular schwannomas from neurinomas, which are made up of all components of the nerve. Acoustic tumors typically are composed of two types of proliferating elements: Antoni type A and Antoni type B cells (Fig. 5: see color plate 34 following page 484). Antoni A tumors consist of compact, elongated spindle cells with long oval

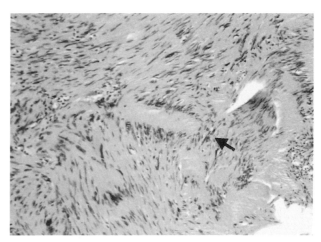

FIG. 5. Typical schwannoma. Note spindle cells distributed in alternating Antoni A areas (compact and more cellular) and Antoni B areas (loose and less cellular). Parallel rows of Schwann cells *(arrow)* known as Verocay bodies are highly characteristic of this tumor (hematoxylin and eosin, original magnification × 40). (Courtesy of Dr. Pier Luigi Di Patre.)

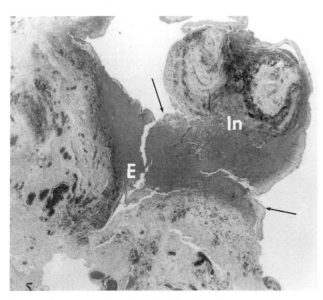

FIG. 3. Low-magnification photograph of an acoustic tumor demonstrating its intracanalicular *(In)* and extracanalicular *(E)* portions. *Arrows* point to plane of separation between the two portions.

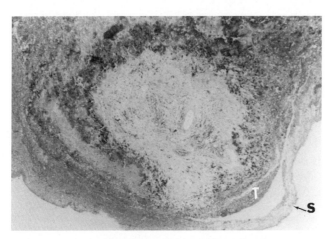

FIG. 4. Higher-magnification photograph of the intracanalicular portion of the lesion shown in Fig. 3 demonstrating the relationships between tumor *(T)* and nerve sheath *(S)*.

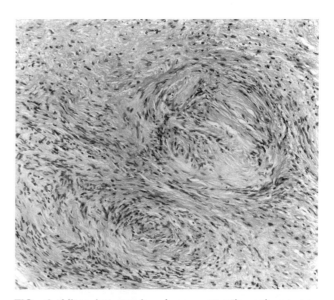

FIG. 6. Microphotograph of an acoustic schwannoma demonstrating interwoven fascicles of spindle-shaped cells characteristic of the Antoni type A configuration (hematoxylin and eosin, original magnification × 60).

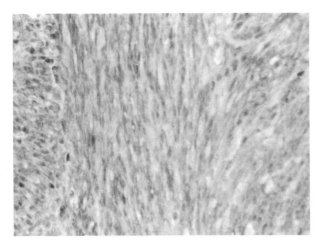

FIG. 7. Section of schwannoma immunostained for S100. Positivity for this marker is useful in the differential diagnosis with meningioma (original magnification × 60). (Courtesy of Dr. Pier Luigi Di Patre.)

nuclei. Antoni B lesions are composed of a loose matrix that stains poorly. Most acoustic tumors contain a substantial portion of type A cells that are necessary for diagnosis (Fig. 6). Occasional Verocay bodies composed of palisading nuclei arranged in pacinian-like rows are found among type A cells. A variable degree of nuclear pleomorphism is seen, and many tumors are quite vascular, with varying amounts of necrosis present. In difficult diagnostic cases, which are infrequent, positive immunostaining with S100 marker differentiates acoustic tumors from meningioma (Fig. 7: see color plate 35 following page 484). Malignant acoustic schwannomas have been described but are rare.

CLINICAL FEATURES

Vestibular Symptoms

Vertigo and Unsteadiness

True vertigo occurs in less than 20% of patients, but 50% will have some balance difficulties, with the majority complaining of unsteadiness (16,21). Because the deficit is chronic, progressive, and nonfluctuating, the loss of peripheral vestibular input caused by the tumor is readily compensated by central vestibular mechanisms. In addition, the vestibular function on the contralateral side usually is intact, which reduces the handicap experienced by the patient during usual activities. The speed of compensation and resulting clinical symptoms are related to the patient's age and presence or absence of visual and proprioceptive deficits. Most patients with a well-compensated peripheral lesion will notice problems only with activities that place stress on the vestibular system, such as rapid movements.

Nystagmus

Three forms of nystagmus may be present in CPA tumors: (a) spontaneous nystagmus, beating away from

the side of the lesion; (b) Bruns' nystagmus; and (c) bilateral horizontal gaze nystagmus (22,23). Bruns' nystagmus is associated with brainstem compression occurring in large CPA tumors. An asymmetric horizontal gaze-evoked nystagmus results, with the larger amplitude appearing when the patient looks toward the side of lesion. It is present in 20% to 40% of patients with tumors larger than 3 cm (22,23). Nedzelski (22) proposed that all three forms of nystagmus are related to varying degrees of tumor compression. Involvement of the nerve produces spontaneous nystagmus, whereas unilateral and bilateral flocculus compression produces bilateral gaze-evoked nystagmus. Variability in the mode of presentation of vestibular symptoms in CPA lesions may be due to differences in the direction of tumor growth. Less prominent findings result from anterior growth, which leaves the flocculus relatively unaffected.

Caloric Testing

In caloric testing, vestibular paresis without signs of brainstem dysfunction usually indicates peripheral disease. The abnormality can be distal in the labyrinth or proximal in the nerve, but a severe unilateral paralysis is more commonly associated with a nerve lesion. Despite this relative specificity, routine caloric testing is not ideal for the assessment of deficits resulting from acoustic neuromas. The test gives information that derives primarily from the lateral semicircular canal and the superior vestibular nerve. Because the inferior vestibular nerve supplies the posterior semicircular canal and saccule, early tumors arising from this branch may be associated with normal caloric responses. Furthermore, because the tumor probably arises with equal frequency from the inferior and superior vestibular nerves, the test is, at best, 50% effective in identifying vestibular damage from small internal auditory canal tumors.

Thomsen and Mirko (16), who evaluated 300 patients with acoustic neuroma, found impaired or abolished caloric responses in 34% and 63% of patients, respectively. However, when they used Fitzgerald and Hallpike's bithermal caloric method without fixation suppression, test results were abnormal in 82% of 50 surgically confirmed cases. Dysfunction varied with tumor location. The test results were abnormal in 97% of patients with superior vestibular lesions and in only 60% of inferior division tumors. These observations are supported by Hoffman et al. (24), who found that the simultaneous binaural, bithermal method increased the ability to identify vestibular dysfunctions to 86%, from 56% when routine caloric testing was used. Linthicum et al. (25) noted this difference was even more pronounced in small tumors.

Rotatory Testing

Rotatory testing may be useful in the assessment of acoustic neuromas because peripheral vestibular lesions produce asymmetric eye gain on bidirectional rotation (ampullofugal and ampullopetal stimulation) of the lateral semicircular canal. This asymmetry also results in phase changes in the vestibular response to a rotatory stimulus. Olson et al. (26) found that 67% of 24 patients with proven acoustic neuroma had abnormal rotatory findings, with acute shifts in phase and asymmetry. The phase shift remained constant over a 3-year period, but the asymmetry normalized over time. Baloh et al. (27) found impaired rotatory test results (sinusoidal and step stimulation) and reduced caloric responses in all patients in a series of acoustic neuromas larger than 1.3 cm. Moretz et al. (28) found that harmonic acceleration was abnormal in all of 18 cases, including seven small tumors of the CPA and internal auditory canal.

Auditory Symptoms

Sensorineural Hearing Loss

Symptoms produced by tumor compression of the auditory nerve are variable. The slow progression of vestibular deficits and their rapid central compensation are responsible for auditory symptoms usually emerging as the first indication of an acoustic neuroma. Patients typically will have an asymmetric sensorineural hearing loss on pure tone audiometry. This asymmetry is currently the most common indication for a retrocochlear pathology workup. A small difference (±5 dB) may be due to technical variability in threshold determination, but greater differences must be evaluated further. Hearing loss in acoustic tumors progresses over time in an unpredictable manner (Fig. 8). Patients also may present with unilateral tinnitus, sometimes with little or no auditory impairment, or with sudden hearing loss (Fig. 9).

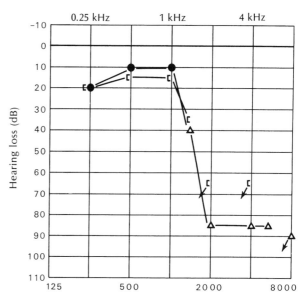

FIG. 9. Initial audiometric evaluation in a 27-year-old patient with a 2 × 2.5 cm right acoustic tumor who presented with sudden hearing loss. ([-[, masked bone conduction; ●-●, unmasked air conduction; Δ-Δ, masked air conduction; Δ *with arrow* and [*with arrow*, no response.)

Auditory Testing

Pure tone thresholds over the mid-frequency range (500 Hz to 2 kHz) have been reported as 21 to 40 dB in 16% of patients with acoustic tumor, 41 to 80 dB in 46%, and greater than 80 dB in 35% (29). Some small acoustic tumors may lack auditory symptoms and have normal pure tone levels (30). In addition to pure tone thresholds, speech discrimination scores and reflex decay test results may be abnormal in patients with retrocochlear disease. Speech

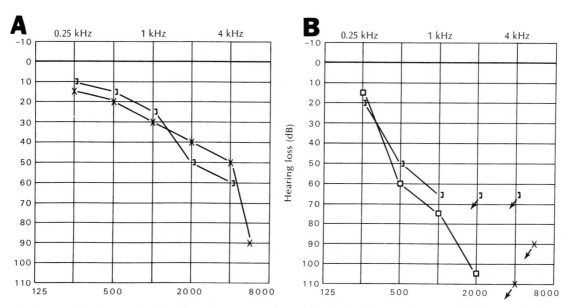

FIG. 8. A: Left ear air–bone conduction curves in a 58-year-old woman with a small acoustic tumor (initial evaluation). **B:** Pure tone audiometry in the same patient 3.5 years after presentation. (]-], masked bone conduction; x-x, unmasked air conduction; □-□, masked air conduction;] *with arrow* and x *with arrow*, no response.)

discrimination scores have two main characteristics in patients with retrocochlear pathology. The most common is a rollover phenomenon, in which increasing levels of loudness of presentation cause a score reduction. Somewhat less frequently, a relatively low discrimination score is seen for a given degree of pure tone loss (31). Interaural asymmetries greater than 10% are significant and should be evaluated with further testing for retrocochlear disease. Stapedial reflexes frequently will be elevated or absent. Reflex decay and increased response latency also may be present (32–35) (see Chapters 12 and 15).

Psychoacoustic tests including alternate binaural loudness balance, tone threshold decay test, and Bekesy speech audiometry have a sensitivity of 50% to 60% and are mentioned only for their historical value, because most investigators have abandoned their use (32).

Auditory brainstem evoked responses (ABR) are the mainstay of audiologic diagnosis in acoustic neuromas (see Chapters 12 and 15). Several clinically useful changes in the ABR commonly are produced by retrocochlear lesions. Among these, increased central conduction time and unequal interaural wave V latencies are the most important. Central conduction time, the interval between waves I and V, frequently is prolonged. However, the probability of detecting changes declines with increasing high-frequency sensorineural hearing loss, which makes this parameter somewhat unreliable.

Interaural wave V latency differences of 0.2 ms are significant, although a correction factor must be applied for sensorineural hearing loss (36). Of note, brainstem compression by large tumors may result in latency prolongation in the contralateral ear (37). Overall, ABR is abnormal in 95% to 98% of all CPA tumors (38). Recently, a false-positive incidence of 2% has been documented (39). These accuracy problems have led most practitioners to primarily use MRI in high suspicion cases. However, because of the high cost of imaging, ABR continues to have a role as the best screening test in cases where the index of suspicion is low. ABR in limited by sensorineural mid-frequency hearing losses greater than 70 dB, because wave I cannot be identified with this degree of impairment. When available, this difficulty can be circumvented with the use of electrocochleography.

Facial Nerve Dysfunction

The facial nerve is in direct contact with acoustic tumors, and the growth of these tumors results in significant compression of the facial nerve fibers. However, the slow growth rate of these lesions and the nerve's tolerance to gradual stretching accounts for the nerve's normal function, even when it is in contact with very large tumors. When present, facial nerve dysfunction usually is gradual in onset and incomplete. In general, facial nerve paralysis in a patient with a CPA mass is suggestive of a lesion other than an acoustic neuroma (40).

A considerable number of facial nerve fibers must be compromised to produce dysfunction. Kartush et al. (41) used electroneurography to investigate subclinical involvement of the facial nerve and found no prognostic value to this test. Deficits in the sensory component of the facial nerve may give an early indication of its involvement. Hitselberger and Pulec (42) noted conchal hypoesthesia in lesions compressing the facial nerve without producing motor abnormalities. Facial nerve dysfunction is more likely to occur in acoustic neurofibromas. Eckermeier et al. (18) showed that the facial nerve frequently is infiltrated in these cases and demonstrated invasion of the geniculate ganglion in 11 of 30 tumors, only two of which were schwannomas.

Cerebellopontine Angle Syndrome

As the tumor expands into the CPA, it grows superiorly toward the trigeminal nerve and inferiorly toward the lower cranial nerves and the foramen magnum. Medial extension results in progressive brainstem displacement. The sequence of neurologic events resulting from tumoral growth has been termed CPA syndrome and is divided into four stages (43).

Stage 1. Symptoms are limited to the eighth cranial nerve. Unilateral hearing loss, tinnitus, and unsteadiness are present.

Stage 2. Marked by the progression of stage 1 deficits and the onset of facial, trigeminal, and cerebellar symptoms. The following are relatively common: hypoactive corneal reflex; facial hypoesthesia, which may be intermittent; segmental or diffuse facial nerve weakness; loss of the acoustic reflex; gait unsteadiness; deviation to the affected side when walking; and impairment of precise hand coordination.

Stage 3. Characterized by further worsening of prior deficits, loss of function of lower cranial nerves, and brainstem compression. Vocal cord, palatal paralysis, and shoulder weakness may develop. Long tract signs such as contralateral extensor plantar responses and decreased sensation and motor strength are present. A positive Romberg sign and mild-to-moderate hydrocephalus are common.

Stage 4. Characterized by increased intracranial pressure along with worsening of previous deficits. Persistent headache and papilledema are prominent.

RADIOGRAPHIC DIAGNOSIS

MRI with contrast is the method of choice for evaluation of CPA pathology. Lesions of this region have a characteristic MRI appearance (see Chapter 18). Acoustic neuromas typically show enhancement on T2-weighted images and with the paramagnetic agent gadolinium-DTPA (44), which allows diagnosis of extremely small intracanalicular tumors (Fig. 10) and accurate delineation

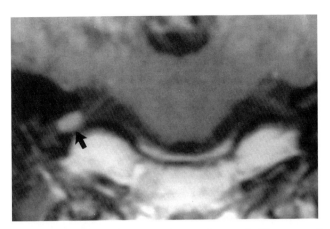

FIG. 10. Magnetic resonance image demonstrating a small left intracanalicular tumor *(arrow)* in a 43-year-old patient.

of their interface with cerebellum and brainstem in larger tumors (Fig. 11). Acoustic tumors may have areas of cystic degeneration or be uniform in appearance. Contrast enhancement permits differentiation of recurrent or residual tumor from surrounding scar, loculated cerebrospinal fluid, and brain tissue; however, false-positive findings may occur. Areas of nerve edema and nonneoplastic pathology can enhance and have the appearance of mass lesions (45). Facial nerve neuromas and meningiomas show contrast enhancement and often cannot be differentiated from acoustic tumors (46). Therefore, MRI findings must be interpreted in conjunction with a carefully obtained clinical history and physical examination.

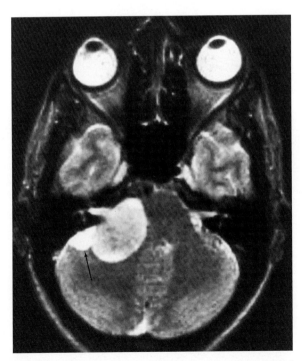

FIG. 11. Magnetic resonance imaging study with gadolinium contrast in an advanced acoustic neuroma. Note associated pseudocyst *(arrow).*

Computed tomographic (CT) scans are valuable in the preoperative assessment of temporal bone anatomy when planning specific approaches to the CPA. Preoperative knowledge of the position of the semicircular canals, cochlea, and sigmoid sinus are especially important when hearing preservation operations are planned. Contrast CT also is helpful when MRI is contraindicated or not feasible, such as in patients who are obese, claustrophobic, or who have implanted metallic devices or pacemakers. Arteriography is not routinely required in the evaluation of CPA pathology, but it may be indicated in the assessment of large tumors.

DIFFERENTIAL DIAGNOSIS

The differential diagnosis of acoustic tumors is based on the clinical history, physical findings, and imaging characteristics. It includes meningioma, cholesteatoma, hemangioma, lipoma, arachnoid cysts, metastatic disease, schwannoma of other cranial nerves, and primary central nervous system neoplasm (14) (see following section on Nonacoustic Tumors of the Cerebellopontine Angle).

PRESENT WORKUP RECOMMENDATIONS

Patients with asymmetric hearing loss, unilateral tinnitus, speech discrimination differences greater than 10%, rollover, reflex decay, or reflex absence should be evaluated for retrocochlear pathology.

Welling et al. (47) used decision-tree analysis and suggested the early use of MRI and ABR, bypassing all other tests except basic audiometry, as a cost-effective approach to the diagnosis of acoustic tumors. MRI is recommended in patients with highly suspicious symptoms, such as unilateral tinnitus, decreased speech discrimination, or unilateral hearing loss and in those patients with intermediately suspicious symptoms, such as sudden hearing loss. In patients with a low index of suspicious symptoms, such as isolated vertigo or historically explainable unilateral hearing loss, ABR is recommended, with follow-up MRI as needed. A more cost-effective alternative, which is not universally available, is MRI screening consisting of imaging limited to the internal auditory canal.

TREATMENT

The treatment of acoustic neuroma is primarily surgical. Stereotactic radiotherapy is an alternative in selected cases, and observation may be elected in elderly and debilitated patients without signs of progressive disease. In general, early removal is advocated for small lesions, because when hearing is present its preservation is more feasible and because morbidity increases with larger tumors. The translabyrinthine, middle cranial fossa, and suboccipital/retrosigmoid approaches currently are used.

Translabyrinthine Approach

Indications

The translabyrinthine approach is best suited for patients without serviceable hearing. Tumors of any size may be removed with this approach, especially when combined with retrosigmoid craniotomy or transcochlear extension. Facial nerve preservation is enhanced with this approach.

Technique

Electromyographic facial nerve monitoring is used throughout the operation. The operation begins with a

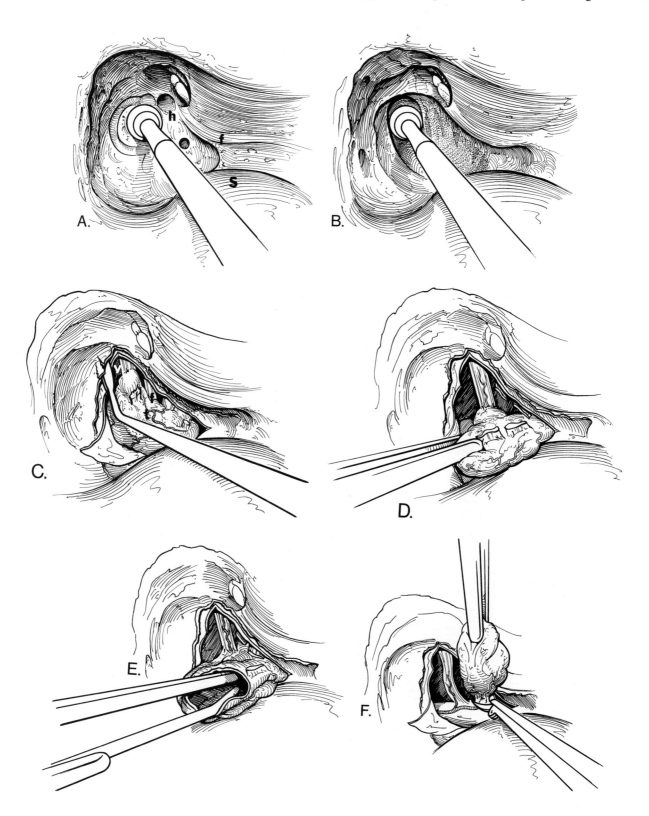

canal-wall-up mastoidectomy and dissection of the posterior and middle fossa plates. The jugular bulb and the sigmoid sinus are exposed. The sinus plate may be partially or totally removed, depending on exposure needs. A labyrinthectomy is performed following identification of the semicircular canals, vertical facial canal, and attic (Fig. 12A). Care must be taken to avoid damage to the facial nerve when opening the superior canal ampulla, as the labyrinthine portion of the nerve is just deep to this structure. The vestibule is entered and all neuroepithelium removed. Dissection of the internal auditory canal is performed, exposing approximately 180 degrees of its circumference (Fig. 12B). The posterior fossa dura is exposed to the level of the jugular bulb. The endolymphatic sac is identified. Prior to opening the dura, the labyrinthine portion of the facial nerve and the vertical crest (Bill's bar) are identified. Unroofing the labyrinthine portion of the facial nerve is performed, because doing so may decrease the incidence of postoperative delayed facial paralysis (48). The dura is opened at a location medial to the fundus, and the facial nerve is identified visually and electrically (Fig. 12C). The distal portions of the superior and inferior vestibular nerves and cochlear nerve are avulsed from the fundus of the internal auditory canal (Fig. 12D). Debulking of the center of the tumor is accomplished using the Greenwood suction cautery instrument, Nd-YAG or CO_2 laser, Cavitron, or other dissection tool (Fig. 12E). After decompression, the tumor capsule can be gently rolled posteriorly from the facial nerve while any capsular vessels encountered are cauterized. In this fashion, the tumor gradually is debulked and devascularized but the surrounding neurovascular structures are preserved (Fig. 12F). During the course of the dissection, the posterior fossa dura may be opened to allow further access to the tumor. Following resection, the tumor bed is irrigated and bleeding controlled. The defect is obliterated with muscle and adipose tissue. The dissected periosteum is reapproximated to maintain the grafts in place. Following skin closure, a mastoid dressing is placed and left on for 5 days.

Limitations

Exposure of the internal auditory canal through this approach is restricted posteriorly by the sigmoid sinus and anteriorly by the facial nerve. Inferior internal auditory canal exposure occasionally may be limited by a high jugular bulb that makes inferior pole dissection of the tumor difficult.

Extensions

The translabyrinthine technique may be combined with a transcochlear approach to allow resection of tumors extending anteriorly to involve the brainstem. The cochlea is resected, leaving a thin layer of bone over the internal carotid artery. The fallopian canal is skeletonized throughout its temporal course, but the facial nerve does not need to be transposed. Further exposure may be obtained by combining retrosigmoid craniectomy with the translabyrinthine approach. The skin incision is modified to permit exposure of occipital bone posterior to the sigmoid sinus. Incision of the dura will allow access to the medial aspect of the posterior extent of the tumor after the cerebellum is medially retracted.

Conclusions

The main advantage of the translabyrinthine approach is that it enhances the surgeon's ability to preserve the facial nerve. This structure can be identified in the labyrinthine portion of the fallopian canal before tumor work is begun, then followed into the internal auditory canal and on the surface of the tumor mass. Because hearing is sacrificed, this approach is preferred in patients with limited or nonserviceable hearing. Modifications of the translabyrinthine technique aimed at hearing preservation are currently under study (49).

Middle Cranial Fossa Approach

Indications

This approach is favored for patients with serviceable hearing and with tumors confined to the internal auditory canal. Tumors with limited CPA extension can be resected with the expanded middle cranial fossa approach.

Technique

A craniectomy is performed just above the floor of the middle cranial fossa. The temporal lobe dura is elevated until the arcuate eminence (prominence of the superior semicircular canal) is located. Several modalities can be used to find the internal auditory canal (50), but we favor the approach reported by Fish (51). The superior semicircular canal is blue lined and aligned with a 60-degree triangle with its apex oriented anteriorly (Fig. 13A: see color plate 36A following page 484). The internal auditory canal is found along the posterior limb of the triangle. Care must be

---

FIG. 12. Translabyrinthine resection of acoustic tumors. **A:** Mastoidectomy is completed and labyrinthectomy is initiated. **B:** Initial exposure of the internal auditory canal. **C:** Tumor *(t)* arising from the superior vestibular nerve *(v)* is exposed after opening the internal auditory canal. **D:** Tumor is partially dislodged by avulsing the vestibular and cochlear nerves. **E:** The center of the tumor is debulked. **F:** Tumor removal is completed. *f,* facial nerve; *h,* lateral canal; *s,* sigmoid sinus.

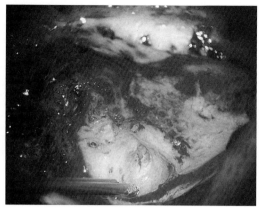

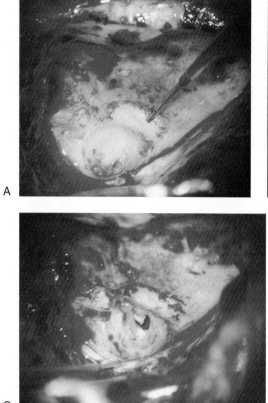

FIG. 13. Middle cranial fossa approach to acoustic tumors. **A:** Pointer is on the superior semicircular canal (SC); temporal lobe is retracted. **B:** SC is blue lined; geniculate ganglion is exposed; initial opening of the internal auditory canal (IAC). **C:** Dura of the IAC has been opened and tumor partially resected.

taken not to enter the cochlea. Approximately 120-degree circumference of the canal circumference is removed, giving special attention to the area near the medial wall of the porus acusticus (Fig. 13B: see color plate 36B following page 484). Prior to opening the canal dura, the labyrinthine segment of the facial nerve and the vertical crest are identified (Fig. 13C: see color plate 36C following page 484). The cochlear and facial nerves are located in the anterior portion of the canal and preserved. The tumor is removed using standard techniques of central debulking followed by peripheral cautery and dissection. Closure of the defect is accomplished with a temporalis muscle plug, along with sealing of any exposed mastoid air cells with bone wax.

Extensions

The extended or middle cranial fossa technique used extensively by Kanzaki et al. (52) and Wigand et al. (53) allows resection of tumors with up to 3.0 cm of CPA involvement. In this modification, the superior petrosal vein, which limits extension of the dissection into the middle fossa, is divided to expose the CPA. Further exposure is obtained by removal of bone anterior and posterior to the internal auditory canal, as well as the labyrinth when serviceable hearing is not present (54).

Glasscock et al. (55) described a combined, hearing preservation middle fossa/suboccipital procedure for patients with large tumors. The middle fossa approach

allows identification of the auditory and facial nerves in the internal auditory canal, and the posterior suboccipital approach permits rapid removal of the tumor (56).

Limitations

This approach requires significant experience and is restricted to small tumors. Treatment of lesions with extension into the CPA is difficult. The facial nerve occasionally is in the way of tumor resection.

Conclusions

The middle cranial fossa approach is favored for small intracanalicular tumors with serviceable hearing. It is most useful when the tumor does not extend into the fundus of the internal auditory canal. The extended middle cranial fossa approach can be used for tumors with medial extension.

Suboccipital/retrosigmoid Approach

Indications

This approach frequently is utilized for large tumors or for smaller ones with serviceable hearing. Tumors of any size can be approached, as it provides a wide view of the CPA and its structures. It is especially useful for lesions with inferior extension.

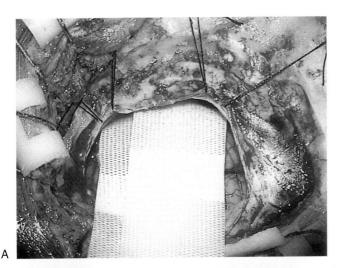

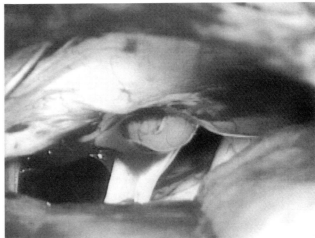

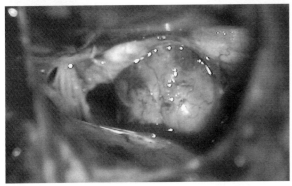

FIG. 14. Retrosigmoid approach to acoustic tumors. **A:** Retrosigmoid craniotomy/craniectomy is completed; sigmoid is exposed; initial dural opening. **B:** Small tumor extending just out of the internal auditory canal. Cranial nerve VIII bundle is clearly seen. **C:** Medium-size tumor. Branches of cranial nerves IX and X are seen to the left (inferior) of the tumor.

Technique

The posterior portion of the mastoid cortex is removed, exposing the sigmoid plate. The sigmoid sinus is exposed superior to the jugular bulb and to the level of the transverse sinus. All exposed mastoid cells are thoroughly obliterated with bone wax. Two bur holes usually are needed, one suboccipitally and one just under the edge of the transverse sinus. Following separation of the underlying dura, a circumferential craniotomy approximately 3 to 4 cm in diameter is performed, although some surgeons prefer to perform a craniectomy. The dura is incised parallel to the sigmoid and transverse sinuses, exposing the cerebellum. With release of cerebrospinal fluid from the cisterna magna and gentle cerebellar retraction, the CPA is exposed revealing the tumor (Fig. 14A–C: see color plates 37A–C following page 484). The internal auditory canal is skeletonized and then opened, taking care not to enter the posterior semicircular canal or the cochlea as dissection approaches the fundus. Removal proceeds with central debulking of the tumor followed by peripheral dissection to free its capsule from surrounding neurovascular structures. In this maneuver, careful identification of the arachnoid intervening between the lesion and underlying structures is helpful in achieving preservation of cranial nerve function (Fig. 15).

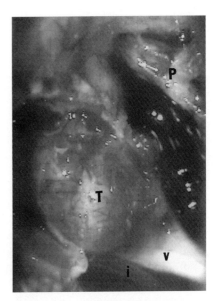

FIG. 15. Tumor exposure via the retrosigmoid approach. The internal auditory canal has been opened to the fundus. *i,* Labyrinthine artery; *p,* petrosal vein; *T,* tumor; *v,* vestibular nerve.

Limitations

Dissection of the internal auditory canal fundus may be restricted. The facial nerve usually is deep to the lesion and, except for very small tumors, it tends to be flattened so that its identification demands great care and frequent electrical stimulation.

Conclusions

The suboccipital/retrosigmoid approach permits wide exposure of the CPA. It is preferred as a hearing preservation technique in small tumors or for large tumors (Fig. 15).

Electrophysiologic Monitoring

Intraoperative facial nerve monitoring and ABR recordings are used routinely in acoustic neuroma surgery (56a). The discharge pattern of the electromyographic monitor can be used to assess facial nerve status on a real-time basis and alerts the surgeon to traumatic maneuvers during the dissection. In addition, electrical stimulation permits identification of the nerve when attenuation by tumor pressure has made visual identification difficult. Other nerves monitored on a selected basis are the hypoglossal, vagal, and spinal accessory. Intraoperative ABR is critical in cases where hearing preservation is attempted. Chapters 17 and 44 present a detailed discussion of the indications and techniques of intraoperative monitoring.

Surgical Complications

Complications vary according to the surgical approach used. Overall mortality currently is less than 1% (57,58), and morbidity is generally greater for large tumors (>3 cm). As complete tumor resection now is routinely achieved and mortality reduced, preservation of facial and auditory functions have increased in priority in acoustic tumor surgery. Since the advent of intraoperative monitoring, small tumors usually can be removed with no significant facial nerve dysfunction. In general, facial nerve preservation depends on tumor size, tumor consistency, and the surgeon's technical skills. In tumors limited to the internal auditory canal, 90% to 100% nerve preservation with a House grade I to II result may be obtained (59–61). In tumors with less than 2 cm of CPA extension, a grade I to II result may be expected in 80% to 90% of cases. In medium-size tumors (2–3.9 cm), a grade I to II functional result is expected in 60% to 75%, and in large tumors (>4.0 cm), a grade I to II result is expected in 28% to 57% (62–64). Tumors that infiltrate the facial nerve or fibrous tumors, which are more difficult to dissect, have an adverse impact on postoperative facial nerve function.

Facial nerve preservation rates are comparable for the translabyrinthine and suboccipital approaches (58,59). The rate of nerve preservation with grade I to II results for the middle cranial fossa approach is greater than 95% (65–68), in part due to the small size of the tumors treated. When the facial nerve is interrupted restoration is best achieved, when possible, by end-to-end anastomosis (69). If the defect is too large, cable grafting using the greater auricular nerve is used. If this is not possible or the condition of the nerve is unclear, a hypoglossal-facial transfer is recommended at a second stage.

Hearing preservation is often an elusive goal in acoustic neuroma surgery. As in facial nerve preservation, retention of serviceable hearing is influenced by tumor size, and many surgeons do not attempt it for tumors larger than 2 cm (66,70). Other surgeons use a hearing-sparing approach in nearly all cases (71). The preoperative hearing level is important in hearing preservation, although the definition of salvageable hearing is controversial. Many surgeons have adopted the 50-50 rule (at least 50-dB speech reception threshold and 50% speech understanding) of Gardner and Robertson (72), but others apply more stringent criteria. In a large, multiinstitutional study, Gardner and Robertson reported hearing preservation in 33% of 600 tumors removed by the suboccipital or middle cranial fossa approach. Long-term hearing preservation results may be even less favorable, because further hearing deterioration has been noted in some patients followed beyond the first few postoperative years (73–75).

After cranial nerves VII and VIII deficits, cerebrospinal fluid leaks are the most common complication of acoustic neuroma surgery. The incidence of this complication is approximately 8% regardless of the approach used. Cerebrospinal fluid can exit through the wound or nasally, and it may foster the development of retrograde meningitis. Several technical steps can be taken to prevent this complication. Pressure dressing should be maintained for the first 5 postoperative days to prevent accumulation of cerebrospinal fluid in the subcutaneous spaces dissected during surgery. When the translabyrinthine approach is used, the defect should be obliterated in several layers. The antrum is plugged first with temporalis muscle and fascia. Temporalis muscle fascia is placed over the defect in the IAC followed by small (1 cm³) adipose tissue grafts. Fascia lata can be used if the temporalis fascia is not thick enough. It is important to eliminate routes of cerebrospinal fluid egress by carefully blocking with bone wax all opened air cells.

In the suboccipital/retrosigmoid technique, attention first must be given to the internal auditory canal. Opened air cells are obliterated with bone wax. The defect is closed with a free muscle graft, morsellized, and cut to fit. Autologous glue is used sometimes, but its adhesive capacity and benefits in leak prevention are not clear. In this approach, the many mastoid air cells that are opened during the initial exposure should be obliterated carefully with muscle and bone wax. The dural closure should be water tight.

Cerebrospinal fluid leaks may occur during the first few days or, infrequently, several weeks or even months after surgery. In the translabyrinthine approach, they tend to occur through the open dural defect and extrude through the suture line or appear as clear rhinorrhea. In the suboccipital/retrosigmoid approach, failure to obliterate defects, either at the internal auditory canal or in the posterior mastoid air cell system (Fig. 16), can result in postoperative cerebrospinal fluid leaks. Once identified clinically and, if necessary, by glucose level determination (>40 mg/mL) or β-transferrin analysis (76), the leaks first are treated conservatively. Bed rest, head elevation, and pressure dressing are the basic initial steps. Transcutaneous leakage is addressed with resuture of the wound using a sterile technique. A lumbar drain is inserted to decompress the subarachnoid space and maintained for 5 days. Subcutaneous collections of fluid that accumulate after pressure dressing removal are managed in a similar manner. Prophylactic antibiotics often are used, but they are somewhat controversial because of the risk of fostering the development of resistant bacterial strains. Overall, most leaks respond to conservative measures. Persistence of the leak beyond 5 days and delayed leaks usually are indications for reexploration (77).

Epidural blood accumulation occurs rarely. Progression leads to brain compression with functional loss. Excessive retraction may produce *cerebellar edema* and infrequently parenchymal hemorrhage or necrosis, which may lead to increased intracranial pressure and cerebellar dysfunction. *Subdural hematoma* is a serious complication that is best prevented by meticulous attention to operative hemostasis. *Cranial nerve injuries* other than

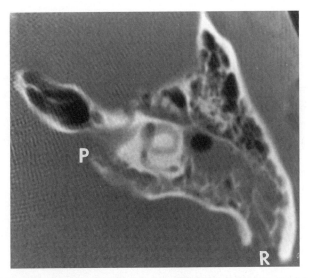

FIG. 16. Routes of escape of cerebrospinal fluid leaks following suboccipital resection of acoustic tumors. Note open *(R)* retrosigmoid and petrosal *(P)* cells.

cochlear and facial are unusual but can occur in large tumors. The trigeminal nerve is tolerant of surgical manipulation and rarely is injured. The lower cranial nerves (glossopharyngeal, spinal accessory, and hypoglossal) may be displaced by inferior extending tumors and are at risk during the resection, but they seldom are injured (78).

RADIOTHERAPY

Conventional external beam radiotherapy has no current role in the management of acoustic neuromas. It has been used to treat incompletely resected tumors, but the low tolerance of the central nervous system limits its usefulness in primary therapy. To circumvent this problem, Leksell (79) pioneered a stereotactic method that allows for precise radiation control and protection of normal structures. Stereotactic radiotherapy and "gamma knife surgery" differ from the conventional methods of deliverance in that ionizing radiation from several hundred external sources (typically cobalt 60) converge on the area to be treated, thus minimizing the energy received by the surrounding normal tissues. The treatment may be done in one session, and current generation devices can focus a beam of 300 to 400 cGy/min over a 5- to 24-mm area. A recent retrospective review reports growth arrest or size reduction in 98% of acoustic neuromas treated with stereotaxic radiotherapy (80). In a study of 40 patients followed for 10 years, Noren et al. (81) reported increased tumor size in 17.5%, no change in 17.5%, and tumor size reduction in 65%. In a group of 10 patients followed for 24 months, Lunsford and Linskey (82) reported decrease in tumor size in 42%, no change in 58%, and no instances of further tumor growth. These results are supported by Linskey et al. (83), who also reported a 50% rate of hearing preservation at 6 months and 30% 1 year after treatment. Facial paralysis occurred in 34% of patients and typically appeared 5 to 6 months after therapy. In an attempt to limit the complication rate of stereotactic radiotherapy, reduced tumor doses have been recommended (84). Although no long-term follow-up data are available from centers using lower irradiation regimens, the incidence of complications appears to have decreased. For tumors smaller than 30 mm, facial weakness is seen in approximately 16% to 29% of patients (85,86), with all intracanalicular tumors regaining preoperative levels of function within 25 months (87). Hearing conservation rates remain variable but similar (approximately 35%) to those reported in microsurgical series of small tumors (71,86).

Mortality attributable to radiotherapy has not been reported, but surgeons have noted increased morbidity in patients requiring surgery for tumor control after radiation. The facial nerve is particularly difficult to preserve in radiated patients (88). In a careful review (with rebuttal comments from microsurgical and radiotherapy advocates), Sekhar et al. (71) concluded that although early results on morbidity are similar for both microsurgery and radiotherapy, the long-term results with recently adopted radiotherapy protocols are still incomplete, thus making it difficult to fully define its role in the treatment of acoustic neuromas. It does have a clear role in patients with contraindications to surgery, such as those with bilateral tumors, contralateral deafness, residual tumor after surgery, and in those who refuse surgical therapy. Contraindications include posterior fossa compression symptoms and previous irradiation.

OTHER TREATMENTS

Jahrsdoerfer and Benjamin (89) reported on two patients with neurofibromatosis who were treated with a regimen of doxorubicin, dacarbazine, and cyclophosphamide and followed for approximately 2 years. Hearing was stabilized and no growth of tumor was observed over this period. However, the high toxicity of these agents and the unpredictability of their growth patterns preclude their consideration in the routine management of acoustic neuromas.

The effect of hormones is being investigated as a potential therapeutic tool. Siglock et al. (90) recently found progesterone receptors in 10 of 19 tumor specimens. However, there is no evidence that the administration of sex hormones alters tumor growth rate, and other investigators have not been able to detect estrogen or progesterone receptors in these tumors (91).

MANAGEMENT OF BILATERAL ACOUSTIC TUMORS

The management of bilateral acoustic tumors is very complex. The majority of patients in this group have NF2, the variant of von Recklinghausen's disease associated with axial neoplasms. These tumors tend to invade the cochlear and facial nerves much more frequently than isolated acoustic neuromas. More than 90% of patients with NF2 have bilateral acoustic tumors, and hearing preservation in these cases should be considered at the outset (92). However, attempts at sparing auditory function in patients with NF2 often are unsuccessful, thereby making the decision as to when to intervene more difficult. In patients with small tumors and symmetric hearing, some surgeons advocate operating on the smaller tumor first, as it may offer the best chance for hearing preservation. In patients with unilateral deafness, the tumor on the nonfunctioning side can be removed using any of the standard approaches. Observation or alternative therapies then may be considered for the second tumor. Stereotactic radiotherapy, chemotherapy, internal auditory canal decompression (93), and subtotal resection (94) are all possibilities, but insufficient data make utilization of these forms of therapy uncertain. In consideration of the poor results with long-term hearing preservation in these patients, early involvement in alternative hearing strategies, such as lip reading, is encouraged. Recent work on direct neural stimulation implants for brainstem auditory nuclei may eventually be of value for patients with bilateral disease (95).

TREATMENT OF ELDERLY PATIENTS

In the elderly patient who is not a good surgical risk or in other nonoperative situations, tumor growth may be followed with yearly MRI. The average growth rate in acoustic neuroma varies between 1 and 2 mm per year, although acute size changes sometimes can be caused by hemorrhage into the substance of the tumor. In cases of incomplete resection, there are no factors to predict growth. Residual tumor may remain dormant for years (96). In many cases, changes in symptoms will force some type of intervention, ranging from shunt placement for hydrocephalus to more extensive surgical procedures. Nedzelski et al. (97) found in a group of elderly patients (mean age 71 years) that 20% required surgery within one third of their expected survival time (14.3 years). Older patients with poor vestibular compensation are likely to have greater morbidity and mortality (15% at 1 year) from the hip replacement surgery they ultimately may need than from acoustic neuroma surgery (98).

Decompression by subtotal resection remains a viable alternative in the elderly patient. Kemink et al. (99) showed in a group of 20 patients undergoing subtotal (<95%) and near-total (>95%) resection that tumor regrowth was noted in only one patient in the subtotal group after a mean follow-up of 5 years. In addition, satisfactory rates of facial nerve preservation and low surgical morbidity were obtained in this group of suboptimal candidates. Other authors, however, have found high recurrence rates following subtotal resection, which, coupled with higher complication rates for reintervention, have made this approach unpopular (92).

CONCLUSION

The diagnosis of acoustic neuroma is increasingly being made when the tumor is still small. Using modern microscopic skull base techniques aided by intraoperative monitoring, total extirpation of the tumor is feasible, with anatomic preservation of the facial nerve in the majority of cases and, in selected cases, maintenance of serviceable hearing. Stereotactic radiotherapy plays a role in selected cases. Its value in the primary treatment of acoustic neuroma is still being defined.

NONACOUSTIC TUMORS OF THE CEREBELLOPONTINE ANGLE

In 1902, Henneberg and Koch introduced the term "cerebellopontine angle" (13), and in 1917, Cushing (3) defined the clinical features of lesions involving this area. The following is a list of the most frequent CPA lesions.

1. Acoustic neuroma (80%–90%)
2. Meningioma (3%)
3. Cholesteatoma (epidermoid tumor)
4. Cholesterol granuloma
5. Facial nerve schwannoma
6. Metastasis
   A. Breast
   B. Kidney
   C. Lung
   D. Stomach
   E. Larynx
   F. Prostate
   G. Thyroid
   H. Yolk sac tumor
7. Miscellaneous
   A. Other cranial nerve neuroma
   B. Arachnoid cyst
   C. Dermoid
   D. Leiomyoma
   E. Medulloblastoma
   F. Chordoma
   G. Chondrosarcoma
   H. Teratoma
   I. Melanoma
   J. Hemangioma
   K. Malignant nerve sheath tumor
   L. Lipoma
8. Nonneoplastic
   A. Xanthogranuloma
   B. Lyme disease
   C. Hematoma
   D. Vascular loop
   E. Multiple sclerosis

Meningioma

Meningiomas are histologically benign, nonencapsulated, locally invasive tumors. They arise from endothelial lining cells of the arachnoid villi, which are found in the walls of the cranial venous sinuses and their tributary veins. A small number of these tumors arise from perineural or choroid plexus arachnoidal tissue, or from

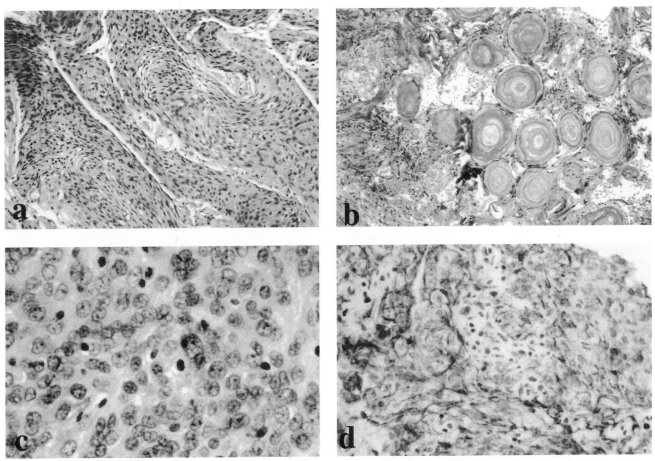

FIG. 17. A: Typical meningioma consisting of spindle-shaped cells arranged in fascicles and whorls (hematoxylin and eosin, original magnification × 40). **B:** Psammoma bodies are characteristic of meningiomas and may be abundant (original magnification × 60). **C:** Loss of whorling pattern and presence of mitotic activity characterize atypical anaplastic meningiomas (original magnification × 90). **D:** Section of meningioma immunostained for epithelial membrane antigen (EMA). Meningiomas are consistently immunoreactive for vimentin and EMA. (Courtesy of Dr. Pier Luigi Di Patre.)

dural fibroblasts. Monosomy and deletions of chromosomes 17 and 22 have been implicated in the pathogenesis of both the sporadic form and in NF2, the primary disease entity associated with meningioma tumor formation (100). Although these lesions comprise 19% of all brain tumors, only about 7% arise in the CPA (100). Occasionally, a meningioma originates within the internal auditory canal and, rarely, in the middle ear (arachnoid villi may be found in the geniculate ganglion and in the roof of the attic). Meningiomas usually appear grossly as ovoid, dense, well-circumscribed masses of the dura. Less commonly, they are plaquelike, with little elevation above the dural surface, enveloping and infiltrating nerves and underlying bone. Microscopically, meningiomas are made up of endothelial cells with large, uniform nuclei occurring in whorls. Psammoma bodies are characteristic. These tumors usually are highly vascular, with a fibromatous or angiomatous stroma (Fig. 17A–D: see color plate 38A–D following page 484).

Symptoms of meningioma depend on their location. Tumors arising along the surface of the petrous pyramid and tentorium cause trigeminal symptoms, facial and eye pain, sensorimotor changes, and, depending on the predominant side, aphasia (101). Meningiomas arising from the posterior surface of the petrous pyramid produce the CPA syndrome (see earlier). When they develop in the internal auditory canal they may be unrecognizable from acoustic neuromas (22). More often, these tumors originate outside the meatus, thereby involving other cranial nerves and the cerebellum earlier than the eighth cranial nerve. The tendency for meningiomas to infiltrate bone results in petrous bone invasion. If the primary site is the middle ear, symptoms include conductive hearing loss, otorrhea, polyps, and granulation (100).

The diagnostic steps for CPA meningiomas are similar to those for acoustic neuromas. However, audiometry usually does not help the differential diagnosis, whereas MRI and CT frequently are definitive. On CT, meningiomas tend to be more dense than acoustic neuromas and more sessile in their attachment to the temporal bone. They are not centered on the porus acusticus and do not enlarge the IAC (Fig. 18). They can cause significant edema of the surrounding brain tissue.

Although radiotherapy can be effective in the management of microscopic or scant postoperative residual disease, it usually is not recommended as primary treatment for meningiomas. Surgical removal is the treatment of choice in most cases; however, the lack of tumor encapsulation and its tendency to infiltrate bone often make complete removal difficult. Lesions confined to the CPA are best treated via the suboccipital/retrosigmoid approach. If hearing is impaired, a translabyrinthine approach is an option. If the lesion is in the far-anterior portion of the CPA, an extended retrolabyrinthine approach provides an excellent view of this region. Wigand et al. (53) described a modified middle cranial fossa approach to these lesions (see earlier).

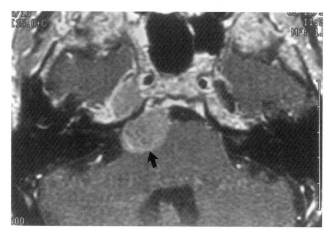

FIG. 18. Magnetic resonance T1-weighted image of right cerebellopontine angle meningioma *(arrow)*.

Epidermoid Tumor

Congenital cholesteatomas arise from epithelial rests and should be distinguished from acquired cholesteatomas and congenital lesions that develop behind an atresia plate. They can be divided into four anatomic groups: mesotympanic, perigeniculate, petrous apex, and CPA. Congenital middle ear and mastoid cholesteatomas are discussed in Chapter 25. Epidermoids are histologically identical to acquired cholesteatomas. They possess a lining of keratinizing, stratified squamous epithelium containing dry, usually sterile, odorless masses of keratin (Fig. 19: see color plates 39A–B following page 484). Perigeniculate and petrous apex cholesteatomas present with progressive facial weakness and sensorineural hearing loss (secondary to fistulization into the internal auditory canal or labyrinth). Posterior fossa epidermoids may be asymptomatic for many years and then present with a clinical picture similar to that of other cerebellopontine tumors (102).

CPA cholesteatomas represent one third of all intracranial epidermoid tumors. They tend to occur in young adults and often cause fifth cranial nerve symptoms when they become symptomatic. Progressive enlargement may result in a complete CPA syndrome. Neurologic findings depend on the direction of growth, as the matrix insinuates into the crevices of the brainstem. Weakness or paralysis of the facial nerve is relatively common (102,103). Diagnosis usually is confirmed by MRI. Typically, these lesions are nonenhancing and less dense than brain, with irregular borders on CT scan. On MRI, they appear gray on T1 and white on T2 sequences (Fig. 20). Petrous apex and perigeniculate cholesteatomas may be managed via radical mastoidectomy, with opening of several tracts into the petrous apex. However, when only a limited opening is achieved, recurrence is frequent. If hearing is poor, labyrinthectomy aids with the exposure, prevents recurrence, and facilitates postoperative care, which is lifelong. When hearing is to be preserved, middle fossa and suboccipital approaches may be considered for total

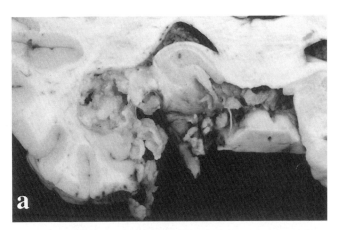
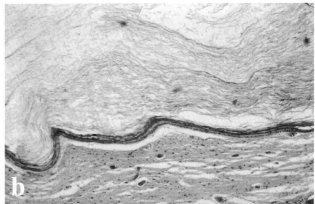

FIG. 19. Epidermoid tumor. **A:** Coronal slice of a brain from a patient with a large epidermoid tumor of the left cerebellopontine angle. The patient died of pulmonary thromboembolism after surgery. Residual tumor is present within the hippocampal fissure, compressing the hippocampus medially and the temporal lobe laterally. **B:** Photomicrograph of the epidermoid tumor. The cyst cavity is filled with keratin, and the wall consists of stratified squamous epithelium. Reactive gliosis is present in the surrounding brain (hematoxylin and eosin). (Courtesy of Dr. Pier Luigi Di Patre.)

removal. CPA cholesteatomas often are managed via the suboccipital/retrosigmoid approach. The matrix usually cannot be entirely removed from the brainstem, but decompression relieves symptoms. Patients with this ailment usually require multiple procedures.

Cholesterol Granuloma

Cholesterol granuloma results from nonspecific tissue reaction to a foreign body, i.e., cholesterol crystals (see Chapter 25). Breakdown of local tissue or blood appears to be the source of cholesterol. Although most commonly seen in the mastoid, these granulomas may arise within a pneumatized petrous apex, secondarily to blocked air cell tracts resulting from eustachian tube obstruction, mucosal edema, trauma, or tumor.

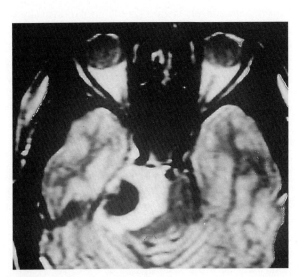

FIG. 20. Magnetic resonance image of a large right cerebellopontine angle epidermoid tumor.

Like other lesions, cholesterol granulomas grow silently until they exert pressure on cranial nerves. Most commonly, they produce diplopia (sixth cranial nerve involvement), unilateral hearing loss, tinnitus, vertigo, and facial weakness. Physical examination usually is unremarkable. The finding of a cystic lesion of the petrous apex that does not enhance with intravenous contrast and is isodense with brain on CT scan suggests cholesterol granuloma. On MRI, this lesion is bright on T1 and T2 sequences, as opposed to cholesteatoma, which is bright only on T2.

Treatment of cholesterol granuloma is surgical drainage with establishment of permanent aeration to prevent recurrence. The surgical approach will depend on the state of hearing and may involve translabyrinthine, infralabyrinthine, or middle fossa approaches (102,103).

Facial Nerve Tumors

Facial nerve neurilemomas originate from Schwann cells and may develop anywhere along the course of the nerve. In a review, Nelson and House (104) noted that of 23 patients with facial neuromas, 13 presented in the internal auditory canal and CPA. The remaining 10 tumors were infratemporal, with 6 developing in the middle ear and mastoid. Extratemporal tumors are infrequent and present as a parotid mass. Most patients are in the fourth decade of life. They are rare in children. There is an even distribution between male and female. Although most symptoms depend on tumor location, the most frequent complaint at presentation (except for parotid lesions) is hearing loss. Tinnitus is second in frequency (105–107). When located in the CPA, facial neuromas may mimic the symptoms of acoustic neuroma. Facial palsy usually does not appear until the tumor becomes large, but synkinesis may be present. Primary malignant tumors of the facial nerve are extremely rare (108).

Diagnosis is made with gadolinium-enhanced MRI. Imaging may show findings identical to those of acoustic neuroma or may show an enlarged geniculate ganglion or fallopian canal. Treatment is with mastoidectomy, translabyrinthine, suboccipital, or middle fossa approach, depending on the location of the tumor. Small lesions may be dissected off the nerve. However, in most cases, the facial nerve needs to be excised with the tumor and repaired with an interposition graft.

Metastasis

The most common sites of origin of metastatic tumors to the temporal bone are, in order of frequency: breast, kidney, lung, stomach, larynx, prostate, and thyroid. Usually, the duration of retrocochlear symptoms will be short. The rapid development of hearing impairment in association with other cranial neuropathies and/or brainstem dysfunction suggests a malignant neoplasm of the posterior fossa. These symptoms, when seen in conjunction with a history of malignancy, are highly suspicious for metastatic tumor. Usually, CT and MRI will delineate the lesion. In a minority of uncertain cases, such as those where a primary lesion appears to have been under control or cured, exploration may be needed to confirm the diagnosis. Prognosis is poor with or without treatment, which may be limited to palliative radiation therapy (109).

Miscellaneous

Several uncommon lesions may originate in the petrous apex and produce the CPA syndrome. These lesions include other cranial nerve neuromas and malignant tumors, arachnoid cysts, hemangiomas, dermoids, leiomyomas, medulloblastomas, chordomas, chondrosarcomas, yolk sac tumors, xanthogranulomas, and teratomas (110–121). Lesions of the regional arterial system can produce symptoms suggestive of neoplasia. Among these, a vascular loop in the internal auditory canal pressing on the vestibular nerves may be a rare cause of vertigo and motion intolerance. Vertebral artery aneurysms and arteriovenous malformations of the posterior fossa also can mimic neoplasms of the CPA. Anterior-inferior cerebellar artery aneurysms can present with acute subarachnoid hemorrhage or as a CPA mass lesion. Hearing loss, vertigo, and erosion of the internal auditory canal may all be seen. Vertebrobasilar angiography usually is diagnostic.

SUMMARY POINTS

- Acoustic neuromas account for 10% of all intracranial neoplasms and are the most common tumors of the CPA.
- Acoustic neuromas typically arise from the internal auditory canal portion of one of the vestibular nerves.
- Acoustic neuromas are more precisely termed vestibular schwannomas.
- Hearing loss and tinnitus usually emerge as the first indication of acoustic neuroma.
- In addition to pure tone thresholds, speech discrimination scores and reflex decay test results tend to be abnormal in patients with acoustic neuroma.
- The most significant ABR abnormalities in patients with acoustic neuromas are increased central conduction time and unequal interaural wave V latencies (>0.2 ms).
- Approximately 50% of patients with acoustic neuroma experience gait unsteadiness.
- Impaired or abolished caloric responses are found in approximately 35% to 65% of patients with acoustic neuroma.
- Facial nerve dysfunction is found infrequently in patients with acoustic neuroma.
- MRI is the method of choice for evaluation of CPA pathology.
- The treatment for acoustic neuroma is primarily surgical; stereotactic radiotherapy is an alternative in selected cases.
- Currently the translabyrinthine, suboccipital/retrosigmoid, and middle cranial fossa approaches are used for acoustic neuroma resection.
- The overall mortality for acoustic neuroma resection is less than 1%. Morbidity is higher for larger tumors (>3 cm).
- In acoustic neuroma resection, facial nerve preservation depends on tumor size, tumor consistency, and the surgeon's skill. In tumors smaller than 2 cm, grade I to II postoperative function can be expected.
- Hearing preservation is possible in approximately 30% of patients with acoustic neuromas that do not reach the fundus of the internal auditory canal and who have good preoperative thresholds.
- After cranial nerve VII and VIII deficits, cerebrospinal fluid leaks are the most common (8%) complication of acoustic neuroma surgery.
- Decompression by subtotal resection is a treatment alternative for elderly patients with acoustic neuroma.
- Many nonacoustic benign and malignant lesions may arise in the CPA. These include cholesteatomas, cholesterol granulomas, facial neuromas, metastatic tumors, and others.
- Following acoustic neuroma, meningiomas are the most common (3%) tumors of the CPA.

REFERENCES

1. Sandifort E. *Observation anatomico-pathologicale.* Lugduni Botavorom: Apud P.v.d. Eyk et D. Vygh, 1777.
2. Leveque-Lasource A. Observation sur un amaurosis et un cophosis, avec parte diminution de la voix, de movements, etc. par suite de lesion organique apparente de plusiers parties du cerveau. *J Gen Med Chir Pharm* 1810;37:368–373.
3. Cushing H. *Tumors of the nervus acoustics and the syndrome of the cerebellopontine angle.* Philadelphia: WB Saunders, 1917:244–272.
4. Bell C. The nervous system of the human body. London: *Appendix of cases.* 1830:112–114.
5. Cruveilhier J. *Anatomie pathologique du corps humain.* Paris: Chez J.B. Boillière, 1829.
6. Oppenheim H. Uber mehrene Falle von endocraniellen tumor in Welchen es gelang eine genavere local diagnose zu stellen. *Berl Klin Wehnschr* 1890;27:38–40.
7. Sternberg C. Beitrag zur Kenntnis der sogenannten Geschwulste des N. *Acusticus Z Heilk* 1900;21:163–186.
8. Fraenkel J, Hunt J. Tumors of the ponto-medullo-cerebellar space. *Acoust Neuromata (Central Neurofibromatosis) Med Rec Ny* 1903;64:100–1013.
9. Ballance C. *Some points in the surgery of the brain and its membranes.* London: MacMillian & Co., 1907:276.
10. House WF. Evolution of trans-temporal bone removal of acoustic tumors. *Arch Otolaryngol* 1964;80:731–741.
11. House WE. Surgical exposure of the internal auditory canal and its contents through the middle cranial fossa. *Laryngoscope* 1961;71:1363–1385.
12. Rand RW, Kurze T. Microneurosurgical resection of acoustic tumors by a transmeatal posterior fossa approach. *Bull Los Angeles Neurol Soc* 1965;30:17–20.
13. House WF. A history of acoustic tumor surgery. In: House WF, Luetje CM, eds. *Acoustic tumors.* Baltimore: University Park Press, 1979;1–44.
14. Brackmann DE, Bartels LJ. Rare tumors of the cerebellopontine angle. *Otol Head Neck Surg* 1980;88:555–559.
15. Brackmann DE, Kwartler JA. A review of acoustic tumors: 1983–1988. *Am J Otol* 1990;11:216–232.
16. Thomsen J, Mirko T. Diagnostic strategies in search for acoustic neuromas. *Acta Otolaryngol Suppl* 1988;452:16–25.
17. Dutton JEM, Ramsden RT, Lye RH, et al. Acoustic neuroma (schwannoma) surgery 1978–1990. *Laryngol Otol* 1991;105:165–173.
18. Eckermeier L, Pirsig W, Mueller D. Histopathology of 30 non-operated acoustic schwannomas. *Arch Otolaryngol* 1979;222:1–9.
19. Schuknecht HF. *Pathology of the ear,* 1st ed. Cambridge, MA: Harvard University Press, 1974:425–436.
20. Clemis JD, Ballad WJ, Baggot PJ, Lyon ST. Relative frequency of inferior vestibular schwannoma. *Arch Otolaryngol Head Neck Surg* 1986;112:190–194.
21. Erickson LS, Sorenson GD, McGavran MH. A review of 140 acoustic neurinomas (neurilemmoma). *Laryngoscope* 1965;75:601–627.
22. Nedzelski JM. Cerebellopontine angle tumors: bilateral flocculus compression as cause of associated oculomotor abnormalities. *Laryngoscope* 1983;93:1251–1260.
23. Croxson GR, Moffat DA, Baguley D. Bruns' bidirectional nystagmus in cerebellopontine angle tumors. *Clin Otolaryngol* 1988;13:153–157.
24. Hoffman RA, Brookler KH, Baker AH. The accuracy of the simultaneous binaural bithermal test in the diagnosis of acoustic neuromas. *Laryngoscope* 1979;89:1046–1052.
25. Linthicum FH, Khalessi MH, Churchill D. Electronystagmographic caloric bithermal vestibular test (ENG): results in acoustic tumor cases. In: House WF, Luetje CM, eds. *Acoustic tumors.* Baltimore: University Park Press, 1979:237–240.
26. Olson JE, Wolfe JW, Engelken EJ. Responses to low frequency harmonic acceleration in patients with acoustic neuromas. *Laryngoscope* 1988;91:1270–1277.
27. Baloh RW, Konrad HR, Dirks D, Honrubia V. Cerebellar-pontine angle tumors. *Arch Neurol* 1976;33:507–512.
28. Moretz WH, Orchik DJ, Shea JJJ, Emett JR. Low-frequency harmonic acceleration in the evaluation of patients with intracanalicular and cerebellopontine angle tumors. *Otolaryngol Head Neck Surg* 1986;95:324–332.
29. Harner SG, Laws ERJ. Clinical findings in patients with acoustic neurinoma. *Mayo Clin Proc* 1983;58:721–728.
30. Beck HJ, Beatty CW, Harner SG. Acoustic neuromas with normal pure tone hearing levels. *Otolaryngol Head Neck Surg* 1986;94:96–103.
31. Hirsch A, Anderson H. Elevated stapedius reflex threshold and pathologic reflex decay: clinical occurrence and significance. *Acta Otolaryngol Suppl* 1980;369:1–26.
32. Jerger J, Jerger S. Diagnostic significance of PB word functions. *Arch Otolaryngol* 1971;93:572–580.
33. Johnson EW. Results of auditory tests in acoustic patients. In: WF House, CM Luetje, eds. *Acoustic tumors.* Baltimore: University Park Press, 1979:209–224.
34. Clemis JD, Sarno CN. The acoustic reflex latency test: clinical application. *Laryngoscope* 1980;90:601–611.
35. Jerger J, Hayes D. Latency of the acoustic reflex in eighth-nerve tumors. *Arch Otol* 1983;109:1–5.
36. Selters WA, Brackmann DE. Brainstem electric response audiometry in acoustic tumor detection. In: House WF, Luetje CM, eds. *Acoustic tumors.* Baltimore: University Park Press, 1979:225–235.
37. Moffat DA, Baguley D, Hardy DG, Tsui YN. Contralateral auditory brainstem response abnormalities in acoustic neuroma. *J Laryngol Otol* 1989;103:835–838.
38. Barrs DM, Brackmann DE, Olson JE, House WF. Changing concepts of acoustic neuroma diagnosis. *Arch Otolaryngol* 1985;111:17–21.
39. Telian SA, Kileny PR, Niparko JK, Kemink JL, Graham MD. Normal auditory brainstem response in patients with acoustic neuroma. *Laryngoscope* 1989;99:10–14.
40. Neely JG, Neblett CR. Differential facial nerve function in tumors of the internal auditory meatus. *Otol Rhinol Laryngol* 1983;92:39–41.
41. Kartush JM, Niparko JK, Graham MD, Kemink JL. Electroneurography: preoperative facial nerve assessment of tumors. *Otolaryngol Head Neck Surg* 1987;97:257–261.
42. Hitselberger WE, Pulec JL. Trigeminal nerve (posterior root) retrolabyrinthine selective section—operative procedure for intractable pain. *Arch Otolaryngol* 1972;96:412–415.
43. Eidelman BH. Clinical syndromes of the posterior fossa. In: Sekhar LN, Schramm VL, eds. *Tumors of the cranial base: diagnosis and treatment.* Mount Kisco, NY: Futura Publishing Co., 1987:541–543.
44. Jackler RK, Shapiro MS, Dillon WP, Pitts L, Lanser MJ. Gadolinium-DTPA enhanced magnetic resonance imaging in acoustic neuroma diagnosis and management. *Otolaryngol Head Neck Surg* 1990;102:670–677.
45. Han MH, Jabour BA, Andrews JC, et al. Nonneoplastic enhancing lesions mimicking intracanalicular acoustic neuroma on gadolinium-enhanced MR images. *Radiology* 1991;179:795–796.
46. Tien R, Dillon WP, Jackler RK. Contrast enhanced MR imaging of the facial nerve in 11 patients with Bell's palsy. *Am Radiol* 1990;11:735–741.
47. Welling DB, Glasscock ME, Woods CI, Jackson CG. Acoustic neuroma: a cost-effective approach. *Otolaryngol Head Neck Surg* 1990;103:364–370.
48. Kartush JM, Graham MD, LaRouere MJ. Meatal decompression following acoustic neuroma resection: minimizing delayed facial palsy. *Laryngoscope* 1991;101:674–675.
49. McElveen JT, Wilkins RH, Erwin AC, Wolford RD. Modifying the translabyrinthine approach to preserve hearing during acoustic tumor surgery. *Laryngol Otol* 1991;105:34–37.
50. House WF, Shelton C. Middle fossa approach for acoustic tumor removal. *Otolaryngol Clin North Am* 1992;25:347–359.
51. Fish U. Transtemporal surgery of the internal auditory canal. *Adv Otol Rhinol Laryngol* 1970;17:203–240.
52. Kanzaki J, Kawase T, Sano K, Shiobara R, Toya S. A modified extended middle cranial fossa approach for acoustic tumors. *Arch Otorhinolaryngol* 1977;217:119–121.
53. Wigand ME, Haid T, Berg M. The enlarged middle cranial fossa approach for surgery of the temporal bone and of the cerebellopontine angle. *Arch Otorhinolaryngol* 1989;246:299–302.
54. Kanzaki J, Shiobara R, Toya S. Classification of the extended middle cranial fossa approach. *Acta Otolaryngol Suppl (Stockh)* 1991;487:6–16.
55. Glasscock ME, Poe DS, Johnson GD. Hearing preservation in surgery of cerebellopontine angle tumors. In: Fish U, Valavanis A, Yosargil MG, eds. *Neurological surgery of the ear and skull base. Proceedings of the sixth international symposium on neurological surgery of the ear and skull base.* Zurich: Schmon Kruger, 1989:207–216.
56. Wade PJ, House W. Hearing preservation in patients with acoustic neuromas via the middle fossa approach. *Otolaryngol Head Neck Surg* 1984;92:184–193.

56a. Kartush JM, Bouchard KR, eds. *Neuromonitoring in otology and head and neck surgery.* New York: Raven Press, 1992.

57. Mangham CA. Complications of translabyrinthine vs suboccipital approach for acoustic tumor surgery. *Otolaryngol Head Neck Surg* 1988;99:396–400.

58. DiTullio MV Jr, Malkasian D, Rand RW. A critical comparison of neurosurgical and otolaryngological approaches to acoustic neuromas. *J Neurosurg* 1978;48:1–12.

59. Nadol JB, Chiong CM, Ojemann RG, et al. Preservation of hearing and facial nerve function in resection of acoustic neuroma. *Laryngoscope* 1992;102:1153–1158.

60. Haines SJ, Levine SC. Intracanalicular acoustic neuroma: early surgery for preservation of hearing. *J Neurosurg* 1993;79:515–520.

61. House JW, Brackmann DE. Facial nerve grading system. *Otolaryngol Head Neck Surg* 1985;93:146–147.

62. Glasscock ME, Kveton JF, Jackson CG, Levine SC, McKenna KX. A systematic approach to the surgical management of acoustic neuroma. *Laryngoscope* 1986;96:1088–1094.

63. Ojemann RG. Management of acoustic neuromas (vestibular schwannomas). *Clin Neurosurg* 1993;40:493–535.

64. Ebersold MJ, Harner SG, Beatty CW, Harper CM, Quast LM. Current results of the retrosigmoid approach to acoustic neurinomas. *J Neurosurg* 1992;76:901–909.

65. Gantz BJ, Parnes LS, Harker LA, McCabe BF. Middle cranial fossa acoustic neuroma excision: results and complications. *Ann Otol Rhinol Laryngol* 1986;95:454–459.

66. Glasscock ME III, McKenna KX, Levine SC. Acoustic neuroma surgery: the results of hearing conservation surgery. *Laryngoscope* 1987;97:785–789.

67. Sanna M, Zini C, Mazzoni A, Gandolfi A, Pareschi R, Gamaletti R. Hearing preservation in acoustic neuroma surgery. Middle fossa versus suboccipital approach. *Am J Otol* 1987;8:500–506.

68. Shelton C, Brackmann DE, House WF, Hitselberger WE. Middle fossa acoustic tumor: results in 106 cases. *Laryngoscope* 1989;99:405–408.

69. Fisch U, Dobie RA, Gmor A, Felix H. Intracranial facial nerve anastomosis. *Am J Otol* 1981;8:23–29.

70. Cohen NL, Hammerschlag P, Berg H, Ransohoff J. Acoustic neuroma surgery. An eclectic approach with emphasis on preservation of hearing. The New York University–Bellevue Experiences. *Ann Otol Rhinol Laryngol* 1986;95:21–27.

71. Sekhar LN, Gormley WB, Wright DC. The best treatment for vestibular schwannoma (acoustic neuroma): microsurgery or radiosurgery? *Am J Otol* 1996;17:676–682.

72. Gardner G, Robertson JH. Hearing preservation in unilateral acoustic neuroma surgery. *Ann Otol Rhinol Laryngol* 1988;97:55–66.

73. Shelton C, Hitselberger WE, House WF, Brackmann DE. Hearing preservation after acoustic tumor removal: long term results. *Laryngoscope* 1990;100:115–119.

74. Jannetta PJ, Moller AR, Moller MB. Technique of hearing preservation in small acoustic neuromas. *Ann Surg* 1984;200:513–523.

75. Palva T, Troupp H, Jauhianinen T. Hearing preservation in acoustic neurinoma surgery. *Acta Otolaryngol (Stockh)* 1985;99:1–7.

76. Skedros DG, Cass SP, Hirsch BE, Kelly RH. Beta 2 transferrin assay in clinical management of cerebral spinal fluid and perilymphatic fluid leaks. *J Otolaryngol* 1993;22:341–344.

77. Bryce GE, Nedzelski JM, Rowed DW, Rappaport JM. Cerebrospinal fluid leaks and meningitis in acoustic neuroma surgery. *Otolaryngol Head Neck Surg* 1991;104:81–87.

78. Deleted in proof.

79. Leksell L. A note on the treatment of acoustic tumors. *Acta Chir Scand* 1971;137:763–765.

80. Lunsford LD, King TT, Morrison AW. Stereotactic radiosurgery for acoustic neuromas. *Arch Otolaryngol Head Neck Surg* 1990;116:907–909.

81. Noren G, Greitz D, Hirsch A, Lax I. Gamma knife surgery in acoustic tumors. *Acta Neurochir Suppl (Wein)* 1993;58:104–107.

82. Lunsford LD, Linskey ME. Stereotactic radiosurgery in the treatment of patients with acoustic tumors. *Otolaryngol Clin North Am* 1992;25:471–491.

83. Linskey ME, Lunsford LD, Flickinger JC, et al. Stereotactic radiosurgery for acoustic tumors. *Neurosurg Clin North Am* 1991;3:191–205.

84. Flickinger JC, Kondziolka D, Pollock BE, Lunsford LD. Evolution in technique for vestibular schwannoma radiosurgery and effect on outcome. *Int J Radiat Oncol Biol Phys* 1996;36:275–280.

85. Mendenhall WM, Friedman WA, Bova FJ. LINAC radiosurgery for acoustic schwannomas. *Int J Radiat Oncol Biol Phys* 1994;28:803–810.

86. Flickinger JC, Lunsford LD, Linskey ME, Duma CM, Kondziolka D. Gamma knife radiosurgery for acoustic neuroma: multivariate analysis of four year results. *Radiother Oncol* 1993;27:91–98.

87. Ogunrinde OK, Lunsford DL, Kondziolka DS, Bissonette DJ, Flickinger JC. Cranial nerve preservation after stereotactic radiosurgery of intracanalicular acoustic tumors. *Stereotact Funct Neurosurg Suppl* 1995;64:87–97.

88. Slattery W, Brackmann DE. Results of surgery following sterotactic irradiation for acoustic neuromas. *Am J Otol* 1995;16:315–321.

89. Jahrsdoerfer RA, Benjamin RS. Chemotherapy of bilateral acoustic neuromas. *Otolaryngol Head Neck Surg* 1971;98:572–580.

90. Siglock TJ, Rosenblatt SS, Finck F, House WF, Hitselberger WE. Sex hormone receptors in acoustic neuromas. *Am J Otol* 1990;11:237–239.

91. Klinken L, Thomsen J, Rasmussen BB, Wiet RJ, Tos M. Estrogen and progesterone receptors in acoustic neuromas. *Arch Otolaryngol Head Neck Surg* 1990;116:202–204.

92. Neurofibromatosis. Conference Statement. National Institute of Health Consensus Development Conference. *Arch Neurol* 1988;45:575–578.

93. Gadre AK, Kwartler JA, Brackmann DE, House WF, Hitselberger WE. Middle fossa decompression of the internal auditory canal in acoustic neuroma surgery: a therapeutic alternative. *Laryngoscope* 1990;100:948–952.

94. Wigand ME, Goertzen W, Berg M. Transtemporal planned partial resection of bilateral acoustic neurinomas. *Acta Neurochir (Wien)* 1988;92:50–54.

95. Otto SR, Brackmann DE, Staller S, Menapce CM. The multichannel auditory brainstem implant. Six month coinvestigator results. *Adv Otorhinolaryngol* 1997;52:1–7.

96. Wazen J, Silverstein H, Norrell H, Besse B. Preoperative and postoperative growth rates in acoustic neuromas documented with CT scanning. *Otolaryngol Head Neck Surg* 1985;93:151–155.

97. Nedzelski JM, Canter RJ, Kassel EE, Rowed DW, Tator CH. Is no treatment good treatment in the management of acoustic neuromas in the elderly? *Laryngoscope* 1986;96:825–829.

98. Kenzora JE, McCarthy, RE Lowell JD, et al. Hip fracture mortality. *Clin Orthop* 1984;186:45–56.

99. Kemink JL, Langman AW, Niparko JK, Graham MD. Operative management of acoustic neuromas: the priority of neurologic function over complete resection. *Otolaryngol Head Neck Surg* 1991;104:96–99.

100. Leonetti JP, Reichman H, Smith PG, Grubb RL, Kaiser P. Meningiomas of the lateral skull base: neurotologic manifestations and patterns of recurrence. *Otolaryngol Head Neck Neck Surg* 1990;103:972–980.

101. Persing JA, Muir A, Becker DG, Jankovic JJ, Anderson RL, Edlich RF. Blepharospasm-oromandibular dystonia associated with a left cerebellopontine angle meningioma. *J Emerg Med* 1990;8:571–574.

102. Hasegawa T, Komai T, Kitabayashi M, Raymano K. Cerebellopontine angle epidermoid tumor extending into the upper cervical spinal canal. *Neurol Med Chir (Tokyo)* 1989;29:614–618.

103. Sabin HI, Bordi LT, Symon L. Epidermoid cysts and cholesterol granulomas centered on the posterior fossa. Twenty years of diagnosis and management. *Neurosurgery* 1987;21:798–805.

104. Nelson RA, House WF. Facial nerve neuroma in the posterior fossa: surgical considerations. In: Graham MD, House WF, eds. *Disorders of the facial nerve.* New York: Raven Press, 1982:403–406.

105. King TT, Morrison AW. Primary facial tumors within the skull. *J Neurosurg* 1990;72:1–8.

106. Inoue Y, Tabuchi T, Hakuba A, et al. Facial nerve neuromas: CT findings. *J Comput Assist Tomogr* 1987;11:942–947.

107. Lee KS, Britton BH, Kelly DL Jr. Schwannoma of the facial nerve in cerebellopontine angle presenting with hearing loss. *Surg Neurol* 1989;32:231–234.

108. Muhlbauer M, Clark WC, Robertson JH, Gardner LG, Dohan FC Jr. Malignant nerve sheath tumor to the facial nerve: case report and discussion. *Neurosurgery* 1987;21:68–73.

109. Anderson C, Krutchkoff D, Ludwig M. Carcinoma of the lower lip with perineural invasion to the middle cranial fossa. *Oral Surg Oral Med Oral Pathol* 1990;69:614–618.

110. Asano N, Oka H, Takase K, et al. Intracranial and intraspinal dissemination from a pineal yok sac tumor treated by PVB therapy. *Neurol Med Chir (Tokyo)* 1990;30:483–488.

111. Bordi L, Compton J, Symon L. Trigeminal neuroma. *Surg Neurol* 1989;31:272–276.

112. Braga FM, Tella OI, Ferreira A, Jordy CF. Malignant melanoma of the cerebellopontine angle region. *Arq Neuro-Psiquiat (Sao Paulo)* 1989; 47:496–500.

113. Gouvea VM, Hahn MD, Chimelli L. Lipoma of the midbrain. *Arq Neuro-Psiquiat (Sao Paulo)* 1989;47:371–374.

114. Ito M, Tajima A, Sato K, Ishii S. Calcified cerebellopontine angle hematoma mimicking recurrent acoustic neurinoma. *Clin Neurol Neurosurg* 1988;90:65–70.

115. Mokry M, Flashka G, Kleinert R, Fazekas F, Kopp W. Chronic Lyme disease with an expansive granulomatous lesion in the cerebellopontine angle. *Neurosurgery* 1990;27:446–451.

116. Nagatani K, Waga S, Takeuchi J, Takebe Y, Hohda K, Hirano A. Multiple intracranial xanthogranulomas: case report. *Neurol Med Chir (Tokyo)* 1990;30:960–965.

117. Nishiura I, Koyama T, Handa J, Amono S. Primary intracranial epidermoid carcinoma: case report. *Neurol Med Chir (Tokyo)* 1989;29: 600–605.

118. Nishizawa S, Yokoyama T, Ohta S, et al. Lipoma in the cerebellopontine angle: case report. *Neurol Med Chir (Tokyo)* 1990;30:137–142.

119. Pappas DG, Scheiderman TS, Brackmann DE, Simpson LC, Chandra-Sekar B, Sofferman RA. Cavernous hemangiomas of the internal auditory canal. *Otolaryngol Head Neck Surg* 1989;101:27–32.

120. Yoshii K, Yamada S, Aiba T, Myoshi S. Cerebellopontine angle lipoma with abnormal body structure: case report. *Neurol Med Chir (Tokyo)* 1989;29:48–51.

121. Vassilakis D, Phylaktakis M, Selviaridis P, Karavelis A, Sirmos C, Vlaikidis N. Symptomatic trigeminal neuralgia. *J Neurol Sci* 1988;32: 117–120.

The Ear: Comprehensive Otology,
edited by R. F. Canalis and P. R. Lambert.
Lippincott Williams & Wilkins, Philadelphia © 2000.

CHAPTER 54

An Eye to the Future of Otology

Jeffrey T. Corwin

What Changes Should We Expect from Molecular Biology?	**What Should We Expect from Regeneration Research?**
Genetic Testing of Tumors	**Potential Strategies to Protect Hair Cells**
Genetic Screening	**Improved Prosthetic Devices**
Technology for Reading Genes	**Opportunities in Vestibular System Research**
Impact of Molecular Biology on Otologic Research	

Every great advance in science has issued from a new audacity of imagination. —John Dewey

Would practitioners from 50 years ago have expected the continued growth and importance of otology in the period since the discovery of antibiotics? Fifty years ago, who would have expected that patients would be diagnosed with the help of far-field responses from the brain that can be less than one-millionth of a volt at scalp recording sites? Who would have expected that sounds emitted from the cochlea would be used to screen the hearing of thousands of newborn infants each year? In the operating room, the use of microscopes, the role of video imaging in surgical training, the development and use of cochlear implants, the electrical monitoring of nerve activity, and the bold aims and remarkable outcomes of the surgical procedures themselves would have been unthinkable just a few decades ago.

The pace of developments in the laboratory has been equally impressive. Just 55 years ago, Avery et al. transformed bacteria by incubating them in an extract that contained only the DNA from a strain that had smooth coats, and the transformants passed that coat property on to their decendants. In 1953, a two-page article by Watson and Crick presented the solution to the structure of DNA, revealed an inherent mechanism for complementary replication of its nucleotide sequence, and set in motion the revolutionary development of molecular

biology. Now, we are poised to know the entire nucleotide sequence for the human genome.

In view of the remarkable changes that have occurred during the past 50 years it seems impractical to try to predict what otology may be like 50 years in the future. Serendipity plays too great a role in scientific discoveries and clinical progress over such a period. Therefore, this chapter focuses on the next 20 years by considering developments that we might reasonably expect on the basis of recent discoveries. In the past otologists made significant advances in two ways: through research focused on the ear itself and through adaptation of technologic developments from molecular biology, cell biology, electronics, and other fields for use in otology. How might such discoveries and developments be applied over the coming years?

WHAT CHANGES SHOULD WE EXPECT FROM MOLECULAR BIOLOGY?

In the near future it should be possible to routinely identify the exact genetic composition of pathogens that have caused individual infections and the specific mutations that have caused individual tumors so that therapies can be targeted much more specifically than is now possible. In addition, a patient's genetic makeup will become accessible in ways that are comparable to current access to the patient's CBC and enzyme levels. Such genetic determinations already are possible on a limited scale. Powerful genetic diagnostic capacities will develop and spread quickly. They will greatly improve outcomes, but they also will present challenging ethical and legal issues for physicians, patients, and hospitals.

J. T. Corwin: Departments of Otolaryngology–Head and Neck Surgery and Neuroscience, University of Virginia School of Medicine, Charlottesville, Virginia 22908

An account of recent progress in molecular biology may help to assess how and when such developments are likely to affect otology. An international effort has already sequenced approximately 12% of the human genome and entered that sequence in public databases. Many genes have been fully sequenced, but the majority of the human data still come from short sequences that have not been identified with the specific genes that they partially encode. As the Human Genome Project approaches its planned completion in 2003, the intervening segments will be filled in to stitch together the complete sequence of the human genome (1).

GenBank and other sequence databases are growing at an accelerating rate (Fig. 1). The entire genomes of *Escherichia coli*, yeast, and the nematode, *Caenorhabditis elegans* already have been sequenced. By the time this book is in print, sequencing of *Drosophila's* genome will be 1 to 2 years away from completion. The mouse genome will be completely sequenced by 2005. Sequencing of the genomes of the rat, the zebra fish, the guinea pig, the chicken, and other organisms will follow in the coming decade. Progress reports, sequence data, links to

protein data and the literature, and other molecular genetic resources are available at the National Library of Medicine's web site (www.ncbi.nlm.nih.gov).

The haploid human genome comprises about 3 billion base pairs of DNA and is believed to code for approximately 100,000 genes that are interspersed with noncoding sequence. The gene-coding regions themselves are typically interrupted by substantial amounts of noncoding sequence. Average messenger RNAs (mRNAs) transcribed from the genes of eukaryotes are 1,000 to 2,000 bases long but can be much larger, ranging up to at least the size of the dystrophin message, which is 17 kilobases long. The locations of many genes and thousands of polymorphic markers have been mapped to specific positions on the 23 pairs of human chromosomes. This map provides a critical resource for identifying the specific mutations responsible for inherited disorders. The current version of that map is available at www.ncbi.nlm. nih.gov/genemap. Related regions of human and mouse chromosomes also have been identified. Those maps and linkage analyses contributed to recent identifications of the mutations that cause Alport's syndrome, Usher's syn-

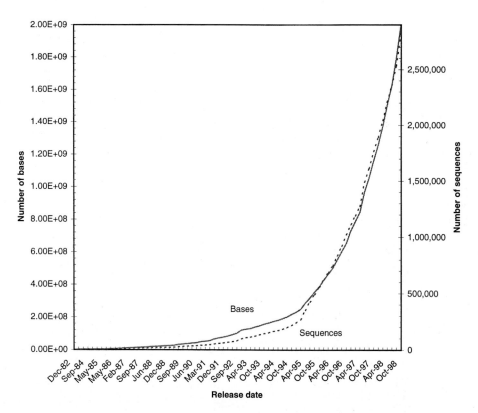

FIG. 1. The growth of nucleotide sequence information in the public database GenBank. The *solid line* traces the data measured as total nucleotide bases sequenced, which reached 2 billion in 1998. The *broken line* traces the number of individual segments of sequence, which grew to more than 2.5 million in 1998. This valuable resource for biomedical research continues to grow at an accelerating rate because of technologic advances in the speed of sequence determination. (Courtesy of Dr. Jacques Retief.)

drome, Pendred's syndrome, and many nonsyndromic forms of inherited hearing impairment and dysequilibrium (Fig. 2) (see Van Camp G, Smith RJH. Hereditary Hearing Loss Homepage at http://dnalab-www.uia.ac.be/dnalab/hhh/) (2,3).

One child in 2,000 is born with inherited hearing impairment, and genetic analysis has indicated that more than 100 mutations give rise to hearing impairment (http://www.ncbi.nlm.nih.gov/omim) (4). In the coming decade the mutated genes responsible for many of the inherited forms of congenital and progressive hearing loss and dysequilibrium will be identified. Otologists can contribute to this progress by improving diagnostic criteria and ascertaining which families have inherited disorders that may be informative. Results from the identification of mutated genes can provide the basis for relatively straightforward tests to identify individuals who carry mutations that are transmitted as recessive traits and those who have mutations that may lead to progressive disorders. Such tests can provide objective information for patients who seek genetic counseling, and in theory they can be used to screen the genome of a fetus in utero, two capacities that highlight some of the ethical concerns associated with genetic testing. Early identification of genetic propensities for hearing or balance disorders should allow some patients to make behavioral changes or seek clinical intervention to avert

or delay some disorders. Identification of mutated genes responsible for inherited otologic disorders is also certain to contribute to improved understanding of the origins of those conditions and better understanding of the normal ear. In some instances identification of mutations may reveal opportunities for gene therapy to prevent or reverse disorders.

GENETIC TESTING OF TUMORS

Sequence databases provide resources that can be used in the way that many of us use dictionaries, encyclopedias, and libraries. Knowledge of normal gene sequences can serve as references for spell checking and for searches to identify variants of sequence that may be linked to propensities for particular diseases. Searches can be used to compare all normal genes against just those genes expressed within a tissue. This is useful in pathology, because at any moment each cell in the body expresses only a limited subset of the 100,000 genes that are contained in the complete genome within its nucleus. Most cells are believed to express 10,000 to 20,000 different proteins, which would be encoded by 10% to 20% of the human genome. Differences between the subsets of the genes that different cells and tissues express, by making the mRNAs and the proteins that they encode, cause all the recognizable differences in the nature of different cells

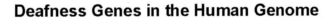

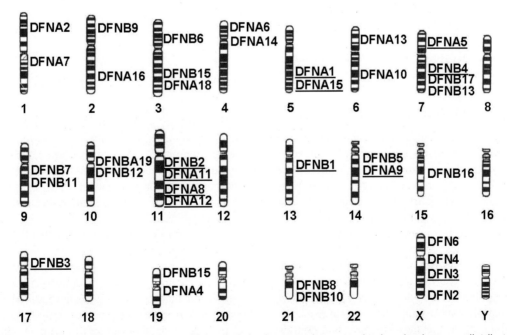

FIG. 2. Loci for nonsyndromic forms of inherited deafness and progressive hearing loss are distributed throughout the 23 pairs of human chromosomes. Dominant loci are represented by the designation *DFNA*, recessive loci by *DFNB*, and X-linked loci by *DFN*. Each *underscored* locus has been identified with a cloned gene. For the other loci only the chromosomal locations are known. (Courtesy of Dr. Karen Avraham. From Avraham KB. Hear come more genes! *Nat Med* 1998;4:1238–1239, with permission.)

and tissues. The courses of pathologic conditions are determined by just which genes are expressed over time as cells respond to pathogens, trauma, or homeostatic imbalances, or when they change from within because of somatic mutations that have affected one or a few genes.

Biopsies provide access to the genes expressed within a tissue, and the sequences of those genes can be compared with sequences in databases to find the mutations responsible for the abnormal growth of cells in a specific tumor. Limited tests of this type are in use now, but this type of test will become much more powerful in the next decade as data on mutations accumulate and as assay methods become faster. At the same time, information about the structure of the proteins that can be affected by different mutations in tumor cells is being developed and used to identify drugs that can intervene in the control mechanisms that have been affected in the abnormal cells. Such approaches to cancer diagnosis and treatment hold the promise of much more specific and effective therapies that should be brought to fruition in the coming decade.

GENETIC SCREENING

In the 1960s, cloning of frogs confirmed that nearly all the cells in an organism retain the full genome, and the cloning of sheep and mice confirmed that principle. Therefore, it is possible to sample blood or other cells from a patient and use those cells to assess the patient's entire complement of genes. Even now, the polymerase chain reaction (PCR) can be used to achieve millionfold amplifications of almost any gene fragment in an afternoon if one knows a small part of the sequence at each end of the fragment. Such methods permit screening for specific mutations, such as defects in the gene for connexin 26, which recently were found to cause many cases of inherited deafness (5,6).

TECHNOLOGY FOR READING GENES

A number of biotechnology companies are developing tests that can provide global assessments of a person's genetic makeup. Searching through the 3 billion base pairs of sequence in our chromosomes is too time consuming to be practical with current serial procedures, so parallel searching methods are under development. Some tests utilize arrays of custom-made sequences that are complementary to genes or portions of genes. Those complementary sequences can be used in chemical binding reactions that are somewhat analogous to the Watson-Crick base pairing that occurs within cells. DNA or RNA from a tissue sample can be amplified, cut into pieces, and tested for binding to the sites in arrays that contain perfect complementary matches to specific gene sequences. Such test arrays now are available in the form of sheets and chips on which thousands of genes or short segments of sequence have been placed or directly syn-

thesized. Each sequence is mapped to a specific position in the array.

Genomic screening will have profound effects in all medical specialties during the coming decade. Sequence sampling arrays that are currently available for research purposes have the capacity to simultaneously assess thousands of genes in a single tissue sample. Limited assessment of a patient's genome is now possible, but such assessment will be possible with fine resolution through the entire genome after the completion of the Human Genome Project. Such specific genetic information will allow quantitative evaluation of a patient's statistical prospect for development of age-related hearing loss, age-related dysequilibrium, cancers, cardiovascular disease, and other conditions. Because, chance events and behavior profoundly influence most inherited traits, an individual patient's actual incidence of disease would not be directly predictable from such genetic information, but future assessments of a patient's genotype should reveal the quantitative probability of developing any of 100 or more diseases and dysfunctions.

It is not unreasonable to expect such testing to become commonplace in developed countries. The power of the methods may allow prediction of life expectancy in the absence of trauma. The methods would also help to alert patients to changes in behavior that may be recommended on the basis of their individual inherited vulnerability to specific environmental hazards, for example their individual susceptibility to noise and sensorineural hearing loss. Such a capacity for knowledge carries both opportunities and hazards. Decisions about how such information will be protected, who will have access to it, and under what circumstances they will have access are needed in the near future.

IMPACT OF MOLECULAR BIOLOGY ON OTOLOGIC RESEARCH

The capacity to readout the specific composition of genes is providing broad insights into the functional elements of proteins. Many genes are mosaics comprising segments of unique sequence interspersed with segments of sequence similar or identical to segments in other genes. The less unique regions often are recognizable on the basis of the sequence of amino acids they code for, and they typically code for domains within proteins that have specific functional properties. Individual proteins often are comprised of a series of different domains. For example, a protein can contain a sequence of amino acids that served as a domain for binding to a signaling intermediate within the cytoplasm. Another sequence of amino acids in that protein might serve as a domain that targets the protein for transport into the nucleus, and a third domain might cause that protein to bind with another protein normally present within the nucleus. The recognizably similar elements of sequence within genes that encode these domains can appear repeatedly within one gene and they can appear over and over again in different genes throughout the genome. Wherever they occur they can code for that particular type of functional domain within a protein. Those regions also can be recognized across species. For instance, many genes code for domains within proteins that are similar to short segments in fibronectin, an extracellular matrix protein. The nucleotide codes for these domains, called type III fibronectin repeats, are readily recognizable in various genes in species ranging from flies to humans.

Biomedical research has identified many elements of genes at that level, and others are being identified and used to continually improve recognition software for searching the sequence databases. That knowledge and the enhancement of searching effectiveness that will develop as the normal sequences of more of our genes are determined will provide the potential to improve understanding of the molecular processes that underlie the normal functions of our ears. Such knowledge also will be applicable to understanding inherited disorders, somatic (e.g., tumorigenic) mutations, and dysfunctional responses to trauma.

Transcription of genes determines just what proteins are present to interact within cells, and it is proteins that most directly determine how one hears, thinks, and functions. Proteins in the form of receptors, signaling intermediates, and transcription factors directly determine how the body responds to pharmaceutical agents. Understanding how that occurs requires knowledge of protein structure, but that currently cannot be predicted from the amino acid sequences in their peptide chains. Protein structure can be determined by means of x-ray crystallography which requires pure crystals of proteins and a large number of mathematical calculations. Structural determinations for proteins are many times more difficult than sequence determinations for nucleic acids. Fortunately, the transfection of certain eukaryotic cells with the gene that encodes the sequence of a protein now can readily lead to the production of a quantity of the pure protein. Computers needed for the many calculations in crystallography are becoming faster. A massively parallel computer recently achieved 1 trillion calculations per second. Application of such developments to the determination of protein structures will contribute to a new level of understanding cell function. It will allow insight into chemical interactions at the exposed surfaces of proteins that are folded into complex structures. Those interactions most directly determine what occurs in cells.

The complex folding pattern that is characteristic of a protein's structure reveals which amino acids are at the surface of the protein and in what positions on the surface. When that structure is known it is possible to determine how and where chemical interactions may occur between that protein and others and between that protein and smaller molecules within cells. Progress in determining protein structures is already contributing to understanding the chemical interactions that underlie the normal regula-

tion of metabolism, growth and differentiation signaling, intracellular transport, cell motility, and other functions in cells. Structural information also can be used to analyze the interactions between pharmaceutical agents and catalytic sites in proteins to allow rational design of highly specific new drugs.

It is to be expected that rational drug design will eventually supplant drug discovery by screening of natural and synthetic products in bioassays. However, the recent development of gene sequence arrays has provided pharmaceutical researchers with tools for assaying the multitude of gene expression changes that occur when cells respond to any new drug. Many pharmaceutical companies are already using such arrays in drug discovery efforts, in effect performing automated bioassays at the level of global gene expression. Like rational drug design that is based on structural data, this new pharmacogenetic approach to drug discovery should lead to accelerated progress in identifying more effective treatments for many disorders.

Molecular biology holds many other promises for progress in otology. The identification of temporal gene expression changes that regulate the development of the ear is already progressing and should continue to provide insights into the development of this complex organ, the causes of congenital defects, and the potential for some forms of repair. Identification of genes that are only expressed in cells of the inner ear and the subsequent identification of ear-specific promoter sequences will allow targeted expression of engineered genes under the control of such a promoter. Differences in gene expression between inner and outer hair cells of the cochlea, differences in gene expression between cochlear and vestibular hair cells, and differences in gene expression between hair cells and supporting cells should all be identified through the extension of current efforts in molecular biology. Targeted deletions of genes in mice already have been very informative in the case of Int-2 and the transcription factors Brn 3.1 and Thyroid Receptor β (7,8). Such gene knockouts will continue to be important for unambiguous demonstration of the functional importance of the products of specific genes. Conditional targeted deletion protocols should be even more informative in the future when it becomes possible in cells of the ear after specific promoters have been identified. Gene therapy also may hold promise for otology, in part because the inner ear's fluid spaces provide a point for viral inoculations that is limited to the target organ, but such therapeutic methods probably will be applicable in only a limited set of disorders.

WHAT SHOULD WE EXPECT FROM REGENERATION RESEARCH?

It would be wonderful if self-repair could heal patients hearing impairments and balance disorders in the way that cells regenerate to heal wounds in skin. That is the ultimate objective for research on hair cell regeneration, and there are reasons for some optimism. It is now established that the ears of most vertebrates retain the capacity to produce new hair cells throughout postembryonic life (see reference 9). Many species progressively accumulate new hair cells as they age and grow. In sharks millions of new hair cells are added to the ear during postembryonic life. In birds new hair cells are continually being produced in the vestibular organs as older hair cells die in a process of turnover, but in the cochlea there is little if any production of new cells during postembryonic life under normal conditions. However, new hair cells are produced in the avian cochlea on demand when preexisting hair cells have been killed by trauma or poisoning. The new hair cells arise from the divisions of supporting cells near the site of the trauma. The proliferative response of the supporting cells provides the avian cochlea with the capacity to heal and recover function after trauma that would result in permanent impairment if it occurred in a patient. Similar proliferative regeneration occurs in the vestibular organs of birds and in various hair cell epithelia in the ears of fish and amphibians (Fig. 3).

What characteristics of the ears of fish, amphibians, and birds underlie this capacity for regeneration of hair cells?

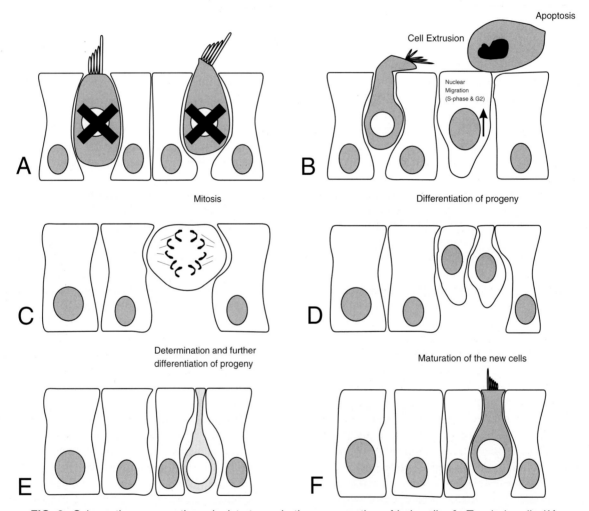

FIG. 3. Schematic cross sections depict stages in the regeneration of hair cells. **A:** Two hair cells (*X*) and four supporting cells are shown in their normal positions and as they would appear after trauma. **B:** Severely injured hair cells often are extruded from the epithelium and die by means of apoptosis. Loss of the hair cells is followed by a proliferative response in some nearby supporting cells, which begin to replicate their chromosomes as the cell nucleus rises toward the luminal surface. **C:** Replicated chromosomes of a surviving supporting cell separate in mitosis, and the cell divides into two new cells at the luminal surface of the epithelium. **D:** Both cells produced from a supporting cell division initially appear to have the ability to become either supporting cells or replacement hair cells when they develop at sites where hair cells are missing. **E:** Each cell becomes committed to differentiating as either a supporting cell or as a replacement hair cell. **F:** The cells pass through stages of differentiation similar to the stages of embryonic development of the epithelium and become innervated. Regeneration can largely reconstitute the structure of hair cell epithelia in fish, amphibians, and birds, and it can lead to functional recovery of hearing and balance sensitivity. Limited regeneration appears to occur in the vestibular epithelia of mammals.

An adequate answer should identify the signals and receptors of the growth control mechanisms that operate throughout life in the ears of fish, amphibians, and birds. Such mechanisms must include extracellular growth factors that trigger and regulate cell proliferation by binding to specific receptors and activating intracellular signaling cascades within the supporting cells. Other controls that also may depend on extracellular factors must regulate how and when hair cells and supporting cells differentiate from progeny produced by the divisions of supporting cells. Both types of control mechanisms are fundamental to the control of cell growth in vertebrates, and such mechanisms are clearly functional in otic epithelia in most vertebrate classes during postembryonic life, even in the absence of trauma. It is reasonable to expect that the same controls would influence the response to trauma in the ears of those species.

What causes the mammalian ear's response to trauma to be so different? That question awaits an adequate answer. When the differences between the ears of mammals and nonmammalian vertebrates have been identified, they may account for the permanence of sensory deficits that typically occur in humans after a loss of hair cells. Even though permanent sensorineural hearing loss and balance disorders are common clinical outcomes, the mammalian ear has some limited capacities for self-repair. This was first demonstrated in juvenile guinea pigs that were given gentamicin for 10 days (10). Structural examinations of those animals after different periods of recovery demonstrated a depletion and reappearance of hair bundles in some parts of the utricle and saccule. Other experiments (11) in which the utricles from juvenile and adult guinea pigs were exposed to gentamicin in culture demonstrated that loss of hair cells in those epithelia could evoke renewed proliferation of supporting cells. The numbers of supporting cells that divided were limited as would be expected from the clinical permanence of hair cell loss in mammals, but during the weeks after trauma a few of the newly produced cells moved into the positions normally occupied by hair cells.

Utricles from 50- and 60-year-old patients who were undergoing acoustic neuroma resection demonstrated that at least 100 supporting cells could be caused to reenter the proliferative state in each sensory epithelium exposed to such chemical trauma in similar *in vitro* experiments (11). In contrast to the conclusions of an earlier report based on questionable data (Rubel et al., comments letter, *Science* 1995), recent *in vivo* experiments with mammals have once more confirmed that rodent vestibular epithelia have the capacity to undergo limited cell proliferation that leads to the formation of new hair cells (12). This evidence and the results of tests of mitogenic growth factors (13–15) support optimism about the potential for the eventual development of therapeutic regeneration of hair cells in the vestibular epithelia.

It is of considerable interest that in the utricles of mature guinea pigs approximately one hair bundle in 1,000 is distinctly smaller than the bundles of neighboring cells and that intermediate sized bundles are about six times more frequent (16). The occurrence of those small bundles suggests the possibility that new hair cells may be added to the sensory epithelia of mature mammals at a very low rate during postembryonic life. The observations of the cells were made in tissues from control animals suggesting that such small bundles may form even in the absence of trauma. It remains to be determined whether the small bundles represent new hair cells produced from divisions of supporting cells that occurred during the postembryonic life of the guinea pigs. Certainly, that seems a possibility. Would careful examination of the vestibular epithelia from adult humans also reveal the presence of such small hair bundles?

How might regenerative therapies be developed? What needs might they meet? How would they change clinical and research practice? None of these questions can be answered with certainty, but it is possible to predict some of the likely developments in this aspect of otology. Many areas of biomedical progress have depended on the development of useful cell lines. Mammalian supporting cell lines would be particularly useful for screening growth factors and small molecules for their potential to enhance the proliferative capacity of their counterparts in the human ear. Supporting cell lines would also be useful to screen for agents that could temporarily suspend the antiproliferative effects of the products of tumor suppressor genes and for screening for agents that would regulate cell differentiation and dedifferentiation. Construction, subtraction, and screening of complementary DNA (cDNA) libraries and other types of molecular biology experiments have made great contributions to our understanding of cancer and other areas of cell biology. Those methods have the capacity to contribute to the identification of the key elements in the signal mechanisms that remove or suppress the proliferative capacities of mammalian hair cell epithelia during development and may help to guide efforts to bring those mechanisms under pharmacologic modulation.

Many other methods from cellular and molecular biology hold potential for investigation of hair cell regeneration in mammals and other species. Much remains to be learned, and there are considerable difficulties inherent in working with cells that are so limited in number, but the potential clinical payoff of investigating the self-repair processes of the ear justifies efforts to overcome the difficulties.

POTENTIAL STRATEGIES TO PROTECT HAIR CELLS

The rates of cell turnover in the vestibular epithelia of the avian ear were recently measured and indicate that on average those hair cells have life spans of one month or less even in the absence of trauma (17). The life spans of those cells contrast dramatically to those of their counterparts in the cochlear sensory epithelia that are less than 500 μm away. Evidence indicates that in the absence of trauma the cochlear hair cells are likely to live for the entire life of the bird. The short life span of the vestibular hair cells in birds focuses attention on questions about factors that influence the life spans of hair cells.

The apparent longevity of hair cells in mammalian ears is remarkable. Hearing and equilibrium sensation at the age of 100 years are believed to depend on the same individual sensory cells that heard that person's first vocalizations and detected his or her movements as a newborn. What factors and regulatory mechanisms underlie the difference in hair cell life spans between birds and mammals? Is the accepted view of the life spans of mammalian hair cells accurate? These questions should be answered in the coming decades. Their answers may lead to treatments that could protect hair cells from age-related loss and trauma. Treatments with growth factors and cell death inhibitors already have extended the life of hair cells in ears from laboratory animals.

IMPROVED PROSTHETIC DEVICES

The development of cochlear prostheses and their successful implantation in thousands of patients are undoubtedly among the most impressive achievements in otology. It would be highly desirable if more patients could benefit from the remarkable recovery of auditory capabilities that some patients attain after receiving a cochlear implant, but ossification of the cochlear lumen can limit the depth of insertion or prevent implantation. If methods could be developed to prevent or reverse the ossification of the cochlea that is a common sequela of meningitis, then it might be possible to increase the number of patients who would have access to cochlear implants. An accurate understanding of the responses and signaling cascades of osteocytes that react to meningeal infection should present opportunities to block such neoossification. Improved understanding of the processes of bone remodeling might even lead to the capacity to reverse ossification of the cochlea via therapeutic control over resorption of the new bone.

Computed tomography can identify ossified cochleae less suitable for implants, but there is a need for methods that could judge the potential outcomes for implantation in other cochleae. Of course, psychologic factors influence the performance that individual patients attain with cochlear implants, but anatomic and physiologic differences in the peripheral and central pathways can limit the maximum performance attainable. More effective methods for predicting the outcome of implant procedures would be of considerable use. Stimulation delivered via transtympanic electrodes can provide positive indications of cochlear nerve survival in some patients, but the method is only partially successful in predicting which patients will receive significant benefits from an implant.

Effective electrical stimulation of nerves depends on at least three factors: the pattern of current spread from the electrode and the resultant pattern and magnitude of the voltage gradients around the neuron, the time constant of the system, and the level of interference from other sources of voltage gradients. Biomedical engineers have continually improved those characteristics of cochlear implant devices, and it is anticipated that such improvements will continue.

Unfortunately, inadequate neuronal survival can limit the effectiveness of even the best device. When hair cells die, that often leads to the death of auditory and vestibular neurons, because the neurons depend on hair cells for a constant source of secreted survival factors. The development of the complex innervation of the sensory epithelia of the ear appears to be regulated through the interplay of that neuronal dependence and trophic support. Different types of cochlear and vestibular neurons express high-affinity receptors for Brain Derived Neurotrophic Factor (BDNF) or Neurotrophin-3 (NT-3), and other types express both receptors (18). Soon after the growing processes from those neurons have reached the embryonic ear, the neurons become dependent for their survival on a constant supply of those neurotrophic factors. Therefore, when the hair cells that supply those factors in the mature ear have been killed, many of the dependent neurons die.

It is now clear from experiments that neuronal survival can be achieved in the absence of hair cell epithelia when the appropriate neurotrophic factors are supplied to eighth-nerve neurons by infusion into the ear or by other means (10). It seems likely that some forms of trophic factor administration will be of value in clinical situations in which patients may be at risk of losing neurons that might be stimulated by a cochlear implant. It remains to be determined just how useful such survival promotion might be, but another form of growth factor administration seems particularly promising. Evidence from a range of studies indicates that the developing and regenerating processes of neurons can use many different types of cues to guide the path of their growth, including gradients of certain growth factors, gradients of substrate adhesion, and voltage gradients (19). It appears likely that there might be beneficial effects to be gained through modification of cochlear implant electrode arrays to allow infusion or slow release of the specific growth factors that might cause neuronal processes to grow toward the sites of stimulating electrodes. There is also the potential for using electrical activity itself as a means to stimulate neuronal process growth and improved neuronal survival.

In some instances implantation of electrode arrays directly into the brain or on its surface provides benefits to patients who might not otherwise be candidates for prostheses. The further effectiveness of these implants depends on many factors that remain to be explored, including long-term tolerance of indwelling electrode arrays, appropriate placement, the development of effective stimulation parameters, etc. At present it is difficult to predict the potential for development of such devices, but there are reasons to suspect that central implants could have important applications in otology as well as in other clinical specialties. As advances are made in the development of faster, more compact computer and optimized biocompatible materials, areas of opportunity that once were the exclusive domain of science fiction authors may come into areas of medical practice.

OPPORTUNITIES IN VESTIBULAR SYSTEM RESEARCH

Since the start of the twentieth century life expectancy in the United States has increased from 47 to 76 years. The fastest growing segment of the United States population is persons 85 years and older. There now are 3.8 million members of this group, and they are at greatest risk for balance disorders, which increase with age. Over 50% of elderly patients interviewed at home complain of balance disorders, and these disorders are the most common reason for patients 75 years of age and older to seek the help of a physician (NIDCD National Strategic Research Plan, 1993) (20). Progressive loss of hair cells occurs in most patients as they age and that cellular loss is accompanied by deterioration of the vestibuloocular reflex with concomitant deterioration of the ability to stabilize visual gaze during movement of the head (Fig. 4) (21). These losses become most pronounced after 70 years of age.

The prevention, early detection, and improved treatment of heart disease, stroke, cancer, and other life-threatening conditions will contribute to still greater longevity in the future. As life spans are extended, even more patients will be at risk for age-related balance disorders. Basic epidemiologic research is needed to assess the current prevalence of these disorders. Improved methods of diagnosis are also needed.

The challenges of diagnosing balance problems result in part from inadequate methods for evaluating the elements of the many different systems that contribute to our perception of position in space and our postural and dynamic stability. Small mismatches in magnitude or timing in the complex interplay of sensory inputs from the vestibular organs and proprioceptors in the neck and body can cause patients to feel dizzy. Mismatches in the normally coordinated contractions of the muscles that control visual gaze and head and body position also can result in imbalance, as can changes in blood pressure and peripheral neuropathies. Even if we consider only cases of dizziness that originate from otic causes, those cases can result from impaired functions in any of six semicircular canals and four otolithic detectors and from impairments in the brain centers that process their sensory inputs. The difficulty of assessing the potential impairments in the many separate elements of the complex systems that contribute to balance often make it impractical to reach a definitive diagnosis of the singular or multifactorial causes of balance disorders.

Technologically advanced rotary chairs, eye-tracking systems, and posturography stations can provide objective measures, but the size and expense of those instru-

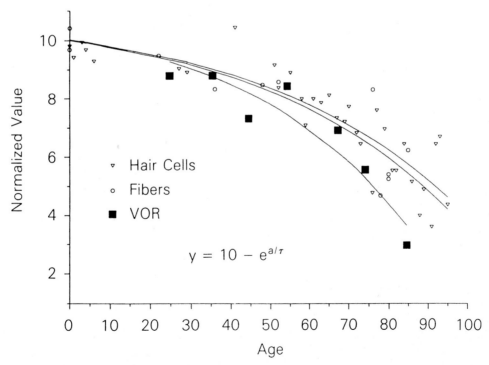

FIG. 4. Anatomic and physiologic measures of vestibular deterioration as functions of age. Anatomic measurements include the number of hair cells and nerve fibers in the vestibular epithelia. The physiologic measurement is transformation of the vestibuloocular phase lead for patients tested in a rotary chair at 0.25 Hz, 300 degrees per second peak head velocity. Data are normalized to a value of 10 at birth. *Curves* depict the best fit of the equation to each data set. (Courtesy of Dr. Gary Paige. From Paige GD. Senescence of human visual-vestibular interactions, 1: Vestibulo-ocular reflex and adaptive plasticity with aging. *J Vestib Res* 1992;2:133–151, with permission.)

ments have limited their use in diagnosis. The development of more accessible instruments and methods for evaluation of freely moving patients could increase the use of objective diagnostic testing. If more patients were thoroughly tested by objective means, then specific disorders might be recognized from patterns of symptoms. Objective and standardized diagnostic criteria would also be of use in identifying genetic predispositions likely to influence susceptibility to age-related and drug-induced balance disorders. Genetic screens of animals that incorporate vestibuloocular reflex measurements and other functional assays of vestibular performance are likely to help identify mutated genes responsible for balance disorders and for differences in susceptibility to those disorders. A clear understanding of the developmental and genetic influences that contribute to the heterogeneous susceptibility of individuals to motion sickness should be a goal for future investigation. Objectively measurable evaluation of various forms of balance therapy is another goal for the future.

SUMMARY POINTS

- Substantial hearing loss affects 16% of the general population (22), surpassing the combined economic impact of multiple sclerosis, stroke, epilepsy, spinal injury, Huntington's disease, and Parkinson's disease and accounting for $50 billion dollars in costs annually in the United States (23).
- Balance disorders affect untold lives, and it is to be expected that these otologic conditions will become even more prevalent.
- Progressive improvements in medicine since the turn of the twentieth century have been accompanied by extension of the average life span from 47 to 76 years.
- There is every reason to believe that future research and applications of the knowledge gained through biomedical research will result in improved therapy for life-threatening cardiovascular disease, cancer, and stroke that will extend life spans even further.
- Otologists are challenged to acquire knowledge that may be applied to the prevention and management of hearing loss and dysequilibrium.
- The challenges are substantial, but future research and audacious efforts may contribute to fulfilling the hopes of patients.

ACKNOWLEDGMENT

The author thanks Dr. Jacques Retief of the University of Virginia for constructing Fig. 1, Dr. Karen Avarham of Tel Aviv University for permission to reprint Fig. 2, and Dr. Gary Paige of the University of Rochester for permission to reprint Fig. 4. Work in the author's laboratory is supported by grant RO1-DC0200 from the National Institute on Deafness and Other Communication Disorders.

REFERENCES

1. Collins FS, Patrinos A, Jordan E, Chakravarti A, Gesteland R, Walters L. New goals for the U.S. Human Genome Project: 1998–2003. *Science* 1998;282:682–689.
2. Avraham KB. Hear come more genes! *Nat Med* 1998;4:1238–1239.
3. Corwin JT. Identifying the genes of hearing, deafness, and dysequilibrium. *Proc Natl Acad Sci U S A* 1998;95:12080–12082.
4. Morton NE. Genetic epidemiology of hearing impairment. *Ann N Y Acad Sci* 1991;630:16–31.
5. Denoyelle F, Weil D, Maw MA, et al. Prelingual deafness: high prevalence of a 30delG mutation in the connexin 26 gene. *Hum Mol Genet* 1997;6:2173–2177.
6. Denoyelle F, Lina-Granade G, Plauchu H, et al. Connexin 26 gene linked to a dominant deafness. *Nature* 1998;393:319–320.
7. Mansour SL, Goddard JM, Capecchi MR. Mice homozygous for a targeted disruption of the proto-oncogene int-2 have developmental defects in the tail and inner ear. *Development* 1993;117:13–28.
8. Erkman L, McEvilly RJ, Luo L, et al. Role of transcription factors Brn-3.1 and Brn-3.2 in auditory and visual system development. *Nature* 1996;381:603–606.
9. Corwin JT, Oberholtzer JC. Fish n' chicks: model recipes for hair-cell regeneration? *Neuron* 1997;19:951–954.
10. Forge A, Lin L, Corwin JT, Nevill G. Ultrastructural evidence for hair cell regeneration in the mammalian inner ear. *Science* 1993;259:1616–1619.
11. Warchol ME, Lambert PR, Goldstein BJ, Corwin JT. Regenerative proliferation in inner ear sensory epithelia from adult guinea pigs and humans. *Science* 1993;1619–1622.
12. Kuntz AL, Oesterle EC. Transforming growth factor alpha with insulin stimulates cell proliferation in vivo in adult rat vestibular sensory epithelium. *J Comp Neurol* 1998;399:413–423.
13. Lambert, PR. Inner ear hair cell regeneration in a mammal: identification of a triggering factor. *Laryngoscope* 1994;104:701–718.
14. Yamashita H, Oesterle EC. Induction of cell proliferation in mammalian inner-ear sensory epithelia by transforming growth factor alpha and epidermal growth factor. *Proc Natl Acad Sci USA* 1995;92:3152–3155.
15. Zheng JL, Helbig C, Gao WQ. Induction of cell proliferation by fibroblast and insulin-like growth factors in pure rat inner ear epithelial cell cultures. *J Neurosci* 1997;17:216–226.
16. Lambert PR, Gu R, Corwin JT. Analysis of small hair bundles in the utricles of mature guinea pigs. *Am J Otol* 1997;18:637–643.
17. Kil J, Warchol ME, Corwin JT. Cell death, cell proliferation, and estimates of hair cell life spans in the vestibular organs of chicks. *Hear Res* 1997;114:117–126.
18. Fritzsch B, Silos-Santiago I, Bianchi LM, Farinas I. The role of neurotrophic factors in regulating the development of inner ear innervation. *Trends Neurosci* 1997;20:159–164.
19. Zigmond MJ, Bloom FE, Landis SC, Roberts JL, Squire LR. *Fundamental neuroscience.* San Diego: Academic Press, 1998.
20. Mahoney D, Restak R. *The longevity strategy: how to live to 100 using brain-body connection.* New York: John Wiley and Sons, 1998.
21. Paige GD. Senescence of human visual-vestibular interactions, 1: Vestibulo-ocular reflex and adaptive plasticity with aging. *J Vestib Res* 1992;2:133–151.
22. Davis AC. The prevalence of hearing impairment and reported hearing disability among adults in Great Britain. *Int J Epidemiol* 1989;18:911–917.
23. Hudspeth AJ. How hearing happens. *Neuron* 1997;19:947–950.

Subject Index

879